AF669514

Spinal Disorders and Treatments

The NYU-HJD Comprehensive Textbook

Spinal Disorders and Treatments

The NYU-HJD Comprehensive Textbook

Editors

Thomas J Errico MD
Professor of Orthopaedic surgery
Professor of Neurosurgery
Chief, Division of Spine Surgery
Hospital for Joint Diseases
New York University Langone Medical Center
New York University School of Medicine
New York, New York, USA

Thomas Cheriyan MD PGDHM
Research Scientist
Division of Spine Surgery
Hospital for Joint Diseases
New York University Langone Medical Center
New York University School of Medicine
New York, New York, USA

Gerard P Varlotta DO
Associate Professor of Rehabilitation Medicine
Nonoperative Spine Care
Sports, Spinal, and Pain Rehabilitation
New York, New York, USA

JAYPEE The Health Sciences Publisher
New Delhi | London | Philadelphia | Panama

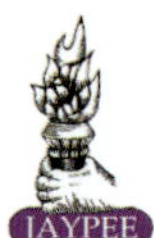

Jaypee Brothers Medical Publishers (P) Ltd

Headquarters
Jaypee Brothers Medical Publishers (P) Ltd.
4838/24, Ansari Road, Daryaganj
New Delhi 110 002, India
Phone: +91-11-43574357
Fax: +91-11-43574314
E-mail: jaypee@jaypeebrothers.com

Overseas Offices
J.P. Medical Ltd.
83, Victoria Street, London
SW1H 0HW (UK)
Phone: +44-20 3170 8910
Fax: +44(0)20 3008 6180
E-mail: info@jpmedpub.com

Jaypee-Highlights Medical Publishers Inc.
City of Knowledge, Bld. 237, Clayton
Panama City, Panama
Phone: +1 507-301-0496
Fax: +1 507-301-0499
E-mail: cservice@jphmedical.com

Jaypee Medical Inc.
The Bourse
111, South Independence Mall East
Suite 835, Philadelphia, PA 19106, USA
Phone: +1 267-519-9789
E-mail: jpmed.us@gmail.com

Jaypee Brothers Medical Publishers (P) Ltd.
17/1-B, Babar Road, Block-B, Shaymali
Mohammadpur, Dhaka-1207
Bangladesh
Mobile: +08801912003485
E-mail: jaypeedhaka@gmail.com

Jaypee Brothers Medical Publishers (P) Ltd.
Bhotahity, Kathmandu, Nepal
Phone: +977-9741283608
E-mail: kathmandu@jaypeebrothers.com

Website: www.jaypeebrothers.com
Website: www.jaypeedigital.com

Inquiries for bulk sales may be solicited at: jaypee@jaypeebrothers.com

Spinal Disorders and Treatments: The NYU-HJD Comprehensive Textbook

First Edition: **2015**

ISBN: 978-93-5152-495-3

Printed at Replika Press Pvt. Ltd.

Dedicated

To

Countless people at New York University who dedicate their professional careers to the care of patients and to improving the lives of those afflicted with disorders and deformities of the spine through research and education.

Thomas J Errico MD

To

My brother, Jerry, for his support, inspiration and love.

Thomas Cheriyan MD

To

* *All of those who have provided me with support, direction and inspiration.*
* *My parents, Gerard Sr and Isabel for setting an example with their tireless work ethic.*
* *My wonderful children, Caroline, Chris and Stephen for always making me smile and their eternal love.*
* *Mark D Brown, MD, PhD, who, early in my career, inspired my pursuit of knowledge of orthopedics and nonoperative care of patients with back pain.*
* *Thomas Errico, for being my supporter and friend.*
* *Most importantly I would like to thank Angela, my supportive and loving wife of 25 years, for standing beside me throughout my career and our journey.*

Gerard P Varlotta DO

Contributors

Robert J Ames BA
Medical Student
Temple University School of Medicine
Philadelphia, PA, USA

Rohan Bannis MD
Pain Medicine Fellow
Department of Anesthesiology
New York University Langone
Medical Center
New York, NY, USA

John A Bendo MD
Director, Spine Service
Associate Professor of
Orthopedic Surgery
Hospital for Joint Diseases
New York University Langone
Medical Center
New York University School of
Medicine
New York, NY, USA

Kristina L Bianco BA
Division of Spine Surgery
Department of Orthopaedic Surgery
Hospital for Joint Diseases
New York Langone Medical Center
New York, NY, USA

Ludmilla Bronfin MD
Assistant Professor of Neurology
New York University School of
Medicine
New York, NY, USA

Steven Calvino MD
Assistant Professor of Anesthesiology
Assistant Professor of
Rehabilitation Medicine
New York University Langone
Medical Center
New York, NY, USA

Andy L Chang BS
Medical College of Georgia
Augusta, Georgia, USA

Jerry Cheriyan MD MRCS
Resident Physician
Department of Surgery
Marshfield Clinic
Wisconsin, USA

Thomas Cheriyan MD PGDHM
Research Scientist
Division of Spine Surgery
Hospital for Joint Diseases
New York University Langone
Medical Center
New York University School of
Medicine
New York, NY, USA

Gina A Ciavarra MD
Assistant Professor of Radiology
New York University School of
Medicine
New York, NY, USA

Pierre Devos BE
Division of Spine Surgery
Hospital for Joint Diseases
New York University Langone
Medical Center
New York, NY, USA

Thomas J Errico MD
Professor of Orthopaedic Surgery
Professor of Neurosurgery
Chief, Division of Spine Surgery
Hospital for Joint Diseases
New York University Langone
Medical Center
New York University School of
Medicine
New York, NY, USA

Jean-Pierre Farcy MD
Clinical Professor of
Orthopedic Surgery
Division of Spine surgery
Hospital for Joint Diseases
New York University Langone
Medical Center, New York, NY, USA

Brian Forzani MD
Resident Physician
Department of Physical Medicine
and Rehabilitation
New York University Langone
Medical Center
New York, NY, USA

Brian Freed DO
Resident Physician
Department of Physical Medicine and
Rehabilitation
New York University Langone
Medical Center, New York, NY, USA

Anthony K Frempong-Boadu MD FACS FAANS
Associate Professor of Neurosurgery
Chief, Division of Spinal Surgery
Director, Neurosurgical Spine
Fellowship Training Program
New York University Langone
Medical Center
New York, NY, USA

Michael C Gerling MD
Assistant Professor of Orthopedics
New York University Langone
Medical Center
Chief of Spine Surgery, New York
University Lutheran Medical Center
Brooklyn, NY, USA

Christopher Gharibo MD
Associate Professor of Anesthesiology
Associate Professor of Orthopaedics
Director, Chronic Pain Management
Hospital for Joint Diseases
New York University Langone
Medical Center
New York University School of
Medicine
New York, NY, USA

Brian D Golden MD
Clinical Associate Professor of
Medicine
Division of Rheumatology
New York University School of
Medicine
New York, NY, USA

Jeffrey A Goldstein MD
Director of Spine Service—Education
Director of Spine Fellowship
Clinical Professor of
Orthopaedic Surgery
Hospital for Joint Diseases
New York University Langone
Medical Center
New York University School of
Medicine
New York, NY, USA

Vadim Goz MD
Resident Physician
Department of Orthopaedic Surgery
University of Utah, Salt Lake City
Utah, USA

Bartosz T Grobelny MD
Resident Physician
Department of Neurosurgery
New York University Langone
Medical Center
New York, NY, USA

Marianne T Guschwan MD
Clinical Assistant Professor of
Psychiatry
New York University School of Medicine
New York, NY, USA

Jane S Hoashi MD MPH
Fellow, Division of Spine Surgery
Department of Orthopaedic Surgery
Hospital for Joint Diseases
New York University Langone
Medical Center
New York, NY, USA

Stephen Honig MD
Clinical Associate Professor of
Medicine
Division of Rheumatology
Director, Osteoporosis Center
Hospital for Joint Diseases
New York University Langone
Medical Center
New York, NY, USA

Qasim M Husain MD
Fellow, Division of Spine Surgery
Department of Orthopaedic Surgery
Hospital for Joint Diseases
New York University Langone
Medical Center
New York, NY, USA

M Fahad Khan MD MSPH
Assistant Professor of Anesthesiology
New York University Langone
Medical Center
New York University School of Medicine
New York, NY, USA

Irene Kim MD
Resident Physician
Department of Neurosurgery
New York University Langone
Medical Center
New York, NY, USA

Yong H Kim MD
Clinical Assistant Professor of
Orthopedic Surgery
Associate Director of Spine Fellowship
Hospital for Joint Diseases
New York University Langone
Medical Center
New York, NY, USA

Kiril Kiprovski MD
Clinical Associate Professor of
Neurology
New York University School of
Medicine
New York, NY, USA

Jeffrey D Klein MD
Clinical Instructor of
Orthopaedic Surgery
Division of Spine Surgery
Hospital for Joint Diseases
New York University Langone
Medical Center
New York, NY, USA

Jeffrey B Knox MD
Assistant Professor of Surgery
Orthopedic Surgery Service
Tripler Army Medical Center
Honolulu, Hawaii, USA

Virginie Lafage PhD
Research Director
Division of Spine Surgery
Department of Orthopaedic Surgery
Hospital for Joint Disease
New York University Langone
Medical Center
New York, NY, USA

Barthelemy Liabaud MD
Research Fellow
Division of Spine Surgery
Departments of Orthopedic Surgery
Hospital for Joint Diseases
New York University Langone
Medical Center
New York, NY, USA

Angela Lis PhD PT
Associate Clinical Director
Occupational & Industrial
Orthopaedic Center
Hospital for Joint Diseases
New York University Langone
Medical Center
New York, NY, USA

Jackson William Liu MD
Clinical Instructor of
Rehabilitation Medicine
New York University Langone
Medical Center
Attending Physician, Physical Medicine
and Pain Management Orthopedic
Associates of Lancaster
Lancaster, PA, USA

Athena M Lolis MD
Assistant Professor of Neurology
New York University Langone
Medical Center.
New York, NY, USA

Baron S Lonner MD
Chief, Division of Spine Surgery
Mount Sinai Beth Israel Hospital
Director of the Spine Institute of
New York
Director of Scoliosis and
Spine Associates
Professor of Orthopaedic Surgery
Mount Sinai School of
Medicine
New York, NY, USA

Stephen P Maier II BA
Division of Spine Surgery
Hospital for Joint Diseases
New York University Langone
Medical Center
New York, NY, USA

Michael B Mechlin MD
Assistant Professor of Radiology
New York University Langone
Medical Center
New York University School of
Medicine
New York, NY, USA

Alex Moroz MD FACP
Associate Professor of
Rehabilitation Medicine
Director of Integrative Sports Medicine
Rusk Rehabilitation
New York University Langone
Medical Center
New York University School of
Medicine
New York, NY, USA

Jesse Ng MD
Assistant Professor of Anesthesiology
New York University Langone
Medical Center
New York, NY, USA

Robert P Norton MD
Fellow, Division of Spine Surgery
Department of Orthopaedic Surgery
Hospital for Joint Diseases
New York University Langone
Medical Center
New York, NY, USA

Donato Pacione MD
Clinical Assistant Professor of Neurosurgery
New York University Langone Medical Center
New York, NY, USA

Brian Park MD
Resident Physician
Department of Orthopaedics
Hospital for Joint Diseases
New York University Langone Medical Center
New York, NY, USA

Peter G Passias MD
Assistant Professor of Orthopaedic Surgery
Division of Spine Surgery
Hospital for Joint Diseases
New York University Langone Medical Center
New York, NY, USA

Justin C Paul MD
Resident Physician
Department of Orthopaedics
Hospital for Joint Diseases
New York University Langone Medical Center
New York, NY, USA

Noel I Perin MD FRCS FAANS
Director Minimally Invasive Neurosurgery
Professor of Neurosurgery
New York University Langone Medical Center
New York, NY, USA

Jeffrey Perry DO
Clinical Instructor of Orthopaedic Surgery
Hospital for Joint Diseases
New York University Langone Medical Center, Clinical Instructor of Rehabilitation Medicine
New York University Langone Medical Center, Adjunct Clinical Assistant Professor of Medicine
New York College of Osteopathic Medicine
Director of NYCOM/NUMC Physical Medicine and Rehabilitation Residency Training Program
Nassau University Medical Center
New York, USA

Anthony M Petrizzo DO
Clinical Assistant Professor of Orthopaedic Surgery
Division of Spine Surgery
Hospital for Joint Diseases
New York University Langone Medical Center
New York, NY, USA

Dimitris Placantonakis MD PhD
Assistant Professor of Neurosurgery
Director, Neurosurgical Laboratory for Stem Cell Research
New York University Langone Medical Center
New York, NY, USA

Themistocles Protopsaltis MD
Assistant Professor of Orthopaedic Surgery
Division of Spine Surgery
Hospital for Joint Diseases
New York University Langone Medical Center
New York, NY, USA

Rachel N Rattenni BA
Division of Spine Surgery
Hospital for Joint Diseases
New York University Langone Medical Center
New York, NY, USA

Faruk Razzak DO
Resident Physician
Department of Physical Medicine and Rehabilitation
New York University Langone Medical Center, New York, NY, USA

Juan C Robles MD
Diplomate of the American Board of Physical Medicine and Rehabilitation
Clinical Instructor of Rehabilitation Medicine, New York Langone Medical Center
Staff Physician
Department of Medicine—Division of Physical Medicine and Rehabilitation
The Brooklyn Hospital Center
New York, NY, USA

Devon J Ryan BA
Division of Spine Surgery
Hospital for Joint Diseases
New York University Langone Medical Center
New York, NY, USA

Leon D Rybak MD
Assistant Professor of Radiology
New York University Langone Medical Center
New York University School of Medicine
New York, NY, USA

Frank Schwab MD
Clinical Professor of Orthopedic Surgery
Division of Spine surgery
Hospital for Joint Diseases
New York University Langone Medical Center
New York, NY, USA

Sachin K Shah MD
Pain Medicine Fellow
Department of Anesthesiology
New York University Langone Medical Center
New York, NY, USA

Kseniya Slobodyanyuk BA
Division of Spine Surgery
Hospital for Joint Diseases
New York University Langone Medical Center
New York, NY, USA

Matthew B Smith MD
Clinical Assistant Professor of Psychiatry
New York University School of Medicine
New York, NY, USA

Michael L Smith MD
Assistant Professor of Neurosurgery
New York University Langone Medical Center
New York University School of Medicine
New York, NY, USA

Jeffrey M Spivak MS MD
Director, New York University Hospital for Joint Diseases Spine Center
Associate Professor of Orthopaedic Surgery
New York University Langone Medical Center
New York University School of Medicine
New York, NY, USA

Jonathan Stieber MD
Clinical Assistant Professor of Orthopaedic Surgery
Hospital for Joint Diseases
New York University Langone Medical Center, New York, NY, USA

Wayne Stokes MD
Associate Professor of Rehabilitation Medicine, Director of Sports Medicine
Rusk Rehabilitation, New York University Langone Medical Center
New York University School of Medicine
New York, NY, USA

Jamie S Terran BS
Division of Spine Surgery
Hospital for Joint Diseases
New York University Langone Medical Center
New York, NY, USA

Courtney S Toombs BA
New York University School of Medicine
New York, NY, USA

Antonio Valdevit PhD
Assistant Professor
Department of Biomedical Engineering
Schaefer School of Engineering and Science
Stevens Institute of Technology
Hoboken, New Jersey, USA

Gerard P Varlotta DO
Associate Professor of Rehabilitation Medicine
Nonoperative Spine Care
Sports, Spinal, and Pain Rehabilitation
New York, NY, USA

Sherri Weiser PhD
Director of Clinical Services and Research
Occupational and Industrial Orthopaedic Center
Hospital for Joint Diseases
New York University Langone Medical Center, New York, NY, USA

Tony Wong MD
Assistant Professor of Radiology
Columbia University Medical Center
New York, NY, USA

Hiroyuki Yoshihara MD PhD
Assistant Professor of Orthopaedic Surgery and Rehabilitation Medicine
SUNY Downstate Medical Center
Brooklyn, NY, USA
Attending Spine Surgeon
Nassau University Medical Center
NY, USA

Preface

The treatment of spine disorders has evolved rapidly over the past few decades. In order to provide high-quality, evidence-based care and maximize patient outcomes, a multidisciplinary patient care team should include primary care physicians, radiologists, neurologists, psychiatrists, internists, rheumatologists, physiatrists, anesthesiologists, neurosurgeons and orthopedic surgeons.

This textbook provides its readers with a basic understanding of the principles that underlie the vast field of spinal disorders. It does so by highlighting the fundamental aspects of anatomy, biomechanics, diagnoses and management of spinal disorders. The textbook is organized into four sections that correspond to the four stages of the spine care continuum: Basic Science and Spinal Assessment, Non-Invasive Therapeutic Intervention, Spinal Injection and Surgical Management. Each section focuses on evidence-based, patient-centric applications of therapeutic modalities. Particular emphasis has been placed on both the operative and nonoperative management of spinal conditions.

This textbook is intended to help both medical professionals and patients to further their understanding and knowledge of spinal conditions. With the advent of new technologies, techniques and treatment modalities, the management of these challenging conditions will continue to evolve. By contrast, the basic principles and tenets of spine disorders will endure, and this textbook will remain relevant and educational for its readers over time.

Thomas J Errico
Thomas Cheriyan
Gerard P Varlotta

Acknowledgments

I would like to acknowledge my teachers, especially John Kostuik MD, Roy Camille MD, Joseph Ransohoff MD and Theodore Waugh MD, who helped influence my career and therefore the writing of this book.

Thomas J Errico

I would like to acknowledge and thank my parents, Annie and Jimmy, for all their support. I also thank my friends and colleagues for their advice, insight and support. Special thanks to my mentor and teacher, Dr Thomas Errico, for his invaluable help and guidance in molding my career.

Thomas Cheriyan

I would like to acknowledge all the medical students, residents, fellows and research fellows (under the direction of Virginie Lafage) in addition to all the contributors of this book. I also would like to especially thank Dr Thomas Cheriyan for all his hard work and persistence in making the idea of writing this book a reality. Without him this book would not have been completed. And finally we would like to thank M/s Jaypee Brothers Medical Publishers (P) Ltd., New Delhi, India for their assistance in publishing this book.

Gerard P Varlotta

Contents

Section 1: Basic Science and Spinal Assessment

1. Basic Science of Degenerative Disk Disease **3**

Anthony Petrizzo, Kristina Bianco

- Morphology of the Normal IVD *3*
- Morphologic Changes in the Degenerative IVD *4*
- Etiology of IVD Degeneration *5*
- Inflammatory Mediators *7*
- Novel Management Techniques *8*

2. Biomechanics of the Spine **11**

Antonio Valdevit

- The Spinal Column *11*
- Intervertebral Disk *12*
- The Facet Joint and Uncovertebral Joint *12*
- Spinal Motion *13*
- Spinal Loading *13*
- Spinal Arthroplasty *15*
- Mechanical Evaluation and Clinical Implications of Spinal Instrumentation *16*

3. Balance, Posture and Stability in Spinal Disorders **18**

Virginie Lafage, Barthelemy Liabaud, Frank Schwab, Jean-Pierre Farcy

- Balance, Stability and Posture *18*

4. Differential Diagnosis of Spinal Disorders **23**

Michael Gerling, Vadim Goz

- Risk Factors *23*
- Prognosis *23*
- Types of Pain *24*
- Chronic Pain Syndromes and Threshold Modulation *24*
- Differential Diagnosis *24*

5. Neurological Differential Diagnosis of Spinal Disorders **30**

Devon Ryan, Thomas Cheriyan, Ludmilla Bronfin

- Conditions that Mimic Radiculopathy *30*
- Conditions that Mimic Cervical Myelopathy *33*

6. Examination and Evaluation of Neck Pain **36**

Jonathan R Stieber, Robert J Ames

- Prevalence and Natural History *36*
- Anatomy *36*
- Pathophysiology *37*
- History, Physical Examination and Grading *39*
- Imaging and Diagnostic Studies *41*

7. Examination and Evaluation of Low Back Pain **44**

Devon Ryan, Jeffery Perry

- Institutional Guidelines *44*
- Examination and Evaluation of Acute Low Back Pain *45*
- Examination and Evaluation of Chronic Low Back Pain *48*

8. Clinical Examination and Evaluation of Radiculopathy: A Neurological Perspective **49**

Kiril Kiprovski

- History and Physical Examination *49*
- Somatic Referred Pain from the Neck and Lower Back *54*
- Red Flags *57*

9. Evaluation of Adolescent Scoliosis **60**

Stephen P Maier II, Thomas Cheriyan, Baron S Lonner

- Evaluation of Scoliosis *62*
- Classification *67*

10. Evaluation of Adult Spinal Deformity **69**

Jeffrey H Weinreb, Pierre Devos, Frank Schwab

- Evaluation *69*
- Spine Related Measurements in the Setting of Adult Spinal Deformity *71*
- Classification *71*

11. Measurement of Adult Spinal Deformity **75**

Jeffrey H Weinreb, Thomas Cheriyan, Virginie Lafage, Frank Schwab

- Imaging *75*
- Coronal Plane Measurements *75*
- Sagittal Plane Measurements *77*
- Spinopelvic Radiographic Parameters *77*
- Global Alignment *78*
- Criticism of 2D Measurements *78*
- 3D Analysis *78*

12. Assessment of Disability **81**

Juan Carlos Robles

- Functional Assessment Instruments *81*
- Objective Tools *81*
- Subjective Tools *83*

13. Non-MRI Evaluation of the Cervical and Lumbar Spine **85**

Tony Wong, Gina Ciavarra, Leon Rybak

- Radiographs *85*
- Computed Tomography *88*
- Nuclear Medicine *95*
- Ultrasound *100*

14. MRI Evaluation of Cervical and Lumbar Spine Disorders **102**

Michael B Mechlin

- Cervical Spine *102*
- Lumbar Spine *108*

15. Interventional Diagnostic Procedures: Nerve Blocks and Discography **120**

Steven Calvino, Jessie Ng

- Diagnostic Nerve Blocks *120*
- Discography *121*
- Anatomy and Function of the Intervertebral Disk *121*
- Disk Degeneration and Pain *123*
- Procedure *123*
- Complications *123*
- Evidence *124*

16. Rheumatic Diseases and Myofascial Pain **126**

Brian D Golden

- How to tell the Difference between "-ITIS" and "-ALGIA" *126*
- Ankylosing Spondylitis as the Prototypical Inflammatory, Rheumatologic Disease Affecting the Spine *126*
- Fibromyalgia as the Prototypical Noninflammatory Pain Syndrome *128*

17. Diagnosis of Osteopenia and Osteoporosis **130**

Stephen Honig, Stephen P Maier II

- Pathogenesis of Postmenopausal Osteoporosis *132*
- Diagnosing Osteopenia and Osteoporosis *132*

Section 2: Non-Invasive Therapeutic Intervention

18. Multidisciplinary Approach to Spinal Pain **139**

Kseniya Slobodyanyuk, Thomas Cheriyan, Christopher Gharibo

- Spinal Pain Pathophysiology *139*
- Pharmacologic Treatment *139*
- Nonpharmacologic Treatment *141*
- Functional Rehabilitation *141*

19. Pharmacological Management of Spinal Pain: Narcotics **144**

Christopher Gharibo

20. Pharmacological Management of Spinal Pain: Non-narcotics **147**

Juan Carlos Robles, Thomas Cheriyan

- Acetaminophen *147*
- Nonsteroidal Anti-Inflammatory Drugs *147*
- Steroids *147*
- Anticonvulsants *148*
- Tricyclic Antidepressants *149*
- Muscle Relaxants *149*
- Nonopioid Combination Medication *149*
- Topical Medications *150*

21. Prevention and Management of Addiction **151**

Marianne T Guschwan

- The Scope of the Problem with Opioids *151*
- Addiction Management *152*
- Prevention of Addiction *152*

22. Therapeutic Management of Osteoporosis **155**

Stephen Honig

- Aging, Falling, and the Concept of Frailty *155*
- Calcium and Vitamin D Supplementation *156*
- Bone Strengthening Prescription Medications *156*

23. Nonoperative Treatment of Cervical Myelopathy and Radiculopathy **159**

Kristina Bianco, Faruk Razzak, Gerard Varlotta

- Task Force for Neck Pain *159*
- Pathophysiology *160*
- Nonoperative Treatment for Cervical Myelopathy and Cervical Radiculopathy *161*
- Other Nonoperative Treatment Methods *164*

- Nonoperative versus Operative Treatment of Cervical Myelopathy *164*
- Nonoperative versus Operative Treatment of Cervical Radiculopathy *165*

24. Alternative Medicine Treatment in Spinal Disorders: Application of Acupuncture **168**

Alex Moroz, Brian Freed

- Applications of Acupuncture *169*

25. Psychosocial Aspects and Management of Chronic Low Back Pain **171**

Matthew B Smith

- Aversion *171*
- Central Sensitization *172*
- Psychiatric Comorbidity *172*
- Personality Factors *173*
- Interpersonal and Social Factors *173*
- Chronic Illness *174*
- Psychiatric and Psychological Treatment Considerations *174*
- Countertransference *175*

26. A Conservative Care Approach to the Rehabilitation of Patients with Spine Pain **178**

Angela Lis, Sherri Weiser

- Triage Criterion 1: Duration of SP *180*
- Triage Criterion 2: The Presence of Yellow Flags *180*
- Triage Criterion 3: Is the Patient a Candidate for an Intensive Interdisciplinary Conditioning Program? *182*

Section 3: Spinal Injection

27. Introduction to Spinal Injections **187**

Jamie R Terran, Rachel N Rattenni, Faruk Razzak, Gerard P Varlotta

- History *187*
- Trigger Point Injections *187*
- Sacroiliac Injections *188*
- Peripheral Joint Injections *189*
- Sympathetic Nerve Blocks *189*
- Epidural Injections *189*
- Intra-articular Facet Injections *190*
- Median Branch Blocks and Rhizotomy *190*
- Intradiscal Electrothermal Therapy, Nucleoplasty, and Biacuplasty *190*
- Spinal Cord Stimulators *191*
- Complications and Risks *191*

28. Diagnostic and Therapeutic Value of Spinal Injections **193**

Juan Carlos Robles, Vadim Goz

- Discograms *193*
- Epidural Steroid Injections *194*
- Selective Nerve Root Blocks, Facet Joint Blocks, and Medial Branch Blocks *195*

29. Trigger Point Injections **200**

Benjamin Bieber, Devon Ryan

- Diagnosis *200*
- Indications *201*
- Technique *202*

- Preinjection Block *203*
- Evidence *203*

30. Sacroiliac Injections **205**

Jackson Liu, Jeffrey Weinreb, Wayne Stokes

- Anatomy *205*
- Diagnosis *205*
- Injection *208*
- Injection Technique *209*
- Complications *210*
- Newer Techniques *210*

31. Peripheral Joint and Soft Tissue Injections **212**

Warren Young

- Injectables *212*
- Injection Techniques *216*

32. Sympathetic Blocks: Utility in Complex Regional Pain Syndrome **221**

Kseniya Slobodyanyuk, Christopher Gharibo

- Nociceptive and Neuropathic Pain *221*
- Complex Regional Pain Syndrome *221*
- CRPS Management *223*

33. Epidural Steroid Injections **228**

Kseniya Slobodyanyuk, Christopher Gharibo

- Epidural Steroid Injections *228*
- Interlaminar, Transforaminal, and Caudal ESIs *229*
- Complications *231*

34. Intra-articular Facet Injections **233**

Kristina L Bianco, Jeffrey H Weinreb, Gerard P Varlotta

- Facet Joint Anatomy *233*
- Etiology and Pathophysiology *233*
- Grading Scales for Facet Joint Arthropathy *235*
- Diagnosis *235*
- Imaging *236*
- Treatment *236*
- Indications for Injections *237*
- Intra-Articular Facet Joint Injections *237*
- CYST Intervention Results *238*
- Complications *238*
- Differential Diagnosis *238*

35. Complications of Spinal Injections **240**

Brian Forzani, Stephen P Maier II, Kseniya Slobodyanyuk, Thomas J Errico, Thomas Cheriyan, Christopher Gharibo

- Regional/Mechanical Injury *240*
- Needle/Injectate-Related Injuries *241*
- Pressure-Related Injuries *243*
- Infections *244*
- Vascular Injury *244*
- Neural Complications *248*
- Chemical Injury *249*

36. Medial Branch Block and Rhizotomy **253**

Devon Ryan, Jamie Terran, Mohammed Khan

- Medial Branch Block *254*
- Rhizotomy (Medial Branch Neurotomy, Radiofrequency Neurotomy) *256*

37. Intradiscal Electrothermal Therapy, Nucleoplasty and Biacuplasty **259**

Steven Calvino, Rohan Bannis, Sachin Shah

- Intradiscal Electrothermal Therapy *260*
- Nucleoplasty *260*
- Biacuplasty *261*

38. Spinal Cord Stimulators **264**

Brian Park, Yong H Kim

- What are Spinal Cord Stimulators? *264*
- Indications *265*
- Ischemic/Visceral Pain *265*
- Neurogenic Pain *265*
- Spine-Related Conditions *265*
- Technique *266*
- Trial/Screening *266*
- Permanent Implantation *267*
- Complications *268*

Section 4: Surgical Management

39. History of Surgical Management of Spinal Disorders **273**

Justin Paul, Thomas Cheriyan, Thomas J Errico

- Decompression of Spinal Elements *274*
- Stabilization of the Spine *276*
- Antibiotics and Orthopedic Instrumentation *277*
- Posterior Thoracolumbar Instrumentation *278*
- Anterior Thoracolumbar Instrumentation *278*
- Posterior Cervical Instrumentation *280*
- Anterior Cervical Instrumentation *280*
- Interbody Fusion *280*
- Alternatives to Fusion—Total Disk Replacement *282*
- Deformity Correction *282*
- Rods for Distraction and Compression *282*
- Segmental Fixation for Increased Rigidity *283*
- Multiple Hook Rod for Rotation *283*

40. Surgical Management of Lumbar Degenerative Spondylolisthesis **286**

Qasim M Husain, Robert P Norton, Jeffrey M Spivak

- Pathogenesis *286*
- Incidence *286*
- Presentation *287*
- Nonoperative Measures *287*
- Surgical Options *287*
- Case Example *292*

41. Differentiating Cervical Radiculopathy and Peripheral Compressive Neuropathy **294**

Themistocles S Protopsaltis, John A Bendo

- Epidemiology *294*
- Clinical Presentation and Relevant Anatomy *294*
- C8 Radiculopathy vs Cubital Tunnel Syndrome vs T1 Radiculopathy *296*
- Physical Examination *297*
- Electrodiagnostic Studies *299*
- Peripheral Entrapment Neuropathies and NCS *299*
- Treatment *299*
- Surgical Results *300*

42. Surgical Management of Cervical Disk Herniation **301**

Kseniya Slobodyanyuk, Jonathan Stieber

- Epidemiology *301*
- Signs and Symptoms *301*
- Treatment *302*
- Surgical Options *302*
- Anterior Approach *302*
- Posterior Approach *303*
- Selection of Approach *304*
- Complications *306*

43. Surgical Treatment of Cervical Stenosis **310**

Jane S Hoashi, Stephen P Maier II, Jeffrey D Klein

- Cervical Spondylotic Radiculopathy *310*
- Cervical Spondylotic Myelopathy *311*
- Pathogenesis *311*
- Treatment Options *313*
- Anterior Approach *314*
- Posterior Approach *317*
- Laminoplasty *318*
- Posterior Laminoforaminotomy *320*

44. Operative Management of Degenerative Cervical Disorders **324**

Hiroyuki Yoshihara, John A Bendo

- Surgical Indications *324*
- Surgical Options *325*
- Surgical Outcomes *328*
- Complications *329*

45. Newer Motion Preservation Technologies **332**

Kseniya Slobodyanyuk, Rachel N Rattenni, Thomas Cheriyan, Thomas J Errico

- Nucleus Replacement *332*
- Synthetic Nucleus Replacement *332*
- Interspinous Distraction *334*
- Dynamic Stabilization *334*
- Facet Replacement *335*
- Annulus Repair *336*

46. Minimally Invasive Lumbar Spine Fusion **337**

Noel I Perin

- Indications *337*
- Anterior Approaches (ALIF) *337*

- Posterior Approaches *340*
- Discussion *343*

47. Cervical Total Disk Replacement **345**

Robert P Norton, Jeffrey A Goldstein

- Evolution of Implants *345*
- Technical Considerations *346*
- Indications and Contraindications *347*
- Analysis of the FDA IDE Trials *347*
- Further Literature Analysis *347*
- Complications *349*
- Case Example *350*

48. Lumbar Total Disk Replacement Surgery **354**

Hiroyuki Yoshihara, John A Bendo

- Indications for Lumbar Total Disk Replacement *354*
- Surgical Approach and Technique *355*
- Prostheses *355*
- SB Charité III *355*
- Complications *358*

49. Conventional, Microscopic and Endoscopic Surgical Treatment of Lumbar Disk Herniations **361**

Bartosz Grobelny, Michael L Smith

- History *361*
- Modern Techniques *361*
- Comparative Trials *365*

50. Surgical Treatment of Lumbar Spinal Stenosis **369**

Stephen P Maier II, Jane S Hoashi, Jeffrey D Klein

- Clinical Features *369*
- Physical Examination and Differential Diagnosis *370*
- Diagnostic Imaging *370*
- Electrodiagnostic Studies *371*
- Indications for Surgery *371*
- Surgical Treatment *371*
- Surgical Outcomes *373*
- Interspinous Spacer Technology *374*

51. Overview of Spinal Deformity Surgery **378**

Justin Paul, Thomas Cheriyan, Anthony Petrizzo, Thomas J Errico

- Anatomy and Biomechanics *379*
- Clinical Evaluation *381*
- Radiologic Evaluation *381*
- Classification *382*
- Treatment *383*

52. Operative Management of Pediatric Deformities **388**

Justin C Paul, Baron S Lonner, Courtney S Toombs

- Scoliosis *388*
- Anatomy/Biomechanics *388*
- Clinical Evaluation *389*
- Radiologic Evaluation *392*
- Classification *393*
- Nonoperative Treatment *394*

- Operative Treatment *395*
- Surgical Technique *395*
- Outcomes/Complications *397*
- Kyphosis *399*
- Spondylolisthesis *400*

53. Surgical Treatment of Adult Degenerative Deformity **406**

Jeffrey B Knox, Justin Paul, Frank Schwab

- Surgical Indications *406*
- Presurgical Considerations *407*
- Surgical Planning *407*
- Surgical Techniques *407*
- Staged Operations *410*
- Complications *410*

54. Surgical Interventions in Osteoporosis and Compression Fracture **414**

Peter G Passias, Andy Chang

- Osteoporotic Compression Fractures *414*
- Conservative Management *414*
- Surgical Treatment *415*
- Adverse Events for Vertebroplasty and Kyphoplasty *417*

55. Surgical Management of the Rheumatoid Spine **420**

Ronald Moskovich, Jeffrey Knox

- Spine Manifestations *420*
- Clinical Evaluation *421*
- Natural History *421*
- Grading *421*
- Imaging *421*
- Treatment *423*
- Surgical Options *425*

56. Traumatic Cervical Spinal Fracture Surgery **429**

Justin C Paul, Robert Norton, Themistocles Protopsaltis

- Cervical Spine *429*
- Classification *434*
- Nonoperative Treatment *437*
- Operative Treatment *438*
- Classification *444*
- Operative Care to Optimize Function *445*

57. Thoracolumbar and Sacral Fracture Surgery **448**

Robert Norton, Justin C Paul, Themistocles Protopsaltis

- Anatomy and Mechanism of Injury *448*
- Clinical Evaluation *448*
- Radiologic Evaluation *448*
- Classification *449*
- Compression Fractures *449*
- Burst Fractures *450*
- Flexion-Distraction Injuries *451*
- Fracture-Dislocation Injuries *451*
- Low Lumbar Injuries *452*
- Treatment Goals *452*

58. Tumors of the Spine **456**

Donato Pacione, Irene Kim, Dimitris Placantonakis, Anthony Frempong-Boadu

- Primary Extradural Spinal Tumors *456*
- Intradural Extramedullary Spinal Tumors *461*
- Intradural Intramedullary Spinal Tumors *463*
- Spinal Metastases *468*

59. Intraoperative Monitoring in Spine Surgery **482**

Thomas Cheriyan, Rachel N Rattenni, Jerry Cheriyan, Athena M Lolis, Thomas J Errico

- Stagnara Wake-Up Test *482*
- Somatosensory Evoked Potential *482*
- Motor Evoked Potentials *483*
- Spontaneous EMG *484*
- Triggered EMG *485*
- Multimodal Intraoperative Monitoring *486*

Index **489**

SECTION

1

Basic Science and Spinal Assessment

CHAPTER 1

Basic Science of Degenerative Disk Disease

Anthony Petrizzo, Kristina Bianco

INTRODUCTION

The intervertebral disk (IVD) is a unique, multifunctional structure that plays a key role in spine biomechanics.[1] The IVD allows for movement of a spinal segment and acts as a connection between vertebrae. It provides a stabilizing structure for the spine by dissipating compressive loads, while enabling spine flexibility.[2] Degenerative changes to the chemical and mechanical composition of IVD are universal and increase with age. These changes result in degenerative disk disease (DDD), which detrimentally affects spinal function, leading to progressive degeneration of the spine.

Most patients presenting to healthcare professionals with back pain have no identifiable cause. A small subgroup of these patients has pain originating from the disk. However, it is difficult to differentiate between patients who present with discogenic-type back pain and patients presenting with back pain for other reasons. While DDD is very painful for some patients, disk degeneration may be a benign pain process for others. There are no pathologic findings for this pain syndrome on the history or physical presentation; this represents an enigma for practitioners treating patients with low back pain.

Research done over the past decade has helped better understand the mechanical, traumatic, immunologic, and genetic etiologies of DDD. This chapter reviews the morphology of a normal disk and describes the pathologic changes that occur in the degenerative disk. In addition, we examine the etiology, molecular mechanisms, and novel therapeutic modalities that may potentially provide a therapeutic option for patients with DDD.

MORPHOLOGY OF THE NORMAL IVD

The normal IVD is an avascular, fibrocartilaginous structure located between adjacent vertebrae (Fig. 1.1). The IVD is divided into three different regions: the nucleus pulposus (NP), annulus fibrosus (AF), and cartilaginous endplates. Each region has a different structural composition and function. The cells of the inner NP are characterized as chondrocyte-like, and the cells of the outer AF are fibroblast-like. Due to the lack of vascularity in the disk, the cells depend on the diffusion from blood vessels in the disk margin for the supply of nutrients and removal of metabolic waste. The disk matrix is a framework of macromolecules, specifically collagens and proteoglycans, which regulate the amount of water in the disk matrix (Fig. 1.2). Proteoglycans have a much larger affinity for water than collagens.

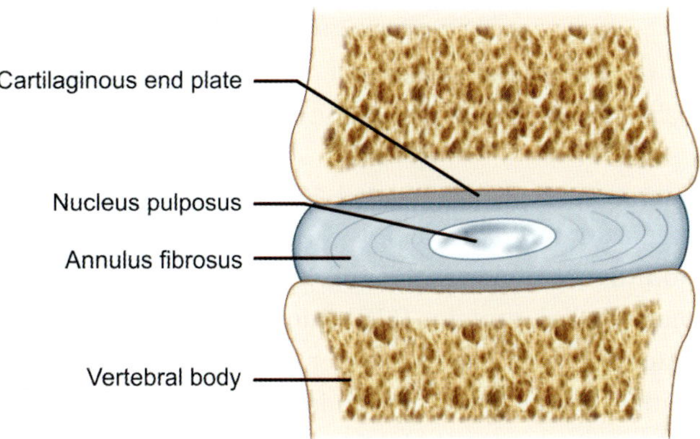

Fig. 1.1: The anatomy of a healthy intervertebral disk, including the nucleus pulposus, annulus fibrosus, and cartilaginous endplates.

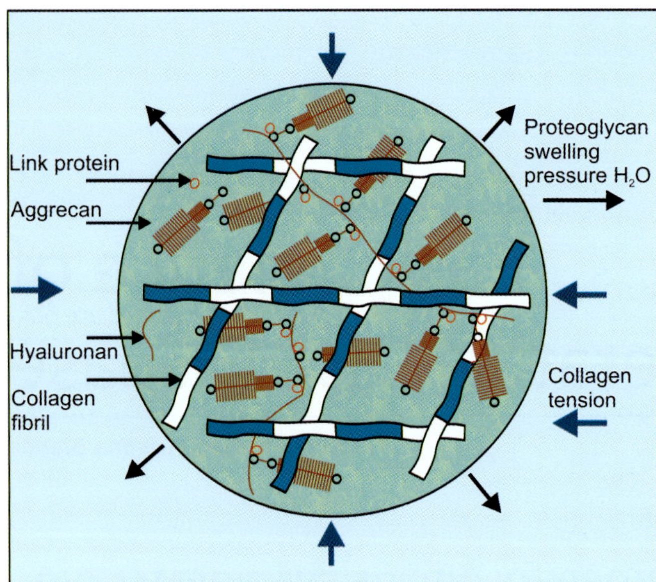

Fig. 1.2: The matrix of a healthy intervertebral disk, containing proteoglycans and collagen.

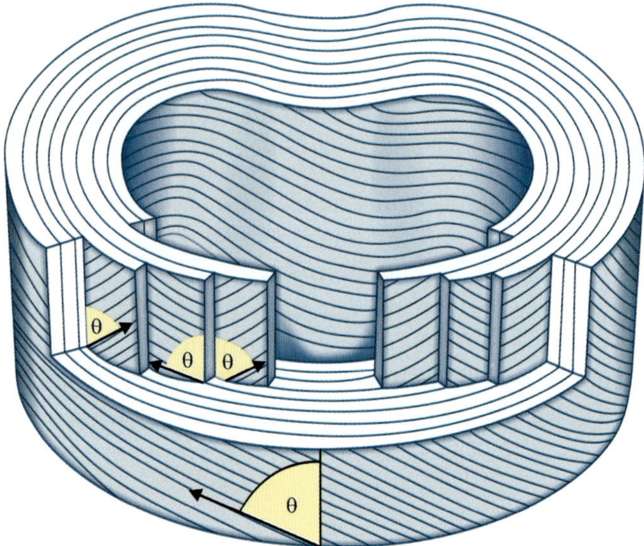

Fig. 1.4: The structural arrangement of collagen fibers in the disk. Collagen fibers are more tightly bound in the outer annulus.

The gelatinous NP, located at the core of the IVD, is formed from remnants of the notochord. The NP contains an abundance of proteoglycans, which are bound to hyaluronate via link proteins (LP) which facilitate the binding of water (Fig. 1.3).[1] The high water content allows the NP to essentially act as a fluid, which is critical in handling and distributing compressive loads.

The NP is surrounded by a stiff AF composed of collagen fibers oriented in a specific structural arrangement

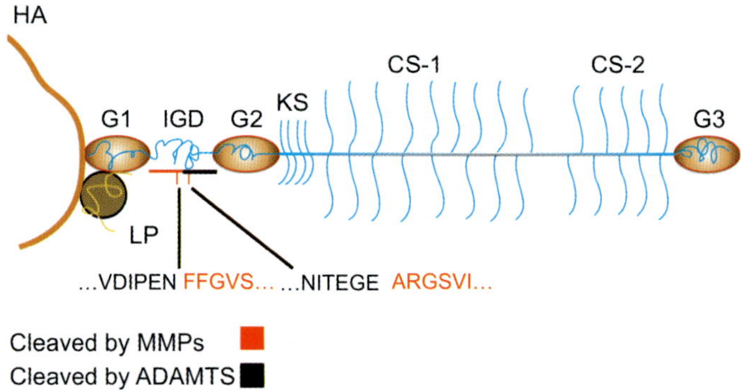

Fig. 1.3: A proteoglycan unit. Proteoglycans are attached to hyaluronate by link proteins (LP). Proteoglycans are composed of keratin sulfate (KS) or chondroitin sulfate (CS).

(Fig. 1.4). The annulus is made up a series of 15–25 concentric rings, or lamellae with the collagen fibers lying parallel within each lamella.[1] The fibers are oriented at approximately 60° vertically, alternating from left to right with each layer.[3] The majority of the collagen in the disk is type I or type II collagen. The outer annulus is composed of highly packed and densely organized collagen fibrils, which attach to the cartilaginous endplates on either side of the IVD, which facilitate its spine stabilizing capabilities.[2] In addition to the collagen fibrils, the outer annulus is also composed of a small amount of elastin, which helps with elastic recoil after stretching. The inner AF is neither as dense nor as organized as the outer annulus. The inner annulus is composed of a small amount of proteoglycan; thus, it has higher water content than the outer annulus.

The cartilaginous endplates separate the IVD from the vertebral body on both sides. The endplates are attached by a thin calcium layer, which are absent near the perforated areas of the bony plate, allowing for the diffusion of nutrients into the IVD.[2] The IVD is the largest avascular structure in the body; thus, nutrient diffusion through the cartilaginous endplates is imperative for cell survival and disk homeostasis.

MORPHOLOGIC CHANGES IN THE DEGENERATIVE IVD

In 1983, Kirkady—Wallis and Farfan described three clinical and biomechanical stages of spine degeneration: dysfunction, instability, and stabilization.[4] A spinal segment is composed of an anterior IVD and two posterior facet joints, referred to as a "three-joint complex".[5] These joints are intimately linked and damage to one ultimately inflicts damage on the other two joints. In the classic degenerative cascade, disk desiccation initiates intervertebral narrowing. This narrowing changes the orientation of the superior and inferior facets, resulting in incongruent facet loading, abnormal translation, facet hypertrophy, ligamentous infolding and hypertrophy, and osteophyte formation. Spinal stenosis can also present with or without foraminal compromise.

It is widely accepted that disk degeneration starts in the NP. In an aging disk, the rate of proteoglycan synthesis decreases, resulting in a diminished ability for the NP to absorb water.[6] Fragmentation of the large aggregated proteoglycans occurs, leading to more nonaggregated proteoglycans. This change in proportion results in a promotion of keratin sulfate (KS) as opposed to chondroitin sulfate (CS) in proteoglycans. KS is much smaller in molecular size and cannot attract water as well as CS. Increased collagen–proteoglycan binding also results in dehydration of the nucleus due to fewer polar groups and a decreased ability to bind water. This results in drying, cracking, and granulation of the nucleus. Cracks also appear in the annulus, which becomes increasingly fibrillated. A tear in the annulus initiates a "repair" process marked by an inflammatory response.

In the annulus, disk degeneration results in an increased concentration of both type I and type II collagen. With further degeneration, phenotypic changes also lead to more collagen of types III, V, and VI. Lastly, posttranslational modifications occur, which leads to cross-linking and nonenzymatic glycation, resulting in a change to a "less-efficient" collagen. This results in a more fibrous NP and a decreased ability to handle the normal compressive loads of the disk.

ETIOLOGY OF IVD DEGENERATION

Disk degeneration has a multifactorial etiology. Risk factors of disk degeneration include age, gender, genetic, environmental, and mechanical factors.[7] However, despite extensive research, the exact mechanism of disk degeneration is not fully understood.

Age

Aging results in the natural degeneration of the IVD. As the disk ages, changes occur to the molecular composition of the disk, resulting in significant structural and functional alterations. Although disk degeneration is predominantly a condition affecting adults, DDD is also seen in young patients. Juvenile disk degeneration is highly associated with spinal deformities and vertebral endplate changes.[8]

Gender

Disk space narrowing and osteoporosis are two factors that influence IVD degeneration. It has been found that disk space narrowing is more frequent in women than in men, and osteophyte formation is more frequent in men than in women.[9] Although degenerative changes are observed in both sexes, a study showed that female elderly patients have a mild tendency to develop more severe disk degeneration than their male counterparts.[10]

Genetic Factors

Susceptibility genetics is an active area of research for understanding the etiology of disk degeneration. Past research has indicated a familial aggregation of disk degeneration, and current studies aim to identify whether genetic factors or environmental factors play a more important role in the development of DDD. It is speculated that interactions among genes have presumably small individual effects, but a combination of genetic factors likely have significant additive effects.[11,12] In addition, gene–environment interactions, effects of genes on disease, and risks for individuals with different exposures to environmental factors are also likely.[12,13]

Current research uses polymerase chain reaction (PCR) to identify single nucleotide polymorphisms (SNPs) among genetic samples. An SNP is a sequence variation that occurs within DNA fragments of an individual. These SNPs are noted when compared to genome wide scans with either normal individuals or patients with phenotypes of DDD. Several gene loci have been identified to play an important role in the development of DDD. There are numerous genes that affect every step in the structural and functional environment of the disk. Genes that code for collagens I, IX, and XI, interleukins 1 and 6 (IL-1 and IL-6), aggrecan, the vitamin D receptor (VDR), matrix metalloproteinase 3 (MMP-3), and other proteins have been found to contribute to the degeneration of disks.[11] These candidate genes have been placed into four major categories of gene polymorphisms that lead to the development of disk degeneration (Fig. 1.5).[14]

Genes Associated with Disk Structure

Collagen I is a major protein found in bone and in the outer layer of the AF of the IVD. A guanine (G) to thymine (T) Sp1 polymorphism in intron 1 of the collagen type I

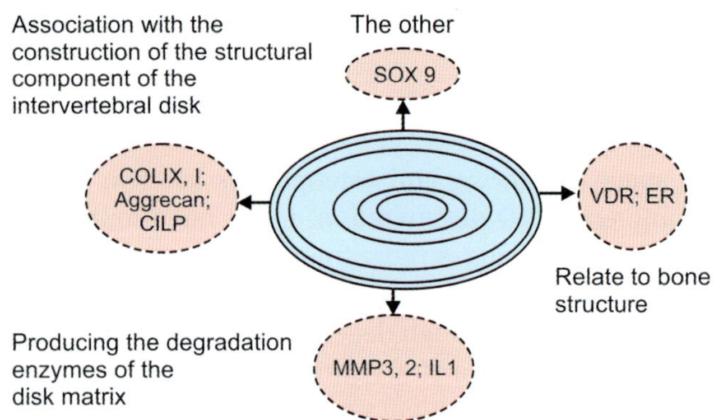

Fig. 1.5: Four main categories of genes associated with degenerative disk disease.

α1 gene (COLIA1) has been found to be associated with increased risk of IVD degeneration due to low mineral density, increased bone loss, higher bone turnover, and increased fracture risk.[11] A study by Pluijim et al. found that individuals with TT genotype had a higher risk of developing disk degeneration than individuals with GG and GT genotypes (OR 3.6, 95% CI 1.3–10).[15] Genes coding for collagen IX, which acts as a bridge between collagenous and noncollagenous proteins in tissue, have also been associated with increased risk of IVD degeneration.[14] Additionally, studies have found that a gene coding for collagen XI, COL11A2, is associated with an increased risk of bulges and degenerative stenosis, which can be caused by disk degeneration.[16,17]

Genes that Produce Matrix Degrading Enzymes

IL-1 is a cytokine produced in response to infection or injury, and plays a regulatory role in the health of the disk. A polymorphism of the IL-1 gene has been found to increase the risk of developing disk degeneration by inducing enzymes that destroy proteoglycan.[18] It has also been speculated that IL-6 contributes to IVD degeneration due to its role in inflammation, collateral tissue destruction, and pain.[19]

Aggrecan is a proteoglycan that binds to hyaluronic acid. The ability of the NP to dissipate loads is largely due to chondroitin sulfate chains, which exist in two domains of the aggrecan core protein, termed the CS1 and CS2 domains. In humans, the CS1 domain has been found to exhibit allele size polymorphism, which can change the properties of aggrecan and result in IVD degeneration.[20] A study by Kawaguchi et al. found that there was a significant difference between the distribution of allele sizes and the severity of disk degeneration, as analyzed by magnetic resonance imaging (MRI).[21] The correlation between shorter CS1 lengths and the presence of disk degeneration has been found; however, it has yet to be replicated in large sample study groups.[20]

Other enzymes that are crucial to the homeostasis of the disk environment are MMPs, which are synthesized and secreted by the connective tissue cells. MMPs play a fundamental role in the inflammation of the disk and are induced in response to local conditions such as mechanical loading and inflammation. The genetic expression and alteration of this gene is also fundamentally important. MMP-3 is a proteoglycan-degrading type of MMP that has been found to play an essential role in the degeneration of disks.[22] A common polymorphism in the promoter region of the MMP-3 gene may be a key risk factor for the acceleration of IVD degeneration.

Genes Related to Bone Structure

VDR is known to play a significant role in the mineralization and remodeling of bones.[11] Gene polymorphisms of VDR have been demonstrated to contribute to disorders such as osteoporosis, arthritis, and DDD.[11] A study of male monozygotic twins showed that an intragenic polymorphism in the VDR gene was associated with increased risk of developing disk degeneration.[23] Furthermore, a study by Kawaguchi et al. showed that allelic variation in the VDR receptor gene was associated with IVD degeneration.[24] Though there is still uncertainty as to how the genetic variants of the VDR affect disk generation, it is speculated that polymorphisms of the VDR may alter the structural composition of the disk.

All Other Genes Identified

Genes that code for other proteins, such as keep SOX 9, cartilage intermediate layer protein, tissue inhibitor of metalloproteinase 1, cyclooxygenase 2, and thrombospondin, and a gene referred by the acronym SPARC (secreted protein, acidic, rich in cytosine) have shown potential for increased risk of disk degeneration.[11] Further research is needed to fully understand the genetic components contributing to disk degeneration.

Environmental Factors

Although it is widely recognized that environmental factors are secondary to genetic factors in the development of DDD, environmental factors still play a pivotal role in the degenerative process. Occupational factors, exposure to toxins, nutrient availability, increased body mass, and obesity all contribute to the environmental component of disk degeneration. Mechanical stresses, such as manual handling of heavy materials, frequent bending or twisting, and whole body vibration have all been associated with a higher risk of developing DDD.[25] Mechanical overload of the disk can also lead to annular or endplate injury.

Exposure to toxins and smoke has also been associated with increased risk of developing DDD. A study by Battié et al. found that for groups of identical twins who were discordant for cigarette smoking, disk degeneration scores were 18% higher for smokers than nonsmokers.[26] The higher risk of disk degeneration among smokers is likely due to impaired blood flow to the disk, resulting in decreased oxygen tension and decreased synthesis of proteoglycan and collagen.[27]

Nutrient availability is a microenvironmental factor that has been found to lead to the development of DDD. The activity of the disk cells is very sensitive to extracellular oxygen and pH levels. Inefficient anaerobic metabolism leads to increased lactic acid levels, lowering the pH within the disk and making the environment more acidic. When the pH is decreased, proteoglycan synthesis is decreased. Since the IVD is an avascular tissue, nutrients must diffuse to the nucleus and inner annulus through a complicated path extending from the blood vessels of the vertebral body, through the endplate. The endplate is composed of a thin layer of cortical bone covered by hyaline cartilage. In a healthy disk, nutrients pass through the porous endplates into the disk. A reduction in the transport of nutrients into the disk and decreased ability of waste products to exit the disk space contribute to disk degeneration. Calcification of the endplate results in a loss of endplate permeability and a barrier to the transport of nutrients.[28] Calcification has been correlated with loss of nutrition and the death of cells in the IVD.

Finally, excess body weight and obesity has been found to play an important role in the development of IVD degeneration. A study by Samartzis et al. found that juvenile disk degeneration is strongly associated with an increase in body mass index.[14] Individuals regarded as overweight or obese were found to have a 14-fold greater prevalence of disk degeneration than underweight and normal-weight individuals. The exact mechanism by which obesity relates to disk degeneration is not fully understood; it may be mechanical or due to an inflammatory component that may incite inflammatory responses in the disk.[29] Studies have also shown that various metabolic disorders, such as diabetes mellitus, result in disk degeneration due to a change in the biochemical and vascular properties of the disk matrix.[30]

INFLAMMATORY MEDIATORS

The release of inflammatory mediators plays an important role in the development of discogenic back pain (Flowchart 1.1). Degenerated disks display heightened

Flowchart 1.1: A schematic representation of how inflammatory mediators play a role in the development of degenerative disk disease.

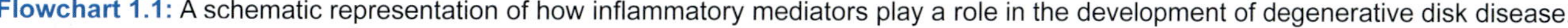

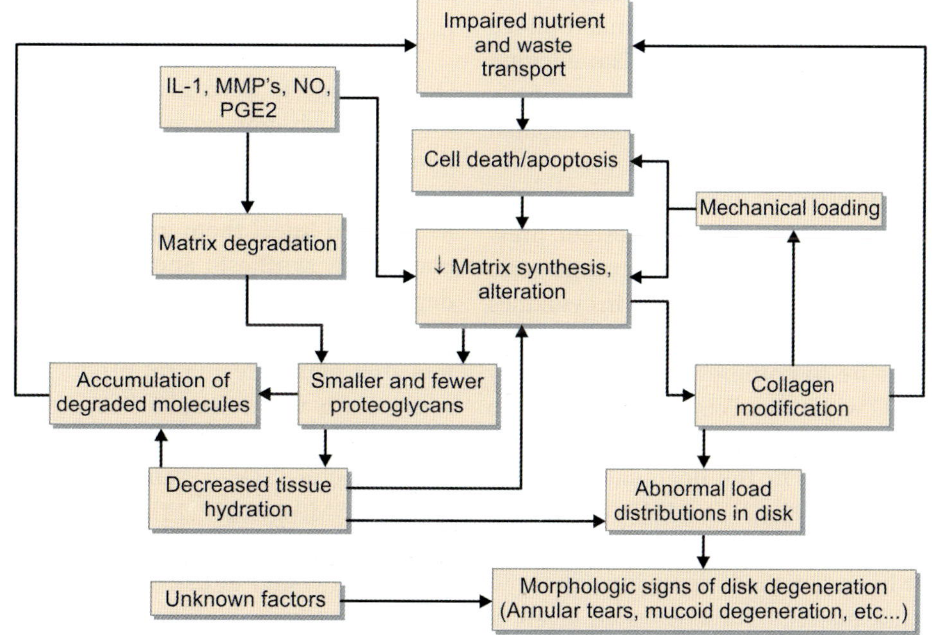

amounts of inflammatory mediators, suggesting their role in DDD.[31] ILs are a class of cytokines produced in response to infection, injury, or exposure of previously immune-privileged mesenchymal stem cells of the NP.[1] IL-1 directly regulates the breakdown of proteoglycan synthesis and activates IL-6, nitric oxide (NO), and prostaglandin E2 (PGE2), resulting in a further inhibition of proteoglycan synthesis. IL-1 also increases the synthesis of MMPs.

The inflammatory cascade exhibited by a herniated disk differs from the immune activation profile observed in IVD degeneration. In patients with disk herniations, there is a greater presence of tumor necrosis factor α (TNF-α), IL 1B, IL-6 compared with controls. A variety of these inflammatory mediators have also been suggested to play a role in the degenerative process. IL-1 and IL-6, NO, MMPs, TNF-α, PGE2, and cytokines are all present in the environment of the degraded IVD.[31] Chemical mediators of inflammation are elevated in both annular and nuclear tissue of painful IVDs. Inflammatory mediators influx with degeneration of the disk, inciting collateral inflammation of the juxtaposed nerve root. Inflammatory mediators can sensitize the nerve endings or result in nerve and blood vessel ingrowth into the degenerative disk.

There appears to be greater IL-12 and interferon-γ (IFNγ) expression in herniated disk fragments compared with bulging disks that remain contained within the disk space by an intact annulus fibrosus.[32] These cytokines are mostly macrophage products that can promote lymphocyte activation and differentiation while also recruiting additional macrophages and activating phagocytosis and secretion of proteolytic enzymes. Activated Th1 lymphocytes produce IFNγ that assists in further macrophage recruitment and activation, and the mechanism eliciting the heightened IFNγ expression in herniated disk fragments may represent a specific immune response against herniated NP tissue.[32]

NO production is the result of degradation of proteoglycan in the lumbar IVD in response to hydrostatic pressure.[31] Mechanical stress due to prolonged compressive loading has been found to result in an increase in cytokines within the IVD, which upregulate the production of NO. Thus, prolonged exposure to compressive loading likely results in increased NO within the IVD, and is a measure of inflammation and destruction.

MMPs are key mediators in the degradation of the extracellular matrix. In a healthy IVD, MMPs are necessary for matrix turnover. In a degenerated disk, elevated levels of MMPs have been recorded, signifying enhanced degradation of the disk matrix.[31] These elevated levels of MMPs are likely due to increased levels in cytokines. The increased level of MMPs in the degenerated disk also appears to be directly associated with the increase in ILs in the IVD.

In addition, phospholipase A2 is abundant in disk tissue and induces prostaglandin and MMP activity, promoting matrix degeneration. Phospholipase A2 levels correlate closely with the symptoms of sciatica in patients who have herniated or extruded disk fragments but less to patients who have an exacerbation of back pain secondary to degenerative disks.

NOVEL MANAGEMENT TECHNIQUES

Currently, there are a variety of procedures targeted to manage and treat disk degeneration. Traditional approaches, such as fusion of spinal segments, partial discectomies, disk replacement, intradiscal heating, and intradiscal neurolytics, have varying clinical outcomes. While a spinal fusion may limit pain, it does not halt the underlying degeneration cascade and may even increase the risk of degeneration in adjacent spinal motion segments.[12] Novel approaches, such as protein factors, gene transfers, cell therapy, and tissue engineering, aim at targeting the underlying causes of disk degeneration. The goal of these therapies is to achieve cellular repair of the degenerative disk matrix. Current advances in genomics, nanotechnology, stem cell biology, and gene therapy have the potential to significantly contribute to therapeutic efforts to treat patients with DDD.[12]

Protein Growth Factors

One strategy to reverse disk degeneration attempts to initiate rehydration by stimulating proteoglycan production, and/or inhibit cytokines that degrade proteoglycans in the disk.[33] Another approach aims to modulate growth factors and inject them into aging cells in order to stimulate DNA synthesis and reverse the aging process of degenerative disks. Growth factors can increase rates of matrix synthesis by up to fivefold. Common growth factors that stimulate matrix production are platelet-derived growth factor insulin-like growth factor, fibroblast growth factor, epidermal growth factor, transforming growth factor (TGF-β), and bone morphogenic proteins (BMP-2, BMP-7, BMP-14).[34] Furthermore, protease inhibitors, transcription factors, and platelet-rich plasma have been tested to assess the ability to promote extracellular matrix production.[28] Though there are a variety of growth factors that seem to be viable for the management of DDD, coadministration of multiple growth factors may provide synergistic effects. A limitation in the clinical use of protein factors is a relatively short duration of therapeutic activity.

Gene Transfers

Gene transfer has the potential to provide sustained synthesis of therapeutic proteins. In a gene transfer technique, genes triggering a therapeutic effect can be introduced into the targeted disk by injection of transplanted cells using a viral or nonviral vector.[28] Gene transfer may be a cheaper and longer lasting way to deliver protein factors aimed at the management of DDD.

Cell Therapy

Introducing cells capable of regenerating disk tissue has the potential to reverse degeneration of the IVD. Autologous sources for cell-based therapies include native disk cells that could be harvested during the therapeutic discectomy and mesenchymal stem cells from bone marrow. In addition, autologous articular chondrocytes may also serve as a source of cell therapy. Current studies are in their infancy and long-term effects are not established.

Tissue Engineering

Strategies that aim to repair disks through tissue engineering may be optimal for restoring proper biomechanical and biochemical behavior of the disk. Annular and nuclear tissue-engineering techniques have been studied.[28] However, the insufficient biomechanical properties of engineered tissues are an inherent shortcoming to tissue engineering techniques.

CONCLUSION

Degeneration of the IVD is estimated to be the most prevalent source of low back pain; however, DDD is still poorly understood.[28] The etiology of disk degeneration is multifactorial and is a combination of extrinsic, intrinsic, and genetic factors. The natural history of this degenerative process can be affected by trauma, vascular disease, and the normal aging process. There are currently a few management techniques that can alter the course of progressive degeneration. However, further research on protein factors, gene transfers, cell therapy, and tissue engineering is needed in order to develop an optimal management technique to treat DDD.

Since disk degeneration is a natural process that occurs with age, shifting demographics and aging populations will likely result in an increased amount of patients suffering from disk degeneration in future years. Thus, it is imperative for physicians and patients alike to understand the risk factors associated with DDD and possible prevention and treatment methods to address DDD.

REFERENCES

1. Buckwalter JA, Einhorn TA, Simon SR. Orthopaedic basic science: biology and biomechanics of the musculoskeletal system. Rosemont: Amer Academy of Orthopaedic; 2000.
2. Benzel, EC. Spine surgery: techniques, complication avoidance, and management. Philadelphia: Elsevier Saunders; 2012.
3. Urban J, Roberts S. Degeneration of the intervertebral disk. Arthritis Res Ther. 2003;5(3):120-8.
4. Kirkaldy-Willis W, Farfan H. Instability of the lumbar spine. Clin Orthop Relat Res. 1982;165:110.
5. Yong-Hing K, Kirkaldy-Willis W. The pathophysiology of degenerative disease of the lumbar spine. Orthop Clin North America. 1983;14(3):491.
6. Johnstone B, Bayliss MT. The large proteoglycans of the human intervertebral disc. Changes in their biosynthesis and structure with age, topography, and pathology. Spine. 1995;20(6):674.
7. Hadjipavlou A, Tzermaidianos M, Bogduk N, et al. The pathophysiology of disc degeneration: a critical review. J Bone Joint Surg Br. 2008;90:1261-70.
8. Guiot BH, Fessler RG. Molecular biology of degenerative disc disease. Neurosurgery. 2000;47(5):1034-40.
9. de Schepper EIT, Damen J, van Meurs JBJ, et al. The association between lumbar disc degeneration and low back pain: the influence of age, gender, and individual radiographic features. Spine. 2010;35(5):531.
10. Wang YXJ, Griffith J, Ma H, et al. Relationship between gender, bone mineral density, and disc degeneration in the lumbar spine: a study in elderly subjects using an eight-level MRI-based disc degeneration grading system. Osteoporos Int. 2011;22(1):91-6.
11. Kalichman L, Hunter DJ. The genetics of intervertebral disc degeneration. Associated genes. Joint Bone Spine. 2008;75(4):388-96.
12. Taher F, Essig D, Lebl DR, et al. Lumbar degenerative disc disease: current and future concepts of diagnosis and management. Adv Orthop. 2012;2012.
13. Zhang Y, Sun Z, Liu J, et al. Advances in susceptibility genetics of intervertebral degenerative disc disease. Int J Biol Sci. 2008;4(5):283.
14. Samartzis D, Karppinen J, Mok F, et al. A population-based study of juvenile disc degeneration and its association with overweight and obesity, low back pain, and diminished functional status. J Bone Joint Surg (Am). 2011;93(7):662-70.

15. Pluijm S, Van Essen H, Bravenboer N, et al. Collagen type I α1 Sp1 polymorphism, osteoporosis, and intervertebral disc degeneration in older men and women. Ann Rheum Dis. 2004;63(1):71-7.
16. Solovieva S, Lohiniva J, Leino-Arjas P, et al. Intervertebral disc degeneration in relation to the COL9A3 and the IL-1ss gene polymorphisms. Eur Spine J. 2006;15(5):613-9.
17. Noponen-Hietala N, Kyllönen E, Männikkö M, et al. Sequence variations in the collagen IX and XI genes are associated with degenerative lumbar spinal stenosis. Ann Rheum Dis. 2003;62(12):1208-14.
18. Solovieva S, Kouhia S, Leino-Arjas P, et al. Interleukin 1 polymorphisms and intervertebral disc degeneration. Epidemiology. 2004;15(5):626.
19. Noponen-Hietala N, Virtanen I, Karttunen R, et al. Genetic variations in *IL6* associate with intervertebral disc disease characterized by sciatica. Pain. 2005;114(1):186-94.
20. Roughley P, Martens D, Rantakokko J, et al. The involvement of aggrecan polymorphism in degeneration of human intervertebral disc and articular cartilage. Eur Cell Mater. 2006;11(1):7.
21. Kawaguchi Y, Osada R, Kanamori M, et al. Association between an aggrecan gene polymorphism and lumbar disc degeneration. Spine. 1999;24(23):2456.
22. Goupille P, Jayson IV M, Valat JP, et al. Matrix metalloproteinases: the clue to intervertebral disc degeneration? Spine. 1998;23(14):1612.
23. Videman T, Leppävuori J, Kaprio J, et al. Intragenic polymorphisms of the vitamin D receptor gene associated with intervertebral disc degeneration. Spine. 1998;23(23): 2477.
24. Kawaguchi Y, Kanamori M, Ishihara H, et al. The association of lumbar disc disease with vitamin-D receptor gene polymorphism. J Bone Joint Surg (Am). 2002;84(11):2022-8.
25. Lötters F, Burdorf A, Kuiper J, et al. Model for the work-relatedness of low-back pain. Scand J Work, Environ Health. 2003;29(6):431.
26. Battié MC, Videman T, Gill K, et al. 1991 Volvo Award in clinical sciences. Smoking and lumbar intervertebral disc degeneration: an MRI study of identical twins. Spine. 1991;16(9):1015.
27. Iwahashi M, Matsuzaki H, Tokuhashi Y, et al. Mechanism of intervertebral disc degeneration caused by nicotine in rabbits to explicate intervertebral disc disorders caused by smoking. Spine. 2002;27(13):1396.
28. DePalma MJ, Ketchum JM, Saullo T. What is the source of chronic low back pain and does age play a role? Pain Med. 2011;12(2):224-33.
29. Das U. Is obesity an inflammatory condition? Nutrition. 2001;17(11):953-66.
30. Robinson D, Mirovsky Y, Halperin N, et al. Changes in proteoglycans of intervertebral disc in diabetic patients: a possible cause of increased back pain. Spine. 1998; 23(8): 849.
31. Podichetty VK. The aging spine: the role of inflammatory mediators in intervertebral disc degeneration. Cell Mol Biol (Noisy-le-Grand, France). 2007;53(5):4.
32. Shamji MF, Setton LA, Jarvis W, et al. Proinflammatory cytokine expression profile in degenerated and herniated human intervertebral disc tissues. ArthritisRheum. 2010; 62(7):1974-82.
33. DePalma M. Biologic treatments for discogenic low back pain. SpineLine. 2012;19-26.
34. Chrastil J, Patel AA. Complications associated with posterior and transforaminal lumbar interbody fusion. J Am Acad Orthop Sur. 2012;20(5):283-91.

CHAPTER

2

Biomechanics of the Spine

Antonio Valdevit

THE SPINAL COLUMN

The spine column is comprised of four sections: cervical, thoracic, lumbar, and the sacrum/coccyx (Fig. 2.1).

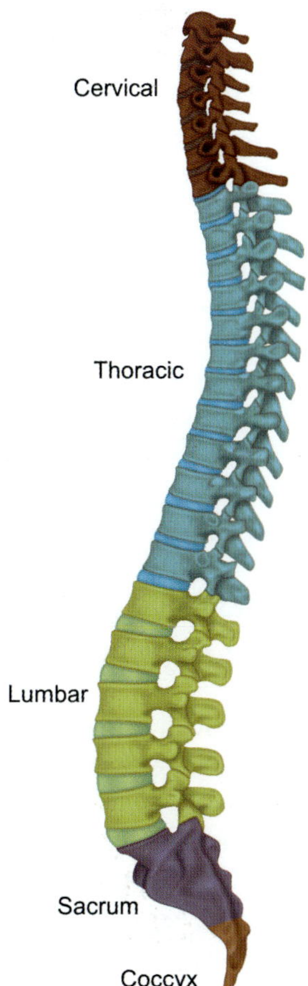

Fig. 2.1: Regions of the spinal column.

The cervical, thoracic, and lumbar are flexible; however, their individual contributions to the range of motion (ROM) do vary significantly (Fig. 2.2).[1]

The spine displays four functions: support, protection, mobility, and motion. The spinal column forms a major support structure in the human body and can sustain heavy loads particularly in the lumbar region. Not only does it carry the weight of our upper body but anything being carried or lifted, as well. The spinal canal houses and protects; the spinal cord and nerves as they pass from the brainstem to the limbs. The muscles and ligaments associated with the spine contribute toward the stability and overall ROM. These soft tissues are involved in the active (muscles) and passive (ligaments and tendons) loading of the spine that permits control of motion. Without these elements, the spine is inherently unstable. For example, Olympic weightlifters can support over

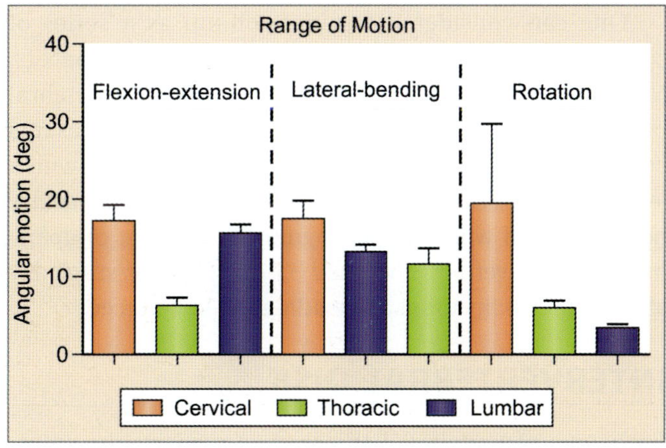

Fig. 2.2: Contribution to overall range of motion by region.[1]

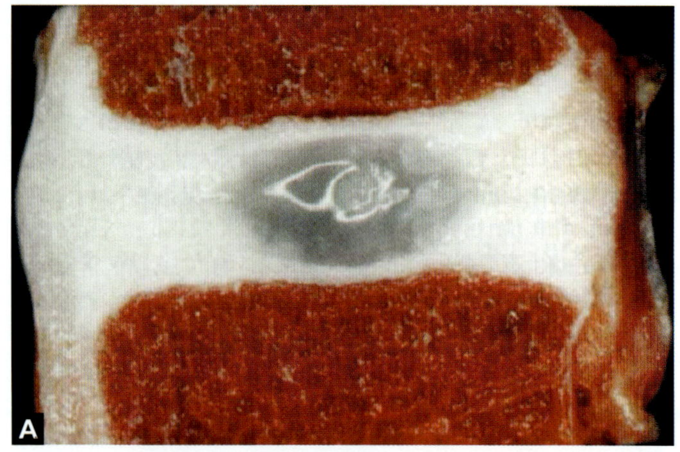

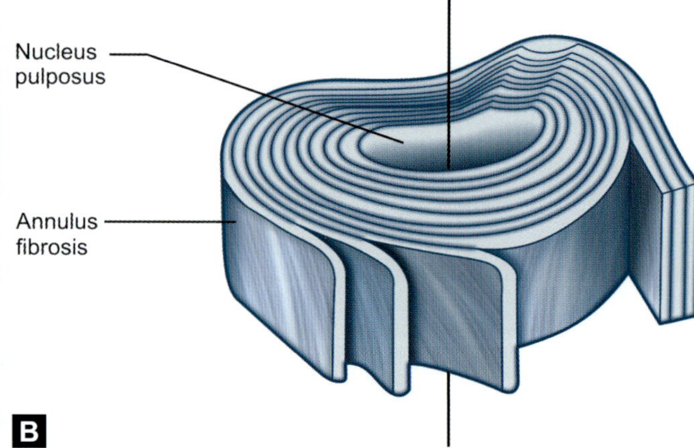

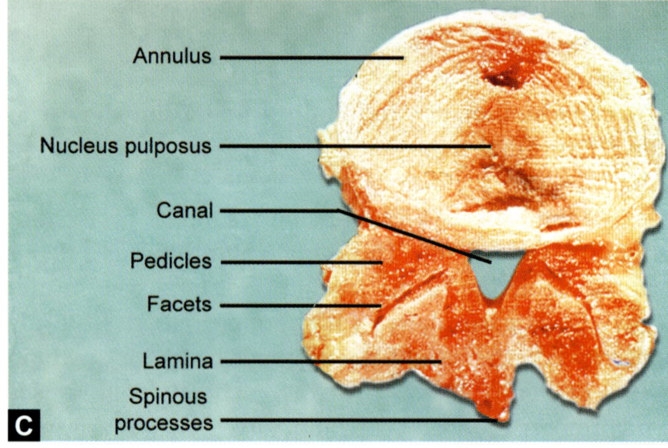

Figs. 2.3A to C: (A) Longitudinal section along the spine representing a functional spinal unit (FSU); (B) Schematic diagram of the intervertebral disk comprised of concentric rings of collagen fibers oriented at ±30° to the horizontal; (C) Cross-section of the spinal column at the level of an intervertebral disk.

30,000 N of load. However, in a laboratory setting, the spine collapses under a 200 N force when surrounding soft tissue is removed. One thing that should be emphasized is that the motions and articulations of spine (or any anatomical joint) is actually caused by moments (that is a force action via a lever arm) rather than direct forces such as those generated by the muscular contractions.

One can consider the spinal column as a series of connected hard elements connected with soft spacers. More specifically, one can use the analogy of the vertebral body as a can of soda. The dense outer layer represents cortical bone (the aluminum) and is filled internally with a less dense material (the soda) representative of trabecular bone. The can will sustain a significant amount of deformation. However, when opened (i.e. fractured or surgically altered) the ability to sustain loading will be reduced.

INTERVERTEBRAL DISK

Each pair of vertebral body is separated by the intervertebral disk and such a configuration is termed a functional spinal unit (FSU). The disk is comprised of concentric rings of collagen fibers oriented at ±30° to the horizontal (Figs. 2.3A to C). At the center of this ring structure is the nucleus pulposus, a gelatinous structure that aids is hydrostatic resistance to loading.[2] At any one spinal level, the disk structure contributes to about 50% of torsional stability and supports about 80% of the axial load with minimal resistance to flexion and extension.

THE FACET JOINT AND UNCOVERTEBRAL JOINT

The facet joints are synovial joints formed between the superior articular process of one vertebra and the inferior articular process of the vertebra directly above it. The facet joints provide the remaining 50% of torsional stability. In lumbar region, the facet joints support approximately 20% of the weight-bearing capacity with one of the prime functions being resistance to shear.

With specific reference to the cervical spine (Fig. 2.4), the uncovertebral joints, also called joints of Luschka, are

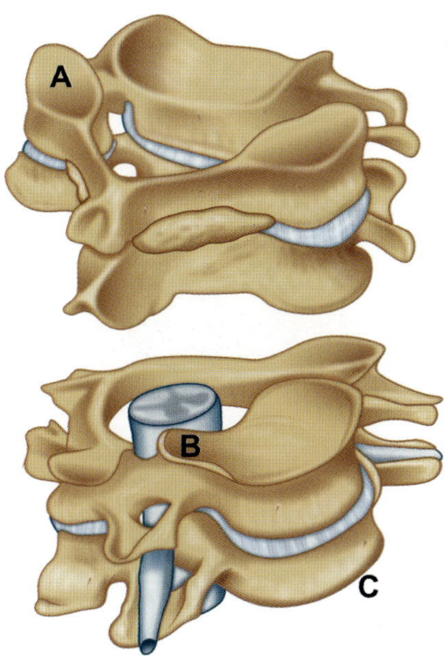

Fig. 2.4: The cervical spine: (A) facet joints, (B) two uncovertebral joints are also seen, and (C) the intervertebral disk.[1]

seen between C3 and C7. The joint is formed between the uncinate process above and uncus below and function to limit lateral translation of the cervical spine.[3]

SPINAL MOTION

The upper cervical spine supports the head and is naturally positioned in flexion and the act of rotation is such that the motion occurs coaxially with the spinal canal so as to permit safe rotation of the skull without danger of cord damage. Cervical spine motions are different as compared to the lumbar and thoracic spine. In cervical flexion, the facet joints slide over each other and resulting in some vertebral translation. In extension, the spinous processes physically come into contact thereby limiting the range of maximum extension. In this plan of motion, the center of rotation is located in the distal vertebral body (Fig. 2.5A).

In lateral bending, the motion is guided by the uncovertebral joints, which act as a rail to minimize lateral shear. Simultaneously, the center of rotation in this mode of motion is located in the superior vertebral body and is determined by the overall radius of the two uncovertebral joints (Fig. 2.5B).

While the motion displayed in the thoracic/lumbar section of the spine displays similar characteristics with respect to the motion planes, these physical values in range are reduced, especially in the thoracic region. In the lumbar region, overall range in increased relative to

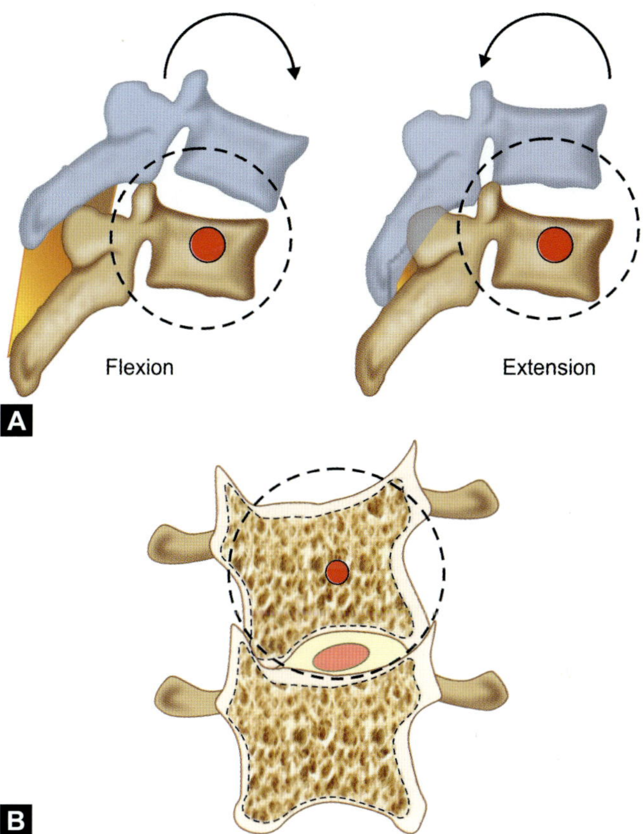

Figs. 2.5A and B: (A) In flexion-extension, the center of rotation resides in the inferior vertebral body and (B) in lateral bending, the center of rotation resides in the superior vertebral body.

the thoracic region but is less than that displayed by the cervical spine. The dominant role of the lumbar region is load bearing and as such a propensity toward stability is warranted, which comes as a trade-off for mobility.

SPINAL LOADING

Spinal loading is in fact quite complex and considered to be a combination of several, if not all, types of loading: tension, bending, shear, compression, and torsion (Fig. 2.6). The overall motion is dependent upon which loading type is dominant.

Unlike other anatomical joints, the spine exhibits what is termed "coupled motion",[4] implying motion in one plane will display reactions in other directions other than the dominant motion in the lumbar region. At L5, a combination of torsion and lateral bending is displayed. In the cervical spine, you do get axial distraction beyond 2° or 3° of rotation. At C2, for example, one would see 2°

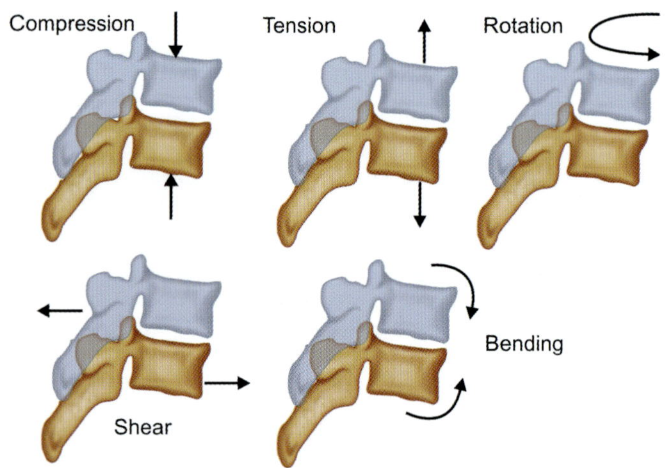

Fig. 2.6: The true loading mechanism in the spine is a combination of many types, though one dominates in any one motion.

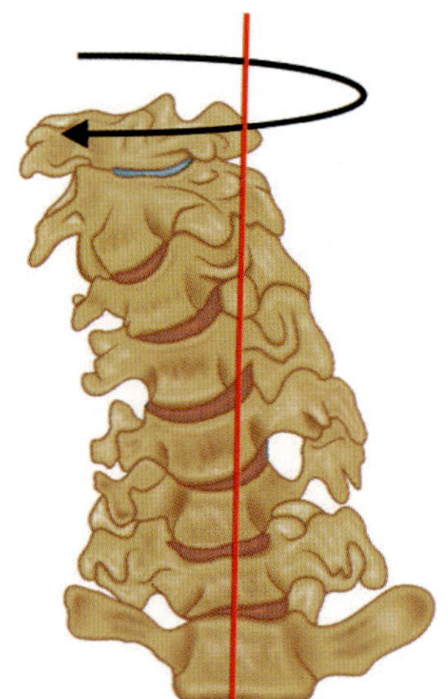

Fig. 2.7: All spinal segment display coupled motion. That is motion in one plane also displays motion in other planes.

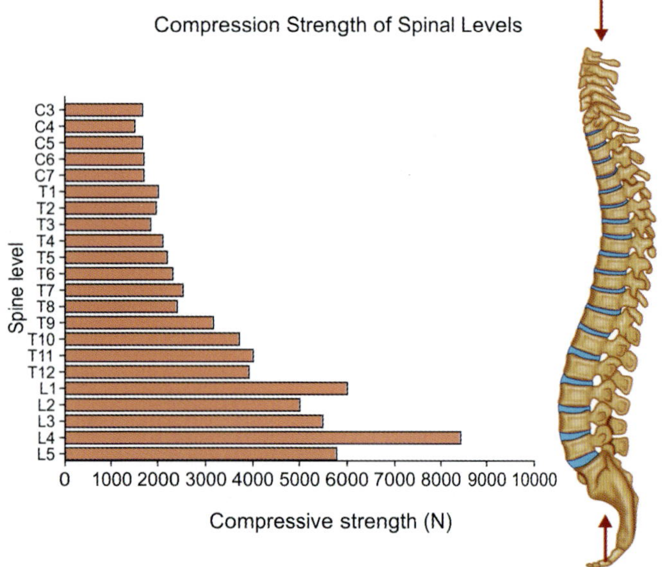

Fig. 2.8: Compressive strength variations in the spinal column.[4]

of coupled axial rotation for every 3° of lateral bending, or a ratio of (2:3). However, at C7, this ratio drops to about two parts in 15 (Fig. 2.7).

There are similarities and differences between the cervical and lumbar spine. They have similar shape and curvature; a posterior tension band effect to restrict the amount of forward flexion; display anterior support and the respective FSU mobility displays similar characteristics. One of the main differences between the two regions is the load-bearing capacity. The cervical spine carries about 100 N of load while the lower lumbar region can sustain over 2000 N. The cervical spine is equipped to account for acceleration via a geometrically reduced size and the load sharing between the anterior and posterior regions that are approximately 64:36 versus 80:20 in the lumbar spine.

We must recognize that lumbar and cervical mechanics are different and results in different demands being placed upon the instrumentation employed in each region. For example, in considering treatment options, the compressive strength of the vertebrae in the lumbar region it is well over 5500 N as compared to 1800 N in the cervical region (Fig. 2.8). The lumbar region actually takes most of the large physiological loads we encounter during activities of daily living.

When considering implants one should also address the resulting stiffness characteristic of the resulting construct and the introduction of stress shielding. This condition occurs when an overly stiff implant or construct is employed and the loading is such that the implant/construct bears all of the physiological loading. This situation can result in delayed fusion as well as bone resorption according to Wolff's law. At the same time, a construct or implant that displays a stiffness value that is insufficient can lead to strain microfractures, delayed healing and callus. When one obtains a construct stiffness that induces load sharing between the implants and the host bone, faster healing, good vascularity and good bone orientation can result.

In considering intervertebral devices, whether they be in conjunction with posterior instrumentation or used in isolation, clinicians must consider that one can have load sharing when you have an intervertebral implant with

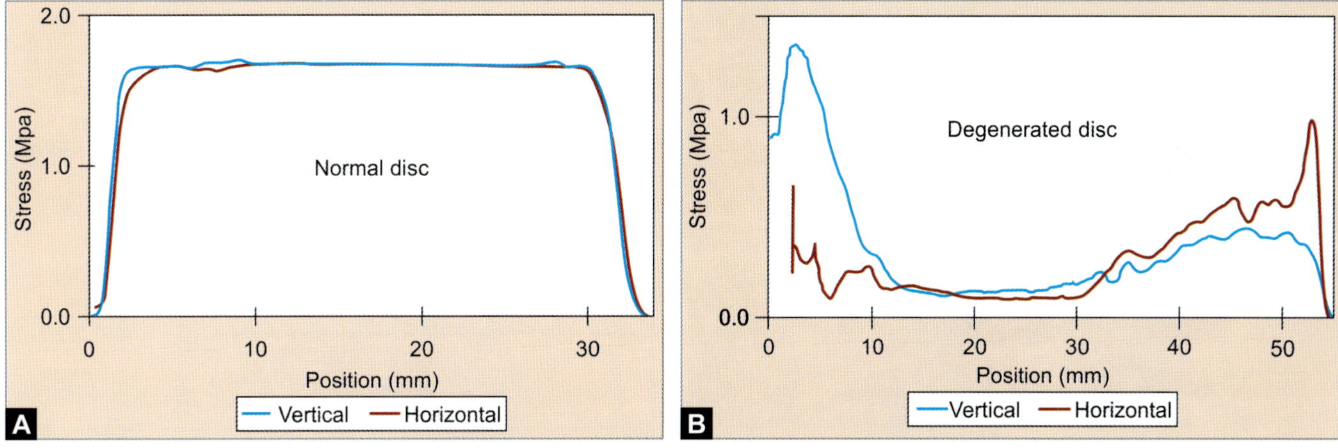

Figs. 2.9A and B: Loading patterns within the disk under (A) normal and (B) degenerated conditions.[5]

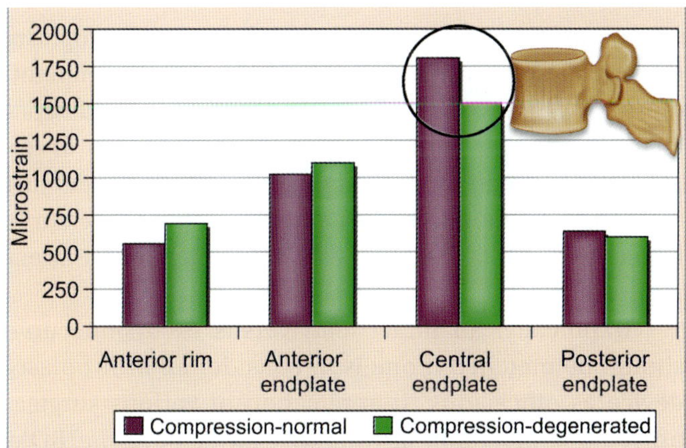

Fig. 2.10: Changes in endplate strain due to degeneration.[6]

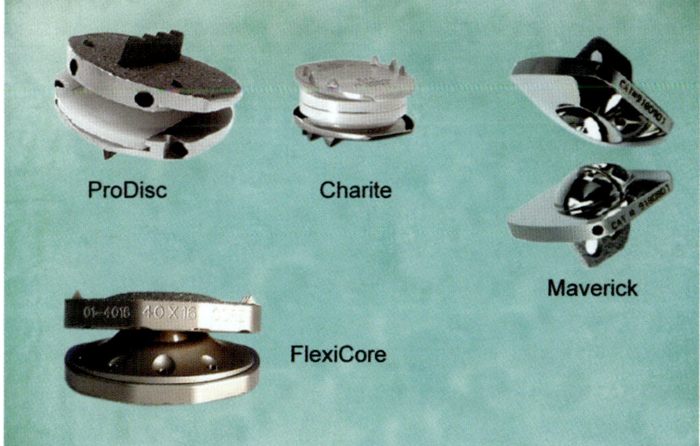

Fig. 2.11: Lumbar intervertebral disk prostheses under development or in the market.

posterior screws, whereas the stand-alone device gives you load bearing. The ultimate decision as to which route is best is based on clinical findings and comorbidities of the patient. Regardless of final approach if intervertebral devices are to be employed, endplate preservation following a discectomy is important. This is especially crucial in cases where the intervertebral device is acting in a stand-alone configuration as it is in a load-bearing condition.

Mechanically, degeneration is presented with high annular loading in compression and increased shear and facet loading.[6] Examining the loading patterns along the disks in the position for anterior and posterior depicts changes primarily in axial rotation and lateral bending (Figs. 2.9A and B).

In examining the endplate under degenerative conditions with respect to strain, the central region is most affected with similar findings also seen in the mediolateral and anterior and posterior directions. This is important to recognize, as the central plate is the region that should be avoided clinically when placing intervertebral devices as this region is known to be the weakest region of the endplate. Placement should encompass the vertebral rim that is stronger and contains more cortical bone (Fig. 2.10).

SPINAL ARTHROPLASTY

The goal of any arthroplasty device is to restore normal kinematics and joint function in addition to reducing pain. Spinal arthroplasty might be more advantageous than spinal fusion, offsetting complications like possible adjacent segment degeneration and prolonged postoperative rehabilitation and pain.

Figure 2.11 shows a few spinal arthroplasty devices either on the market or under development. Among them are metal-polymer devices such as the ProDisc and Charite, and metal-metal devices such as the Maverick

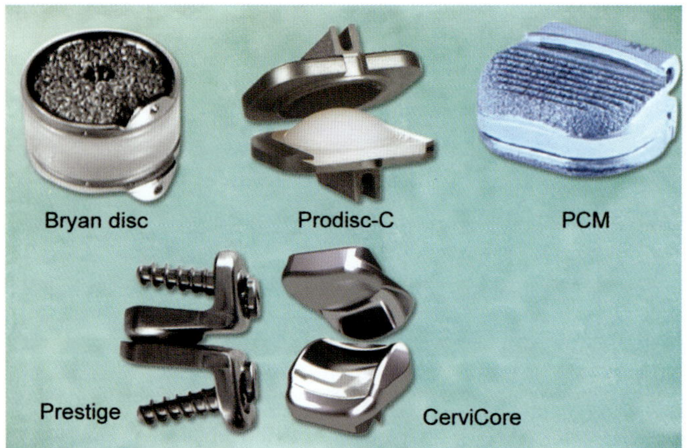

Fig. 2.12: Cervical intervertebral disk prostheses under development or in the market.

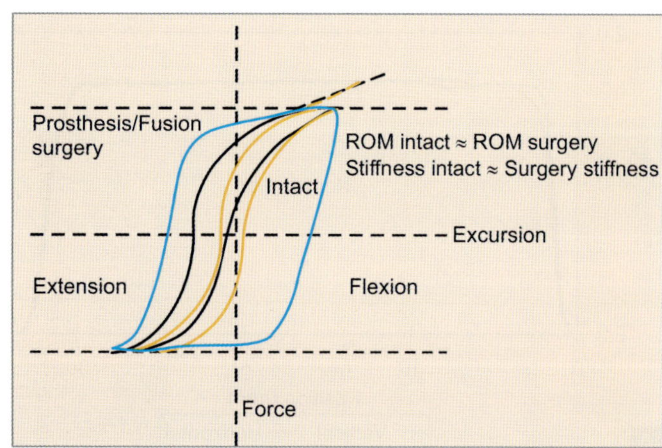

Fig. 2.13: ROM can be misleading if one only considers the endpoint and not the nature of the motion path.

and FlexiCore. Some have a mobile polymer core, while other designs have a fixed center of rotation. All of the designs have a textured surface for bonding to bone and incorporate some form of immediate fixation such as contours, keels, or teeth. Each device displays a unique set of motion parameters but as to which device does in fact replicate the motions encountered in the lumbar spine is still unknown. To some degree, all may be acceptable as the body will adapt when only small deviations from the physiological normals are manifested with the introduction of arthroplasty.

Cervical metal on plastic combinations include Bryan disk, Prodisc-C and PCM and metal-metal designs that are Prestige and CerviCore. All of the devices encompass a bone ingrowth surface (Fig. 2.12).

MECHANICAL EVALUATION AND CLINICAL IMPLICATIONS OF SPINAL INSTRUMENTATION

One of the current areas of concern is the method used to evaluate, not just artificial disks and constructs, in general. This is not with respect to the standardized testing methods set forth by American Society for Testing and Materials or International Organization for Standardization. Rather, there is a significant variation in the methods and criteria to evaluate spinal arthroplasty devices in an in-vitro setting. A common question has been to determine if the ROM is appropriate. While the ROM is important, perhaps more so is the path or tracking required to achieve the ROM. That is, should one be investigating the quality associated with the ROM? The ROM is in fact patient specific and may not be appropriate to evaluate the efficacy of arthroplasty devices. If one is to achieve a proper functioning implant, the motion track through the ROM should avoid rapid changes and stay within an acceptable deviation of the physiological motion path. It is insufficient to consider just the endpoints motion curves and the profile of the curve would dictate that the analysis would entail a non-linear approach.

Graphically, an intact load versus excursion curve should be matched if one is to consider an arthroplasty device as efficacious. If application of various surgical procedures including arthroplasty all achieve the ROM seen under intact conditions, one would conclude that all surgical interventions are efficacious and hence equivalent (Fig. 2.13).

The pertinent question is to investigate the motion tracking between the ROM endpoints, where one would predominantly reside. Use of nonlinear methods could be utilized to consider and characterize the entire motion path in an effort to compare the path of a native disk to that of an arthroplasty device. Another important component of the motion track is the area between the flexion to extension and the extension to flexion curve components. The area between those curves is the work done during the motion covering the ROM. Certainly one would not wish to design an arthroplasty device that would require a significant amount of work to be expended by the patient in order to achieve the ROM.

A study by Kuroda et al. indicated that < 2% energy loss was required to move the knee through a full ROM.[7] In other words, the dominant motion should be very energy efficient. This could be a new way of establishing

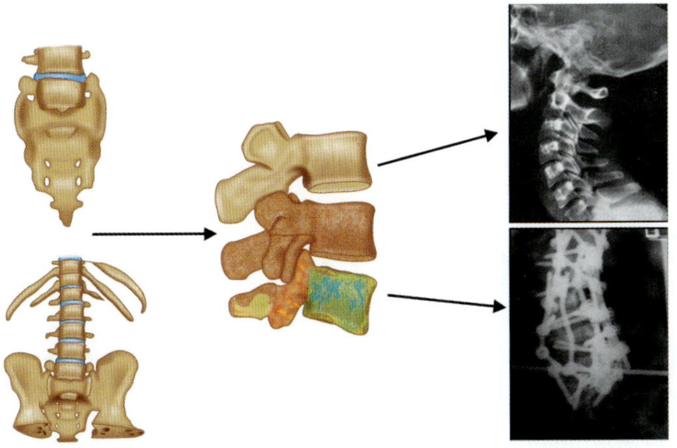

Fig. 2.14: A patient-specific generated computational models that can be used to plan and evaluate surgical outcomes.
Courtesy: Materialize LLC, using Mimics Software.

the longevity associated with arthroplasty devices and degeneration effects on adjacent segments. As was stated, the spine displays coupled motion. In considering the motion path, one should also examine at motion occurring out of the plane of dominant motion. That is, we should consider the "wobble" or tilting perpendicular to the dominant motion.

The tools exist to produce patient-specific computational models (Fig. 2.14). While perhaps application of these methods to customized spinal implants may not be economically or clinically viable, their use as a predictive tool for outcomes may be a vehicle by which clinical interventions can be assessed pre- and postoperatively.

REFERENCES

1. Augustus AW III, Panjabi MM. Clinical biomechanics of the spine, 2nd edn. Philadelphia, PA: Lippincott Williams and Wilkins; 1990.
2. Robert SF. Manipulation under anesthesia: pathomechanics in international MUA academy of physicians. New York, NY, USA: Taylor and Francis; 2005.
3. Boreadis AG, Gershon-Cohen J. Luschka joints of the cervical spine. Radiology. 1956; 66(2):181-7.
4. Panjabi MM. Experimental determination of spinal motion segment behavior. Orthop Clin N Am. 1977;8(1): 169-80.
5. McNally DS, Adams MA. Internal intervertebral disc mechanics as revealed by stress profilometry. Spine. 1992; 17(1): 66-73.
6. Frei H, Oxland TR, Rathony GC, Nolte LP. The effect of nucleotomy on lumbar spine mechanics in compression and shear loading. Spine (Phila Pa 1976). 2001;26(19):2080-9.
7. Kuroda R, Kambic H, Valdevit A, et al. Articular cartiage contact pressure after tibial tuberosity transfer: a cadaveric study. Am J Sports Med. 2001;29(4):403-9.

CHAPTER

3

Balance, Posture and Stability in Spinal Disorders

Virginie Lafage, Barthelemy Liabaud, Frank Schwab, Jean-Pierre Farcy

INTRODUCTION

A comprehensive understanding of spinal disorders demands an appropriate interpretation of a patient's symptomatology within the landscape of the patient's functional domain. Pain and decreased ability become most symptomatic when a patient loses his or her ability to perform activities of daily living (ADLs). ADLs require the most basic of human functions: standing, balance and stability.

Balance and stability represent a more dynamic understanding of patient's dysfunction. Some patients remain functional despite observed local or regional deformity. While these patients have pathologic entities, they are capable of compensation by altering their alignment in attempts to increase their stability. Other patients have significant deformity that they may have tolerated for decades, but then, rather quickly, lose their compensatory mechanisms.

A better understanding of the vital role of pelvic parameters and the static interrelationship of these parameters in predicting the fate of multiple spinal disorders has been elucidated from research done in the past few decades. When a patient presents with back pain, spine specialists see the end result of a failed mechanism. A good understanding of the complex interplay of muscle, fascia, joint mechanics, vestibular and somatosensory systems will help better predict which spinal deformities will ultimately benefit from surgical intervention.

Subsequent chapters address specific normal parameters of regions of the spine and the examination of deformities. This chapter reviews the concepts of the spinal parameters with the juxtaspinal regions such as the pelvis, and lower extremities for a clear understanding of the interplay of a balanced spine and its role in posture, leading to balance and stability. The complexity of standing and the definitions of balance, stability, and posture as well as novel ways of assessing the spinal influences of maintaining this equilibrium will be discussed.

BALANCE, STABILITY AND POSTURE

The understanding and analysis of human standing is quite complex. Balance, posture, and stability are some of the terms used to describe this state; each representing a distinct aspect. Balance is a state of equilibrium. Stability is the state or quality of maintaining equilibrium and self-restoring as needed. Posture is the relative disposition of the parts of the body (Fig. 3.1).

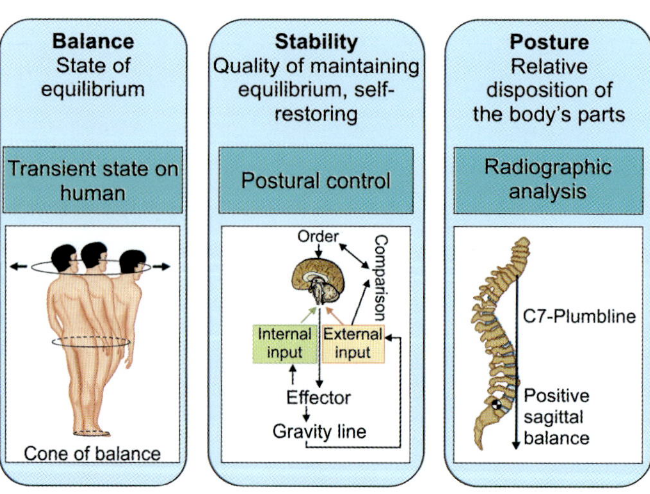

Fig. 3.1: Balance, stability and posture.

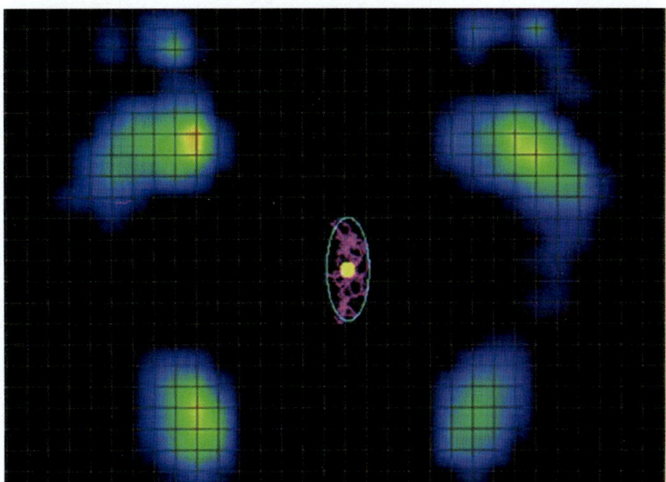

Fig. 3.2: An example of a stabilometry platform localizing the center of pressure. The graph obtained from this stabilometry platform can help the clinician to quantify the subject stability and also may permit the characterization of the postural control system (speed and acceleration of the COP travel, surface covered by the COP).

Balance and Stability

In stance, the body is submitted to the force of gravity and to the ground reaction. These forces are, respectively, applied on the center of mass (COM) and center of pressure (COP). As defined by Brisson[1] in 1803, "[In a state of equilibrium ...] the body is positioned between two aligned, equal and opposite forces". In other words, the body is balanced only when the COM and the COP are aligned on the same vertical line. Standing itself may be classified as a simple activity, but maintenance of balance, posture and stability requires a rapid processing of signals from the visual, vestibular, and somatic systems[2] (Fig. 3.1).

Because our body is made of different moving parts all leading to a dynamic COM, this perfect alignment is almost never reached. And as soon as the COM is not aligned with the COP, a moment is created that would cause the body to fall in the absence of a sophisticated control system (nervous system and muscles). In order to stay as close as possible to a state of balance, two stabilization mechanisms, which have been described by Gagey et al.,[3] come into play: the COM maneuver and the COP maneuver depending on whether the COM or COP is mobilized to reach the balance state. In the COM maneuver, the body parts are moved in space in order to localize the COM above the COP. In the COP maneuver, the feet pressures are adjusted in such a way to bring the COP below the COM. Both maneuvers help in maintaining the standing position.

Historically, the first measurement device for human posture was proposed by Vierordt[4] in 1860. A quill was placed on the head of a subject to record the body sways on a piece of paper. Evolution of technology and understanding of balance has lead to current devices, which precisely quantify the standing stability. This group of devices is called stabilometry platforms. These platforms measure, for a given sampling rate, the location of the COP (i.e. the ground reaction, Figure 3.2). In a dynamic condition, the COP does not coincide with the projection on the gravity line (GL). It has been demonstrated[5-7] that the signal measured may be dissociated in two components: a controlled slow sway that represents the motion of the COM and a noncontrolled quick sway around the GL projection that represents the displacement of the COP around the projected GL.

Posture

In the context of an orthopedics evaluation, X-ray images are the most common way to quantify a subject's posture. Although radiographs permit an evaluation of vertebral alignment and pelvic landmarks, current standard techniques using 36-inch cassettes only offer a limited view and do not capture foot position or the global alignment of a person in space.

The authors of the chapter combined the technology of full-length radiographs with force plate acquisition to further improve our understanding of human standing sagittal alignment.[8] This technique presents not only the advantages of a standard radiographic analysis but also offer the ability to investigate the relative location of the body parts in regard to the GL and to the feet location (Fig. 3.3).

Based on the hypothesis that the mean location of the COP is a good estimation of the projected GL on the floor in the neutral (static) standing position,[9] the compensatory mechanisms required to maintain a standing posture in the setting of age-related changes and spinal deformity were investigated and are summarized hereafter.

How Does New Technology Help us in to Better Assess Patients with Spinal Deformity?

Age-related Changes

The aging process and deformity of the spinal column can lead to altered sagittal plane alignment. Despite the expanded use of radiographic parameters, optimal spinal alignment remains currently poorly defined. However, a number of radiographic parameters have been developed as guides of sagittal alignment. Values of thoracic kyphosis by Cobb measurements and lumbar lordosis are commonly used to measure regional alignment. Global spinal alignment is commonly assessed by the plumb line method drawn onto full-length radiographs.[10-13] The plumb line represents a common and convenient visual display of apparent sagittal plane alignment but its value as a marker of true postural balance has been questioned.[14] Even though radiographs can capture the alignment of osseous structures, they do not place them in relation to the distribution of forces and do not capture the association to position of the feet in a standing subject.[8] More recently pelvic parameters have been examined in order to improve the evaluation of sagittal plane alignment.[15-17]

While numerous teams have investigated age-related changes in asymptomatic subjects based on radiographic measurements, little is known regarding the overall posture adopted by those aging subjects. Through force plate analysis, foot position and transmission of forces across the feet can be analyzed. The center of these recorded pressures on a force plate, in the still standing position, reflects the projected center of gravity (GL). This GL may enhance our understanding of spinopelvic alignment in patients with spinal deformity. As Dubousset has noted in the "cone of economy" concept, ideal balance, and lowest

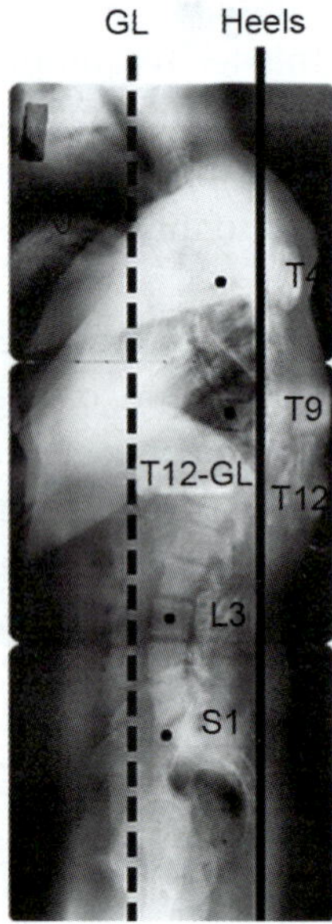

Fig. 3.3: Projection of anatomical landmarks, gravity line (GL, dotted line), and heel line on digital X-rays. The gravity line and heels line are projected on each X-ray to evaluate offsets between these lines and radiological landmarks.

energy use is noted in a state of minimal displacement of the entire body GL over the feet. Through an analysis of pelvic and spinal column offsets from the projected GL (and foot position), norms of alignment in a healthy population can be established, and pathologic states of spinal deformity can be studied in reference to such a benchmark population.[8] By combining force plate technology and standard radiographic analysis, it has been demonstrated that radiographic changes (with age, the trunk tilts forward) are compensated by a posterior translation of the pelvis. This basic mechanism allows for maintenance of a fixed offset between the GL and the heels, independently of the subject age[8] (Figs. 3.4A to C).

Global head-to-feet analysis brings to light the limitation of standard X-rays and the interest of the EOS system and/or force plate that would allow a better understanding of the role of the lower extremity in the setting of spinopelvic alignment.

Spinal Deformity

Lafage et al.[18] evaluated the impact of sagittal vertebral axis (SVA) offset on GL, pelvic parameters and spinopelvic position relative to the feet in standing subjects. The SVA is the distance from a plumb line drawn from C7 and the posterosuperior corner of S1. An offset > 2.5 cm anteriorly or posteriorly is considered beyond the normal range.[12]

By using varying SVA values, three distinct groups were created (neutral, sagittal backward, and sagittal forward). Significant differences between groups were noted for a number of radiographic and GL parameters. Increasing SVA leads to a posterior pelvic shift in relation to the feet. Increasing pelvic incidence was also noted in the sagittal forward displaced SVA group. However, no significant difference in the GL-heels offset (GHO) was noted across subject groups (Figs. 3.5A to C). It appears that pelvic shift is a key component in maintaining a fixed GHO even in the setting of a variable SVA and trunk inclination. This study highlights the role of the pelvis as a compensatory mechanism (translation and rotation).[18]

Findings related to the higher pelvic incidence in the setting of sagittal deformity raise the question of whether pelvic morphology can predispose a patient to sagittal plane malalignment, whether changes can occur in the sacral endplate or, as suggested by Skalli et al., sagittal malalignment can lead to compensatory motion in the sacroiliac joint.[19] Lafage et al. findings were consistent with

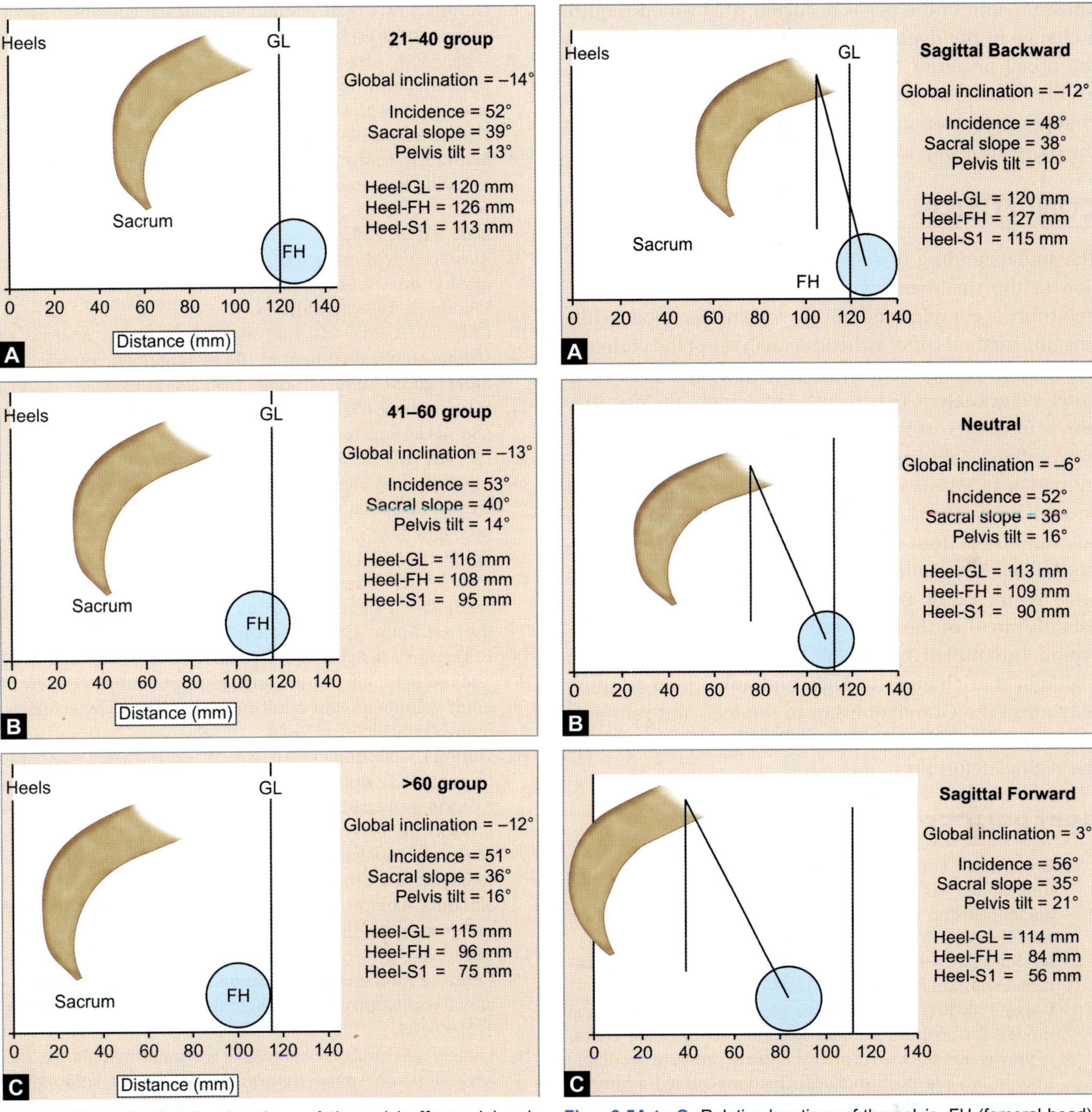

Figs. 3.4A to C: Relative locations of the pelvis [femoral heads (FH) and sacrum] in regard to the gravity line (GL) and heel line. This comparison of age-related changes in asymptomatic subjects illustrates the posterior translation of the pelvis with advance age and the rather fixed offset between gravity lines and heal line.

Figs. 3.5A to C: Relative locations of the pelvis, FH (femoral head), GL (gravity line), and heel line.

those studies focusing on adult asymptomatic population,[8] meaning the same global mechanisms of compensation can take place in both asymptomatic and symptomatic populations.

It appears that even wide variations in SVA can be tolerated so long as compensatory mechanisms come into play to maintain standing alignment. It is evident from the data in Lafage et al.'s study that the role of the lower extremities and pelvis are critical in understanding spino-pelvic posture as well as malalignment observed in pathologic states. As SVA offset increased, a posterior shift of the pelvis occurred. This would require a change in the degree of hip flexion or extension given the noted posterior translation of the pelvis in relation to the feet with increasing SVA offset. Furthermore, changes in knee and ankle joint positioning may affect the GL relationship to the feet.

CONCLUSION

The understanding of optimal balance and its application in the treatment of patients suffering from spinal deformity is complex and not yet fully understood. While imaging methods offer structural analyses of the vertebral column, the ability to evaluate spinal balance is limited. Force plate analysis may be used to analyze the distribution of forces across the feet and to estimate the GL, which may enhance our understanding of balance in deformity patients. Norms of balance in a healthy population should be established by assessing pelvic and spinal column offsets from the projected GL. Establishing healthy balance guidelines may improve the identification and treatment of pathogenic spinal deformities. The establishment of the relationship between truncal inclination (quantified by the SVA) and pelvis translation highlight that changes in knee and ankle joint position may affect the GL relationship to the feet, and reinforce the importance of a full-body evaluation when assessing the sagittal deformity of the spine.

REFERENCES

1. Brisson MJ. Traité élémentaire ou Principes de Physique, fondés sur les connaiasances les plus certaines, tant anciennes que modernes, et confirmés par l'expérience, 4th edn. Paris: Masson et Besson; 1803.
2. Nashner LM. Adapting reflexes controlling the human posture. Exp Brain Res.1976;26(1):59-72.
3. Gagey PM, Bizzo G, Ouaknine M, et al. Two mechanical models for postural stabilization: the tactics of the center of gravity and the tactics of the center of pressure. Available from http://ada-posturologie.fr/TactiqueDuPied-a.htm
4. Vierordt Kv. Grundriss der Physiologie des Menschen. Laupp H. Frankfurt AM, Meidinger Sohn u. Comp. 1860:p. 561.
5. Collins JJ, De Luca CJ. Open-loop and closed-loop control of posture: a random-walk analysis of center-of-pressure trajectories. Exp Brain Res.1993;95(2):308-18.
6. Gurfinkel EV. Physical foundations of stabilography. Agressologie. 1973;14(Spec No C):9-13.
7. Gagey PM, Bizzo G, Debruille O, et al. The one Hertz phenomenon. In: Igarashi M, Black FO (eds), Vestibular and visual control on posture and locomotor equilibrium. Karger: Basel; 1985. pp. 89-92.
8. Schwab F, Lafage V, Boyce R, et al. Gravity line analysis in adult volunteers: age-related correlation with spinal parameters, pelvic parameters, and foot position. Spine. 2006; 31(25):E959-67.
9. Zatsiorsky VM, King DL. An algorithm for determining gravity line location from posturographic recordings. J Biomech. 1998;31(2):161-4.
10. Gelb DE, Lenke LG, Bridwell KH, et al. An analysis of sagittal spinal alignment in 100 asymptomatic middle and older aged volunteers. Spine. 1995;20(12):1351-8.
11. Hammerberg EM, Wood KB. Sagittal profile of the elderly. J Spinal Disord Tech. 2003;16(1):44-50.
12. Jackson RP, McManus AC. Radiographic analysis of sagittal plane alignment and balance in standing volunteers and patients with low back pain matched for age, sex, and size. A prospective controlled clinical study. Spine. 1994;19(14):1611-8.
13. McLean IP, Gillan MG, Ross JC, et al. A comparison of methods for measuring trunk list. A simple plumbline is the best. Spine. 1996;21(14):1667-70.
14. El Fegoun AB, Schwab F, Gamez L, et al. Center of gravity and radiographic posture analysis: a preliminary review of adult volunteers and adult patients affected by scoliosis. Spine. 2005;30(13):1535-40.
15. During J, Goudfrooij H, Keessen W, et al. Toward standards for posture. Postural characteristics of the lower back system in normal and pathologic conditions. Spine. 1985;10(1):83-7.
16. Jackson RP, Peterson MD, McManus AC, et al. Compensatory spinopelvic balance over the hip axis and better reliability in measuring lordosis to the pelvic radius on standing lateral radiographs of adult volunteers and patients. Spine. 1998;23(16):1750-67.
17. Legaye J, Duval-Beaupere G, Hecquet J, et al. Pelvic incidence: a fundamental pelvic parameter for three-dimensional regulation of spinal sagittal curves. Eur Spine J. 1998; 7(2):99-103.
18. Lafage V, Schwab F, Skalli W, et al. Standing balance and sagittal plane spinal deformity: analysis of spinopelvic and gravity line parameters. Spine. 2008;33(14):1572-8.
19. Skalli W, Zeller RD, Miladi L, et al. Importance of pelvic compensation in posture and motion after posterior spinal fusion using CD instrumentation for idiopathic scoliosis. Spine (Phila Pa 1976). 2006;31(12):E359-66.

CHAPTER

4

Differential Diagnosis of Spinal Disorders

Michael Gerling, Vadim Goz

INTRODUCTION

Back pain is one of the most common presenting complaints of patients in the United States. It accounts for about $200 billion in annual cost due to direct medical expenditures and indirect loss of productivity.[1] Back pain is the second most common symptom for physician visits and is the most common reason for disability in those under 45 years of age. By some estimates over 90% of people will experience back pain at some point in their lives.[2] The prevalence of back pain is continuing to increase, more than doubling over a 14-year time period.

RISK FACTORS

A number of risk factors have been associated with development of acute and chronic back pain. These risk factors include smoking, obesity, older age, female gender, physically strenuous work, sedentary work, psychologically strenuous work, low educational attainment, workers' compensation insurance, job dissatisfaction, and psychological factors such as somatization disorder, anxiety, and depression.[3-5] It is important to note that while some factors are mechanical in nature, others are socioeconomic and psychological.

PROGNOSIS

The majority of acute back pain complaints will resolve without intervention. However recurrence is common and long-term disability is difficult to predict. Anatomic findings on imaging studies have not been found to be reliable predictors of long-term pain and often do not correlate with the clinical picture.[6] Psychosocial factors including psychiatric comorbidities and the presence of nonorganic or Waddell's signs are correlated with long-term persistence of back pain.[7] Back pain is a remarkably nonspecific symptom, the etiology of which can range from benign musculoskeletal injury to malignancy or infection. While full recovery can be expected in over 85% of patients with acute axial pain in the absence of radicular symptoms, certain red flag symptoms warrant immediate evaluation.[8]

Signs of potentially serious underlying etiologies of back pain must be followed up with immediate radiographic evaluation. A number of red flag symptoms and signs have been recognized.[9] Recent significant trauma with acute onset of axial pain with or without radiculopathy may indicate a potential fracture. Osteoporosis and prolonged corticosteroid use increase this risk. Back pain in the setting of unexplained weight loss or in a patient with a history of cancer should raise suspicion for malignancy. Fever, immunosuppression, injection drug use, and current infection are significant risk factors for a potential infection spreading to the spinal canal and surrounding structures. Saddle anesthesia, bowel or bladder incontinence may be signs of cauda equina syndrome. And progressive neurologic deficits raise concerns for a potential expanding hematoma, abscess, or tumor. While these symptoms may aid in identifying specific etiologies, it is often impossible to isolate a particular underlying diagnosis since multiple pathologies may cause similar types of pain.

TYPES OF PAIN

A useful tool in differentiating the potential causes of back pain is separating it in three general types: local pain, referred pain, and radicular pain. The type of pain is identified based on the characteristics reported by the patient, and most spinal pathologies can cause multiple types of pain.

Local Pain

Local or axial pain is caused by excitation of nociceptive sensory neurons that innervate the musculoskeletal structures surrounding the spine. Nociceptive nerve endings can be found in the periosteum of the vertebral body, capsule of apophyseal joints, annulus fibrosis, as well as ligaments and muscles surrounding the spine.[10] Axial pain is typically steady, aching, and can range from sharp to dull. A key-defining feature is that this pain is felt in the same region as the affected part of the spine, and intensifies with movement of the part or direct palpation.

Referred Pain

Referred pain is a dull, deep pain that is projected between two sites that are embryologically related. The convergent sensory innervation hypothesized to be responsible for this mechanism is a result of the multiple structures arising from a single somite during embryologic development.[11,12] Tissue migration and rearrangement is most notable in the limbs allowing for more distant referral of pain, e.g. from lumbar spine to the hip or knee.

A separate type of referred pain is one that is viscerogenic in nature. The mechanism is hypothesized to be similar to that referred to above and involves convergent visceral sensory innervation with innervation of axial or somatic structures at the same vertebral level.[8] This allows for pain secondary to visceral pathology to be misinterpreted as axial pain.

Radicular Pain

of the L5 or S1 nerve roots. The pain originates in the buttock with distribution down the posterolateral thigh along the path of the sciatic nerve. If impingement is solely of the dorsal roots then sensory symptoms will predominate, sometimes accompanied by paresthesia of the overlying skin of the dermatome supplied by the impinged roots. Motor symptoms including weakness, atrophy, and fasciculations may be present if the lesion involves the anterior roots that contain secondary or lower motor neurons. An understanding of these three types of pain is the fundamental basis for creating a functional differential diagnosis.

CHRONIC PAIN SYNDROMES AND THRESHOLD MODULATION

The symptoms of back pain are often chronic in nature and occur in the absence of clear precipitating factors such as trauma or muscle strain. These chronic pain syndromes must be considered separately from their acute counterparts. Chronic pain leads to neuromodulation and central sensitization of the involved sensory neurons, thereby lowering their excitatory threshold. Central sensitization is the mechanism involved in the lowering of action potential threshold of sensory neurons in the dorsal horn due to repeated depolarization. A pathology such as degenerative disk disease or disk herniation can lead to repeat firing of nociceptive fibers, which through central sensitization can continue to produce pain even after the resolution of the initial pathology. Sensitization of nociceptors also occurs in the setting of inflammation through cytokines, leukotrienes, and altered pH in the local environment of the nociceptive nerve endings.[14]

DIFFERENTIAL DIAGNOSIS

Keeping in mind the typical symptom patterns encountered during evaluation of spinal disorders, a differential diagnosis can be formulated. The causes of neck and back pain are typically grouped into three categories: mechanical, nonmechanical, and viscerogenic (Table 4.1).

Mechanical Etiologies of Back Pain

Mechanical back pain is secondary to pathology of the musculoskeletal components of the axial skeleton. It intensifies with activity, worsening by end of day. When inflammation sets in, patients have increased symptoms in the morning and after prolonged rest. They should be able to point to specific site of pain.

One study estimated that 98% of primary care patients with axial pain have a mechanical etiology.[15] This includes muscle strains, ligamentous injury, degenerative disk disease (spondylosis), degenerative facet joint disease, fractures, spinal stenosis, spondylolisthesis, and many other factors. Over 90% of such patients will have a full recovery over a period of 6 weeks, and do not warrant an

Table 4.1: Potential etiologies of back pain categorized into three groups: mechanical, nonmechanical, and viscerogenic

Mechanical	*Nonmechanical*	*Viscerogenic*
Degenerative disk disease	Malignancy (primary or metastatic)	Abdominal aortic aneurysm
Spondylosis	Vertebral osteomyelitis	Cardiac ischemia
Spondylolysis	Perivertebral abscess	Nephrolithiasis
Vertebral compression fractures	Rheumatic disease of the spine (rheumatoid arthritis, ankylosing spondylitis, Reiter's syndrome, etc.)	Pyelonephritis
Spinal stenosis		Cholelithiasis
Muscle strain		Pelvic inflammatory disease
Ligamentous injury		Endometriosis

Table 4.2: "Red flag" symptoms suggesting the need for early radiographic evaluation

Finding	*Rationale for plain radiography or advanced imaging*
Major trauma (e.g. fall from height, motor vehicle crash)	Possible fracture
Age >50 years	Greater risk of malignancy, osteoporotic fractures
History of cancer	Greater risk of underlying malignancy
Unexplained weight loss	Greater risk of malignancy or infection
Fever, immunosuppression, immunodeficiency, injection drug use, or active infection	Risk for spinal infection
Saddle anesthesia, bladder, or bowel incontinence	Possible cauda equina syndrome
Severe or progressive neurologic deficit	Possible cauda equina syndrome or severe nerve root compression

extensive workup upon initial presentation in the absence of previously mentioned red flag symptoms (Table 4.2). A careful history and physical is essential to guide the diagnostician toward identifying the potential site of the lesion, but will rarely provide a specific diagnosis. A few important causes of mechanical back pain are discussed below.

Spondylolysis and Spondylolisthesis

Spondylolysis is a defect at the pars interarticularis located between the lamina and pedicle of a vertebra. This defect can be congenital, often found in children between 5 years and 7 years of age.[16] It can also occur in adults secondary to trauma. Spondylolysis can present as unilateral or bilateral axial pain. Bilateral fractures of the pars interarticularis predispose to anterior displacement of one vertebral body in relation to the adjacent vertebra. Once this anterior motion occurs the condition is termed spondylolisthesis, and can lead to severe spinal stenosis, a frequent cause of radiculopathy and or neuroclaudication. Though less common in the cervical and thoracic spine, at these levels the associated narrowing of the spinal canal can impinge on the spinal cord and result in a myelopathy. Severe or progressive neurologic symptoms require immediate evaluation for surgical correction.

Spinal Stenosis

Spinal and foraminal stenosis cause pain secondary to narrowing of the central canal and intervertebral foramen, respectively. Narrowing can occur secondary to a number of etiologies including osteophyte formation, thickening of the ligamentum flavum, disk herniation, or degenerative and osteoarthritic changes of the canal commonly referred to as spondylosis.[17] Central canal stenosis in the cervical spine causes spinal cord compression and myelopathy, foraminal stenosis causes a radiculopathy. Lumbar spinal stenosis typically causes neuroclaudication, "the onset of sciatica, leg pain and numbness, while walking that is relieved by sitting down or leaning forward".

Radicular or root level symptoms result in pain, sensory and motor symptoms at the level of the lesion. Specifically, patients may experience sharp pains in a dermatomal distribution at the level of the lesion, as well as lower motor neuron symptoms including weakness and fasciculations.[18] Radicular symptoms indicate a nerve root level lesion such as foraminal stenosis.

In contrast to radiculopathy, myelopathy typically presents with diffuse symptoms at and below the level of the lesion secondary to impingement of the spinal cord. Depending on the location of the lesion a combination of sensory and motor symptoms may be present. Myelopathy may present as pain, weakness, numbness, loss of balance, or increased tone in one or all four limbs. The involvement of multiple levels such as weakness in upper and lower extremities indicates a cord level lesion such as central canal stenosis. Pathologic reflexes or upper motor neuron signs, and hyper-reflexia are common, but may be absent or blunted by simultaneous radiculopathy or chronic peripheral stenosis.

Vascular claudication secondary to peripheral vascular disease can present in a similar manner to the neurogenic claudication of spinal stenosis. Peripheral vascular disease includes etiologies such as atherosclerotic disease of the distal aorta and iliac arteries. Intermittent claudication induced by exercise and relieved by rest is a classic sign of atherosclerotic disease.[19] Pain is worse while supine in bed at night, when arterial blood pressure decreases in the extremities. Patients will often hang their foot over the edge of the bed for relief. Signs include diminished distal pulses, decrease in body hair of the affected area, atrophic skin changes and ulceration of the skin overlaying the lateral malleolus. Pain and cramping can be unilateral, with the calf musculature most typically affected. Bilateral cramping in the hips and buttocks is possible with atherosclerosis of the distal aorta known as Leriche syndrome.

Vascular claudicatory symptoms closely mimic the neurogenic claudication associated with spinal stenosis. A key differentiating factor is that the symptoms of spinal stenosis are dependent on flexion of the spine. Pain relief associated with walking up hill or assuming a hunched over posture (allowing for lumbar flexion) is more consistent with spinal stenosis as the etiology as opposed to atherosclerotic disease.

Disk Herniation

Disk herniation is a common condition causing chronic axial and neurologic symptoms. This condition most often occurs at the L5-S1 intervertebral disk, but can occur anywhere in the spine.[20] Disk herniations in the lumbar and cervical spine are more common than those of the thoracic spine. Herniation involves the tearing of the annulus fibrosus and extrusion of the gelatinous nucleus pulposus.[21] This can occur secondary to trauma, but often occurs in the absence of a recognizable traumatic event. The latter scenario likely involves degeneration of the intervertebral disk over time and weakening the integrity of the annulus fibrosis, or outer ring of the disk. Once the integrity of the disk is sufficiently weakened a typically benign stress placed on the disk by sneezing or regular movements may result in herniation.

The annulus fibrosus contains sensory innervation that produces the axial pain at the level of the lesion associated with annular tears and subsequent disk herniation.[10] The extruded nucleus pulposus can impinge on surrounding neurologic structures, causing radiculopathy from the nerve roots and myelopathy when the spinal cord is affected (Fig. 4.1). A careful motor and sensory exam can further identify the level of the lesion. Imaging has also been particularly helpful in identifying herniated disks. However, degenerative changes are a common finding amongst asymptomatic individuals leading to difficulty in attributing clinical significance to radiographic findings.[22]

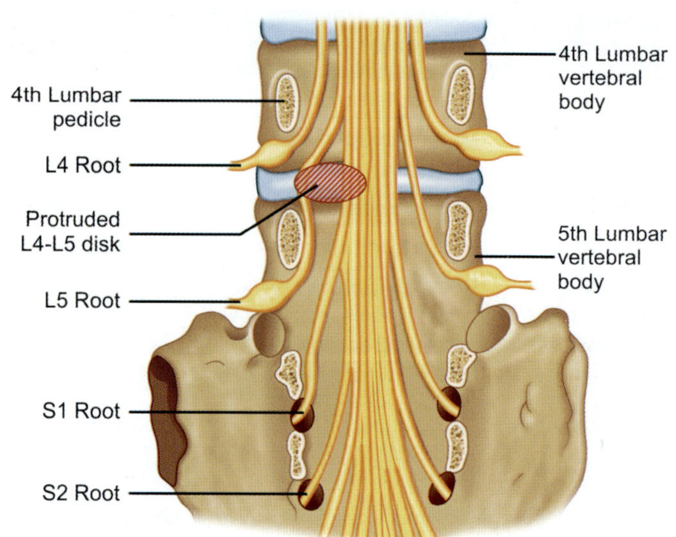

Fig. 4.1: Protrusion of the L4-L5 disk impinges the surrounding nerve roots.

Nonmechanical Etiologies of Axial Pain

This category of back pain refers to etiologies that fall into one of three categories: malignancy, infectious, or rheumatologic conditions. A number of the aforementioned red flag symptoms are aimed at quickly and efficiently identifying axial pain of nonmechanical etiology.

Malignancy of the spine can be primary or metastatic. The most common spinal tumors are metastatic carcinoma (from breast, lung, and prostate), multiple myeloma, and lymphoma.[23-25] A number of significantly more rare sarcomas can occur in the spine as well. Pain associated with spinal malignancy is often constant, unrelieved by rest, worse or of similar intensity at night comparing to daytime. The pain can be axial if generated by irritation of the nociceptors of the vertebral body and periosteum. Referred pain and radicular pain are also possible depending on the extent of the lesion. A previous history of malignancy, recent unexplained weight loss and heavy tobacco use are red flags in the history that raise the suspicion for malignancy. In such cases, a timely CT scan, MRI, or radioactive isotope scan is warranted to rule out a malignant process.

Infection is a cause of nonmechanical back pain that must be identified in a timely manner. Pain associated with infection of the paraspinal structures can be subacute or chronic in nature; it is exacerbated by movement and often not completely alleviated by rest. Percussion-induced axial pain over the involved vertebral level is consistent with an infectious process. Staphylococcal infections are most common; however, infections with gram-negative bacilli and mycobacteria are also possible.[26] Axial pain is common with infectious etiology; however, peripheral symptoms may occur if abscess or granulomas impinge on nerves or the spinal cord.

Paraspinal infections can be difficult to detect. The clinical presentation varies from nonspecific constitutional symptoms including general malaise and fever to completely asymptomatic. Leukocytosis is not a reliable indicator. C-reactive protein levels and erythrocyte sedimentation rates are two indicators that have a higher sensitivity for identifying infection.[27] A detailed history plays a pivotal role in identifying patients at high risk of vertebral infections. Patients with documented sepsis, osteomyelitis, endocarditis, or any other potential sources of infection are at increased risk of seeding the vertebra and surrounding spinal structures with the preexisting infection. Rarely, an infection can be introduced from lumbar puncture, epidural, or recent spinal surgery. Those with a history of intravenous drug use are at a significantly increased risk of spinal infections. Suspicion of an infectious etiology for a patient presenting with back pain warrants immediate evaluation with a CT scan or MRI.

Rheumatologic conditions can present as nonmechanical back pain. Rheumatoid arthritis often affects the cervical spine, especially the atlantoaxial joint; however, the disease is rarely limited to the spine and the involvement of multiple joints can be a strong indication of this process. Seronegative arthropathies commonly affect the spine. Ankylosing spondylitis is an inflammatory arthropathy that can be limited to the spine, predominantly affecting the lumbar spine of young men.[28] Axial back pain is typically the dominant symptom early in the disease, as the condition progresses morning stiffness and limitation in movement become more pronounced. Referred pain from the afflicted spinal level to the posterior thighs and hips can be present. Radicular pain, marked by a sharp radiation of pain typically in a dermatomal pattern, is rare early in the disease but may potentially occur as the disease progresses.[29] Symptoms of impingement on surrounding structures, including radiculopathy, are common complications from proliferation of connective tissue after years of chronic inflammation. Ankylosing spondylitis can be accompanied by other autoimmune and rheumatologic conditions including Reiter's syndrome, psoriasis, or inflammatory bowel disease. Seronegative spondyloarthropathies of the spine are associated with HLA-B27 histocompatibility complex. Plain radiographs of patients with ankylosing spondylitis may show the stereotypical vertebral bridging or "bamboo spine". This is a late finding in the disease process.

Viscerogenic Etiologies of Back Pain

Pain of viscerogenic origin can manifest itself as back pain (Fig. 4.2). This is made possible by afferent nociceptive neurons from visceral organs that converge on the same pain sensing pathways in the spine as nociceptive afferent somatic innervation.[30] This convergence is hypothesized to hinder the brain's ability to differentiate somatic from visceral pain of the same level. A large number of visceral etiologies can present as back pain.

Peptic ulcer disease and carcinoma of the stomach can present as thoracic level back pain.[31] This is more common with involvement of the posterior stomach wall, as well as extension of disease into the retroperitoneum. A detailed history can help differentiate back pain of gastric etiology from musculoskeletal pain. Symptoms of peptic ulcer disease will often be related to food consumption, are relieved by antacids, and may be associated with other symptoms typical of peptic ulcer disease such as epigastric pain, nausea/vomiting, and weight loss. The presence of risk factors for peptic ulcer disease such as cigarette smoking, NSAID use, large consumption of coffee and mints, may direct the differential diagnosis toward peptic ulcer disease.

Pancreatic pathologies can also produce symptoms of back pain. Due to anatomic location, involvement of the pancreatic head can present as right-sided back pain, and involvement of the body or tail will produce pain to the left of the spine. Neoplasms of the kidney can produce pain in the lower thoracic region that radiates toward the groin if the lesion extends to the iliopsoas. Pain in a similar thoracolumbar distribution can also be produced by retroperitoneal bleeding, or aneurysm disease of the abdominal aorta. Physicians must keep a high degree of suspicion for abdominal aortic aneurysms due to the significant potential for mortality associated with this disease.

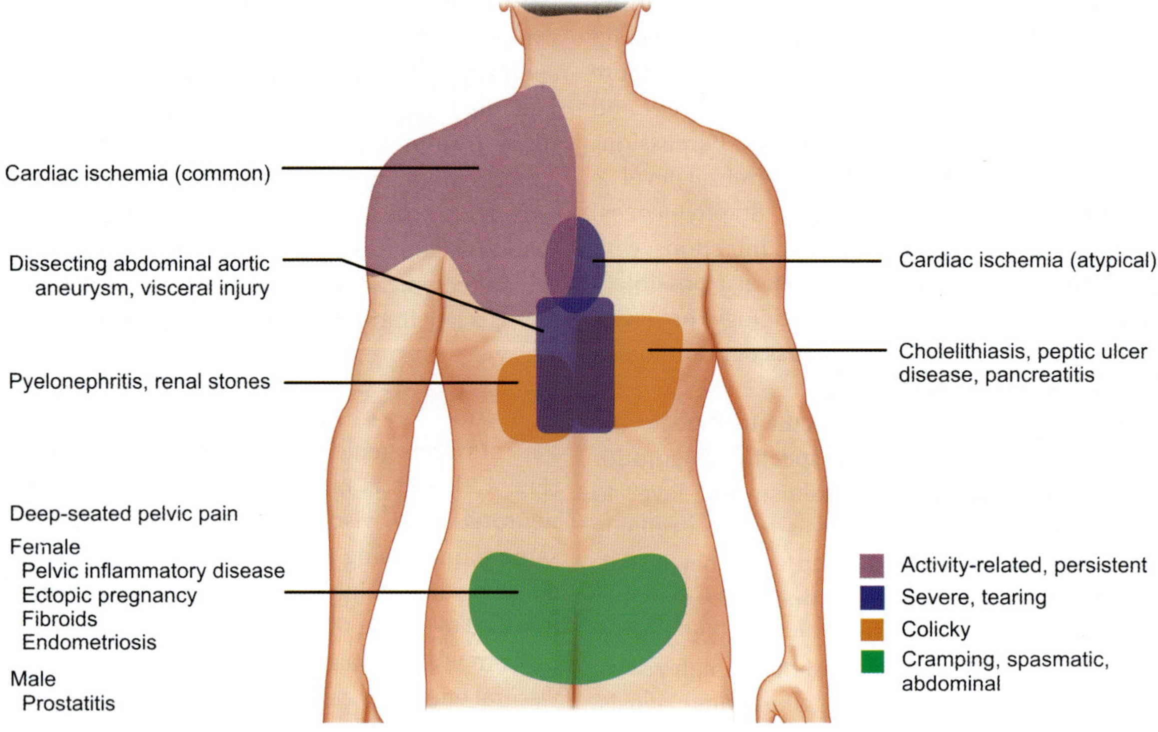

Fig. 4.2: Location of potential back pain secondary to medical conditions.

CONCLUSION

Back pain can be the presenting symptom of a wide range of mechanical, nonmechanical, and visceral etiologies. Keeping in mind the potential emergent and nonemergent causes, it is vital that clinicians develop an organized differential diagnosis and systematic evaluation plan for patients with back pain.

REFERENCES

1. Andersson G, Bouchard J, Bozic KJ et al. United States Bone and Joint Initiative: The Burden of Musculoskeletal Diseases in the United States, 2nd Edition. Rosemont, IL: American Academy of Orthopaedic Surgeons; 2011.
2. Hicks GS, Duddleston DN, Russell LD, et al. Low back pain. Am J Med Sci. 2002;324(4):207-11.
3. Cassidy JD, Carroll LJ, Côté P. The Saskatchewan health and back pain survey: the prevalence of low back pain and related disability in Saskatchewan adults. Spine. 1998;23 (17):1860.
4. Skovron M, Szpalski M, Nordin M, et al. Sociocultural factors and back pain: a population-based study in Belgian adults. Spine. 1994;19(2):129.
5. Katz JN. Lumbar disc disorders and low-back pain: socioeconomic factors and consequences. J Bone Joint Surg. 2006;88(suppl 2):21-4.
6. Chou R, Huffman LH. Medications for acute and chronic low back pain: a review of the evidence for an American Pain Society/American College of Physicians clinical practice guideline. Ann Intern Med. 2007;147(7):505.
7. Chou R, Shekelle P. Will this patient develop persistent disabling low back pain? JAMA: J Am Med Assoc. 2010;303(13):1295-1302.
8. Engstrom JW. Back and neck pain. In: Dennis L Kasper (Ed). Harrison's Principles of Medicine, 16th illustrated edition. McGraw-Hill; 2005. p. 94.
9. Deyo RA, Weinstein JN. Low back pain. N Engl J Med. 2001;344(5):363-70.
10. Coppes MH, Marani E, Thomeer RT, et al. Innervation of annulus fibrosis in low back pain. Lancet. 1990;336(8708): 189-90.
11. Rawls JA, Fisher RE. Development and functional anatomy of the spine. In: Kusumi K, Sally L Dunwoodie (Eds). The Genetics and Development of Scoliosis, New York: Springer; 2010. pp. 21-46.
12. Jinkins J. The pathoanatomic basis of somatic and autonomic syndromes originating in the lumbosacral spine. Neuroimaging Clin North Am. 1993;3:443-63.
13. Garfin SR, Rydevik B, Lind B, et al. Spinal nerve root compression. Spine. 1995;20(16):1810.
14. Schwartzman RJ, Grothusen J, Kiefer TR, et al. Neuropathic central pain: epidemiology, etiology, and treatment options. Arch Neurol. 2001;58(10):1547.

15. Wheeler AH. Diagnosis and management of low back pain and sciatica. American family physician 52, no. 5 (1995): pp. 1333-1341.
16. Hu SS, Tribus CB, Diab M, et al. Spondylolisthesis and spondylolysis. J Bone Joint Surg. 2008;90(3):656-71.
17. Amundsen T, Weber H, Lilleås F, et al. Lumbar spinal stenosis: clinical and radiologic features. Spine. 1995;20(10):1178.
18. Porter RW. Spinal stenosis and neurogenic claudication. Spine. 1996;21(17):2046.
19. Liao SL, Luthra M, Rogers KM. Leriche Syndrome. J Am Coll Cardiol. 2009;54(19):e11.
20. Kuisma M, Karppinen J, Niinimäki J, et al. Modic changes in endplates of lumbar vertebral bodies: prevalence and association with low back and sciatic pain among middle-aged male workers. Spine. 2007;32(10):1116-22.
21. Del Grande F, Maus TP, Carrino JA. Imaging the intervertebral disk: age-related changes, herniations, and radicular pain. Radiol Clin N Am. 2012;50(4):629.
22. Powell MC, Wilson M, Szypryt P, et al. Prevalence of lumbar disc degeneration observed by magnetic resonance in symptomless women. Lancet. 1986;2(8520):1366-7.
23. Heller J, Pedlow Jr F. Tumors of the spine: orthopaedic knowledge update. Spine. 1997:235-56.
24. Murphey MD, Andrews CL, Flemming DJ, et al. From the archives of the AFIP. Primary tumors of the spine: radiologic pathologic correlation. Radiographics. 1996; 16(5):1131-58.
25. Schaberg J, Gainor BJ. A profile of metastatic carcinoma of the spine. Spine. 1985;10(1):19.
26. Darouiche RO. Spinal epidural abscess. NEJM. 2006;355 (19):2012-2020.
27. Nussbaum ES, Rigamonti D, Standiford H, et al. Spinal epidural abscess: a report of 40 cases and review. Surg Neurol. 1992;38(3):225-31.
28. Brent LH. Inflammatory Arthritis. Postgrad Med. 2009; 121(2).
29. Kataria RK, Brent LH. Spondyloarthropathies. Am Fam Physician. 2004;69(12):2853.
30. McLeod J. The physiology of visceral sensation and referred pain. Aust N Z J Surg. 1961;30(4):298-305.
31. Klineberg E, Mazanec D, Orr D, et al. Masquerade: medical causes of back pain. Cleve Clin J Med. 2007;74(12): 905-13.

CHAPTER

5

Neurological Differential Diagnosis of Spinal Disorders

Devon Ryan, Thomas Cheriyan, Ludmilla Bronfin

INTRODUCTION

Neurological symptoms in patients with spinal disorders usually manifest themselves as a result of compression of neural elements. Radiculopathy and myelopathy, two classifications of nerve impingement, may be seen concomitantly, but they are distinct conditions. Radiculopathy refers to irritation of a nerve root as it exits the spine. It might be caused by compression from a herniated disk that inflames the root, for example. Symptoms can include pain, weakness, numbness, tingling, and hyporeflexia along the affected nerve.[1] Radiculopathy occurs most frequently in the cervical and lumbosacral regions of the spine, which would correspond with symptoms in the upper and lower extremities, respectively. Radiculopathy in the thoracic region is possible but is much rarer.[2] Myelopathy refers to a syndrome due to compression of the spinal cord itself. In contrast to radiculopathy, symptoms are typically bilateral, and can include numbness and clumsiness of the hands, weakness or spasticity in upper or lower extremities, leg stiffness, and loss of balance.[3] Most commonly, myelopathy is caused by natural degeneration of the spine—or spondylosis—in the cervical region, in which case the disorder is referred to as cervical spondylotic myelopathy. Table 5.1 presents salient aspects of the two conditions.

Typically, the symptoms described above are indeed caused by relatively routine spinal disorders: disk herniation, spinal stenosis, spondylosis, scoliosis, or trauma, for example. However, there are also serious neurological disorders that can present with similar symptoms and, although rare, need to be considered as differential diagnoses. This chapter aims to describe several important neurological conditions that can mimic radiculopathy (cervical or lumbosacral) or cervical myelopathy. Where possible, methods of distinguishing a given condition from spinal disease are also discussed.

CONDITIONS THAT MIMIC RADICULOPATHY

There are several neurological conditions that can present with symptoms akin to those of cervical or lumbosacral radiculopathy caused by a spinal disorder.

Table 5.1: Differences between radiculopathy and myelopathy

	Radiculopathy	*Myelopathy*
Location of compression	Nerve root	Spinal cord
Spinal region	Cervical, lumbosacral	Cervical
Common etiologies	Herniated disk, acute injury, spondylosis	Spondylosis, tumor
Symptoms	Pain, numbness, tingling, muscle weakness	Gait imbalance, muscle weakness, tingling, pain
Bilateral	No	Yes

Multiple Sclerosis

Multiple sclerosis (MS), a progressive demyelinating disorder, is the most common of these maladies. Its causes are unknown, although there are thought to be both genetic and environmental components. Patients with a family history of the disease are more susceptible, and it more commonly afflicts women than men. As the myelin sheath is damaged in patients with MS, nerve conduction is hindered, producing a variety of symptoms depending on the precise location of the lesions. Presentation is highly variable; patients may have intermittent or progressive symptoms. About 4% of those diagnosed with MS exhibit the primary symptom of acute motor radiculopathy, and the majority of these patients report pain in one or more extremities.[4,5] In such cases, the clinical picture is indistinguishable from radiculopathy caused by, e.g. a herniated disk.

Magnetic resonance imaging (MRI) is the most useful diagnostic tool for identifying and monitoring MS. Scans of both the brain and spinal cord should be obtained, although about 12% of patients who meet the criteria for MS have lesions only in the spinal cord.[6] Spinal lesions generate increased signal in T2-weighted images (Fig. 5.1). This is due to increased water content, which in turn is caused by the pathological features of the disease: swelling, inflammation, demyelination, and axonal loss. Gadolinium enhancement can help detect active MS lesions. Typically, plaques are fewer than two vertebral body segments in length and found in the cervical region.[7] An analysis of cerebrospinal fluid (CSF) can also be utilized to confirm diagnosis. Eighty percent of patients with MS have increased levels of IgG or oligoclonal IgG bands in the CSF, although patients with recent onset of symptoms may not present with this characteristic.[8]

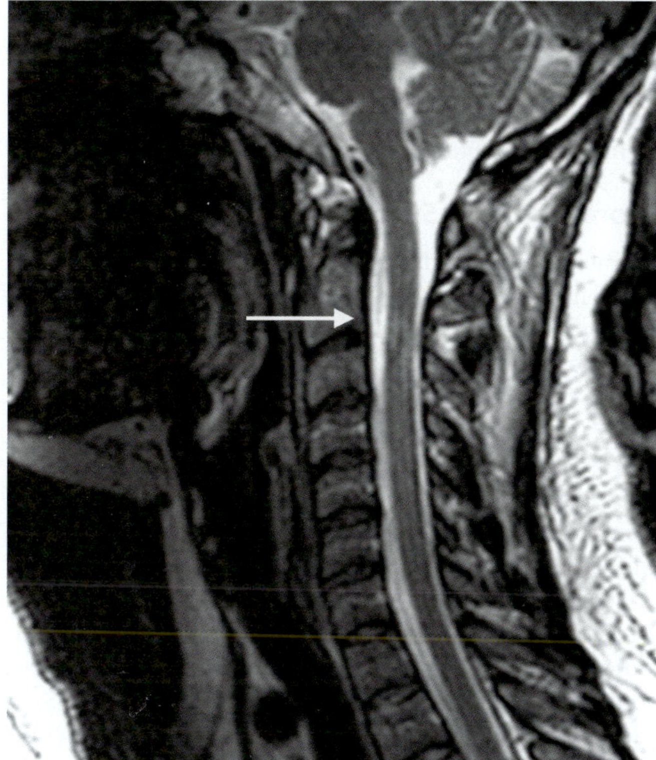

Fig. 5.1: Lesion (arrow) indicative of MS on T2-weighted spinal MRI.

Peripheral Neuropathy

Peripheral neuropathy is a broad classification that refers to the damaging or irritation of nerves after they have exited from the spinal cord instead of at the root level as with radiculopathy. This damage could be due to a wide variety of causes. Symptoms are identical to those of radiculopathy—pain, weakness, tingling, and numbness—and could manifest themselves in upper or lower extremities depending on the location of the affected nerve(s). Carpal tunnel syndrome, in which inflammation causes compression of the median nerve leading the hand, is a common condition of this type.

Differentiating between peripheral neuropathy and radiculopathy can be difficult, and doing so often hinges on linking symptoms to either a single nerve branch or to a nerve root distribution. This is usually done through nerve conduction studies, which are abnormal in patients with peripheral neuropathy but normal in those with radiculopathy. Tinel's test is noninvasive and can be used to estimate the site of nerve entrapment, although inconsistency between clinicians in the testing procedure seems to limit its diagnostic value.[9] The neurological examination may also include electromyography (EMG) studies, and targeted MRI should be used in conjunction to confirm the diagnosis.[10]

Plexopathy

Plexopathy is essentially a subset of the peripheral neuropathy category, referring specifically to damage done to the brachial or lumbosacral plexus. Such damage is most often the result of traumatic injury—from contact sports or an automobile accident, for example. The exception to this rule is Parsonage-Turner syndrome (acute brachial plexitis), which refers to a rare disease in which the brachial plexus becomes inflamed without a known cause.

In patients with plexopathy, pain is often followed by weakness after a period of days or weeks, while with radiculopathy, onset of pain and weakness is usually simultaneous. Differential diagnosis is made in the same manner as with other types of peripheral neuropathy.

Thoracic Outlet Syndrome

Thoracic outlet syndrome (TOS) refers to a related disorder in which there is abnormal compression of the neurovascular bundle that passes through the superior thoracic outlet, the aperture at the top of the thoracic cavity. The condition most often affects the nerves that make up the brachial plexus, and can be caused by trauma, overuse, or the existence of an extra cervical rib above what is normally the first rib. Symptoms of TOS include pain, tingling, and numbness in the neck, shoulders, and arms. These are very similar to signs of cervical radiculopathy, but often patients with TOS will exhibit symptoms in a C8-T1 distribution, which is rare with radiculopathy. There are several provocative tests, but none is a so-called "gold standard" for diagnosing TOS. In addition, the neurological examination, nerve conduction studies, and EMG are often normal or inconclusive, so some combination of MRI, CT, and radiography is usually necessary for differential diagnosis.[11]

Pancoast Tumor

Pancoast tumor (superior pulmonary sulcus tumor) is a relatively rare cancer located at the apex of one of the lungs. It can cause radiating pain in the neck and upper extremities as well as weakness and paresthesia in a C8-T1 distribution. These symptoms are attributable to the tumor's encroachment on the brachial plexus, intervertebral foramens, or vertebral bodies, and again mean that the syndrome closely mirrors certain features of cervical radiculopathy. Differential diagnosis of Pancoast tumor relies on a combination of history, physical examination, and imaging studies. Patients with this syndrome typically have a shorter history of pain than patients with cervical radiculopathy. Often they do not exhibit pain upon palpation or restricted range of motion in the neck and have a negative result with Spurling's test. They may present with Horner's syndrome (ipsilateral ptosis, miosis, anhidrosis, and enophthalmos) and constitutional symptoms such as fever or unexplained weight loss. Most importantly, anterior-posterior cervical radiographs reveal a lack of pulmonary air at the top of the affected lung (Fig. 5.2), and diagnosis can be confirmed using MRI, computed tomography (CT), or biopsy.[12]

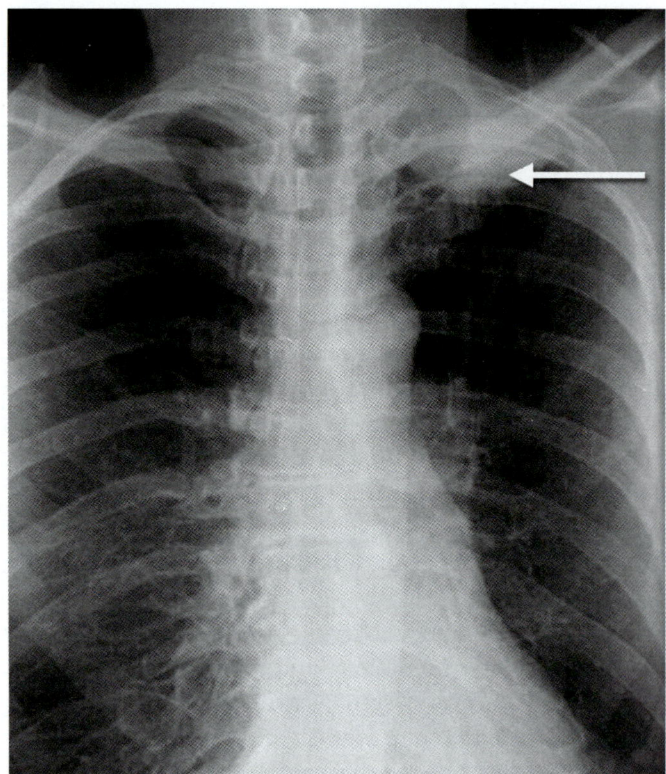

Fig. 5.2: Chest radiograph showing pancoast tumor (arrow) decreasing lung capacity on the left side.

Complex Regional Pain Syndrome

Complex regional pain syndrome (CRPS) is a rare chronic condition characterized by intense pain in an upper or lower limb. In the vast majority of CRPS patients, the pain develops following trauma to the involved extremity, but it is not commensurate with the severity of the initial injury and remains long after resolution of that malady.[13] The etiology of the disorder is not well known. While the pain may be consistent with cervical or lumbosacral radiculopathy, a neurological examination in a patient with CRPS is typically normal. Further, other symptoms that are often seen in the affected limb in CRPS—such as swelling, change in temperature or color, hyperesthesia, and allodynia—are not typically seen with radiculopathy.

Herpes Zoster

Herpes zoster, commonly known as shingles, is a disease caused by the same varicella zoster virus that is responsible for chickenpox. After resolution of an initial chickenpox infection as a child, the virus typically remains latent in some nerve cells and can become active later in life for reasons that are not known. Initially, patients with herpes zoster present with pain, burning, tingling, numbness, or itching in a dermatomal distribution—symptoms that are very similar to those of radiculopathy. The appearance of a red rash accompanied by blisters within a period of days or weeks is the telltale sign of herpes zoster, but the condition is often misdiagnosed because the skin irritation usually presents only after the neurological symptoms.

Intracranial Tumor

Intracranial tumors have been described as presenting in a similar manner as cervical or lumbosacral radiculopathy. Often, patients with brain cancer will exhibit symptoms such as headache, dizziness, and seizures, but that need not be the case. In one instance, e.g. a patient who was eventually diagnosed with a glioblastoma initially complained of numbness in the fingers of one hand. He subsequently reported muscle weakness in that arm and eventually in one of his legs.[14] Thus, his symptoms that were at first consistent with cervical radiculopathy. In another case, a patient presented with muscle weakness and foot drop in one leg, characteristic of lumbosacral radiculopathy, and was ultimately found to have an oligoastrocytoma.[15] In such scenarios, radiculopathy is typically deemed unlikely due to a normal neurological assessment, and the intracranial tumor can be visualized using MRI.

CONDITIONS THAT MIMIC CERVICAL MYELOPATHY

Cervical myelopathy is most commonly caused by spondylosis, a natural process of aging in which disk degeneration causes osteophyte formation, which in turn narrows the spinal canal. In fact, visual evidence of spondylosis can be found in about 95% of people by age 65. The majority of these individuals, however, remain asymptomatic.[16] This can make diagnosis difficult, as an MRI showing spondylosis in a patient with symptoms of cervical myelopathy does not necessarily determine cause and effect. In other words, the patient could have asymptomatic spondylosis and a different condition that is generating the symptoms of myelopathy. As with radiculopathy, there are a number of neurological disorders that can mimic the symptoms of myelopathy.

Multiple Sclerosis

Multiple sclerosis, a relatively common demyelinating disorder, was outlined in considerable detail in the preceding section. To reiterate, presentation of the disorder is highly variable. Primary symptoms could include loss of balance, trouble walking, and bilateral muscle weakness.[17] In such cases, MS would closely mimic cervical myelopathy. Differential diagnosis should be made in the same manner as explained previously.

Amyotrophic Lateral Sclerosis

Amyotrophic lateral sclerosis (ALS), or Lou Gehrig's disease, is a disorder of progressive upper and lower motor neuron degeneration, leading eventually to paralysis and death. The cause of the disease is not known in more than 90% of cases; in the others, a specific genetic defect is responsible. In most patients, ALS may be classified as "bulbar onset," in which the first symptoms are slurred speech, difficulty swallowing, and drooling, or "limb onset" in which the first symptom is muscle weakness in one or more extremities.[18] Patients with the latter presentation may have symptoms that closely mimic those of cervical myelopathy. In such cases, MRI is of limited use because ALS can neither be confirmed nor rejected visually, and the vast majority of elderly patients show some evidence of cervical spondylosis. Patients with ALS, however, are more likely than those with cervical myelopathy to present with fasciculations, and ALS typically progresses much more rapidly than myelopathy, leading to more pronounced muscle degeneration. Electrophysiological studies are also important in making a diagnosis, as EMG can demonstrate the denervation that is characteristic of ALS but not myelopathy.

Subacute Combined Degeneration

Subacute combined degeneration (SCD) is a disorder that affects the spine, brain, and peripheral nerves and is caused by vitamin B12 deficiency. Pernicious anemia, a condition in which individuals have trouble absorbing vitamin B12 in the intestines, is predictably the most common cause of this deficiency. Nitrous oxide anesthesia, however, has also been known to cause SCD, as the gas exerts its effects by interfering with vitamin B12's activity. This does not occur regularly, but rather in patients who, unbeknownst to their physicians, already had low levels of B12.[19] Symptoms of SCD are often similar to those of cervical myelopathy: bilateral weakness, numbness, or tingling in the upper or lower extremities, along with gait imbalance and clumsiness. Patients with SCD may also present with mental status changes or decreased vision.

Lesions in the spinal cord can usually be visualized, and diagnosis confirmed by measuring vitamin B12 levels in the blood.[20]

Hereditary Spastic Paraplegias

Hereditary spastic paraplegias (HSPs) are a group of genetic neurodegenerative disorders. All are characterized by the primary symptom of progressive lower limb spasticity and weakness, meaning that HSP may mimic cervical myelopathy. There have been about 50 different forms of HSP identified, each associated with a mutation in a different gene, and secondary symptoms and age of onset are highly variable between these forms. HSP could of course be suggested by a family history of the disease, and only genetic testing for a known mutation can confirm diagnosis.[21]

Tropical Spastic Paraparesis

Tropical spastic paraparesis (TSP) is a chronic spinal cord infection caused by the human T-lymphotropic virus (HTLV-I), which gives it the alternate name HTLV-I-associated myelopathy (HAM). The disease is characterized by slowly progressing weakness in the legs; spasticity, hyperreflexia, and muscle stiffness are also common. The primary risk factor for TSP is, as its name suggests, time spent in tropical regions of the world where the disease is most common. TSP is indicated by the presence of HLTV-I antibodies in the blood and CSF, although other conditions should also be ruled out to confirm diagnosis.[22]

Normal Pressure Hydrocephalus

Normal pressure hydrocephalus (NPH) is a disorder in which an accumulation of CSF in the ventricles of the brain first causes an increase in ICP. The ICP then gradually declines, however, to the point that it is either normal or only slightly elevated. The condition can be either idiopathic or secondary to another disease. NPH is characterized by a classic triad of symptoms: gait impairment, dementia, and urinary incontinence. Gait impairment often appears before the others, meaning that the symptoms can, at least initially, present as similar to those of cervical myelopathy. Ventricular enlargement can be seen on MRI in cases of NPH, and invasive tests that measure the dynamics of CSF can be performed to establish diagnosis with a reasonable degree of certainty.[23]

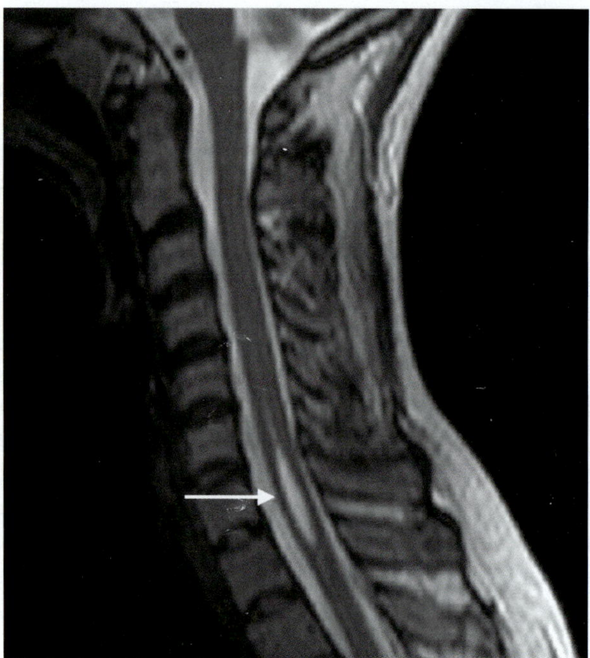

Fig. 5.3: MRI showing syrinx in spinal canal.

Syringomyelia

Syringomyelia refers to a condition in which a fluid-filled cavity (syrinx) forms in the spinal canal. In adults, it occurs most frequently because of a birth defect called Chiari malformation I, but it can also arise due to trauma or a spinal cord tumor. Syringomyelia of idiopathic origin has also been noted. The syrinx typically forms in the cervical spine and slowly expands, compressing the spinal cord and causing progressive symptoms similar to those of myelopathy: bilateral weakness, numbness, and gait imbalance. Often, these symptoms appear in a cape-like pattern in the shoulders, arms, and upper back. Pain may also be present, and can be consistent with radiculopathy. MRI allows for visualization of the syrinx and is thus the most reliable diagnostic tool for syringomyelia (Fig. 5.3).[24]

Spinal Infarction

Spinal infarction is rare condition in which blood supply to the spine is cut off. It is much rarer than cerebellar infarction, accounting for about 1% of all strokes.[25] The disorder can occur via two general mechanisms: (1) extensive spinal hypoperfusion due to arterial insufficiency and hypotension and (2) occlusion of a particular arterial branch in the spine. Spinal infarction typically presents with bilateral weakness and paraparesis; however, unlike with myelopathy, symptoms typically appear very rapidly, often within a matter of minutes. Further, pain is often reported, either in the spine and neck or radiating outwardly into the limbs. Diagnosis is typically confirmed using MRI.[26]

Spinal Tumor

Spinal neoplasms can be classified as either intramedullary (within the spinal canal) or extramedullary (outside the canal). They are often metastatic but can be primary. Details of the types of cancerous growths that can cause spinal disease are outside the scope of this chapter. In all cases, however, the tumor can cause compression of the spinal cord, generating symptoms identical to those of cervical spondylotic myelopathy. Often, patients experience pain characteristic of radiculopathy as well.[27] MRI allows for visualization of the neoplasm and can thus be used for diagnosis, followed by biopsy to confirm the identity of the abnormal cells.

SUMMARY

There are several neurological disorders that can generate symptoms of radiculopathy and cervical myelopathy, thereby mimicking common spinal disorders. While the referenced neurological conditions are relatively rare, they should still be considered by the clinician and ruled out, as they are often progressive and necessitate immediate attention. To do so, the physician must adhere closely to studied differential diagnosis mechanisms. Only in that manner can serious disorders with highly variant presentation be reliably identified.

REFERENCES

1. Lauder TD. Musculoskeletal disorders that frequently mimic radiculopathy. Phys Med Rehabil Clin N Am. 2002; 13:469-86.
2. O Connor RC, Andary MT, Russo RB, et al. Thoracic radiculopathy. Phys Med Rehabil Clin N Am. 2002;13:623-44.
3. Nikolaidis I, Fouyas IP, Sandercock P, et al. Surgery for cervical radiculopathy or myelopathy. Cochrane Database Syst Rev. 2010;1.
4. Lavallee P, Apartis E, Vidal JS, et al. Acute motor radiculopathy as a first symptom of MS: Anatomic–radiologic correlation. Neurology. 2001;56:1603-4.
5. Ramirez-Lassepas M, Tulloch JW, Quinones MR, et al. Acute radicular pain as a presenting symptom in multiple sclerosis. Arch Neurol. 1992;49:255.
6. Honig LS, Sheremata W. Magnetic resonance imaging of spinal cord lesions in multiple sclerosis. J Neurol Neurosurg Psychiatry. 1989;52:459-66.
7. Braverman DL, Lachmann EA, Tunkel R, et al. Multiple sclerosis presenting as a spinal cord tumor. Arch Phys Med Rehabil. 1997;78:1274-6.
8. Miller DH, Leary SM. Primary-progressive multiple sclerosis. Lancet Neurol. 2007;6:903-12.
9. Lifchez SD, Means Jr KR, Dunn RE, et al. Intra- and inter-examiner variability in performing Tinel's test. J Hand Surg. 2010;35:212-6.
10. Nardin RA, Patel MR, Gudas TF, et al. Electromyography and magnetic resonance imaging in the evaluation of radiculopathy. Muscle Nerve. 1999;22:151-5.
11. Aralasmak A, Cevikol C, Karaali K, et al. MRI findings in thoracic outlet syndrome. Skeletal Radiol. 2012:1-10.
12. Gu R, Kang M, Gao Z, et al. Differential diagnosis of cervical radiculopathy and superior pulmonary sulcus tumor. Chin Med J. 2012;125:2755-7.
13. Goebel A. Complex regional pain syndrome in adults. Rheumatology. 2011;50:1739-50.
14. Clar SA, Cianca JC. Intracranial tumor masquerading as cervical radiculopathy: a case study. Arch Phys Med Rehabil. 1998;79:1301-2.
15. Lee YS, Wang PY. Foot drop caused by a brain tumor: a case report. Acta Neurol Taiwanica. 2009;18:130-1.
16. Shedid D, Benzel EC. Cervical spondylosis anatomy: pathophysiology and biomechanics. Neurosurgery. 2007;60:S1.
17. Calabresi PA. Diagnosis and management of multiple sclerosis. Am Fam Physician. 2004;70:1935.
18. Wijesekera LC, Leigh PN. Amyotrophic lateral sclerosis. Orphanet J Rare Dis. 2009;4:3.
19. Beltramello A, Puppini G, Cerini R, et al. Subacute combined degeneration of the spinal cord after nitrous oxide anaesthesia: role of magnetic resonance imaging. J Neurol Neurosurg Psychiatry. 1998;64:563.
20. Tajima Y, Mito Y, Owada Y, et al. MR appearance of subacute combined degeneration of the spinal cord. Psychiatry Clin Neurosci. 1994;48:611-4.
21. Schüle R, Schöls L. Genetics of hereditary spastic paraplegias. Seminars in neurology; 2011: © Thieme Medical Publishers. p. 484-93.
22. Castro-Costa CMD, Araújo AQC, Barreto MM, et al. Proposal for diagnostic criteria of tropical spastic paraparesis/HTLV-I-associated myelopathy (TSP/HAM). AIDS Res Hum Retroviruses. 2006;22:931-5.
23. Kiefer M, Unterberg A. The differential diagnosis and treatment of normal-pressure hydrocephalus. Dtsch Ärzteblatt Int. 2012;109:15.
24. Roy AK, Slimack NP, Ganju A. Idiopathic syringomyelia: retrospective case series, comprehensive review, and update on management. Neurosur Focus. 2011;31:1-9.
25. Novy J, Carruzzo A, Maeder P, et al. Spinal cord ischemia: clinical and imaging patterns, pathogenesis, and outcomes in 27 patients. Arch Neurol. 2006;63:1113.
26. Wang VY, Chou D, Chin C. Spine and spinal cord emergencies: vascular and infectious causes. Neuroimaging Clin N Am. 2010;20:639.
27. Hammack J. Spinal cord disease in patients with cancer. Continuum (Minneapolis, Minn.). 2012;18:312.

CHAPTER

6

Examination and Evaluation of Neck Pain

Jonathan R Stieber, Robert J Ames

INTRODUCTION

Axial neck pain is a common and challenging complaint for both clinicians and patients. This chapter provides an overview of the natural history, basic anatomy, pathophysiology and evaluation of axial neck pain. The concomitant presence of cervical myelopathy and/or radiculopathy in patients with axial neck pain may strongly influence their evaluation and treatment, potentially necessitating surgical intervention. As such, their clinical course is distinct from the management of patients who suffer exclusively from axial neck pain.

PREVALENCE AND NATURAL HISTORY

Many adults will experience neck pain at some point in their lives.[1] One study reported the age-standardized lifetime prevalence of neck pain at 66.7%, with the point prevalence at 22.2%.[2] The same study reported the 6-month prevalence of low-intensity and low-disability neck pain at 39.7%. Significantly disabling neck pain within the past 6 months was reported in 4.6% of individuals, with more women experiencing high-disability neck pain than men. A best evidence review of the current literature revealed up to 50% annual prevalence of neck pain with upwards of 11.5% of pain being described as "activity-limiting".[3] While certainly frustrating, neck pain is generally a self-limiting condition and will often improve with little or no intervention. In a systematic review of the clinical course of nonspecific neck pain, several studies reported a range of general improvement between 36% and 95%.[4] However, Gore et al. report that between 22% and 32% of patients will go on to experience persistent pain.[5]

ANATOMY

A comprehensive understanding of neck and cervical spine anatomy is essential to the evaluation and management of patients presenting with axial neck pain. Cervical anatomy may be divided into the bony structures of the vertebral column, the articulating joints, the intervertebral disks, ligamentous and muscular anatomy, vasculature, as well as the neurological elements. The cervical spine includes the seven most cephalad vertebrae, C1 through C7. The normal curvature of the cervical spine is a slight inward arc of the vertebral column. Normal lordosis in this region of the spine is typically between 34° and 42° (Fig. 6.1).[6]

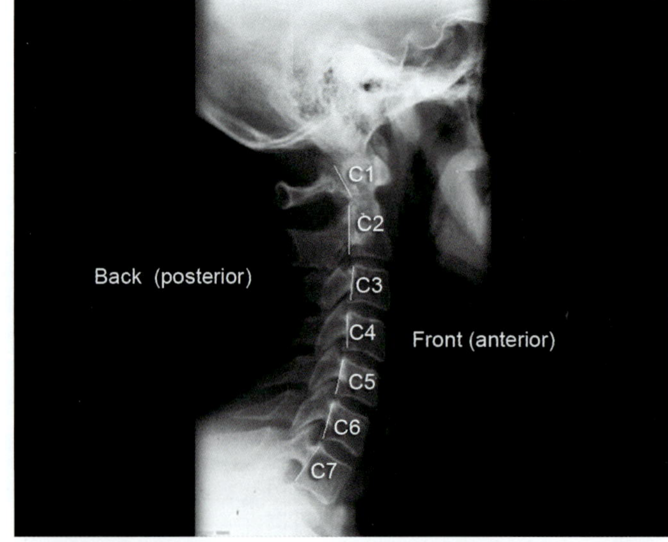

Fig. 6.1: Lateral radiograph of cervical spine showing normal lordosis, between 34° and 42°.

In the subaxial spine, extending from C2-3 to C6-7, intervertebral disks are located between the vertebral bodies in the anterior column of the spine. The disks are constructed of fibrocartilaginous material (principally type I collagen) and are relatively avascular, receiving their blood supply from the adjacent endplates of the vertebral bodies. The nucleus pulposus (consisting mostly of type II collagen) is the inner mucoid part of the disk and the annulus fibrosus is the outer multilayered portion of the disk. Coupled with the uncovertebral and facet joints, the intervertebral disks permit six degrees of freedom for each motion segment: flexion, extension, lateral bending, and lateral rotation.

Uncinate processes protrude superiorly from the lateral margins of the vertebral bodies of the subaxial cervical spine (C3-C7). These processes articulate with the adjacent superior vertebral bodies forming the uncovertebral joints, or joints of Luschka, and provide additionally stability to the motion segments. At each level of the subaxial spine from C2 through C7, a pair of diarthrodial facet joints provides stability as part of the posterior elements.

The ligamentous structures of the cervical spine are extensive. When motion segments are stressed to a maximum range of motion, the spinal ligaments help serve to protect the spine from exceeding normal physiologic motion and subsequent injury. The anterior longitudinal ligament runs along the anterior aspect of the vertebral column and prevents hyperextension of the cervical spine. A combination of posterior ligamentous structures provides stability and help to prevent hyperflexion of the spine. The posterior longitudinal ligament is situated posterior to the vertebral bodies on the ventral aspect of the spinal canal. The ligamentum flavum (yellow ligament) runs longitudinally between adjacent laminae along the dorsal aspect of the spinal canal. Lastly, the interspinous and supraspinous ligaments run in between the spinous processes and along the posterior aspect of the spinous processes, respectively. They serve to act as a posterior tension band, resisting hyperflexion and kyphosis.

The spinal cord itself is contained within the spinal canal just posterior to the vertebral bodies and the intervertebral disks. Eight pairs of nerve roots exit the spinal cord at the cervical level. Spinal nerves one through seven exit the spinal cord via the neural foramina at the level above their named vertebrae. Spinal nerve C8 exits below C7 and above T1. Due to the close proximity of the musculoskeletal anatomy, it is important to appreciate the potential for pathologic compression or irritation of the neurological elements.

PATHOPHYSIOLOGY

Muscle and Soft Tissue Pain

Axial neck pain is most commonly associated with the regional soft tissue surrounding the cervical spinal column.[7] Muscular neck pain can be brought on by heavy lifting, a whiplash type injury, sleeping in an unusual position, or by certain muscular pathologies such as torticollis. It is important to keep in mind that while inciting event may be useful in understanding the pathogenesis of neck pain, in most cases no specific cause can be identified.[4]

Whiplash type injuries may be a cause of axial neck pain in patients who have suffered a trauma such as a motor vehicle accident. Contrary to popular belief, a whiplash injury is not a flexion-extension injury. Studies have shown that whiplash is a compression injury due to the trunk of the body being forced upward toward the head.[8] Pain may be generated as a result of a sagittal deformity that can occur postinjury, or via direct injury to the facet joints or intervertebral disks.[9]

Sprains or strains may cause significant discomfort or pain. Occasionally, high-tension stress on the neck can initiate injury of the tendinous attachments of muscles to bone, or even rupture of the muscles themselves. Muscle sprains or whiplash type injuries may initially present as a sharp or stabbing pain acutely via stimulation of unmyelinated pain fibers. Often, acute pain is followed by more prolonged aching pain. This may be due to alterations in the physiologic thresholds of afferent pain fibers caused by the release of chemical mediators in a protracted inflammatory response.[10] In most cases, symptoms resulting from soft tissue injury of the cervical spine will resolve themselves within 6 weeks with conservative treatment alone.[11] Other patients, however, will continue to experience symptoms for a prolonged duration. It has been reported that 10–34% of patients will go on to experience chronic axial neck pain lasting longer than 1 month.[1,12,13]

Torticollis is a condition associated with severe lateral flexion contracture of the cervical spine musculature, causing the head to be tilted and laterally rotated to one side. Often the sternocleidomastoid or trapezius muscles are involved. Torticollis may be congenital or acquired.

Congenital torticollis is usually associated with certain anatomical deformities or anomalies. Acquired torticollis can be due to trauma, muscle injury, neoplasm, or infection.[10]

Degenerative Pain

In addition to muscle and ligament strain, degeneration of the spinal elements is also a common source of pain. Degenerative causes of pain include cervical spondylosis, osteophyte formation, uncovertebral or facet joint arthritis, segmental instability, and cervical disk herniation.

Cervical Spondylosis

Cervical spondylosis is believed to be related to natural degenerative changes in the intervertebral disks of the spine. Biomechanical and metabolic changes in cartilaginous structure of the disks play a role in the pathogenesis of cervical spondylosis. These changes include, but are not limited to, desiccation of the nucleus pulposus, loss of disk height, and decreased annular competence. Moreover, disk degeneration can also lead to segmental instability, endplate stress and spurring/osteophyte formation, in addition to uncovertebral and facet joint arthritis. Most commonly, patients who present with cervical spondylosis are over 40 years old and may complain of neck pain and occasional headache. Disk degeneration can undoubtedly cause axial neck pain. However, the pain is often poorly localized and referred to other areas such as the shoulder, the interscapular zone or the anterior chest wall. This type of pain can also be exacerbated with movement.[10] Investigations have shown that degenerative changes of the cervical disks are quite common even among asymptomatic individuals. One study reported asymptomatic disk degeneration in 86–89% of people aged 60 and older.[14] Therefore, assignment of cervical spondylosis as a primary pain generator should be considered with caution.[15]

Zygapophyseal/Uncovertebral Joint Arthritis

The zygapophyseal joints are the diarthrodial synovial joints between the superior and inferior articular processes of two adjacent vertebrae. In an experiment employing cervical medial branch blocks in patients experiencing neck pain, Bogduk and Marsland demonstrated the validity of facetogenic pain. Complete temporary relief of all symptoms was obtained in 17 out of 24 consecutive patients with idiopathic neck pain.[16] Osteoarthritis or hyperextension injuries of the zygapophyseal joints may account for the pain originating from this area.[17] Clinically, patients experiencing pain from a degenerative facet joint will most likely present with localized pain over the involved joint.[18] Spondylolisthesis or retrolisthesis (most commonly associated with peripheral neuropathic pain) can present secondary to progressive degeneration of the zygapophyseal joints, and may also be sources of axial neck pain.

Osteoarthritis of the uncovertebral joints can be part of the cervical spondylosis milieu.[19] A recent cadaveric study utilizing immunohistochemical and histological techniques revealed that the uncovertebral joints are, indeed, synovial in nature; the authors therefore suggest that the joints of Luschka are likely pain generators in the cervical spine.[20]

Acute Cervical Disk Herniation

Over time, alterations in the biomechanics and biochemistry of the intervertebral disks lead to degenerative changes that negatively impact disk function. Acute herniation of the nucleus pulposus may occur and frequently leads to radicular symptoms. In the cervical spine, herniation may lead to compression of the spinal cord and myelopathy as well.[21] The anatomy of the intervertebral disks, their position, and proximity to the neurological elements lead to clear pathophysiological patterns of herniation. Most disk herniations occur in the posterolateral direction and may impinge upon exiting nerve roots. However, there are patients who experience little or no radicular or myelopathic symptomatology and present with axial neck pain.[10] While little biomechanical data exists, some authors speculate that just as other ligamentous tears or disruptions in the body are painful, a tear or herniation of the intervertebral disk (even without radicular or myelopathic disturbances) should certainly be painful as well.[22] With disk herniations, problems exist again in assigning accountability to any particular radiographic finding. Boden et al. reported abnormal disk findings in 14% of people who were <40 years old, and 28% of people who were older than forty. Of these patients, 10% under 40 years old and 5% over 40 years old demonstrated a herniated nucleus pulposus on MRI.[23]

Rheumatologic Disorders

The cervical spine can be affected by a number of rheumatologic disorders including rheumatoid arthritis and ankylosing spondylitis. When rheumatoid arthritis or ankylosing spondylitis affects the neck, it generally does so in patients in which disease has already manifested itself in the peripheral skeleton (such as the appendicular joints in rheumatoid arthritis, or sacroiliac joints in ankylosing spondylitis).[24] Rheumatoid arthritis rarely presents as neck pain without any appendicular symptoms.[25]

Referred Pain

For many sources of neck pain, patterns of somatic referred pain have been well documented. Pain can be referred from the cervical spine to various regional areas including the head, upper limbs, anterior chest wall or interscapular regions. Referred pain may be due to a convergence in the nervous system of afferent fibers from deeper structures (e.g. the facet joints or intervertebral disks) that join with neurons innervating structures in other regions.[26] Common patterns of referred pain can be seen in Figure 6.2.

Myelopathy and Radiculopathy

Cervical level radiculopathy and myelopathy are also potential sources of neck pain. While peripheral neurological pain and/or deficits associated with these conditions often eclipse axial neck pain, it is important, nevertheless, to understand that these conditions can be sources of axial pain as well. Degenerative changes of the spine occur during the natural course of aging.[27] Sometimes, these changes can include a narrowing of the vertebral canal and a slow, progressive compression of the spinal cord. Often, an insidious onset of manual sensation changes, coupled with reports of decreased manual dexterity, clumsiness, or gait disturbance, is seen in patients suffering from cervical myelopathy.[10,28]

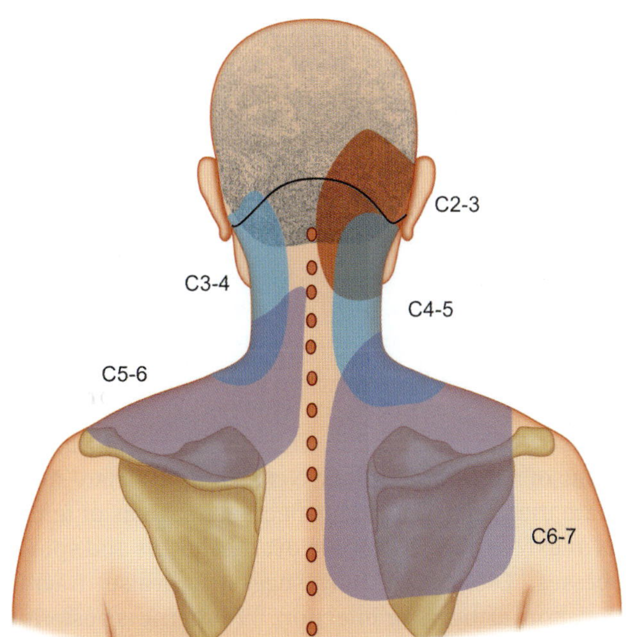

Fig. 6.2: Cervical pain referral patterns.

Cervical radiculopathy, colloquially referred to as a "pinched nerve", involves compression or irritation of a spinal nerve. This commonly occurs as a result of degenerative or traumatic changes to the intervertebral disks. When these changes occur, the intervertebral disks can bulge or herniate. As mentioned previously, due to the anatomy of the spinal ligaments and the disks themselves, herniation often occurs in the posterolateral direction, making compression of the exiting nerve root a likely outcome. Patients report pain that descends from the neck along the distribution of the nerve in the upper limb. Along with paresthesias, radiculopathy may be associated with predictable patterns of weakness, pins and needles, and/or numbness.

Other Pain Syndromes

Though less common, there are quite a number of other pathologies that may result in axial neck pain. These sources include but are not limited to; fibromyalgia, fracture, spinal cord tumors, vertebral tumors, epidural hematoma, diffuse idiopathic skeletal hyperostosis, Paget's disease, discitis, osteomyelitis, crystal arthropathies (gout), thoracic outlet syndrome, and psychogenic pain.[24]

HISTORY, PHYSICAL EXAMINATION AND GRADING

Neck pain is often self-limiting within a few weeks; however, 40% of patients with axial neck pain will contact their general practitioner for an evaluation. Of these patients, 30% are referred for further diagnosis to a medical specialist, and 32% to physiotherapy or some other type of conservative therapy.[29,30]

According to the findings reported by the bone and joint decade task force on neck pain and its associated disorders, patients who present to a primary care physician for evaluation of neck pain should undergo a screening history and physical in order to be triaged into four broad categories to help direct care. The assigned grade should dictate the appropriateness of clinical investigations and management.[31] Grading is assigned using levels I–IV according to severity of the patient's condition, and is discussed in greater detail shortly.

History

A careful and thorough history is of paramount importance in the assessment of patients who present with axial neck pain. Initial questioning should focus on location, quality, severity and radiation of the pain, timing (onset and duration), any aggravating or alleviating factors, as well as associated symptoms. It is important to question the patient about any neurologic deficits they may be experiencing in association with their neck pain. Patients should be questioned specifically about sensory and ataxic changes in the upper and lower limbs, gait abnormalities, bowel or bladder disturbances, weakness, or clumsiness. Any number of these symptoms may be a sign of a more serious condition such as cervical myelopathy or radiculopathy. Patients with these conditions may often present with axial neck pain as their chief complaint, but when thoroughly evaluated are found to suffer from significant neurological deficits.[18]

Red Flags

The screening history and physical examination will be able to help the clinician triage the patient into one of the four categories. While taking the patient's history, it is important to recognize any "red flags" that potentially indicate a more serious condition. Pain associated with a history of trauma must be investigated for fracture and/or instability. Neoplasm must also be included in the differential diagnosis when pain is associated with a history of cancer, night pain, unexplained weight loss, constitutional symptomatology, or failure to improve with a reasonably duration of therapy. A rheumatologic evaluation may be warranted if there is sufficient suspicion of systemic inflammatory disease such as rheumatoid arthritis, ankylosing spondylitis, or inflammatory arthritis. Discitis and/or osteomyelitis should be investigated in the context of recent or ongoing systemic infection, immunosuppression, or a history of intravenous drug use. Any previous spinal surgery should be explored as well for pseudoarthrosis; however, a comprehensive discussion of this topic is beyond the scope of this chapter. Again, any neurologic pathology including cervical myelopathy or radiculopathy should be ruled out.[32]

After these "red flag" symptoms have been excluded or investigated, the clinician should query the patient about the location, intensity, severity, and character of the pain. The physician may choose to use a visual analog scale or solicit a numerical pain rating. It is likewise important to investigate if the pain is episodic, remitting and relapsing, or unremitting. The clinician should explore the history of previous episodes, as well as any inciting, exacerbating, or ameliorating factors. The clinician should solicit information from the patient on the level of interference in daily activities that is caused by their neck pain. This may be obtained by administering the "Neck Disability Index" questionnaire that investigates ten areas of possible disability due to neck pain, including pain intensity, personal care, lifting, reading, headaches, concentration, work, driving, sleeping, and recreation.[33] In a healthy patient, severe or unremitting pain of extended duration is always a concern and serious underlying pathology should be excluded as an etiology.

Physical Examination

The physician should then complete a thorough physical examination of the cervical spine. This begins with inspection and palpation of the patient. Inspection of the patient includes assessing the coronal and sagittal alignment of the spine, paying attention to confirm that the patient has normal lordosis of the cervical region. If deformity of the cervical spine is suspected, it should not be automatically considered the source of the pain. While a true kyphotic deformity can certainly be a pain generator, no studies have shown loss of normal physiologic kyphosis to be related to neck pain, and this finding may be only incidental to the actual pain generator.[22] While not necessarily diagnostic, recognizing a deformity is important as it may assist the clinician in building a more complete understanding of the patient's condition.

Active and gentle passive range of motion of the neck should be assessed. This includes flexion, extension, lateral bending to the right and left, as well as right and left rotation of the neck. The clinician should note any decreased range of motion or pain elicited during this portion of the examination. Next, the physician should palpate the patient's neck inspecting for areas of tenderness or excess pain, including over the facets and spinous processes. Tenderness may suggest a bruise, fracture, dislocation, arthritis, or infection.[34] Tenderness posteriorly over the facet joints (located approximately one inch lateral to the spinous processes of C2 through C7) may be an important indicator of facet arthrosis or degeneration.[18] The clinician should also assess any paraspinal muscular spasm that may be present, and palpate for any potential soft tissue masses.

Lastly, a complete neurological examination for reflexes, muscle strength, and sensory deficits should be administered. It is important to recognize that some neurological symptoms may not always be apparent to the patient. As such, the clinician should perform an exhaustive examination to rule out any evidence of myelopathy, radiculopathy or other neurologic disorders. Provocative tests including Lhermitte's sign and Spurling's test should be performed to help evaluate for cervical cord compression and nerve root compression, respectively.[31] Hoffman's sign, finger escape sign, and inverted radial reflex are useful tests when investigating upper motor neuron symptomatology. Neurologic examination should also include the Rhomberg maneuver, assessment of gait, manual dexterity, and dysdiadochokinesia when warranted.

Grading

As previously mentioned, a four-tiered grading system has been proposed in order to clinically assess and manage patients who present with neck pain (Table 6.1).[31] Patients with *Grade I* neck pain show no signs or symptoms of structural pathology such as fracture, spinal cord or nerve injury, neoplasm, infection, or systemic disease. Patients in this category present with little or no interference in their daily activities. These patients are likely to respond to minimal intervention and reassurance and are less likely to require further investigation or continued treatment.

Grade II patients also do not show signs of serious pathology (structural or otherwise); however, they do present with significant interference in their daily activities. These patients will require pain relief and early nonoperative treatment aimed at preventing long-term difficulties.

Grade III patients do not present with any significant structural pathology; however, they exhibit neurologic deficits such as decreased deep tendon reflexes, weakness, and/or sensory deficits. These symptoms generally require further investigation and ongoing or more aggressive treatment.

Grade IV patients present with major pathology. This category includes spinal fracture, myelopathy, neoplasm, or systemic diseases such as inflammatory arthropathies. It is important to perform a thorough history and physical examination in order to identify these patients. If such a classification is appropriate then rapid and thorough investigation and treatment is required.

IMAGING AND DIAGNOSTIC STUDIES

Imaging studies can be utilized to rule out any structural instability or compromise of neurological elements. Plain film X-rays provide the most basic and useful initial screening.[35] Lateral, anteroposterior, and open mouth views can be used to assess the following: spinal alignment, degenerative changes, gross pathologic processes, fractures, vertebral or facet subluxation/dislocation, facet arthrosis, disk degeneration or loss of disk height, uncovertebral arthrosis, relationship of C1 and C2 to the occiput, congenital deformity or stenosis, and space available for the cord.[18,36,37] Importantly, plain radiographs are not sufficiently sensitive for the diagnosis of malignancy or infection, especially in their early stages.

Computed tomography (CT) and CT myelography may be utilized to evaluate patients presenting with radiculopathy or myelopathy. In the absence of trauma, no data exist in the literature supporting the use of CT

Table 6.1: Grading of patients with axial neck pain

Grade	*Presentation*	*Management*
I	• No signs or symptoms of fracture, spinal cord injury, nerve injury, neoplasm, infection, systemic disease or other serious pathology • No disruption in daily activities	• No further investigation required • Minimal intervention/self-care • Reassurance
II	• No signs of serious pathology (structural or otherwise) • Significant interference in daily activities	• Early nonoperative treatment • Provide options for short term pain relief
III	• No significant structural pathology • Patient exhibits neurologic deficits (e.g. decreased deep tendon reflexes, weakness, and/or sensory deficits)	• Further investigation required • Consider MRI and referral • Ongoing and more aggressive treatment
IV	• Major pathology (e.g. spinal fracture, myelopathy, neoplasm, or systemic disease)	• Rapid and thorough investigation • Referral required

in patients who present with primary axial neck pain. Indications for CT include neurologic signs, myelopathy, progressive motor deficits, and suspicion or cancer/infection.[38] Magnetic resonance imaging (MRI) may be used in the diagnosis of cervical pathology. MRI is useful in visualizing intervertebral disk or joint degeneration, spinal stenosis, discitis/osteomyelitis, spinal column neoplasm, effects of demyelinating disease, or trauma.[39] As with CT, however, there is no indication for MRI in patients with uncomplicated neck pain.[40]

Presently, there is no gold standard or validated sequence of imaging or diagnostic studies for the treatment of axial neck pain.[37] If "red flags" exist it is important to recognize that further investigation and treatment is imperative, and the clinician should proceed with plain radiography at the initial encounter with subsequent imaging studies if warranted. Initial management is universally nonoperative for patients who present with axial neck pain in the absence of more serious findings. Consequently, imaging studies such as MRI will seldom provide information that will alter the treatment algorithm.[41] If, after 6 weeks, a patient returns with symptoms that have failed to resolve despite nonoperative treatment or the patient's pain is intractable, then further radiographic evaluation is recommended.[18]

SUMMARY

The evaluation of axial neck pain is a frequent and potentially challenging task for clinicians. Moreover, the morbidity and disability associated with neck pain is a significant issue for both the individual patient and society. This overview of neck pain and its natural history, basic anatomy, pathophysiology, and evaluation lays a foundation for successive chapters as they explore in depth various diagnostic modalities and treatment options.

REFERENCES

1. Bovim G, Schrader H, Sand T. Neck pain in the general population. Spine. 1994;19(12):1307-9.
2. Cote P, Cassidy JD, Carroll L. The Saskatchewan health and back pain survey: the prevalence of neck pain and related disability in Saskatchewan adults. Spine. 1998;23 (15): 1689-98.
3. Hogg-Johnson S, van der Velde G, Carroll LJ, et al. The burden and determinants of neck pain in the general population: results of the Bone and Joint Decade 2000-2010 Task Force on Neck Pain and Its Associated Disorders. Spine. 2008;33(4 Suppl):S39-51.
4. Borghouts JA, Koes BW, Bouter LM. The clinical course and prognostic factors of non-specific neck pain: a systematic review. Pain. 1998;77(1):1-13.
5. Gore DR, Sepic SB, Gardner GM, et al. Neck pain: a long-term follow-up of 205 patients. Spine. 1987;12(1):1-5.
6. Harrison DD, Janik TJ, Troyanovich SJ, et al. Comparisons of lordotic cervical spine curvatures to a theoretical ideal model of the static sagittal cervical spine. Spine. 1996;21(6):667-75.
7. Ahn NU, Ahn UM, Ipsen B, et al. Mechanical neck pain and cervicogenic headache. Neurosurgery. 2007;60(1 Suppl 1): S21-7.
8. Whiplash: mechanics of injury. In: Bogduk N, McGuirk B. Management of Acute and Chronic Neck Pain, 1st edition. Philadelphia, PA: Elsevier; 2006. pp. 125-31.
9. Hammacher ER, van der Werken C. Acute neck sprain: "whiplash" reappraised. Injury. 1996;27(7):463-6.
10. Mechanical disorders of the spine. In: Borenstein DG, Wiesel SW, Boden SD. Low Back and Neck Pain, 3rd edition. Philadelphia, PA: Saunders; 2004. pp. 229-300.
11. Walter O, Spitzer, Francis E LeBlanc. Scientific approach to the assessment and management of activity-related spinal disorders. A monograph for clinicians. Report of the Quebec Task Force on Spinal Disorders. Spine. 1987;12(7 Suppl):S1-59.
12. Dvorak J. Epidemiology, physical examination, and neurodiagnostics. Spine. 1998;23(24):2663-73.
13. Makela M, Heliovaara M, Sievers K, et al. Prevalence, determinants, and consequences of chronic neck pain in Finland. Am J Epidemiol. 1991;134(11):1356-67.
14. Matsumoto M, Fujimura Y, Suzuki N, et al. MRI of cervical intervertebral discs in asymptomatic subjects. J Bone Joint Surg Br Vol. 1998;80(1):19-24.
15. Grob D. Surgery in the degenerative cervical spine. Spine. 1998;23(24):2674-83.
16. Bogduk N, Marsland A. The cervical zygapophysial joints as a source of neck pain. Spine. 1988;13(6):610-7.
17. Chronic neck pain: causes. In: Bogduk N, McGuirk B (Eds). Management of Acute and Chronic Neck Pain. Philadelphia, PA: Elsevier; 2006. pp. 95-8.
18. Rhee JM. Evaluation of axial neck pain. Who is a surgical candidate and who isn't: how to manage the nonoperative treatment, how to work up the pathology. In: Keith H, Dewald RL (Eds). Textbook of Spinal Surgery. Philadelphia, PA: Lippincott Williams and Wilkins; 2011. pp. 185-95.
19. Cervical spondylosis. In: Michael Benatar (Ed). Neuromuscular Disease. Totowa: New Jersey Humana Press; 2006. pp. 61-78.
20. Brismee JM, Sizer PS, Jr, Dedrick GS, et al. Immunohistochemical and histological study of human uncovertebral joints: a preliminary investigation. Spine. 2009;34(12): 1257-63.
21. Hunt WE, Miller CA. Management of cervical radiculopathy. Clin Neurosurg. 1986;33:485-502.
22. Chronic neck pain: assessment. In: Bogduk N, McGuirk B (Eds). Management of Acute and Chronic Neck Pain, 1st edition. Philadelphia, PA: Elsevier; 2006. pp. 95-8.

23. Boden SD, McCowin PR, Davis DO, et al. Abnormal magnetic-resonance scans of the cervical spine in asymptomatic subjects: a prospective investigation. J Bone Joint Surg Am Vol. 1990;72(8):1178-84.
24. Sources and causes of neck pain. In: Bogduk N, McGuirk B (Eds). Management of Acute and Chronic Neck Pain, 1st edition. Philadelphia, PA: Elsevier; 2006. pp. 9-20.
25. Sharp J, Purser DW, Lawrence JS. Rheumatoid arthritis of the cervical spine in the adult. Ann Rheum Dis. 1958; 17(3):303-13.
26. Bogduk N. The anatomy and pathophysiology of neck pain. Phys Med Rehabil Clin N Am. 2003;14(3):455-72, v.
27. Friedenberg ZB, Miller WT. Degenerative disc disease of the cervical spine. J Bone Joint Surg Am Vol. 1963;45:1171-8.
28. Crandall PH, Batzdorf U. Cervical spondylotic myelopathy. J Neurosurg. 1966;25(1):57-66.
29. Borghouts JA, Koes BW, Vondeling H, et al. Cost-of-illness of neck pain in The Netherlands in 1996. Pain. 1999;80(3): 629-36.
30. Picavet HS, Schouten JS. Musculoskeletal pain in the Netherlands: prevalences, consequences and risk groups, the DMC(3)-study. Pain. 2003;102(1-2):167-78.
31. Guzman J, Haldeman S, Carroll LJ, et al. Clinical practice implications of the Bone and Joint Decade 2000-2010 Task Force on Neck Pain and Its Associated Disorders: from concepts and findings to recommendations. Spine. 2008;33(4 Suppl):S199-213.
32. Nordin M, Carragee EJ, Hogg-Johnson S, et al. Assessment of neck pain and its associated disorders: results of the Bone and Joint Decade 2000-2010 Task Force on Neck Pain and Its Associated Disorders. Spine. 2008;33(4 Suppl):S101-22.
33. Vernon H, Mior S. The Neck Disability Index: a study of reliability and validity. J Manipulative Physiol Ther. 1991; 14(7):409-15.
34. Malone J HJ, Sharan AD, Eichenbaum MD, et al. Physical examination of the spine. In: Albert T, Vaccaro A (Eds). Spine, 1st edition. Philadelphia, PA: Elsevier Mosby; 2005. pp. 14-32.
35. Kaiser JA, Holland BA. Imaging of the cervical spine. Spine. 1998;23(24):2701-12.
36. Radiographic evaluation. In: Borenstein DG, Wiesel SW, Boden SD (Eds). Low Back and Neck Pain, 3rd edition. Philadelphia, PA: Saunders; 2004. pp. 146-76.
37. Clarke MJ, Krauss WE, Pichelmann MA, et al. Axial neck pain: a surgeon's perspective. Therapy;8(6):763-70.
38. Yinggang ZKL, Edward S. Diagnostic imaging of painful cervical discs. In: MJ DePalma (Ed). ISpine: Evidence Based Interventional Spine Care. New York, NY: Demos Medical Publishing; 2011. pp. 298-301.
39. Modic MT, Masaryk T, Paushter D. Magnetic resonance imaging of the spine. Radiol Clin N Am. 1986;24(2):229-45.
40. Bogduk N, McGuirk B. Acute neck pain: imaging. Management of Acute and Chronic Neck Pain, 1st edition. Philadelphia, PA: Elsevier; 2006. pp. 51-66.
41. Nachemson Alf L, Jonsson E. Neck and back pain: the scientific evidence of causes, diagnosis and treatment. Philadelphia, PA: Lippincott Williams & Wilkins; 2000.

CHAPTER 7

Examination and Evaluation of Low Back Pain

Devon Ryan, Jeffery Perry

INTRODUCTION

Low back pain is the fifth most common reason for physician visits in the United States.[1] It is also the most frequent type of pain in adults, with over one quarter of respondents in a 2002 survey noting at least one daylong episode of low back pain in the preceding 3 months.[2] And, over the course of their lifetimes, approximately two-thirds of Americans will experience at least one episode of low back pain,[2] with the figure increasing to 90% when all types of back pain are considered.[3] Given its high incidence rate, the economic burden of low back pain is considerable, both in terms of cost of treatment and income lost due to missed workdays.[4] It can also be debilitating, preventing those afflicted from enjoying their usual activities.

Low back pain is classified as acute, subacute, or chronic. These distinctions are based on duration of activity intolerance due to symptoms in the low back: acute refers to periods of fewer than 6 weeks, subacute to periods of between 6 weeks and 3 months, and chronic to periods of longer than 3 months.[5] The distinction between acute and chronic pain is clinically meaningful, as a majority (up to 90%) of patients with nonspecific acute low back pain spontaneously regain activity tolerance within 4–6 weeks without medical intervention.[6] There is some dispute over which metric best captures recovery, but studies generally agree that most patients improve rapidly in the first few weeks following onset of symptoms.[7] Recurrences of pain are not uncommon; however, each new episode is typically treated as if it were the first instance of pain.[8] The etiology and course of chronic, unremitting nonspecific pain are not well-understood, but may relate in large part to psychosocial factors.[9]

INSTITUTIONAL GUIDELINES

Current guidelines for the evaluation and examination of low back pain—such as those issued by the New York Workers' Compensation Board—are based largely upon two important publications.[10] First, in 1994, the United States Agency for Health Care Policy and Research (AHCPR) issued guidelines that address examination and treatment of acute low back pain in adults.[6] Second, in 2007, Chou et al. published a paper that prescribed seven recommendations for the treatment of patients presenting with low back pain.[11] The overlap between these two works is substantial; aspects of each form the basis for current physician practices.

The AHCPR's guidelines call for a detailed medical history and physical examination with the goal of identifying "red flags" that could point to a serious underlying condition as the source of the patient's low back pain. Examples of such conditions are spinal fracture, cancer, severe infection, and cauda equina syndrome.[6] Different conditions are associated with different red flags (Table 7.1). In the absence of a red flag, no further action (imaging or treatment) is suggested.[6] The logic behind this recommendation is that the presence of red flags should identify the minority of patients that will not regain activity tolerance on its own; these are the patients who require immediate follow-up or referral.

The AHCPR guidelines were the primary reference for clinicians until 2007, when the American College of

Physicians (ACP) and the American Pain Society (APS) issued joint clinical practice guidelines based on the study led by Chou. Chou's paper outlines seven recommendations: four for evaluation of low back pain and three for treatment of such pain (Box 7.1).[11] The recommendations incorporate many of the general principles that formed the foundation of the AHCPR guidelines, in many cases expanding upon them. Again, there is an emphasis on utilizing the history and physical examination and avoiding unnecessary imaging.

Table 7.1: Serious medical conditions and associated red flags[6]

Condition	*Red flag(s)*
Spinal fracture	• Major trauma (e.g. vehicle accident and fall) • Minor trauma or heavy lifting (if patient is older/osteoporotic)
Spinal tumor	• History of cancer • Constitutional symptoms (e.g. unexplained weight loss, fever, and fatigue) • Pain when supine, severe night-time pain
Spinal infection	• Constitutional symptoms (e.g. unexplained weight loss, fever, and fatigue) • Recent bacterial infection (e.g. UTI), IV drug use, immune suppression • Pain when supine, and severe night-time pain
Cauda equina syndrome	• Saddle anesthesia • Bladder dysfunction (e.g. urinary retention and increased frequency) • Laxity of anal sphincter and perianal/perineal sensory loss • Significant neurologic or motor deficit in low extremities

EXAMINATION AND EVALUATION OF ACUTE LOW BACK PAIN

As indicated by the institutional guidelines discussed above, the key to effective evaluation of low back pain is ruling out serious underlying conditions by taking a detailed patient history and performing a physical examination.

Patient History

It is very important to establish rapport with the patient in the initial visit. While this may seem to be common sense, it is especially critical when one considers that the majority of patients with low back pain will be sent home without any diagnostic imaging studies or invasive treatment, a situation that can lead to patient anxiety if not handled properly. Clinicians should ask about the specific location, frequency, and duration of pain, as well any history of similar symptoms and treatment. Patients should also be asked about the characteristics about their pain—Is it sharp or dull? Is there associated tingling or numbness? Is it local or radiating; dermatomal or nondermatomal?

A number of risk factors for serious conditions can be addressed in the patient history, and if such a disorder is suspected, relevant tests should be performed, and referred to a specialist if necessary. Mechanism of injury, if applicable, is important and potentially indicative of a spinal fracture if the patient experienced trauma. The possibility of a compression fracture should be

Box 7.1: American college of physicians (ACP)/American pain society (APS) recommendations[11]

1. Clinicians should take a detailed history and perform a physical examination with the goal of categorizing patients' pain into one of three categories: nonspecific low back pain, back pain potentially associated with radiculopathy (Fig. 7.1) or spinal stenosis, or back pain associated with a different specific cause.
2. Clinicians should not perform imaging or other diagnostic tests on patients presenting with nonspecific low back pain.
3. Clinicians should perform diagnostic imaging and other relevant tests on patients who have progressive neurologic deficits or who present with a potentially serious underlying condition.
4. Clinicians should perform magnetic resonance imaging (MRI) or computed tomography (CT) scans on patients with persistent low back pain or who present with signs of radiculopathy or spinal stenosis only if they are candidates for surgery or, in the case of radiculopathy, epidural steroid injection.
5. Clinicians should provide patients with evidence-based information relevant to their expected course, advise patients to remain active as much as their pain permits, and provide information about potential self-care options.
6. Clinicians should consider the use of medications with proven benefits for patients with low back pain; acetaminophen and nonsteroidal anti-inflammatory drugs (NSAIDs) are the most common of these drugs.
7. For patients who do not improve with these two recommendations, practitioners should consider the addition of nonpharmacological therapy, such as spinal manipulation, intensive interdisciplinary rehabilitation, exercise therapy, acupuncture, massage therapy, yoga, cognitive-behavioral therapy, or progressive relaxation.

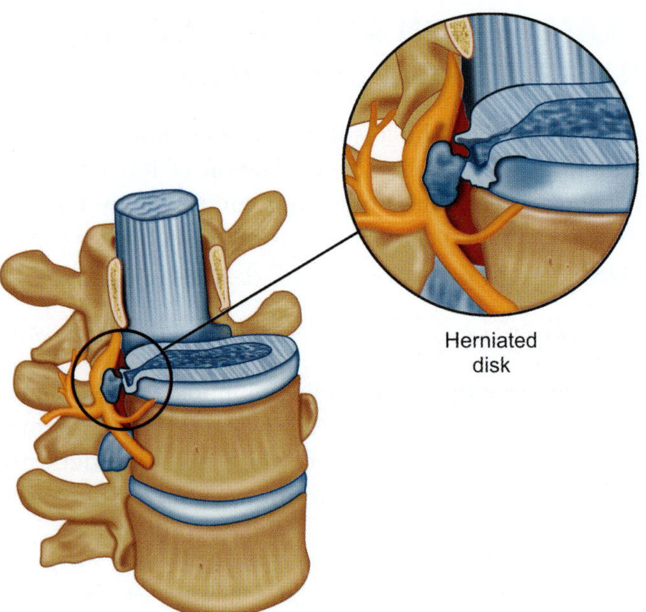

Fig. 7.1: Schemata of herniated disk causing radiculopathy.

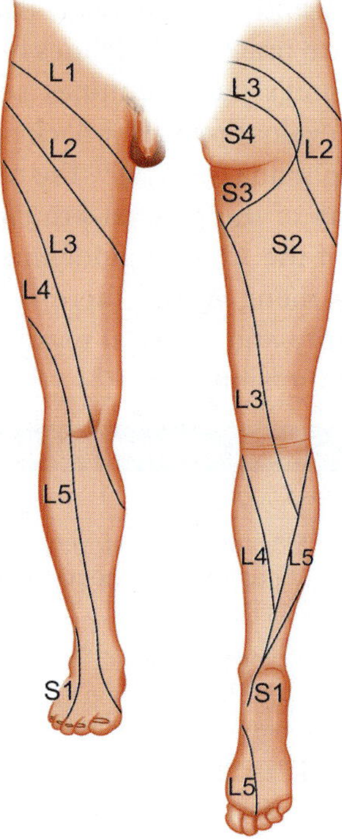

Fig. 7.2: Nerve root distribution of the lower limb.

considered even without trauma if the patient is older and potentially osteoporotic. Concerns about a vertebral fracture can be effectively addressed using a plain lumbosacral radiograph.

The prevalence of cancer in the low back pain population is estimated to be only 0.7%, and a history of cancer is overwhelmingly the largest risk factor—or red flag—for the condition.[12] That indication, especially if combined with constitutional symptoms or unexpected weight loss, should be probed using radiography or magnetic resonance imaging (MRI). The possibility of vertebral infection is indicated by fever, recent infection, intravenous drug use, and the use of immunosuppressants, although the prevalence of such infection in low back pain patients is just 0.01%.[13] MRI is the best imaging paradigm to detect spinal infection. In addition, the clinician should consider the possibility of the infectious symptoms (as well as the back pain) being caused by a problem outside the back, such as pancreatitis, nephrolithiasis, aortic aneurysm, endocarditis, or viral syndromes.[11]

Practitioners should also inquire about bladder and bowel function. Cauda equina syndrome is rare (0.04% of patients presenting with low back pain), but urinary retention has large predictive value due to its high specificity. In patients with low back pain but not bladder symptoms, the prevalence of cauda equina syndrome is just 1 in 10,000.[14] MRI is also the most useful imaging modality for this condition due to its ability to detail soft tissue structure.

In addition to a history tailored to the patient's symptoms, it is important that the clinician assess the patient's state of mind, as mental factors have been shown to affect both severity and duration of pain. Psychological factors, such as depression or distress, can identify which patients with acute back pain are likely to develop chronic pain.[15] And psychosocial factors, such as workplace social support and job satisfaction, are risk factors for more severe or more enduring back pain.[16] Identifying at-risk patients in these categories might point to those who are unlikely to spontaneously recover within a short period of time.

Physical Examination

The physical examination tests neurological function, and, like the history, is designed to identify those patients who have a serious condition that may not resolve itself—primarily radiculopathy. More than 90% of lower extremity radiculopathy caused by disk herniation occurs at the L4/L5 or L5/S1 levels,[11] so the examination should focus on these nerve roots, assessing muscle strength, reflexes, and sensory function. For sensory tests, a light touch at the relevant location should be sufficient (Fig. 7.2). Table 7.2 lists important tests by nerve root level. It should be noted that there is no reliable reflex test for the L5 nerve root. Additionally, the validity of reflex testing can be affected

Table 7.2: Summary of basic neurological examination

Nerve root	*Muscle strength test (muscles used)*	*Reflex test*	*Sensory test location*
L4	Squat and rise (quadriceps)	Knee jerk	Medial foot
L5	Heel walking (ankle and toe dorsiflexors)	None	Dorsal foot
S1	Toe walking (calves and toe flexors)	Ankle jerk	Lateral foot

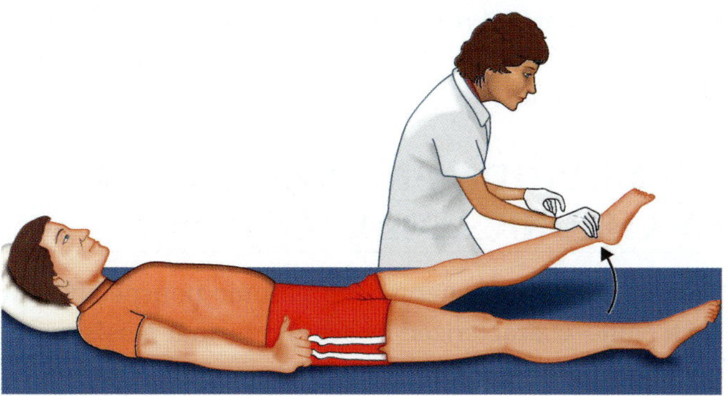

Fig. 7.3: Straight-leg raise test demonstration.

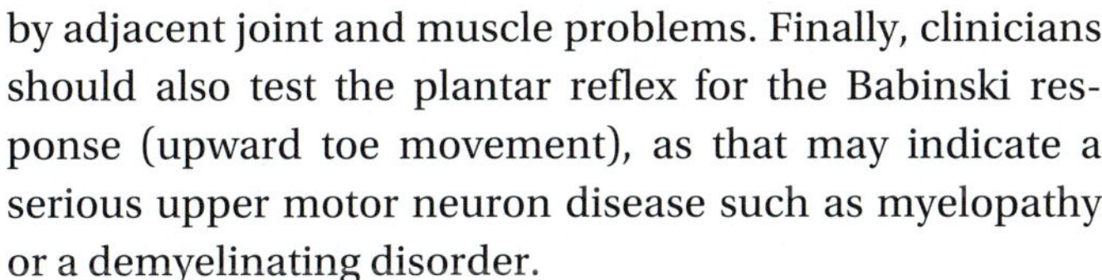

by adjacent joint and muscle problems. Finally, clinicians should also test the plantar reflex for the Babinski response (upward toe movement), as that may indicate a serious upper motor neuron disease such as myelopathy or a demyelinating disorder.

The straight-leg raise (SLR) test is another useful procedure that can identify irritation of the L5 or S1 nerve roots (due to disk herniation) by stretching them. The existence of standardized methods and interpretation across clinicians is very important for consistent diagnosis. The following is an outline of the suggested procedure (Fig. 7.3):[14]

- Have the patient lie as straight as possible in a supine position on the table
- Place one hand above the knee on the leg being examined, exerting enough pressure to keep the knee fully extended. Ask the patient to remain relaxed
- Cup the other hand around the heel and slowly raise the straightened leg, telling the patient to notify you when the procedure becomes uncomfortable
- Monitor for any pelvic movement before a complaint is elicited; true sciatic tension should cause pain before the hamstring is stretched enough to move the pelvis
- Estimate the angle of leg elevation that elicits a complaint, and note the most distal area location of pain: back, hip, thigh, knee, or below the knee.

A positive test is defined as reproduction of the patient's sciatica at between 30° and 70° of elevation, but the exact point at which pain is reproduced should be reported to ensure clear interpretation by other clinicians. As outlined, the test is highly sensitive for herniated disk (91%) but not very specific (26%). The "crossed" SLR test, in which the leg opposite from the one in which the patient feels symptoms is raised, by contrast, is quite specific (88%) for herniated disk but not very sensitive (29%).[11] There are also several modifiers that may be performed that increase the diagnostic value of the test.

Severe or quickly progressing neurological deficits should be immediately attended to using MRI and, if indicated, electrodiagnostic studies. However, in patients who show signs of radiculopathy but whose condition is not debilitating, imaging should only be performed if the patient is a strong candidate for surgery or other targeted treatment (such as an epidural steroid injection). Patients with radiculopathy or spinal stenosis have a good prognosis without invasive treatment: one study found that nearly three in four patients presenting with sciatica (an indication of radiculopathy or stenosis) reported reasonable to major improvement within 12 weeks without surgery.[17] And, if a patient is not a candidate for surgery, imaging would have no value in terms of deciding on a more aggressive therapeutic approach.

Routine Imaging

Most patients who present with acute low back pain will not have any red flags indicative of serious disorders. These patients have nonspecific back pain—due perhaps to problems with muscles or ligaments in the back—and are likely to recover within 4–6 weeks. In this population, no routine imaging should be performed.[18] Signs of spinal degeneration in radiography are common in the general population—even in those without low back pain; as a result, it is not possible to discern what, if any, visual abnormalities are symptomatic.[19] In fact, evidence has shown that radiography for nonspecific back pain is not associated with better outcomes in terms of pain or disability.[20] Thus, patients with nonspecific low back pain should be assured that there is no serious malady present and advised to resume normal activity levels as soon as possible, which is associated with better outcomes than bed rest, even if the bed rest is as short as 2 days in duration.[21,22] Nonprescription analgesics may also prove useful.

EXAMINATION AND EVALUATION OF CHRONIC LOW BACK PAIN

The evaluation of patients with chronic nonspecific low back pain—characterized by symptoms that persist without improvement for at least 6 weeks, and often much longer—is less straightforward. As mentioned previously, psychological and psychosocial factors seem to feature prominently in chronic pain. The physical examination is exactly the same as with acute pain. Emphasis should be placed on changes in the patient's symptoms, and tests can be utilized somewhat more liberally than with acute pain if a specific diagnosis is suspected or if a patient's presentation changes.

CONCLUSION

Modern guidelines for the evaluation of low back pain may vary slightly depending on the publishing institution, but they are generally conservative. Clinicians should take a detailed patient history and perform a thorough physical examination with the goal of identifying a serious underlying medical condition that would require immediate attention. A majority of patients without such an indication will recover rapidly on their own, and these patients should be advised to resume normal activities as soon as possible. Routine imaging on patients with nonspecific back pain is not recommended and does not improve outcomes.

REFERENCES

1. Hart LG, Deyo RA, Cherkin DC. Physician office visits for low back pain: frequency, clinical evaluation, and treatment patterns from a US national survey. Spine. 1995;20:11.
2. Deyo RA, Mirza SK, Martin BI. Back pain prevalence and visit rates: estimates from US national surveys, 2002. Spine. 2006;31:2724.
3. Winters ME, Kluetz P, Zilberstein J. Back pain emergencies. Med Clin N Am. 2006;90.
4. Luo X, Pietrobon R, X Sun S, et al. Estimates and patterns of direct health care expenditures among individuals with back pain in the United States. Spine. 2004;29:79.
5. Koes B, Van Tulder M, Thomas S. Diagnosis and treatment of low back pain. BMJ. 2006;332:1430.
6. Bigos S, Bowyer O, Braen G. Acute low back problems in adults. Clinical Practice Guideline No. 14. AHCPR Publication No. 95-0642. Rockville, MD: Agency for Health Care Policy and Research, Public Health Service, U.S. Department of Health and Human Services; 1994.
7. Hestbaek L, Leboeuf-Yde C, Manniche C. Low back pain: what is the long-term course? A review of studies of general patient populations. Eur Spine J. 2003;12:149-65.
8. Pengel LHM, Herbert RD, Maher CG, et al. Acute low back pain: systematic review of its prognosis. BMJ. 2003;327:323.
9. Airaksinen O, Brox J, Cedraschi C, et al. European guidelines for the management of chronic nonspecific low back pain. Eur Spine J. 2006;15:192-300.
10. The New York State Workers' Compensation Board. New York Mid and Low Back Injury Medical Treatment Guidelines. 2010.
11. Chou R, Qaseem A, Snow V, et al. Diagnosis and treatment of low back pain: a joint clinical practice guideline from the American College of Physicians and the American Pain Society. Ann Int Med. 2007;147:478-91.
12. Deyo RA, Diehl AK. Cancer as a cause of back pain. J Gen Int Med. 1988;3:230-8.
13. Jarvik JG, Deyo RA. Diagnostic evaluation of low back pain with emphasis on imaging. Ann Int Med. 2002;137:586-97.
14. Deyo RA, Rainville J, Kent DL. What can the history and physical examination tell us about low back pain? JAMA. 1992;268:760-5.
15. Pincus T, Burton AK, Vogel S, et al. A systematic review of psychological factors as predictors of chronicity/disability in prospective cohorts of low back pain. Spine. 2002;27:E109.
16. Hoogendoorn WE, van Poppel MNM, Bongers PM, et al. Systematic review of psychosocial factors at work and private life as risk factors for back pain. Spine. 2000;25:2114.
17. Vroomen PCAJ, De Krom M, Knottnerus J. Predicting the outcome of sciatica at short-term follow-up. Br J Gen Pract. 2002;52:119.
18. Davis PC, Wippold II FJ, Brunberg JA, et al. ACR appropriateness criteria on low back pain. J Am College Radiol. 2009;6:401-7.
19. Chou R, Deyo RA, Jarvik JG. Appropriate use of lumbar imaging for evaluation of low back pain. Radiol Clin N Am. 2012;50:569.
20. Kerry S, Hilton S, Dundas D, et al. Radiography for low back pain: a randomised controlled trial and observational study in primary care. Br J Gen Pract. 2002;52:469.
21. Malmivaara A, Häkkinen U, Aro T, et al. The treatment of acute low back pain - bed rest, exercises, or ordinary activity? N Engl J Med. 1995;332:351-5.
22. Dahm KT, Brurberg KG, Jamtvedt G, et al. Advice to rest in bed versus advice to stay active for acute low-back pain and sciatica. Cochrane Database Syst Rev. 2010;6.

CHAPTER

8 Clinical Examination and Evaluation of Radiculopathy: A Neurological Perspective

Kiril Kiprovski

INTRODUCTION

Radiculopathy is defined as a nerve root dysfunction or any disease of the nerve roots, which usually causes symptoms of pain associated with sensory loss or paresthesias, weakness, atrophy, and depressed or absent tendon reflexes in the distribution of the affected nerve root. Radiculopathy is commonly caused by degenerative spine disease or disk herniation. Less frequently, radiculopathies can also be caused by neoplasms like metastases, leptomeningeal carcinomatosis, lymphoma, primary schwannoma or meningioma; infections including epidural abscess, Lyme disease, herpes zoster, CMV, HIV; traumatic injuries and other diseases of the spine such as epidural hematoma, lipomatosis, arachnoiditis, ankylosing spondylitis, Paget's disease, sarcoidosis, cysts, tethered cord syndrome or diabetes. The first detailed description of radiculopathy and differentiating radiculopathy from other diseases was published in 1943 by Semmes and Murphey.[1]

Radiculopathies from various etiologies cause similar clinical symptoms. Fully developed radiculopathy manifest with radicular pain, dermatomal sensory positive or negative symptoms, weakness in the same myotome, and decreased or absent muscle stretch reflex in the affected nerve root. Physiologically, the pain in radiculopathy is evoked by ectopic discharges emanating from a dorsal root or its ganglion. Radicular or nerve root pain has neuropathic characteristics and is described as knife-like, lancinating, burning, stinging or aching in a narrow band-like distribution and is projecting in sclerotomal distribution (such as muscles and bones innervated by the same nerve root). Paresthesias in the specific dermatomal distribution, especially to the distal regions of the dermatomes, usually accompany the pain. Presence of paresthesia is helpful in the differential diagnosis of the source of the pain and suggests that the pain has neurogenic origin. Radicular pain is aggravated by Valsalva maneuver, coughing, sneezing, and straining. Sensory loss caused by the compromise of a single root may be difficult to ascertain because of the overlapping territories of adjacent roots. In most cases, the patient's history and physical examination are sufficient to make the diagnosis. Careful clinical examination remains the best tool for diagnosing a radiculopathy.

HISTORY AND PHYSICAL EXAMINATION

The history should focus first on features of the pain and associated symptoms: mode of onset, the quality, distribution, duration, severity, time of the appearance, associated motor and sensory symptoms, bladder and bowel control, exacerbating and remitting factors, and history of predisposing factors. Symptoms of the radiculopathy are more sensitive than specific. Physical examination findings are more specific than sensitive except the straight leg raise test. The examination of the patients with radiculopathy should include general physical examination and meticulous neurological examination.[2]

General physical examination includes assessment of the general appearance and behavior related to the reported pain. Do patients seem to be in pain? Do patients seem calm? are they in distress? It also includes inspection, palpation, active and passive range of motion of the spine and the joints of the symptomatic extremities.

Table 8.1: Manual muscle strength testing for individual nerve roots and segment-pointer muscles

Segment	*Movement*	*Segment-pointer muscles*
C5	Shoulder abduction and external rotation, elbow flexion	Deltoid, biceps brachii
C6	Elbow flexion, wrist dorsiflexion	Extensor carpi radialis longus
C7	Elbow extension, wrist flexion, fingers dorsiflexion	Triceps, extensor carpi ulnaris, extensor digitorum communis
C8 and/or T1	Index finger dorsiflexion, fingers abduction/adduction/flexion	Extensor indicis, dorsal interossei, finger flexors
L2	Hip flexion	Iliopsoas
L3	Knee extension, hip adduction	Quadriceps femoris
L4	Knee extension, ankle dorsiflexion	Quadriceps femoris, tibialis anterior
L5	Ankle dorsiflexion, great toe dorsiflexion, ankle inversion/eversion, hip abduction	Extensor hallucis longus, gluteus medius
S1	Ankle plantar flexion, hip extension, knee flexion	Gastrocnemius
S2	Toes abduction	Abductor hallucis

Table 8.2: Medical Research Council (MRC) muscle power recording

0	No muscle contraction is detected
1	A trace contraction is noted in the muscle by palpating the muscle while the patient attempts to contract it. No joint motion
2	The patient is able to actively move the muscle when gravity is eliminated
3	The patient may move the muscle against gravity but not against resistance from the examiner
4	The patient may move the muscle group against some resistance from the examiner
5	The patient moves the muscle group and overcomes the resistance of the examiner. This is normal muscle strength

Neurological examination of radiculopathy is not different from the neurological examination that we use for other neurological conditions. Components of the neurological examination for radiculopathies include motor examination, sensory examination, reflexes examination, and gait examination. Not to forget the cranial nerve examination, particularly in the setting of lower cervical radiculopathies. For example, the cranial nerve examination can detect Horner syndrome associated with lower cervical radiculopathy.

Motor Examination

Motor examination includes the systematic examination all of the major muscle groups. This includes evaluation of the appearance of the muscles, looking for atrophy, hypertrophy, or normal muscle bulk; evaluation of the muscle tone, flaccid, spastic, or normal; observation for involuntary movements and manual and functional muscle strength testing. Patients who are experiencing pain and sensory symptoms related to the radiculopathy can also report subjective weakness of the extremity, which might not be detected on the clinical examination.

Testing the strength of particular muscles may indicate which nerve root is involved. Segment-pointer muscles are frequently used in clinical practice to determine to level of the radicular involvement (Table 8.1).

During the manual muscle strength testing, the grade of the weakness needs to be determined. The grading of the weakness will help to compare the examination between different examiners and to be used as a baseline for further follow-up and monitoring of the treatment. Manual muscle testing should be performed bilaterally in upper and lower extremities. The most commonly used grading system is the 0–5 grading system outlined by the Medical Research Council (MRC), with 0 being no movement, 3 representing antigravity strength, and 5 representing normal strength (Table 8.2).[3] The examiner should try to determine if the patient is applying full effort. It may be helpful to test the asymptomatic side first to help the patient understand the task before testing the painful extremity. Modification of this grading system to four response categories (0-paralysis; 1-severe weakness; 2-slight weakness; and 3-normal strength) was recently proposed, in order to improve the ability of clinicians to differentiate degrees of weakness with greater precision.[4]

Nearly every muscle receives motor nerve fibers from more than one spinal level. Although many muscles have a dominant innervating nerve root, to consider a muscle to be innervated by a single spinal level is inaccurate. Weakness may not be present even in a radiculopathy with severe pain and sensory symptoms. The reason might be that the radiculopathy often involves only a fraction of the motor fibers contained in the nerve root and it would require denervation or conduction block of a relatively large proportion of axons contributing to the innervation of a particular muscle before weakness is observed clinically. In addition, nearly all muscles receive innervation from more than one nerve root. Weakness in the radicular distribution without pain is usually secondary to compression of the ventral nerve rootlets.

Sensory Examination

Prior to starting the sensory examination the examiner should determine whether the patient is aware of subjective sensory loss or has abnormal spontaneous sensation. The patient should be asked whether she or he notices any numbness or sensation of tingling, burning, "pins and needles", itching, constriction, electric like sensation into any part of the body. Sensory examination in radiculopathies should include testing the light touch, pinprick, temperature, vibration and position sense. Performing Romberg's test can help to evaluate the dorsal columns and aid us in the differential diagnosis. The findings on sensory examination are not that well defined in radiculopathies compared to peripheral nerve lesions because there is so much dermatomal overlap and there is no point of the skin that does not fall within the territory of at least two nerve roots. Therefore, in monoradicular lesions, no loss of modality can be always demonstrated, so the patients can have normal sensory examination because of this overlap.

Sensory evaluation in radiculopathies as in any other nervous system disease includes determining positive and negative sensory symptoms. The positive sensory symptoms include paresthesia, dysesthesia, hyperesthesia, and allodynia. The negative sensory symptoms include hypoesthesia and anesthesia.

There are various tools that are used to assess the sensation. Sterile cotton swab on a wooden stick is excellent tool for this purpose. The cotton tip can be used to test the light touch or contact allodynia and the opposite wooded end is excellent for testing the plantar response. The stick can be split in half, and the pointy end is used to test the pinprick sensation. There are other tools that we can use to assess the sensory examination. The monofilament is used for sensory quantification of light touch. A brush can be used to assess light touch or for hyperpathia or other type of neuropathic pain. Sterile single use pinwheel is used to assess the pinprick. Reusable rollers are used to assess cold or warm sensation (Figs. 8.1A to C).

Both the upper and lower extremities and the torso should be examined, and comparison made between the left and right sides, distal to proximal distribution and adjacent dermatomes (Figs. 8.2A and B). The examination should proceed from the center of the area of maximum abnormality toward the normal area to define the borders of the area of altered sensation.

The history will usually determine whether examination of dermatomal sensation is required. It is usually not necessary to test all dermatomes, with the examination focusing instead on the region suggested by the history. A lesion of a nerve root may produce a much smaller area of sensory loss than a dermatome map might suggest. The dermatomal maps are approximations and we need to be aware of the considerable shortcomings of the methods used to derive the maps. They should serve merely as a guide as they have limitations, such as variation between individuals, as well as overlap between dermatomes.

Reflex Testing

Testing the reflexes is integral part of the neurological examination. In patients with suspected radiculopathies essentially two categories of reflexes are tested, the muscle stretch (or tendon) reflexes and the plantar cutaneous response. The following is the accepted gradation of the muscle stretch reflexes:

0: Complete absence
+: Diminished
++: Normal reflex
+++: Hyperactive reflex
++++: Markedly hyperactive, often with clonus.

For appropriate reflex testing appropriate well-weighted reflex hammer is needed. Preferred hammers are the queen square hammer or Trömner hammer (Fig. 8.3). Lighter hammers are used in the pediatric population. The light hammer might not deliver enough force to stretch the tendon in some adults, and therefore, it will fail to elicit the muscle stretch reflex and provide the examiner with false information.

As with much of the physical examination, the pattern of the reflex abnormalities helps in localization of the neurogenic dysfunction (Table 8.3). Hyperactive reflexes

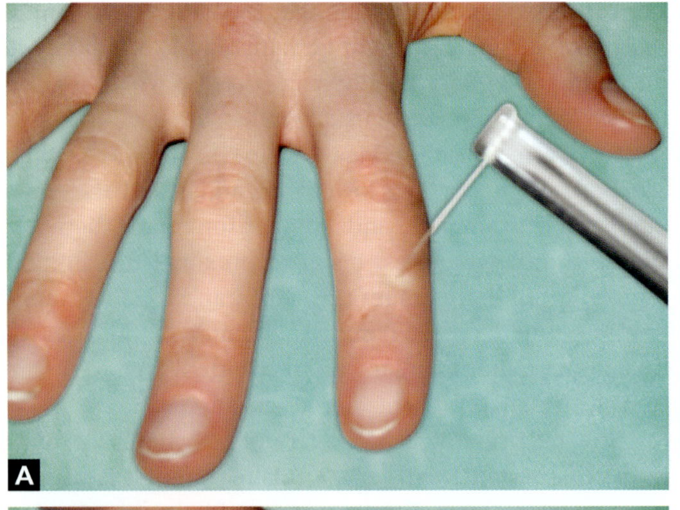

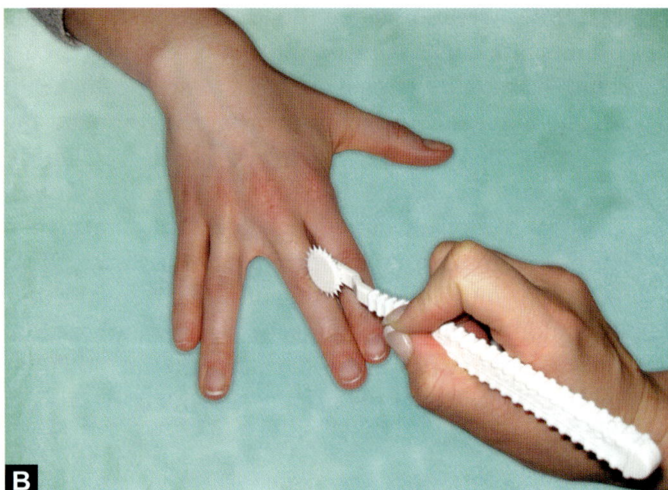

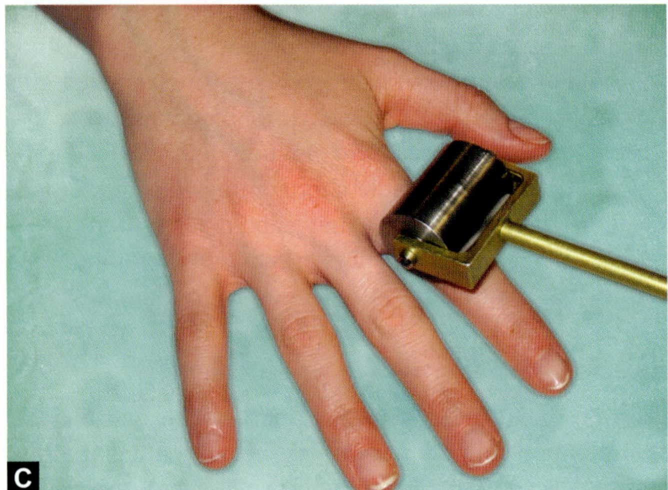

Figs. 8.1A to C: Tools used for sensory examination: (A) monofilament used to test the light touch threshold; (B) Pinwheel used to test pinprick sensation; (C) Roller used to test temperature sensation.

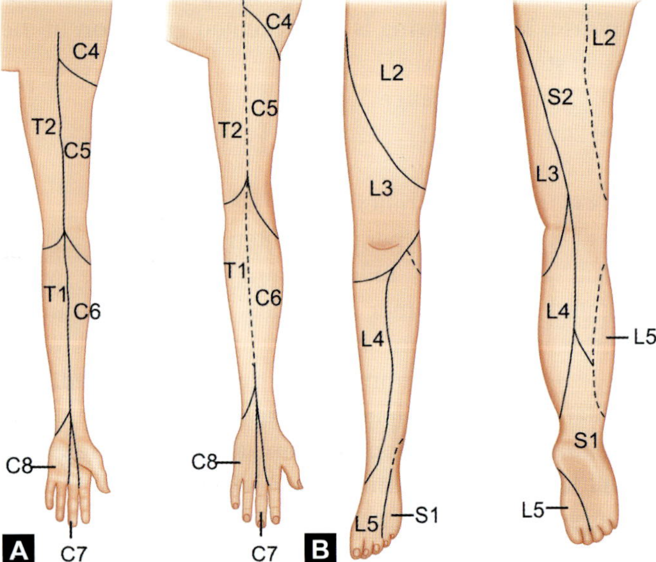

Figs. 8.2A and B: (A) Dermatomes—Upper extremity; (B) Dermatomes—Lower extremity.

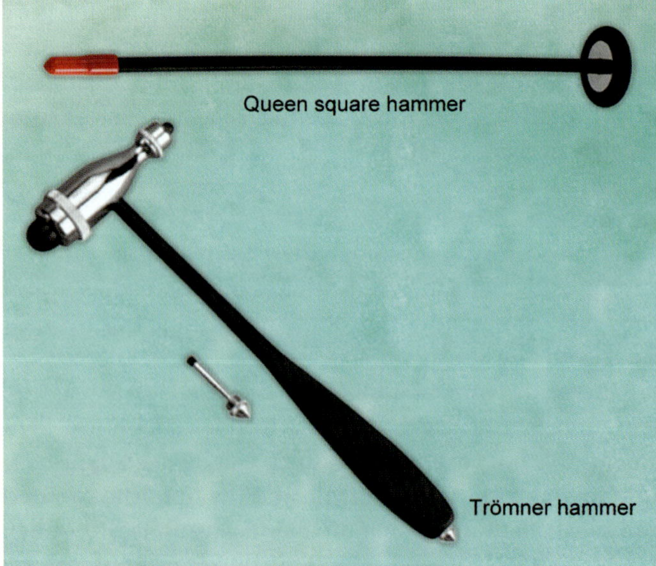

Fig. 8.3: Hammers used to test the tendon reflexes: queen square hammer and Trömner hammer.

Table 8.3: Deep tendon reflex

Reflex	*Nerve root*
Biceps	C5/C6
Triceps	C7
Brachioradialis	C5/C6
Patellar	L4
Achilles	S1
Peroneal	L5

and the presence of a Hoffman or Babinski reflex suggest myelopathy or other diseases affecting the upper motor neuron.

Gait

The gait evaluation is probably the single most useful test in examining the patient with a possible radiculopathy in the lower extremities. Clinical assessment of the gait typically include observing of the posture, stance base, patient's ability to walk short distances, initiation of stepping, velocity, stride length, cadence, trajectory (shallow, shuffling or high stepping), turning while walking and getting in and out of chair or bed. Patient is also asked to perform other maneuvers such as tandem walking, walking backwards, walking on toes and heels, and sometimes even running. Patients with lumbar or radicular leg pain will have antalgic gait. Astasia-abasia would indicate functional gait impairment.

L5 radiculopathy can cause foot drop due to weakness of the ankle dorsiflexion. In this case the patient will develop typical steppage gait. The patient lifts the leg and foot high above the ground with each step in order to improve the clearance because of weakness of ankle dorsiflexion. Identical gait impairment could be also seen in a common peroneal or sciatic nerve palsy. In case of S1 radiculopathy, weakness of ankle plantar flexion produces a shallow stepped gait. The patient will have poor heel lift on walking and will not be able to stand on the toes. The L3 and/or L4 radiculopathies can produce weakness of knee extension and buckling of the knee when walking or standing. This may first be evident when walking down stairs.

Neuromechanical or Provocative Tests

Examination of patients with suspected radiculopathies also includes neuromechanical or provocative tests. There is a wide variety of provocative tests and signs described in the literature regarding physical examination of the cervical or lumbar radiculopathies. In addition to the variance in the nomenclature of these tests, there are multiple descriptions on how these tests should be properly performed.

One of the best recognized is Lasègue's sign or straight leg raise test and its variations. The patient is in supine position. The examiner slowly raises the patient's leg with the knee in extension until the patient feels pain. The examiner then assesses the distribution and the quality of the pain and estimates the degree of maximum pain-free angle that can be achieved. A positive straight leg-raising test result is a sensitive indicator of L5 or S1 nerve root involvement. The test is deemed positive when the patient complains of pain radiating from the back into the buttock and thigh with leg elevation between 30° and 70°. The test result is positive in 95% of patients with a proven disk herniation at surgery. A less sensitive but highly specific test is the crossed straight leg-raising test when the patient complains of radiating pain on the affected side with elevation of the contralateral leg (contralateral Lasègue's sign; well-leg-raising test).

Bragard's test is performed at the onset of the Lasègue's signs, when the examiner lowers the patient's leg just enough so will not trigger the pain. The examiner then passively dorsiflexes the patient's ankle to elicit the typical radicular pain. The Bragard's test increases the specificity of the Lasègue's sign for radiculopathy. The Lasègue's sign can be also tested with the patient seated. Contralateral leg should be always examined in the same manner for comparison and differentiation from other possible pathologies.

Reverse Lasègue test (femoral nerve Lasègue test) is done with the patient is in prone position. The examiner passively raises the leg that is flexed at the knee and with hip extension. Pain in the groin and hip with radiation into the anterior medial thigh indicates an L3 radiculopathy and pain extension to the medial lower leg indicates L4 radiculopathy.

The shoulder abduction (Bakody) test demonstrates involvement of the C4 and C5 nerve roots. Patients experience ipsilateral pain relief by placing their hands on their heads with shoulder abduction and external rotation.

Manual traction test is performed by the examiner placing one hand on the occiput and the other on the chin of the patient while slowly pulling the head of the patient. A positive finding is noted when the pain is diminished during the traction.

Valsalva test (cough impulse test) is performed with asking the patient to cough. The test is positive if it will increase the radicular symptoms. The coughing or other Valsalva maneuvers increases the intrathecal pressure, which can accentuate radicular pain.

Neck compression test is also known as the Spurling's test or Jackson's compression test.[5] The idea in this test is to compress the nerve root in the foramen and to reproduce the radicular pain. The neck is passively tilted toward the symptomatic side and the examiner applies pressure on the top of the head. Positive test will reproduce the pain. Sometimes just tilting of the neck to the symptomatic side, even without additional pressure by the examiner will intensify or reproduce the patient's typical pain and/or positive sensory symptoms.

SOMATIC REFERRED PAIN FROM THE NECK AND LOWER BACK

When taking care of patients with radiculopathies it is important to differentiate the source of pain they experience, e.g. is it related to nerve root compression or it is originating from the other spinal structures, which can sometimes coincide together. The source of spinal somatic referred pain lies in the somatic tissues of the spine. The pain spreads into the extremities, and is perceived in regions innervated by nerves other than those that innervate the site of noxious stimulation. Somatic referred pain is perceived in regions that share the same segmental innervation as the source.

Somatic referred pain is not caused by compression of nerve roots, and therefore, there are no neurological signs. It is produced by noxious stimulation of nerve endings within spinal structures such as disks, zygapophysial joints or sacroiliac joints. The pattern of the somatic referred pain is not dermatomal, but it is sclerotomal and corresponds to the segmental innervation of deep tissues in the limbs, such as muscles, tendons, or joints. The proposed mechanism of referral is convergence of nociceptive afferents on second-order neurons in the spinal cord that also innervate regions of the limb. Somatic referred pain is dull, aching or pressure like and extends into wide distribution and the boundaries can be difficult to delineate. The distribution of the somatic referred is usually fixed in location and tends to follow relatively constant and recognizable patterns (Figs. 8.4 and 8.5).

Patients can have combinations of various pains. It is possible for a patient to have nociceptive back pain, somatic referred pain, and radicular pain.

Cervical Radiculopathy

Cervical nerve roots emerge above the vertebra that shares the same numerical designation. Therefore C7 exits between C6 and C7, and spondylotic changes with or without additional acute disk herniation would be expected to compress the C7 nerve root. Similarly, disk protrusion at C5-C6 and C7-T1 would compress the C6 and C8 roots, respectively. In the cervical region, it is likely that the greater mobility at levels C5-C6 and C6-C7 promotes the development of degenerative

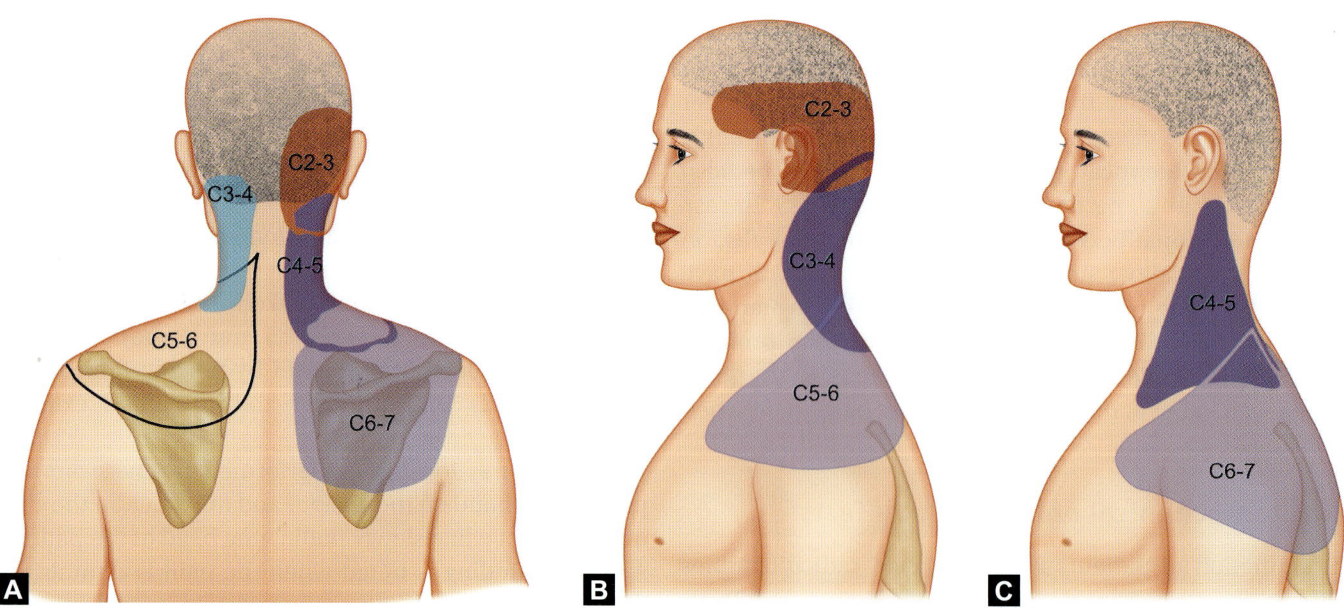

Figs. 8.4A to C: Referred cervical pain.
Source: Adapted from Dwyer.[6]

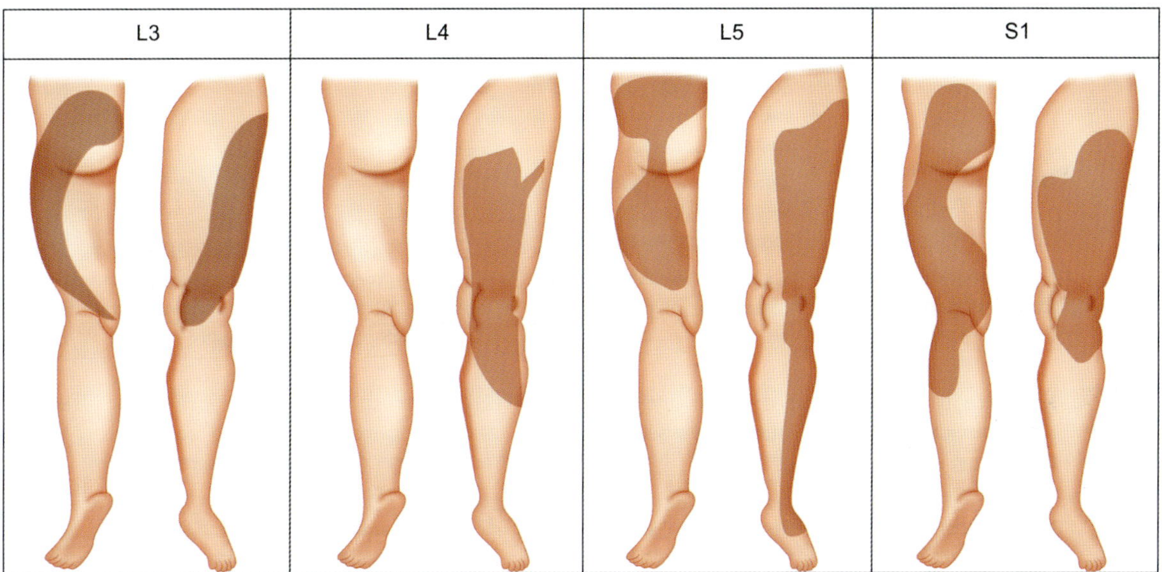

Fig. 8.5: Referred lumbar pain.
Source: Adapted from Bogduk.[7]

process in the same levels and that leads to subsequent most common cervical nerve root compression and radiculopathies. Most common cervical radiculopathy is C7 (70%), followed by C6 (19–25%), uncommonly at C8 (4–10%) and C5 (2%) and rarely involving the T1 root.

Involvement of C6 is associated with pain at the tip of the shoulder radiating into the upper part of the arm, lateral side of the forearm, and thumb. Paresthesias are felt in the thumb and index finger. The brachioradialis and biceps reflexes are diminished or absent. Weakness may occur in the muscles of the C6 myotome including the biceps brachii, deltoid, and pronator teres. The clinical features of C5 radiculopathies are similar, except that the rhomboids and supra and infraspinatus muscles are more likely to be weak. When the C7 root is compressed, pain radiates through the shoulder, to the upper chest, into the dorsal forearm, and hand. Paresthesias would usually involve the dorsal surface of the middle finger. The triceps reflex is usually reduced or absent. Weakness usually involves one or more muscles of the C7 myotome, especially the triceps and the flexor carpi radialis. Less common C8 root involvement presents a similar clinical picture with regard to pain. Paresthesias, however, are experienced in the fourth and fifth digits, and weakness may affect the intrinsic muscles of the hand, including finger abductor and adductor muscles, thumb abduction and opposition, index finger extension and finger flexion (Table 8.4). History and clinical examination will also help to establish the initial differential diagnosis and appropriately direct further investigations or care (Tables 8.5 and 8.6).

Lumbosacral Radiculopathies

Lumbosacral radiculopathies are about 62–90% of all are radiculopathies. More than 75% of all herniated disks compressing nerve roots involve the L5 and S1 nerve root. L3 and/or L4 radiculopathies are uncommon. The L4 root exits beneath the pedicle of L4 through the L4-L5 foramen and L5 exits through the L5-S1 foramen, one might predict that disk herniation roots, respectively. In about only 10% of cases of the disk herniating far laterally at these levels would compress the L4 and L5 exiting nerve root. More commonly, posterolateral disk herniation compresses the nerve root passing through the foramen below that disk, so L4-L5 and L5-S1 herniations usually produce L5 and S1 radiculopathies, respectively.

In an S1 radiculopathy, pain radiates to the buttock and down the back of the leg, extending below the knee with paresthesias in the lateral ankle and foot. The ankle jerk is diminished or absent, and weakness may be detected in the gastrocnemius and gluteus maximus. In an L5 radiculopathy, the distribution of pain is similar, but paresthesias involve the dorsum of the foot and the lateral aspect of the calf. The peroneal reflex and/or medial hamstring reflex might be diminished or absent. Weakness may be present in L5 innervated muscles

Table 8.4: Cervical radiculopathy presentation of the symptoms and examination

Nerve root	*Pain*	*Dermatome*	*Myotome*	*Reflex*
C3	Upper neck	Supraclavicular, suboccipital, and posterior auricular regions	Diaphragm	None
C4	Upper neck	Infraclavicular and posterior cervical regions, posterior shoulder (cape distribution)	Diaphragm	None
C5	Neck, medial scapula, shoulder and lateral upper arm	Superolateral aspect of the upper arm	Pectoralis major, rhomboids, levator scapulae, supraspinatus, infraspinatus, deltoid, biceps, brachioradialis	Deltoid, Pectoralis, Biceps
C6	Neck, scapula, shoulder, lateral arm and forearm, thumb, and index	Lateral arm and forearm, thumb and index finger	Biceps, brachioradialis, extensor carpi radialis longus, supinator, pronator teres, flexor carpi radialis, triceps	Biceps, brachioradialis
C7 (most common)	Neck, medial scapula, posterior arm, and dorsum of the forearm	Posterolateral arm and forearm, and middle finger	Triceps, latissimus dorsi, pronator teres, flexor carpi radialis, extensor carpi ulnaris, extensor digitorum	Triceps
C8	Neck, medial scapula, medial aspect of the arm, forearm and 4th and 5th digits	Medial arm and forearm, fourth and fifth digits	Flexor digitorum superficialis and profundus, pronator quadratus, flexor pollicis longus, flexor carpi ulnaris, lumbricals 3 and 4	None
T1	Axilla, proximal medial arm	Axillary and pectoral region, medial arm and proximal medial forearm	Adductor pollicis, abductor pollicis brevis, opponens pollicis, flexor pollicis brevis, interossei, lumbricals 1 and 2. Horner's syndrome may be present	None

Table 8.5: Neurogenic conditions that can mimic specific cervical radicular syndromes

C5	Suprascapular neuropathy	This is not associated with weakness of all C5 innervated muscles
C6 or C7	Carpal tunnel syndrome	Nocturnal dysesthesias, and hypoesthesia in median nerve distribution, weakness and atrophy of the thenar muscles (C8 and T1 innervated). Positive Phalen's and Tinel's signs
C7	Posterior interosseous nerve syndrome	Not associated with sensory findings and does not affect the triceps, pronator teres, and flexor carpi radialis
C8 and/or T1	Anterior interosseous nerve entrapment	Mild pain over the proximal anterior forearm, positive "pinch sign" and "straight thumb sign" with absent sensory symptoms
	Ulnar entrapment at the elbow	Not associated with weakness of the pronator quadratus and flexor digitorum superficialis and of the first two flexor digitorum profundus muscles. Sensory symptoms and findings do not extend proximal to the wrist in ulnar nerve entrapment
	Thoracic outlet syndrome	Rare syndrome, slowly developing, intermittent paresthesias in the hand, slowly progressing atrophy and weakness of the intrinsic hand muscles. Can be painless or only with mild pain

Contd...

Contd...

	Pancoast syndrome	Pain in the arm, sensory symptoms in the medial forearm and hand, weakness in the lower cervical segments innervated muscles. Horner's syndrome
Multiple	Neuralgic amyotrophy (Parsonage–Turner syndrome)	Acute severe pain in neck, shoulder, and arm, followed within several days by marked arm weakness and atrophy (usually not in a single myotome) as the pain recedes. Associated paresthesias or sensory loss that are not in a dermatomal distribution
Any	Herpes zoster	Acute severe neuropathic pain in a dermatomal distribution, followed within several days by the appearance of the typical vesicular rash
Multiple	Flail arm syndrome (ALS)	Gradual onset, multiple myotomes, no sensory symptoms and painless. Associated symptoms of ALS might be present

Table 8.6: Musculoskeletal conditions that can mimic cervical radiculopathy

Condition	*Clinical symptoms/signs*
Fibromyalgia syndrome	Generalized myofascial pain, fatigue, tenderness to palpation over multiple muscles
Shoulder joint arthropathy, bursitis, impingement syndrome, tendonitis, rotator cuff tear	Pain in anterior chest, localized shoulder pain and with shoulder movements, pain on palpation, positive impingement signs, normal sensory exam, normal reflexes, antalgic weakness, there is no weakness of all C5 innervated muscles, mainly antalgic weakness and pain aggravated by shoulder movements, normal sensory exam, normal reflexes
Elbow pain, lateral epicondylitis	Pain in the elbow or lateral forearm, pain with palpation and resisted wrist extension, antalgic weakness and pain aggravated by elbow movements, normal sensory exam, normal reflexes
De Quervain's syndrome	Lateral wrist and forearm pain and edema and pain on palpation, difficulty flexion the thumb, positive Finkelstein test

including the extensor hallucis longus, tibialis anterior and peroneus longus, as well as the tibialis posterior and the gluteus medius weakness may be restricted to the extensor hallucis longus only. The less common L4 radiculopathy is characterized by pain and paresthesias along the lateral thigh, at the knee and down to the medial aspect of the knee and lower leg.

The patellar reflex is diminished or absent. Weakness may be present in the quadriceps and hip adductors (Tables 8.7 to 8.9).

RED FLAGS

The examiner should be also aware of possible "red flags" when caring for patients with radiculopathy. Constitutional symptoms, fever, chills, preceding bacterial infections, unexplained weight loss, unremitting night pain, history of cancer, history of trauma, recent procedures or surgical interventions, immunocompromised state, chronic steroid use, history of alcohol or drug abuse, skin rash, or failure to improve with treatment should alert the clinician to the possibility of a serious and/or urgent medical condition such as infection or neoplasm. Sudden onset of acute lumbosacral pain with radicular pain, sensory loss and weakness in the lower extremities and associated urinary dysfunction should raise suspicion of cauda equina syndrome that will require urgent evaluation and treatment.

SUMMARY

Ability to make diagnosis of radiculopathy depends on capacity to understand the patient history to carry out reliable examination and to interpret the symptoms and signs.

Table 8.7: Lumbosacral radiculopathy presentation of the symptoms and examination

Nerve root	*Pain*	*Dermatome*	*Myotome*	*Provocative tests*	*Reflex*
L1	To groin	Inguinal region	None	None	None
L2	To groin and anterior thigh	Anterolateral thigh	Hip flexion	Reversed SLT	None
L3	To anterior thigh and knee	Groin and medial thigh	Hip flexion and adduction and knee extension	Reversed SLT	Knee jerk
L4	To anterior thigh, knee and medial foreleg	Anterior thigh and medial leg	Knee extension, hip adduction and ankle dorsiflexion	Reversed SLT	Knee jerk
L5	To buttock, lateral thigh and leg and dorsal foot	Lateral leg, dorsal foot and big toe	Toe and ankle dorsiflexion, inversion and eversion, gluteus medius, TFL	SLT	Hamstrings
S1	To buttock, posterior thigh and leg and lateral foot	Posterior thigh, lateral foot and little toe	Plantar flexion, toe flexion, hamstrings, Gluteus maximus	SLT	Ankle jerk
S2-4	Medial buttocks	Medial buttocks, perineal, and perianal region	Sphincters	None	Bulbocavernosus Anal wink

Table 8.8: Neurogenic conditions that can mimic specific lumbosacral radicular syndromes

L2, L3, L4	Femoral neuropathy	Only femoral nerve innervated muscles involved with sensory symptoms and findings. Hip adductors and tibialis anterior will be spared
L3, L4	Meralgia paresthetica (lateral femoral cutaneous nerve dysfunction)	Pain and loss of sensation of lateral femoral cutaneous nerve
L5	Peroneal mononeuropathy	Pronounced sensory symptoms in peroneal distribution, ankle dorsiflexion, and eversion weakness
	Foot drop as early ALS symptom	Progressive ankle weakness without pain or sensory symptoms
L5, S1, S2	Claudication	Exertional pain/claudications in thigh and lower leg without back pain. Normal neurological examination
	Peripheral neuropathy	Stocking-like bilateral symmetrical sensory loss, absent bilateral ankle reflexes
S1 and S2	Tarsal tunnel syndrome	Rare syndrome Neuropathic pain localized at the ankle and/or sole of the foot and sensory impairment in the sole
Multiple	Lumbosacral plexopathy	Pronounced weakness in multiple myotomes and multidermatomal sensory loss
Any	Herpes zoster	Acute severe neuropathic pain in a dermatomal distribution, followed within several days by the appearance of the typical vesicular rash

Table 8.9: Musculoskeletal conditions that can mimic lumbosacral radiculopathy

Condition	*Clinical symptoms/signs*
Fibromyalgia syndrome	Generalized myofascial pain, fatigue, tenderness to palpation over multiple muscles
Hip arthritis	Pain in groin, anterior thigh, pain with weight bearing, positive Patrick's test
Trochanteric bursitis, Iliotibial band syndrome	Lateral hip pain, pain with palpation along lateral hip
Knee arthritis	Pain localized to the knee, knee edema, limited range of movements, tenderness on palpation, pain with weight bearing

Contd...

Contd...

Condition	*Clinical symptoms/signs*
Hamstring strain, tendinitis	Posterior thigh pain, worse on knee extension
Plantar fasciitis	Pain in sole of foot, worsened with weight bearing, local tenderness to palpation
Trices surae strain, Achillis tendinitis	Calf pain, tendon pain, local tenderness on palpation, worsened with walking or running, limited range of movement of the ankle dorsiflexion.

REFERENCES

1. Semmes RE, Murphey F. The syndrome of unilateral rupture of the sixth cervical intervertebral disk with compression of the seventh cervical nerve root: a report of four cases with symptoms simulation coronary disease. JAMA. 1943;121:1209-14.
2. Warlow C. Why I have not stopped examining patients. Pract Neurol. 2010;10:126-8.
3. Aids to the examination of the peripheral nervous system. The Guarantors of Brain. Edinburgh, New York: Saunders Elsevier; 2010.
4. Vanhoutte EK, Faber CG, van Nes SI, et al. Modifying the Medical Research Council system through Rasch analyses. Brain. 2012;135:1639-49.
5. Spurling RG, Scoville WB. Lateral rupture of the cervical intervertebral discs. Surg Gynecol Obstet. 1944;78:350-8.
6. Dwyer A, Aprill C, Bogduk N. Cervical zygapophysial joint pain patterns I: a study in normal volunteers. Spine. 1990;15:453-7.
7. Bogduk N. On the definitions and physiology of back pain, referred pain, and radicular pain. PAIN. 2009;147:17-9.

CHAPTER

9

Evaluation of Adolescent Scoliosis

Stephen P Maier II, Thomas Cheriyan, Baron S Lonner

INTRODUCTION

Scoliosis is a deformity defined as lateral curvature of the spine that exceeds 10° measured by the Cobb angle method on radiographs, which is most apparent in the coronal plane, and is associated with vertebral rotation (Figs. 9.1A to C). Normal alignment and biomechanics of the spine has been described in detail in Chapters 2 and 3 (Fig. 9.2).

Scoliosis affects people of all ages, but is more commonly seen in young, growing teenagers. Based on etiology, scoliosis may be classified into idiopathic, congenital, neuromuscular, post-traumatic, postirradiation, thoracogenic, or related to connective tissue disorders. So-called olisthetic scoliosis is a result of severe spondylolisthesis and may lead to rotation of the spinal column, consequently resulting in scoliosis emanating out of the pelvis. Scoliosis can also be classified into structural or nonstructural forms. Structural scoliosis is an irreversible spine curvature with rotation, which can be idiopathic or be due to an underlying disease or condition. Nonstructural scoliosis is a reversible spinal curvature having no

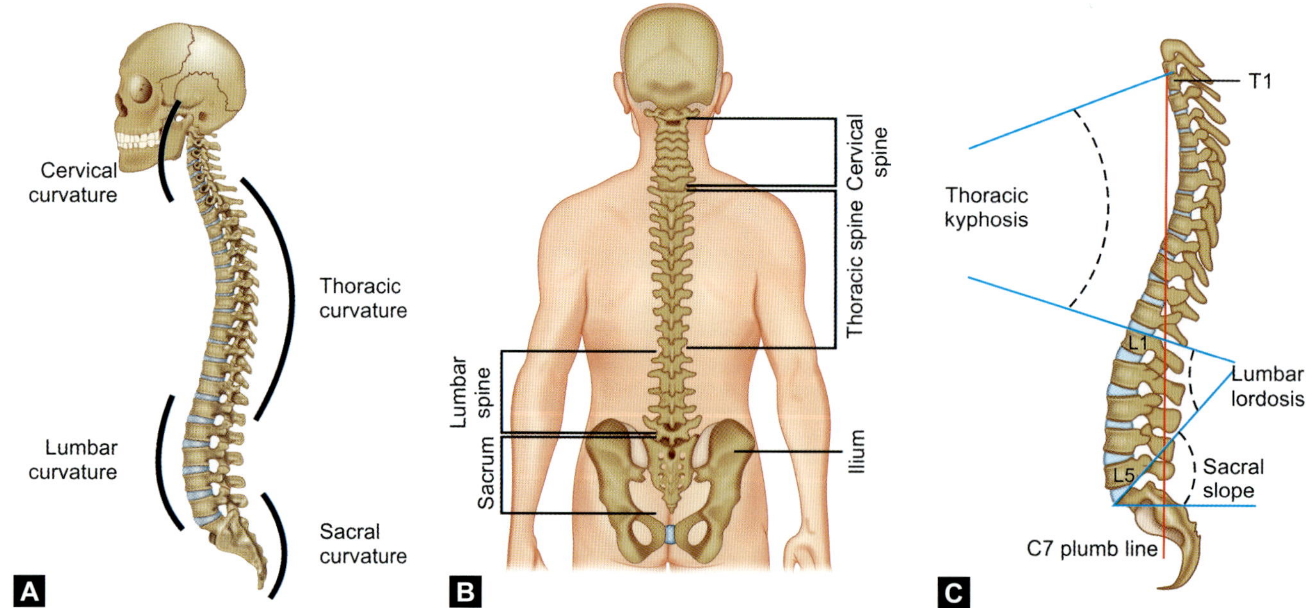

Figs. 9.1A to C: (A) A schematic illustration of the normal alignment and natural curvature of the spine in the sagittal and (B) coronal views. (A and C)The thoracic and sacral segments of the spine are normally kyphotic, while the cervical and lumbar spine is normally lordotic.

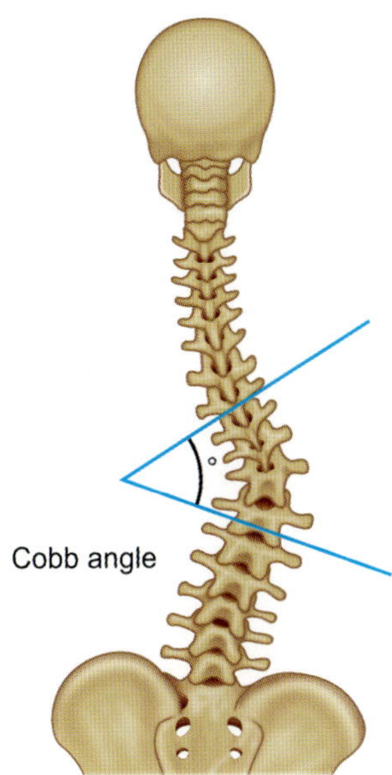

Fig. 9.2: The Cobb angle is the angle formed between a line drawn parallel to the superior end plate of one vertebra above the fracture and a line drawn parallel to the inferior end plate of the vertebra.

rotation and is caused by conditions like pain, muscle spasm or leg length discrepancy.

Based on age at diagnosis, the Scoliosis Research Society (SRS) categorizes scoliosis in children into congenital, infantile, juvenile, and adolescent. Congenital scoliosis as refers to deformity caused by malformation of vertebrae during embryonic development, usually in the first 6 weeks of gestation. Infantile scoliosis is diagnosed in children younger than 3 years old and accounts for 2–3% of idiopathic scoliosis in children. Juvenile idiopathic scoliosis is diagnosed in children between 4 years and 10 years old, accounting for 10–15% of idiopathic scoliosis cases, and both of these so-called early onset forms of scoliosis can be highly progressive although small curvature in the infantile group often resolves spontaneously. Adolescent idiopathic scoliosis (AIS) patients are between 10 years and 18 years and comprise the large majority of idiopathic scoliosis cases.

Scoliosis occurs in 0.5–3% of adolescents.[1-5] The prevalence decreases with curve magnitude. For example, the prevalence of a 10°, 20°, and 40° curve are 2–3%, 0.3–0.5%, and 0.1%, respectively.[6] While overall prevalence is equal between genders, girls are seven to 10 times more likely to have curves more than 30°.[7] Females are also more likely to experience more progressive deformity than males. The etiology of AIS is not clearly understood. Hereditary factors have shown to be an important contributing factor, although the molecular mechanism by which this entity occurs is not known. The incidence of scoliosis is 11% in first-degree relatives.

It is important to diagnose scoliosis early and manage patients optimally as curve progression may lead to severe physical consequences. For example, increasing progression may cause vertebral and subsequent rib cage rotation. This can lead to pulmonary and cardiac compromise in the most severe cases. Patients may experience shortness of breath, pulmonary dysfunction, or respiratory failure from restrictive and, more recently recognized, obstructive lung disease. Scoliosis in the lumbar spine may lead to premature intervertebral disk degeneration and facet arthrosis and debilitating pain. In cases of neuromuscular deformity, loss of trunk stability and balance may cause seating difficulties in nonambulators. Furthermore, a distortion in a patient's appearance may affect his/her psychological self-perception. Adolescent teens are particularly predisposed to the psychological trauma associated with the deformity of scoliosis including large rib humps, waistline and breast asymmetry, and truncal decompensation or shift to one side or the other.

Scoliosis curves can be left or right, single, double, or triple, and may be associated with significant sagittal (lateral view) deformity. Single thoracic curves present most commonly with a right-sided apex, while left-sided apexes are associated with increased incidence of neural element abnormalities (Fig. 9.3).[8,9] Patients also commonly present with a right thoracic, left lumbar "S"-shaped double curve (Fig. 9.4).[7] Initial curvature may begin at puberty and be exacerbated during the adolescent growth spurt.

Most curves between 0° and 20° in adolescents do not progress (Table 9.1). Patients with the highest magnitude of curvature at diagnosis have the highest probability of progression both before and after maturity. Curves more than 50° with the apex located in the thoracic spine, or curves more than 35° with an apex in the thoracolumbar spine have the highest tendencies to progress. In an effort to evaluate the severity of the scoliosis, mathematical models have been developed by several researchers to predict the risk of progression. Lonstein and Carlson first published their progression factor model in 1984,[10] and Peterson and Nachemson later established their own prognostic model in 1995 that predicted the progressivity of curves.[11]

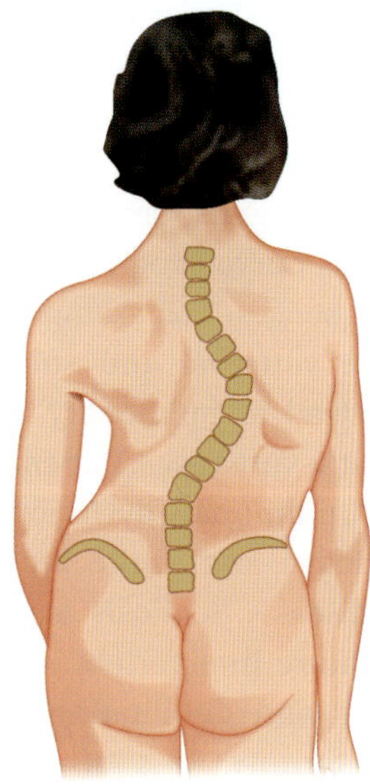

Fig. 9.3: Single curves in scoliosis patients most commonly feature right-sided apexes, as displayed in the figure. Single curves that feature a left-sided apex are associated with more severe symptoms, particularly neurologic symptoms.

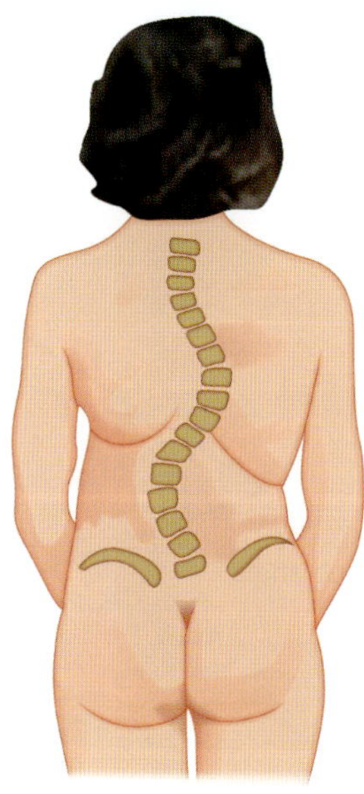

Fig. 9.4: Patients commonly present with an S-shaped pattern of scoliosis. Such cases are usually the result of a right thoracic, left lumbar double curve.

Table 9.1: Percentage of curve progression

	10–12 Years	*13–15 Years*	*16 Years*
< 19	25%	10%	0%
20–29	60%	40%	10%
30–39	90%	70%	30%
> 40	100%	90%	70%

Source: Lonstein JE. Patient evaluation. In: Bradford DS, et al. (Eds). Moe's Textbook of Scoliosis and Other Spinal Deformities, 2nd edition Philadelphia, PA: WB Saunders Co; 1987. pp. 47-88.

EVALUATION OF SCOLIOSIS

Evaluation of adolescent scoliosis consists of four distinct but collaborative steps. The physician first conducts a patient interview to learn of the patient's condition. Second, the physician completes a full physical examination, particularly measuring flexibility of the spine in various planes. Third, diagnostic radiographs are taken, and finally, additional studies may be performed. Comprehensive evaluation of scoliosis facilitates optimal treatment.

Patient Interview

A comprehensive, thorough history is a critical component of the patient interview. Patients often present with spinal deformity, pain, altered pulmonary function, or neurologic impairment, though the latter is less common. Pain is often a minor component of the patient's history, although patients often present with some degree. Onset of the deformity and associated symptoms and underlying medical history and family history should be documented.

Back pain is often due to the overactivity of the paraspinal muscles in their efforts to compensate for the spinal curvature. The force generated by the back muscles leads to typical fatigue pain or aching associated with scoliosis. Pain may also emanate from impingement of the curve at the costopelvic junction.[12]

It is important to note that patients may not necessarily be symptomatic when they first present with scoliosis. Asymptomatic patients often present due to deformity or suspected spine deformity that is documented during a screening (i.e. nurse screen at school) or a routine physical examination with one's primary care physician. Patient psychological and emotional deficits are a major component in the evaluation and treatment of scoliosis. Patients frequently present with self-image and body image disturbance issues. Although it is uncommon for a patient to complain that his/her body looks different than those of peers and for that patient to conclude that there is something wrong with him/her, outcomes instruments such as the SRS-22, Spinal Appearance Questionnaire, and Body Image Disturbance Questionnaire may reveal these concerns.

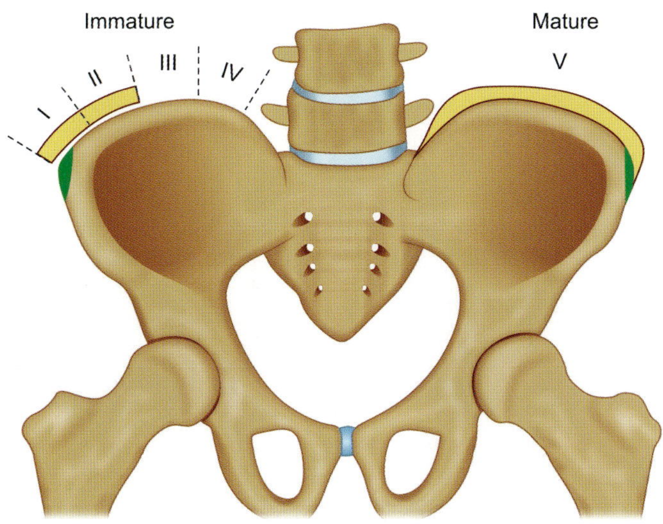

Fig. 9.5: Schematic representation of the Risser classification for skeletal maturity.

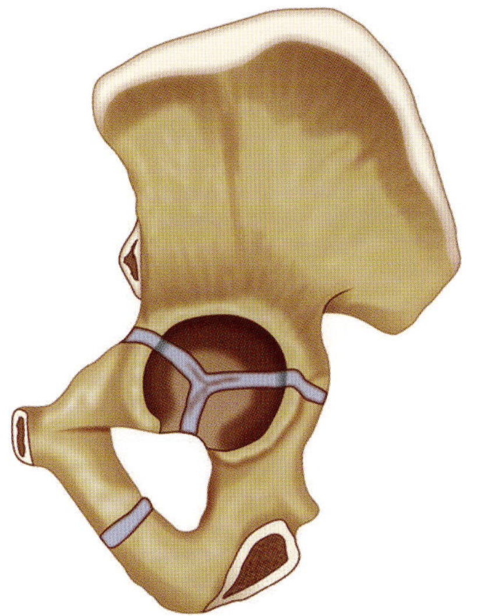

Fig. 9.6: An immature pelvis with the triradiate cartilage still apparent prior to fusion. As one reaches skeletal maturity, the acetabulum forms when bony contributions from the ilium, ischium, and pubis come together.

It is important to assess for menarcheal status in girls, predicted age of skeletal maturity, curve size, and location of curve apex. The patient's sex and age at diagnosis are also factors that may aid in predicting curve progression. Adolescents with the greatest room for skeletal growth have the highest risk of progression.[4] Prepubescent adolescents experience increasing growth velocity, while postpubescent adolescents experience declining growth velocity. Menarche in females and voice-deepening in males as well as body hair are the indicators of the onset of puberty. Skeletal maturity can be assessed by means of Risser staging, vertebral ring apophysis, and triradiate cartilage closure. The Risser stages are used to classify the degree of ossification in a patient's iliac crest, which aid the physician in determining the extent of a patient's future growth (Fig. 9.5). When the apophyses of the iliac spine fuse to the pelvis, a patient is classified as Risser stage 5 and the skeleton is considered to be completely mature, though limited growth may occur after stage 5.[13] The vertebral ring apophyses are thin ossification centers at the superior and inferior vertebral end plates that are not fused to the vertebral bodies until skeletal maturity; therefore, when the ring apophyses fuse with the vertebral bodies, then cessation of vertebral body growth is indicated and skeletal maturity has been reached.[14] Open triradiate cartilage of the acetabulum as measured on radiographs indicate a great deal of remaining growth that continues even after closure of the growth plate.[13] The Sanders Classification as measured by a left-hand X-ray give very objective information about the stage of growth of the individual[15] (Fig. 9.6).

The physician should record prior spine surgery, neuromuscular symptoms, history of recurrent urinary tract or pulmonary infections, genitourinary symptoms, which are particularly of concern in neuromuscular disease such as cerebral palsy and muscular dystrophy as well as in myelomeningocele, and if relevant, pregnancy history in females. The patient's functionality status is also important to consider during evaluation. Any deficits or limitations in activities of daily living including sports should be noted.

Physical Examination

Following the completion of the patient interview, the physician should conduct a meticulous physical examination. Patients should be dressed in lightweight clothing, specifically an open-backed gown and underwear, allowing the physician the greatest visibility of the spine.[16] All supplemental garments, including socks and shoes, should be removed. Record the patient's standing, barefoot height and weight. Arm span measurements may also be useful for calculating percent predicted values of pulmonary function based on true expected height, which is approximated by an arm span measurement.

The physician should closely examine the target areas that were highlighted during the patient interview and medical history. The patient's skin is to be examined for

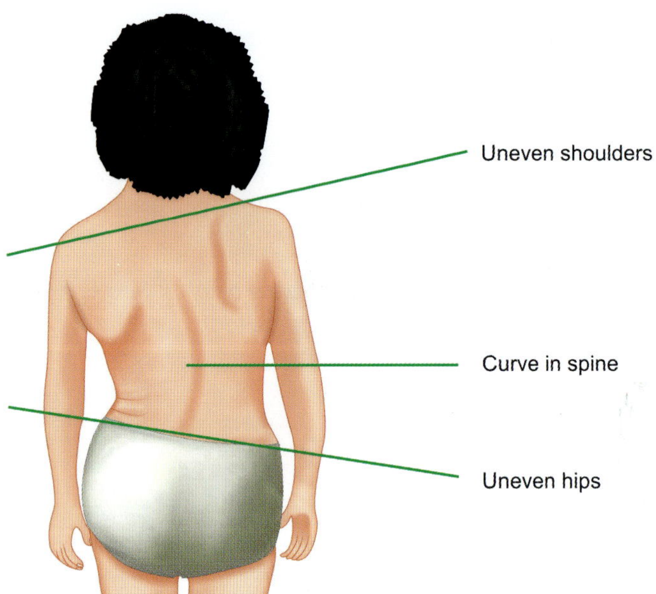

Fig. 9.7: Some of the common, obvious symptoms of scoliosis include an unevenness in the shoulders and/or hips and a curve in the spine.

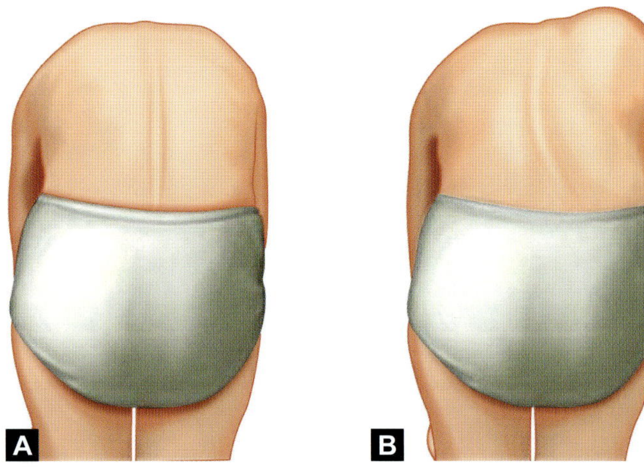

Figs. 9.8A and B: The Adams forward bend test reveals coronal curvature of the spine (right) in patients with scoliosis. A normal spine will remain straight as the patient bends forward (left).

café au lait spots, hairy patches, or skin dimples over the spine, which may point to underlying causes of scoliosis.[17] The patient's stance should be noted. His/her arms should be at the sides, knees straight, and feet placed symmetrically but not touching. The patient should first be evaluated for alignment, levelness of shoulders and pelvis, and waist crease asymmetry in a posterior upright position (Fig. 9.7). Alignment is determined by the location of the patient's head in relation to his/her gluteal cleft and he/she is considered normally balanced if the deviation from the mid-sagittal plane is less than 1.5 cm. Waist crease asymmetry is determined by extending a line from the greatest prominence of the greater trochanter or the lateral aspect of the iliac crest and measuring the distance to the deepest indentation of the waist. The difference between the measurement on the left and the right is recorded as the waist crease asymmetry. Waist crease asymmetries less than 2 cm are considered normal. It is critical to remove limb length inequality as a confounding factor, thus allowing for the true measurement of lumbar asymmetry as opposed to asymmetry secondary to lower extremity differences. If a leg length asymmetry exists, a lift can be place under the shorter limb and the examination performed. Improvement in subtle curvatures is often seen when limb length differences exist.

A standing forward flexion by the patient, called an Adams Forward Bend Test (Figs. 9.8A and B), is essential to a complete examination. Such positioning is necessary to detect subtle scoliotic curves measuring less than 25°. The posterior upright position may not provide enough visibility for the clinician to identify minimal curves, therefore, the patient should flex at the waist keeping the knees straight allowing the head and arms to hang freely toward the floor and the trunk should be maintained parallel to the floor. Patients should avoid pressing their hands together as it may lead to false-positive diagnosis due to physiologic upper extremity asymmetry. Fingers should extend to or beyond the inferior region of the patella; patients with the inability to do so should be suspected of spinal cord pathology.[10]

The patient should be examined from the back with particular focus on the rib cage. Rib cage asymmetry in the thoracic spine and asymmetry of the paraspinal muscle mass in the lumbar spine should be noted. Small curves may be detectable by this examination.[16] Thoracic asymmetry measured as more than 0.8 cm or lumbar asymmetry between sides more than 0.5 cm are of concern and should be continuously monitored.[16] A scoliometer, or inclinometer, may also be used to determine the magnitude of asymmetry by measuring the degree of truncal rotation. Accurate results leading to diagnosis are reliant upon proper use of the scoliometer (Fig. 9.9).

Patients who are unable to touch their toes should bend their knees enabling them to do so, a task essential

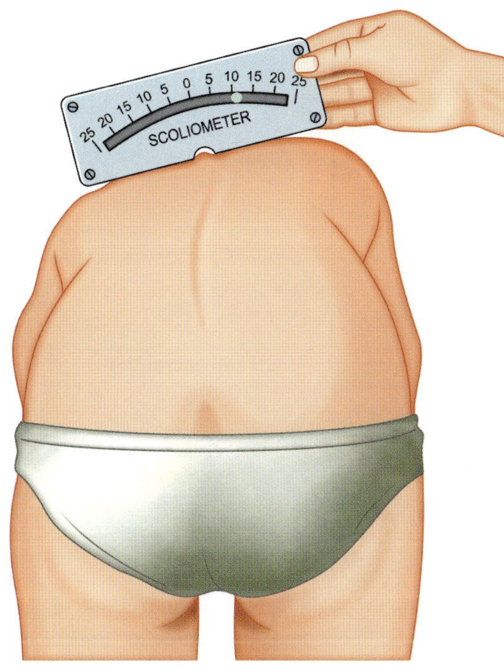

Fig. 9.9: To measure the degree of a patient's coronal deformity, he/she is asked to bend forward toward the floor so the back is parallel to the ground. A scoliometer is then positioned directly above the spine to determine the degrees of curvature.

for lumbar positioning for measurement. Truncal rotation more than 7° is considered abnormal.

The patient is then asked to return to an upright position and bend backward at the waist. If the attending physician notes any difficulty or pain in reverse bending, then an abnormality in the lumbosacral junction may exist, such as a stress fracture in the region of the pars interarticularis known as spondylolysis. Lateral standing upright evaluation follows for assessment of abnormal sagittal alignment, such as hyperkyphosis or roundback.

Neurological evaluation is essential to rule out any underlying neurological deficits that may indicate neural pathology such as syrinx or tethered cord. Neurological abnormalities may be evaluated by means of gait observation and thorough motor, sensory, and reflex examination, particularly including the Patrick's test (Fig. 9.10).

Patients with increased lumbar lordosis should be examined for hip flexion contractures using the Thomas test. Contracture of the abductor muscles in either hip may lead to disturbances in biomechanics and oblique positioning of the pelvic bone possibly resulting in secondary scoliosis.[18] If the patient presents with pelvic obliquity, limb lengths should be taken as this is not an infrequent cause of lumbar scoliosis.[19]

It is often possible to make a preliminary diagnosis following the patient interview and physical examination. Referrals to a specialist are often made following school screenings for scoliosis. Mild curvatures are treated non-operatively. Frequent use of radiographs may subject children to unnecessary doses of radiation in addition to the high costs incurred. Factors including stage of developmental maturity, sex, and physical complaints should be considered while formulating a treatment plan and determining follow-up intervals.

Imaging

Consistent radiography is both appropriate and necessary in evaluating young patients with scoliosis. Spinal deformity may progress without treatment, thus the earliest recognition of progression will allow for appropriate intervention. Supine, push-prone, lateral pressure, traction, side-bending, and fulcrum-bending radiographs have all been utilized in assessing the preoperative coronal flexibility of scoliotic patients.[20] Standing posteroanterior and lateral radiographs of the entire spine are the preferred views.[13] Supine, push-prone, lateral pressure, traction, side-bending, and fulcrum-bending radiograph are useful in assessing curve flexibility, generally as part of a preoperative evaluation.

An accurate assessment of spinal parameters, namely diagnosis, location, levels, classification, and curve magnitude, is critical. Characteristics to note are the presence of truncal shift, vertebral rotation, and skeletal maturation of the patient, and if the patient has undergone prior surgery, then the amount of correction and type of instrumentation should be described.[13]

Curve location, i.e. proximal thoracic, main thoracic, thoracolumbar or two or all three of these, is noted and curve magnitude via the Cobb method are assessed, as is the sidedness of the apex of each curve. Thoracic or thoracolumbar kyphosis is also assessed and presence of sagittal plane abnormalities such as excessive kyphosis, lordosis, or spondylolisthesis is noted.

The Cobb angle is the standard technique to measure deformities in both the sagittal and coronal planes. The curve with the greatest Cobb angle is termed the major curve. The Cobb angle is defined as the angle formed between the two most tilted spinal vertebrae. It can be measured manually by marking radiographs and analyzing using a protractor, or electronically by means of digital computer-assisted (semiautomatic), automatic,

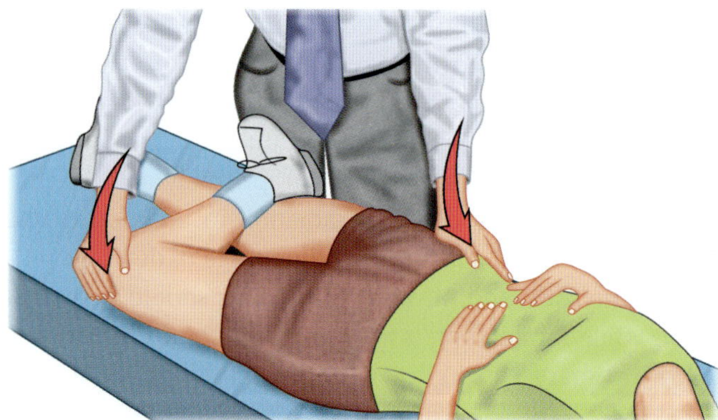

Fig. 9.10: Patrick's test is a component of the neurologic examination in patients who present with low back pain.

and smartphone application procedures.[21] The apical vertebra is first identified in order to define the location of the curvature. The apical vertebra is the most displaced and rotated vertebra having the least tilted end plate. The end/transitional vertebrae are then identified. An apex between T1 and the T11/12 disk defines a thoracic curve, between T12 and L1, thoracolumbar, and below L1, lumbar. The end vertebrae are the most superior and inferior vertebra that are least displaced and rotated and have the maximally tilted end plate. A line is drawn along the superior end plate of the superior end vertebra and a second line drawn along the inferior end plate of the inferior end vertebra. A line drawn through the pedicles may be used if the end plates are not visible. The angle between these two lines (or lines drawn perpendicular to them) is the Cobb angle (Fig. 9.2). For S-shaped curves, the lower end vertebrae of the upper curve will reflect the upper end vertebrae of the lower curve and is called the inflection vertebrae.

Normal measurements for lumbar lordosis range from approximately 35° to 70°,[22] and those for thoracic kyphosis from T5–12 range from 10° to 40°.[23] The central sacral vertical line (CSVL) is used to assess truncal balance, in addition to identifying the lower level vertebral body to be instrumented in patients requiring surgery and determining the deviation of the lumbar curvature from the midline[13] (Fig. 9.11). The CSVL is a vertical line drawn downward from the S1 spinous process. The vertebral body that is most bisected by the perpendicular plumb line is designated as the stable lower level vertebral body, which historically was used to determine the lowest instrumented vertebrae although that rule is only followed for certain curve types in which a selective fusion of the thoracic curvature is performed leaving the lumbar curvature unfused.[13]

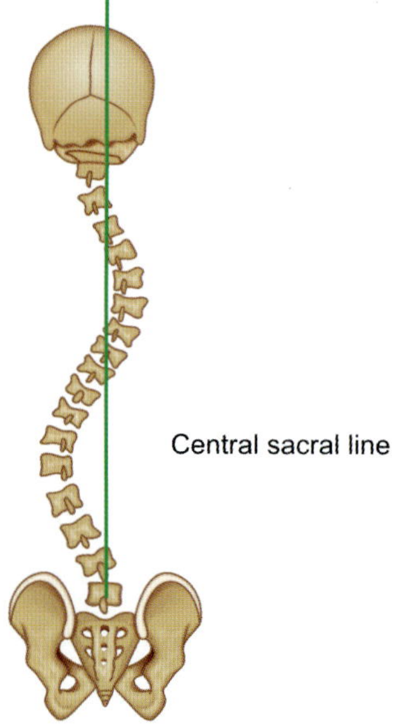

Fig. 9.11: The central sacral line is a plumb line that bisects the S1 spinous process and measures the degree of truncal imbalance. It also aids the surgeon during surgical planning by indicating the lowest, most stable vertebral body to be instrumented.

Perhaps the most significant component of scoliosis is transverse plane deformity, in particular vertebral body rotation. The characteristic rib hump, or back asymmetry, associated with scoliosis is caused by vertebral body rotation taking the rib cage with each individual rotated vertebra and resulting in asymmetric rib growth and deformity. Rotation is easily recognizable on radiographs by the change in alignment of spinous processes or pedicles; however, CT scans and MR imaging are the most demonstrative method of displaying vertebral body rotation and the newer EOS imaging now, as well.

Pulmonary Function

Pulmonary function should be assessed in patients with severe deformity through spirometry for those who are able to cooperate with the testing.[24,25] In very young or severely cognitively impaired individuals, arterial blood gas testing maybe useful, particularly in patients with a history of recurrent pneumonia, bronchitis, or dyspnea.[24]

Genetic Testing

Genetic testing may also aid in making decisions on future treatment of AIS patients. Launched in 2010, the ScoliScore AIS Prognostic Test was designed to assess the progression of curvature in younger patients with mild cases of AIS.[26] A simple saliva-based DNA sample can provide details necessary for determining whether bracing or surgery is necessary.[26] ScoliScore recognizes single nucleotide polymorphisms that are associated with risk of AIS progression, and the test denotes a patient as low, intermediate, or high risk with high negative predictive value.[26] However, the disadvantages of ScoliScore are the high cost and strict inclusion criteria (ages between 9 years and skeletal maturity, Cobb angle 10°–25°, and self-reported Caucasian race). The test has not yet been validated in other races. Further validation is required. Genetic testing is also useful for patients suspected of having a genetic syndrome due to chromosomal abnormalities. There are numerous syndromes. Marfans syndrome is often diagnosed by genetic testing in individuals with a defective gene for fibrillin and have tall stature, scoliosis, and other musculoskeletal manifestations, as well as deficient aortic arch and cardiac valves due to collagen abnormalities and superior lens of the eye dislocations.

CLASSIFICATION

In 2001, Lenke and colleagues published a comprehensive classification of AIS. Three components are utilized in analyzing a patient's degree of scoliosis, namely, curve type, a sagittal thoracic modifier, and a lumbar spine modifier[27] (Fig. 9.12). This system embodies both the sagittal and coronal planes of the spine and addresses thoracic, lumbar, and thoracolumbar deformities. It has demonstrated high inter- and intraobserver reliabilities, and is simple to use. The Lenke classification has enhanced the analysis of AIS, allowing for a more rigid assessment of the deformity and a more global understanding of its effect on the spine for surgical decision making.[28]

CONCLUSION

The overarching goal in treating scoliosis is to prevent, stop, or correct progression of the deformity, normalize spinal function, and minimize associated pain in doing so. An appropriate treatment only follows a thorough and meticulous evaluation. The physician must be diligent in completing the patient interview, examination, diagnostic radiography, and all necessary tests in order to elicit a treatment plan for the individual patient with a specific disorder.

	Curve Type (1–6)					
Lumbar spine modifier	Type 1 (Main thoracic)	Type 2 (Double thoracic)	Type 3 (Double major)	Type 4 (Triple major)	Type 5 (TL/L)	Type 6 (TL/L-MT)
A	1A*	2A*	3A*	4A*		
B	1B*	2B*	3B*	4B*		
C	1C*	2C*	3C*	4C*	5C*	6C*

*"T5–T12 Sagittal Alignment Modifier" which measures the amount of lateral curvature in the thoracic region. It can be graded as –, N, or +

"–" < 10°

"N" : 10–40°

"+" > 40°

Fig. 9.12: The Lenke classification system establishes a simple schema to universally describe scoliotic curves by addressing three components of the deformity: the curve type (1-6), the sagittal thoracic modifier (–, N, +), and the lumbar spine modifier (A to C).

REFERENCES

1. Reamy BV, Slakey JB. Adolescent idiopathic scoliosis: review and current concepts. Am Fam Phys. 2001;64(1): 111-6.
2. Greiner KA. Adolescent idiopathic scoliosis: radiologic decision-making. Am Fam Phys. 2002;65(9):1817-22.
3. Jaramillo D, Poussaint TY, Grottkau BE. Scoliosis: evidence-based diagnostic evaluation. Neuroimaging Clin N Am. 2003;13(2):335-41.
4. Cote P, Kreitz BG, Cassidy JD, et al. A study of the diagnostic accuracy and reliability of the Scoliometer and Adam's forward bend test. Spine (Phila Pa 1976). 1998;23(7):796-802; discussion 803.
5. Goldberg CJ, Dowling FE, Fogarty EE, et al. Adolescent idiopathic scoliosis as developmental instability. Genetica. 1995;96(3):247-55.
6. Errico TJ, Lonner BS, Moulton AW (Eds). Surgical Management of Spinal Deformity. Philadelphia, PA: Saunders Elsevier; 2009.

7. Barnes PD, Brody JD, Jaramillo D, et al. Atypical idiopathic scoliosis: MR imaging evaluation. Radiology 1993;186(1): 247-53.
8. Goldberg CJ, Dowling FE, Fogarty EE. Left thoracic scoliosis configurations. Why so different? Spine (Phila Pa 1976). 1994;19(12):1385-9.
9. Goldberg CJ, Moore DP, Fogarty EE, et al. Left thoracic curve patterns and their association with disease. Spine (Phila Pa 1976). 1999;24(12):1228-33.
10. Lonstein JE, Carlson JM. The prediction of curve progression in untreated idiopathic scoliosis during growth. J Bone Joint Surg Am. 1984;66(7):1061-71.
11. Peterson LE, Nachemson AL. Prediction of progression of the curve in girls who have adolescent idiopathic scoliosis of moderate severity: logistic regression analysis based on data from The Brace Study of the Scoliosis Research Society. J Bone Joint Surg Am. 1995;77(6):823-7.
12. Berven S, Bradford DS. Neuromuscular scoliosis: causes of deformity and principles for evaluation and management. Semin Neurol. 2002;22(2):167-78.
13. Gilmore A, Thompson GH. Radiographic evaluation of children and adolescents with a spinal deformity. Semin Musculoskelet Radiol. 2000;4(3):349-59.
14. Pathria M. Radiologic perspective: imaging of the spine in sports medicine. In: Pedowitz R, Chung C, Resnick D (Eds). Magnetic Resonance Imaging in Orthopedic Sports Medicine. Springer; 2008. p. 126.
15. Sanders JO, Khoury JG, Kishan S, et al. Predicting scoliosis progression from skeletal maturity: a simplified classification during adolescence. J Bone Joint Surg Am. 2008;90(3):540-53.
16. Asher MA. Scoliosis evaluation. Orthop Clin North Am. 1988;19(4):805-14.
17. Janicki JA, Alman B. Scoliosis: review of diagnosis and treatment. Paediatr Child Health. 2007;12(9):771-6.
18. Karski T, Kalakucki J, Karski J. 'Syndrome of contractures' (according to Mau) with the abduction contracture of the right hip as causative factor for development of the so-called idiopathic scoliosis. Stud Health Technol Inform. 2006;123:34-9.
19. Karski T. Etiology of the so-called 'idiopathic scoliosis.' Biomechanical explanation of spine deformity. Two groups of development of scoliosis: New rehabilitation treatment; possibility of prophylactics. Stud Health Technol Inform. 2002;91:37-46.
20. Klepps SJ, Lenke LG, Bridwell KH, et al. Prospective comparison of flexibility radiographs in adolescent idiopathic scoliosis. Spine (Phila Pa 1976). 2001;26(5):E74-9.
21. Langensiepen S, Semler O, Sobottke R, et al. Measuring procedures to determine the Cobb angle in idiopathic scoliosis: a systematic review. Eur Spine J. 2013.
22. Giglio CA, Volpon JB. Development and evaluation of thoracic kyphosis and lumbar lordosis during growth. J Child Orthop. 2007;1(3):187-93.
23. Schroerlucke SR, Akbarnia BA, Pawelek JB, et al. How does thoracic kyphosis affect patient outcomes in growing rod surgery? Spine (Phila Pa 1976). 2012;37(15):1303-9.
24. Weber B, Smith JP, Briscoe WA, et al. Pulmonary function in asymptomatic adolescents with idiopathic scoliosis. Am Rev Respir Dis. 1975;111(4):389-97.
25. de Torres Garcia I, de Cabo Moreno P, Ramirez AM. Extrinsic bronchial obstruction caused by scoliosis. Spine (Phila Pa 1976). 2013;38(13):E840-3.
26. Carlson B. Scoli score AIS prognostic test personalizes treatment for children with spinal curve. Biotechnol Healthc. 2011;8(2):30-31.
27. Lenke LG, Betz RR, Harms J, et al. Adolescent idiopathic scoliosis: a new classification to determine extent of spinal arthrodesis. J Bone Joint Surg Am. 2001;83-A(8):1169-81.
28. Silva F, Lenke LG. Adolescent idiopathic scoliosis. In: Errico T, Lonner BS, Moulton AW (Eds). Surgical Management of Spinal Deformities. Philadelphia, PA: Saunders Elsevier; 2009. pp. 97-104.

CHAPTER

10

Evaluation of Adult Spinal Deformity

Jeffrey H Weinreb, Pierre Devos, Frank Schwab

INTRODUCTION

In the adult, the etiology of scoliotic deformity can be varied but frequently is grouped as either adolescent idiopathic scoliosis in an adult or degenerative/de novo scoliosis. Adolescent idiopathic scoliosis (AIS) is the most common form of pediatric scoliosis and refers to spinal deformity in a child older than age 9 with no etiologic explanation. Adult idiopathic scoliosis is the result of untreated AIS. However, nonidiopathic types of scoliosis from childhood can be observed in adults, which may have resulted from neurologic, idiopathic, and traumatic sources. Neurologic sources include poliomyelitis, spina bifida, cerebral palsy, and spinal muscular atrophy.[1]

Degenerative, or de novo, adult scoliosis is a consequence of the aging processes such as loss of muscle tension and volume, osteoporosis and disk or facet joint degeneration. Although childhood scoliosis evaluation and treatment are based primarily on radiographic measurements and concerns over progression, adult scoliosis is evaluated primarily by assessment of pain and disability.

Although adult scoliosis refers to curvature in the coronal plane, abnormal curvature may occur in the sagittal plane (kyphosis and lordosis) and in the axial plane. Adult spinal deformity (ASD) refers to spinal deformity in any plane and more completely describes abnormality in the adult spine than adult scoliosis.[2,3] In the adult, many cases of deformity may be asymptomatic, and patients with deformities may not be aware of their condition. Research suggests that more than 60% of adults over 60 have a spinal deformity.[4] This chapter examines how ASD is evaluated and classified, with attention to recent developments regarding clinically relevant radiographic parameters applied to the evaluation and treatment of ASD.

EVALUATION

History and Physical

An evaluation of an adult with suspected ASD begins with a complete history and physical examination. A history of idiopathic scoliosis indicates that present deformity is most likely not degenerative/de novo scoliosis.[5] The patient is questioned regarding changes in gait, habits, or clothing fit. Additionally, pain location (axial vs. radicular), quality, severity, provocations, and previous treatments are examined.[5] As back pain is the most frequent clinical symptom of ASD, pain at the site of the curve should be localized either at the apex or in its concavity.[6]

The patient is evaluated to assess for trunk-shift, coronal and sagittal balance, and relationship of the head and pelvis, with specific attention paid to asymmetry. Curve rigidity is assessed with lateral and anterior-posterior bending maneuvers. If leg-length discrepancy is observed, a shoe-lift is performed to see if the curve can be corrected. Neurological examination is performed to assess cranial nerve and sensory function, reflexes, and gait. Finally, cardiopulmonary nutritional and general health statuses are determined to evaluate operative candidacy.[5]

Imaging

Diagnostic imaging is an important element in the evaluation and management of patients with ASD. Several

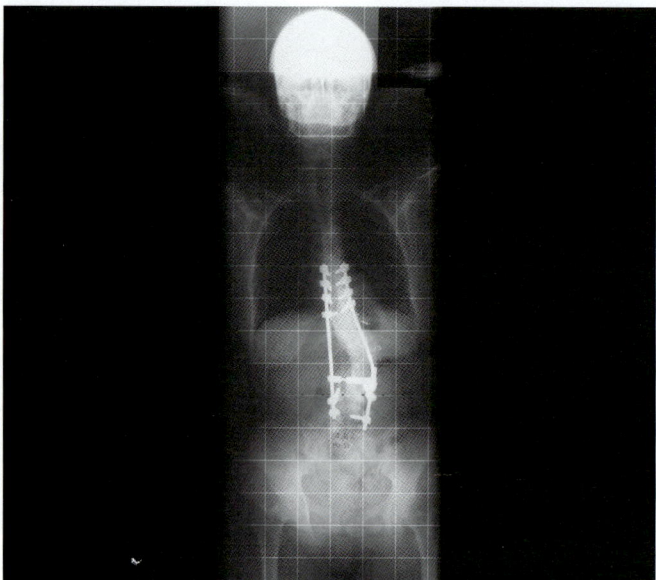

Fig. 10.1: Conventional radiography allows for imaging in a weight-bearing position with standard resolution. However, as X-ray utilizes radiation, long or frequent exposure may increase the risk of cancer.

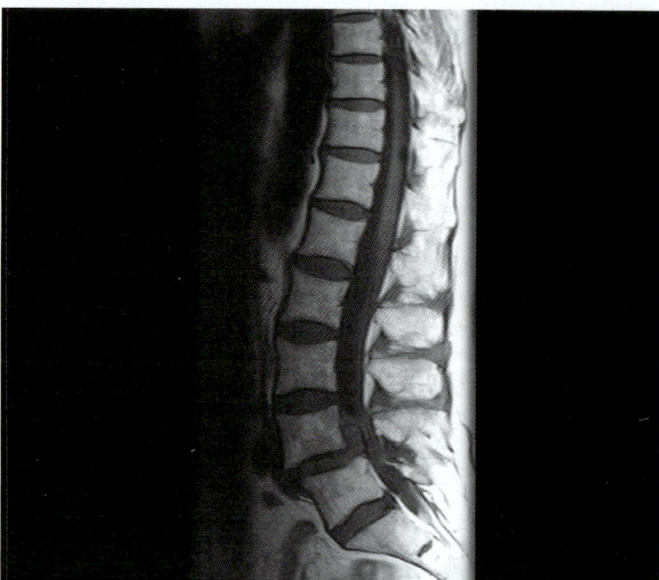

Fig. 10.2: Magnetic resonance imaging is beneficial in diagnosing ASD as it provides clear imaging with no radiation. However, the patient is supine in a standard MRI machine and global deformity or truncal inclination can be underestimated and may lead to erroneous patient evaluation and treatment. Additionally, most patients with implanted medical devices, such as pacemakers, cannot get an MRI. Careful selection of MRI type may aid in evaluation.

imaging techniques are used to evaluate ASD, including conventional radiography, magnetic resonance imaging (MRI), computed tomography (CT), and the EOS imaging system.

Conventional Radiography

Whole spine radiographs of the standing frontal (anteroposterior) and sagittal (lateral) views are required for evaluation of the patient's deformity. Radiographs should include the occiput superiorly and the femoral heads inferiorly. This process allows spinal assessment in a position of function because the patient is upright and bearing weight. However, this method utilizes ionizing radiations and can be harmful with prolonged exposure (Fig. 10.1).

Magnetic Resonance Imaging

Magnetic resonance imaging is particularly useful for the visualization of soft tissue structures: the disk space and adjacent soft tissues. Major limitations of this process include the length of procedure, which requires the full cooperation of the patient during the examination, and the use of a strong magnetic field which may be problematic for patients which electronic devices such as a pacemaker or spinal cord stimulator.[5] Moreover, patients are supine with conventional MRI, thus certain information is not obtained in the most relevant fashion from a clinical perspective (stenotic areas' instabilities and deformity will not be accurately captured compared to a loaded/upright trunk position) (Fig. 10.2).

Computed Tomography

Computed tomography produces tomographic slices of specific area of the body through the axial plane, which allows an excellent representation of the spinal anatomy. Results of this combination provide better osseous and joint anatomy than the highest quality MRI. However, as with conventional radiographs, this method utilizes ionizing radiations that may be dangerous for patients (Fig. 10.3).

EOS

EOS is a relatively new 2D and 3D radio imaging technology based on Georges Charpak's Nobel Prize winning work in 1992 on particle detectors, specifically the multiwire proportional chamber. The machine is constructed from two pairs of units comprising an X-ray tube and a Charpak detector, and is capable of biplanar capture of high-quality digital images of an area of 180 × 45 cm within 10–25 seconds. The slot-scanning radiograph

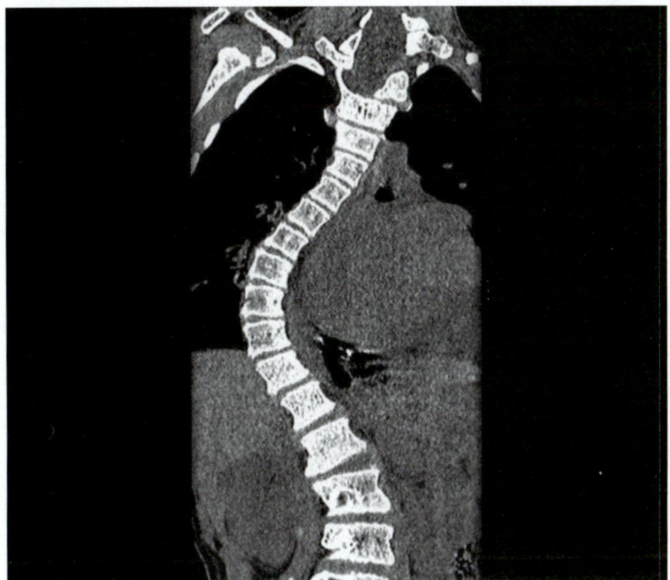

Fig. 10.3: Computed tomography provides high-resolution images in slices that may be used to evaluate ASD. However, CT is not generally taken in a weight-bearing position and utilizes radiation and may increase risk for cancer. Reprinted with permission from Ha HI, Seo JB, Lee SH, et al. Imaging of Marfan syndrome: multisystemic manifestations. Radiographics. 2007;27(4):989-1004.

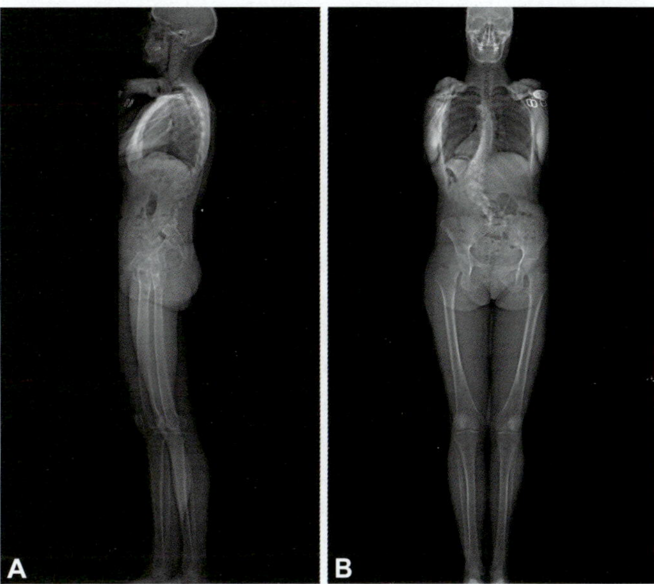

Figs. 10.4A and B: EOS imaging provides high-quality, low-radiation and weight-bearing images that can be used to effectively evaluate ASD. However, the prevalence of EOS imaging technology is not currently widespread.

imager allows the acquisition of radiograph images of a patient in a weight-bearing position, which has inherent benefits for ASD evaluation. The EOS machine is capable of high-quality images with less irradiation than standard imagers. Collimation of both the beams and detectors minimizes the scattered radiation and increases the signal-to-noise ratio.[7,8] The EOS 3D images are comparable to similar CT images at a lower dose and with similar reproducibility and produce full-body images, which is essential to adequately evaluate ASD (Figs. 10.4 A and B).[9,10]

SPINE RELATED MEASUREMENTS IN THE SETTING OF ADULT SPINAL DEFORMITY

Adult scoliosis is a spinal curvature in the coronal plane more than 10° as measured by the Cobb angle (*see* Chapter 11).[11] There are several key measurements that have emerged as being essential in the evaluation of ASD. These measurements include the pelvic incidence (PI), pelvic tilt (PT), sacral slope (SS), sagittal vertical axis (SVA), and T1/T9 spino-pelvic inclination (T1/T9SPI). For information regarding specific spine-related measurements, *see* Chapter 11. Radiographic measurements require that images are obtained in a free-standing patient position. This is essential to adequately capture key aspects of a deformity and potential compensatory mechanisms that a patient may be recruiting. If a patient is not free-standing then global deformity, truncal inclination, or compensatory mechanisms can be underestimated and lead to erroneous patient evaluation and treatment. The ideal position for obtaining standing radiographs (or EOS images) involves natural foot position, shoulder forward flexion, and elbow flexion to bring fingertips onto the face (cheekbones) or mid-clavicles.

CLASSIFICATION

Spinal deformity classification systems are important in evaluation and treatment of patients for a variety of reasons. Classification allows easy case comparison and can provide treatment and management guidelines.[12] AIS has a widely accepted classification system, first proposed by King et al.[13] and updated by Lenke et al.[14] to include sagittal plane parameters and surgical fusion level guidelines based on the classification. Evaluation for pediatric spinal deformity, such as AIS, is based on radiographic data as these pediatric patients are often asymptomatic but progression of deformity is anticipated.

Adult spinal deformity classification, however, is significantly more complicated due to varying etiologies, symptoms, and treatment goals. The need for a distinct adult system has been recognized.[2,14] A comprehensive adult classification system must address high variability in the segmental, regional, and global deformity parameters of the spine and pelvis.[15]

Adult spinal deformity evaluation, however, is generally based on functional concerns and pain, which must take into account radiographic data from a disability perspective and not simply progression risk. Interestingly, treatment is stratified within the adult population, with younger adults (with generally larger Cobb angles) more likely to receive treatment based on radiographic data while older patients are more likely to receive treatment based on pain and disability.[16] An ASD classification system must account for the different considerations of age groups and drivers of treatment.

Numerous studies have examined the average radiographic measurements in the asymptomatic and healthy adult population.[4,17] However, these data have little clinical significance without comparison to the symptoms that cause a patient to seek treatment. A 947 adult patient prospective study by Schwab et al. analyzed the correlation between radiographic parameters and health-related quality of life (HRQOL) questionnaire scores.[18] Questionnaires administered included the Oswestry Disability Index (ODI)[19] and the Scoliosis Research Society (SRS) instrument.[20] These studies demonstrate that the contributions of loss of lumbar lordosis and lumbar vertebra obliquity are more closely correlated with self-assessed pain scores than the Cobb angle on frontal radiographs. Other important radiographic factors include SVA offset, apical level of scoliotic deformity, and intervertebral subluxation.[12]

Schwab et al. proposed a classification system in 2006 that takes HRQOL score into consideration.[15] This classification system is based on high impact clinically significant radiographic parameters, determined by the previously discussed patient self-assessment.[21–23] The classification system categorizes patients into six groups based on location of the apex of the primary curve on standing radiograph. The patient is then further classified by two modifiers that account for degree of lumbar lordosis and subluxation on either frontal or sagittal radiographs. A global balance modifier subdivides the classification (Fig. 10.5).[12,15]

The study did not include the previously discussed pelvic parameters. An ensuing study by Lafage et al. demonstrated significant correlation between certain pelvic parameters and HRQOL scores.[24] The three most important parameters, from most significant to least, are PI minus LL, SVA/T1SPI, and PT. In light of the recently illuminated importance of the spino-pelvic parameters by Lafage et al.,[24] Schwab et al. described at new classification system that includes curve type and sagittal radiographic parameters such as PI-LL, SVA, and PT (Fig. 10.6). These modifiers are clinically correlated with disability and were used to determine the modified SRS-Schwab threshold (Table 10.1).[25] The curve type is determined based on the maximal Cobb angle in the coronal plane. Curve types include thoracic curve only (apical

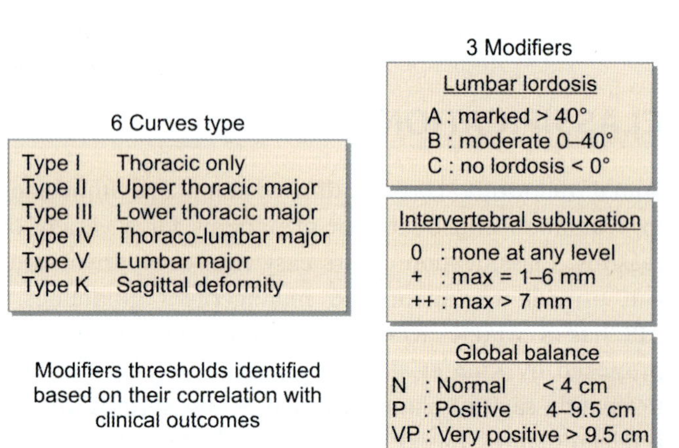

Fig. 10.5: Previously defined adult spinal deformity classification. This classification system was created prior to the inclusion of spino-pelvic parameter criteria.

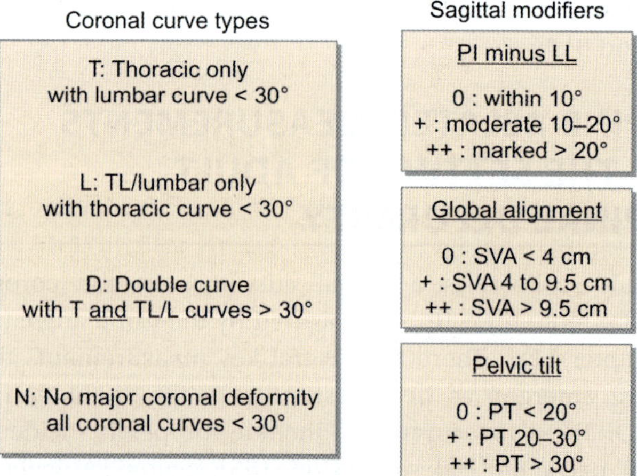

Fig. 10.6: The SRS-Schwab adult spinal deformity classification system, updated to include the sagittal modifiers based on work by Lafage et al.[24]

Table 10.1: Radiographic parameter thresholds that predict an Oswestry Disability Index (ODI) score of 40. These parameters were used to define the radiographic modifiers of the updated SRS-Schwab ASD, classification

Radiographical parameter	*Radiographical threshold*	*Correlation coefficient, r*
Pelvic incidence/lumbar lordosis	11°	0.45
Sagittal vertical axis	46 mm	0.47
Pelvic tilt	22°	0.38

Adapted from Schwab et al.[26]

level of T9 or higher), lumbar or thoracolumbar (apical level of T10 or lower), double (both thoracic and lumbar/thoracolumbar), and no marked coronal curve. Sagittal modifiers are then added to the classification to indicate global alignment, pelvic compensation, and spino-pelvic harmony (PI minus LL). This new classification system has high inter and intrarater reliability.[26] Considering the parameters of the rating system, is it thus essential to obtain proper full-length radiographs (or EOS scans) of the spine and pelvis.[25]

Based on previous HRQOL studies, the threshold for disability, defined as an ODI score more than 40, is an SVA more than 47 mm, a PT more than 22° and absolute value of PI minus LL more than 11°.[25] Considering the radiographic parameter correlation with pain and disability, Schwab et al. define realignment objectives in the sagittal plane as an SVA less than 50 mm, a PT less than 20° and LL equal to PI ± 9° (Fig. 10.7).[27] Surgical correction to these values seeks to reestablish level gaze, physiologic standing posture, effective ambulation and appropriate lordotic alignment. The SRS-Schwab classification system provides realistic clinical goals for both operative and nonoperative patients. A recent study by Smith et al. demonstrates that the SRS-Schwab classification modifiers are responsive to changes in disease state and a change in classification indicates a significant change in patient reported outcomes.[28]

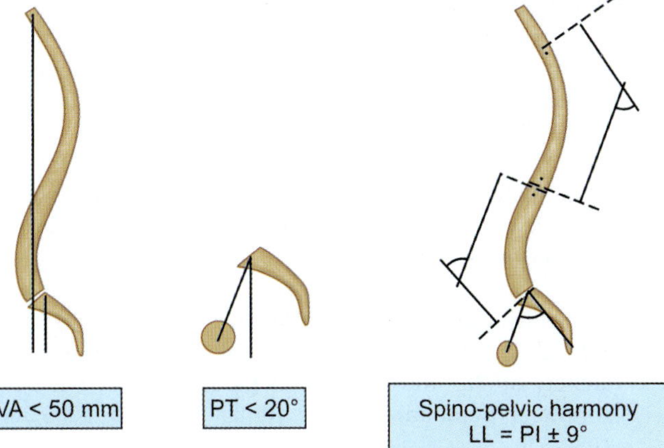

Fig. 10.7: The SRS-Schwab adult spinal deformity surgical realignment goals, based on disability threshold and spino-pelvic parameter correlation with Oswestry Disability Index (ODI) scores.
(SVA: Sagittal vertical axis; PT: Pelvic tilt; LL: Lumbar lordosis; PL: Pelvic incidence).

CONCLUSION

Adult spinal deformity has various etiologies and degrees of clinical presentation. The drivers of treatment, and thus keys to evaluation of the patient, must be based on disability and pain. Imaging studies, in addition to HRQOL measures, are thus critical. Decisions regarding imaging technique should take into account the potential benefits of the obtained information, as well as potential harm to the patient. The discussed classification systems offer the clinician a common language and valuable systematic approach to ASD. Through a common classification, it is possible to identify the essential aspects of a deformity and parameters that should be taken into account when considering treatment.

A recent study predicted outcomes in operative patients using variables including age group, type of surgery, baseline HRQOL scores, and subluxation presence as predictors of whether a patient will reach a minimal clinically important difference (MCID). Patients with thoracolumbar deformity, intervertebral subluxation, osteotomy, sacrum fixation, and worse baseline HRQOL scores were more likely to reach MCID, while patients with thoracic deformity, absence of subluxation, negative sagittal alignment, and better baseline HRQOL scores were less likely to reach the MCID.[29] Additionally, nonsurgical patients have greater preoperative medical risk factors, while surgical patients have more frequent leg pain, higher level of daily back pain and more frequent moderate-to-severe back pain.[30] These factors should be taken into consideration during surgical planning. Different approaches, including nonoperative management, should be considered for patients less likely to reach the MCID. Nevertheless, the SRS-Schwab Classification provides standardization and evidence based clinical goals for both operative and nonoperative patients and should be utilized for improved clinical outcomes in the evaluation of ASD.

REFERENCES

1. Kouwenhoven JWM, Castelein RM. The pathogenesis of adolescent idiopathic scoliosis: review of the literature. Spine. 2008;33(26):2898.
2. Bess S, Schwab F, Lafage V, et al. Classifications for adult spinal deformity and use of the scoliosis research society-Schwab adult spinal deformity classification. Neurosurg Clin N Am. 2013;24(2):185-93.
3. Good C, Auerbach J, O'Leary P, Schuler T. Adult spine deformity. Curr Rev Musculoskelet Med. 2011;4(4):159-167.
4. Schwab F, Dubey A, Gamez L, et al. Adult scoliosis: prevalence, SF-36, and nutritional parameters in an elderly volunteer population. Spine (Phila Pa 1976). 2005;30(9): 1082-5.
5. Silva FE, Lenke LG. Adult degenerative scoliosis: evaluation and management. Neurosurgical Focus. 2010;28(3):E1.
6. Aebi M. The adult scoliosis. Eur Spine J. 2005;14(10):925-48.
7. Illés T, Tunyogi-Csapó M, Somoskeöy S. Breakthrough in three-dimensional scoliosis diagnosis: significance of horizontal plane view and vertebra vectors. Eur Spine J. 2011; 20(1):135-43.
8. Deschênes S, Charron G, Beaudoin G, et al. Diagnostic imaging of spinal deformities: reducing patients radiation dose with a new slot-scanning X-ray imager. Spine. 2010;35(9):989.
9. Glaser DA, Doan J, Newton PO. Comparison of 3-dimensional spinal reconstruction accuracy: biplanar radiographs with EOS versus computed tomography. Spine. 2012;37(16):1391-7.
10. Rousseau MA, Laporte S, Chavary-Bernier E, et al. Reproducibility of measuring the shape and three-dimensional position of cervical vertebrae in upright position using the EOS stereoradiography system. Spine. 2007;32(23):2569.
11. Benzel EC, Steinmetz MP, Lenke LG. Spine Deformity and Correction,: The Fundamentals" in Spine surgery: techniques, complication avoidance, and management, 3rd edition. Philadelphia, PA: Gulf Professional Publishing; 2005.
12. Benzel EC, Heller JE, Fu KMG, et al. Adult Thoracic and Lumbar Deformity" in Spine surgery: techniques, complication avoidance, and management, 3rd edition. Philadelphia, PA: Gulf Professional Publishing; 2005.
13. King HA, Moe JH, Bradford DS, et al. The selection of fusion levels in thoracic idiopathic scoliosis. J Bone Joint Surg Am. 1983;65(9):1302-13.
14. Lenke LG, Betz RR, Harms J, et al. Adolescent idiopathic scoliosis: a new classification to determine extent of spinal arthrodesis. J Bone Joint Surg Am. 2001;83-A(8):1169-81.
15. Schwab F, Lafage V, Farcy JP, et al. Surgical rates and operative outcome analysis in thoracolumbar and lumbar major adult scoliosis: application of the new adult deformity classification. Spine. 2007;32(24):2723.
16. Bess S, Boachie-Adjei O, Burton D, et al. Pain and disability determine treatment modality for older patients with adult scoliosis, while deformity guides treatment for younger patients. Spine (Phila Pa 1976). 2009;34(20):2186-90.
17. Vialle R, Levassor N, Rillardon L, et al. Radiographic analysis of the sagittal alignment and balance of the spine in asymptomatic subjects. J Bone Joint Surg Am. 2005;87(2):260-67.
18. Schwab F, Farcy JP, Bridwell K, et al. A clinical impact classification of scoliosis in the adult. Spine. 2006;31(18):2109.
19. Fairbank JCT, Pynsent PB. The Oswestry disability index. Spine. 2000;25(22):2940.
20. Lowe T, Berven SH, Schwab FJ, et al. The SRS classification for adult spinal deformity: building on the King/Moe and Lenke classification systems. Spine. 2006;31(19S):S119.
21. Glassman SD, Berven S, Bridwell K, et al. Correlation of radiographic parameters and clinical symptoms in adult scoliosis. Spine (Phila Pa 1976). 2005;30 (6):682-8.
22. Schwab F, Dubey A, Pagala M, et al. Adult scoliosis: a health assessment analysis by SF-36. Spine (Phila Pa 1976). 2003;28(6):602-6.
23. Schwab F, el-Fegoun AB, Gamez L, et al. A lumbar classification of scoliosis in the adult patient: preliminary approach. Spine (Phila Pa 1976). 2005;30(14): 1670-73.
24. Lafage V, Schwab F, Patel A, et al. Pelvic tilt and truncal inclination: two key radiographic parameters in the setting of adults with spinal deformity. Spine. 2009;34(17):E599.
25. Schwab FJ, Blondel B, Bess S, et al. Combined assessment of pelvic tilt, pelvic incidence/lumbar lordosis mismatch and sagittal vertical axis predicts disability in adult spinal deformity: a prospective analysis: paper #20*; 2011. p. 65.
26. Schwab F, Ungar B, Blondel B, et al. SRS-Schwab adult spinal deformity classification: a validation study. Spine. 2011.
27. Schwab F, Patel A, Ungar B, et al. Adult spinal deformity - postoperative standing imbalance: how much can you tolerate? An overview of key parameters in assessing alignment and planning corrective surgery. Spine. 2010;35(25):2224.
28. Smith JS, Klineberg E, Schwab F, et al. Change in classification grade by the SRS-Schwab adult deformity classification predicts impact on health-related quality of life measures: prospective analysis of operative and non-operative treatment. Spine (Phila Pa 1976). 2013;38(19):1663-71.
29. Schwab FJ, Lafage V, Farcy JP, et al. Predicting outcome and complications in the surgical treatment of adult scoliosis. Spine (Phila Pa 1976). 2008;33(20):2243-7.
30. Glassman SD, Schwab FJ, Bridwell KH, et al. The selection of operative versus nonoperative treatment in patients with adult scoliosis. Spine. 2007;32(1):93.

CHAPTER 11

Measurement of Adult Spinal Deformity

Jeffrey H Weinreb, Thomas Cheriyan, Virginie Lafage, Frank Schwab

Adult spinal deformity (ASD) curve measurement allows standardization and reproducibility in the treatment and management of ASD. For these reasons, ASD treatment should always include some form of curve measurement. This chapter addresses the methodology behind measuring ASD, and additional measurements that have been adopted in other planes, important parameters including the recently examined spinopelvic parameters, as well as the limitations and critiques of ASD measurement.

IMAGING

Diagnostic imaging is the most precise and accurate way to measure spinal deformity. Proper radiographic images are obtained in a freestanding patient position. This is essential to adequately capture key aspects of a deformity and potential compensatory mechanisms that a patient may be recruiting. If a patient is not freestanding then global deformity or truncal inclination can be over or underestimated and lead to erroneous patient evaluation and treatment. The ideal position for obtaining standing images involves natural foot position, shoulder forward flexion, and elbow flexion to bring fingertips onto the face or mid-clavicles. For additional information regarding these imaging techniques, *see* Chapters 11 and 13.

Two-dimensional Analysis

Simple two-dimensional (2D) measurements are widely used to quantify ASD and to determine reference values in symptomatic and asymptomatic conditions. The angles used to measure ASD can be determined with a simple protractor on printed radiographs or using software specifically designed to assist the user with measuring.[1-3] It has been suggested that digital imaging measuring techniques reduce intrinsic errors in hand measurement including variability introduced by using different manual protractors, lost information between multiple printed copies of a radiograph, and the use of wide-diameter radiographic markers.[2]

CORONAL PLANE MEASUREMENTS

Ferguson Method

One of the first methods to determine the extent of scoliosis in the coronal plane was described by Ferguson et al.[4] This method evaluates the angles formed between two straight lines that connect the centers of end vertebra with the center of the apical vertebra.[5] The end vertebrae that define the ends of a curve in a frontal or sagittal projection. Cephalad end vertebra is the first vertebra in the cephalad direction from a curve apex whose superior surface is tilted maximally toward the concavity of the curve.

Caudad end vertebra is the first vertebra in the caudad direction from a curve apex whose inferior surface is tilted maximally toward the concavity of the curve.

The apical vertebra in a curve is most deviated laterally from the vertical axis that passes through the patient's sacrum, i.e. from the central sacral line.

The center of these three vertebrae is marked with a dot and lines are drawn from the apical vertebra to each of the end vertebra.

Cobb Angle

The Cobb angle measurement technique, originally described by John Cobb in 1948, is a commonly utilized measurement technique to determine the extent of thoracic and lumbar scoliosis in the coronal plane.[7] From a free-standing anteroposterior radiograph, the vertebrae maximally tilted into the curve are selected and lines are drawn parallel to the superior plate of the rostral vertebra and the inferior end plate of the caudal vertebra. The angle formed from the bisection of perpendicular lines drawn from each end-plate plane line determines the Cobb angle.[8] The literature has reported a high correlation between the Cobb and Ferguson techniques, with the Cobb measurement generally overvaluing the Ferguson angle.[9] It has also been suggested that the Ferguson method is best suited to curves <50°, while the Cobb method is best suited to curves >50° (Figs. 11.1A and B).[6]

Rotatory Subluxation

Coronal subluxations including lateral olisthesis and rotatory subluxation have been implicated as factors in the development of ASD, curve progression, and pain, and are defined as lateral translations or rotation of the vertebral body.[11,12] To measure subluxation, a line perpendicular to the superior end-plate plane is erected from the superior corner of the caudal vertebra and another perpendicular line is drawn from the inferior end-plate plane at the inferior corner of the cephalad vertebra. The distance between these two lines defines the degree of subluxation in millimeters. In lateral olisthesis the axial rotation of adjacent vertebrae are relatively neutral in relation to each other while in rotatory subluxation the cephalad vertebra is rotated. The initial ASD classification system described by Schwab et al. included a subluxation modifier, as greater subluxation measurements correlate with worse pain, function, and disability scores.[13]

Coronal Alignment

Coronal alignment (CA) is assessed using standing coronal radiographs. CA is the horizontal distance in centimeters between a vertical line dropped from the middle of the C7 vertebral body and the central sacral vertical

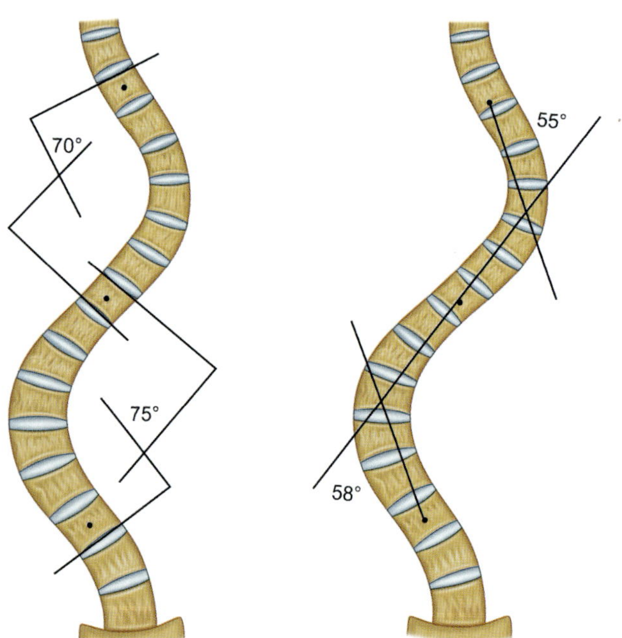

Fig. 11.1A: From a free-standing anteroposterior radiograph, the vertebrae maximally tilted into the curve are selected and lines are drawn parallel to the superior plate of the rostral vertebra and the inferior end plate of the caudal vertebra. The angle formed from the bisection of perpendicular lines drawn from each end-plate plane line determines the Cobb angle (left). The ferguson angle (right) is formed between two straight lines that connect the centers of end vertebra with the center of the apical vertebra.

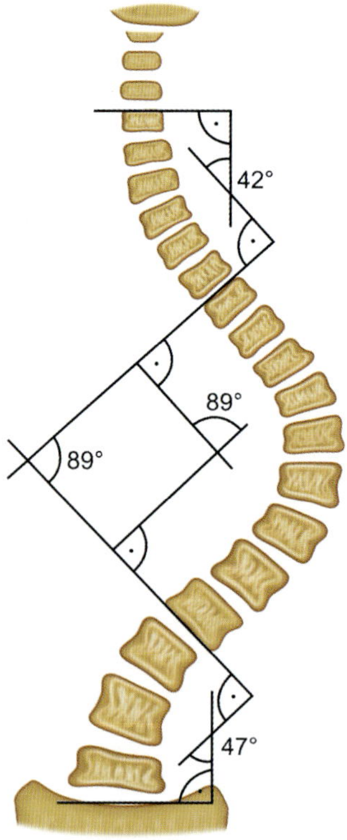

Fig. 11.1B: An example of a Cobb angle evaluation. The Cobb angle provides an efficient way to categorize and compare scoliosis across the population. However, recent research suggests the Cobb angle does not correlate with pain and disability as closely as spinopelvic parameters.[10]

line, the vertical line that passes through the center of the sacrum. A CA of 0 is designated as neutral. Misalignments to the left of the center are represented as a negative value and decompensation to the right are represented as a positive value.[14]

SAGITTAL PLANE MEASUREMENTS

Spinal Curvature

Although scoliosis was initially considered deformity in the coronal plane, research in the past few decades has been focused on redefining scoliotic deformity parameters.[15] The medical community now recognizes that deformity may occur in several planes, and sagittal deformity may correlate with the symptoms of coronal scoliosis.[15-20] The lumbar sagittal curve is known as lumbar lordosis (LL), while the thoracic curve is known as thoracic kyphosis (TK). Either of these curves may exist to a lower or higher extent than the general population, and may be symptomatic or asymptomatic.[20]

The Cobb angle in the lateral plane is known as the modified Cobb and is measured in the same manner as the coronal Cobb angle. The modified Cobb, however, uses the superior L1 end plate and the sacral end plate to constitute the LL measurement, while the Cobb angle drawn utilizing the inferior end plate of T12 and the superior end plate of T4 constitutes TK (Fig. 11.2).[5,7,22]

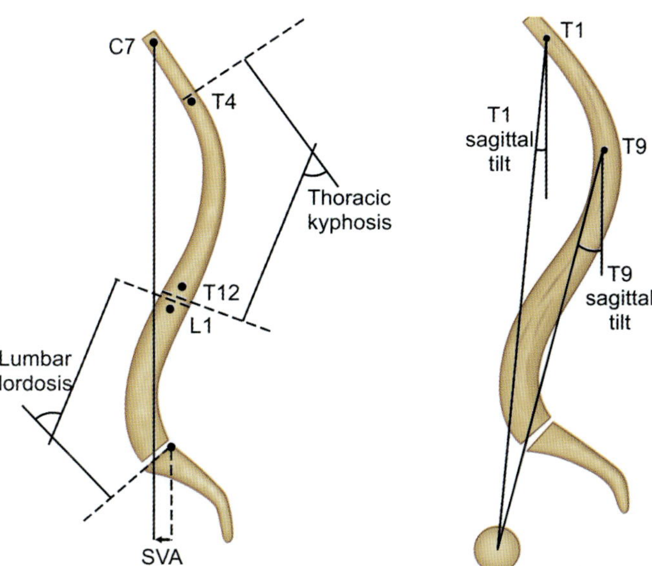

Fig. 11.2: (Lateral view) Examples of thoracic kyphosis and lumbar lordosis as measured by the Cobb angle, the C7 plumbline and the corresponding sagittal vertical axis measurement: T1 sagittal tilt and T9 sagittal tilt.[21]

SPINOPELVIC RADIOGRAPHIC PARAMETERS

The pelvis has recently been shown to play an essential role related to ASD evaluation.[23-28] Several key parameters, including the pelvic incidence (PI), pelvic tilt (PT), and sacral slope (SS), have been examined to determine their relation to function and disability in the setting of ASD (Table 11.1 and Fig. 11.3).[24,25]

Table 11.1: Average radiographic parameter measurement in the asymptomatic adult and adolescent population with no prior spinal disorder between 20 and 85 years old[18,19,21,29,30]

Parameter	*Average value in the asymptomatic adult (Degrees)*
Pelvic tilt	36–42
Sacral slope	12–18
Thoracic kyphosis	41–48
Lumbar lordosis	43–61
	Average value in the asymptomatic adolescent (Degrees)
Pelvic tilt	0.2–15.6
Sacral slope	32.9–49.9
Thoracic kyphosis	33.9–54.5
Lumbar lordosis	36.8–61.6

Source: Adapted from Mehta et al.[31]

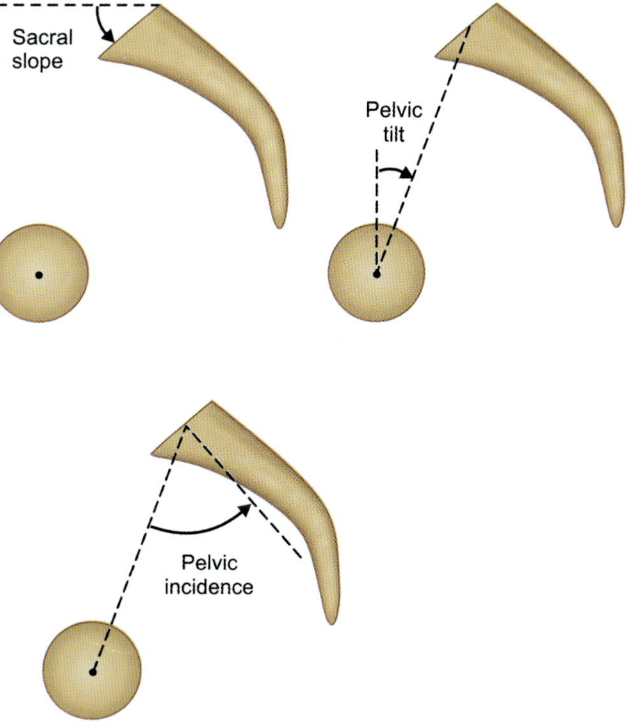

Fig. 11.3: A depiction of the spinopelvic parameters.

Pelvic Incidence

Defined as the angle between a line drawn from the center of the femoral head axis to the midpoint of the sacral plate and the perpendicular to the sacral plate. Pelvic incidence (PI) is a morphologic parameter and does not change much throughout adulthood. However, PI increases between childhood and adulthood.[32]

Pelvic Tilt

Defined as the angle between a line drawn from the center of the femoral head axis to the midpoint of the sacral plate and the vertical. Pelvic tilt (PT) is a positional parameter and is determined by the position of the pelvis with respect to the body. Like PI, PT increases from childhood to adulthood. PT often increases during old age for reasons that will be discussed.

Sacral Slope

Defined as the angle between plane of the sacral plate and the horizontal. Like PT, SS is a positional parameter and changes based on the position of the pelvis with respect to the body.

Pelvic incidence is equal to the sum of PT and SS. By definition, changing either of the positional parameters alters the other inversely. The pelvis plays a fundamental regulatory role within the chain of correlation between the spine and lower limbs.[33]

GLOBAL ALIGNMENT

The coronal and sagittal measurements, when examined together, compose the global alignment (GA). GA is measured in several ways, including the sagittal vertical axis and T1/T9 spinopelvic inclination.[22]

Sagittal Vertical Axis

Defined as the distance between the plumb line from the midpointt of the C7 vertebra and its offset from the posterior-superior corner of the sacral end plate.[34]

T1/T9 Spinopelvic Inclination

Defined as the angle between the vertical and a line connecting the center of the T1 or T9 vertebra and the femoral head axis.

These factors have been shown to be related to spinal parameters such as LL and TK in what is known as the "chain of correlation," as abnormal pelvic parameters may prompt compensatory spinal dimensions to maintain the head over the pelvis or vice versa.[24] It has been shown that PI, SS, PT, LL, and TK are closely linked and balance themselves, by muscular activity, to maintain global alignment.[35]

CRITICISM OF 2D MEASUREMENTS

It should be noted there has been criticism regarding 2D measurement, as the technique is based on the noncuboidal vertebral shape.[36] The end plates of maximally tilted vertebrae may appear indistinct, cup-shaped, or biconcave, making it more challenging to define the appropriate planes.[3] The Ferguson method has been reported to have a 5.6° intraobserver error and 6.6° interobserver error.[37] The Cobb technique is believed to have an inherent error of 3° to 5°, an intraobserver error range between 1% and 5%, and interobserver error can be as high as 10°.[3,8] The modified Cobb technique has a reported intraobserver variability of 0.95° and interobserver variability of 0.92°.[36] End plates are three-dimensional (3D) structures, so 2D analysis itself introduces uncertainty into the evaluation and is a source or error.[1] Both the Cobb and Ferguson methods are based on manual identification of the end vertebrae, therefore increasing the variability and unreliability.[5]

3D ANALYSIS

The complex 3D deformity of the spine cannot be fully appreciated in 2D. Technological advances, including CT, MRI, and stereoradiographic reconstruction based on anatomical landmarks, have been applied to the spine to better evaluate ASD.[38, 39] Harmonic functions, splines, polynomials, and statistical interpolation techniques have been used to model the scoliotic spine in three dimensions.[5, 40-44] Although 3D evaluation is able to better depict the spine than 2D measurement, information extraction, 3D navigation and methods originally designed for 2D analysis make 3D evaluation difficult. Clinically relevant 3D measurements for the spine have yet to be developed and put into practice.[5] Ultimately, 3D analysis will be completely automated; therefore, avoiding the inherent errors of manual evaluation. However, manual settings determination is the most challenging aspect in the development of computerized models.[5]

CONCLUSION

Despite critique, the Cobb angle for measuring the extent of deformity in both the coronal and sagittal planes allows for standardization and comparison across the population. When combined with spinopelvic parameter measurement, the spinal parameters help to contextualize the extent of deformity. Management and treatment of spinal deformity is challenging because patients may be symptomatic or asymptomatic, young or old and with a variety of etiologies. Although 2D spinal deformity measurement is imperfect, it is currently the simplest and most clinically relevant way to simplify diagnosis and to help create treatment and management goals. Hopefully, as 3D modeling becomes more effective and widespread, its implementation will reduce human variability and error to help develop more clinically effective deformity diagnosis and treatment.

REFERENCES

1. Gstoettner M, Sekyra K, Walochnik N, et al. Inter-and intraobserver reliability assessment of the Cobb angle: manual versus digital measurement tools. Eur Spine J. 2007;16(10):1587-92.
2. Shea KG, Stevens PM, Nelson M, et al. A comparison of manual versus computer-assisted radiographic measurement. Intraobserver measurement variability for Cobb angles. Spine (Phila Pa 1976). 1998;23(5):551-5.
3. Morrissy R, Goldsmith G, Hall E, et al. Measurement of the Cobb angle on radiographs of patients who have scoliosis: evaluation of intrinsic error. J Bone Joint Surgery Am. 1990;72(3):320.
4. Ferguson AB. The study and treatment of scoliosis. South Med J. 1930;23(2):116-20.
5. Vrtovec T, Pernus F, Likar B. A review of methods for quantitative evaluation of spinal curvature. Eur Spine J. 2009;18(5):593-607.
6. Kittleson AC, LIM LW. Measurement of scoliosis. Am J Roentgenol. 1970;108(4):775-7.
7. Cobb J. Outline for the study of scoliosis, IN: Instructional Course Lectures. Am Acad Orthop Surg. 1948;5:261-75.
8. Benzel EC. Spine Surgery: Techniques, Complication Avoidance, and Management. 3rd edn, Saunders; Philadelphia 2012
9. Stokes IAF, Aronson DD, Ronchetti PJ, et al. Reexamination of the Cobb and Ferguson angles: bigger is not always better. J Spinal Disord. 1993;6:333-8.
10. Schwab F, Ungar B, Blondel B, et al. SRS-Schwab adult spinal deformity classification: a validation study. Spine. 2011.
11. Toyone T, Tanaka T, Kato D, et al. Anatomic changes in lateral spondylolisthesis associated with adult lumbar scoliosis. Spine. 2005;30(22):E671-E675.
12. Tribus CB. Degenerative lumbar scoliosis: evaluation and management. J Am Acad Orthop Surg. 2003;11(3):174-83.
13. Schwab F, Farcy JP, Bridwell K, et al. A clinical impact classification of scolios is in the adult. Spine (Phila Pa 1976). 2006;31(18):2109-14.
14. Ames CP, Smith JS, Scheer JK, et al. Impact of spinopelvic alignment on decision making in deformity surgery in adults: a review. J Neurosurg Spine. 2012;16(6):547-64.
15. Stokes IAF, Bigalow LC, Moreland MS. Three dimensional spinal curvature in idiopathic scoliosis. J Orthop Res. 1987;5(1):102-113.
16. Deacon P, Flood B, Dickson R. Idiopathic scoliosis in three dimensions: a radiographic and morphometric analysis. J Bone Joint Surg Br Vol. 1984;66(4):509-512.
17. Barrey C, Roussouly P, Perrin G, et al. Sagittal balance disorders in severe degenerative spine: can we identify the compensatory mechanisms? Eur Spine J. 2011:1-8.
18. Qiu Y, Yin G, Cao X. The influence of thoracic kyphosis on sagittal balance of the lumbosacral spine in thoracic idiopathic scoliosis patients]. Zhonghua wai ke za zhi [Chin J Surg]. 2008;46(16):1237.
19. Jackson RP, Phipps T, Hales C, et al. Pelvic lordosis and alignment in spondylolisthesis. Spine. 2003;28(2):151.
20. Schwab F, Patel A, Ungar B, et al. Adult spinal deformity—postoperative standing imbalance: how much can you tolerate? An overview of key parameters in assessing alignment and planning corrective surgery. Spine. 2010;35(25):2224.
21. Peleg S, Dar G, Steinberg N, et al. Sacral orientation and spondylolysis. Spine. 2009;34(25):E906.
22. Lafage V, Ames C, Schwab F, et al. Changes in thoracic kyphosis negatively impact sagittal alignment after lumbar pedicle subtraction osteotomy: a comprehensive radiographic analysis. Spine (Phila Pa 1976). 2012;37(3):E180-7.
23. Schwab F, Dubey A, Gamez L, et al. Adult scoliosis: prevalence, SF-36, and nutritional parameters in an elderly volunteer population. Spine (Phila Pa 1976). 2005;30(9): 1082-5.
24. Duval-Beaupere G, Marty C, Barthel F, et al. Sagittal profile of the spine prominent part of the pelvis. Stud Health Technol Inform. 2002;88:47-64.
25. Legaye J, Duval-Beaupere G, Hecquet J, et al. Pelvic incidence: a fundamental pelvic parameter for three-dimensional regulation of spinal sagittal curves. Eur Spine J. 1998;7(2):99-103.
26. Roussouly P, Gollogly S, Berthonnaud E, et al. Classification of the normal variation in the sagittal alignment of the human lumbar spine and pelvis in the standing position. Spine (Phila Pa 1976). 2005;30(3):346-53.
27. Vialle R, Levassor N, Rillardon L, et al. Radiographic analysis of the sagittal alignment and balance of the spine in asymptomatic subjects. J Bone Joint Surg Am. 2005;87(2): 260-67.
28. Schwab F, Lafage V, Boyce R, et al. Gravity line analysis in adult volunteers: age-related correlation with spinal parameters, pelvic parameters, and foot position. Spine (Phila Pa 1976). 2006;31(25):E959-67.
29. Betz RR. Kyphosis of the thoracic and thoracolumbar spine in the pediatric patient: normal sagittal parameters and scope of the problem. Instr Course Lect. 2004;53:479-84.

30. Mac-Thiong JM, Berthonnaud E, Dimar JR, 2nd, et al. Sagittal alignment of the spine and pelvis during growth. Spine (Phila Pa 1976). 2004;29(15):1642-7.
31. Mehta VA, Amin A, Omeis I, et al. Gottfried ON. Implications of spinopelvic alignment for the spine surgeon. Neurosurgery. 2012;70(3):707.
32. Mac-Thiong JM, Berthonnaud É, Dimar JR, et al. Sagittal alignment of the spine and pelvis during growth. Spine. 2004;29(15):1642.
33. Lafage V, Schwab F, Patel A, et al. Pelvic tilt and truncal inclination: two key radiographic parameters in the setting of adults with spinal deformity. Spine. 2009;34(17):E599.
34. Van Royen B, Toussaint H, Kingma I, et al. Accuracy of the sagittal vertical axis in a standing lateral radiograph as a measurement of balance in spinal deformities. Eur Spine J. 1998;7(5):408-12.
35. Labelle H, Roussouly P, Berthonnaud E, et al. The importance of spino-pelvic balance in L5-s1 developmental spondylolisthesis: a review of pertinent radiologic measurements. Spine (Phila Pa 1976). 2005;30 (6 Suppl):S27-34.
36. Harrison DE, Harrison DD, Cailliet R, et al. Cobb method or Harrison posterior tangent method: which to choose for lateral cervical radiographic analysis. Spine (Phila Pa 1976). 2000;25(16):2072-8.
37. Diab KM, Sevastik JA, Hedlund R, Suliman IA. Accuracy and applicability of measurement of the scoliotic angle at the frontal plane by Cobb's method, by Ferguson's method and by a new method. Eur Spine J. 1995;4(5):291-5.
38. Suh CH. The fundamentals of computer aided X-ray analysis of the spine. J Biomech. 1974;7(2):161-9.
39. Saraste H, Östman A. Stereophotogrammetry in the evaluation of the treatment of scoliosis. Int Orthop. 1986;10(1):63-7.
40. Drerup B, Hierholzer E. Assessment of scoliotic deformity from back shape asymmetry using an improved mathe matical model. Clin Biomech (Bristol, Avon). 1996;11 (7):376-83.
41. Huysmans T, Haex B, Van Audekercke R, et al. Three- dimensional mathematical reconstruction of the spinal shape, based on active contours. J Biomech. 2004;37(11): 1793-8.
42. Berthonnaud E, Dimnet J. Analysis of structural features of deformed spines in frontal and sagittal projections. Comput Med Imaging Graph. 2007;31(1):9-16.
43. Peng Z, Zhong J, Wee W, Lee JH. Automated Vertebra Detection and Segmentation from the Whole Spine MR Images. Conf Proc IEEE Eng Med Biol Soc. 2005;3:2527-30.
44. Poncet P, Trochu F, Dansereau J. Curvilinear Three-dimensional modeling of spinal curves with dual Kriging. Comput Methods Biomech Biomed Engin. 1999;2(4):295-308.

CHAPTER

12

Assessment of Disability

Juan Carlos Robles

INTRODUCTION

Disability, as defined by the American Medical Association, is "an alteration of an individual's capacity to meet personal, social, or occupational demands because of impairment". Disability evaluation takes into consideration whether a patient's pathological process or physiological impairment results in a disability that interferes substantially with the performance of daily tasks, especially occupational and work-related activities. There are multiple assessment tools used in the evaluation of functional disability, some more widely used than others.[1,2]

The previously used World Health Organization (WHO) model of disability assessment failed to recognize the complexity of chronic musculoskeletal pain and disability. In the past, assessment of disability had been made based on an oversimplified model. For this disability assessment, patients were evaluated with questions such as, "Do you think that you are ready to go back to work?" or "What do you think you won't be able to do if you go back to work?" Key factors not included in assessment were the patient's perception of pain, knowledge of his/her disability and incentives or motivations for the patient to return to work. Furthermore, the patients' functional abilities in relation to the functional requirements necessary for a particular work were not evaluated.

This lack of key information in the WHO disability assessment led to the development of improved functional assessment evaluations. Functional status after injury has been shown to be a reliable predictor of future disability and return to work. Thus, in order to support the clinical assessment of function and determine a patient's level of disability, functional status after injury was incorporated into the improved disability assessment.[3]

FUNCTIONAL ASSESSMENT INSTRUMENTS

Although there is no "gold standard" for the assessment of disability, there are many functional assessment instruments. These include both objective and subjective assessment tools. Objective tools include functional capacity evaluations (FCE), such as the physical work performance evaluation, while subjective tools are based mainly on questionnaires and surveys. The questionnaires are used to obtain the patient's perceptions of their own disabilities. Examples include the Oswestry Disability Index, the Roland-Morris patient questionnaire, McGill pain questionnaire, and the Medical Outcome Study short form-36.

OBJECTIVE TOOLS

Functional Capacity Evaluation

Functional capacity evaluation is defined as a direct measurement of work capacity designed to evaluate an individual's functional abilities or limitations in the context of safe, productive work tasks. Such an assessment can then be translated into a performance-potential, which considers the individual's body functions and structures, environmental factors, personal factors, and status.[4,5]

The usefulness of FCE has been acknowledged by many agencies including the Social Security Administration and Occupational Safety and Health Administration

(OSHA). Regulatory agencies, such as OSHA, are promoting the use of FCEs in an effort to ensure employee health and safety in job placement. In addition, the Americans with Disabilities Act places emphasis on identifying an individual's physical abilities and limitations for employment and accommodation considerations.[6]

The FCE provides a performance-based assessment of an individual's functional abilities that can lead professionals to conclude what the patient can do or cannot do when he/she returns to work. FCEs help guide treatment, facilitate return to work decisions, and determine level of disability. Additionally, the FCE has the potential to match a specific type of work to a worker that has been evaluated.

Physical Work Performance Evaluations

There are many FCEs available. Our institution uses the physical work performance evaluation (PWPE), an evaluation developed by Lechner at the University of Alabama at Birmingham.[7] The PWPE uses a psychophysical and kinesiophysical approach. It tests the subject's safe maximal performance level, which is the highest level the patient can perform his/her job without compromising safety. It takes into account the client's behavior, that is, the patient can stop the test at any point for any reason, including pain, fear of pain, anxiety, or lack of motivation. The PWPE is a 4-h, 1-day evaluation. It has a structured scoring system and must be performed by certified professionals, such as a licensed physical therapist.

The PWPE is divided into 36 tasks in seven sections. The most important tasks are dynamic strength, position tolerance, mobility, fine motor, balance, coordination, and endurance. The outcomes of these tasks determine the maximum safety level of performance in each task. An overall level of work for each section can be determined which then are combined together for the overall level of work.

The PWPE combines inputs from many tasks into a categorical overall level of work—very heavy, heavy, medium, light, sedentary, and unable to perform even sedentary work. These levels are used as defined by the US Department of Labor in the dictionary of occupational titles (Table 12.1). Even though it is a 3–4 h test, it can project performance of an 8-h workday. Most importantly, it takes into account the overall level of client participation and self-limiting behavior, which is what the patient feels that he can do versus a maximal effort of work. For example, if we assess that the patient is able to go back to work, but only at a new lower level of work: light or sedentary, and his job description recommends heavy or very heavy work, then the patient cannot go back to his former level of work. This assessment helps guide return to work decisions and to make a final disability assessment.

Table 12.1: Classification of occupational work as defined by the US Department of Labor

Classification	*Description*
V-Very heavy work	Exerting in excess of 100 lb of force occasionally, and/or in excess of 50 lb of force frequently, and/or in excess of 20 lb of force constantly to move objects. Physical Demand requirements are in excess of those for heavy work.
H-Heavy work	Exerting 50–100 lb of force occasionally, and/or 25–50 lb of force frequently, and/or 10–20 lb of force constantly to move objects. Physical Demand requirements are in excess of those for medium work.
M-Medium work	Exerting 20–50 lb of force occasionally, and/or 10–25 lb of force frequently, and/or greater than negligible up to 10 lb of force constantly to move objects. Physical demand requirements are in excess of those for light work.
L-Light work	Exerting up to 20 lb of force occasionally, and/or up to 10 lb of force frequently, and/or a negligible amount of force constantly (constantly: activity or condition exists 2/3 or more of the time) to move objects. Physical demand requirements are in excess of those for sedentary work. Even though the weight lifted may be only a negligible amount, a job should be rated light work: (1) when it requires walking or standing to a significant degree; or (2) when it requires sitting most of the time but entails pushing and/or pulling of arm or leg controls; and/or (3) when the job requires working at a production rate pace entailing the constant pushing and/or pulling of materials even though the weight of those materials is negligible. Note: The constant stress and strain of maintaining a production rate pace, especially in an industrial setting, can be and is physically demanding of a worker even though the amount of force exerted is negligible.
S-Sedentary work	Exerting up to 10 lb of force occasionally (occasionally: activity or condition exists up to 1/3 of the time) and/or a negligible amount of force frequently (frequently: activity or condition exists from 1/3 to 2/3 of the time) to lift, carry, push, pull, or otherwise move objects, including the human body. Sedentary work involves sitting most of the time, but may involve walking or standing for brief periods of time. Jobs are sedentary if walking and standing are required only occasionally and all other sedentary criteria are met.

New York University, among other institutions, uses this FCE because it is feasible, user-friendly and safe. An advantage is the 1-day, 4-h evaluation structure, as opposed to evaluations where the patient has to return for a second or even third day. Subjects using this assessment have a user-friendly procedure manual, complete with summary reports. The equipment used to carry out the evaluation is portable; however, some minor assembly is required. Parameters like overall strength, pushing, pulling, and handgrip strength are measured. Individual tasks may also be administered for job-specific or injury-specific testing.

Since PWPE primarily measures physical abilities, it cannot be used to assess complex behavioral factors, like self-limiting behaviors. One should not imply or assume that these behavioral, psychosocial, or motivational factors may influence the patient when he returns to work. This must be carefully taken into consideration. Even though the self-limiting behavior is not measured, if the patient subjectively communicates that he cannot complete 10 out of the 18 tasks, for example, it can be presumed that some physical or other limitations are present. One could conclude that if the patient goes back to work, he will not be able to do his job even though in reality he may be functionally able to do so.

SUBJECTIVE TOOLS

The Oswestry Disability Index: Low Back Pain Disability Questionnaire

Most functional assessment questionnaires are based on the patient's own perception of the pain. The Oswestry Disability Index is a disease-specific functional assessment questionnaire used specifically for low back pain. It has ten questions on a 0 to 5 ordinary scale and evaluates how low back pain impacts the activities of daily living. It covers pain related to daily activities, such as sleeping, sex life, social life, and traveling (Table 12.2). The total sum of responses is used to grade level of disability, with a higher score signifying a greater disability (Table 12.3). The questionnaire has good validity and responsiveness.

Roland Morris Questionnaire

The Roland Morris Questionnaire is another disease-specific functional assessment for low back pain. It contains 24 "yes" or "no" questions with items directed at functional limitations, i.e. difficulty getting out of an easy chair, pain, sleep, appetite, and mood. It has strong validity and responsiveness and is shown to predict long-term functional limitations, secondary to back pain. It is helpful in evaluating improvement over time. However, unlike the Oswestry Disability Index, which grades the type of disability by level, the questionnaire does not provide a descriptive level.

The McGill Pain Questionnaire

The McGill pain questionnaire reflects three primary dimensions of pain:

Table 12.3: Scoring rubric of the Oswestry Disability Index

Raw score	*Level of disability*
0–10	Minimal disability – no treatment necessary
11–20	Mild disability – conservative treatment recommended
21–30	Severe disability – detailed investigation required
31–40	Crippling disability – severe intervention required
41–50	Bed bound

Table 12.2: Question topic and example with respective score on the Oswestry Disability Index

Question	*Topic*	*Example*	*Score*
1	Pain intensity	Painkillers give complete relief from pain	2
2	Personal care	I need help every day in most aspects of self-care	4
3	Lifting	I can lift only very lightweights	4
4	Walking	Pain prevents me walking more than 1 mile	1
5	Sitting	I can sit in any chair as long as I like	0
6	Standing	Pain prevents me from standing at all	5
7	Sleeping	Pain prevents me from sleeping at all	5
8	Sex life	My sex life is severely restricted by pain	3
9	Social life	My social life is normal but increases the degree of pain	1
10	Traveling	I can travel anywhere without extra pain	0

1. Sensory - discriminative
2. Motivational - effective
3. Cognitive - evaluative

It has a high reliability and good validity. The maximum pain score is a 78, with higher scores corresponding to greater levels of pain. The McGill Pain Questionnaire can be used to evaluate a person experiencing significant pain, to monitor pain over time or to determine an effectiveness of any intervention.

Medical Outcomes Study SF-36

The Medical Outcomes Study short form-36 is not a disease-specific evaluation. It evaluates general health status and can be used effectively for specific conditions when paired with another disease-specific measure. It has eight domains—physical functioning, bodily pain, and role imitation caused by physical health issues, role imitations caused by emotional issues, energy fatigue, mental health, social functioning, and general health perceptions. This measure also has good reliability and validity.

In summary, early focus on disability as a direct effect of impairment has given way to new approaches that are acknowledging subjective factors. In addition to evaluating the underlining permanent pathology, assessment of individual functional status should be incorporated in disability evaluations. Inclusion of subjective information into disability determinations, using a patient centered approach, may provide unknown factors that are imperative for patient prognosis and return to work determinations.

REFERENCES

1. Pransky GS, Dempsey PG. Practical aspects of functional capacity evaluations. J Occup Rehabil. 2004;14(3):217-29.
2. Gibson L, Strong J, Wallace A. Functional capacity evaluation as a performance measure: evidence for a new approach for clients with chronic back pain. Clin J Pain. 2005;21(3):207-15.
3. Koval KJ, Skovron ML, Aharonoff GB, et al. Predictors of functional recovery after hip fracture in the elderly. Clin Orthop Relat Res. 1998;348:22-8.
4. Soer R, van der Schans CP, Geertzen JH, et al. Normative values for a functional capacity evaluation. Arch Phys Med Rehabil. 2009;90(10):1785-94.
5. King PM, Tuckwell N, Barrett TE. A critical review of functional capacity evaluations. Phys Ther. 1998;78(8):852-66.
6. Isernhagen SJ. Principles of prevention for cumulative trauma. Occup Med. 1992;7(1):147-53.
7. Lechner DE, Jackson JR, Roth DL, et al. Reliability and validity of a newly developed test of physical work performance. J Occup Med. 1994;36(9):997-1004.

CHAPTER

13

Non-MRI Evaluation of the Cervical and Lumbar Spine

Tony Wong, Gina Ciavarra, Leon Rybak

INTRODUCTION

Magnetic resonance imaging (MRI) has revolutionized spine imaging, allowing for exquisite detailed evaluation of both osseous and soft tissue structure in a multiplanar format without the use of ionizing radiation. However, MRI has several limitations. First, MR images can underestimate the degree of osseous contributions in cases of stenosis. Second, patients are limited to being prone or supine during imaging, as high-field systems do not allow for recreation of the weight-bearing or dynamic positions that may have resulted in clinical symptoms. Third, patients who are claustrophobic or have certain implants are not MRI candidates. Fourth, while some investigators are using MRI for interventional guidance, the logistics of using this modality in spinal procedures are so complex that most practitioners continue to use fluoroscopy or computed tomography (CT) in the majority of their procedures. Due to these drawbacks of MRI, other imaging modalities—including plain radiographs, CT, and nuclear imaging—still play an important role in the diagnosis and treatment of patients with spine disease.

RADIOGRAPHS

Due to their widespread availability, ease of acquisition, and low cost, radiographs are often the first line imaging study obtained when evaluating the spine. Plain films can be particularly valuable in the evaluation of acute trauma, complicated low back pain, instability, and postoperative patient followup.[1]

There is evidence supporting the use of CT for initial imaging of the cervical spine trauma patient when the scenario meets either the National Emergency X-Radiography Utilization Study (NEXUS) or the Canadian C-Spine Rule (CCR) criteria.[1-3] However, if clinical suspicion is low, radiographs are sometimes used instead. For such a patient, flexion and extension views should only be used to address specific clinical concerns, as their routine use is of low yield and may aggravate an existing injury.[4] Instead, the most important view for the evaluation of cervical trauma is the lateral view, where the smooth continuity of the anterior vertebral, posterior vertebral, and spinolaminar lines can be assessed (Fig. 13.1); the disruption of any of these lines may be indicative of an injury.

Radiographs can provide a general assessment of the spine for patients with complicated low back pain (Box 13.1), possibly revealing nondegenerative or traumatic

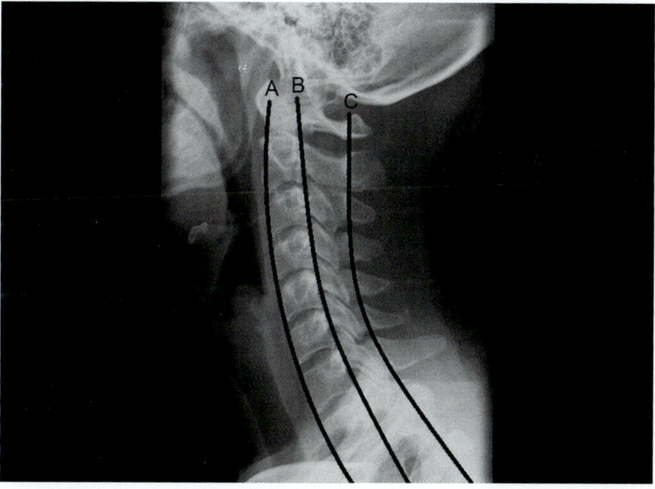

Fig. 13.1: (A) The anterior vertebral, (B) posterior vertebral, and (C) spinolaminar lines should have a smooth contour without disruption.

causes of pain. For example, the presence of compression fractures can indicate underlying osteoporosis or malignancy, and the presence of syndesmophytes can signify ankylosing spondylitis. Limited evaluation of portions of the pelvis may also demonstrate the presence of hip disease, sacroiliitis, or sacral insufficiency fractures, all of which can mimic lumbar spine disease. Intervertebral disk space narrowing, end-plate osteophyte formation, and facet arthrosis can all be easily identified with respect to degenerative changes (Fig. 13.2). Flexion and extension radiographs offer a distinct advantage in allowing for a dynamic assessment of instability that can be occult on other static imaging modalities (Figs. 13.3A and B); this abnormal motion between vertebral bodies may be a cause of pain and ultimately require surgical fusion. Although variable thresholds exist defining the normal range of motion, a grading scheme based on degree of translation of one vertebral body upon another can be applied (Box 13.2).[8,9]

Box 13.1: Indications of complicated low back pain

- Trauma
- Unexplained weight loss, insidious onset
- Age >50 years, especially women, and males with osteoporosis or compression fracture
- Unexplained fever, history of infection
- Immunosuppression, diabetes mellitus
- History of cancer
- Intravenous drug use
- Prolonged use of corticosteroids, osteoporosis
- Age >70 years
- Focal neurologic deficit(s), cauda equina syndrome
- Duration longer than 6 weeks
- Prior surgery

Adapted from ACR appropriateness criteria on low back pain.[5-7]

Dynamic images can also be useful in evaluating the spine for the presence of intervertebral disk vacuum phenomenon. This frequent incidental finding seen in the radiographs of many patients can be elicited by extension, which generates negative pressure resulting in the extraction of nitrogen gas from the extracellular fluid into the disk space (Fig. 13.4).[10] It is a reliable indicator of a degenerated disk and, more importantly, makes the presence of concomitant infection highly unlikely.[11]

Oblique radiographs can be very useful in the setting of spondylolisthesis. The Wiltse-Newman classification outlines the many causes of spondylolisthesis (Box 13.3). Type II, or isthmic, spondylolisthesis is commonly seen in young athletes, due to acute or repetitive microtrauma, and is associated with fractures of the pars interarticularis. Pars defects, which are usually difficult to detect on routine anteroposterior (AP) and lateral views, may be more apparent on oblique views, appearing as the abnormal lucencies described in the literature as the "collar" around the neck of the Scottie Dog (Figs. 13.5 and 13.6).

Box 13.2: Spondylolisthesis grading

- Grade 1: 0–25%
- Grade 2: 26–50%
- Grade 3: 51–75%
- Grade 4: >75%

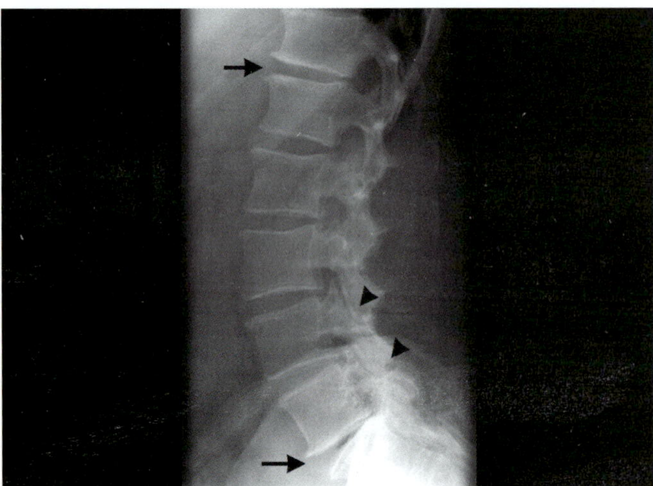

Fig. 13.2: Disk space narrowing and sclerosis with end-plate osteophyte formation (arrows) and facet arthrosis (arrow heads).

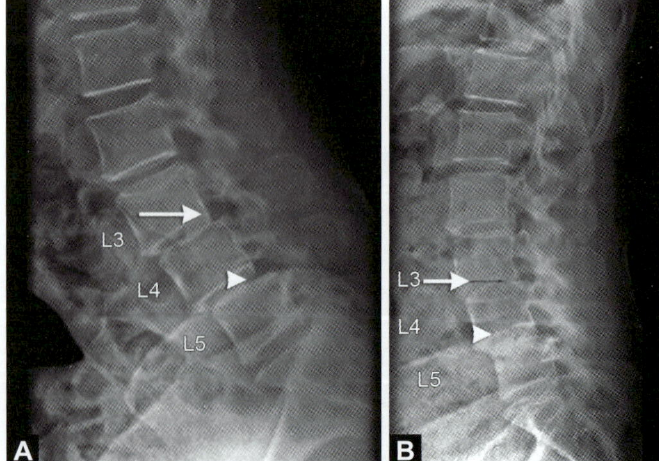

Figs. 13.3A and B: Dynamic instability with increased degree of anterolisthesis of L3 on L4 (arrows) and stable anterolisthesis of L4 on L5 (arrowheads) between (A) flexion and (B) extension.

Box 13.3: Wiltse–Newman classification of spondylolisthesis[12]

- Dysplastic
- Isthmic
  - pars disruption from stress fracture
  - pars elongation without disruption from repetitive healed microfractures
  - acute pars fracture
- Degenerative
- Traumatic
- Pathologic

Plain radiographs are indispensable to the evaluation of both coronal and sagittal alignment, as well as disk space narrowing and listhesis elicited only upon weight bearing, as they may be obtained in the standing position. Both AP and lateral standing views of the spine are necessary for the evaluation of scoliosis (Fig. 13.7). Lateral bending films and films obtained with the use of a bolster can both be used in differentiating rigid structural curves from secondary flexible curves, and in determining the number of levels to be included in corrective surgeries; possible associated segmentation anomalies can also be identified (Fig. 13.8).

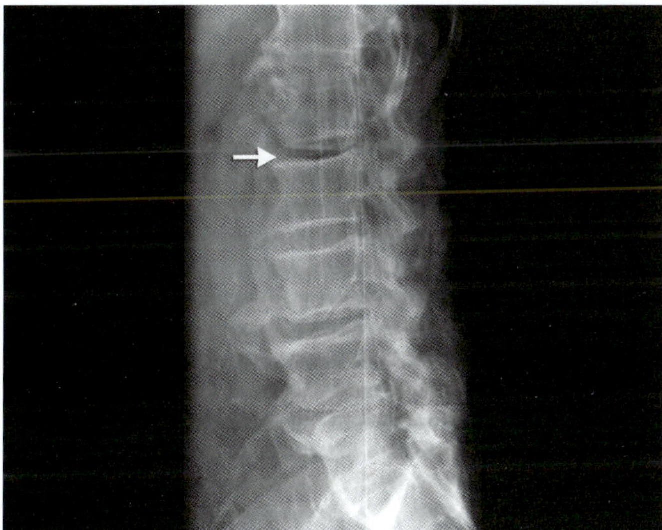

Fig. 13.4: Multilevel discogenic degenerative change with a vacuum disk (arrow).

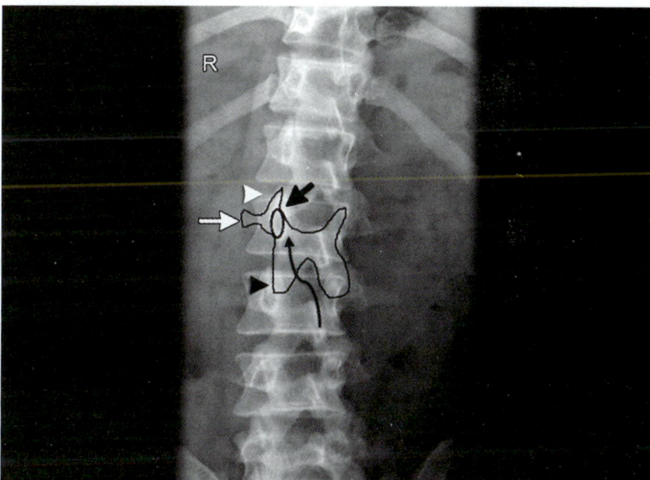

Fig. 13.5: Scottie dog: right pedicle (black arrow); right inferior articular process (white arrowhead); right transverse process (white arrow); right superior articular process (black arrowhead); right pars (squiggly black arrow).

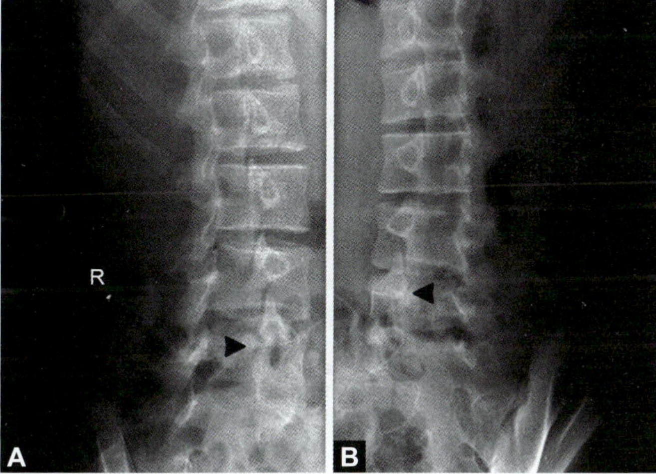

Figs. 13.6A and B: Bilateral pars fractures (arrowheads) through the neck of the Scottie dog.

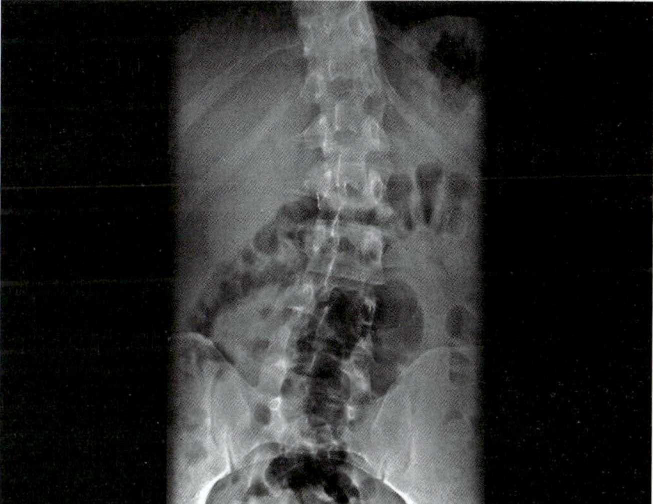

Fig. 13.7: Idiopathic lumbar scoliosis with leftward curvature.

The development of the EOS machine has enabled the acquisition of high-resolution scoliosis films. The standing X-ray unit, which looks a bit like a phone booth, operates in part on Nobel Prize winning detector technology that allows for the rapid, biplanar acquisition of low-dose, full-body images in 25 seconds or less. Slot scanning technology, employing a pressurized gas detector, minimizes scatter radiation, thus maximizing the signal-to-noise ratio and allowing for equal or greater image quality at lower doses as compared to plain radiograph (Figs.13.9A and B). Additionally, an internal calibration system optimizes the dynamic contrast range over all portions of the images; this uniform high image quality can reduce the repeat rate for nondiagnostic studies. When assessing pediatric scoliosis, where the nature of the disease may call for multiple follow-up examinations to assess progression, the dose savings provided by the EOS machine over time can be substantial. Additional postprocessing software allows for the creation of 3D images that may make the assessment of new clinical parameters a reality. However, imaging with the EOS is limited to patients who can assume the standing position.

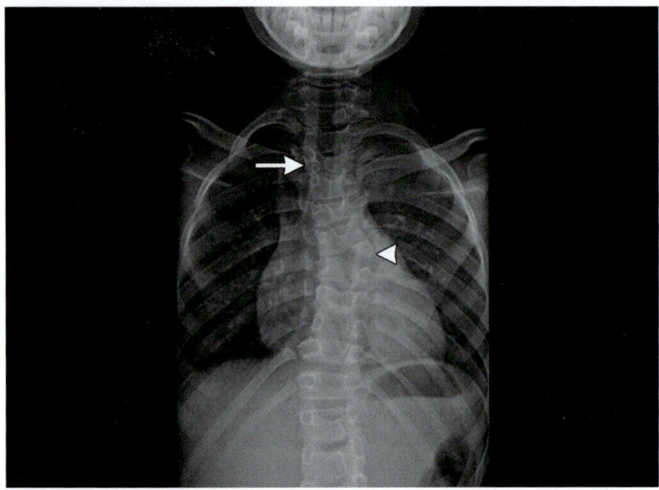

Fig. 13.8: Thoracic scoliosis caused by butterfly (arrow) and hemivertebrae (arrowhead) segmentation anomalies.

Spinal hardware does not generate problematic artifacts on plain radiographs, as it does on CT and MRI (Fig. 13.10). Thus, radiographs are valuable in the assessment of both alignment and instability in postoperative patients presenting with back pain, as well as in initial hardware documentation postoperatively. Later on, the development of hardware failure or adjacent segment disease in the setting of fusion can be detected with sequential radiographs (Figs. 13.11 and 13.12).[13] Infection may also be indicated by lucency surrounding the hardware and erosion of the end plates. Abnormalities noted on radiographs may be further evaluated by MRI when necessary.

COMPUTED TOMOGRAPHY

Computed tomography can be useful when cross-sectional imaging is indicated for further evaluation of findings from plain radiographs, particularly when there are contraindications to MRI. CT may also be used to clarify equivocal MRI findings. Though MRI generally provides higher soft tissue resolution, bony abnormalities

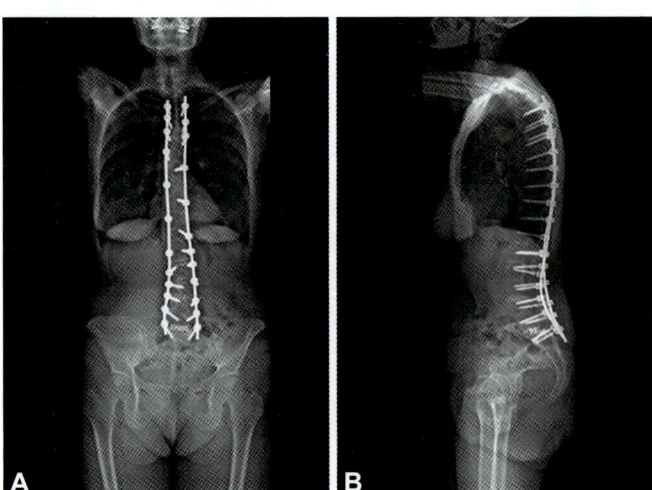

Figs. 13.9A and B: (A) AP and (B) lateral whole body images obtained on the EOS machine following surgery for scoliosis.

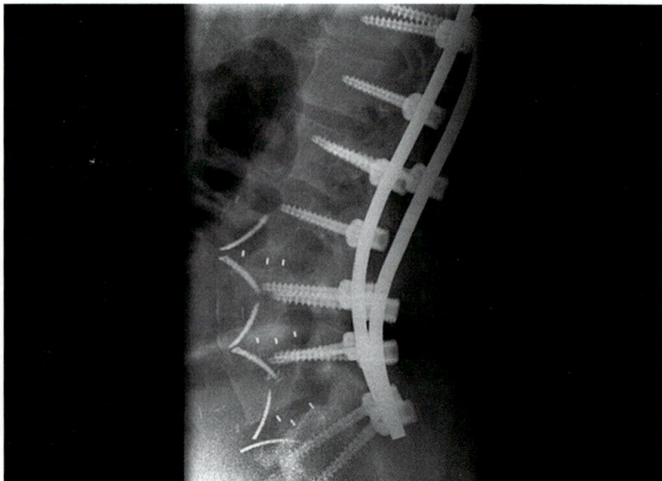

Fig. 13.10: No hardware related artifact in a postoperative patient with lumbar fusion.

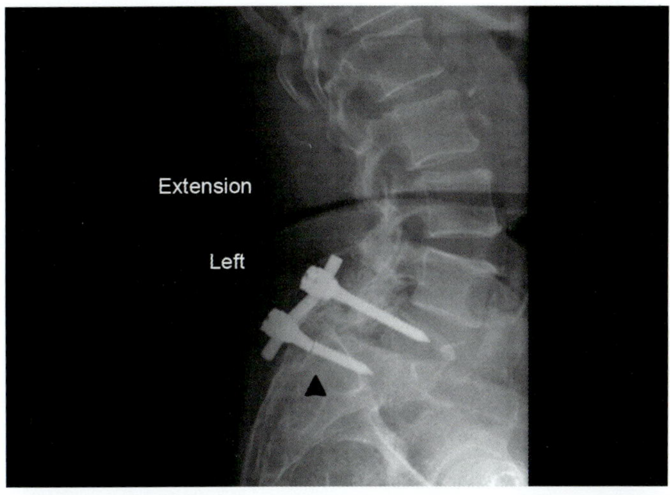

Fig. 13.11: Fracture of an S1 pedicle screw following posterior instrumentation (arrowhead).

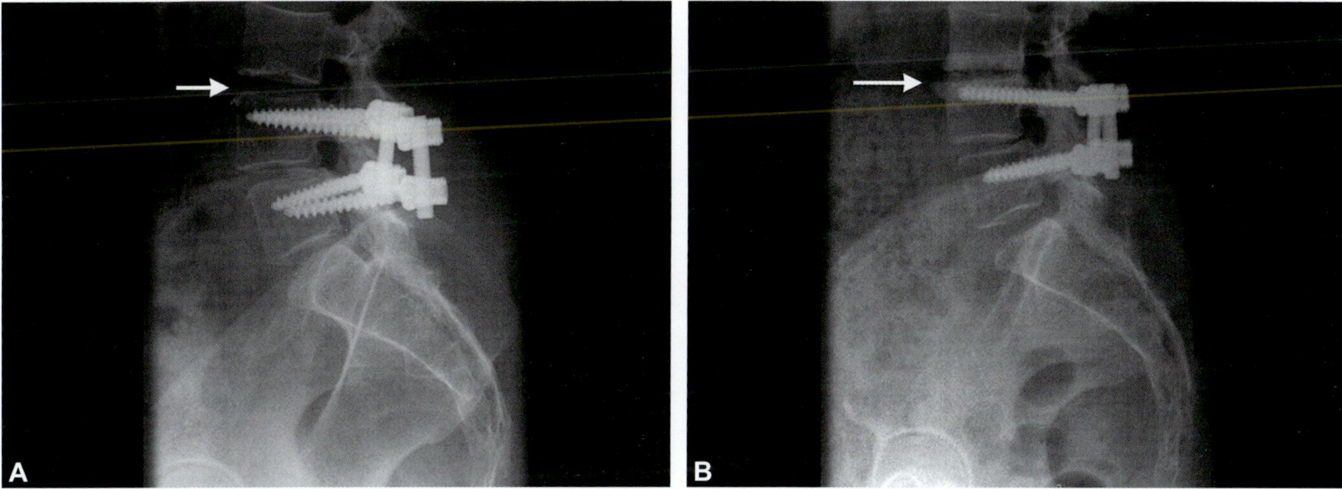

Figs. 13.12A and B: Development of adjacent segment disease (arrow) above the level of fusion (from A to B) with disk space narrowing, end-plate sclerosis, and osteophyte formation.

are better characterized by CT. Other advantages of CT over MRI include faster acquisition speed and lower cost.

As discussed previously, CT is used for post-traumatic evaluation of the spine in patients with significant clinical findings (Figs. 13.13A to C). CT can also be used in the further analysis of equivocal findings from plain radiographs, or as the first line of imaging in an obtunded or unresponsive patient. While CT is excellent for demonstrating the nature of fractures, MRI may still be necessary to evaluate associated soft tissue abnormalities or trauma to the spinal cord.

For patients with back pain suspected to be related to degenerative spine changes or disk herniation, CT may be used in lieu of MRI if it is contraindicated. Degenerative disk disease associated with loss of disk height, end-plate changes, facet hypertrophy, and malalignment can be assessed in three planes. The abnormalities of disk contour—including bulges and herniations—though visible, are not as conspicuous as on MRI because of the lack of contrast between herniated disk material and surrounding soft tissues (Figs. 13.14A and B). Additionally, although CT can identify the degree of central canal and neural foraminal stenosis with similar accuracy to MRI (Figs. 13.15A and B), potential mass effect on the spinal cord or individual nerve roots has to be inferred, since it is not directly visualized.[14] Still, CT remains superior to MRI in delineating the contribution of bone hypertrophy to stenosis (Figs. 13.16A to D). CT also provides added sensitivity in detection of both gas and calcification within the disk or surrounding soft tissues.

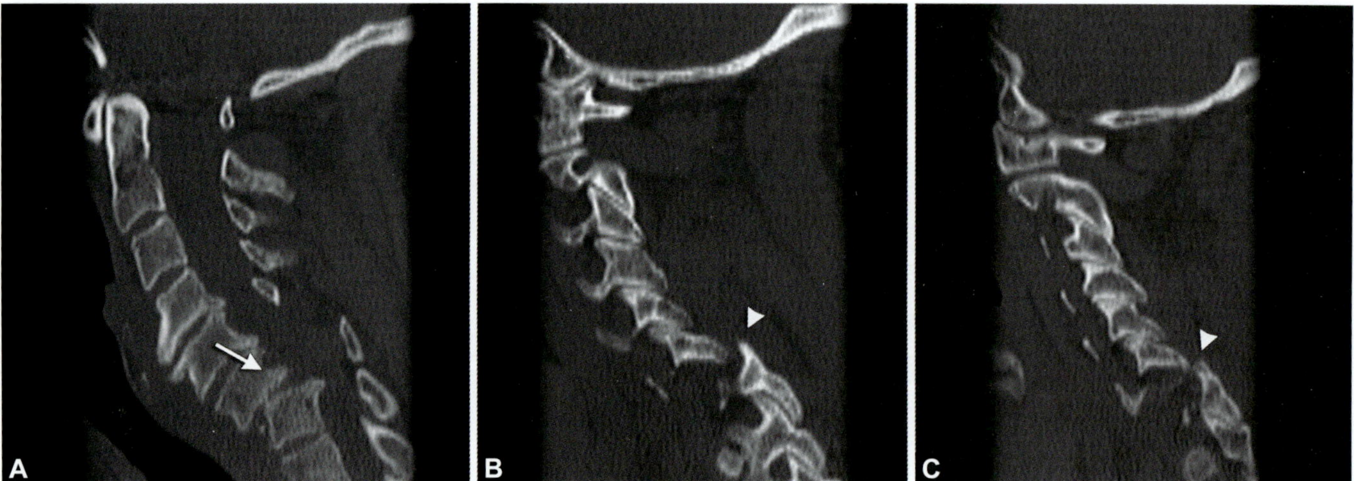

Figs. 13.13A to C: (A) Sagittal midline, (B) right parasagittal, and (C) left parasagittal CT images showing post-traumatic kyphosis with anterolisthesis of C6 on C7 (arrow) and bilateral jumped facets (arrowheads).

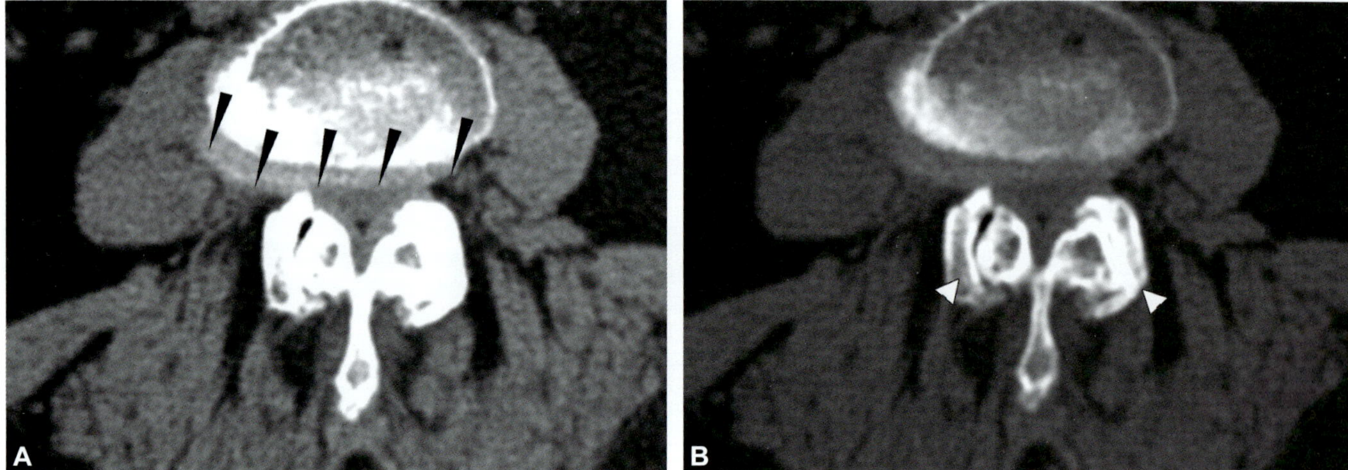

Figs. 13.14A and B: (A) Circumferential disk bulge, eccentric towards right neural foraminal region. (B) Same level showing severe bilateral facet arthrosis with a vacuum right facet.

In the pediatric population, CT can be a useful tool for confirming and further evaluating pars defects identified both on plain radiographs and MRI. CT is the most accurate method for following these patients to assess fracture healing (Figs. 13.17A and B). Thorough evaluation of complex congenital scoliosis with accurate depiction of segmentation anomalies and critical findings like bony bars is also provided (Figs. 13.18A to C).

Computed tomography is valuable in the postoperative setting for the assessment of hardware position and complications. Although metallic hardware can cause a certain amount of artifact on CT imaging, this can be minimized with parameter optimization. The trade-off, unfortunately, can be an increased radiation dose to the patient. Using these techniques, the integrity, positioning, and stability of hardware can be assessed much like on radiographs, but with the added benefit of multiplanar reconstruction. Failure of the hardware including fractures of pedicle screws and stabilization rods is not an uncommon occurrence (Fig. 13.19). Malpositioning of the hardware may result in unintended injury to vital structures. Pedicle screws can encroach upon the spinal canal or terminate in close proximity to major vessels such as the aorta (Figs. 13.20A and B). Graft material can also be displaced into critical areas (Fig. 13.21). Finally, instability or loosening can be diagnosed when more than 2 mm of lucency surrounds the hardware (Figs. 13.22B and 13.24B).[15] The cause of loosening, either septic or aseptic, can ultimately be difficult to differentiate and may require a more extensive workup (Figs. 13.22A and B).

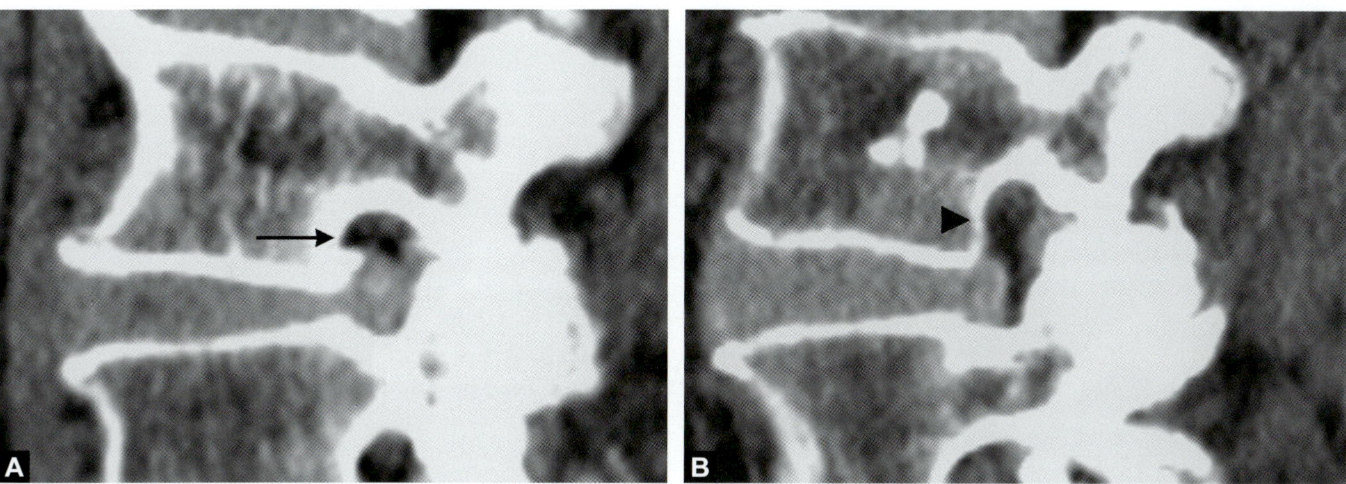

Figs. 13.15A and B: Same level as Figure 13.14 showing moderate to severe right (A) and mild left (B) neural foraminal narrowing due to a disk bulge and facet arthrosis.

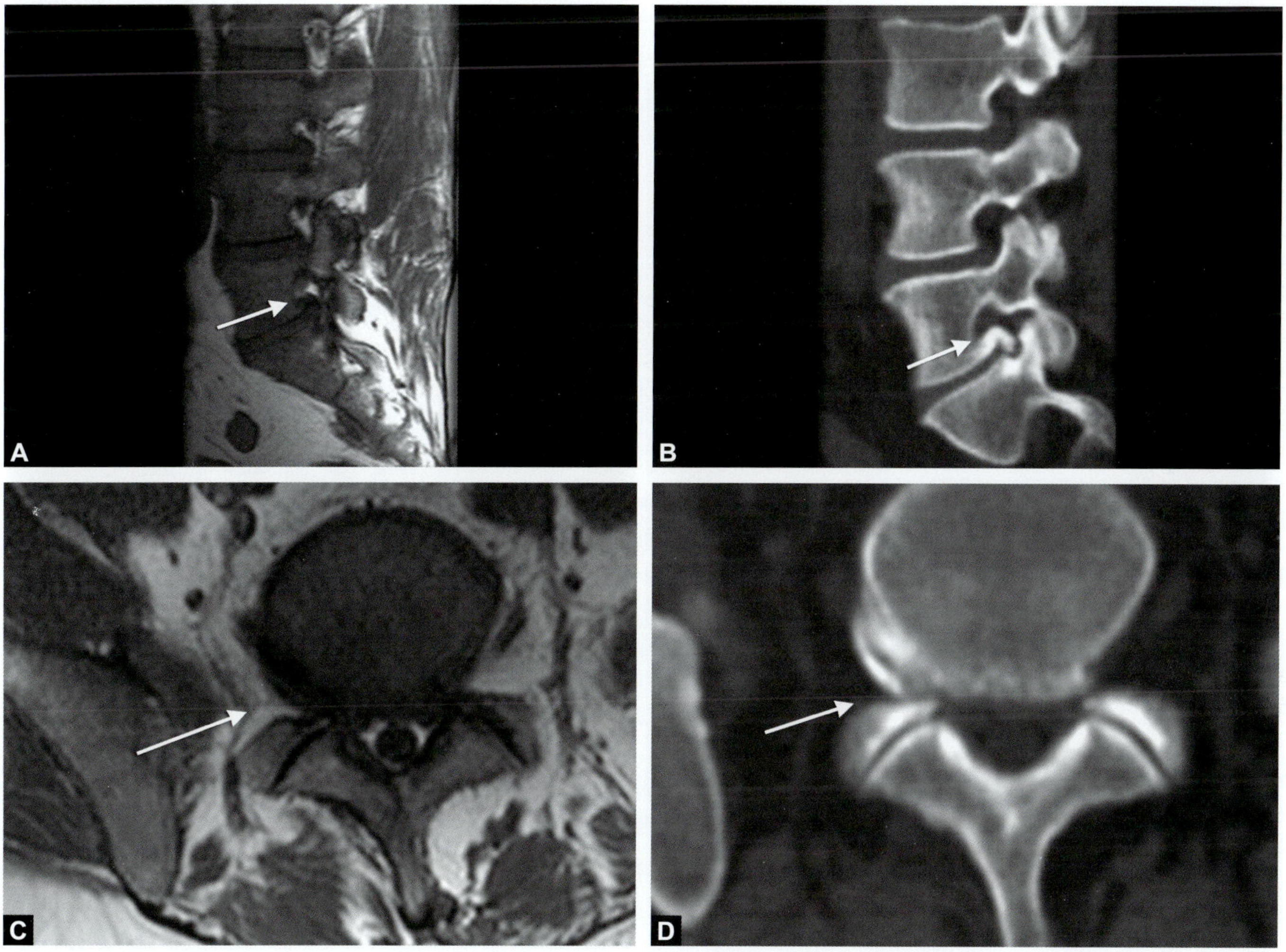

Figs. 13.16A to D: (A) Sagittal and (C) axial T1 weighted MRI images showing an underestimation of the contribution of osseous spurs to right-sided neural foraminal stenosis. Compare with (B) sagittal and (D) axial images from a CT scan of the same patient, which better depicts the bony hypertrophic change causing stenosis.

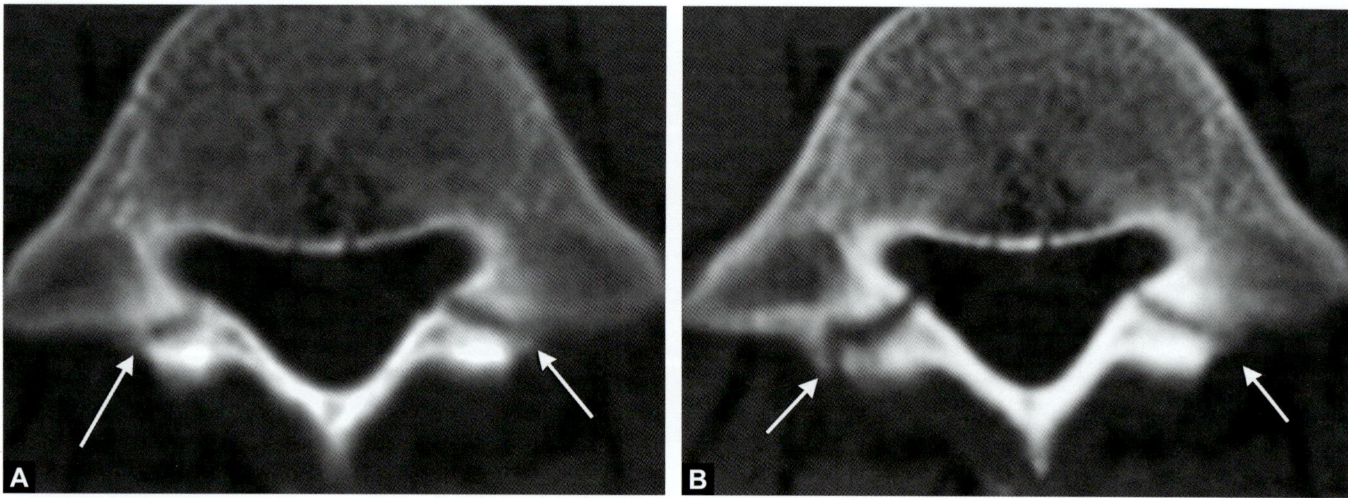

Figs. 13.17A and B: Nonhealing bilateral pars fractures at 1-year CT followup (from A to B).

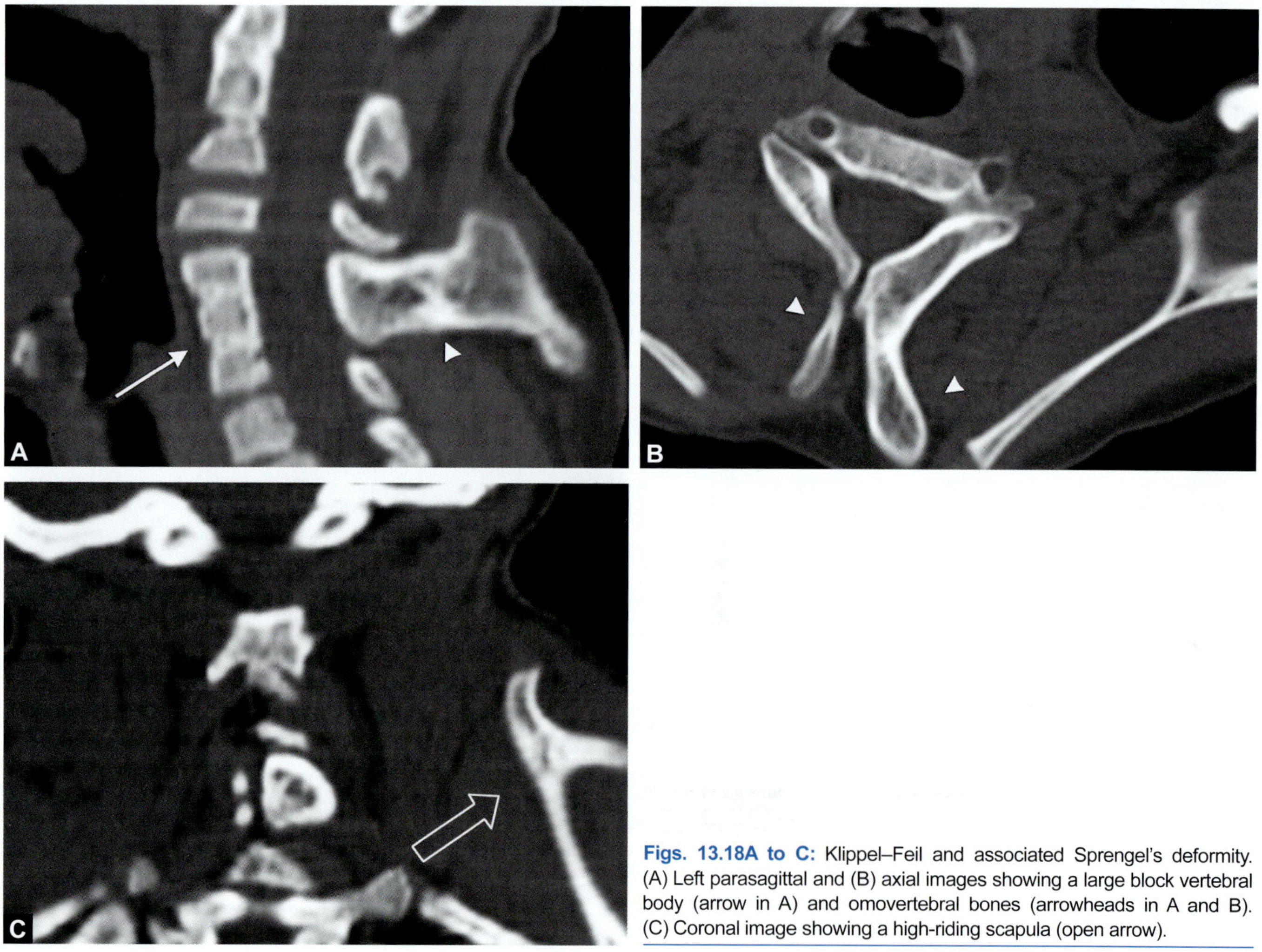

Figs. 13.18A to C: Klippel–Feil and associated Sprengel's deformity. (A) Left parasagittal and (B) axial images showing a large block vertebral body (arrow in A) and omovertebral bones (arrowheads in A and B). (C) Coronal image showing a high-riding scapula (open arrow).

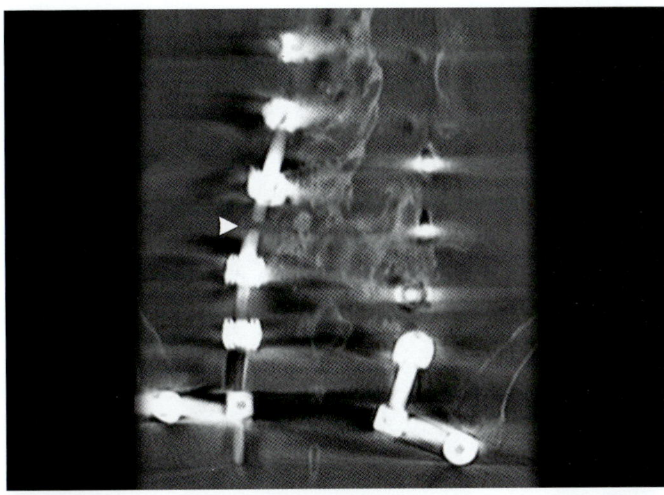

Fig. 13.19: Fracture of the right-sided stabilization rod.

Besides potential hardware complications, assessing the success or failure of fusion after spinal instrumentation is another common indication for imaging. Most fusions involve both hardware to facilitate early stability, and osseous graft material to provide longer term results. If incorporation of the osseous material is not successful, the hardware may in turn be at risk for failure. Thus, it is important not only to assess the hardware but also the formation of a solid fusion mass (Fig. 13.23). An unsuccessful fusion, or pseudoarthrosis, can be a source of postoperative pain that is well evaluated on CT, where the coronal and sagittal planes in particular, can help detect defects in the osseous fusion mass (Figs. 13.24A and 13.25).[16]

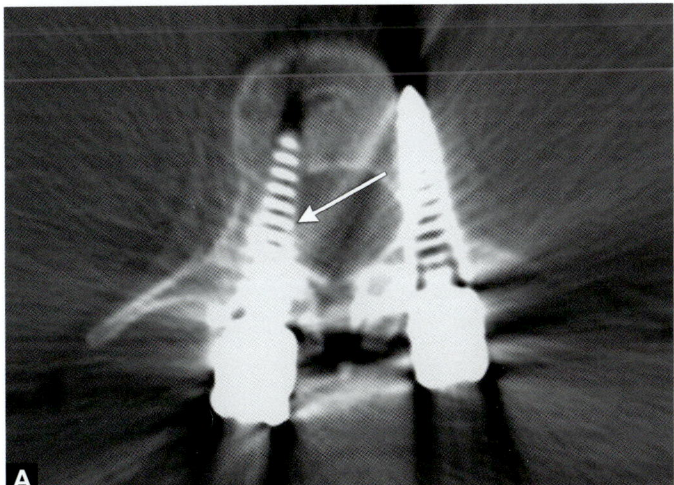

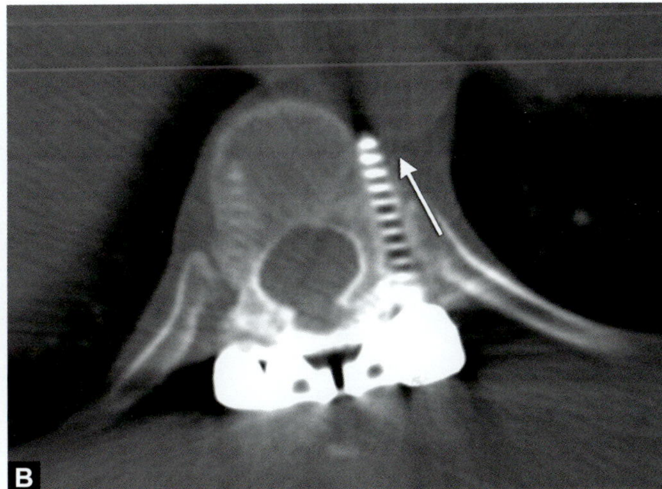

Figs. 13.20A and B: (A) Right-sided pedicle screw encroaching upon the spinal canal. (B) Left-sided pedicle screw going through the anterior vertebral cortex and terminating in close proximity to aorta.

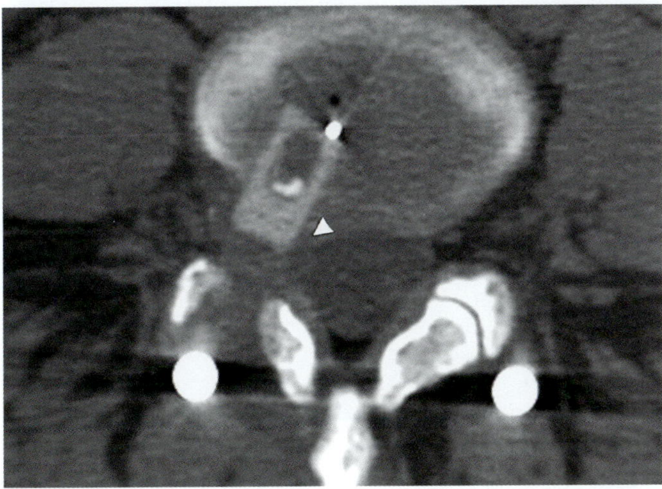

Fig. 13.21: Graft material displaced into right neural foramen following transforaminal lumbar interbody fusion (arrowhead).

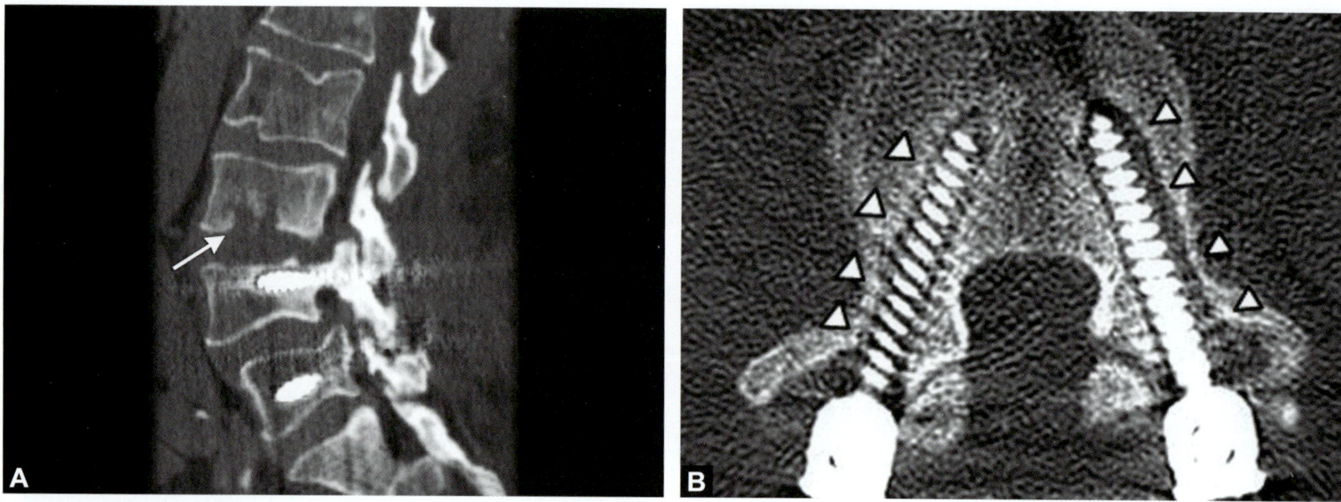

Figs. 13.22A and B: Postoperative infection with erosion of the adjacent end plate (arrow in A) and loosening of the pedicle screws (arrowheads in B).

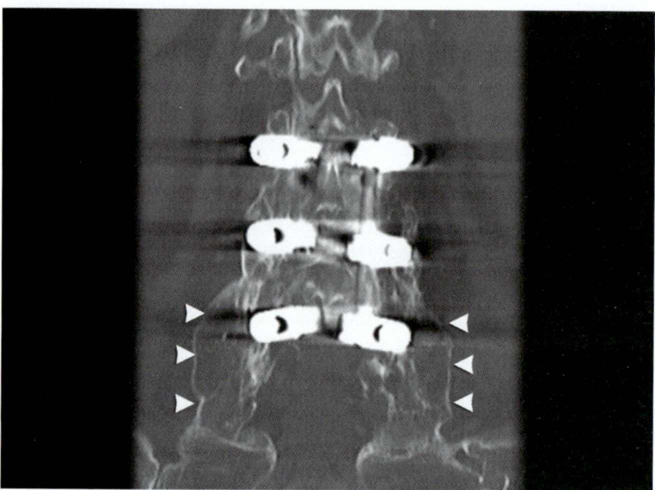

Fig. 13.23: Solid mature posterolateral bony fusion following posterior decompression and instrumentation.

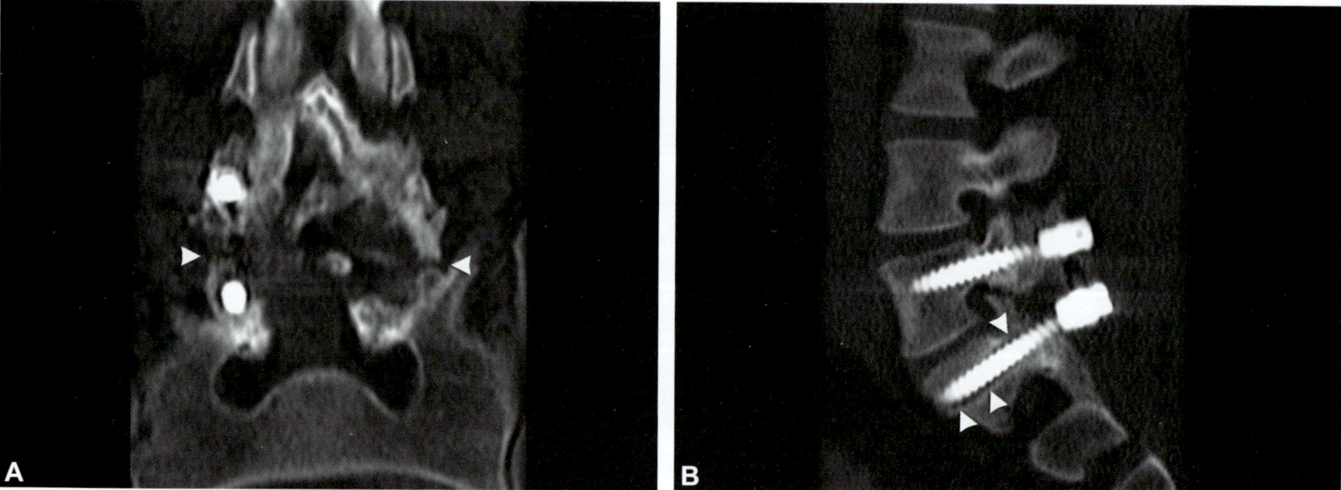

Figs. 13.24A and B: Lack of fusion (arrowheads in A) with associated loosening of inferior pedicle screw (arrowheads in B). Compare with the normal pedicle screw one level above.

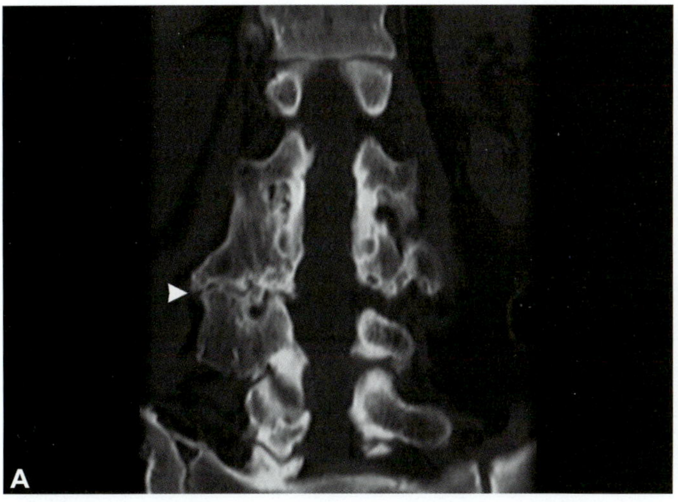

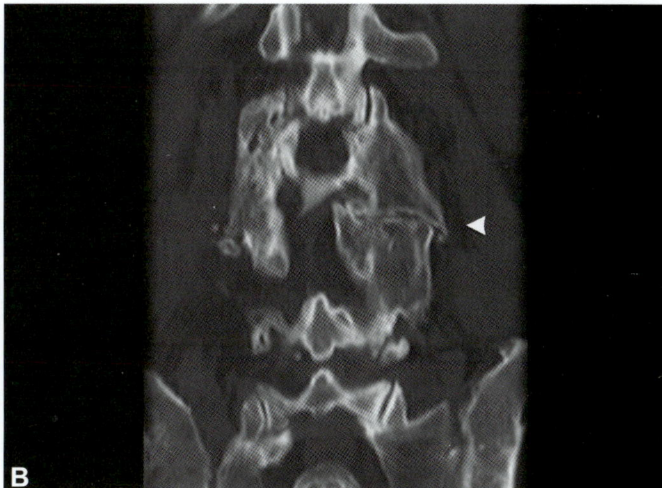

Figs. 13.25A and B: Incomplete fusion resulting in pseudoarthrosis.

Computed tomography can also be used as a problem-solving tool when equivocal findings for certain types of osseous lesions, such as vertebral body hemangiomas, are noted on plain film or MRI. Hemangiomas can have variable signal intensity on MRI, and atypical hemangiomas may be mistaken for more ominous lesions such as metastases. Hemangiomas have a characteristic appearance on CT with vertical struts of bone resulting in a "polka-dot" configuration on axial images or a "corduroy" pattern on coronal and sagittal reconstructions that allows for greater confidence in the diagnosis (Figs. 13.26A to D).[17] Another example of improved bony lesion characterization on CT is with osteoid osteomas. These small tumors can incite a large amount of reactive edema making diagnosis difficult on MRI. However, on CT scan, they have a characteristic appearance of a small lucent nidus, often with a tiny central calcification.[18] Radiofrequency ablation, which is now frequently being used for treatment, is performed under CT guidance (Figs. 13.27A and B).[19]

Computed tomography myelography was once considered the gold standard for diagnosis of nerve compression and disk pathology. But CT myelography is invasive in nature, requiring the installation of intrathecal contrast, and has been largely replaced by MRI.[20] Nevertheless, CT myelography remains a valuable diagnostic tool in situations when MRI is contraindicated. Myelography can also be particularly useful for patients with spinal hardware, as the contrast material outlines the neural structures and demonstrates compression to a greater advantage than conventional CT (Figs. 13.28A and B). Some data even suggest that CT myelography surpasses MRI in evaluation of nerve compression in the lateral recess.[21]

The invasiveness of CT discography makes it a controversial diagnostic tool, but it is the only direct means of evaluating discogenic pain and possible level(s) of origin.[22] Discography can help a surgeon determine which levels need to be addressed during surgery, especially in cases where the clinical findings and imaging are discordant or where there are multiple levels of abnormality (Figs. 13.29A to E). One caveat of discography is that it has only been shown to be of clinical value in patients with an abnormal MRI.[23]

The main drawback of CT use is the amount of radiation involved. With the increasing recognition of CT radiation exposure, judicious use is advised; there should always be a risk-benefit analysis, with special consideration given to younger patients, and females, because of the high potential dose delivered to the breasts and ovaries.[24–26]

NUCLEAR MEDICINE

There are several nuclear medicine tests that can be useful in work up of the spine. The most common and widely used is the bone scan, while other less utilized tests include gallium, tagged white blood cell (WBC), and indium diethylenetriaminepentaacetic acid (In-DTPA) scans. The one common advantage to these, and all other nuclear medicine tests, is that they provide physiologic information.

A bone scan is typically performed to assess for fracture, infection, or neoplasm (Figs. 13.30 and 13.31). Bone scan agents are taken up at sites of bone formation, but activity depends on the degree of regional blood perfusion. Bone formation is a reactive response to any

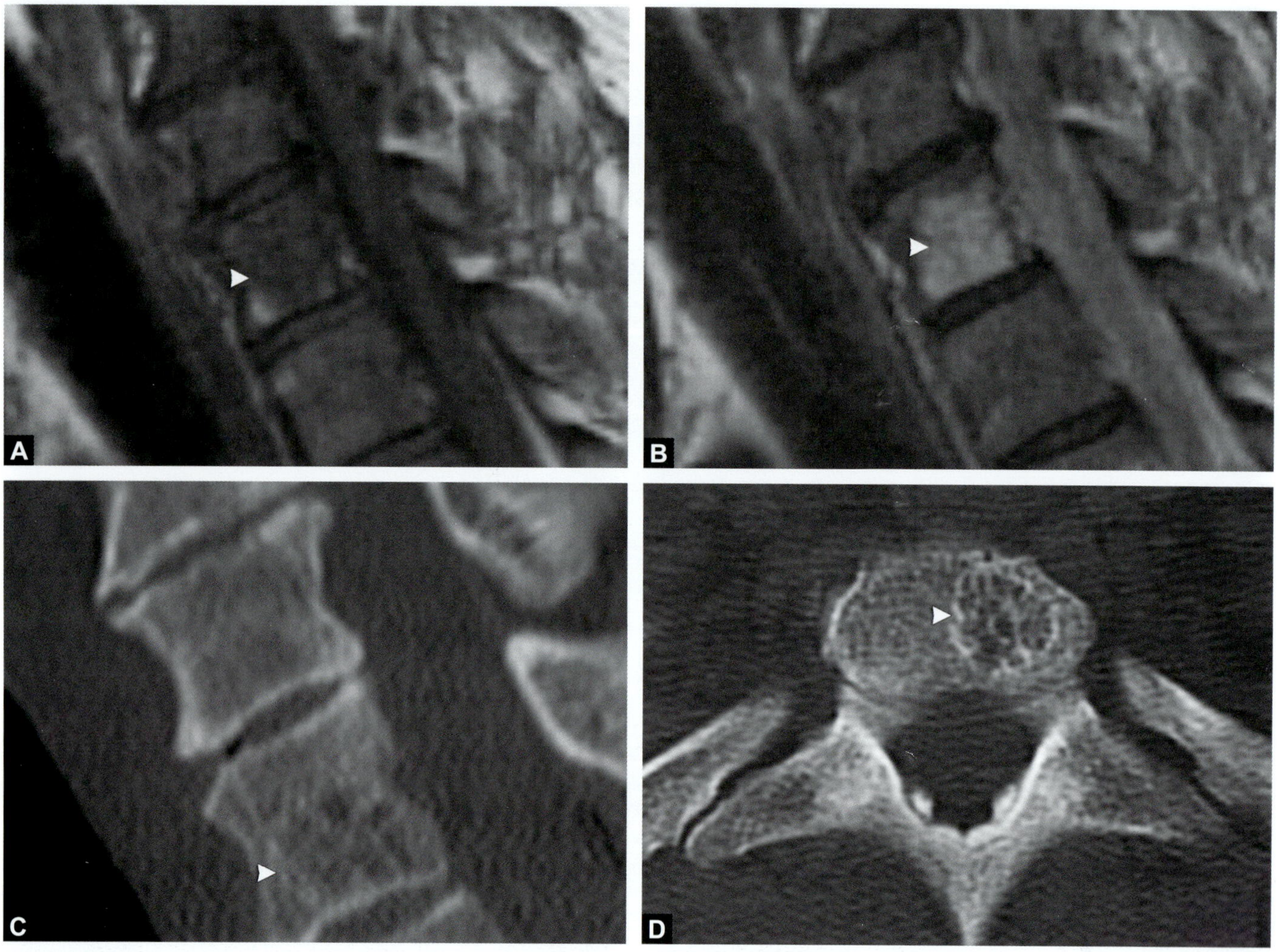

Figs. 13.26A to D: (A) Suspected atypical hemangioma on MRI is hypointense on the T1-weighted image and (B) hyperintense on T2-weighted image. (C and D) CT confirms the diagnosis with the typical appearance of a well-circumscribed lesion containing thickened vertical struts.

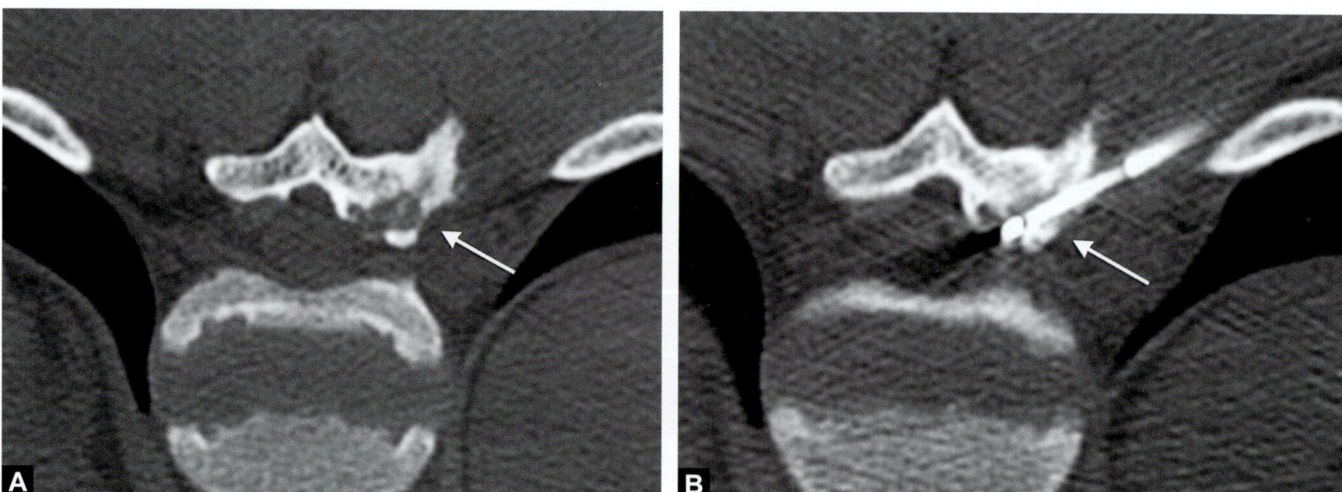

Figs. 13.27A and B: (A) An osteoid osteoma in the lamina with the characteristic appearance of a small lucent nidus and central calcification. (B) CT guided radiofrequency ablation with probe tip positioned in the nidus.

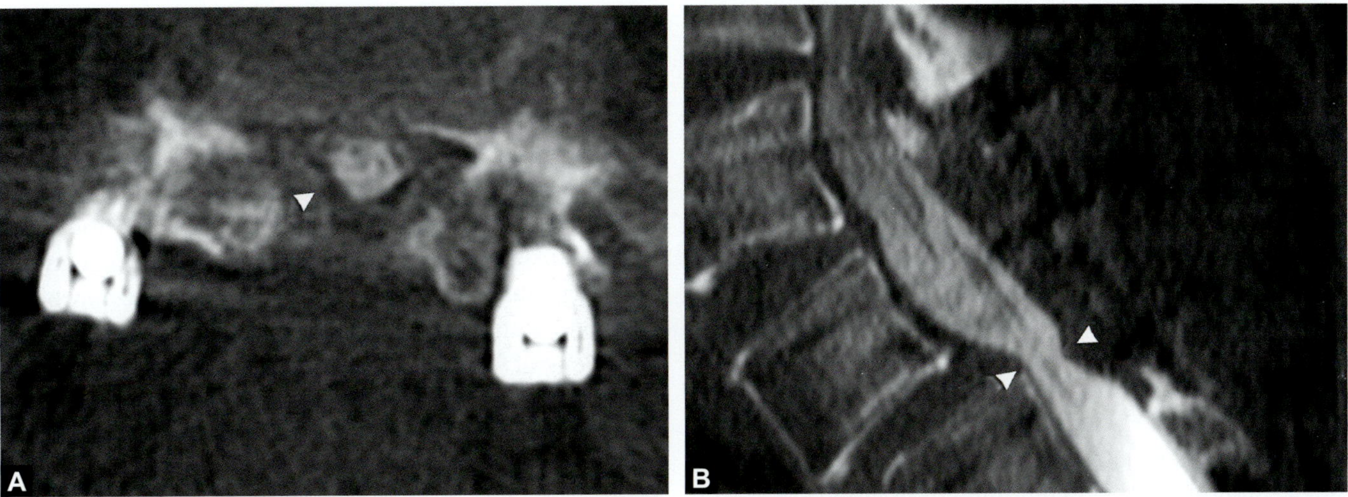

Figs. 13.28A and B: Lumbar myelogram following posterior decompression and instrumentation showing Grade 1 anterolisthesis of L5 on S1 (B) with associated central canal stenosis (A and B).

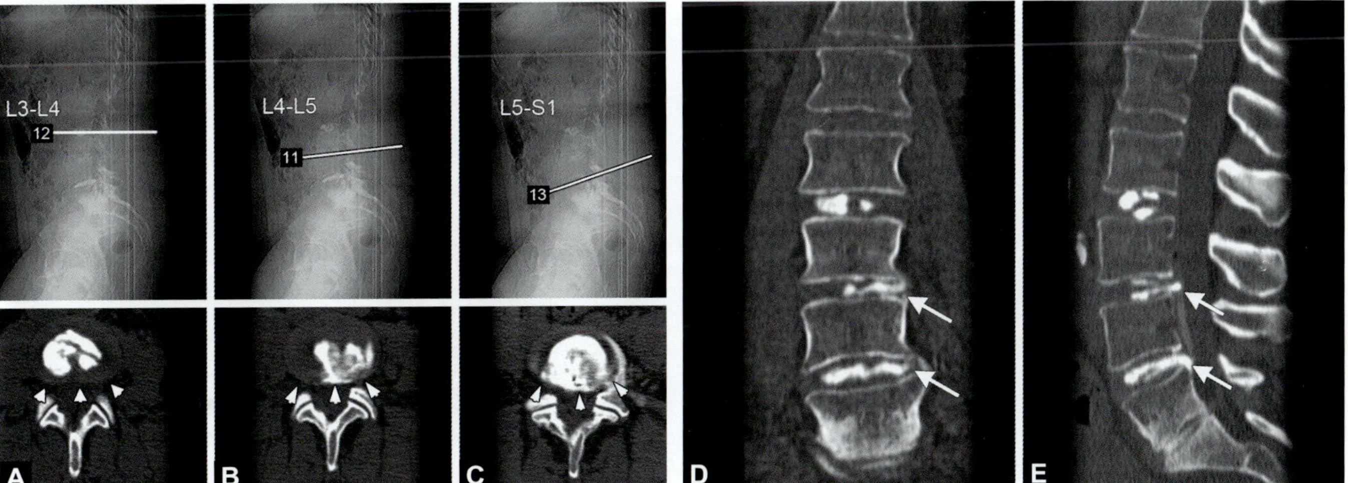

Figs. 13.29A to E: Multilevel CT discography. Normal injection at L3-L4 with contrast confined by annulus fibrosis (arrowheads in A). Annular tears at L4-L5 and L5-S1 with contrast extruding through tears of the annulus fibrosis (arrowheads in B and C, respectively). Coronal and sagittal reconstructions again demonstrating annular tears (arrows in D and E).

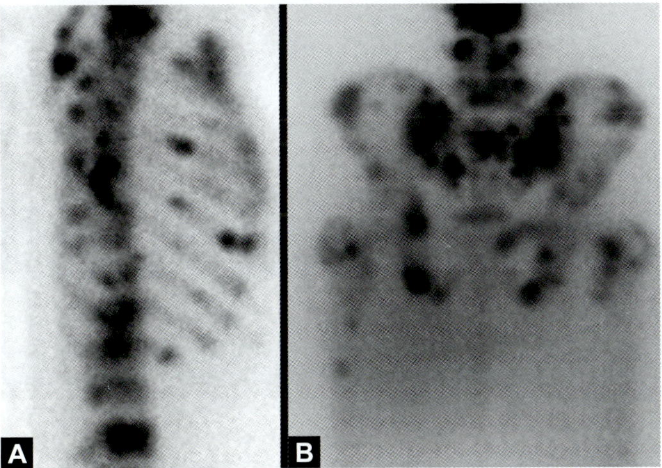

Figs. 13.30A and B: (A) Bone scan (Tc 99m-MDP) showing numerous skeletal metastases in the vertebral bodies and ribs on the lateral view and (B) throughout the lower spine and pelvis on the coronal view.

of the aforementioned entities that, in general, lead to high sensitivity and low specificity with routine imaging. Specificity, though, can be increased when the triple-phase scan replaces the single-phase bone scan.

Bone scans are often obtained in the setting of suspected trauma when radiographs are negative. A fracture typically becomes positive after 24 hours, with activity persisting on subsequent evaluation for up to 2 years.[27] Although the specificity for a fracture may be lacking, there are several characteristic patterns that allow for a confident diagnosis. A sacral insufficiency fracture, for example, classically appears as a 'Honda sign' (Figs. 13.32A and B).[28] A pars fracture can be easily identified once activity is localized to the pars with the addition of single-photon emission computed tomography (SPECT), which provides cross-sectional analysis (Figs. 13.33A and B).

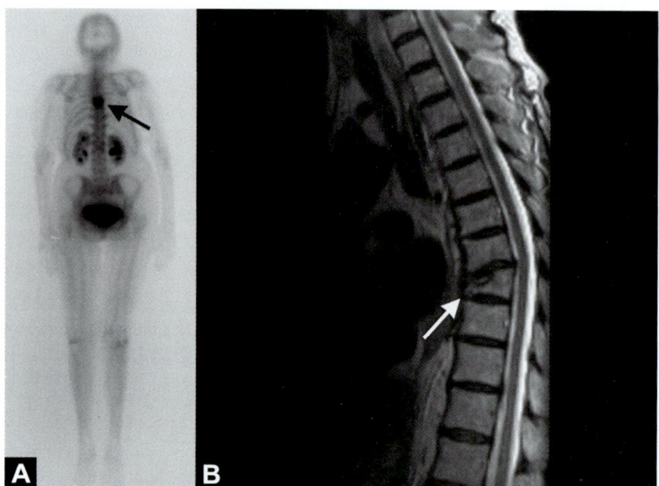

Figs. 13.31A and B: (A) Bone scan (Tc 99m-MDP) showing increased radiotracer activity (B) corresponding to a vertebral body compression fracture on MRI.

Infection in the spine can be detected using a variety of tests, each with varying degrees of sensitivity and specificity. A bone scan is typically not sufficient when performed in isolation. A gallium scan interpreted in conjunction with the bone scan provides a more accurate diagnosis than a bone scan alone. Osteomyelitis is likely when there is either greater gallium uptake in the same area as the bone scan uptake, or if there is an incongruent area of gallium activity. A gallium SPECT alone may be an even better alternative, offering a sensitivity of 91% and a specificity of 92% (Figs. 13.34A to D).[29] One disadvantage of a gallium scan, however, is that it is performed over multiple days, which may create a delay in diagnosis. Patient compliance can also be an issue, as several returns to the nuclear medicine department may be necessary. Tagged WBC scans are not typically used because both increased and decreased activity occurs at nearly equal rates, making interpretation difficult.[30]

Dural tears resulting in cerebrospinal fluid (CSF) leaks are one complication that can occur following spinal instrumentation. One series found an incidence for dural tears of 2% following placement of 648 pedicle screws in 91 total patients.[31] Although its use in detecting a leak in the postoperative setting has not been investigated, In-DTPA scans have a sensitivity ranging from 50% to 100% with a specificity of nearly 100% in detecting CSF leaks in other

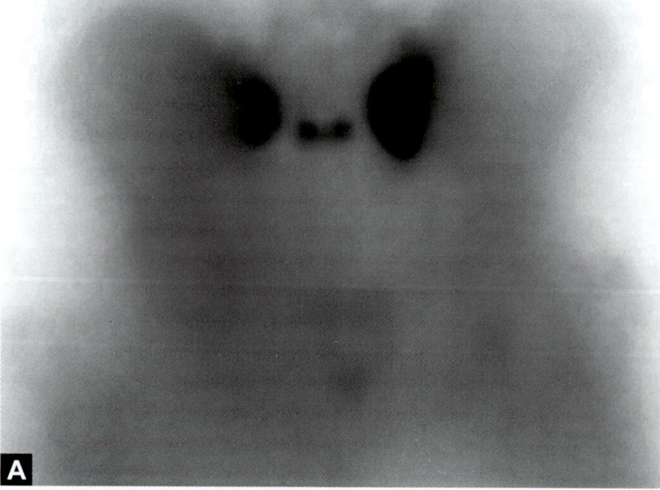

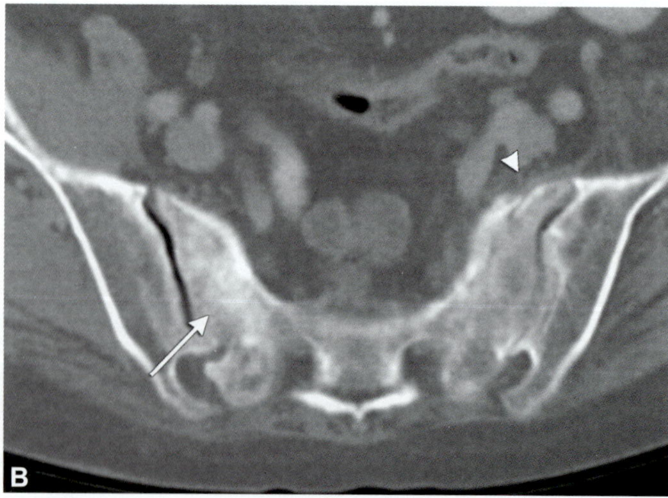

Figs. 13.32A and B: (A) Bone scan (Tc 99m-MDP) showing "Honda sign" with uptake in the sacrum in an H shape. (B) Corresponding CT scan showing sacral insufficiency fracture with abnormal sclerosis in the right sacrum (arrow) and cortical break in left sacrum (arrowhead).

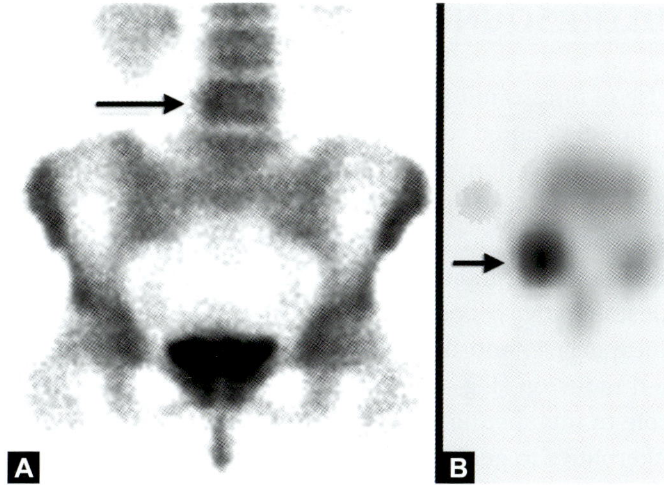

Figs. 13.33A and B: (A) Bone scan (Tc 99m-MDP) showing a right-sided pars fracture with increased uptake at the right side of the L5 vertebral body, (B) which localizes to the pars on the axial SPECT.

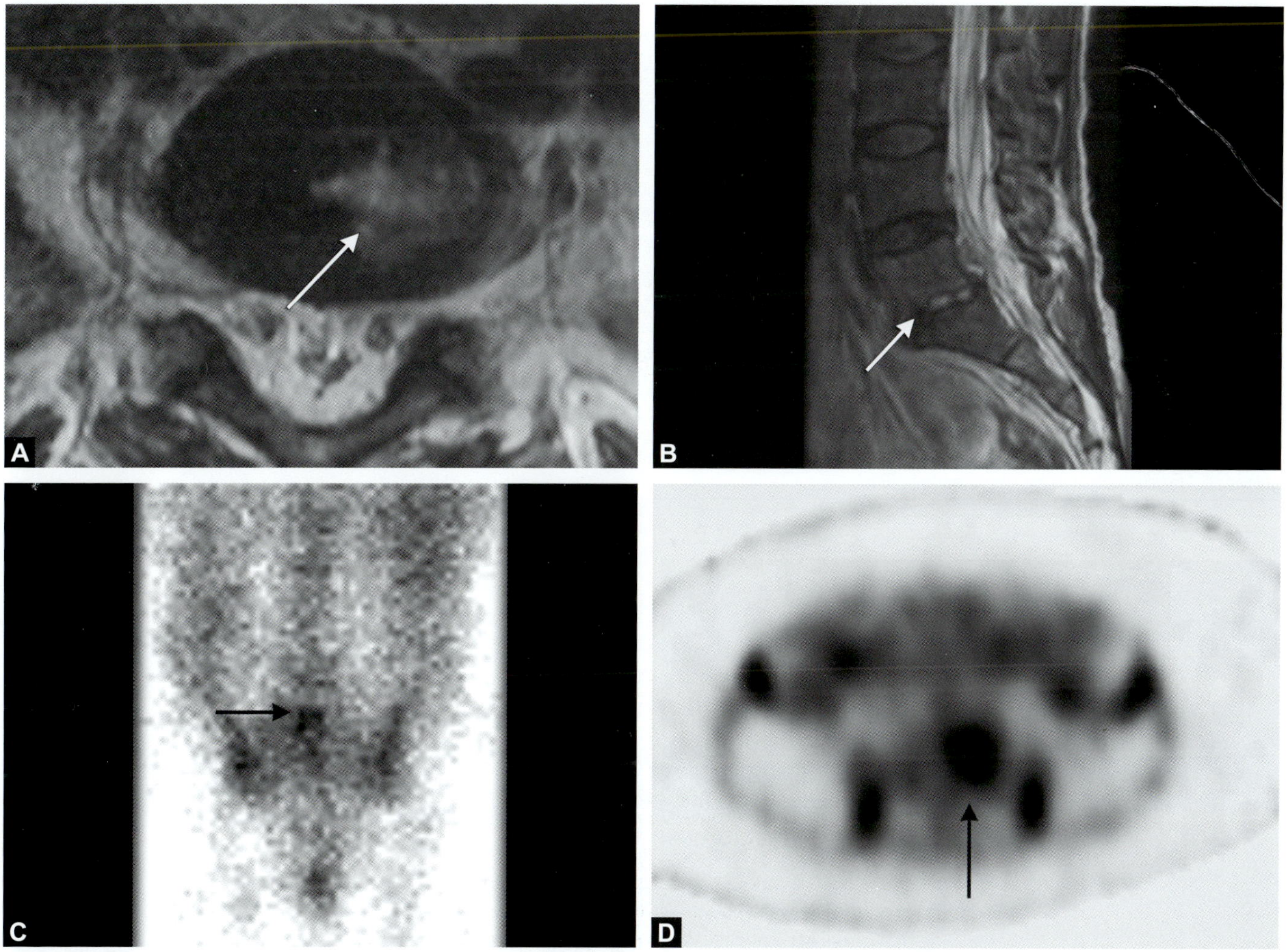

Figs. 13.34A to D: (A and B) T2 hyperintensity in the L5-S1 disk space on MRI suspicious for discitis/osteomyelitis. (C) Findings confirmed on 48-hours delayed gallium scan with increased corresponding uptake on the posterior planar view and (D) the axial SPECT.

scenarios.[32-34] In-DTPA scans require a lumbar puncture for intrathecal administration of the radiotracer and are performed over multiple days.

Despite having the advantage of providing physiologic information, there are several drawbacks to nuclear medicine tests. First, there is radiation exposure, as in CT, with varying doses delivered to organs based upon the physiologic and biologic half-life of the radiotracer, as well as its route of clearance. Second, resolution can be lacking, thus sometimes limiting diagnosis. Although SPECT by itself can improve diagnostic accuracy, fusion techniques including SPECT-CT and positron emission tomography (PET) combined with either CT or MRI, all provide an overlay of nuclear medicine data with correlative anatomic imaging for even better localization of abnormalities.

ULTRASOUND

Use of ultrasound for diagnostic spine imaging is predominantly limited to the pediatric population, since complete ossification of the posterior elements in an adult inhibits the acoustic window. However, ultrasound can evaluate the more superficial tissues, particularly following surgery. Draining and following the resolution of postoperative collections with ultrasound is fast, relatively inexpensive, and does not subject the patient to repeated radiation (Figs. 13.35A and B). Ultrasound also has a role in therapeutic joint injections, as it can offer a good alternative to guidance with CT or fluoroscopy. One such example is a sacroiliac joint injection (Fig. 13.36).

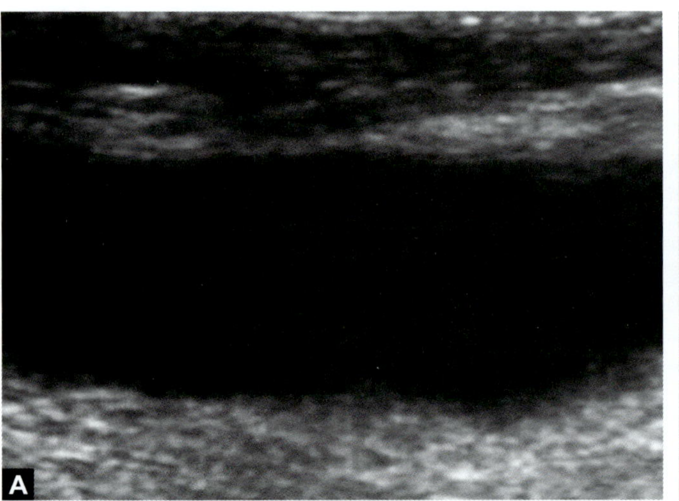

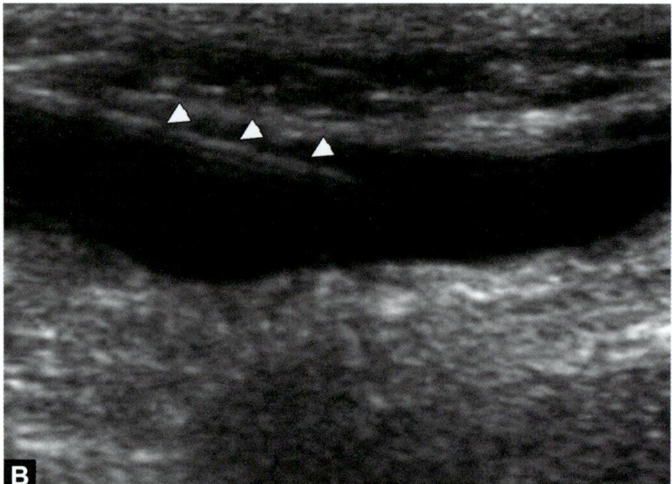

Figs. 13.35A and B: (A) Hypoechoic collection superficial to spine is a postoperative seroma. (B) Real-time decrease in size with drainage under US guidance. Needle indicated by arrowheads in (B).

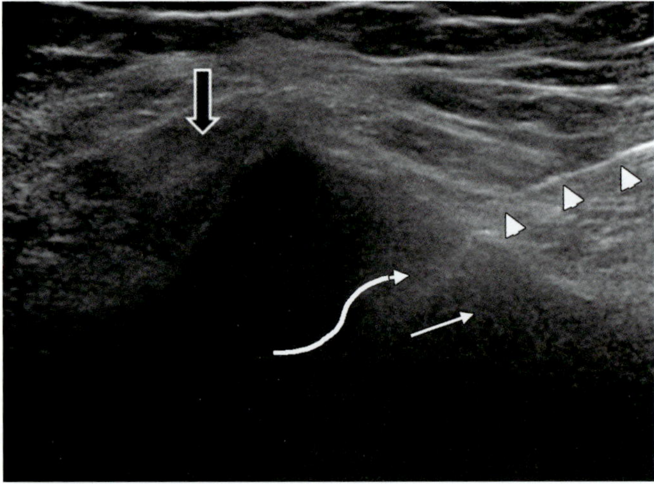

Fig. 13.36: Therapeutic sacroiliac joint injection with US guidance. Ilium (black arrow), sacrum (white arrow), sacroiliac joint (squiggly white arrow), and needle (arrowheads).

SUMMARY

While MRI is an important modality in imaging of the spine, other imaging techniques including radiographs, CT, nuclear imaging, and ultrasound play a significant role in the diagnosis and assessment of spinal disorders.

REFERENCES

1. Radiology ACo. ACR Appropriateness Criteria®: suspected spine trauma. Reston (VA): American College of Radiology (ACR); 2012. 20 p.
2. Hoffman JR, Mower WR, Wolfson AB, et al. Validity of a set of clinical criteria to rule out injury to the cervical spine in patients with blunt trauma. National Emergency X-Radiography Utilization Study Group. N Engl J Med. 2000;343(2): 94-9.
3. Stiell IG, Wells GA, Vandemheen KL, et al. The Canadian C-spine rule for radiography in alert and stable trauma patients. JAMA. 2001;286(15):1841-8.
4. Pollack CV, Jr, Hendey GW, Martin DR, et al. Use of flexion-extension radiographs of the cervical spine in blunt trauma. Ann Emerg Med. 2001;38(1):8-11.
5. Radiology ACo. ACR Appropriateness Criteria®: low back pain. Reston (VA): American College of Radiology (ACR); 2008. P.7.
6. Scientific approach to the assessment and management of activity-related spinal disorders. A monograph for clinicians. Report of the Quebec Task Force on Spinal Disorders. Spine. 1976;12(7 Suppl):S1-59.
7. Staiger TO, Paauw DS, Deyo RA, et al. Imaging studies for acute low back pain. When and when not to order them. Postgrad Med. 1999;105(4):161-2.
8. White AA PM. Clinical Biomechanics of the Spine. Philadelphia, PA: JB Lippincott Co.; 1990.
9. Sonntag VK, Marciano FF. Is fusion indicated for lumbar spinal disorders? Spine. 1976;20(24 Suppl):138S-142S.
10. Ford LT, Gilula LA, Murphy WA, et al. Analysis of gas in vacuum lumbar disc. AJR Am J Roentgenol. 1977;128(6): 1056-7.
11. Bielecki DK, Sartoris D, Resnick D, et al. Intraosseous and intradiscal gas in association with spinal infection: report of three cases. AJR Am J Roentgenol. 1986;147(1):83-6.
12. Wiltse LL, Newman PH, Macnab I. Classification of spondylolysis and spondylolisthesis. Clin Orthop Relat Res. 1976;117:23-9.
13. Park P, Garton HJ, Gala VC, et al. Adjacent segment disease after lumbar or lumbosacral fusion: review of the literature. Spine. 1976;29(17):1938-44.
14. Douglas-Akinwande AC, Rydberg J, Shah MV, et al. Accuracy of contrast-enhanced MDCT and MRI for identifying the severity and cause of neural foraminal stenosis in cervical radiculopathy: a prospective study. AJR Am J Roentgenol. 2010;194(1):55-61.
15. Ohashi K, El-Khoury GY, Bennett DL, et al. Orthopedic hardware complications diagnosed with multi-detector row CT. Radiology. 2005;237(2):570-7.
16. Young PM, Berquist TH, Bancroft LW, et al. Complications of spinal instrumentation. Radiographics. 2007;27(3): 775-89.
17. Cross JJ, Antoun NM, Laing RJ, Xuereb J. Imaging of compressive vertebral haemangiomas. European Radiology. 2000;10:997-1002.
18. Chai JW, Hong SH, Choi JY, et al. Radiologic diagnosis of osteoid osteoma: from simple to challenging findings. Radiographics. 2010;30(3):737-49.
19. Rybak LD. Fire and ice: thermal ablation of musculoskeletal tumors. Radiol Clin North Am. 2009;47(3):455-69.
20. Ozdoba C, Gralla J, Rieke A, et al. Myelography in the Age of MRI: Why We Do It, and How We Do It. Radiol Res Pract. 2011;329017(10):6.
21. Bartynski WS, Lin L. Lumbar root compression in the lateral recess: MR imaging, conventional myelography, and CT myelography comparison with surgical confirmation. AJNR Am J Neuroradiol. 2003;24(3):348-60.
22. Lim CH, Jee WH, Son BC, et al. Discogenic lumbar pain: association with MR imaging and CT discography. Eur J Radiol. 2005;54(3):431-7.
23. Gill K, Blumenthal SL. Functional results after anterior lumbar fusion at L5-S1 in patients with normal and abnormal MRI scans. Spine. 1976;17(8):940-2.
24. Hall EJ. Lessons we have learned from our children: cancer risks from diagnostic radiology: Pediatr Radiol. 2002;32(10):700-6. Epub 2002 Jul 19.
25. Brenner DJ, Hall EJ. Computed tomography—an increasing source of radiation exposure. N Engl J Med. 2007;357 (22):2277-84.
26. Parker MS, Hui FK, Camacho MA, et al. Female breast radiation exposure during CT pulmonary angiography. AJR Am J Roentgenol. 2005;185(5): 1228-33.
27. Love C, Din AS, Tomas MB, et al. Radionuclide bone imaging: an illustrative review. Radiographics. 2003;23(2): 341-58.
28. Fujii M, Abe K, Hayashi K, et al. Honda sign and variants in patients suspected of having a sacral insufficiency fracture. Clin Nucl Med. 2005;30(3):165-9.
29. Love C, Patel M, Lonner BS, et al. Diagnosing spinal osteomyelitis: a comparison of bone and Ga-67 scintigraphy and magnetic resonance imaging. Clin Nucl Med. 2000;25(12): 963-77.
30. Palestro CJ, Kim CK, Swyer AJ, et al. Radionuclide diagnosis of vertebral osteomyelitis: indium-111-leukocyte and technetium-99m-methylene diphosphonate bone scintigraphy. J Nucl Med. 1991;32(10):1861-5.
31. Faraj AA, Webb JK. Early complications of spinal pedicle screw. Eur Spine J. 1997;6(5):324-6.
32. Flynn BM, Butler SP, Quinn RJ, et al. Radionuclide cisternography in the diagnosis and management of cerebrospinal fluid leaks: the test of choice. Med J Aust. 1987;146(2):82-4.
33. Park JI, Strelzow VV, Friedman WH. Current management of cerebrospinal fluid rhinorrhea. Laryngoscope. 1983;93(10):1294-300.
34. Oberson R. Radioisotopic diagnosis of rhinorrhea. Radiol Clin Biol. 1972;41(1):28-35.

CHAPTER

14 MRI Evaluation of Cervical and Lumbar Spine Disorders

Michael B Mechlin

INTRODUCTION

For many patients with cervical and lumbar spine disorders, magnetic resonance imaging (MRI) helps in establishing an accurate and precise diagnosis. MRI uses nonionizing electromagnetic fields to generate high-quality images that provide excellent soft tissue contrast resolution.[1] MRI is useful for diagnosis and evaluation of degenerative disk disease (DDD), disk herniation, cord and nerve root compression, spinal fractures and injuries, tumors, congenital defects, and other spine disorders.

The MRI sequence that is most helpful in spine imaging is the T2-weighted or fluid sensitive sequence. On T2-weighted images, water or cerebrospinal fluid (CSF) shows up bright, while on T1-weighted images, water or CSF appears dark. Thus, T2-weighted images are very helpful for visualization of edema.

CERVICAL SPINE

Normal disks in the cervical spine will have intermediate to bright signal on T2-weighted sagittal sequences (Fig. 14.1A). Also in the cervical spine, on the axial images normal disks are usually concave or straight (Fig. 14.1B) and not convex. MRI can also demonstrate the ligamentous structures about the cervical spine, including the anterior longitudinal ligament, the posterior longitudinal ligament and the interspinous ligaments (Figs. 14.2A and B). This becomes important in assessing for posterior ligamentous abnormalities in the setting of flexion/extension injuries.

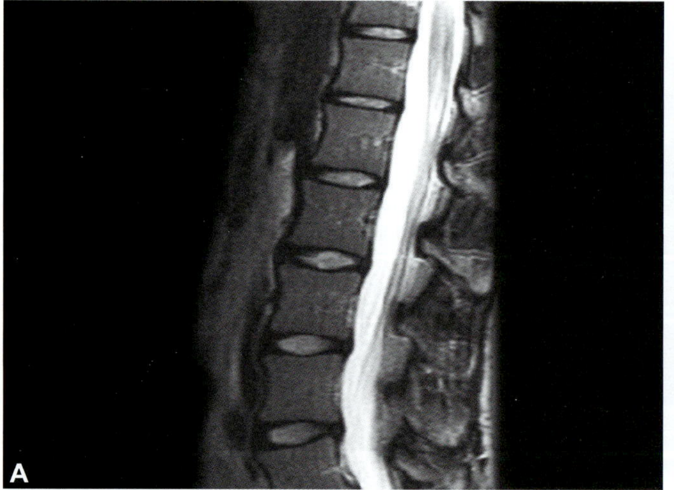

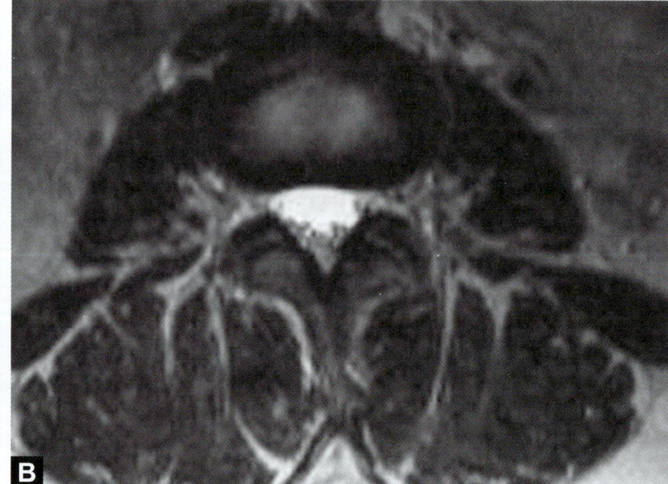

Figs. 14.1A and B: (A) T2-weighted sagittal and (B) T2-weighted axial images of normal cervical disks.

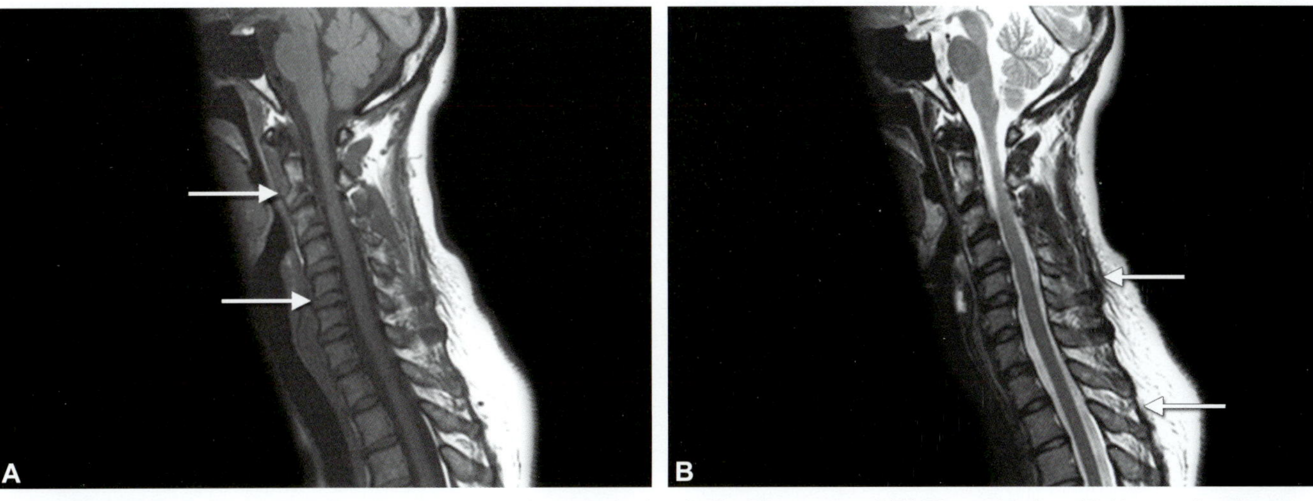

Figs. 14.2A and B: (A) T1-weighted sagittal image showing anterior longitudinal ligament and (B) T2-weighted sagittal image showing supraspinous ligament.

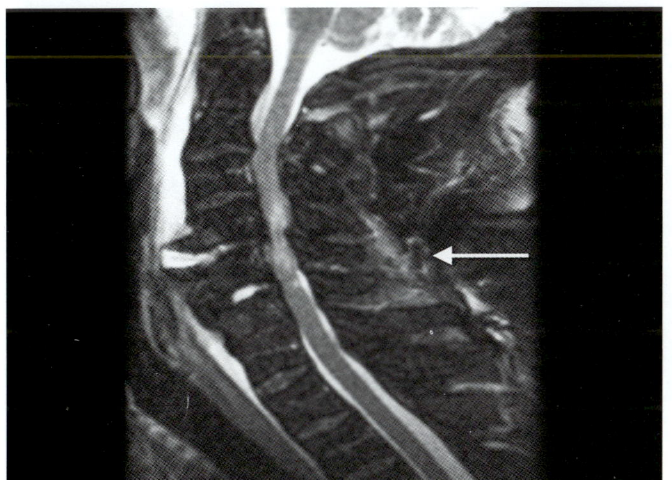

Fig. 14.3: STIR sagittal demonstrating edema in the region of the interspinous ligaments (white arrow).

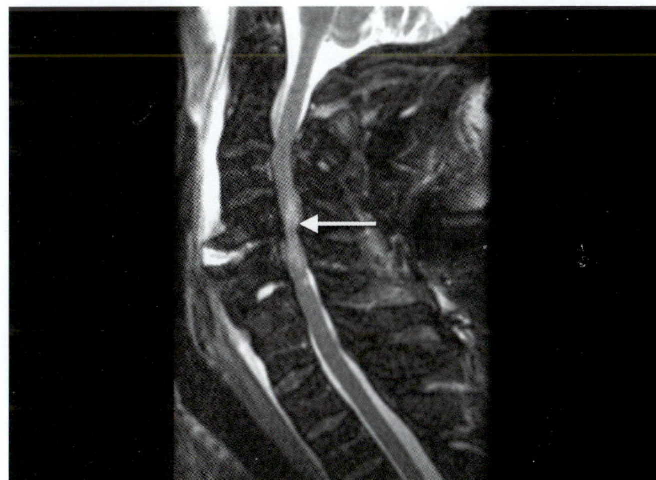

Fig. 14.4: STIR sagittal demonstrating spinal cord T2 hyperintensity (white arrow) due to contusion in the spinal cord at the stenotic C4/5 level.

Injury to the posterior ligaments might manifest as increased distance between spinous processes on X-rays. On MRI, there may be increased signal intensity in the region of the interspinous ligaments. However, this would be best demonstrated on fat saturated T2 or short tau imaging recovery (STIR) sagittal (Fig. 14.3) rather than conventional T2-weighted images. In the setting of trauma, cord signal abnormality can be seen in the cervical cord due to contusion, with preexisting stenotic levels more prone to cord injury because of the decreased CSF around the cord (Fig. 14.4). Syrinx can be the sequelae of previous cord trauma (Fig. 14.5), although it could also be secondary to a tumor in the cord or could be congenital/developmental.

Magnetic resonance imaging can also occasionally show fractures in the cervical spine, although it is not as accurate nor is it as sensitive as CT scanning. Odontoid fractures can be seen on the MRI, but CT will be superior because of its higher spatial resolution and bony detail (Figs. 14.6A and B). Also flexion teardrop fractures can be seen on MRI (Figs. 14.7A and B), but CT will generally better evaluate the associated other bony abnormalities such as locked facets. While one could see sequelae such as anterolisthesis at C5-6 on MRI, CT would better show the etiology in the case of locked facets (Figs. 14.8A to C).

However, the most common indication for MRI of the cervical spine is to assess for DDD, which will manifest as decrease in the signal of the cervical disks on T2-weighted

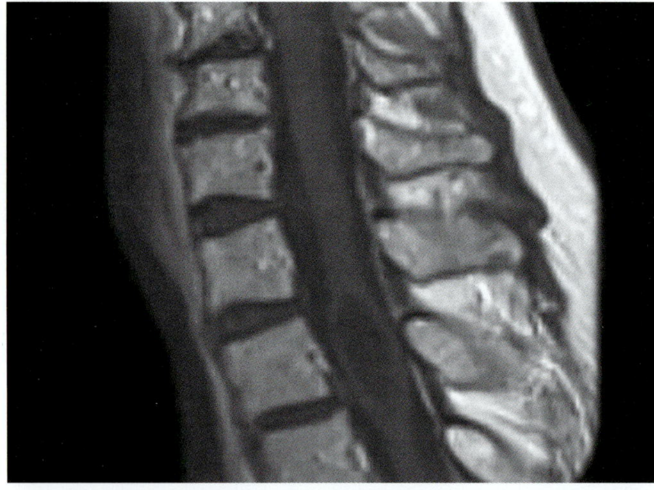

Fig. 14.5: T1-weighted sagittal image showing a large post-traumatic syrinx (white arrows) in the cervical cord.

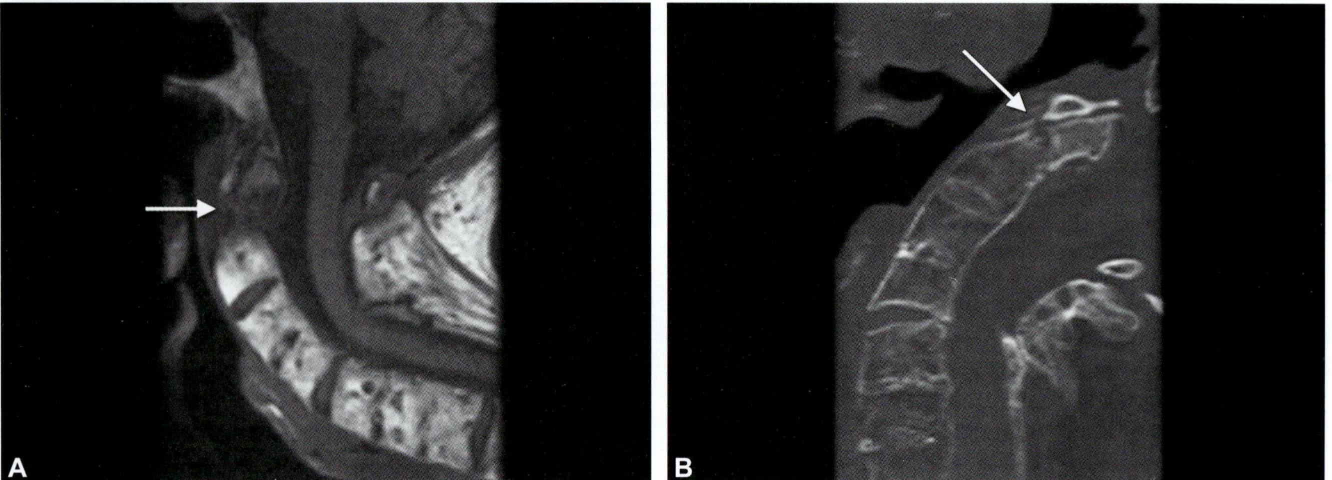

Figs. 14.6A and B: (A) Sagittal T1-weighted MR image and (B) sagittal CT reconstructions both showing the type II odontoid fracture, but seen to better resolution on the CT (arrows).

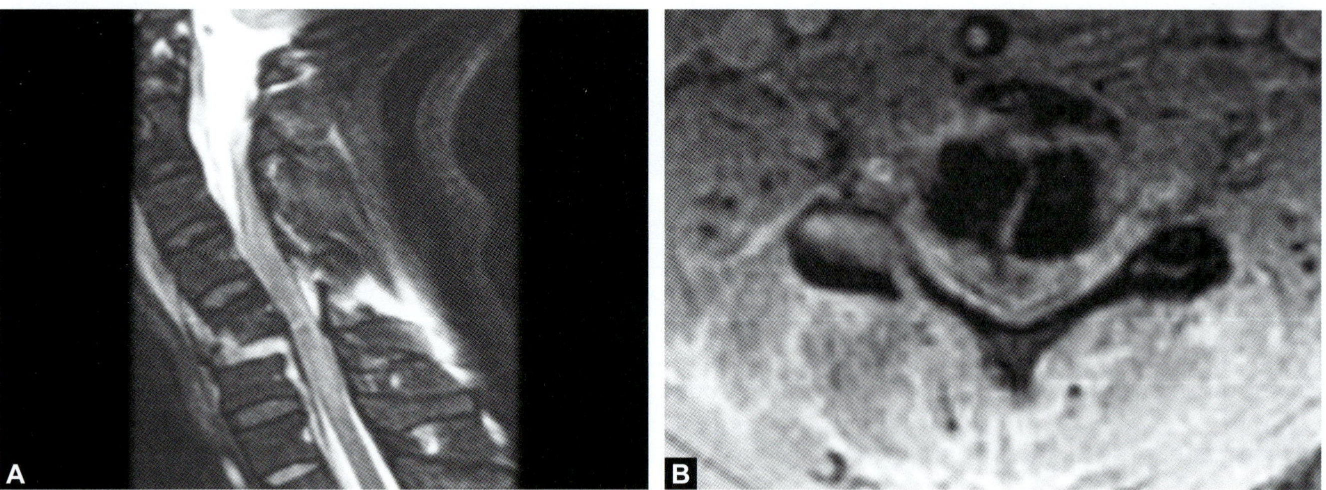

Figs. 14.7A and B: (A) T2 sagittal and (B) gradient echo axial images demonstrating a flexion teardrop fracture at anterior inferior corner of C5.

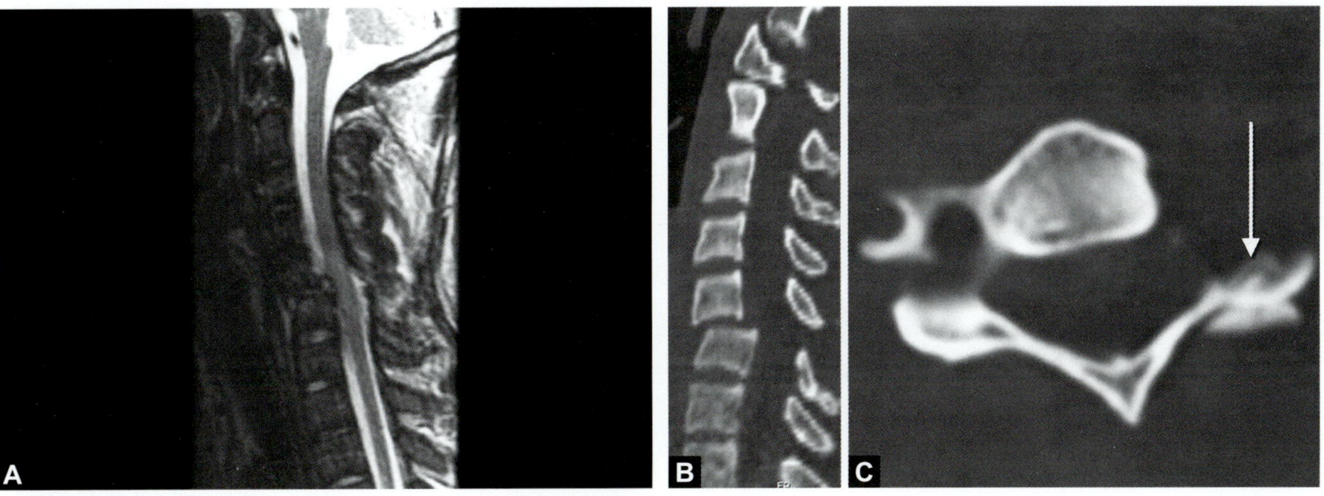

Figs. 14.8A to C: Anterolisthesis of C5 on C6 on the (A) sagittal MRI and (B) sagittal reconstructed CT image, while (C) axial CT image demonstrating that locked facets (arrow) as the etiology.

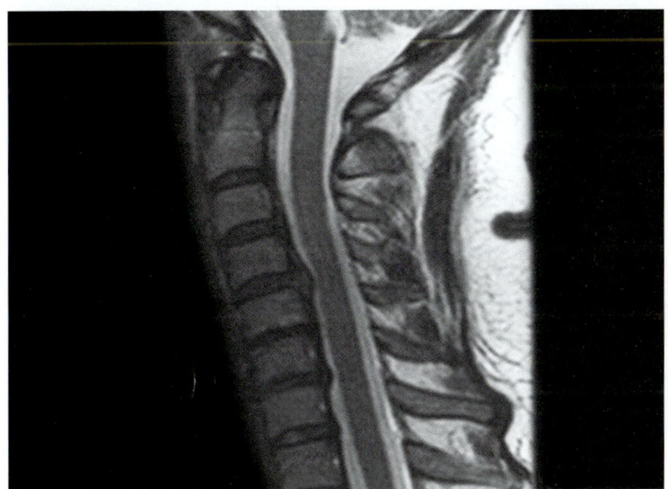

Fig. 14.9: T2 sagittal image demonstrating multilevel degenerative disk disease with multilevel disk herniations.

images (Fig. 14.9). Disk herniations appear convex with focal outpouchings, as seen in Figures 14.10A and B, which shows mild indentation of the ventral thecal sac at C4/5. However, in the cervical spine besides disk herniations, often there are disk/ridge or disk/osteophyte complexes (Figs. 14.11A and B), made up of small amounts of disk material and osseous ridges that can cause compression on the neural structures.

A special type of sequence, a gradient echo sequence is often performed in the cervical spine in order to differentiate disk herniations from disk osteophyte complexes. On the gradient echo axial images, a disk herniation will be seen as a focal area of bright signal (Fig. 14.12) as opposed to a disk osteophyte complex or ridge which will be low signal as seen in Figures 14.13A and B, which demonstrates a right central disk osteophyte complex.

It is important to assess for any cord impression and also to assess for any foraminal narrowing. Both disk herniations and disk osteophyte complexes have the potential to cause cord impression centrally or nerve root compression in the neural foramen, as in Figures 14.14A and B, where a left C5/6 disk osteophyte complex narrows the left neural foramen. Another cause for foraminal narrowing is uncovertebral hyperostosis, as seen in Figure 14.15 where there is severe left foraminal narrowing.

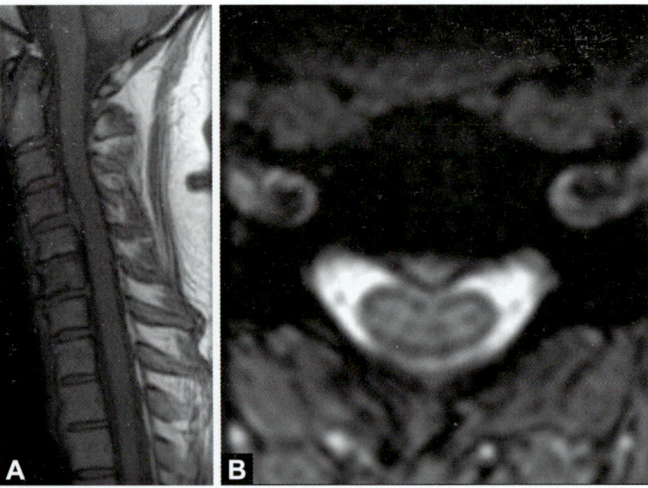

Figs. 14.10A and B: (A) T1-weighted sagittal image and (B) T2-weighted axial image demonstrating a focal disk herniation at C4/5 indenting the ventral thecal sac and flattening the ventral surface of the spinal cord.

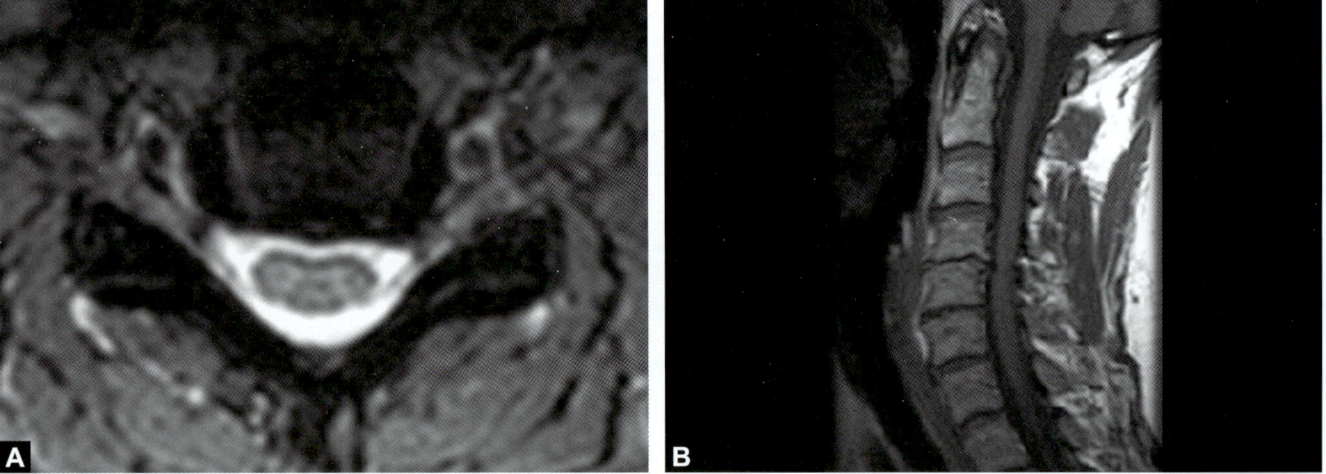

Figs. 14.11A and B: (A) T2-weighted axial and (B) T1-weighted sagittal images demonstrating a disk osteophyte complex at C4/5.

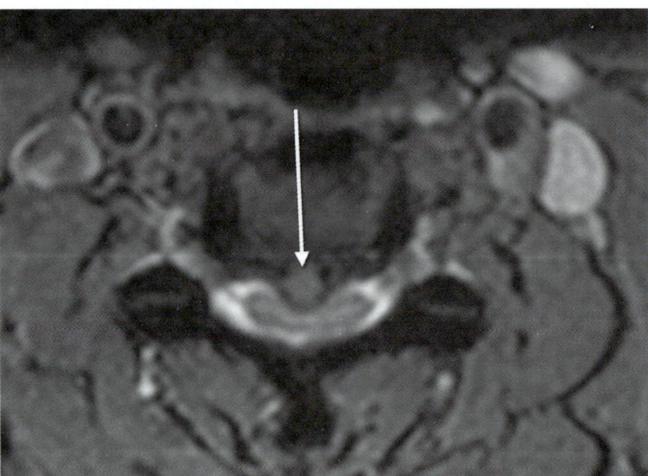

Fig. 14.12: Gradient echo axial image demonstrating a central disk herniation, as manifested by high signal in the displaced disk material (arrow).

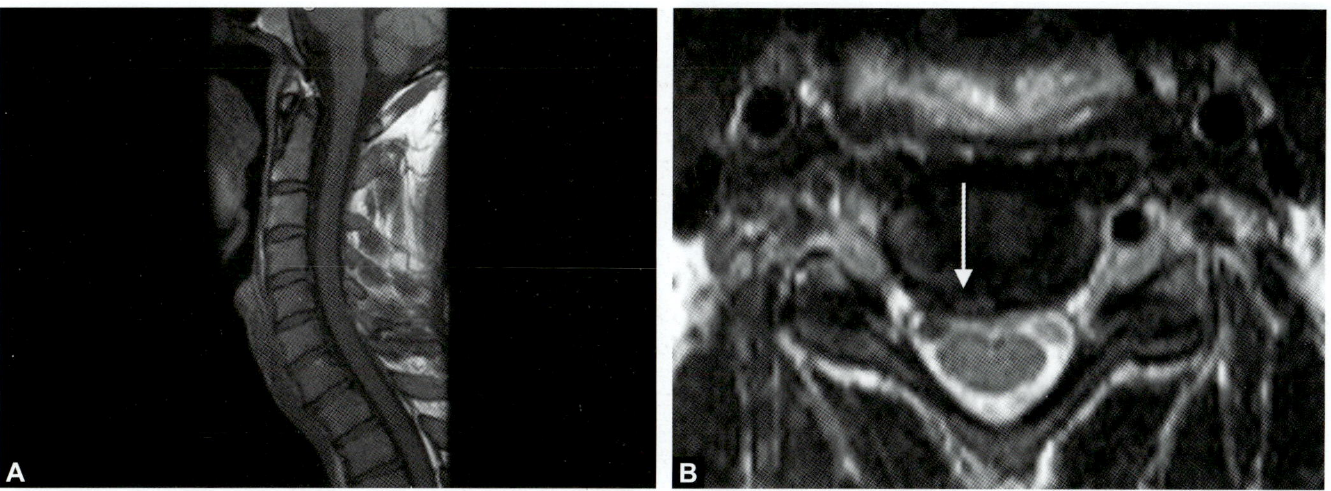

Figs. 14.13A and B: (A) T1-weighted sagittal and (B) T2-weighted axial images demonstrating a right central disk osteophyte complex (white arrow).

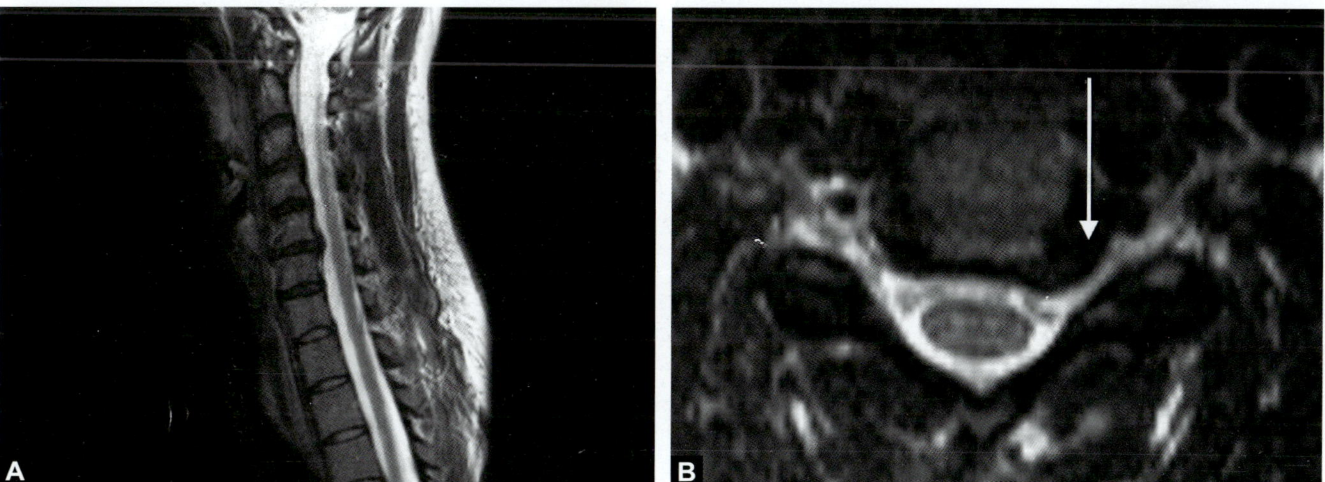

Figs. 14.14A and B: (A) T2-weighted sagittal and (B) T2-weighted axial images showing a left C5/6 disk osteophyte complex narrowing the left neural foramen (white arrow).

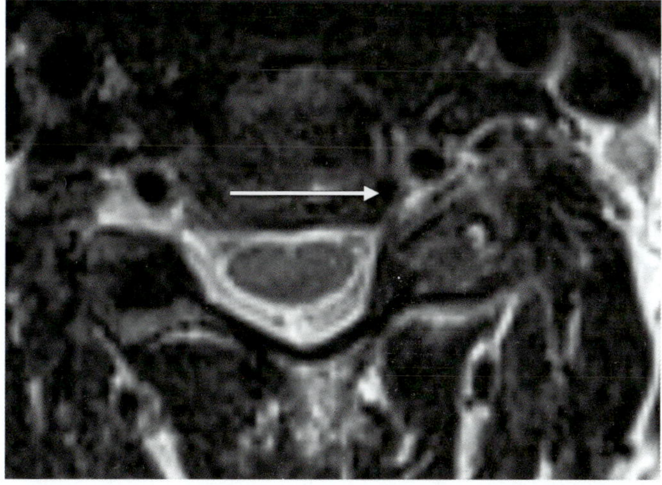

Fig. 14.15: T2-weighted axial image demonstrating left uncovertebral hyperostosis, with resultant narrowing of the left neural foramen (white arrow).

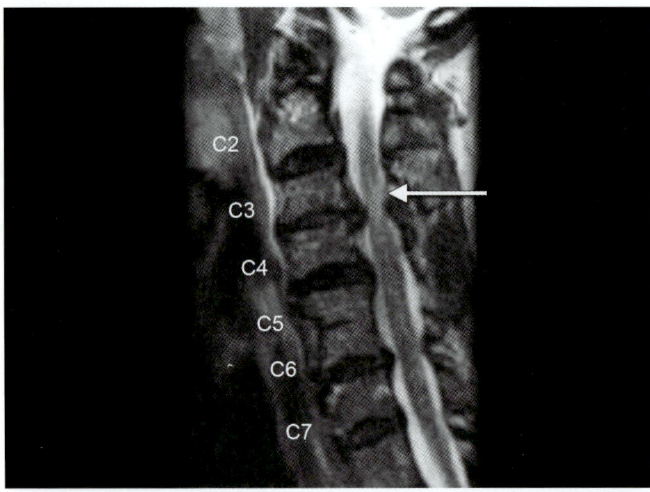

Fig. 14.16: T2-weighted sagittal image demonstrating a disk osteophyte complex in association with facet arthrosis at C3/4 causing central stenosis and cord compression with resultant signal abnormality in the cervical cord (myelomalacia).

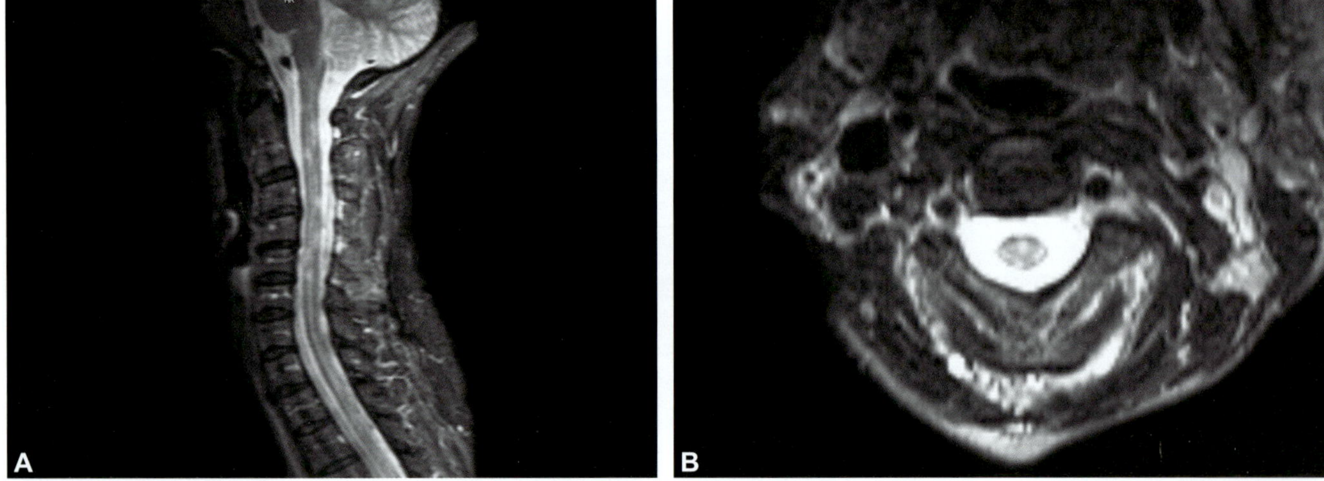

Figs. 14.17A and B: (A) T2-weighted sagittal and (B) T2-weighted axial images demonstrating T2 bright demyelinating plaques throughout the cervical cord in this patient with multiple sclerosis.

Disk osteophyte complexes when large, or in association with facet arthropathy can result in cord compression and signal abnormality in the cord, due to myelomalacia. This is seen in Figure 14.16, where there is a significant disk osteophyte complex at the C3-4 level in association with facet arthropathy causing canal stenosis resulting in cord compression and myelomalacia, manifested by bright signal in the cord.

Another cause for cord signal abnormalities is multiple sclerosis in which MS patients have demyelinating plaques, which are seen as bright areas in the cord on T2-weighted images (Figs. 14.17A and B). These T2 bright lesions do not necessary have to be at the disk level in MS as usually those due to myelomalacia secondary to canal stenosis are, which is one potential way to differentiate. Also, multiple T2 bright areas in the cord are usually due to MS.

Having metal in the cervical spine from prior fusion does not preclude doing an MRI, although interpretation may be limited in those patients with anterior and posterior fusion because of artifact. However, with new metal reduction strategies in order to decrease the amount of artifact, excellent MR images can be obtained especially in those patients who have had a prior anterior cervical discectomy and fusion (ACDF), as in Figures 14.18A and B, where the spinal cord in the canal is well seen.

LUMBAR SPINE

As with the cervical spine, the most common lumbar spine disorder that is evaluated on MRI is degenerative disease of the intervertebral disks. The lumbar disks are important to absorb the compressive load in the spine, which is best accomplished when the disks are normally hydrated. This is seen to greatest advantage on T2-weighted or STIR sequences (fluid sensitive images), such as seen in Figures 14.19A and B, which shows normally hydrated bright disks on the T2-weighted sagittal image and the normal convex nature of the disk on the axial image. On sagittal T2-weighted images, one can see the bright nucleus pulposus surrounded by the low signal annulus fibrosus.

As the disk ages, the nucleus becomes less hydrated, resulting in loss of the bright signal on the T2-weighted images and tears will occur in the peripheral annulus, which results in disk desiccation and disk space narrowing that is evident on MR images (Fig. 14.20).

As time progresses, the disk begins to expand outward.

In the past, there were numerous controversial definitions for disk material displaced beyond the margins of the disk space.

To help clarify this in 2001, a joint task force made up of the North American Spine Society (NASS), the American Society of Spine Radiology (ASSR), and the American Society of Neuroradiology (ASNR) published a document in Spine[2] and on the ASSR and ASNR websites attempting to standardize the nomenclature of DDD. According to that document, the accepted definitions are annular tear (although because tear may imply a traumatic etiology, some people prefer to use annular fissure or a high intensity zone or HIZ instead), disk bulge which is subcategorized as symmetric or asymmetric, and disk herniation which is further subcategorized as disk protrusion, disk extrusion, or disk sequestration.

With an annular fissure or annular tear (also called a high-intensity zone), there is high signal in the posterior annulus fibrosus on T2-weighted images (Fig. 14.21), which may enhance avidly after giving IV contrast. Also, annular fissures although often seen centrally, do not have to be and can be peripheral (Fig. 14.22A). They can also be seen on the axial images, especially if peripheral (Fig. 14.22B).

Disk bulges are defined as a generalized (between 50% and 100%) displacement of disk material in the axial plane beyond the limits of the intervertebral disk space. This displacement can be symmetric (circumferential) which is 100% of the circumference around (Figs. 14.23A and B) or asymmetric which is 50% or more but less than 100% (Fig. 14.24).

Disk herniations are defined as localized displacement of disk material beyond the limits of the intervertebral disk space. They can be focal, which is less than 25% (Figs. 14.25A and B) or can be broad-based which is between 25% and 50% of the disk circumference (Fig. 14.26). Disk herniations are further subcategorized based on the shape of the disk material. A disk protrusion is a herniation where the base of the parent disk is larger than the disk material within the canal. A disk extrusion is a herniation where the disk material in the canal is larger than the base. Disk extrusions may have superiorly or inferiorly migrated fragments as seen in Figures 14.27A and B, where there is disk material extruded all the way down to the inferior aspect of L5, from the L4/5 disk.

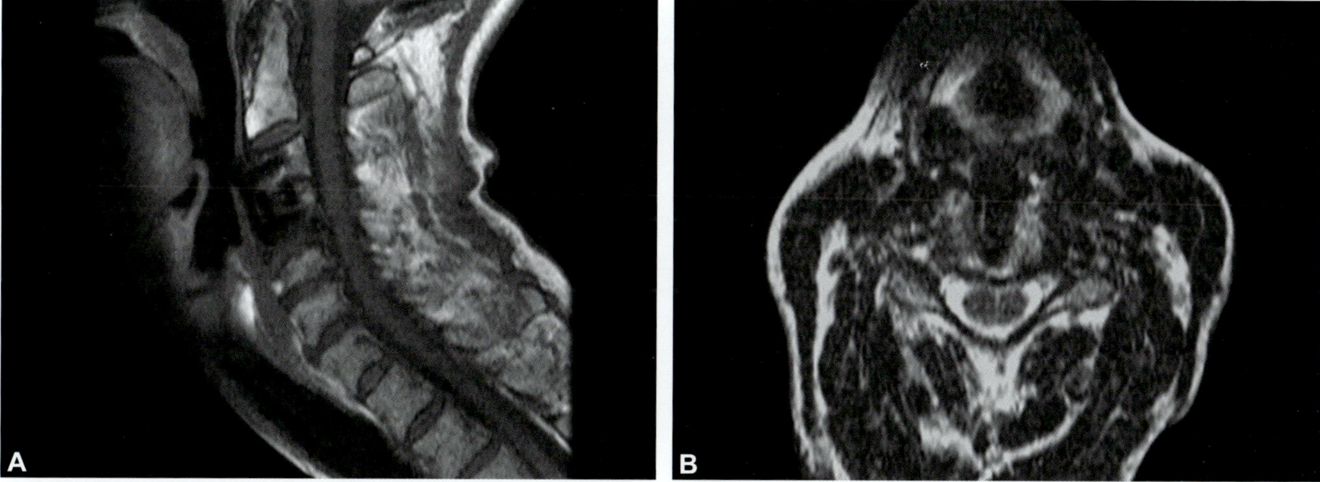

Figs. 14.18A and B: (A) T1-weighted sagittal and (B) T2-weighted axial images in this patient with metal from a prior ACDF. Note that although there is some artifact around the screws, it does not preclude or interfere with evaluation of the cord or canal.

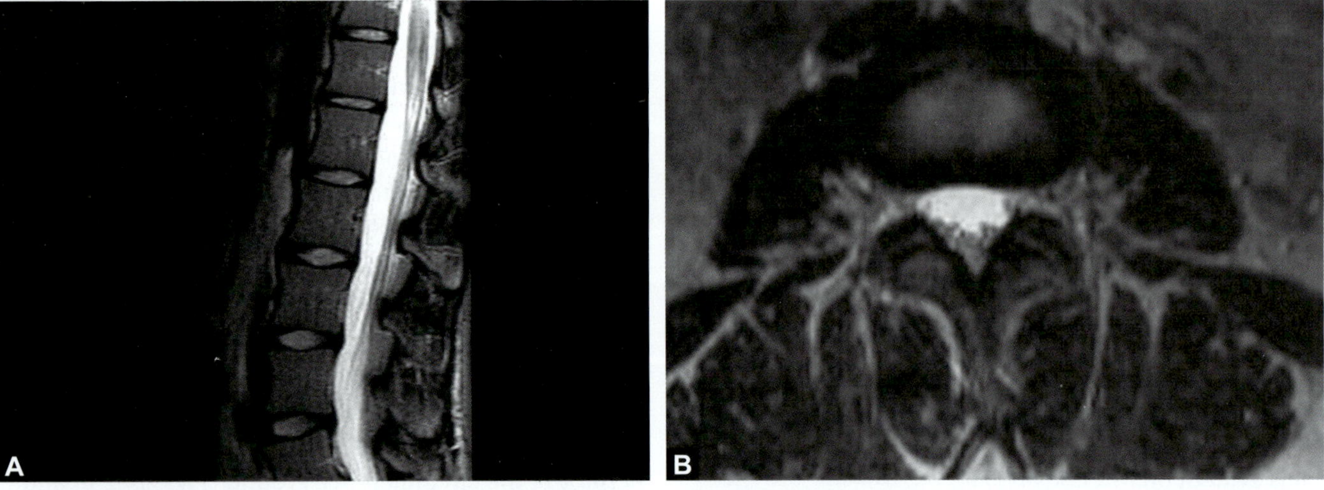

Figs. 14.19A and B: (A) Sagittal and (B) axial T2-weighted images showing normal lumbar disks.

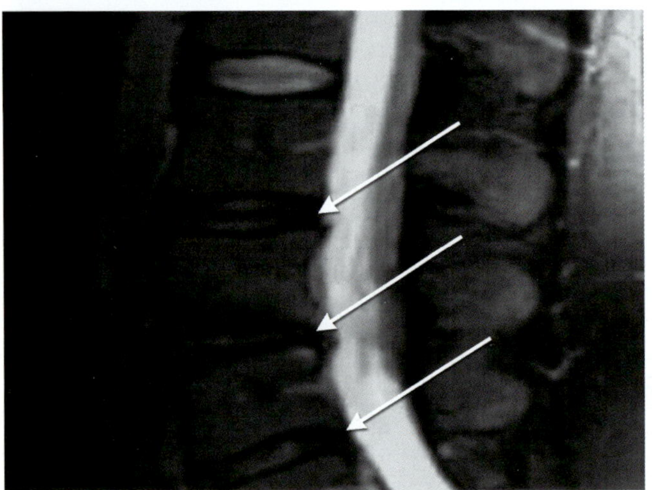

Fig. 14.20: T2-weighted sagittal image showing disk space narrowing and dessicated disks (white arrows) at L3/4, L4/5, and L5/S1.

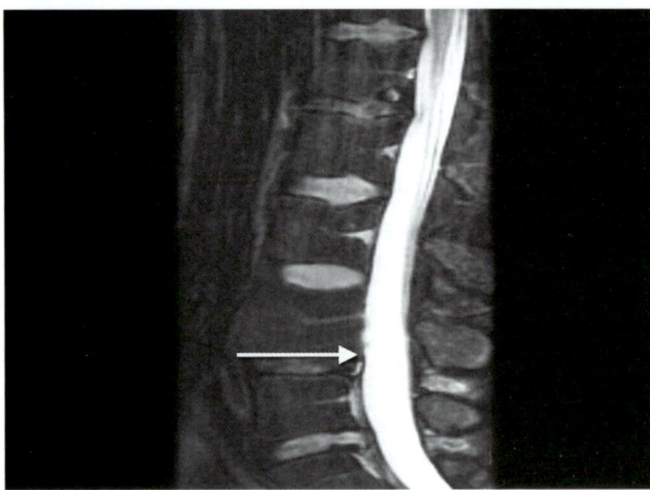

Fig. 14.21: T2-weighted sagittal image showing an annular fissure (arrow).

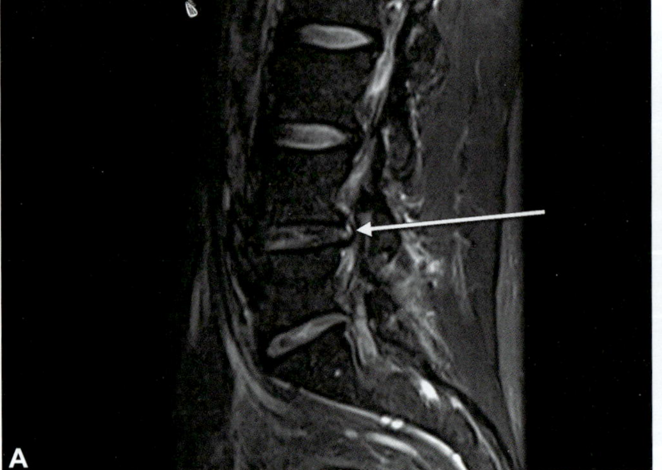

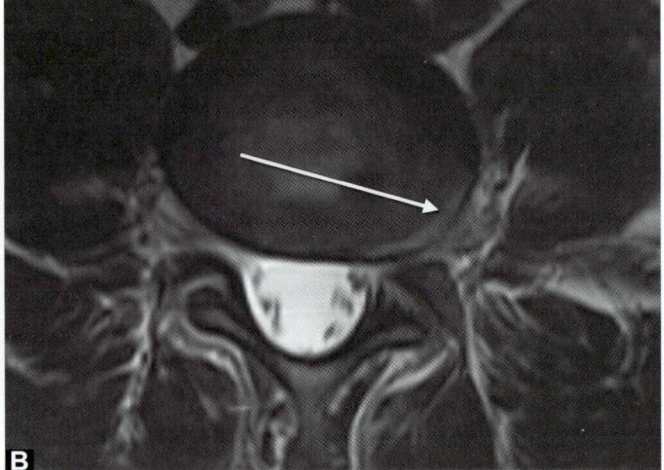

Figs. 14.22A and B: (A) Sagittal and (B) axial T2-weighted images showing peripheral left foraminal annular fissure (arrow).

If the disk material still maintains continuity with the parent disk, it is called an extrusion. However, if the disk material loses continuity with the native parent disk, then it is subcategorized as a sequestration (which is a special type of extrusion). Figure 14.28 shows a disk extrusion cephalad from the L3/4 level, which lost continuity from the parent disk and thus is a sequestration.

When evaluating MR images of the spine, it is important to not just note the disk herniations, but also to evaluate for any nerve root compression, either centrally or in the foramen. Figures 14.29A and B show a left central disk herniation at L5/S1 with caudal extrusion on the sagittal image (Figs. 14.29A and B) which is causing left central canal stenosis and left lateral recess stenosis compressing the descending left S1 nerve root in the canal, seen on the T1-weighted axial image (Figs. 14.29A and B). This might result in a left S1 radiculopathy.

Besides looking for any nerve root compressions in the central canal, it is important to look at the neural foramina as well to evaluate for any exiting nerve root compression. Figures 14.30A and B demonstrate a right L3/4 foraminal disk extrusion with cephalad extrusion compressing the exiting right L3 nerve root, seen best on T1-weighted sagittal images, explaining this patient's right L3 radiculopathy.

Although plain film radiographs will be more sensitive to assess for alignment abnormalities, MRI can give some information with the added benefit of assessing for

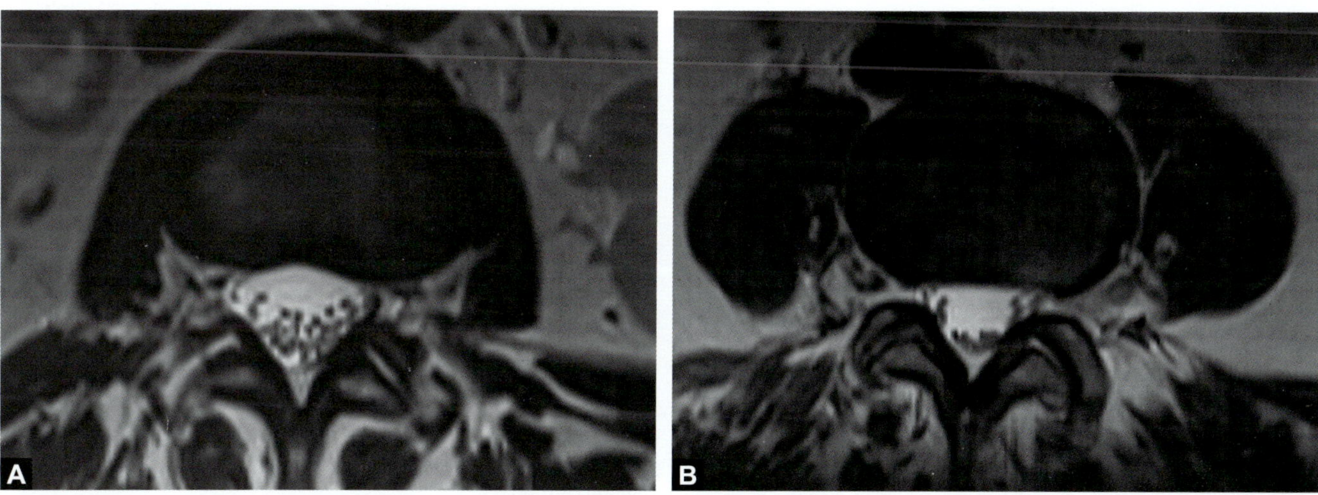

Figs. 14.23A and B: (A) T2-weighted axial image showing normal disk and (B) T2-weighted axial image showing symmetric (circumferential) disk bulge.

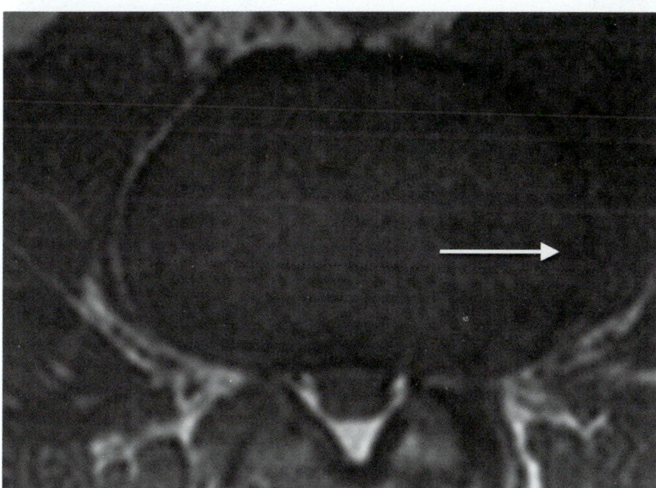

Fig. 14.24: T1 axial image showing asymmetric bulge of the disk to the left (arrow).

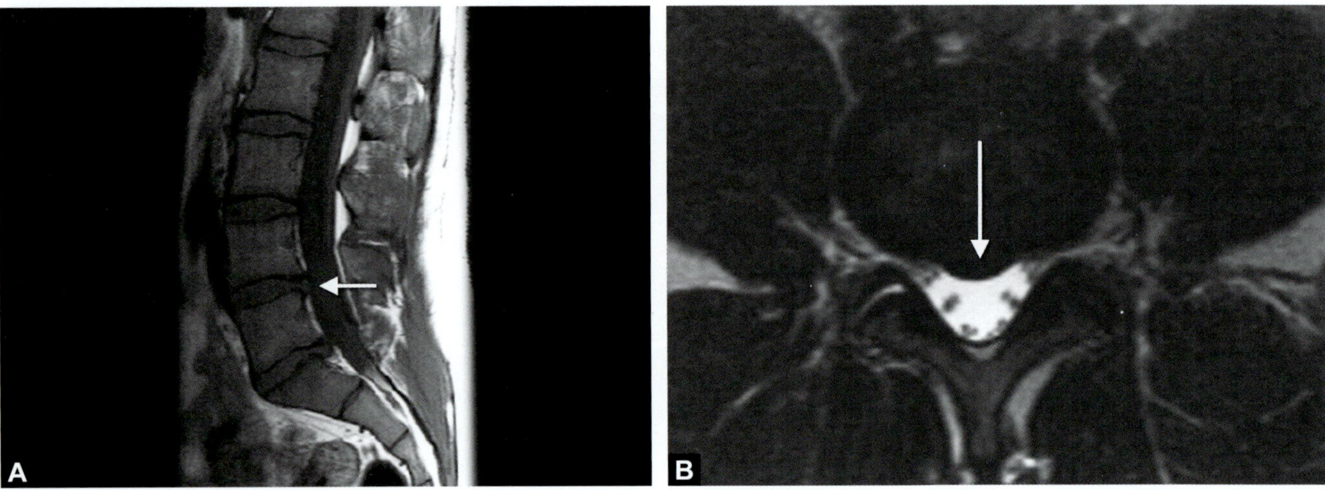

Figs. 14.25A and B: (A) T1-weighted sagittal and (B) T2-weighted axial images showing a focal disk herniation at L4/5 (arrow).

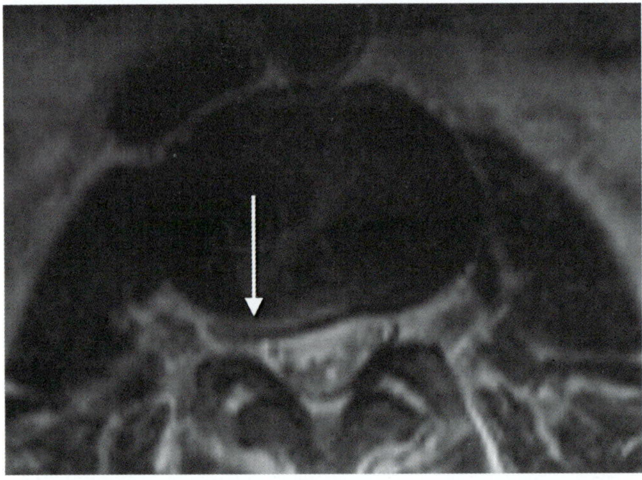

Fig. 14.26: T2-weighted axial image demonstrating a broad based disk herniation (arrow).

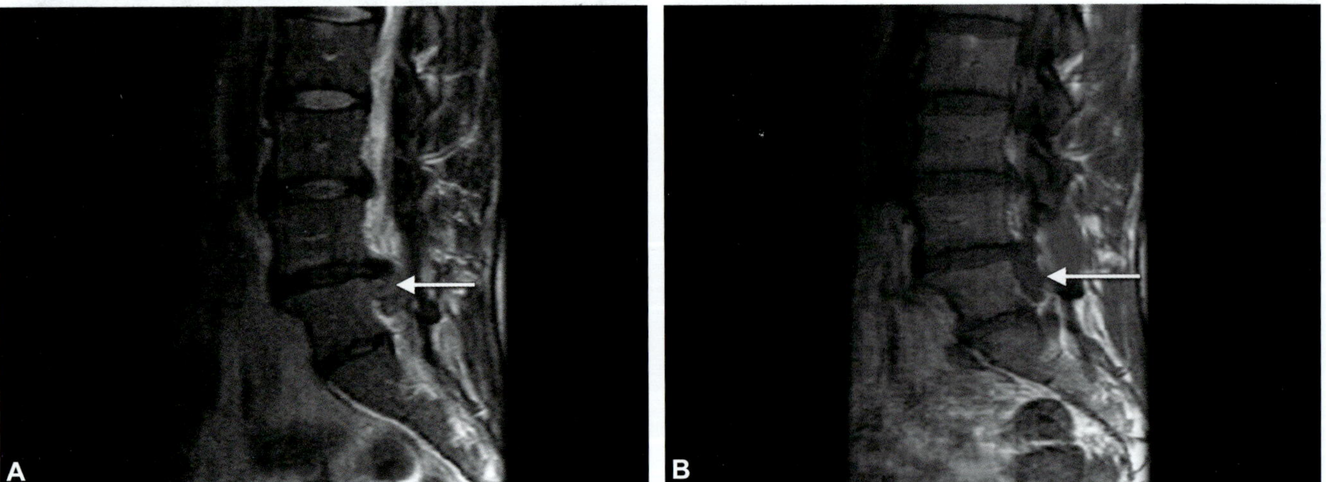

Figs. 14.27A and B: (A) T2- and (B) T1-weighted sagittal images showing an inferior disk extrusion at L4/5 (arrows).

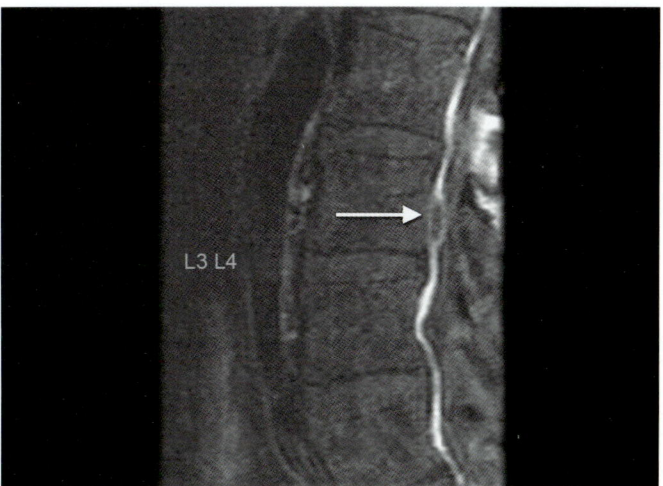

Fig. 14.28: Sagittal image showing a sequestered disk fragment (arrow) superior to L3/4.

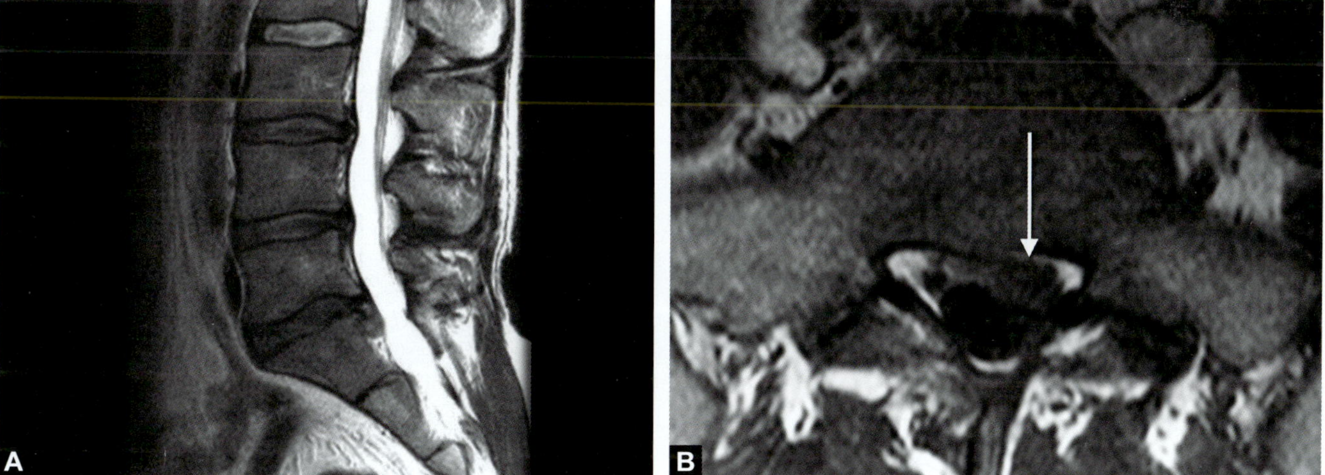

Figs. 14.29A and B: T2-weighted sagittal and (B) T1-weighted axial images showing an inferior disk extrusion from L5/S1 compressing the left S1 nerve root in the left lateral recess (arrow) on the axial image.

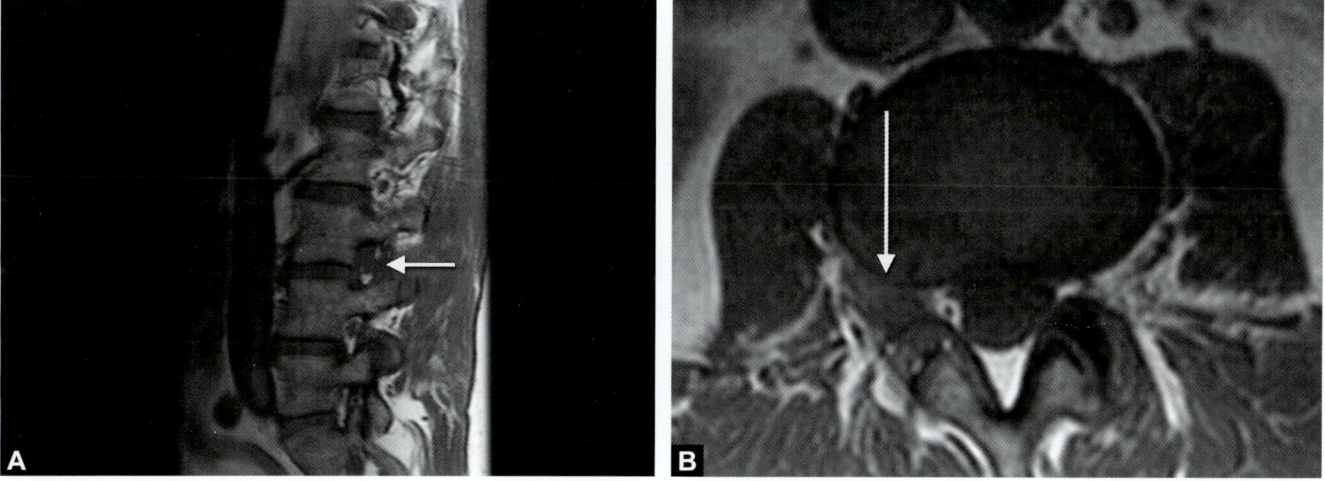

Figs. 14.30A and B: (A) T1-weighted sagittal and (B) axial images demonstrating a cephalad disk extrusion compressing the right L3 nerve root in the right L3/4 foramen (arrow).

any stenosis related to these alignment abnormalities. Figure 14.31 demonstrates such a case, with retrolisthesis of L1 on L2 and anterolisthesis of L4 on L5. In Figures 14.32A and B, there is anterolisthesis of L4 on L5 with evidence of central canal stenosis at L4/5 due to a combination of the anterolisthesis and significant facet hypertrophy. The facet joint is a true synovial joint, which can degenerate and become hypertrophic or can develop fluid in it, as seen in Figures 14.32A and B. In either scenario, spondylolisthesis can develop which can then result in canal and sometimes foraminal stenosis as well.

The most common etiology for spondylolisthesis in the lumbar spine is usually degenerative due to facet arthrosis, especially when it is multilevel. However, occasionally, especially in younger patients, spondylolisthesis can be secondary to spondylolysis that could be posttraumatic due to pars fractures, or could be congenital (isthmic spondylolisthesis). This latter subcategory is somewhat controversial, as it may be that some cases of isthmic spondylolisthesis may be secondary to subclinical trauma. Figures 14.33A and B show an example of anterolisthesis of L5 and S1 due to pars defects. CT would show the bony abnormality of a pars defect with higher bony resolution, but it is still detectable on MRI.

However, MRI is superior to CT in evaluating the acuity of the pars defects. Occasionally, patients who have chronic pars defects can become symptomatic due to refracture or due to motion or further slippage at the pars defect. Figures 14.34A and B demonstrate a patient with a pars defect on T1-weighted image, but with bone marrow edema around the defect best seen on the T2-weighted image, indicating that this is relatively acute, possibly explaining new pain.

Degenerative end-plate changes due to disk disease are commonly seen on MRI, but can have various signal characteristic[3] such as low T1, high T2 (Modic type 1), high T1, isointense to slightly high T2 (Modic type 2), and low T1, low T2 (Modic type 3), with Modic type 1 (Figs. 14.35A and B) being the most common but also potentially the most confusing. When the adjacent end plates have low signal on T1-weighted images and high signal on T2-weighted images, this may indicate a more acute phenomenon, due to bone marrow edema. This is usually not a problem in differential diagnosis, if it is limited to just the end plates.

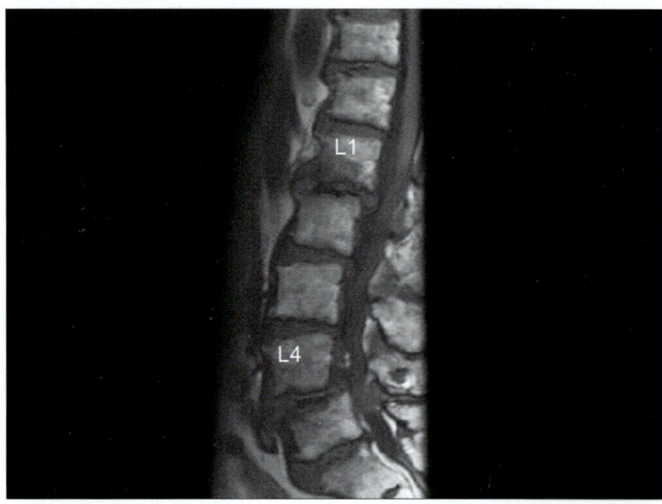

Fig. 14.31: T2-weighted sagittal image showing retrolisthesis of L1 on L2 and anterolisthesis of L4 on L5.

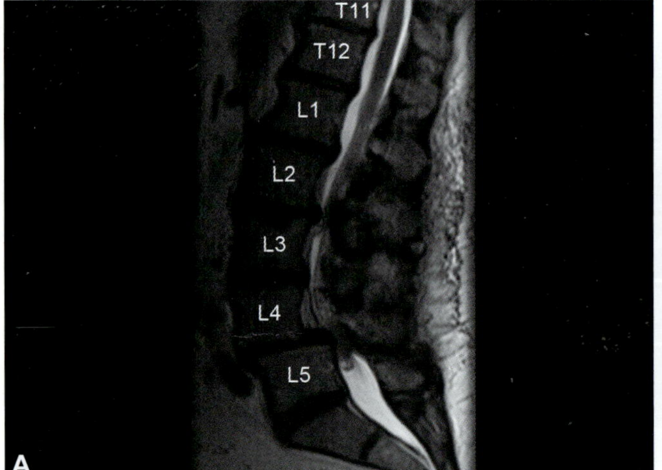

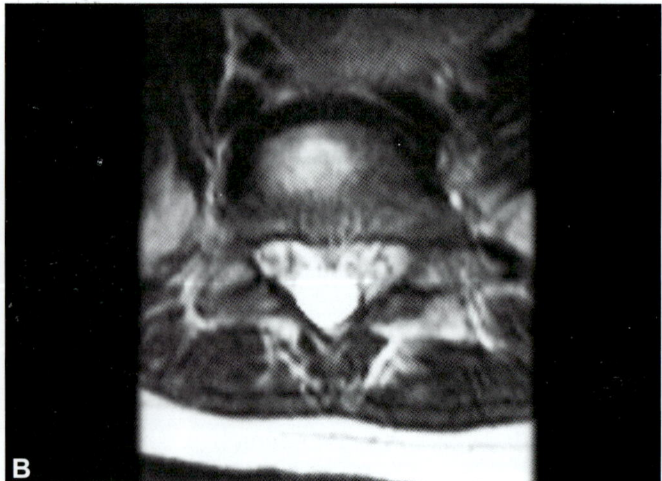

Figs. 14.32A and B: (A) T2-weighted sagittal image showing anterolisthesis of L4 on L5 and (B) T2-weighted axial image showing marked central stenosis and bilateral facet arthrosis with fluid in the right facet joint.

However, occasionally these "end-plate changes" can occupy more than just the end plate, involving a large portion of the vertebral bodies (Figs. 14.36A and B), and/or can enhance following contrast administration (Figs. 14.37A and B). If that would occur, then besides end-plate change, diskitis would have to be in the differential, although still the overwhelming majority will be degenerative end-plate change. A helpful point in trying to differentiate diskitis from end-plate change is that in DDD, usually the disk will be dessicated and low signal on T2-weighted images, while with diskitis, the disk itself may become bright on T2-weighted images (Figs. 14.38A to C). So if there is fluid in what looks like a degenerative disk, then diskitis has to be considered. Also, enhancing paraspinal masses may occur with diskitis (Figs. 14.39A and B) and will not occur with bland DDD, another differentiating point. One type of diskitis, tuberculous (TB) diskitis, is less problematic in differential diagnosis from degenerative end-plate change, as TB often tracks along the anterior longitudinal ligament displacing it (Figs. 14.40A and B) and can occasionally even skip levels.[4] Thus, one may find TB diskitis at one level and then maybe two or three levels above or below it because it tracks along the anterior longitudinal ligament. Also, if an epidural abscess is present, that would help in diagnosing diskitis (Figs. 14.41A and B).

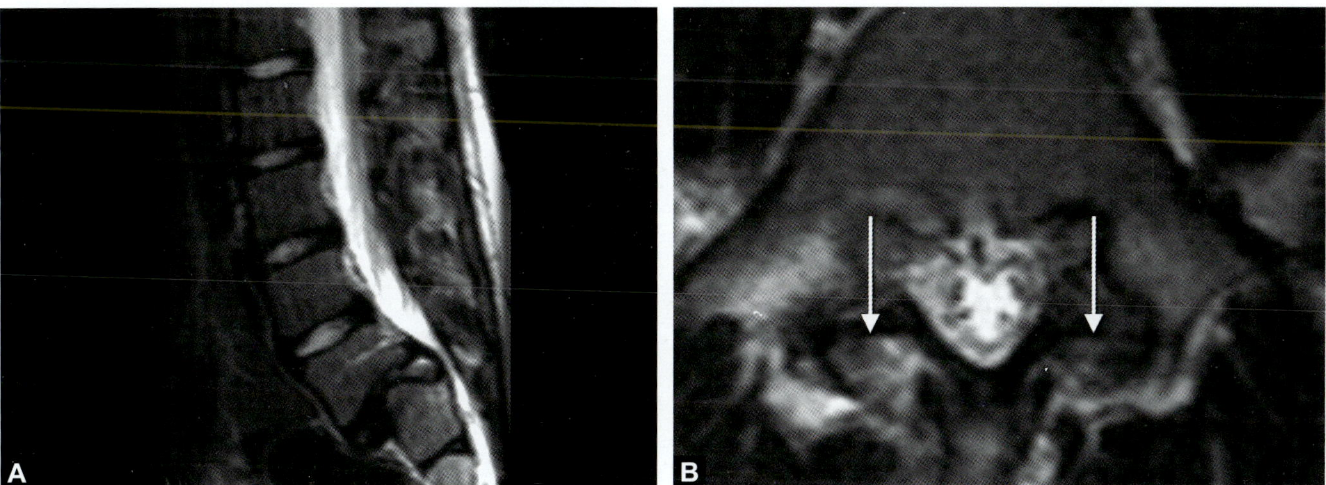

Figs. 14.33A and B: (A) T2-weighted sagittal image showing anterolisthesis on L5 on S1 and (B) T1-weighted axial image demonstrating bilateral pars defects (arrows).

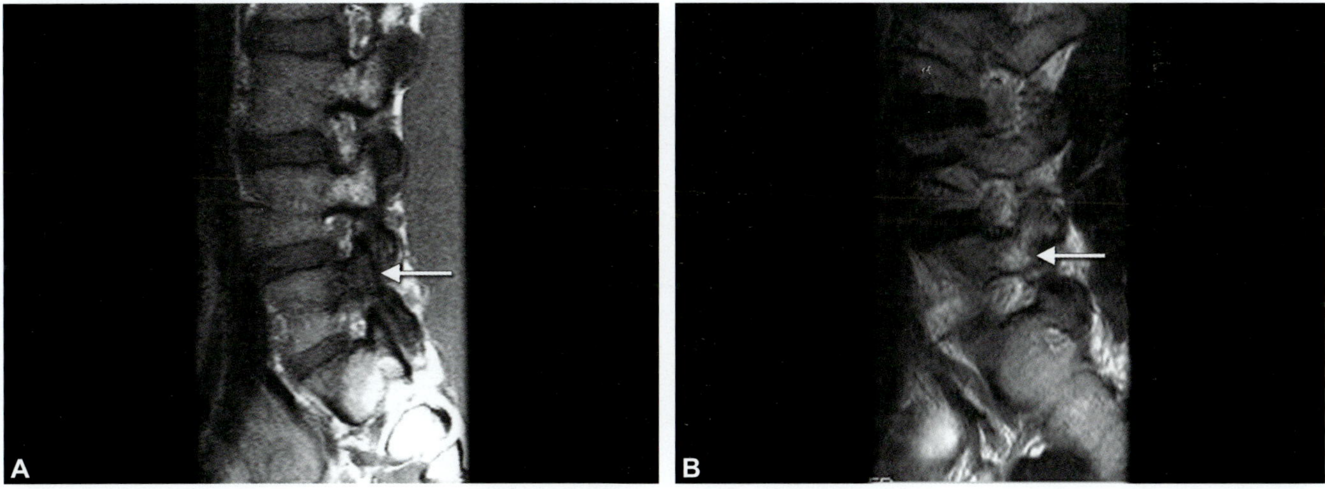

Figs. 14.34A and B: (A) T1-weighted and (B) T2-weighted sagittal images demonstrating a pars defect with edema around it (arrow), suggesting acuity.

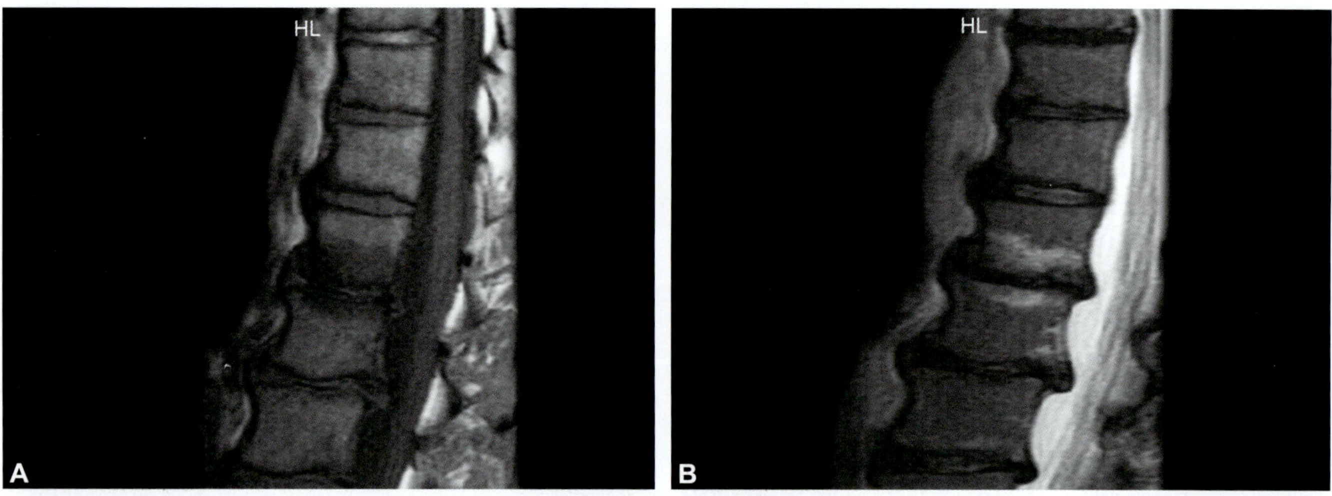

Figs. 14.35A and B: (A) T1-weighted and (B) T2-weighted sagittal images demonstrating Modic Type 1 degenerative end-plate changes at T12/L1.

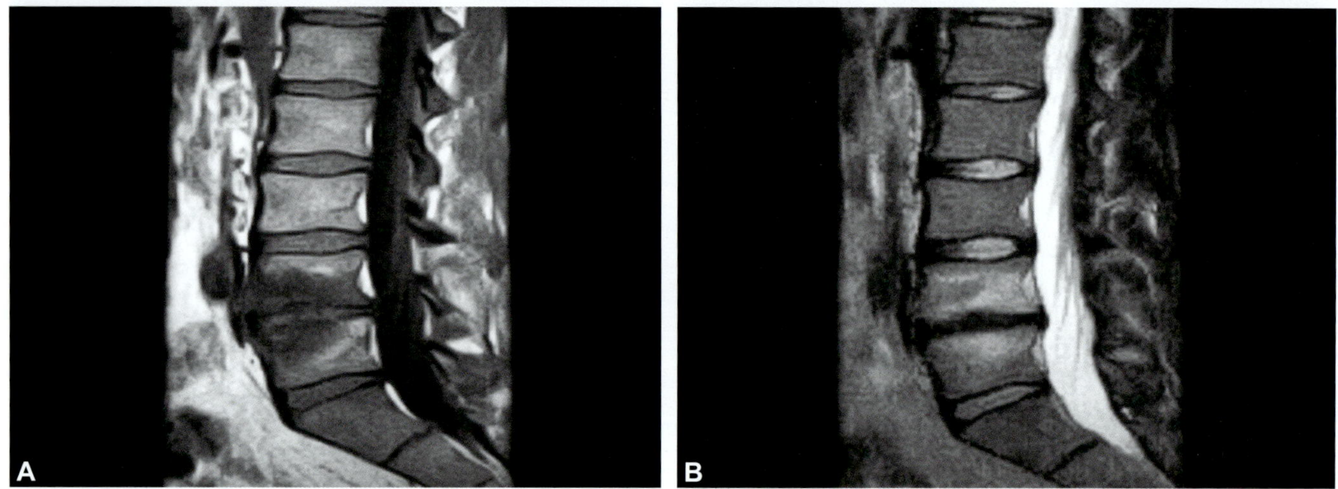

Figs. 14.36A and B: (A) T1-weighted and (B) T2-weighted sagittal images showing degenerative "end-plate changes" at L4/5 that occupy more than just the end plates.

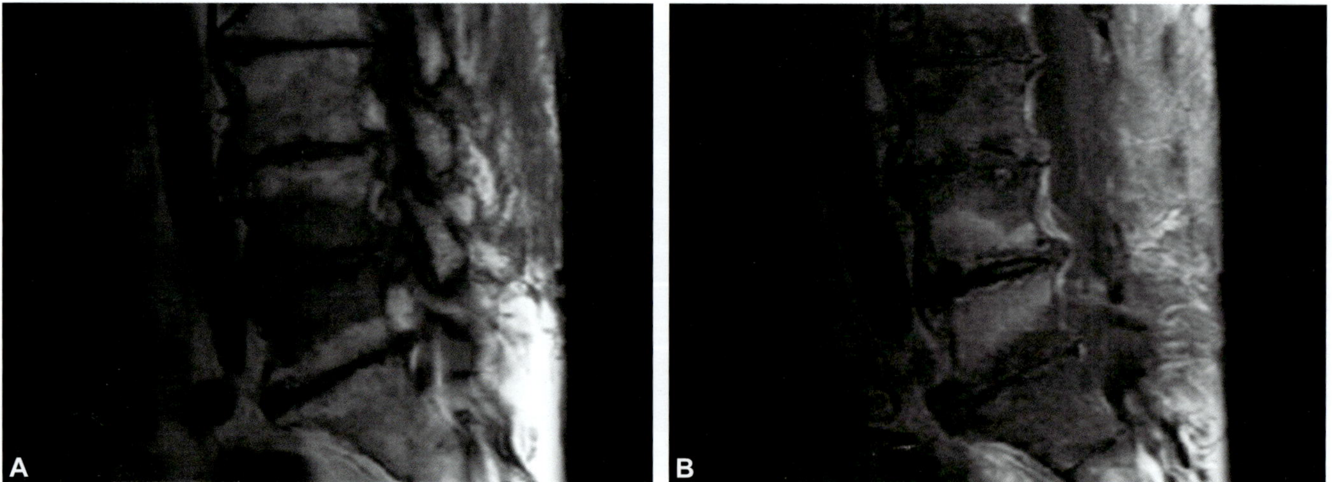

Figs. 14.37A and B: (A) T1-weighted precontrast and (B) T1-weighted postcontrast sagittal images demonstrating enhancement of the degenerative end-plate changes at L4/5.

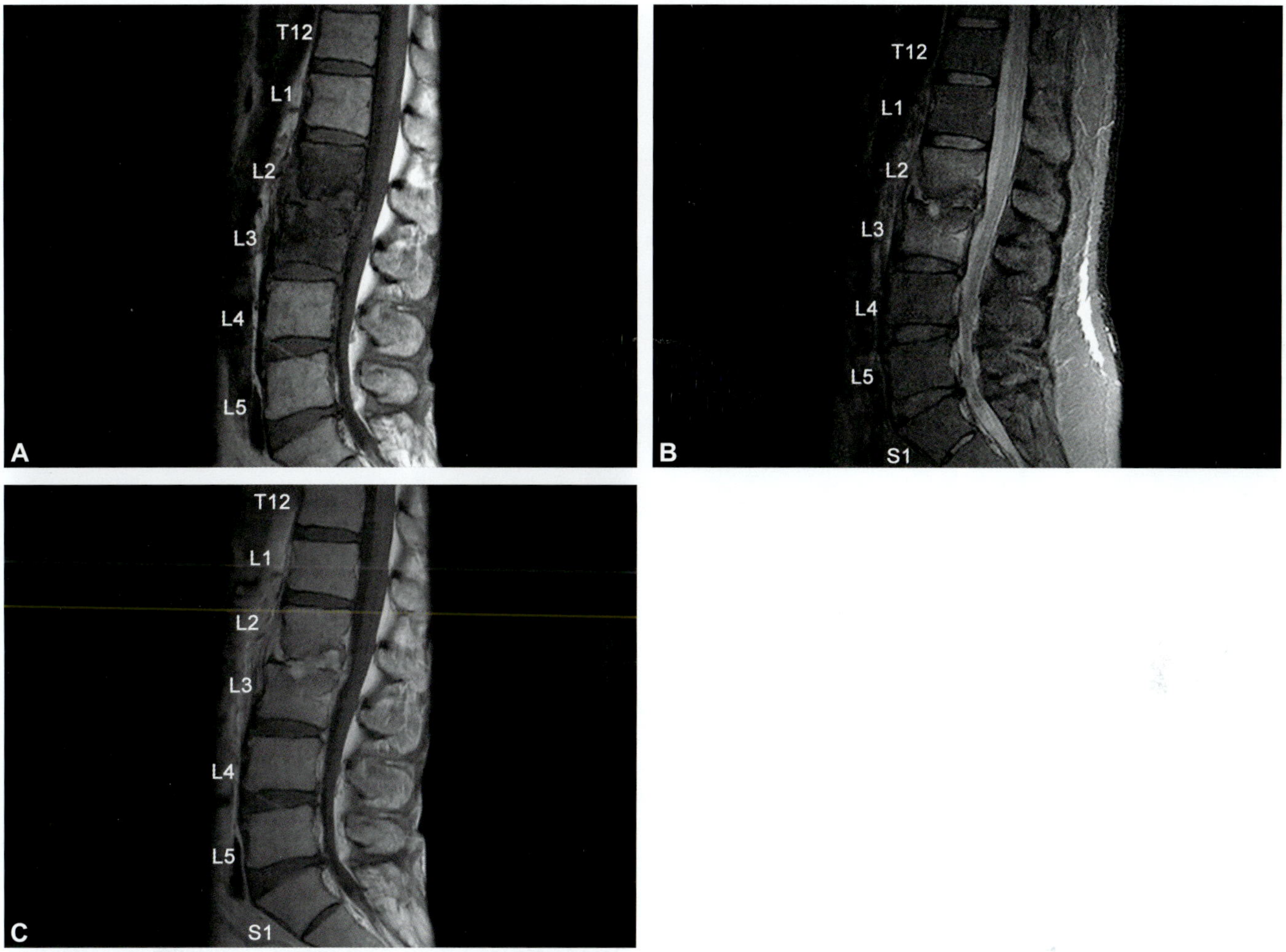

Figs. 14.38A to C: (A) T1-weighted sagittal (B) T2-weighted coronal, and (C) T2 weighed sagittal images demonstrating fluid in the narrowed L3/4 disk suggesting diskitis at the L3/4 level with extensive edema in the L3 and L4 vertebral bodies.

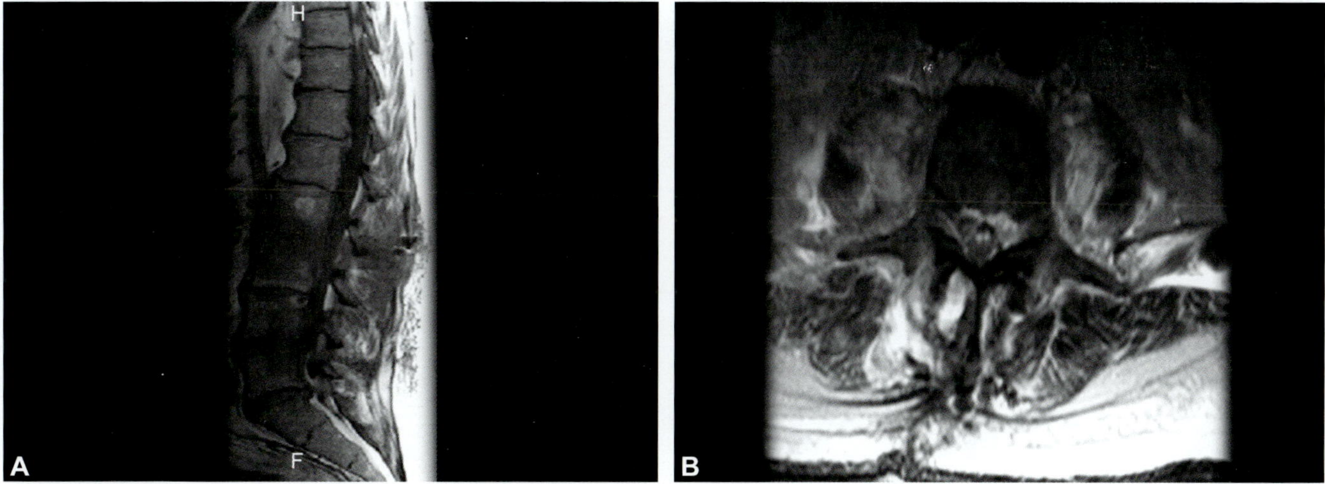

Figs. 14.39A and B: (A) T1-weighted sagittal image showing postsurgical changes and diskitis at L2/3 and (B) T2-weighted axial image showing paraspinal edema in the psoas muscles bilaterally.

Epidural hematomas are much more common than generally previously believed. They can be spontaneous following low-level athletic torsional injuries resulting from tearing of the ventral epidural veins and can clinically present similar to acute disk herniations. These epidural hematomas might be seen in association with disk herniations, which can give a confusing clinical and imaging appearance. CT is usually unable to distinguish disk herniations from epidural hematomas, but MRI can sometimes be helpful in differentiating. On MRI, the epidural hematoma will usually have high signal on T1- and T2-weighted images, best seen on the sagittal images as a fusiform collection (Figs. 14.42A and B). The distinction between disk herniations and epidural hematoma is important because hematomas often resolve spontaneously and can be treated conservatively. While disk herniations can occasionally resorb over time, it is not as common as with epidural hematomas. Thus, it is possible that large apparent disk herniations that subsequently resolve may in part have been epidural hematomas associated with smaller disk herniations (Figs. 14.43A and B).

Imaging of postsurgical cases can be challenging on but MRI can be helpful, especially in cases where the patient had surgery and now has recurrent pain. MRI can be helpful in differentiating recurrent disk herniations from scar and fibrosis. Figures 14.44A and B show an

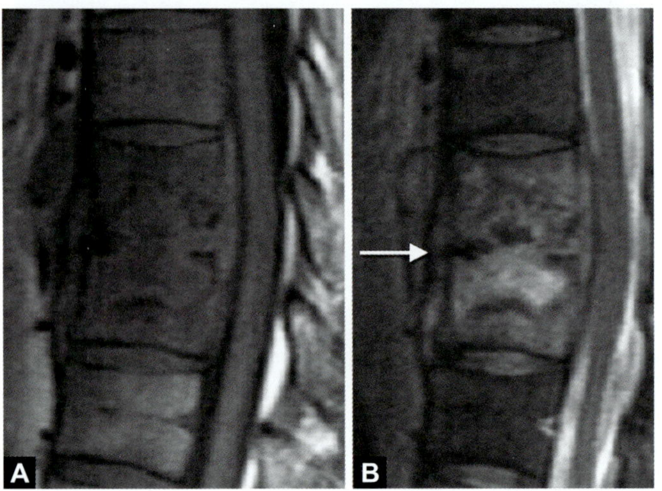

Figs. 14.40A and B: (A) T1-weighted sagittal and (B) T2-weighted sagittal images demonstrating TB diskitis tracking along the anterior longitudinal ligament (arrow).

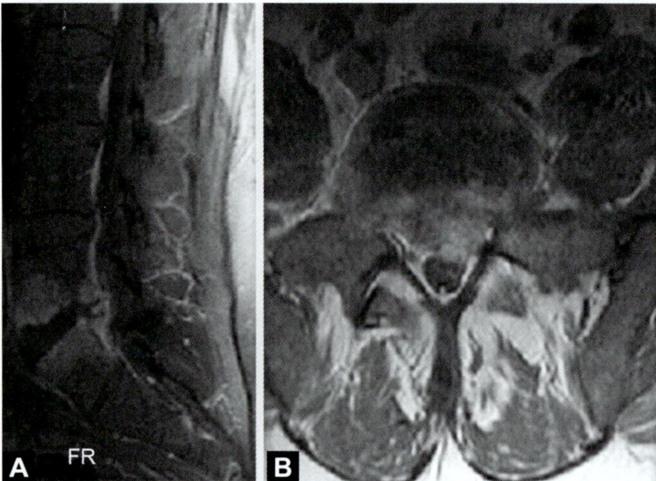

Figs. 14.41A and B: (A) Postcontrast sagittal and (B) postcontrast axial images demonstrating an anterior epidural abscess, indicating that the enhancement around the disk is due to diskitis.

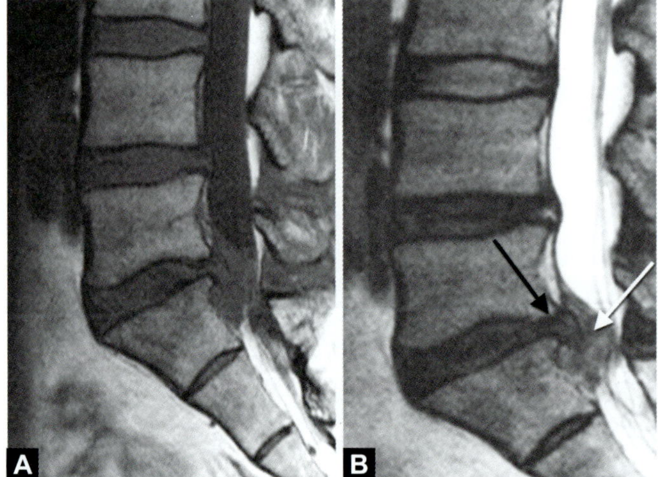

Figs. 14.42A and B: (A) T1-weighted and (B) T2-weighted sagittal images showing an epidural hematoma (white arrow) around a disk herniation (black arrow) at L5/S1.

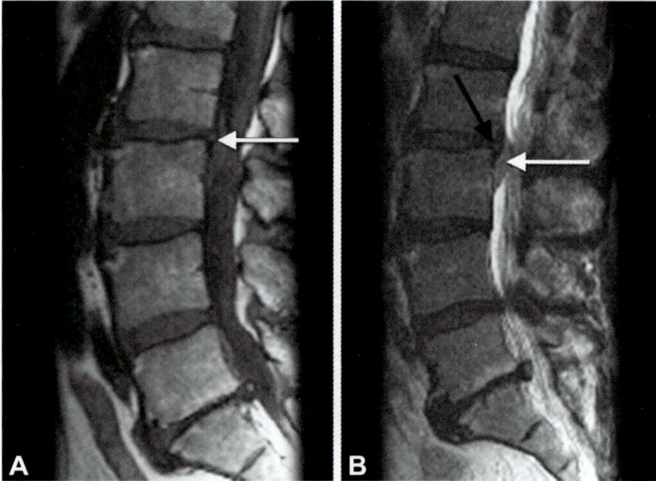

Figs. 14.43A and B: (A) T1-weighted and (B) T2-weighted sagittal images showing a large epidural hematoma (white arrow) around a small disk herniation (black arrow) at L2/3.

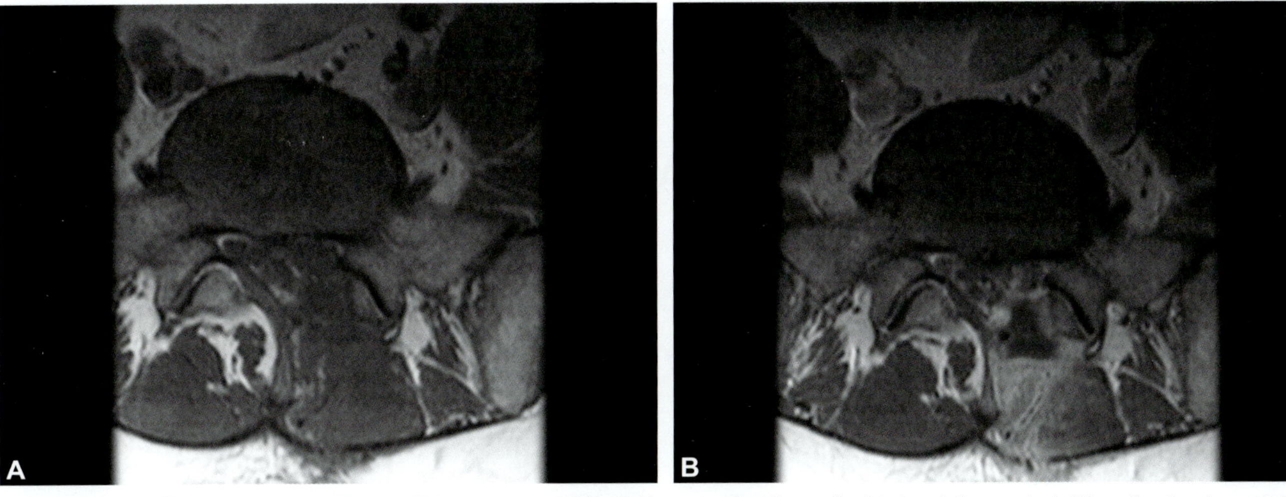

Figs. 14.44A and B: (A) Precontrast T1 and (B) postcontrast T1 axial images showing patient to be status post a left hemilaminectomy at L5/S1 with a postoperative seroma and enhancing scar tissue around the left S1 nerve root without disk herniation.

example of a patient who previously had L5-S1 disk surgery and who developed a progressive left S1 radiculopathy, with the possibility of a recurrent disk herniation in the differential. Postcontrast gadolinium imaging show enhancement around the left S1 nerve root with scar around this left S1 nerve root, ruling out a recurrent disk herniation, obviating the need for additional surgery.

CONCLUSION

Magnetic resonance imaging is an attractive imaging method for evaluating cervical and lumbar disorders as, unlike CT, it provides visualization without ionizing radiation. MRI also has superior soft tissue contrast resolution, relative to CT, because utilization of various sequences such as T2-weighted, T1-weighted, STIR, or gradient echo sequences can help in further differentiating disease processes. Unlike CT, there is no limitation of spatial and contrast detail from signal scatter associated with adjacent bone in MRI.[5] However, due to higher bony resolution, CT produces more detailed images in the case of cervical spine fractures, such as odontoid, and teardrop fractures. Additionally, MRI has been contraindicated in the past when a patient has an implanted medical device such as a pacemaker, although certain modern pacemaker models may be acceptable for MRI.[6]

Also, there may be some limitations in patients who have implanted spinal hardware because of artifact, but newer metal reduction techniques may help in reducing the amount of that artifact.

REFERENCES

1. Edelman RR, Warach S. Magnetic resonance imaging. N Engl J Med. 1993;328(10):708-16.
2. Fardon DF, Milette PC. Nomenclature and classification of lumbar disc pathology: recommendations of the combined task forces of the North American Spine Society, American Society of Spine Radiology, and American Society of Neuroradiology. Spine. 2001;26(5):E93-113.
3. Modic M, Steinberg P, Ross J, et al. Degenerative disk disease: assessment of changes in vertebral body marrow with MR imaging. Radiology. 1988;166(1):193-9.
4. Moorthy S, Prabhu NK. Spectrum of MR imaging findings in spinal tuberculosis. Am J Roentgenol. 2002;179(4):979-83.
5. Norman D, Mills CM, Brant-Zawadzki M, et al. Magnetic resonance imaging of the spinal cord and canal: potentials and limitations. Am J Roentgenol. 1983;141(6):1147-52.
6. Goldsher D, Amikam S, Boulos M, et al. Magnetic resonance imaging for patients with permanent pacemakers: initial clinical experience. IMAJ-RAMAT GAN. 2006;8(2):91-4.

CHAPTER

15 Interventional Diagnostic Procedures: Nerve Blocks and Discography

Steven Calvino, Jessie Ng

INTRODUCTION

The ability to accurately diagnose the etiology of pain is invariably the most important element in treating any individual, because doing so enables one to direct appropriate pharmacologic or interventional therapy. A thorough history and physical examination combined with laboratory and radiological data may not always provide a clear and precise diagnostic conclusion. A well-performed diagnostic block may add an important piece to the clinical "puzzle" that the clinician can use to confirm or disprove his clinical impression.[1]

It is important to note that the vast majority of diagnostic nerve blocks aid in diagnosis by attempting to alleviate a patient's pain. Consider the following brief clinical scenario:

> A 37-year-old male with no significant past medical history presents to your office with a 3 month history of left buttock pain that radiates at times to the posterolateral aspect of the thigh down to the knee. He has failed conservative therapies and radiologic studies report the presence of both lower lumbar facet arthropathy as well as a disk herniation at the L4/5 level indenting the thecal sac in the midline. The physical exam, other laboratory data, and remainder of the history are equivocal.

At this time one may consider the possibility of multiple etiologies including lumbar facet arthropathy, lumbar radiculitis, lumbar discogenic pain, sacroiliitis, or even lateral femoral cutaneous neuropathy. In this instance, a specialized block with local anesthetic to one of those structures or their nerve supply may help the physician in the diagnosis and perhaps allow a targeted therapy, thereby saving time and money and limiting the patient's exposure to painful interventions.

As exemplified above, diagnostic blocks are most often performed when a patient is actively experiencing pain. In such cases, it is the goal of the medical professional to alleviate the pain utilizing local anesthetic medication. However, provocative discography is an exception to this rule. Provocative discography is the only diagnostic nerve block that is performed purely to elicit or reproduce a patient's pain.[2] This chapter aims to guide the physician in the utilization of nerve blocks to aid in the diagnosis of pain. In addition, considering the unique characteristic of provocative discography, this controversial procedure is discussed in greater detail.

DIAGNOSTIC NERVE BLOCKS

In general, a diagnostic nerve block aims to anesthetize a specific structure that the clinician suspects is the source of the patient's pain. A positive result of the block is the elimination, or at least attenuation, of the patient's symptoms. Table 15.1 presents several common blocks.

In performing diagnostic nerve blocks, the clinician should realize that even a technically perfect block is not without limitations. While a diagnostic block may add to the clinical impression, it remains only one part of the overall workup. The patient's history, physical examination, and laboratory and radiographic testing should be considered in combination with results obtained from the diagnostic nerve block. Information obtained from the diagnostic nerve block should not be overly relied upon and contradictory results should be viewed with skepticism.[1]

Technical limitations may also affect the accuracy of diagnostic blocks, as neuroanatomic structure can make the procedure somewhat imprecise. It is thus important

Table 15.1: Types of spinal nerve blocks

Types of spinal nerve block	*Indication*
• Greater and lesser occipital nerve block	• Cervicogenic headache
• Stellate ganglion block	• Upper extremity or facial pain
• Cervical facet block	• Cervicogenic headache and/or neck pain
• Intercostal nerve block	• Chest wall and/or abdominal pain
• Celiac plexus block	• Chest wall, flank and/or abdominal pain
• Lumbar sympathetic block	• Lower extremity pain

that the clinician is familiar with spinal anatomy and has the technical expertise to perform the block so that the potential for false positive or negative results is minimized. In addition, the use of fluoroscopic CT guidance or ultrasound with the addition of radiopaque contrast medium may increase the accuracy of the block.[1]

A diagnostic nerve block should only be performed, while the patient is experiencing pain. For example, in patients who suffer from incident pain, occurring only with certain activities or when certain movements are undertaken, it may be prudent to encourage the patient to attempt to reproduce the pain prior to the diagnostic procedure. It is important to consider pain as a subjective phenomenon related to premedication, placebo effects, the presence of afferent nociceptive input (even in the presence of dense blocks), and modulation of pain sensations along the spinal cord, brain, and higher levels.[3] To provide the most accurate results, the patient should be carefully counseled on the pain in which the diagnostic nerve block is intended to alleviate. In addition, the expected pharmacologic duration of the local anesthetic used should be assessed prior to neural blockade.[1]

In order to properly incorporate the results of the diagnostic block into the clinical impression, the clinician must know the expected results for a positive or negative test. Therefore, prior to performing a block, the clinician must understand the properties of the local anesthetic used, including its time of onset and duration. It is important to note that the duration of action of various local anesthetics was studied in subjects without pain. As such, it is possible for these durations to vary when performing diagnostic blocks in patients with chronic pain.[3,4] Additionally, careful attention should be given to the amount of local anesthetic utilized for the diagnostic block, as too little may produce a false negative result and too much may anesthetize structures that were not intended to be blocked, thereby producing a false positive result.[2] Table 15.2 illustrates commonly used local anesthetics and their expected onset time and duration.

When performing diagnostic nerve blocks of the spine, there are potential complications that may arise both during and after the procedure. These include local anesthetic toxicity, bleeding, and infection; they and other complications will be discussed in greater detail in subsequent chapters.[5]

DISCOGRAPHY

Unlike the previously discussed diagnostic blocks, discography is the only block that is purely diagnostic, and remains a controversial test. This procedure consists of two separate components. The first part involves injection of contrast medium into the nucleus pulposus to study the internal morphology. The second part involves stimulation of the disk by distension of the nucleus pulposus using an injectate to determine whether that specific disk is involved in generating the patient's pain symptoms.[2] The most common pain generators in the axial low back pain population are the intervertebral disk (5–39% of patients), zygapophysial joint (15–40%), and sacroiliac joint (6–13%).[6]

ANATOMY AND FUNCTION OF THE INTERVERTEBRAL DISK

The primary function of the intervertebral disk is to distribute forces/loads to allow motion in the cervical, thoracic, and lumbar regions of the spine. The anatomy and function of intervertebral disks have been described in detail in Chapter 1. The outer annulus consists of fibrous cartilage layered in 15–25 concentric lamellae. Each layer is arranged in the opposite direction as the one opposing it at a 60° angle, and elastin fibers connect the lamellae to each other. The centrally located nucleus pulposus consists of a highly hydrated, aggrecan containing gel that sits in randomly organized collagen fibers and radially arranged elastin fibers.[2]

It is the outer 1/3 of the annulus that receives innervation from both the anterior and posterior plexuses. The anterior plexus is composed of branches of two sympathetic trunks: the proximal ends of the gray rami and the perivascular nerve plexuses of the segmental arteries. The posterior plexus arises mainly from the sinovertebral nerve.[2]

Table 15.2: Clinical profile of local anesthetics

Local anesthetic	*Concentration (%)*	*Clinical use*	*Onset*	*Duration (h)*	*Recommended maximum single dose (mg)*
• Amides					
– Bupivacaine	0.25	Infiltration	Fast	2–8	175/225 + epinephrine
– Levobupivacaine	0.25–0.5	Peripheral nerve block	Slow	4–12	150
	0.5–0.75	Epidural anesthesia	Moderate	2–5	150
	0.03–0.25	Epidural analgesia	NA	NA	NA
	0.5–0.75	Spinal anesthesia	Fast	1–4	20
– Etidocaine	0.5%	Infiltration	Fast	2–8	300/400 + epinephrine
	0.5–1	Peripheral nerve block	Fast	3–12	300/400 + epinephrine
	1–1.5	Epidural anesthesia	Fast	2–4	300/400 + epinephrine
– Lidocaine	0.5–1	Infiltration	Fast	1–4	300/500 + epinephrine
	0.25–0.5	IV regional anesthesia	Fast	0.5–1	300
	1–1.5	Peripheral nerve block	Fast	1–3	300/500 + epinephrine
	1.5–2	Epidural anesthesia	Fast	1–2	300/500 + epinephrine
	1.5–5	Spinal anesthesia	Fast	0.5–1	100
	4	Topical	Fast	0.5–1	300
– Mepivacaine	0.5–1	Infiltration	Fast	1–4	400/500 + epinephrine
	1–1.5	Peripheral nerve block	Fast	2–4	400/500 + epinephrine
	1.5–2	Epidural anesthesia	Fast	1–3	400/500 + epinephrine
	2–4	Spinal anesthesia	Fast	1–2	100
– Prilocaine	0.5–1	Infiltration	Fast	1–2	600
	0.25–0.5	IV regional anesthesia	Fast	0.5–1	600
	1.5–2	Peripheral nerve block	Fast	1.5–3	600
	2–3	Epidural	Fast	1–3	600
– Ropivacaine	0.2–0.5	Infiltration	Fast	2–6	200
	0.5–1	Peripheral nerve block	Slow	5–8	250
	0.5–1	Epidural anesthesia	Moderate	2–6	200
	0.05–0.2	Epidural analgesia	NA	NA	NA
• Mixture					
– Lidocaine + prilocaine	2.5/2.5	Skin topical	Slow	3–5	20 gm
• Esters					
– Benzocaine	Up to 20%	Topical	Fast	0.5–1	200
– Chloroprocaine	1	Infiltration	Fast	0.5–1	800/1,000 + epinephrine
	2	Peripheral nerve block	Fast	0.5–1	800/1,000 + epinephrine
	2–3	Epidural anesthesia	Fast	0.5–1	800/1,000 + epinephrine
– Cocaine	4–10	Topical	Fast	0.5–1	150
– Procaine	10	Spinal anesthesia	Fast	0.5–1	1,000
– Tetracaine	2	Topical	Fast	0.5–1	20
	0.5	Spinal anesthesia	Fast	2–6	20

(IV: Intravenous).

Source: Adapted from Covino BG, Wildsmith JAW. Clinical pharmacology of local anesthetic agents. In: Cousins MJ, Bridenbaugh PO (Eds). Neural Blockade in Clinical Anesthesia and Management of Pain. Philadelphia, PA: Lippincott-Raven; 1998, p. 97, with permission.

DISK DEGENERATION AND PAIN

In the asymptomatic disk, the nerve endings are located in the periphery of the outer annulus, with the central endplate and periannular connective tissue the most densely innervated. In contrast, degenerative disks often have nerve endings that penetrate into the nucleus pulposus. In addition, mechanical stress can contribute to a release of inflammatory enzymes, which may sensitize neural structures within and in close proximity to the disk and result in pain.[2,7]

PROCEDURE (FIG. 15.1)

Indications and contraindications for discography are discribed in Table 15.3. A posterior approach is possible, but more commonly a lateral or extrapedicular approach is used. The patient is placed in prone position on a radiolucent table with support under the abdomen to provide slight flexing of the spine, thereby decreasing the lordotic curve. In order to prevent the patient mistaking the discomfort from needle placement as pain secondary to disk stimulation, the disk is approached from the side opposite the patient's pain. A 22 or 25 gauge, 3.5-inch needle is advanced under fluoroscopic guidance to the level of the superior articular process, with lidocaine injected while the needle is withdrawn. Care should be taken not to inject local anesthetics into the foramen, where the sinovertebral and ramus communicans nerves are located, which could result in a false negative result.[2]

A one-needle (one needle with stylet) or two-needle (introducer needle with a complementary disk puncture needle) technique can be used. The needle is advanced to the intervertebral foramen, where firm resistance will be noted as the needle enters the annulus fibrosis. If radicular pain or dysesthesia is noted, the needle should be partially withdrawn and redirected. The needle is advanced under active fluoroscopy into the center of the disk. Patients may experience axial discomfort with referral into the thigh or buttock due to innervation of the outer third of the annulus. Nonionic myelographic contrast with added antibiotic is injected via a manometer syringe or 3 mL syringe in 0.5 mL aliquots until:

- A 3 mL volume has been attained, or
- Significant pain is noted by the patient, or
- An epidural or vascular pattern is noted, or
- A maximum pressure of 75–100 psi has been reached

A positive result is when concordant pain is experienced with pressure < 15 psi above opening pressures.[2]

COMPLICATIONS

Complications of provocative discography include discitis, pneumothorax (in cervical or thoracic regions), direct nerve injury, and vascular injury (which may result in bleeding). Discitis appears to be the most common complication; however, the literature shows the incidence of this complication to be low: approximately 0.25% by

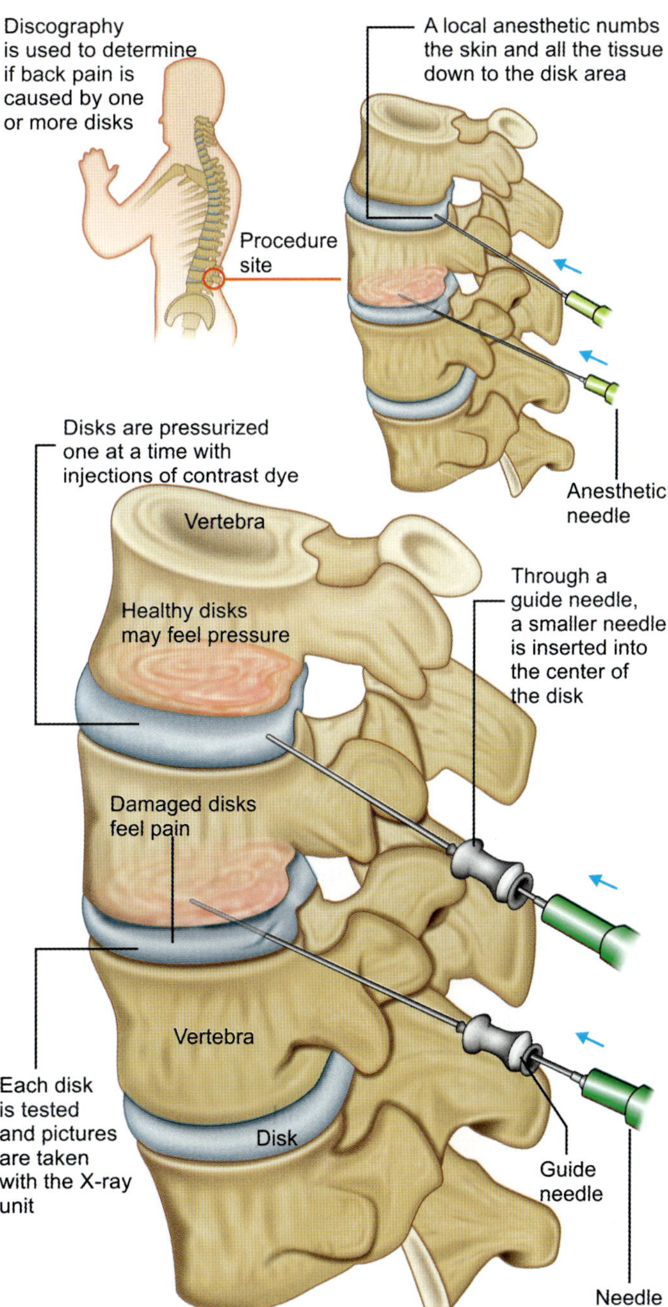

Fig. 15.1: Schematic representation diagram nerve block.

Table 15.3: Indications and contraindications for discography

Indications	*Absolute contraindications*	*Relative contraindications*
• Failure of conservative management for axial low back pain	• Patient is unable to or unwilling to consent for procedure	• Allergy to contrast medium, antibiotics, or local anesthetics
• Pain is not acute or subacute	• Physician is unable to assess patient response during procedure	• Significant or psychological overlay
• Other pain generators have been ruled out	• Patient unable to cooperate	• Beard (cervical)
• Symptoms that may reasonably be expected to be arising from the disk	• Known localized or systemic infection	• Spinal canal AP diameter < 11 mm (cervical)
• Symptoms severe enough to consider surgery or percutaneous treatment	• Pregnancy	• Any other condition, medical, anatomic, or psychological, that would increase the risk of performance of the examination to unsafe levels
• Surgery is planned and the surgeon desires an assessment of the adjacent disk levels regarding internal morphology or pain generation	• Patient receiving anticoagulation therapy or has a bleeding disorder	
• Ability to understand the nature of the technique and participate appropriately during the examination	• Spinal canal AP diameter < 10 mm (cervical)	

Source: Adapted from Waldman SD. Pain Management. Philadelphia, PA: Saunders Elsevier; 2007. p. 123.

patient and 0.14% by disk.[8-10] Other complications have been reported, including meningitis, arachnoiditis, intrinsic disk damage, and headache, which may be related to spinal fluid leak, but these have been reported much less frequently due to improved technique and imaging capabilities.[8]

EVIDENCE

It may seem likely that with advances in imaging technology, a physician could accurately diagnosis a painful disk without the need to perform an invasive procedure that carries potential risks and complications. In fact, the results of several studies suggest that MRI must usually be used in conjunction with provocative discography to successfully diagnose a painful disk.

One such study by Horton et al. (1992) found that MRI was only useful in extremes. They found that a dark or extremely degenerative disk was predictive of a positive provocation and a well-hydrated disk would most likely not have a positive provocation. However, in cases that fall between these extremes, there was no significant correlation between imaging and discography results.[11] In another study, Jensen et al. (1994) performed MRI examinations on 98 asymptomatic people and found that only 36% of those examined had a normal disk at all levels.[12] These results indicate that MRI alone is not sufficient for identifying discogenic pain, and should be used in conjunction with all other available medical data including provocative discography.

There has also been debate over the utilization of discography in the diagnosis of discogenic pain, especially due to the contradictory outcomes of several studies looking at the potential rate of false positives. However, in a recent meta-analysis by Wolfer et al. (2008), it was found that in patients with chronic low back pain, discography is a useful diagnostic test to determine whether or not a particular disk is painful or not. It was reported that a false positive rate of 6% is expected, provided that the International Association for the Study of Pain (IASP) standard is applied when performing the block. Cohen et al. (2005) looked at the accuracy of discography and its relation to outcomes for surgery. Their conclusion was that discography, especially when combined with CT scanning, may be more accurate than other radiologic studies.[7] However, they found no evidence that surgical outcomes are improved following preoperative provocative discography.

CONCLUSION

Diagnostic nerve blocks and discography are invasive procedures that aim to precisely identify the source of a patient's pain. They should be considered after other potential pain generators in the spine have been ruled out, and after all other pertinent medical data including history, physical examination, pertinent laboratory data, and advanced imaging has been performed.

REFERENCES

1. Waldman SD. Neural blockade for the diagnosis of pain. In: Waldman SD (Ed.). Pain Management, 2nd edition. Philadelphia, PA: Saunders; 2011. pp. 149-54.
2. Landers MH. Diskography. In: Waldman SD (Ed.). Pain Management, 2nd edition. Philadelphia, PA: Saunders; 2011. pp. 118-44.
3. Hogan QH, Abram SE. Neural blockade for diagnosis and prognosis: a review. Anesthesiology. 1997;86(1):216-41.
4. Bogduk N. Diagnostic nerve blocks in chronic pain. Best Prac Res Clin Anaesthesiol. 2002;16(4):565-78.
5. Winnie AP, Candido KD. Differential neural blockade for the diagnosis of pain. In: Waldman SD (Ed). Pain Management, 2nd edition. Philadelphia, PA: Saunders; 2011. pp. 155-66.
6. Vora AJ, Doerr KD, Wolfer LR. Functional anatomy and pathophysiology of axial low back pain: disk, posterior elements, sacroiliac joint, and associated pain generators. Phys Med Rehabil Clin N Am. 2010;21(4):679.
7. Cohen SP, Larkin TM, Barna SA, et al. Lumbar discography: a comprehensive review of outcome studies, diagnostic accuracy, and principles. Reg Anesth Pain Med. 2005;30(2): 163-83.
8. Guyer RD, Ohnmeiss DD. Lumbar discography. Spine J. 2003;3(3 Suppl):11S-27S.
9. Sharma SK, Jones JO, Zeballos PP, et al. The prevention of discitis during discography. Spine J. 2009;9(11):936-43.
10. Windsor RE, Storm S, Sugar R. Prevention and management of complications resulting from common spinal injections. Pain Phys. 2003;6(4):473-84.
11. Horton WC, Daftari TK. Which disk as visualized by magnetic resonance imaging is actually a source of pain? A correlation between magnetic resonance imaging and discography. Spine. 1992;17(6 Suppl):S164.
12. Jensen MC, Brant-Zawadzki MN, Obuchowski N, et al. Magnetic resonance imaging of the lumbar spine in people without back pain. N Engl J Med. 1994;331(2):69-73.

CHAPTER 16

Rheumatic Diseases and Myofascial Pain

Brian D Golden

HOW TO TELL THE DIFFERENCE BETWEEN "-ITIS" AND "-ALGIA"

Back pain can arise due to a spectrum of etiologies, including mechanical, inflammatory, and myalgic myofascial mechanisms. The latter two cases may be especially difficult to distinguish from one another. When does spinal/axial pain represent an inflammatory rheumatologic disease, such as ankylosing spondylitis (AS)? And when is it interpretable within the context of a noninflammatory pain syndrome, such as fibromyalgia or myofascial pain syndrome? As a rheumatologist, the most important thing that one can do in diagnosing a patient is drawing that distinction: does he or she have a disease that is characterized by tissue inflammation, an "-itis," or a pain syndrome in the context of an "-algia?"

Patients do not "self-diagnose" very well. They often present with a multitude of symptoms along with back pain. Additional common, nonspecific complaints include stiffness, lack of energy, sleeping problems, lack of concentration, bowel symptoms, fatigue, and generalized pain. Patients who come to see a rheumatologist also have physical signs on objective examination. For example, sometimes patients demonstrate an inability to flex the spine and to reach their feet; they cannot tie their shoes. Their lumbar lordosis may be straightened and irreversible. They may be rather slow and purposeful in how they move. Their demeanor may indicate with drawal. There may be tenderness in certain places on or around the spine or sacroiliac joints/pelvis.

It is important to note that patients may present to a rheumatologist with very similar symptoms but end up with diametrically opposite diagnoses: inflammatory or noninflammatory in etiology. It is critically important to understand this dichotomy and to make the diagnoses properly, as spondylitis and fibromyalgia differ greatly with regard to their respective natural histories and potential for inflammation/injury at the tissue level.

ANKYLOSING SPONDYLITIS AS THE PROTOTYPICAL INFLAMMATORY, RHEUMATOLOGIC DISEASE AFFECTING THE SPINE

Left untreated, and in the years prior to disease-modifying therapy, the natural history of AS[1] is one characterized by progressive inflammatory-type spinal symptoms ("morning stiffness"), slowly progressive spinal deformity (Fig. 16.1) and loss of function, fusion of the sacroiliac joints, vertebral squaring (Fig. 16.2), limited dynamic motion demonstrable on flexion and extension panels, syndesmophyte formation, and ossification of longitudinal ligaments, resulting in classic "bamboo spine (Fig. 16.2)". Generally in AS, patients suffer large joint involvement—hips and shoulders, e.g. not usually small joints like hands, wrists and toes. Radiographically, the obliteration and ankylosis of the sacroiliac joints is usually followed by slow ascension of inflammatory disease cranially, to the thoracic and cervical spines. Peripheral joint inflammatory damage involves large proximal joints, namely, the hips, with resultant concentric cartilage loss and so-called protrusio aceta-buli. Such clinico-radiographic features are pathognomonic of AS.

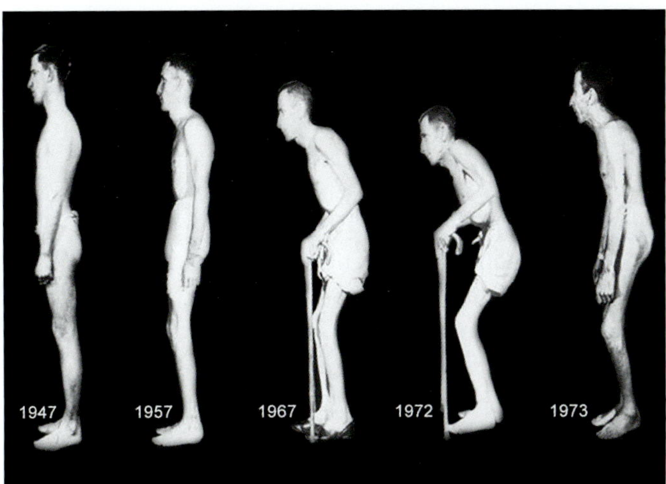

Fig. 16.1: Ankylosing spondylitis is characterised by slow progressive spinal deformity.

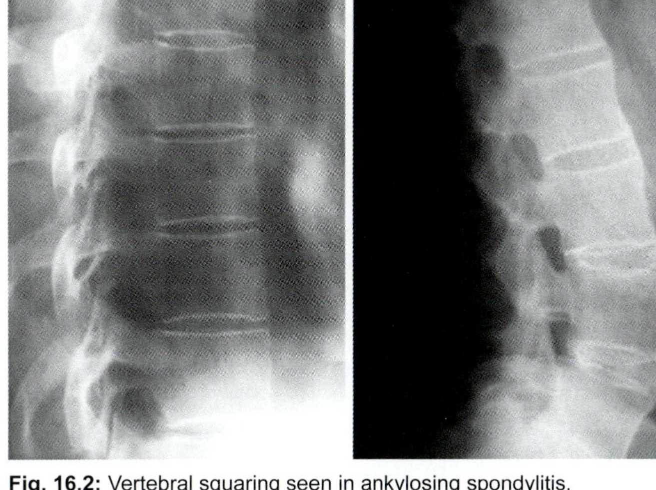

Fig. 16.2: Vertebral squaring seen in ankylosing spondylitis.

Ankylosing spondylitis is a multisystemic inflammatory disease. It is typically characterized by a genetic propensity, family history, and human leukocyte antigen (HLA) association: approximately 90% of patients have the HLA Class I B27 marker. In fact, HLA B27 may be present in a cluster of inflammatory conditions, the seronegative [meaning rheumatoid-factor (RF)-negative] inflammatory arthritides, aka seronegative spondyloarthropathies. This group includes AS, psoriatic arthritis, reactive arthritis (Reiter syndrome), and inflammatory bowel disease (IBD)-associated arthritis. AS is simply the prototype of spinal involvement/spondyloarthropathy. Enthesopathy (inflammation at the site of tendinous insertions into bones) is common among the seronegative arthritides and AS. Often, this manifests as plantar fasciitis.

Bamboo spine is irreversible. Once there has been ossification of the anterior longitudinal ligaments and complete fusion of the posterior spinal elements (facet joints), patients are left with literally no residual motion of the lumbar (and later, thoracic and cervical) spines. As a consequence, in an effort to maintain forward gaze when the normal lumbar lordosis has been fused and lost, patients compensate by flexing at the hip, and a hip flexion contracture may develop (Fig. 16.1). This hip damage is also contributed to by inflammatory arthropathy of the hip joints. Given this prognosis, the best treatment options for AS involve identifying the disease as early in its course as possible, when it may even be possible to slow the progression of the disorder.

The treatment options for AS have expanded in recent years. Nonsteroidal anti-inflammatory drugs (NSAIDs) had been the mainstay of pharmacologic therapy for AS for many years. They exert a great therapeutic effect. They are safe and well tolerated for symptomatic improvement of spinal pain and stiffness. Moreover, there are some data in the literature positing slowing of progression of the inflammatory spinal damage by NSAIDs alone. For some patients, this is good enough. Another treatment option is sulfasalazine. This is not a new drug, as it has been utilized for decades in the treatment of rheumatoid arthritis (RA) and IBD. It is quite helpful for AS, particularly for the inflammatory arthropathy of large joints. It is generally not effective for spinal symptoms (stiffness) or retardation of disease progression, nor for sacroiliitis.

The class of drugs known as antitumor necrosis factor (TNF) biologics has greatly altered treatment of AS. Representative examples, which have been studied for use in AS, include etanercept,[2,3] infliximab,[3] adalimumab,[4] and golimumab.[5] Patients with AS have been shown to benefit tremendously in terms of day-to-day symptom relief by using these drugs.

More importantly, it is believed that the anti-TNF drugs may slow disease progression; that is, they can prevent ankylosis and loss of function over time.[6] There are two components to the key pathogenetic processes of AS: inflammation and bone formation (ankylosis). Inhibitors of TNF effectively block inflammation, as is known from extrapolation from therapies for RA and other small-joint inflammatory polyarthritis, such as psoriatic arthritis. It is also known that AS patients treated with anti-TNF agents display a decrease of serologic inflammatory markers (acute phase reactants such as erythrocyte sedimentation rate (ESR) and C-reactive protein).[6] In terms of ankylosis, studies have shown that treatment of AS reduces early magnetic resonance imaging (MRI) changes (bright T2 signal at the corners of vertebral bodies), and it is believed that the drugs may also prevent erosive damage, e.g. of the SI joints and the hips.[2-5] However, clinical trials are still only a few years in duration at most, making it difficult to truly prove changes in the course of the disease as it presents clinically.[2-5]

However, as indicated previously, ossification and ankylosis cannot be reversed using TNF blockers; they do not exert significant effect upon osteoblasts. It has been suggested that perhaps established bone changes of AS can be addressed or improved by therapy with bisphosphonates, which are antiresorptive, antiosteoclast drugs effective as therapy for osteoporosis and Paget disease of bone. This hypothesis has not presently been borne out in studies, although bisphosphonates as a class have generated some data showing preservation of bone mineral density in patients with AS. Thus, the most important time to prevent structural damage remains early in AS natural history, utilizing effective anti-inflammatory treatment.

Finally, around 40% of AS patients experience ocular inflammatory disease, specifically anterior uveitis: iritis or iridocyclitis. This affects approximately 15–20% of patients with AS and can lead to blindness if untreated. One of the less common clinical manifestations of AS is aortic root inflammation (aortitis) that results in aortic insufficiency.

FIBROMYALGIA AS THE PROTOTYPICAL NONINFLAMMATORY PAIN SYNDROME

To reiterate, AS lies on one end of the spectrum of rheumatic disease as an example of an inflammatory illness that can affect end-organ and widespread tissue damage. On the other end lies fibromyalgia syndrome, a noninflammatory, nondestructive condition characterized by diffuse pain, which most certainly may invoke the spine.[7] The clinical distinction between these entities is often not easy to make.

Fibromyalgia is a syndrome characterized by enhanced sensitivity to pain that affects approximately 4% of the US population. It is characterized by myalgia (muscle pain) or body pain that can be localized, in which case it is termed "myofascial pain." When pain is more generalized and is associated with severe fatigue, fibromyalgia overlaps clinically with chronic fatigue syndrome. These pain diagnoses lie along a continuum. One shared physical examination finding among them is that of tender muscular trigger points. These tender spots may be located in the back, in which case they are termed paraspinal trigger points.

The pathophysiology of fibromyalgia is not well understood, but it is an area of active research. Studies have shown that enhanced pain sensitivity occurs at both the peripheral and central tiers of the nervous system.[8] There is increasing basic science literature positing that central nervous system malfunction results in amplification of pain transmission and interpretation.[8] Genetic investigations have revealed influence of genes for serotoninergic, dopaminergic and catecholaminergic systems in its pathogenesis.[8] What is clear, however, is that the involved painful muscles and joints (including the spine) are themselves not deranged or pathologic.

Clinical features of fibromyalgia are myriad, and it can manifest itself through numerous somatic complaints. Nonetheless, criteria of the syndrome have been accepted by the American College of Rheumatology (ACR).[9] Affected patients generally do not sleep well; there may be frequent nocturnal awakenings and nonrefreshing or nonrestorative sleep. Symptoms include widespread pain. There is a clinical association, in many patients, with depression or anxiety. Some patients have associated "functional" pain conditions, such as irritable bowel syndrome and migraine headaches.

The diagnosis of fibromyalgia is considered by many to be one of exclusion. In other words, many clinical entities, both rheumatologic and nonrheumatologic, may be a primary cause of diffuse pain and myalgias. With regard to the diagnosis of fibromyalgia, the principal role of the rheumatologist is to consider and exclude alternative explanations. Possibilities include the following:

- Mechanical joint pain due to overuse, trauma, or osteoarthritis
- Certain medications (e.g. statins) which can cause myalgia and a toxic myopathy
- Endocrinologic disorders (e.g. hypothyroidism, hypocortisolism, hypogonadism, and diabetes)
- Neurologic disorders (e.g. multiple sclerosis)
- Infectious diseases (e.g. hepatitis C and Lyme disease)
- Inflammatory rheumatic disease (e.g. polymyalgia rheumatica and idiopathic inflammatory myopathy)
- Osteomalacia due to severe vitamin D deficiency

- Steroid tapering or "withdrawal"
- Sleep apnea or other objective sleep disorders.

Treatment of fibromyalgia syndrome includes both nonpharmacologic and pharmacologic approaches.[7] Many patients derive benefit from physical therapy with massage, dedicated aerobic exercise (e.g. swimming), cognitive approaches (such as biofeedback), complementary-alternative medical choices such as yoga and acupuncture, and trigger point injections with corticosteroid +/– lidocaine.

A list of pharmacologic options includes tricyclic antidepressants; NSAIDs; analgesics (both oral and topical); muscle relaxants; selective serotonin reuptake inhibitors (SSRIs) and combined serotonin/norepinephrine reup take antagonists (SNRIs); newer-generation anticonvulsants; soporific agents; and benzodiazepines. These may be tried alone, sequentially, or in combination. Unlike in years past, the clinical use of many of these drugs is now supported by research and clinical trials; FDA-approved drugs for fibromyalgia include duloxetine, milnacipran, and pregabalin.

CONCLUSION

Patients may present to musculoskeletal healthcare providers with certain symptom complexes inclusive of back pain. On some occasions ("-itis"), these symptoms may signal an inflammatory rheumatologic disease capable of causing irreparable spinal damage and organ pathology due to extra-articular disease. On others ("-algia"), the complaints are part of a larger disturbance of pain perception, a syndrome whose aches and pains, though vexing, do not cause destruction at the tissue level. As clinicians, it is important to recognize the distinction between these entities and to tailor appropriate early diagnosis and treatment.

REFERENCES

1. Arnett F. Ankylosing spondylitis. Arthritis and allied conditions. A textbook of rheumatology, 13th edition. Baltimore, MD: Williams & Wilkins; 1997:1197-208.
2. Gorman JD, Sack KE, Davis Jr JC. Treatment of ankylosing spondylitis by inhibition of tumor necrosis factor. N Engl J Med. 2002;346(18):1349-56.
3. van der Heijde D, Dijkmans B, Geusens P, et al. Efficacy and safety of infliximab in patients with ankylosing spondylitis: results of a randomized, placebo-controlled trial (ASSERT). Arthritis Rheum. 2005;52(2):582-91.
4. van der Heijde D, Kivitz A, Schiff MH, et al. Efficacy and safety of adalimumab in patients with ankylosing spondylitis: results of a multicenter, randomized, double-blind, placebocontrolled trial. Arthritis Rheum. 2006;54(7):2136-46.
5. Inman RD, Davis JC, Heijde DVD, et al. Efficacy and safety of golimumab in patients with ankylosing spondylitis: results of a randomized, double-blind, placebo-controlled, phase III trial. Arthritis Rheum. 2008;58(11):3402-12.
6. Appel H, Sieper J. Spondyloarthritis at the crossroads of imaging, pathology, and structural damage in the era of biologics. Curr Rheumatol Rep. 2008;10(5):356-63.
7. Dadabhoy D, Clauw D. Musculoskeletal Signs and Symptoms. In: Klippel J, Stone J, Crofford L, White P (Eds). Primer on the Rheumatic Disease, 13th edition. New York, NY: Springer Science; 2008. pp. 87-93.
8. Buskila D. Developments in the scientific and clinical understanding of fibromyalgia. Arthritis Res Ther. 2009; 11(5):242.
9. Wolfe F, Smythe HA, Yunus MB, et al. The American College of Rheumatology 1990 criteria for the classification of fibromyalgia. Arthritis Rheum. 1990;33(2):160-72.

CHAPTER

17

Diagnosis of Osteopenia and Osteoporosis

Stephen Honig, Stephen P Maier II

INTRODUCTION

Osteoporosis is the most common metabolic bone disease in the United States and most often affects postmenopausal women. In this chapter, the term osteoporosis should be assumed to indicate a low bone mass state affecting postmenopausal woman unless otherwise indicated. Chapter 22 focuses on pharmacologic and non-pharmacologic approaches to fracture prevention for women with postmenopausal osteoporosis. Osteoporosis is, of course, a major public health concern, because of the number of fractures that occur in the population of people with low bone stock. Nearly half of all Caucasian American women age 50 or older will experience a hip, spine, or wrist fracture during the remainder of their lives.[1] In many instances, these fractures permanently and negatively impact an individual's quality and length of life with hip fractures resulting in a significant increase in short-term mortality rates. Nearly 20% of patients who survive the consequences of a hip fracture are no longer able to live independently.[2] Identifying those individuals who are at increased risk of osteoporosis related fractures is a critical imperative for health-care professionals. While bone density testing remains the diagnostic gold standard for osteoporosis, advances in diagnostic imaging including technologies such as peripheral micro-computed tomography (micro-CT) and ultrahigh-resolution magnetic resonance imaging (MRI) are making it possible for investigators to noninvasively assess bone microarchitecture with the hope that these modalities may provide additional insights in identifying individuals at increased fracture risk. This chapter reviews how the diagnosis of osteoporosis has evolved over the past two decades, describes the pathogenesis of postmenopausal osteoporosis, and discusses the role of bone density and other imaging techniques. The chapter also briefly describes the role of FRAX (fracture-risk assessment tool) as a fracture predicting clinical tool.

Population-based fracture prevention strategies depend on the development of cost-effective methods designed to identify individuals at increased risk of fracture. Current guidelines suggest that American women aged 65 and older should have a screening bone density test.[3] The National Osteoporosis Foundation also recommends testing for women younger than 65 if they have certain risk factors that elevate their fracture risk. These risk factors include smoking, a thin body habitus, a history of a previous fracture, and a family history of osteoporosis.[4] Bone density test results are an important part of a number of fracture assessment tools including the web-based FRAX model developed by the World Health Organization (WHO). These tools estimate a person's fracture risk over a finite period of time and that knowledge can help clinicians determine when and if a patient requires bone strengthening medication. Fracture assessment tools emphasize the importance of a patient's age and their fracture history instead of relying only on a static bone density T-score to determine the need to treat. As with all medical care, fracture prevention strategies should help us identify those individuals who are at risk and who will benefit from therapeutic intervention.

DEFINITIONS

The definition of osteoporosis has been evolving over the past two decades in order to more accurately reflect the

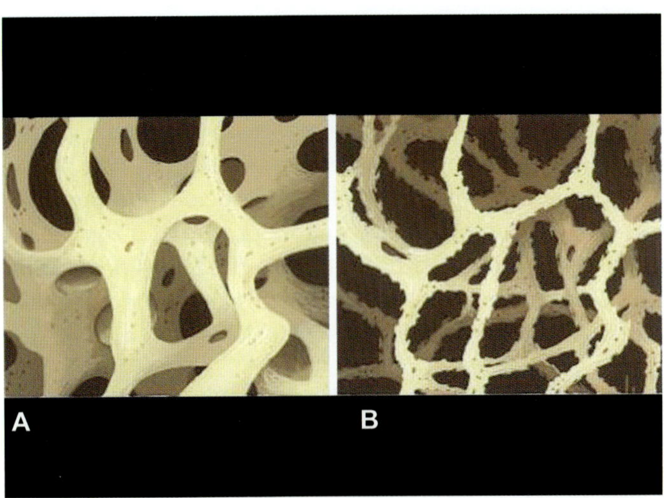

Figs. 17.1A and B: Comparison of bone density and microarchitecture between (A) normal and (B) osteoporotic bone.

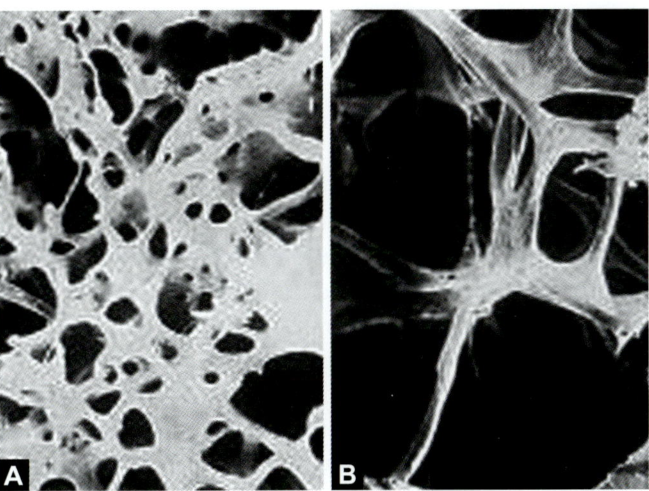

Figs. 17.2A and B: Photomicrograph radiographic images showing microarchitecture of (A) normal bone and (B) osteoporotic bone.

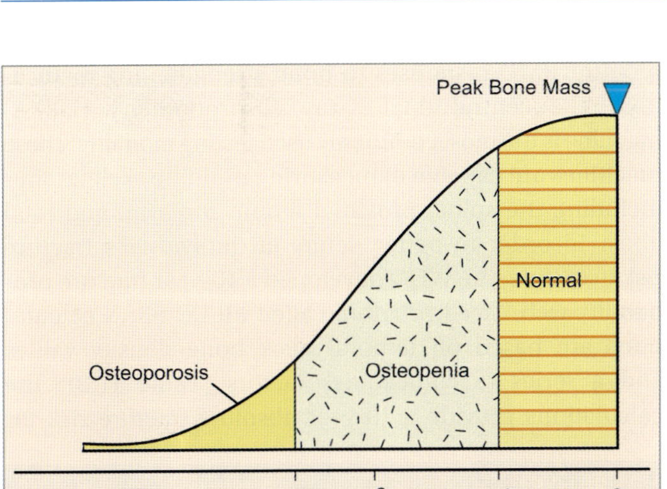

Fig. 17.3: The World Health Organization guidelines for diagnostic categories of bone mass based on bone mineral density values. *Source*: WHO Guidelines for preclinical Evaluation and clinical Trials in Osteoporosis, 1998.

Table 17.1: The standard classification of BMD in normal, osteopenic, and osteoporotic bone

Condition	*Bone mineral density (BMD) in standard deviations from mean healthy BMD*
Normal	> −1.0
Osteopenia	−1.0 to −2.5
Osteoporosis	< −2.5

importance of decreased bone strength and its relationship to fracture susceptibility. Prior to 1994, osteoporosis was defined as a clinical syndrome of low trauma fracture in an elderly patient. In 1994, the WHO introduced an epidemiologic definition of osteoporosis based on a bone density test. The bone density diagnosis of osteoporosis was defined as a bone mineral density (BMD) value more than two and one-half standard deviations (-2.5) below the BMD values of a reference group of 30-year-old women.[5] In 2001, a National Institute of Health (NIH) consensus conference defined osteoporosis as a skeletal disorder characterized by compromised bone strength predisposing a person to an increased risk of fracture.[6] Osteoporosis refers to the condition characterized by low bone mass and microarchitectural deterioration of bone tissue, with a consequent increase in bone fragility and susceptibility to fractures (Figs. 17.1 and 17.2).[7] Osteopenia is a term used to describe a wide range of BMD values that lie between -1.1 and -2.4 standard deviations below the reference group (Fig. 17.3 and Table 17.1). The WHO group chose ≤ 2.5 standard deviations below the reference group as the bone density definition for osteoporosis because it represents the point where the prevalence (percentage of postmenopausal women with those BMD values at the femoral neck) matched the lifetime risk of hip fracture in Caucasian women (16%). According to the National Osteoporosis Foundation, 10 million individuals in the United States are estimated to have osteoporosis, 80% of whom are women. An additional 34 million people are estimated to have some degree of osteopenia. Despite these numbers, a recent survey revealed that most women ages 45–75 have not discussed osteoporosis with their physicians and were unaware that osteoporosis is directly linked to hip fractures in the elderly.[8] African-Americans, because of their higher peak bone mass, have a lower incidence of osteoporosis and fractures than gender and aged-matched Caucasian and Asian-Americans.

PATHOGENESIS OF POSTMENOPAUSAL OSTEOPOROSIS

As a general rule, in the premenopausal years bone remodeling is "balanced" and occurs on a continuous basis in response to signals generated at sites of microfractures and other forms of bone stress. Bone resorption occurs when activated osteoclasts respond to signals from osteoblasts and osteocytes and initiate the process of remodeling. When remodeling is balanced, osteoblasts lay down osteoid and completely fill the newly excavated resorption pit. Over a period of months, the osteoid fully mineralizes into mature bone replacing the older, damaged bone. In the postmenopausal period, estrogen deficiency triggers an increase in both osteoclast number and activity, resulting in an overall increase in the number of active resorption sites affecting both trabecular and cortical bone. However, osteoblasts that are activated in response to the stimulated osteoclasts are not able to fill in the deeper and more numerous resorption pits, resulting in a net loss of bone with each remodeling cycle. In the postmenopausal years, average bone loss can approach 1% of bone mass every year with greater losses seen from trabecular than cortical bone. Postmenopausal bone loss is often further negatively affected by vitamin D deficiency and secondary hyperparathyroidism. Over time, the increase in bone remodeling seen in postmenopausal women results in microarchitectural deterioration of bone leading to increased bone fragility and the greater likelihood of osteoporotic (fragility) fractures. With the aging of the population, osteoporosis-related fractures will likely become a major public health and socioeconomic issue for every country. A recent report projected a significant increase in fracture rates for the United States population ≥50 years of age.[9] A numerical listing of the fracture sites and their incidence by age range is shown in Table 17.2.

DIAGNOSING OSTEOPENIA AND OSTEOPOROSIS

Bone Density Testing and FRAX

Bone density testing for postmenopausal women is done to diagnose osteoporosis, to predict fracture risk, and to monitor BMD responses to bone strengthening medication. The central dual X-ray absorptiometry (DEXA) machine is the most commonly used testing modality. These machines are capable of measuring multiple skeletal sites including the spine, proximal femur, forearm, and total body. In order to better define an individual's fracture risk over time, the WHO developed a 10-year fracture probability web-based program called FRAX. FRAX calculations are based on femoral neck bone density values and a series of clinical risk factors (Table 17.3). The calculations provide a 10-year absolute fracture risk for

Table 17.2: Incident fractures for women by fracture type, age and race in USA (2005)

Number of fractures by fracture type

Stratum	*Hip*	*Vertebral*	*Wrist*	*Pelvis*	*Other*	*Total*
• Woman						
– Age						
50–64	13,420	57,562	136,624	5,532	159,043	372,180
65–74	25,288	85,020	88,072	15,596	84,963	298,938
75–84	84,274	142,892	70,317	43,059	105,394	445,937
≥85	99,771	103,156	31,815	38,469	65,576	338,788
• Race						
– White	201,123	347,739	285,973	88,973	366,360	1,290,168
– Black	6,995	13,838	15,030	5,004	18,057	58,923
– Hisp.	8,175	15,417	15,045	5,276	17,755	61,668
– Other	6,460	11,636	10,781	3,403	12,805	45,085
Total	222,753	388,630	326,828	102,655	414,976	1,455,843

Modified from Burge R, Dawson-Hughes B, Solomon DH, Wong JB, King A, Tosteson A. Incidence and economic burden of osteoporosis-related fractures in the United States, 2005-2025. J Bone Miner Res. 2007;22(3):465-75.

Table 17.3: Clinical risk factors included in FRAX algorithm

• Age	• Current smoking
• Sex	• Glucocorticoid therapy
• Race	• Rheumatoid arthritis
• BMI* (height and weight)	• Secondary osteoporosis
• Personal history of fragility fracture	• Alcohol (>3 units/day)
• Parental history of hip fracture	• Femoral neck BMD*

Table 17.4: Sample bone density report with 10-year absolute fracture risk

• Interpretation	*Fracture risk*: Medium fracture risk *Patient's risk*: 13.0% 10-year risk of osteoporotic fracture *Average risk*: 6.7% 10-year fracture risk for an average 52 year old *NNT*: 154 similar patients would have to be treated for 1 year to prevent one osteoporotic fracture *BMD category*: Osteoporotic
• Results	
– Spine	*Levels*: L1–4 *BMD*: 0.823 g/cm^2 *T-score*: –3.0
– Total hip	*Site*: Left total hip *BMD*: 0.636 g/cm^2 *T-score*: –3.0

Modified from Leslie WD; Manitoba Bone Density Program Committee. Absolute fracture risk reporting in clinical practice: a physician-centered survey. Osteoporos Int. 2008;19(4):459-63.

hip and "major" osteoporotic fractures. Country-specific treatment recommendations based on fracture risk are suggested. In the United States, the National Osteoporosis Foundation recommends initiating treatment if the probability of a hip fracture is 3% or greater, or the risk of a major osteoporotic fracture is 20% or more.[4] The FRAX risk assessment model weighs factors that influence fracture risk beyond that which is provided by bone density testing alone. Increasing age and prior fracture history have very significant impacts on FRAX score and help better define who should be offered bone strengthening treatment to prevent fractures. Many bone density machines are including 10-year fracture-risk assessment estimates in their formal reports (Table 17.4).

Patient History and Physical Examination

A thorough history and physical examination helps to serve as an important tool not only in the diagnosis of osteoporosis but also in assessing frailty, an important component of a fracture-risk assessment. Factors like advanced age, history of previous fracture(s), family history of osteoporosis and parental hip fractures, excess alcohol intake, a smoking history, dietary habits and any history of eating disorders when younger, physical activity, medication history, and other medical concerns predispose some individuals to a greater risk of osteopenia or osteoporosis. Gender-specific factors should also be addressed, including questions regarding age at menarche and menopause and whether a woman has used or is using hormone replacement therapy.[10-12]

On physical examination, any change in height or spinal curvature, the two major indicators of osteoporotic development are to be noted. Vertebral compression fractures most often a result of weak, osteoporotic bone may result in a dramatic change in body habitus including a significant loss of height and the development of a dorsal kyphosis. More than half of all vertebral fractures are painless and require radiographic confirmation; these "morphometric fractures", underline the importance of periodic height and spinal curvature measurements.[13,14]

Laboratory Tests and Biochemical Markers

Laboratory testing may help to identify secondary causes of osteoporosis including celiac disease, inflammatory bowel disease, Cushing's syndrome, hypercalciuria, hypogonadism, multiple myeloma, hyperthyroidism, hyperparathyroidism, and vitamin D deficiency. The treatment of such existing conditions may improve bone health, but in many cases, the source of bone loss or osteoporosis is unknown.[15] Laboratory tests routinely used in the evaluation of individuals with osteoporosis include measurements of serum calcium, 24-hour urine calcium excretion, thyroid function, parathyroid hormone, and testosterone in men (Table 17.5). Decreased testosterone level is associated with bone loss in men. Furthermore, biochemical marker tests, such as osteocalcin, bone specific alkaline phosphatase, urinary collagen type 1 cross-linked N-telopeptide (NTX) and urinary or serum collagen type 1 cross-linked C-telopeptide (CTX), may be ordered to estimate rates of bone formation and resorption.[11,16-20] These tests may also be used to determine how effectively bone is responding to pharmacological treatment.

Standard X-Rays and Vertebral Fracture Assessments

A spinal X-ray is indicated in circumstances including height loss equal to or greater than 0.5 inch in 1 year, height

Table 17.5: Standard testing upon presentation of osteopenia/osteoporosis symptoms, along with each test's normal values and suggestive values for diagnosis

Test	Normal value	Value suggestive of osteopenia/osteoporosis
• Blood calcium levels	8.5–10.5 mg/dL	<8.5 or >10.5 mg/dL
• 24-hour urine calcium levels	100–250 mg	>250 mg
• 25-hydroxy-vitamin D	30–100 ng/mL	<30 ng/mL
• Thyroid function (TSH)	0.5–5.5	≤0.1
• Parathyroid hormone (PTH) levels	10–55 pg/mL	>65 pg/mL
• Testosterone levels (in men)	250–850 ng/dL	<250 ng/dL

loss equal to or greater than 1.5 inches from one's baseline height, presentation of hyperkyphosis, or development of back pain.

Vertebral fracture assessment (VFA) is a relatively new method of diagnosing vertebral deformities. VFA can be a prominent tool for fracture detection due to its demonstrated utility for vertebral visualization. A clinician may order this examination for verification if he or she suspects there is a vertebral compression fracture. The VFA's combination of low radiation exposure and high technical reproducibility renders it an attractive evaluation in groups of patients at increased risk of osteoporosis.[21–23]

Ultrahigh-resolution MRI

Ultrahigh-resolution MRI is an investigational imaging modality that allows evaluation of bone structure and microarchitecture. It can also be used to perform image-based assessments of the mechanical properties of bone that can help define bone strength and a bone's resistance to fracture.[24,25] Since the functioning and structures of the lacunocanalicular network being studied are three-dimensional (3D), they would be best studied in 3D, and may be difficult to analyze in any other way.[26] The scan times are short and there is no radiation exposure to the patient. We are currently using this technology as a complement to standard bone density testing and hope that it may provide information that can help decision making regarding the need to initiate or defer treatment. We are also using high-resolution MRIs before and 1 year after pharmacologic treatment in order to analyze how and if different bone strengthening drugs affect bone architecture as seen by this technique. A high-resolution MRI image of the distal radius of a 76-year-old woman with osteoporosis and a history of fractures detailing a decrease in trabecular bone can be seen in Figure 17.4, which contrasts with the radiological image from a 28-year-old woman with normal bone density seen in Figure 17.5.

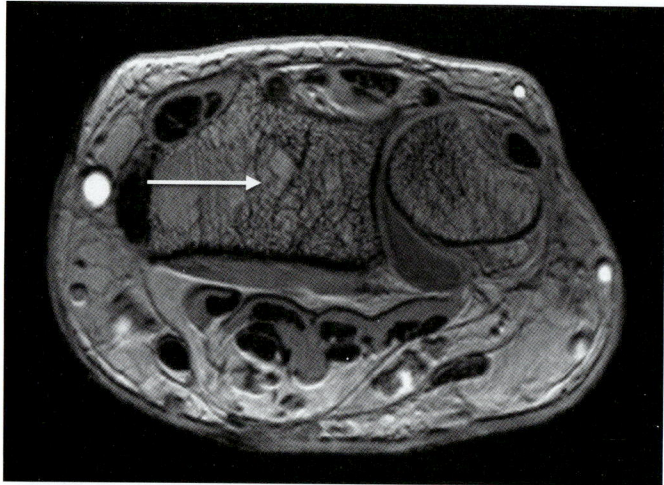

Fig. 17.4: Ultrahigh-resolution MRI of the distal radius of a 76-year-old woman with osteoporosis. White arrow points to area of decreased trabecular bone density.

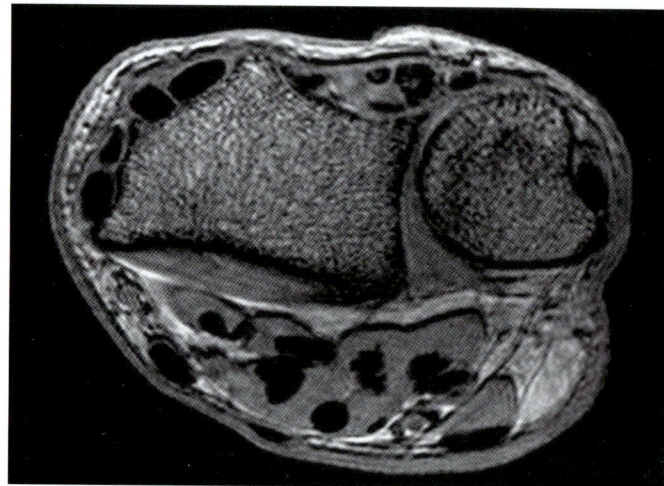

Fig. 17.5: Ultrahigh-resolution MRI of the distal radius of a 28-year-old woman with a normal bone density.

Micro-computed Tomography

Micro-CT can provide ultrahigh-resolution images with resolution of <10 μm, roughly 1,000 times greater resolution than a standard MRI image.[27,28] Micro-CT can be helpful in studying bone pathophysiology and changes in microarchitecture. Detailed 3D images are produced illustrating the orientation, shape, and connectivity of trabeculae, which are critical in understanding complex 3D bone structure. Bone strength is strongly correlated with trabecular microarchitecture, thus micro-CT can be instrumental in analyzing fragility and osteoporotic risk. Ito opined that clinical bone density measurements using DEXA were less useful than high-resolution images using the micro-CT scanner in identifying subjects at high risk of fracture.[29]

CONCLUSION

Bone density testing remains the diagnostic gold standard for osteoporosis. All women 65 and older and postmenopausal women who are younger but have certain risk factors for fracturing should have a screening bone density test. Fracture assessment tools such as FRAX, a web-based program, can help identify which patients have an increased risk for sustaining a fracture over a 10-year period of time and help the clinician who is faced with a decision regarding initiating bone strengthening medication. New modalities such as ultrahigh-resolution MRI and peripheral micro-CT scans may provide further insights into bone architecture and strength and may have a role as a complementary technique to bone density testing. Population-based fracture reduction strategies begin with identifying those individuals who are most likely to benefit from drug treatment. With the increasing aging of the population, such strategies will be increasingly necessary as the incidence of postmenopausal osteoporotic fractures or projected to increase significantly.

REFERENCES

1. Leibson CL, Tosteson AN, Gabriel SE, et al. Mortality, disability, and nursing home use for persons with and without hip fracture: a population-based study. J Am Geriatr Soc. 2002;50(10):1644-50.
2. Cummings SR, Melton LJ. Epidemiology and outcomes of osteoporotic fractures. Lancet. 2002;359(9319):1761-7.
3. Calonge N, Bibbins-Domingo K, Cantu AG, et al. Screening for osteoporosis: U.S. preventive services task force recommendation statement. Ann Intern Med. 2011;154(5):356-64.
4. Watts NB, Lewiecki EM, Miller PD, et al. National Osteoporosis Foundation 2008 Clinician's Guide to Prevention and Treatment of Osteoporosis and the World Health Organization Fracture Risk Assessment Tool (FRAX): what they mean to the bone densitometrist and bone technologist. J Clin Densitom. 2008;11(4):473-7.
5. Assessment of fracture risk and its application to screening for postmenopausal osteoporosis. Report of a WHO Study Group. World Health Organ Tech Rep Ser. 1994;843:1-129.
6. Osteoporosis prevention, diagnosis, and therapy. NIH Consens Statement. 2000;17(1):1-45.
7. Guglielmi G, Muscarella S, Bazzocchi A. Integrated imaging approach to osteoporosis: state-of-the-art review and update. Radiographics. 2011;31(5):1343-64.
8. Czerwinski E, Badurski JE, Marcinowska-Suchowierska E, et al. Current understanding of osteoporosis according to the position of the World Health Organization (WHO) and International Osteoporosis Foundation. Ortop Traumatol Rehabil. 2007;9(4):337-56.
9. Burge R, Dawson-Hughes B, Solomon DH, et al. Incidence and economic burden of osteoporosis-related fractures in the United States, 2005-2025. J Bone Miner Res. 2007;22(3):465-75.
10. Volpe R, Sotis G, Gavita R, et al. Healthy diet to prevent cardiovascular diseases and osteoporosis: the experience of the 'ProSa' project. High Blood Press Cardiovasc Prev. 2012;19(2):65-71.
11. Bours SP, van Geel TA, Geusens PP, et al. Contributors to secondary osteoporosis and metabolic bone diseases in patients presenting with a clinical fracture. J Clin Endocrinol Metab. 2011;96(5):1360-67.
12. Chung M, Lee J, Terasawa T, et al. Vitamin D with or without calcium supplementation for prevention of cancer and fractures: an updated meta-analysis for the U.S. Preventive Services Task Force. Ann Intern Med. 2011;155(12):827-38.
13. Haczynski J, Jakimiuk A. Vertebral fractures: a hidden problem of osteoporosis. Med Sci Monit. 2001;7(5):1108-17.
14. Vlak T. Compression vertebral fracture in osteoporosis—prevention and treatment. Reumatizam. 2004;51(2):50-3.
15. Premaor MO, Compston JE. Diagnosis of secondary etiologies of osteoporosis. Praxis (Bern 1994). 2012;101(1):51-4.
16. Curtis JR, Ewing SK, Bauer DC, et al. Association of intact parathyroid hormone levels with subsequent hip BMD loss: the Osteoporotic Fractures in Men (MrOS) Study. J Clin Endocrinol Metab. 2012;97(6):1937-44.
17. Roberts CG, Ladenson PW. Hypothyroidism. Lancet. 2004;363(9411):793-803.
18. Sandhu SK, Hampson G. The pathogenesis, diagnosis, investigation and management of osteoporosis. J Clin Pathol. 2011;64(12):1042-50.
19. Grados F, Brazier M, Kamel S, et al. Prediction of bone mass density variation by bone remodeling markers in postmenopausal women with vitamin D insufficiency treated with calcium and vitamin D supplementation. J Clin Endocrinol Metab. 2003;88(11):5175-9.
20. Rao SS, Budhwar N, Ashfaque A. Osteoporosis in men. Am Fam Physician. 2010;82(5):503-8.
21. El Maghraoui A, Rezqi A, Mounach A, et al. Prevalence and risk factors of vertebral fractures in women with rheumatoid arthritis using vertebral fracture assessment. Rheumatology (Oxford). 2010;49(7):1303-10.
22. Fuerst T, Wu C, Genant HK, et al. Evaluation of vertebral fracture assessment by dual X-ray absorptiometry in a multicenter setting. Osteoporos Int. 2009;20(7):1199-205.
23. Schousboe JT, Vokes T, Broy SB, et al. Vertebral Fracture Assessment: the 2007 ISCD Official Positions. J Clin Densitom. 2008;11(1):92-108.

24. Chang G, Wang L, Liang G, et al. Reproducibility of subregional trabecular bone micro-architectural measures derived from 7-Tesla magnetic resonance images. MAGMA. 2011;24(3):121-5.
25. Issever AS, Vieth V, Lotter A, et al. Local differences in the trabecular bone structure of the proximal femur depicted with high-spatial-resolution MR imaging and multisection CT. Acad Radiol. 2002;9(12):1395-406.
26. Hannah KM, Thomas CD, Clement JG, et al. Bimodal distribution of osteocyte lacunar size in the human femoral cortex as revealed by micro-CT. Bone. 2010;47(5):866-71.
27. Tommasini SM, Trinward A, Acerbo AS, et al. Changes in intracortical microporosities induced by pharmaceutical treatment of osteoporosis as detected by high resolution micro-CT. Bone. 2012;50(3):596-604.
28. Williams AL, Haughton VM. CT resolution and diagnostic accuracy. AJR Am J Roentgenol. 1979;132(3):353-5.
29. Ito M. Assessment of bone quality using micro-computed tomography (micro-CT) and synchrotron micro-CT. J Bone Miner Metab. 2005;23(Suppl):115-21.

SECTION

2

Non-Invasive Therapeutic Intervention

CHAPTER

18

Multidisciplinary Approach to Spinal Pain

Kseniya Slobodyanyuk, Thomas Cheriyan, Christopher Gharibo

INTRODUCTION

Multidisciplinary rehabilitation of complex pain conditions may include pharmacological, rehabilitative, psychological, interventional, and surgical approaches. Goals include improvement of function, self-sufficiency, problem solving, skills training, maladaptive habit reversal, maintenance, and relapse prevention.[1] There is strong evidence that intensive multidisciplinary rehabilitation improves function and moderate evidence that it reduces pain relative to nonmultidisciplinary treatment. However, single discipline interventions in complex, chronic pain conditions have not been shown to improve functional outcomes.[2]

Beyond restoring lost function, multidisciplinary rehabilitation has been shown to reduce reinjury rate. A 2001 study, randomized 39 patients with acute, first-episode low back pain to medical management and either a control group or specific exercise targeting the spinal multifidus muscles. At 1-year follow-up, only 30% of patients from the specific exercise group experienced recurrence of low back pain, compared to 84% of control; at 3-year follow-up, 35% recurrence was seen in the exercise group, versus 75% in control.[3] More recently, a 2011 prospective cohort of athletes with long-standing groin pain randomized to a strength-training rehabilitation program demonstrated a significant treatment effect among all sports at the end of an 8- to 12-year follow-up period. The authors suggested that recurrent pain from sports injury is a consequence of loss of local muscle support, with resulting defects in spinal proprioception, balance, ability to react to unexpected trunk perturbation, weakness, and poor endurance or ineffective neural control.[4]

Overall, the literature has not supported any single treatment in isolation; rather, it supports treatment that incorporates a variety of approaches, with pain reduction and symptom relief as the key first steps in improving function.

SPINAL PAIN PATHOPHYSIOLOGY

Spinal pain can emanate from anterior column, central canal, or posterior elements. Anterior column pain may be from annular tears, disruption of the internal disk, disk herniation, or spondylolisthesis. Pain from the central canal may originate from the neurological tissue or the dura mater. Pain generators in the posterior elements may be from facet arthropathy, interspinous ligaments, and muscular strain. Structural damage is the initial step of a degenerative cascade perpetuated by the decreased stability of spinal structures that may result from injury. Instability may occur due to culmination of tissue damage, insufficient muscle strength, and poor muscle tone, leading to further damage by increasing load on the spinal segments. Incidence of spinal pain increases with improper exercise practices including sudden increases in exercise or activity, poor or lack of exercise therapy, truncal extension and flexion imbalance, hamstring tightness, and poor technique or equipment.

PHARMACOLOGIC TREATMENT

Adequate pain relief is the initial goal of a pain rehabilitation program. Pharmacologic intervention may include oral medications, spinal injections, nerve blocks, trigger point injections, and botulinum toxin neurolytic injections.

Medications

A 2007 review of acute and chronic low back pain medications found good evidence that nonsteroidal anti-inflammatory drugs (NSAIDs) are moderately effective for short-term pain relief, skeletal muscle relaxants are moderately effective for acute short-term relief, and tricyclic antidepressants have small to moderate effects on pain relief. There is also some evidence in support of acetaminophen, tramadol, benzodiazepines, gabapentin, and opioids. Chronic systemic corticosteroids are not recommended.[5]

Injections

Epidural injections are a common option for radicular pain resulting from neural inflammation and impingement, and facet injections are a common option for pain of lumbar facet arthropathy. A variety of substances may be injected. Anesthetics such as lidocaine bind intracellular sodium channels to block sodium influx and prevent depolarization and neural conductivity. Steroids may have anti-inflammatory and neuromodulatory effects on the spinal structures with duration of effect being dependent on particle size. Proposed mechanisms of steroid action include inhibition of proinflammatory phospholipase A2, membrane stabilization, inhibition of nociceptive C fiber transmission, or simply irrigative washout of the epidural space.

A comprehensive description of various therapeutic injection modalities is discussed in section three of the textbook.

Epidural Steroid Injections

Structural damage to the spine, including tears or herniations of the intervertebral disk, can cause leakage of proinflammatory contents. This inflammatory response provides the rationale for epidural steroid injections (ESIs), which work primarily by inhibiting aggregation, release, and synthesis of proinflammatory substances. Additional mechanisms may include irrigation, prolonged sodium channel blockade, C-fiber neurolysis, lysis of adhesions, relief of muscle spasms, sympathetic block, and central and peripheral sensitization.

Overall, studies of ESI efficacy have been inconclusive. Meta-analysis has been difficult to perform due to heterogeneity of existing studies.[6,7] However, in spite of a lack of definitive clinical evidence, expert clinical opinion tentatively endorses ESIs.[8] Epidural injections can be administered via interlaminar (IL) or transforaminal (TF) and caudal approaches, which differ in location of needle placement and subsequent spread of injectate. TF ESIs generally cover a greater area of nerve root inflammation than can be achieved by IL, and have additional diagnostic utility in foraminal stenosis. They have demonstrated the most efficacy in patients with acute to subacute unilateral radicular pain caused by herniated nucleus pulposus and spinal stenosis, with greatest pain relief in the leg.[7] On the other hand, IL ESIs provide multilevel and potential bilateral spread of injectate, and may be better indicated for patients with multilevel bilateral symptoms. Caudal injections are yet another approach to ESIs. Recently, there has been a renewed interest in this technique, owing to its relative ease and low rate of serious adverse effects.

Complications of ESIs include dural puncture and postdural puncture headache, aseptic meningitis, arachnoiditis, conus medullaris syndrome, direct trauma to the spinal cord, and systemic steroid effects.

Facet Joint Injections

The synovium and capsule of facet joints contain nociceptors. Joint capsule strain and degenerative changes may activate synovial and capsular nociceptors leading to the pain of facet joint syndrome, although the degree of degeneration is unrelated to pain intensity.[9] Furthermore, pain can be referred to adjacent structures including the head, neck, shoulders, chest, buttocks, and proximal lower extremities, making it difficult to distinguish referred facet pain from radiculopathy. Facet joint involvement is widespread, estimated to occur in 15–45% of patients with chronic low back pain, 36–60% with chronic neck pain, and 34–48% with thoracic pain.[10]

In spite of the high prevalence of facet joint involvement in spinal pain, studies of efficacy of facet injections have been inconclusive. In 2007, Boswell suggested that there is some evidence of moderate relief afforded by intra-articular facet injections, medial branch blocks, and neurotomies.[10] However, a review by the author estimated a 20–40% false-positive rate of efficacy with a lack of association between zygapophyseal pain, which is necessary for these injections to work, and patient response.[11] In other words, it appears as if much of the reported efficacy of these techniques is placebo effect. This sentiment is supported in Bogduk's 2005 review, which proposed that only the subgroup of patients with zygapophyseal joint pain could truly benefit from intra-articular injections, with further study of these patients lacking due to cost. Furthermore, while observational data estimates a 47% initial response, stabilizing at 18–22% at 3–6 months, overall benefit is not associated with presence of zygapophyseal pain. Thus, facet joint injections have not been shown to offer more benefit than sham injections.[12] Of all the approaches to the facet joint, the one that has been most studied and with the most evidence-based support is the lumbar medial branch neurotomy.[11]

Trigger Point Injections

Yet another potential target for injections is trigger points that manifest as taut, hypersensitive bands of skeletal muscle. Injection of the trigger point leads to mechanical and chemical disruption of muscle pain, with the final outcome being elongation and relaxation of the muscle fiber as well as pain relief. A recent review concluded that while trigger point injections are felt to be clinically efficacious, there is lack of support in literature that may be due to heterogeneity of diagnosis or technique.[13] Furthermore, rare adverse events have been reported with trigger point injections, including pneumothorax, hematomas, and intravascular injections.

Botulinum Toxin Injections

Injection of botulinum toxin into the muscle suppresses release of acetylcholine at the neuromuscular junction, leading to relaxation of the painful muscle and interruption of the pain generator. The potential benefits of botulinum toxin extend beyond symptom relief; a longer-term reduction in pain would enable the patient to participate in rehabilitation exercises, furthering the healing process. The clinical efficacy of botulinum toxin was investigated in a 2005 crossover study by Graboski.[14] Seventeen patients with diagnosed trigger points in the neck, shoulder girdle, hip girdle, or back regions who have previously demonstrated short-term relief with local anesthetic injections were randomized to either bupivacaine or botulinum toxin. Patients were followed weekly until returning to at least 75% baseline pain level for two consecutive weeks. Following a 2-week washout period, patients were then transferred to the other treatment arm. Primary outcome measures included number of weeks taken to return to 75% baseline pain level and magnitude of relief using the Visual Assessment Scale. Both treatment arms demonstrated a significant decrease in pain intensity over time. However, there was no difference between groups in terms of magnitude and duration of pain relief, onset, or costs outside of the actual materials used. In fact, since average per-patient cost for botulinum toxin is $510, versus less than $1 for bupivacaine, botulinum toxin was deemed a less cost-effective treatment. Furthermore, while botulinum toxin has a theoretical duration of efficacy of 3 months, its actual duration in this study was only 4 weeks.[14] These findings were echoed in a 2012 review which concluded that overall, botulinum toxin has not been shown to be effective, citing poor-quality studies as a possible reason for its lack of demonstrated efficacy.[15]

NONPHARMACOLOGIC TREATMENT

While medications are the mainstay of symptom relief, there is a variety of nonpharmacologic options available including rest, acupuncture, alternative medicine, laser therapy, radio frequency denervation, heat therapies, local exercises, spinal manipulation, and traction. Orthotics, while a popular option, were not found to be more effective than no intervention.[16] Patients with signs of nerve root compression may benefit from use of traction, though it is not recommended that physicians use this option for patients with nonradicular low back pain.[17] Thermal modalities including superficial heat and cold, ultrasound, diathermy, infrared, photophoresis, and iontophoresis have failed to demonstrate a difference in pain or functional outcomes in short-term studies.[18] With regard to electrical modalities, laboratory studies have demonstrated some efficacy, though clinical studies have been inconsistent.[18] Of the physical modalities, manual manipulation has the most concrete evidence-based support.[18,19] Lastly, psychosocial interventions can be incorporated into the treatment plan, including ergonomic modification, behavioral modification, and postural control.

Overall, it appears that the key benefit of nonoperative options is facilitation of a functional rehabilitation program that minimizes adverse consequences of bed rest and natural history of the disease.

FUNCTIONAL REHABILITATION

The rationale behind functional rehabilitation lies in the ability of spinal musculature to compensate for the pain and debilitation of spinal injury. Without muscular support, buckling of the vertebral column occurs with rotation of as little as two kilograms.[20] Patients can be trained to utilize deeper stabilizing muscles and maintain lumbar posture in a neutral position, decreasing the load caused by excessive lordotic and kyphotic postures. The transversus abdominis, quadratus lumborum, and gluteal muscles are key targets of rehabilitation for patients with low back pain.[21-23]

Exercise

Utility of exercise in rehabilitation has been investigated in numerous studies. A 2006 systematic review of trunk strengthening exercise for chronic low back pain found that without surgery, trunk strengthening, similar to other exercise, produced moderate effects for long-term pain relief compared with no exercise. Compared with other treatments, intensive exercise has large, short-term effects on pain and large effects on short- and long-term function. However, while exercise with surgery had a significant effect on short-term pain, there was no difference in function.[24]

Directional Exercise

More specifically, numerous studies have targeted directional exercise as a key approach to functional rehabilitation. A randomized controlled trial of 100 patients with acute low back pain randomized to either unidirectional exercise or education demonstrated superiority of exercise in five of seven outcome measures following a 1-year follow-up period.[25] Numerous other studies have found that pain was significantly reduced with performance of repeated end-range lumbar extension movements, while end-range flexion movements actually increased pain.[26,27]

Core Concepts

The overall sentiment regarding functional rehabilitation is that it is useful in providing at least some degree of relief in patients with acute and chronic back pain. Several core concepts are employed to enhance rehabilitation efficacy. Patients should start with single, pain-free range of motion, and progress to multiple planes. Exercise should be built up gradually, progressing from easy to more challenging. Exercise should also be combined with proprioceptive training in order to prevent reinjury, and the patient should be taught to hold a "neutral" position, without necessitating constant awareness of position in order to minimize strain.

CONCLUSION

In conclusion, it is now well known that immobilization adversely affects most organ systems (Table 18.1). Modern rehabilitation aims for early ambulation and restoration of function and has been shown to reduce pain, improve function, and reduce recurrence in the long term. Symptom and pain relief are the key immediate goals, with available options including medications and injections as well as nonpharmacologic approaches such as orthotics; traction; thermal, electrical, and physical modalities; and psychosocial rehabilitation. Good evidence exists in support of physical exercise to reduce pain, strengthen weakened areas to reduce further degeneration and reinjury, and compensate for physical deficits.

Table 18.1: Effects of prolonged bed rest in various organ systems

Organ system	*Effect*
Joints	• Contractures • Loss of normal range of motion
Muscles	• Disease atrophy—15% loss per week of inactivity
Bone	• Osteoporosis • Pathologic fractures
Urinary tract	• Infection • Calculosis
Heart	• Deconditioning • Decreased cardiac reserve • Decreased stroke volume • Resting and postexercise tachycardia
Circulation	• Orthostatic hypotension • Thrombophlebitis
Lung	• Pulmonary embolism • Atelectasis • Pneumonia
Gastrointestinal	• Anorexia • Hospital-acquired malnutrition
Skin	• Decubitus ulcer
Psyche	• Anxiety • Depression • Disorientation • Learned helplessness

REFERENCES

1. Stanos S. Focused review of interdisciplinary pain rehabilitation programs for chronic pain management. Curr Pain Headache Rep. 2012;16(2):147-52.
2. Guzman J, Esmail R, Karjalainen K, et al. Multidisciplinary rehabilitation for chronic low back pain: systematic review. BMJ. 2001;322(7301):1511-6.
3. Hides JA, Jull GA, Richardson CA. Long-term effects of specific stabilizing exercises for first-episode low back pain. Spine (Phila Pa 1976). 2001;26(11):E243-8.

4. Holmich P, Nyvold P, Larsen K. Continued significant effect of physical training as treatment for overuse injury: 8- to 12-year outcome of a randomized clinical trial. Am J Sports Med. 2011;39(11):2447-51.
5. Chou R, Huffman LH. Medications for acute and chronic low back pain: a review of the evidence for an American Pain Society/American College of Physicians clinical practice guideline. Ann Intern Med. 2007;147(7):505-14.
6. Wilkinson IM, Cohen SP. Epidural steroid injections. Curr Pain Headache Rep. 2012;16(1):50-9.
7. Rho ME, Tang CT. The efficacy of lumbar epidural steroid injections: transforaminal, interlaminar, and caudal approaches. Phys Med Rehabil Clin N Am. 2011;22(1):139-48.
8. Benoist M, Boulu P, Hayem G. Epidural steroid injections in the management of low-back pain with radiculopathy: an update of their efficacy and safety. Eur Spine J. 2012;21(2):204-13.
9. Cavanaugh JM, Lu Y, Chen C, et al. Pain generation in lumbar and cervical facet joints. J Bone Joint Surg Am. 2006;88 (Suppl 2):63-7.
10. Boswell MV, Colson JD, Sehgal N, et al. A systematic review of therapeutic facet joint interventions in chronic spinal pain. Pain Physician. 2007;10(1):229-53.
11. Varlotta GP, Lefkowitz TR, Schweitzer M, et al. The lumbar facet joint: a review of current knowledge: part 1: anatomy, biomechanics, and grading. Skeletal Radiol. 2011;40(1):13-23.
12. Bogduk N. A narrative review of intra-articular corticosteroid injections for low back pain. Pain Med. 2005;6(4):287-96.
13. Wong CS, Wong SH. A new look at trigger point injections. Anesthesiol Res Pract. 2012;2012:492452.
14. Graboski CL, Gray DS, Burnham RS. Botulinum toxin A versus bupivacaine trigger point injections for the treatment of myofascial pain syndrome: a randomised double blind crossover study. Pain. 2005;118(1-2):170-5.
15. Gerwin R. Botulinum toxin treatment of myofascial pain: a critical review of the literature. Curr Pain Headache Rep. 2012;16(5):413-22.
16. van Duijvenbode IC, Jellema P, van Poppel MN, et al. Lumbar supports for prevention and treatment of low back pain. Cochrane Database Syst Rev. 2008(2):CD001823.
17. Delitto A, George SZ, Van Dillen LR, et al. Low back pain. J Orthop Sports Phys Ther. 2012;42(4):A1-57.
18. Rakel B, Barr JO. Physical modalities in chronic pain management. Nurs Clin North Am. 2003;38(3):477-94.
19. Aure OF, Nilsen JH, Vasseljen O. Manual therapy and exercise therapy in patients with chronic low back pain: a randomized, controlled trial with 1-year follow-up. Spine (Phila Pa 1976). 2003;28(6):525-31; discussion 531-2.
20. Morris JM. Biomechanics of the spine. Arch Surg. 1973;107(3):418-23.
21. Nadler SF, Malanga GA, DePrince M, et al. The relationship between lower extremity injury, low back pain, and hip muscle strength in male and female collegiate athletes. Clin J Sport Med. 2000;10(2):89-97.
22. Hodges PW, Richardson CA. Altered trunk muscle recruitment in people with low back pain with upper limb movement at different speeds. Arch Phys Med Rehabil. 1999;80(9):1005-12.
23. McGill SM, Norman RW. Reassessment of the role of intra-abdominal pressure in spinal compression. Ergonomics. 1987;30(11):1565-88.
24. Slade SC, Keating JL. Trunk-strengthening exercises for chronic low back pain: a systematic review. J Manipulative Physiol Ther. 2006;29(2):163-73.
25. Stankovic R, Johnell O. Conservative treatment of acute low-back pain. A prospective randomized trial: McKenzie method of treatment versus patient education in "mini back school". Spine (Phila Pa 1976). 1990;15(2):120-3.
26. Donelson R, Grant W, Kamps C, et al. Pain response to sagittal end-range spinal motion. A prospective, randomized, multicentered trial. Spine (Phila Pa 1976). 1991;16(6 Suppl):S206-12.
27. Delitto A, Cibulka MT, Erhard RE, et al. Evidence for use of an extension-mobilization category in acute low back syndrome: a prescriptive validation pilot study. Phys Ther. 1993;73(4):216-22; discussion 223-8.

CHAPTER

19

Pharmacological Management of Spinal Pain: Narcotics

Christopher Gharibo

INTRODUCTION

Opioid pharmacotherapy should be carefully considered when formulating an analgesic and functional restoration plan for patients with spinal pain. However, the debate regarding opioids is livelier than ever. Appropriate opioid prescribing is a dynamic pendulum that tends to swing from prescribing little or no opioids to overcompensation with opioid pharmacotherapy for patients with spinal pain.[1] The constantly evolving nature of opioid regulations and development of newer formulations including tamper resistant technology makes its essential to keep abreast of advancements.[2]

Opioids are one of the most effective medications for pain. But at the same time, long term and functional outcome studies are lacking. The poor functional outcomes are not just secondary to psychomotor and CNS side effects such as sedation and dizziness that are function limiting. There is also the psychological-dependence risk and the potential for excessive intake of opioids that may lead to progressive misuse, abuse, and diversion.[3]

From a clinical stand point, excessive reliance on opioid pharmacotherapy results in overpresentation of the opioid category to the patient.[4] Rather than present opioid pharmacotherapy as the heart of their analgesic treatment, this modality should be moderated with use of other approaches. Opioids are part of the multimechanistic analgesic plan and should be managed similar to other medications like NSAIDs, anticonvulsants, physical therapy as well as injections. Studies have shown opioids offer no significant advantage over acetaminophen or NSAIDs in relief of symptoms or return to work,[5,6] making it a second/third-line drug for spinal pain.[7] A meta-analysis concluded that there is low-quality evidence that patients who received opioids had greater pain relief and better functional status when compared to placebo.[8] Thus, patients being considered for opioid therapy need to have a robust diagnosis that clinically indicates opioid treatment. Psychological and social circumstances of the patient should be carefully considered, as well. An individual-tailored multimodal treatment plan integrating treatment options including nonopioids, interventional pain management, and physical therapy should be considered.

Pharmacologically, opioids have similar pharmacodynamic profiles. There is multireceptor activation: the μ, κ, δ, chemoreceptor trigger zone albeit at different levels; thus, contributing to the effective analgesia for both nociceptive and neuropathic pain. However, receptor depolarization results in concomitant side effects such as constipation, nausea, dizziness, pruritus, and dysphoria. A whole palette of formulations ranging from ultra rapid acting formulations such as buccal fentanyl in the form of a lozenge (Actiq) and tablet (Fentora) to once a day pills or once every 7-day patch are available.[9-11]

A common misunderstanding with opioid pharmacotherapy is that there are no irreversible end organ effects with opioids; however, this is not completely true. For example, methadone may precipitate cardiac arrhythmia and sudden death.[12] There may also be significant neuroplastic changes in the form of opioid-induced hyperalgesia and physiological dependence in certain individuals that cannot be reversed.[13] End-of-dose pain and withdrawal type symptoms between doses and muscle pain may manifest.[14] There are also hormonal alterations in both sexes that may be persistent with continued therapy.

"No ceiling effect" is another misconception that is commonly associated with opioids.[15] However, opioid response is individual dependent with a wide variations in how individuals respond to an opioid. This is, at least in part, related to genetic factors and related to cytochrome P-450 as well as, age, sex, and ethnicity.[16] For patients not achieving analgesia after a reasonable dose titration, treatment with another opioid compound should be considered.

Opioids differ in their psychosocial risk profiles. Dependence may begin with casual initial treatment. For example, the patient may double up their dose of opioid to dance at their daughter's upcoming wedding and it might work great. However, the next morning they wake up, they are sore and this makes them double up on the short-acting opioid again. So, now patient is developing a noncompliant pill taking behavior pattern that may be deleterious to the patient long term, physiologically and psychosocially. Patient may begin to enjoy the euphoria associated with the opioids that they are taking. They may begin to crush or solubilize the drug and so on. That is the beginning of opioid abuse that started with very innocent misuse of the medication. Therefore, appropriateness of opioid therapy should always be reconsidered.

While certain side effects of opioids resolve with time, some do not. However, even the side effects that resolve with time in most people may not resolve in some. For example, while constipation certainly is refractory, time-resolved symptoms like nausea, sedation, diaphoresis, cognitive changes, and libido decline can be persistent as well. Persistent cognitive changes and side effects indicate the use of an alternative opioid.

Conventionally, when opioid therapy is initiated, a trial of short-acting compounds such as hydrocodone, oxycodone, or codeine is utilized. If the patient is requesting more than several short-acting opioids a day, it is prudent to consider switching to an extended release opioid. Spine patients often have mechanical, daytime pain and are better at night when there is unloading of their spine. In facet osteoarthritis, patients are in pain from the time they wake up; they first have pain for the first couple of hours or so, from which they break out of, followed by ambulatory pain, neurogenic claudication, back pain, radicular symptoms, etc. that stays with them for a large part of the day. Therefore, the lowest dose of long acting compounds should be considered at the onset, rather than a short-acting drug. An opioid qam (every morning) dose may be initiated. However, a narcotic with a 6-hours peak, administered qhs (every night at bedtime) can be considered if qam dose is not effective. Alternatively, a q 12-hours administration may be beneficial. The goal is to provide reliable and consistent analgesia throughout the day when our patients need it the most.

It should be remembered to not over-manage patient and not to keep escalating the doses despite treatment failure. Current guidelines on the use of chronic opioid therapy in chronic noncancer pain suggest maximum daily dose of 120–180 mg of morphine or its equivalent.[18] It is also recommended that patients are referred before increasing opioid dose further.[18,19] Quite frequently, patients may ask: "Well I took one pill, I waited 1 hours and it did not work. Can I go up on the dose?" And the answer to that will be simply "No". A 1–2 week run on the prescribed regimen is required, to make a call on regimen efficacy. Consider about one adjustment a week or every few weeks so that steady state can be established and the patient is not over managed. However, if the patient is not responding to the initial startup dose and one or two adjustments, another opioid compound may be considered.[20]

The equianalgesic tables are highly unreliable and are not as practical as they may appear to be. The patient that needs an opioid adjustment often is in uncontrolled pain on the existing regimen. Such a patient may not benefit from an equianalgesic dose rotation and may need their doses adjusted further. An "equianalgesic conversion" may also be analgesically unreliable since the individual's response to a particular opioid is highly variable. Furthermore, adjusting the nonopioid analgesic plan such as with an antidepressant, anticonvulsant, NSAIDs, or topical agents may be considered.

Once the patient is a reasonable candidate for chronic opioids from a biopsychosocial perspective, supportive documentation should be present in the chart. Pain is undertreated in the United States and opioids as part of an overall plan can play a valuable role in treating pain of the spine patient.

REFERENCES

1. Olsen Y, Daumit GL, Ford DE. Opioid prescriptions by U.S. primary care physicians from 1992 to 2001. J Pain. 2006;7(4):225-35.
2. Bartholomaeus JH, Arkenau-Maric E, Galia E. Opioid extended-release tablets with improved tamper-resistant properties. Expert Opin Drug Deliv. 2012;9(8):879-91.
3. Angst MS, Lazzeroni LC, Phillips NG, et al. Aversive and reinforcing opioid effects: a pharmacogenomic twin study. Anesthesiology. 2012;117(1):22-37.

4. Manchikanti L, Helm Ii S, Fellows B, et al. Opioid epidemic in the United States. Pain Physician. 2012;15(3 Suppl): ES9-ES38.
5. Cifuentes M, Webster B, Genevay S, et al. The course of opioid prescribing for a new episode of disabling low back pain: opioid features and dose escalation. Pain. 2010; 151(1):22-9.
6. Roelofs PD, Deyo RA, Koes BW, et al. Nonsteroidal anti-inflammatory drugs for low back pain: an updated Cochrane review. Spine (Phila Pa 1976). 2008;33(16):1766-74.
7. Kinkade S. Evaluation and treatment of acute low back pain. Am Fam Physician. 2007;75(8):1181-8.
8. Kuijpers T, van Middelkoop M, Rubinstein SM, et al. A systematic review on the effectiveness of pharmacological interventions for chronic non-specific low-back pain. Eur Spine J. 2011;20(1):40-50.
9. Fine PG, Streisand JB. A review of oral transmucosal fentanyl citrate: potent, rapid and noninvasive opioid analgesia. J Palliat Med. 1998;1(1):55-63.
10. Jeal W, Benfield P. Transdermal fentanyl: a review of its pharmacological properties and therapeutic efficacy in pain control. Drugs. 1997;53(1):109-38.
11. Paech MJ, Bloor M, Schug SA. New formulations of fentanyl for acute pain management. Drugs Today (Barc). 2012;48(2):119-32.
12. Modesto-Lowe V, Brooks D, Petry N. Methadone deaths: risk factors in pain and addicted populations. J Gen Intern Med. 2010;25(4):305-9.
13. Low Y, Clarke CF, Huh BK. Opioid-induced hyperalgesia: a review of epidemiology, mechanisms and management. Singapore Med J. 2012;53(5):357-60.
14. Portenoy RK, Bennett DS, Rauck R, et al. Prevalence and characteristics of breakthrough pain in opioid-treated patients with chronic noncancer pain. J Pain. 2006;7(8): 583-91.
15. Khan MI, Walsh D, Brito-Dellan N. Opioid and adjuvant analgesics: compared and contrasted. Am J Hosp Palliat Care. 2011;28(5):378-83.
16. Benzel EC. Spine Surgery: Techniques, Complication Avoidance, and Management, 3rd edition Philadelphia, PA: Churchill Livingstone; 2012.
17. Richarz U, Waechter S, Sabatowski R, et al. Sustained safety and efficacy of once-daily hydromorphone extended-release (OROS((R)) hydromorphone ER) compared with twice-daily oxycodone controlled-release over 52 weeks in patients with moderate to severe chronic noncancer pain. Pain Pract. 2012.
18. Chou R, Fanciullo GJ, Fine PG, et al. Clinical guidelines for the use of chronic opioid therapy in chronic noncancer pain. J Pain. 2009;10(2):113-30.
19. Lee TJ. Pharmacologic treatment for low back pain: one component of pain care. Phys Med Rehabil Clin N Am. 2010;21(4):793-800.
20. Manchikanti L, Abdi S, Atluri S, et al. American Society of Interventional Pain Physicians (ASIPP) Guidelines for Responsible Opioid Prescribing in Chronic Non-Cancer Pain: Part 2 - Guidance. Pain Physician. 2012;15(3 Suppl): S67-S116.

CHAPTER 20

Pharmacological Management of Spinal Pain: Non-narcotics

Juan Carlos Robles, Thomas Cheriyan

INTRODUCTION

Non-narcotic pharmaceutical intervention is an important strategy in the treatment of spinal pain. Commonly used non-narcotics in the management include acetaminophen, nonsteroidal anti-inflammatory drugs (NSAIDs) and cyclooxygenase (COX)-2 inhibitors, steroids, anticonvulsants, antidepressants, muscle relaxants, and nonopioid drug combinations. Careful consideration should be given when prescribing pain medications taking into account the overall benefit to the patient. For example, when combining analgesics with different mechanisms of action the quality of the anesthesia is enhanced, adverse effects are diminished, facilitating lower individual doses, which in turn improve patient compliance.

ACETAMINOPHEN

Acetaminophen, also known as paracetamol in a few countries, is chemically acetyl-para-aminophenol. It is one of the most widely used for drug for antipyresis and analgesia, which also has weak anti-inflammatory effects. The rapid analgesic effect (30–60 min after ingestion), low incidence of adverse effect, low cost and analgesia equivalent to NSAIDs makes it the first-line drug in the treatment of back pain.[1] Though acetaminophen has an exceptional safety profile, hepatotoxicity is encountered in accidental/intentional overdose. Based on reports of liver injury seen close to maximum current recommendation (4000 mg/day), the FDA has revised the maximal recommended dose to 3250 mg/day and even lower for patients taking three or more alcoholic drinks everyday while using acetaminophen.

NONSTEROIDAL ANTI-INFLAMMATORY DRUGS

NSAIDs are nonselective inhibitors of the enzymes cyclooxygenase-1 (COX-1) and cyclooxygenase-2 (COX-2). NSAIDs act by decreasing the production of prostaglandins from arachidonic acid. Prostaglandins play a role in sensitizing the peripheral and the central nervous system to painful stimuli. A Cochrane review by Roelofs et al. concluded that while NSAIDs were effective for short-term treatment of acute and chronic low back pain, they were not more effective than acetaminophen.[1-3]

There is also no evidence to suggest the superiority of any NSAID over the other; however, a different NSAID may be considered if the first is not effective.[4-6] NSAIDs should be administered with caution in patients having pre-existing gastrointestinal, renal, hepatic, and cardiovascular conditions.

Selective COX-2 inhibitors are not more efficacious than non-selective NSAIDs but have less gastrointestinal symptoms.[2,7] Due to a 42% increased incidence of cardiovascular events associated with selective COX-2 inhibitors several drugs in this class has been withdrawn from market (Table 20.1).[8] However, naproxen has a relatively more favorable cardiovascular risk profile.

STEROIDS

Steroids are potent anti-inflammatory drugs that prevent the formation of arachidonic acid, which controls the biosynthesis of prostaglandins and leukotrienes. Though there are no studies that demonstrate the efficacy of oral

Table 20.1: Classification of NSAIDs based on their chemical structure

Salicylates
• Aspirin (acetylsalicylic acid) • Diflunisal • Salsalate • Choline Magnesium Trisalicylate
Propionic acid derivatives
• Ibuprofen • Dexibuprofen • Naproxen • Fenoprofen • Ketoprofen • Dexketoprofen • Flurbiprofen • Oxaprozin • Loxoprofen
Acetic acid derivatives
• Indomethacin • Tolmetin • Sulindac • Etodolac • Ketorolac • Diclofenac (Safety alert by FDA) • Aceclofenac • Nabumetone
Enolic acid (Oxicam) derivatives
• Piroxicam • Meloxicam • Tenoxicam • Droxicam • Lornoxicam • Isoxicam
Anthranilic acid derivatives (Fenamates)
• Mefenamic acid • Meclofenamic acid • Flufenamic acid • Tolfenamic acid
Selective COX-2 inhibitors (Coxibs)
• Celecoxib (FDA alert) • Rofecoxib (withdrawn from market) • Valdecoxib (withdrawn from market) • Parecoxib FDA withdrawn, licenced in the EU • Lumiracoxib TGA cancelled registration • Etoricoxib not FDA approved, licenced in the EU
Sulfonanilides
• Nimesulide (banned by several countries for the potential risk of hepatotoxicity).
Others
• Licofelone acts by inhibiting LOX (lipoxygenase) and COX and hence known as 5-LOX/COX inhibitor.

steroid in the treatment of spinal disorders, it may be indicated for acute episodes of lower neck or back pain. They are prescribed for a short duration, usually not more than 5 days. Treatment options include 10 mg of prednisolone, three to four times a day for 5 days without taper. Another option is the methylprednisolone dose pack, 4-mg pills over a period of 6 days, where the patient takes six pills from day one and by day six they are down to one pill.

Epidural steroid injections may be helpful in patients with radicular symptoms that do not respond to 2–6 weeks of conservative therapy. Long-term improvement in pain and disability with epidural steroid injections has not been demonstrated.

Steroids must be prescribed judiciously taking into consideration drug–drug interactions and high possibility of other harmful side effects. Sudden discontinuation must be avoided, especially if used for more than 7 days to avoid the risk of adrenal insufficiency or crisis. Steroid–warfarin interaction may warrant a decrease in warfarin dosage to maintain optimal international normalised ratio (INR) value. Diabetic patients should be advised about steroid-induced hyperglycemia. Although, steroids that are commonly used for pain are mainly glucocorticoid; all steroids have small mineral corticoid effect that can cause some water retention, potentially sending a patient into heart failure. In addition, a patient with recent myocardial infarct, left ventricular wall rupture is possible, even though rare. Contraindication to steroids use is bacterial infections, measles, varicella, and fungal infections.

ANTICONVULSANTS

The mechanism of action of anticonvulsants is not fully known, but it is thought to suppress the aberrant painful neural activity that is being produced by nerve irritation. They are used in shooting, lancinating pain of neuropathy and radiculopathy. The anticonvulsants have a slow onset of analgesia that requires prolonged titration to take effect, usually weeks to months. The most commonly used for pain are gabapentin and pregabalin. The most common side effects of these medications are drowsiness, dizziness, fatigue, weight gain, nausea, dry mouth, constipation, and depression in some patients experiencing suicidal thoughts. Pregabalin more so than gabapentin can cause low platelet count, increased keratin kinase and muscle pains similar to cholesterol medications.

The mechanism of action of gabapentin is not well understood but is thought to work on the $\alpha 2\delta$ subunit

(1 and 2) of the voltage gated calcium channels, blocking these channels. It mimics the chemical structure of gamma-aminobutyric acid (GABA) but is not believed to act at the same brain receptors as GABA. Gabapentin also increases GABA synthesis and release. The most common indications for gabapentin are post herpetic neuralgia, diabetic neuropathy, peripheral neuropathy and migraine prophylaxis. This medication is usually prescribed three times a day to a maximum dose of 3600 mg daily. It requires an extended titration period of usually 3 weeks to 1 month. The analgesic dose of gabapentin is 900–3600 mg daily divided in t.i.d doses. It can be increased by 100–300 mg every day until effective analgesia is achieved. The analgesic effect needs to be balanced with side-effects like drowsiness and dizziness. It is excreted unchanged in the urine because it is not protein bound. It must be used with precaution in patients with renal failure where the maximum dose should be no more than 200–300 mg daily. Trial of gabapentin may be indicated for chronic lower back pain in patients who have failed first-line drugs.[9]

Pregabalin is FDA approved for diabetic peripheral neuropathy and postherpetic neuralgia. In June of 2007, it became the first medication approved by the FDA for fibromyalgia. It binds to the $\alpha 2\delta$ subunits of the voltage gate calcium channels. It increases the GABA levels and decreases the release of glutamate, noradrenaline, and substance P. The initial analgesic dose of pregabalin is 150 mg daily, 75 mg twice a day, or 50 mg three times a day. It can be increased by 150 mg every week to a maximum dose of 600 mg daily.

TRICYCLIC ANTIDEPRESSANTS

Tricyclic antidepressants are used for the treatment of chronic low back pain. Though a Cochrane concluded that there was no significant evidence that antidepressants was more efficacious than placebo in the treatment of chronic back pain,[10] there have a few meta-analysis that reports a small benefit.[10-12] They are considered to be a second-/third-line therapy due to their high incidence of adverse effects. These medications have a slow onset of analgesia usually more than 2 weeks, and they require a long period of titration until the peak effect is found. They are used once a day for pain and depression. At lower doses, the tricyclic antidepressants inhibit the reuptake of serotonin and at higher doses they inhibit the reuptake of norepinephrine. The most commonly used is amitriptyline, at 10–20 mg at bedtime and can be titrated by 10–25 mg every week to a maximum dose of 150 mg daily. Main indications for this type of medications are neuropathic pain syndromes like complex regional pain syndrome (CRPS) migraine and tension headaches, fibromyalgia, myofascial pain syndrome, cancer pain, and chronic lower pain back. Side-effects include insomnia, anxiety, irritation, seizures, fatigue, nausea, constipation, diarrhea, anorexia, weight gain, decreased libido, impotence, ejaculation disorders, and anorgasmia. The most well-documented side effects are the cardiovascular complications including anemia, hypertension, and orthostatic hypotension. Similar to anticonvulsants, they can also cause suicidal thoughts.

Venlafaxine, duloxetine, and milnacipran are other antidepressants which have been used due to their ability to inhibit the reuptake of norepinephrine.

MUSCLE RELAXANTS

These medications account for 18.5% of all the prescriptions written for chronic pain in the United States.[13] A Cochrane review concluded that there was benefit of use of muscle relaxants in chronic low back pain; however, there was a high incidence of adverse reactions.[14] Most of them are centrally acting and as a group the most common side effects are sedation, drowsiness, dizziness, and dry mouth.

Cyclobenzaprine, a serotonin receptor antagonist, increases stage four sleep, making it very useful for patients having associated insomnia. There is no potential for abuse or dependence with this medication. They may be used in pregnancy but with caution. Life-threatening interaction when combined with MAO inhibitors. The dose for this medication is 5–10 mg three times a day, to a maximum dose of 60 mg daily.

Diazepam is a benzodiazepine that has a potential for dependence and withdrawal symptoms. It binds to the GABA α receptors and produces central nervous system depression. The dose for this medication is 2 mg, 5 mg, or 10 mg, two to four times a day.

Tizanidine can be used for back pain but its main indication for spasticity. It is an α-2 adrenergic agonist, similar to clonidine. It is a short-acting medication and the dose is 2 mg, 4 mg, or 6 mg, three or four times a day to a maximum daily dose of 36 mg.

Other relaxants that may be used are carisoprodol, metaxalone, and methocarbamol.

NONOPIOID COMBINATION MEDICATION

Tramadol alone[15] or in combination with acetaminophen[16] has been used in the treatment of chronic back pain.

Tramadol has a dual mechanism of analgesia. It weakly binds to the μ opioid receptors and also inhibits norepinephrine and serotonin reuptake. It provides synergistic analgesia when combined with acetaminophen. Adverse effects seen with tramadol include seizures and the risk of developing serotonin syndrome when combined with selective serotonin reuptake inhibitors (SSRIs) or selective serotonin norepinephrine reuptake inhibitors (SSNRIs). There is also a mild abuse potential with these medications.

TOPICAL MEDICATIONS

There does not seem to be a significant benefit in pain or function with the application of topical pain medications in patients with spinal pain. Topical medications are available in the form of creams, sprays, patches, ointments, and gels. They include anesthetics, analgesics, and anti-inflammatory drugs. They are quite commonly used as these medications are available over-the-counter.

SUMMARY

When treating a patient with spinal pain, careful consideration to the etiology, duration of symptoms, comorbid conditions and compliance should be considered when formulating an effective and integrative analgesic plan. Due to the lack of high-quality robust data on the pharmacological therapy of patients with spinal pain, it is prudent to use drugs having minimal side effects as the first line of treatment before considering alternatives.

REFERENCES

1. Benzel EC. Spine surgery: techniques, complication avoidance, and management, 3rd edition Philadelphia, PA: Churchill Livingstone; 2012.
2. Roelofs PD, Deyo RA, Koes BW, et al. Non-steroidal anti-inflammatory drugs for low back pain. Cochrane Database Syst Rev. 2008(1):CD000396.
3. Roelofs PD, Deyo RA, Koes BW, et al. Nonsteroidal anti-inflammatory drugs for low back pain: an updated Cochrane review. Spine (Phila Pa 1976). 2008;33(16):1766-74.
4. Hancock MJ, Maher CG, Latimer J, et al. Assessment of diclofenac or spinal manipulative therapy, or both, in addition to recommended first-line treatment for acute low back pain: a randomised controlled trial. Lancet. 2007;370(9599):1638-43.
5. van Tulder MW, Koes BW, Bouter LM. Conservative treatment of acute and chronic nonspecific low back pain. A systematic review of randomized controlled trials of the most common interventions. Spine (Phila Pa 1976). 1997;22(18):2128-56.
6. Casazza BA. Diagnosis and treatment of acute low back pain. Am Fam Physician. 2012;85(4):343-50.
7. Morlion B. Pharmacotherapy of low back pain: targeting nociceptive and neuropathic pain components. Curr Med Res Opin. 2011;27(1):11-33.
8. Kearney PM, Baigent C, Godwin J, et al. Do selective cyclo-oxygenase-2 inhibitors and traditional non-steroidal anti-inflammatory drugs increase the risk of atherothrombosis? Meta-analysis of randomised trials. BMJ. 2006;332(7553):1302-8.
9. Lee TJ. Pharmacologic treatment for low back pain: one component of pain care. Phys Med Rehabil Clin N Am. 2010;21(4):793-800.
10. Urquhart DM, Hoving JL, Assendelft WW, et al. Antidepressants for non-specific low back pain. Cochrane Database Syst Rev. 2008(1):CD001703.
11. Savigny P, Watson P, Underwood M. Early management of persistent non-specific low back pain: summary of NICE guidance. BMJ. 2009;338:b1805.
12. Salerno SM, Browning R, Jackson JL. The effect of antidepressant treatment on chronic back pain: a meta-analysis. Arch Intern Med. 2002;162(1):19-24.
13. Luo X, Pietrobon R, Curtis LH, et al. Prescription of nonsteroidal anti-inflammatory drugs and muscle relaxants for back pain in the United States. Spine (Phila Pa 1976). 2004;29(23):E531-7.
14. van Tulder MW, Touray T, Furlan AD, et al. Muscle relaxants for non-specific low back pain. Cochrane Database Syst Rev. 2003(2):CD004252.
15. Schnitzer TJ, Gray WL, Paster RZ, et al. Efficacy of tramadol in treatment of chronic low back pain. J Rheumatol. 2000;27(3):772-8.
16. Ruoff G, Lema M. Strategies in pain management: new and potential indications for COX-2 specific inhibitors. J Pain Symptom Manage. 2003;25(2 Suppl):S21-31.

CHAPTER 21

Prevention and Management of Addiction

Marianne T Guschwan

INTRODUCTION

As described in the previous chapter, management of spinal pain with narcotics carries the risk of opioid addiction. This chapter reviews the principles of prevention and management of addiction in patients who have been prescribed opioids for pain management.

THE SCOPE OF THE PROBLEM WITH OPIOIDS

The prevalence of nonmedical opioid use has increased significantly in the past two decades. Opioid consumption had a fourfold increase from 1990 to 2002, with teenagers having the highest increase in consumption for all age groups measured.[1] Data from epidemiologic studies of American high school students is reflective of this trend. In 1991, 1% of high school seniors reported having used a prescription opioid for nonmedical use in the 30 days prior to the survey; in 2006, the percentage increased to 4%. Also in 2006, more 12th graders initiated illicit drug use with nonprescription opioids than marijuana.

Another measure of the extent of prescription opioid abuse is the number of deaths per year from opioids. The rate of increase in deaths per year due to opioids from 1979 to 1990 was relatively stable at 5%; however, the rate increased to 18% per year from 1990 through 2002.[2] This increase in deaths trended with increasing sales of the opioid analgesics. Of note, deaths from the synthetic analgesic methadone, which is commonly used as treatment for opioid dependence in replacement therapy, were tracked for analgesic, not therapeutic, use. Therapeutic methadone use is highly regulated and restricted to specially licensed clinics;[3] these restrictions help to minimize diversion.

The increased use of opioids in pain management has likely been a major contributor to the increased misuse of these drugs. In 2000, at a joint meeting of the Joint Commission on the Accreditation of Health Organizations (JCAHO) and the American Pain Society, the following statement was released:

> "The excuses for inadequate pain control appear to have run their course and will no longer be accepted because poor pain controllers, unethical, clinically unsound and economically wasteful. And it came out of good intentions which is recognizing that the pain was under treated and that we should not accept that—that we should do something about that so much so that, that JCAHO added pain as a fifth vital sign in addition to heart rate, temperature, respiratory rate and blood pressure; added a measure for asking patients about pain."[4]

The impetus to adequately treat pain, however, did not come with the concomitant education about addiction risks. In fact, the conference highlighted a common misperception about the risk of addiction pertaining to opioids as pointed out in a 1980 letter to the editor in *The New England Journal of Medicine*.[5] The need for increasing addiction education in medical schools and in other health care profession training programs had been noted since the 1970s, prior to the issues with opioids, when addiction first came under the purview of health care as a result of[6] the National Institutes of Health developing an alcoholism division in 1970. Prior to the inception of the alcoholism division, substance addiction was considered a moral or otherwise nonmedical issue.

Current estimates suggest that upward of 30% of patients who are prescribed opioids may develop a problem with that opioid; some portion of such patients will meet the formal definition of opioid use disorder, as defined by the *Diagnostic and Statistical Manual of Mental Disorders,* version 5 (DSM-5). Early identification of misuse of prescription opioids by a physician may present an opportunity to intervene, potentially preventing future problems.

ADDICTION MANAGEMENT

The goal remains for physicians to adequately treat pain while minimizing the risk of addiction. What is exactly meant by the term addiction? The DSM-5, released in May of 2013 by the American Psychiatric Association, defines addiction in terms of substance use disorder. The diagnosis of a substance use disorder requires the patient meet two or more of the following 11 criteria within a 12-month period:

1. Recurrent substance use leading to a failure to fulfill obligations at home, work, or school
2. Recurrent substance use in situations in which it is physically hazardous (such as while operating an automobile)
3. Recurrent substance use even after social or interpersonal problems resulting from the use of the substance
4. Increased tolerance
5. Withdrawal symptoms
6. Using the substance for a longer period of time or in a larger quantity than was intended
7. A desire or series of unsuccessful attempts to control substance use
8. Allocating significant time to obtaining/using/recovering from the substance
9. Reduced social, occupational, or recreational activities
10. Continued substance abuse despite having a problem likely caused or worsened by the substance
11. Craving the substance[7]

    (Reprinted with permission from the Diagnostic and Statistical Manual of Mental Disorders, Fifth Edition, (Copyright 2013). American Psychiatric Association.)

For opioid use disorder, behaviors four and five are not considered in the diagnosis, as they may be present in many patients using opioids therapeutically for pain management. The benefit of defining the disorder in a given individual is in guiding the level of treatment; the greater the severity of the problems, the more intensive the indicated treatment.

Patients who qualify for opioid use disorder should be referred to formal treatment and/or possibly self-help groups, which can be accomplished by having readily available a resource list of local referrals in addition to self-help groups.[8]

PREVENTION OF ADDICTION

Patients who develop problems with opioids and/or misuse their prescription medication may not meet full criteria for substance use disorder. This situation presents an opportunity to intervene before the patient goes on to develop a disorder.

Prevention is multifactorial. Discussion of risk of addiction prior to taking the medication engages the patient in monitoring his or her use. The practitioner should consider whether the patient and/or his or her family has a history of addiction, as addiction risk has a genetic component (genes are thought to contribute approximately 50% of the risk involved in developing an addiction).[9,10]

However, often patients will not reveal a history of addiction, particularly to opioids. The reasons why patients withhold information regarding their addiction vary, but include a realistic fear of inadequate pain treatment.[11] When patients reveal a history of opioid dependence to a pain management clinician, they are most likely doing so with the intention of having the clinician help him or her limit opioid use in order to minimize the risk of relapse.

When prescribing, clinicians should consider alternative medications first, as well as other adjunctive measures. When there is no alternative to opioids for pain management, prescribing the drugs in small amounts and monitoring prescriptions can help identify potential misuse early in its course, as can setting clear expectations as to how long pain relief will be needed and what to do if that timeframe is exceeded. Establishing periodic follow-up appointments sets up the expectation for the patient that use of the opioids requires monitoring (as opposed to allowing refills with just a phone call). In addition, reviewing progress along the way and setting clear reasons for continuing or increasing doses, as was discussed before starting treatment, can help the physician recognize misuse along the way. If a patient is increasing doses on his or her own, the strategy for pain management should be reviewed; possibly the opioids are not an effective treatment for the patient.[12]

Another important warning sign of potential misuse of opioid medications is lost prescriptions. Requests to call into multiple pharmacies rather than one may also signal a problem. Creating and strictly enforcing policies regarding replacement of prescriptions can potentially prevent problems; such policies may include no replacement for lost prescriptions and having the patient identify one pharmacy that he or she will use.

Another reason a patient may be increasing medications is a phenomenon that has been termed pseudo-addiction. Pseudoaddiction is defined as drug-seeking behavior in a patient who has inadequate pain control.[13] Evaluating the potential for pseudoaddiction is the first step in evaluating prescription misuse. Utilizing longer acting opioids to avoid fluctuations in pain relief and other strategies to effectively address the pain may eliminate the problem.

When a patient appears to be misusing a prescription, a brief intervention may be tried. Studied in primary care practices, a brief intervention is part of an overall approach to addressing behavioral health conditions called SBIRT, or Screening, Brief Intervention, and Referral to Treatment.[14] Research has demonstrated SBIRT to be an effective way to reduce smoking and heavy use of alcohol in patients seen in primary care settings. Data are promising in showing SBIRT's efficacy in addressing prescription drug misuse. It is important to note that brief interventions are not indicated for a patient who meets criteria for a drug use disorder as defined by the DSM-5 criteria. Those patients will need more intensive treatment and should be referred to an addiction specialist or to an addiction program.

Screening for a disorder (the "S" in SBIRT) involves using one of a number of tools (many are described at www.samhsa.gov) to identify individuals at risk for having a substance use disorder. The CAGE-AID (Table 21.1) is a four-item questionnaire administered by a clinician adapted from the widely used alcohol use disorder screening tool—the CAGE. Some criticisms of this tool include that it is less sensitive in women, it is less sensitive in patients with antisocial personality disorder, and one question identifies only late stage alcohol problems. However, CAGE-AID's simplicity makes it easier than lengthier screeners to implement into a busy practice. Even simpler is the use of one particular screening question: "How many times in the past year have you used an illegal drug or used a prescription medication for nonmedical reasons?" This screener has demonstrated comparable sensitivity and specificity in detecting drug use disorders in one primary care setting.[15]

Table 21.1: CAGE-AID questionnaire

When thinking about drug use, include illegal drug use and the use of prescription drugs other than prescribed.
Questions:
• Have you ever felt that you ought to cut down on your drinking or drug use?
• Have people annoyed you by criticizing your drinking or drug use?
• Have you ever felt bad or guilty about your drinking or drug use?
• Have you ever had a drink or used drugs first thing in the morning to steady your nerves or to get rid of a hangover?

Brief Intervention involves reviewing concerns about drug misuse, including information from pertinent laboratory tests (positive urine drug screens, elevated liver function tests) and physical examination findings (withdrawal symptoms), accompanied by suggestions for making changes.[16,17] The acronym FRAMES is helpful in remembering the elements of the intervention.[18] "F" stands for feedback such as "I think you are using more medication than needed for your pain causing you to have some elevation in your liver enzymes. The anxiety, sweating, and insomnia that you are experiencing may be due to withdrawal symptoms". It is important to listen to the patient's reaction. "R" stands for responsibility—that the decision to make a change is up to the patient. "A" stands for advice, "I am recommending that you reduce the pain medications". "M" is for the menu of options given to the patient to begin to address the problem. This menu could include tapering of the opioid medication, while using alternative pain management strategies such as meditation, massage, or acupuncture; the goal is to involve the patient as much as possible in the decision making. "E" represents empathy—reminding the clinician to remain respectful and nonjudgmental, using such statements as "I see that you have really been suffering with pain". "S" stands for supporting self-efficacy, or the ability of an individual to make a change; the clinician should convey optimism that the patient has the ability to change if he or she so chooses.

Once an agreed upon plan is developed, a limited number of short follow-up visits are set to determine if the goals have been achieved (usually a taper or reduction in use of the drug and/or perhaps engaging in alternative pain management strategies). If goals are not met, referral to more intensive treatment is warranted. Remember that prescribing smaller quantities of medication will allow for closer monitoring in the follow-up visits. Importantly, SBIRT has a billable procedure code that can be used. Keep in mind that Medicare has specified the screening instrument that must be used (i.e. AUDIT and/or the DAST) and does not always reimburse for this procedure. Check with specific insurers including Medicare and/or the SAMHSA website for up-to-date billing information.

REFERENCES

1. Sung HE, Richter L, Vaughan R, et al. Nonmedical use of prescription opioids among teenagers in the United States: trends and correlates. J Adolesc Health. 2005;37(1):44-51.
2. Paulozzi LJ, Budnitz DS, Xi Y. Increasing deaths from opioid analgesics in the United States. Pharmacoepidemiol Drug Saf. 2006;15(9):618-27.
3. Fonseca F, de la Torre R, Diaz L, et al. Contribution of cytochrome P450 and ABCB1 genetic variability on methadone pharmacokinetics, dose requirements, and response. PLoS One. 2011;6(5):0019527.
4. Phillips DM. JCAHO pain management standards are unveiled: joint Commission on Accreditation of Healthcare Organizations. JAMA. 2000;284(4):428-9.
5. Porter J, Jick H. Addiction rare in patients treated with narcotics. N Engl J Med. 1980;302(2):123.
6. Miller NS, Sheppard LM, Colenda CC, et al. Why physicians are unprepared to treat patients who have alcohol- and drug-related disorders. Acad Med.. 2001;76(5):410-18.
7. Illness NAoM. NAMI comments on the APA's draft revision of the DSM-V. 2010. http://www.nami.org/Content/ContentGroups/Policy/Issues_Spotlights/DSM5/Substance_Use_Disorder_Paper_4_13_2010.pdf.
8. Whitlock EP, Polen MR, Green CA, et al. Behavioral counseling interventions in primary care to reduce risky/harmful alcohol use by adults: a summary of the evidence for the U.S. Preventive Services Task Force. Ann Intern Med. 2004;140(7):557-68.
9. Volkow ND, Li TK. Drug addiction: the neurobiology of behaviour gone awry. Nature reviews. Neuroscience. 2004;5 (12):963-70.
10. Madras BK, Compton WM, Avula D, et al. Screening, brief interventions, referral to treatment (SBIRT) for illicit drug and alcohol use at multiple healthcare sites: comparison at intake and 6 months later. Drug Alcohol Depend. 2009;99 (1-3):280-95.
11. Liberto LA, Fornili KS. Managing pain in opioid-dependent patients in general hospital settings. Medsurg Nurs. 2013; 22(1):33-7.
12. Ballantyne JC, Mao J. Opioid therapy for chronic pain. N Engl J Med. 2003;349(20):1943-53.
13. Weissman DE, Haddox JD. Opioid pseudoaddiction—an iatrogenic syndrome. Pain. 1989;36(3):363-6.
14. Babor TF, McRee BG, Kassebaum PA, et al. Screening, Brief Intervention, and Referral to Treatment (SBIRT): toward a public health approach to the management of substance abuse. Subst Abus. 2007;28(3):7-30.
15. Smith PC, Schmidt SM, Allensworth-Davies D, et al. A single-question screening test for drug use in primary care. Arch Intern Med. 2010;170(13):1155-60.
16. Srisurapanont M, Sombatmai S, Boripuntakul T. Brief intervention for students with methamphetamine use disorders: a randomized controlled trial. Am J Addict. 2007; 16(2):111-16.
17. Babor TF, Kadden RM. Screening and interventions for alcohol and drug problems in medical settings: what works? J Trauma. 2005;59(3 Suppl):S94-100.
18. Koyyalagunta D, Burton AW, Toro MP, et al. Opioid abuse in cancer pain: report of two cases and presentation of an algorithm of multidisciplinary care. Pain Physician. 2011; 14(4):E361-371.

CHAPTER

22

Therapeutic Management of Osteoporosis

Stephen Honig

INTRODUCTION

The management of osteoporosis focuses on reducing fracture risk and depends on identifying those individuals who are at increased risk for fractures. As discussed in Chapter 17, the FRAX risk assessment model helps quantify risk over a 10-year period of time. This country-specific web-based program projects the likelihood of a hip or major osteoporotic fracture occurring over the next 10 years and suggests treatment thresholds. For the United States, it is recommended that individuals with a 10-year hip fracture risk of 3% or greater and/or a major osteoporotic fracture risk of 20% or greater should be started on bone-strengthening medication. Fall prevention is an important component of a comprehensive fracture reduction strategy, as most fractures are due to falls. This chapter discusses the concept of frailty, particularly in the older patient, and how it relates to fracture risk. Additionally, management of individuals at fracture risk includes attention to exercise requirements, calcium and vitamin D supplementation, and identification of the most effective bone-strengthening medication for patients.

AGING, FALLING, AND THE CONCEPT OF FRAILTY

Falls are a major concern among older adults resulting in significant mortality and morbidity, with one out of three adults age 65 and older falling each year.[1] Almost half of all women age 85 and older will fall at least once in a year (Fig. 22.1). Most fractures among older adults are caused by falls.[2] The major risk factors for falling include muscle weakness, a history of falls, and balance and gait impairments (Table 22.1).[3] Frail women are at increased risk for recurrent falls, hip fracture, any nonspine fracture, and death.[4] A widely accepted definition of frailty introduced by Fried et al. is a condition that has a decreased resistance to stressors, resulting in increased vulnerability to falls, disability, dependency, and mortality. These authors proposed a phenotype of frailty that required three or more components to be present: unintentional weight loss, self-reported exhaustion, weakness, slow walking speed, and low physical activity (Table 22.2).[5] Using these criteria, they estimated that the prevalence of frailty among community-dwelling individuals in 10 European countries was 4.1% among those 50–64 years of age and 17% among those 65 and older.[5] Muscle weakness is increasingly being recognized as a major risk factor for

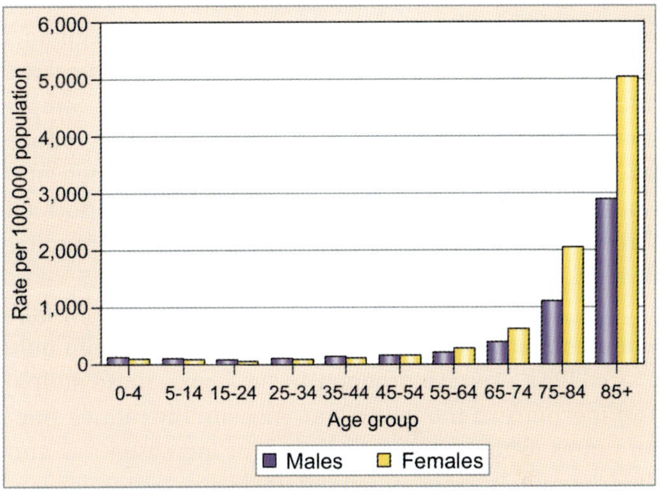

Fig. 22.1: Fall rates grouped by age.

Table 22.1: Risk factors for falls in the elderly population

Rank	Risk factors	Means odd ratio or relative risk
1	Muscle weakness	4.4
2	History of falls	3.0
3	Gait deficit	2.9
4	Balance deficit	2.9
5	Use of assistive device	2.6
6	Visual deficit	2.5
7	Arthritis	2.4
8	Impaired ADLS	2.3
9	Depression	2.2
10	Cognitive impairment	1.8
11	Age > 80 years	1.7

(ADLS: Activities of daily livings).

falls and fractures, and muscle strengthening regimens and balance training exercises should be incorporated into a comprehensive falls prevention strategy. Simple home exercise instructions have been shown to reduce fall rates by 35% among community-dwelling men and women aged 65–97.[6] A study comparing Tai Chi performed three times per week for 6 months among community-dwelling inactive people with a mean age of 77.5 years showed a significant reduction in the incidence of falls when compared to a control group who were given only a stretching exercise program to perform.[7] These simple and inexpensive modalities can measurably reduce fracture rates even among populations at increased risk and they should be recommended to every senior citizen, particularly those who have a history of falling and/or do not engage in regular exercise. Falls prevention activities should be the foundation of a fracture reduction strategy that incorporates both pharmacologic and non-drug approaches such as muscle strengthening and balance training efforts.

CALCIUM AND VITAMIN D SUPPLEMENTATION

There has been much controversy in the past 2 years regarding calcium and vitamin D supplementation and their role as part of an osteoporosis treatment regimen. Concern has been raised that calcium supplements may increase the risk of myocardial infarction and cardiovascular events.[8] However, the meta-analysis data supporting this conclusion has been questioned, and a systematic review of vitamin D and calcium supplements did not find a link between the use of these supplements and cardiovascular events.[9] Our current recommendation for women with postmenopausal osteoporosis is a daily calcium intake of 1200 mg with at least half of that amount derived from dietary sources. Vitamin D deficiency is common among all age groups, especially the elderly. The Institute of Medicine (IOM) reviewed more than a thousand studies and reports and reviewed a range of health outcomes as they relate to vitamin D intake. The IOM general recommendation, which assumed limited amounts of sun exposure, was that 600–800 IU of vitamin D supplementation would meet the needs of almost everyone in the United States and Canada. They suggested the higher dose level for elderly people and a target blood level of 20 ng/mL. They also counseled against daily intake in excess of 4000 IU.[10] We recommend that older adults receive a daily minimum of 1000 IU vitamin D as part of a falls and fracture prevention treatment program.[11]

Table 22.2: Elements involved in operationally defining frailty

Element	Measure
Weight loss, sarcopenia	Unintentional loss of > 10 pounds in previous year
Muscular weakness	Grip strength in lowest quintile adjusted for BMI
Exhaustion, poor endurance	Self-report to exhaustion
Slowness of gait	Time to walk 15 ft in lowest quintile
Low physical activity	Calories expended in physical activity—lowest quintile

BONE STRENGTHENING PRESCRIPTION MEDICATIONS

There are a number of pharmacological options available for patients, once the decision to initiate bone-strengthening medication in a postmenopausal woman has been made (Table 22.3).

Drugs that reduce bone loss are referred to as antiresorptive agents and include the following:

- Bisphosphonates: alendronate, risedronate, ibandronate, zoledronic acid
- Raloxifene, a selective estrogen receptor modulator (SERM)
- Denosumab, a RANK ligand inhibitor
- Calcitonin, a polypeptide hormone secreted by thyroid gland

Table 22.3: FDA approved osteoporosis medications

Antiresorptive drugs	*Anabolic drugs*
• Bisphosphonates	• Teriparatide (subcutaneous)
– Alendronate (oral)	
– Risedronate (oral)	
– Ibandronate (oral, intravenous)	
– Zoledronate (intravenous)	
– Etidronate (oral)	
– Pamidronate (intravenous)	
• Rank-ligand inhibitor	
– Denosumab (subcutaneous)	
• Selective estrogen receptor modulator	
– Raloxifene (oral)	
• Miscellaneous	
– Calcitonin (intranasal, subcutaneous)	

Drugs that increase bone growth are referred to as anabolic agents and includes:

- Teriparatide, a recombinant human parathyroid hormone

The bisphosphonates, the most widely prescribed osteoporosis drugs, include alendronate, risedronate, ibandronate, zoledronate, and etidronate, a first-generation bisphosphonate that is now rarely used.

Bisphosphonates have a strong affinity for hydroxyapatite crystals, the mineral component of bone, binding to these crystals at active resorption sites. Osteoclast-mediated bone resorption is thus reduced or inhibited as bisphosphonates induce osteoclast apoptosis (cell death) at the active binding sites.

The remainder of this chapter summarizes selected aspects of published data from a variety of clinical trials that have established the antifracture efficacy of the osteoporosis medications listed in Table 22.3. An extensive review of these therapeutic agents and a discussion of their clinical utility and adverse effects are beyond the scope of this review chapter.

Alendronate has been shown to increase bone mineral density (BMD) by 8% in the spine and 3.5% in the hip, and reduce vertebral fracture rates by 47% and nonvertebral fracture rates by 50% over 3 years. It is available in a generic version and most commonly used at a weekly dose of 70 mg. It is approved for the prevention and treatment of postmenopausal osteoporosis, osteoporosis in men, and glucocorticoid-induced osteoporosis.

Risedronate increases BMD by 5.4% and 1.6% at the spine and hip, respectively. It has been shown to reduce vertebral fracture rates by 41% and nonvertebral fractures by 39% over 3 years. It has recently become available in a weekly dose that can be taken after a meal, the first bisphosphonate that offers this dosing option. It is approved for the prevention and treatment of postmenopausal osteoporosis, osteoporosis in men, and glucocorticoid-induced osteoporosis.

Ibandronate increases BMD at the spine by 5.7–6.5% and at the hip by 2.4–2.8%. It has been shown to reduce vertebral fracture rates by 50% over 3 years. Its antihip fracture data were shown only in a post-hoc analysis that included clinical trial subjects with lower bone density scores at trial entry. It is available in oral (generic) and intravenous forms. It is approved for the treatment of postmenopausal osteoporosis.

Zoledronic acid is the most potent bisphosphonate available. It has been shown to increase BMD at the spine by 4.3–5.1% and to reduce the incidence of vertebral fractures by 70%, hip fractures by 41% and nonvertebral fractures by 25% over 3 years. It is administered intravenously at a dose of 5 mg annually. It is approved for the treatment of postmenopausal osteoporosis, osteoporosis in men, glucocorticoid-induced osteoporosis, and for prevention of osteoporosis (administered every 2 years).

Teriparatide is a biological compound comprised of the active component of human parathyroid hormone. It is given as a daily subcutaneous injection (20 mcg) and has been shown to both increase bone mass and approve bone microarchitecture. It increases BMD of the lumbar spine by 9–13% and the hip by 3–6% compared to placebo. It reduced the rates of spine fractures by 65% and nonspinal fractures by 54% after an average of 18 months of treatment. It is approved for postmenopausal osteoporosis, osteoporosis in males, and glucocorticoid-induced osteoporosis.

Raloxifene is the only pure SERM with FDA approval in the United States. It increases BMD at the spine and hip and reduces the incidence of spine fractures by 30–55% over 3 years. It has not been shown to reduce the incidence of hip fractures. It is approved for the prevention and treatment of postmenopausal osteoporosis and for the prevention of invasive breast cancer for women at high risk for breast cancer.

Calcitonin is a peptide hormone approved for the treatment and prevention of postmenopausal osteoporosis and has been shown to have some analgesic effects on patients with fractures. It is considered a second-line choice in the treatment for osteoporosis because of its modest effects on bone density and in reducing fracture rates. It has been shown to increase spine BMD by 1–1.5% and to reduce vertebral fracture rates by 33%. It is available in injectable and intranasal forms.

Denosumab binds to RANK ligand, an essential regulator of osteoclast formation, activation, and survival. It reduces bone loss by downregulating osteoclast activity. It is approved for the treatment of postmenopausal osteoporosis women at increased fracture risk. It has been shown to increase BMD by 9.4% at the spine and 6.4% at the hip and to reduce the rates of vertebral (68%), hip (40%), and nonvertebral (20%) fractures. It is administered by subcutaneous injection (60 mg) every 6 months. It can be used in nondialysis patients with creatinine clearances below 35 mL/min without dosage adjustment.

CONCLUSION

A comprehensive fracture reduction strategy begins with identifying those individuals who are at significant enough fracture risk to warrant therapeutic intervention. Low BMD values, increasing age and previous fragility fracture(s) are the most important predictors of future fracture. Most fractures result from falls, and falls prevention programs including balance training and muscle strengthening exercises should be offered to individuals at increased risk. Therapeutic treatment regimens should begin with adequate amounts of calcium and vitamin D and be supplemented with bone-strengthening medications as needed. Individual drug choices depend on a number of factors specific to each patient, and both the type of drug and the length of treatment should be based on an individual's continued risk of fracture tempered by an awareness of potential adverse effects of the drugs used to treat osteoporosis.

REFERENCES

1. Hausdorff JM, Rios DA, Edelberg HK. Gait variability and fall risk in community-living older adults: a 1-year prospective study. Arch Phys Med Rehabil. 2001;82(8):1050-6.
2. Bell AJ, Talbot-Stern JK, Hennessy A. Characteristics and outcomes of older patients presenting to the emergency department after a fall: a retrospective analysis. Med J Aust. 2000;173(4):179-82.
3. Guideline for the prevention of falls in older persons. American Geriatrics Society, British Geriatrics Society, and American Academy of Orthopaedic Surgeons Panel on Falls Prevention. J Am Geriatr Soc. 2001;49(5):664-72.
4. Ensrud KE, Ewing SK, Taylor BC, et al. Frailty and risk of falls, fracture, and mortality in older women: the study of osteoporotic fractures. J Gerontol A Biol Sci Med Sci. 2007;62(7):744-51.
5. Fried LP, Tangen CM, Walston J, et al. Frailty in older adults: evidence for a phenotype. J Gerontol A Biol Sci Med Sci. 2001;56(3):M146-56.
6. Robertson MC, Campbell AJ, Gardner MM, et al. Preventing injuries in older people by preventing falls: a meta-analysis of individual-level data. J Am Geriatr Soc. 2002;50(5):905-11.
7. Li F, Harmer P, Fisher KJ, McAuley E, et al. Tai Chi and fall reductions in older adults: a randomized controlled trial. J Gerontol A Biol Sci Med Sci. 2005;60(2):187-94.
8. Bolland MJ, Avenell A, Baron JA, et al. Effect of calcium supplements on risk of myocardial infarction and cardiovascular events: meta-analysis. BMJ. 2010;341:c3691.
9. Wang L, Manson JE, Song Y, Sesso HD. Systematic review: Vitamin D and calcium supplementation in prevention of cardiovascular events. Ann Intern Med. 2010;152(5):315-23.
10. Ross AC. The 2011 report on dietary reference intakes for calcium and vitamin D. Public Health Nutr. 2011;14(5):938-9.
11. Dawson-Hughes B, Mithal A, Bonjour JP, et al. IOF position statement: vitamin D recommendations for older adults. Osteoporos Int. 2010;21(7):1151-4.

CHAPTER 23

Nonoperative Treatment of Cervical Myelopathy and Radiculopathy

Kristina Bianco, Faruk Razzak, Gerard Varlotta

INTRODUCTION

Spondylosis, a degenerative process increasingly prevalent with aging populations, is one of the leading causes of neural pathologies in the cervical spine.[1] Degenerative changes associated with aging can result in disk herniation, osteophyte formation, hypertrophy of osteoarthritic facet joints, and hypertrophy of ligaments. These conditions are often asymptomatic; however, compression of the cervical spinal cord and nerve roots may occur, resulting in the symptomatic presentation of cervical myelopathy or radiculopathy.[2]

It is essential for physicians to understand how the severity of cervical myelopathy or radiculopathy affects the clinical decision-making process and formulation of an optimal and successful treatment plan. Surgical intervention for myelopathy or radiculopathy is often necessary for patients with progressive neurological symptoms or severe pain and dysfunction. However, for patients with mild to moderate symptoms, invasive surgical techniques should be avoided and nonoperative management is preferred. This may be achieved through symptom control and activity modification, in conjunction with careful clinical and radiographic follow-up. This chapter examines the efficacy of nonoperative treatment options to aid in the clinical decision-making process in the treatment of patients with cervical myelopathy and radiculopathy.

TASK FORCE FOR NECK PAIN

The task force for neck pain was established as a part of the bone and joint decade (2000–2010) initiative by the World Health Organization. The task force performed extensive literature reviews and conducted original research to analyze the prevalence of neck pain and treatment options. This resulted in a four-grade classification system for neck pain, listed below:[3]

- *Grade I neck pain*: No signs of major pathology; little or no interference with activities of daily living (ADLs)
- *Grade II neck pain*: No signs of major pathology; interference with ADLs
- *Grade III neck pain*: No signs of major structural pathology, but presence of neurological signs and symptoms
- *Grade IV neck pain*: Neck pain with major structural pathology, instability or infection

This four-grade classification system considers symptoms as well as functional and neurological involvement. Diagnosis and grading clinically, as suggested, would now parallel decision-making in treatment.

Patients with Grade I and II neck pain do not present with major pathologies or neurological symptoms, so conservative nonoperative treatment is optimal. For patients with Grade III neck pain, clinical judgment and risk stratification is necessary as there is no clear clinical advantage between surgical and conservative treatment in this group. However, surgical interventions are costly and can involve serious risks, such as damage to the spinal cord. Thus, nonoperative treatments are usually the preferred treatment option for patients with Grade III neck pain. Finally, patients with Grade IV neck pain present with major structural pathology or severe myelopathy and radiculopathy. Surgical interventions are needed for these patients, especially for traumatic conditions that have the potential for rapid progression or neurologic deterioration. Surgery is also recommended for patients with severe nontraumatic pathologies, such as spinal infection or neoplasm with airway or neurologic compression.

While patients with Grades I–II and Grade IV neck pain have a clear treatment plan, the treatment plan for patients with Grade III neck pain must be determined on an individual basis. Mild to moderate cervical myelopathy and radiculopathy often present in patients with Grade III neck pain. Thus, the decision to use nonoperative versus operative treatment should be carefully contemplated for patients with mild to moderate cervical myelopathy and radiculopathy.

PATHOPHYSIOLOGY

Cervical myelopathy refers to the compression of the cervical spinal cord that results in neck stiffness and unilateral or bilateral neck, arm, and shoulder pain. The most common type of cervical myelopathy occurs due to spondylitis and degenerative changes of the spine (Fig. 23.1). The development of cervical spondylotic myelopathy (CSM) includes three pathophysiological contributors: (1) static mechanical factors, (2) dynamic mechanical factors, and (3) spinal cord ischemia.[1] Static mechanical factors, such as congenital deformities, degeneration of the intervertebral disk and posterior facet joints, and the development of osteophytes, result in a reduction in the spinal canal diameter. Dynamic mechanical factors and normal motion of the cervical spine can exacerbate the development of CSM. During flexion, the spinal cord may lengthen and stretch over osteophytic regions. During extension, the ligamentum flavum may buckle into the spinal cord and result in the reduction in available space for the spinal cord. Spinal cord ischemia has also been found to play a role in the development of CSM; however, the exact mechanism is not well known.

Cervical radiculopathy (CR) refers to the compression of cervical nerve roots in the neural foramen (Fig. 23.2). CR mostly includes impingement of the anterior ramus, resulting in upper extremity symptoms, such as numbness, weakness, or paresthesia of the arms.[4] Though less prevalent, posterior rami radiculopathy affects the dermatomes and muscles of the upper back and shoulders, resulting in periscapular dysfunction. This may precede the onset of traditional radicular symptoms. CR is the result of nerve root impingement often caused by structural lesions, such as cervical disk herniation, spondylosis, or osteophytosis. Additionally, foraminal stenosis can cause an increase in radicular symptoms. CR caused by degeneration of intervertebral disk or spondylosis often causes radicular pain with or without neurologic compromise. While this pain sometimes subsides over time and without intervention, it often progresses to severe pain and results in disability.

While many cases of cervical myelopathy and radiculopathy occur due to degenerative changes of the spine, they can also be caused by traumatic injuries. Blunt trauma often results in severe spinal cord injury (SCI) followed by a secondary biologic response to the injury that may include significant swelling. Cervical SCI can result in cervical myelopathy or cervical radiculopathy

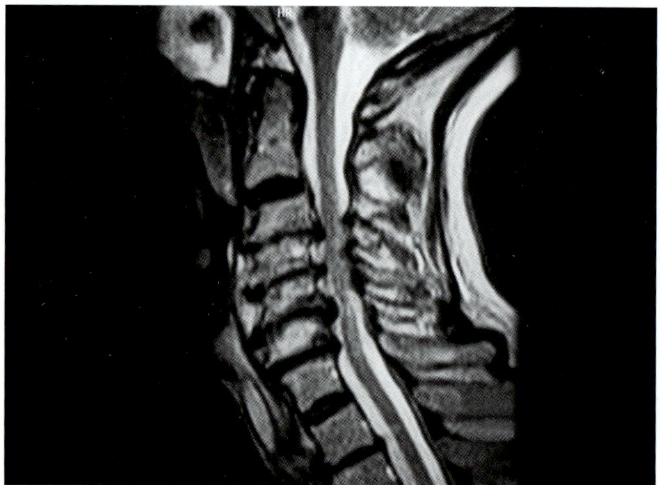

Fig. 23.1: Radiographic image of a patient with cervical spondylotic myelopathy.

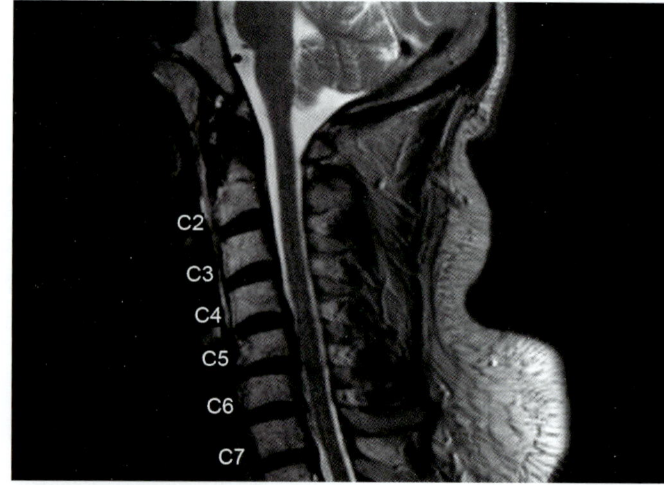

Fig. 23.2: Radiographic image of a patient presenting with cervical radiculopathy.

if there is compression of the spinal cord or nerve roots. The management of patients with SCI from blunt trauma is well studied and defined.[5,6] Patients with SCI are often treated with decompression surgery quickly following the initial injury because blunt trauma often results in very severe cervical myelopathy or radiculopathy.

Nontraumatic neck injuries, such as whiplash-associated disorders (WADs), are also well defined. In the past three decades, the number of individuals reporting to emergency rooms for traffic-related WADs has skyrocketed.[3] WADs are most often treated with nonoperative measures, with an emphasis on regaining function and returning to work as soon as possible. It is unknown if WAD causes an accelerated progression of the natural degenerative or preexisting processes.[7,8]

NONOPERATIVE TREATMENT FOR CERVICAL MYELOPATHY AND CERVICAL RADICULOPATHY

There are various types of nonoperative treatment options for the management of cervical myelopathy and radiculopathy (Table 23.1).

Cervical Immobilization and Cervical Collars

In the United States, cervical immobilization is a commonly used treatment for CSM without rapid progression. However, studies have shown conflicting results for the efficacy of cervical immobilization as a treatment for CSM. While some studies find significant improvement in symptoms with the use of cervical immobilization, others reveal significant deterioration and worsening of symptoms when patients used cervical immobility as the only method of treatment.[9] This highlights the complexity of managing CSM as improvement of symptoms through immobilization often come with reduction in function and strength leading to increased symptoms afterward.

Table 23.1: The efficacy of nonoperative treatment options for cervical myelopathy (CM) and cervical radiculopathy (CR). There are conflicting beliefs about the efficacy of facet injections and acupuncture for the treatment of CR

	CM	*CR*
Immobilization/collars	*No*	*No*
Physical therapy	*Yes*	*Yes*
Manual therapy	*No*	*No*
ART/MFR	*Yes*	*Yes*
Cervical traction	*No*	*Yes*
NSAIDs	*Yes*	*Yes*
Oral steroid drug	Yes	Yes
ESIs	No	Yes
Facet injections	No	Yes/No
Activity modification	Yes	Yes
Posture and erogonomics	Yes	Yes
Acupuncture	Yes	Yes/No
Massage	No	Yes

Cervical immobilization and collars are also used for the treatment and management of radicular pain. Short-term collar use may reduce symptoms of radiculopathy in the inflammatory phase. Although the use of a cervical collar is helpful in alleviating pain and symptoms of radiculopathy, it has not been proven to alter the disease process.[10] In general, hard collars are uncomfortable for patients and while soft collars provide alleviation and muscle relaxation, they do not provide enough support. If cervical immobilization is the chosen treatment plan, semirigid collars are suggested for activities that provoke symptoms.

For patients with cervical myelopathy or radiculopathy from WADs, cervical immobilization has not been found to significantly reduce pain.[11] Soft collars have shown to have no benefit or less benefit when compared with active therapy, rest, and usual care.[12] Furthermore, a randomized study found that patients with WAD experienced pain for 6 weeks after the injury, regardless of collar use.[13] Thus, cervical collars are not the optimal treatment option for patients suffering from WADs, but may be used postoperatively if associated myelopathy or radiculopathy is present.

Physical Therapy

Physical therapy is another conservative treatment option for patients with mild to moderate myelopathy or radiculopathy, with a focus on mobilizing and stabilizing the cervical spine. A prospective, randomized study of various treatment techniques revealed that there were no statistically significant differences between patients treated for CSM with physical therapy and surgery. This suggests that physical therapy can be just as effective as surgical techniques.[14] Thus, for cervical myelopathy and cervical radiculopathy, physical therapy is an effective treatment modality.

Manual Therapy

Manual therapy and spinal manipulation are other nonoperative treatment options. Manual medicine incorporates manipulations to restore postural balance and optimal function and to enhance pain-free movement.[15] It aims to restore disk or facet function, as well as optimal muscular and myofascial range.[16] However, cervical spine manipulation carries risk of complications, including vertebral dissection and spinal cord compression. High velocity manipulation techniques should not be used when patients have cervical disk herniations.[16] Manual therapy intervention should be discouraged for patients with cervical myelopathy or radiculopathy.[17]

Myofascial Release and Active Release Techniques

Soft tissue dysfunction often accompanies the pain and functional deficits imparted by radiculopathy or myelopathy. Conservative adjunctive treatment such as manual therapy includes the use of a practitioner's own hands to palpate dysfunctions and provide treatment through adjustments and manipulation of the patient's body. Myofascial release (MFR) is a type of manual therapy that utilizes concepts introduced by Andrew Taylor Still, the founder of osteopathic medicine, about the influence and changes in the fibrous fascia of the body relating to musculoskeletal injury.[18] Utilizing knowledge of the fascial planes and anatomy, the practitioner stretches and releases adhesive and dysfunctional fascia back into motion. Without active participation on part of the patient, MFR is considered a passive therapy. While manual therapy alone may not address directly the underlying cause of radiculopathy and myelopathy, it has been successful as a supplementary treatment providing symptom relief and functional improvements in patients with soft tissue dysfunctions.

Active release techniques (ARTs) are also another form of manual therapy developed by Dr P Michael Leahy, DC, employing similar concepts and goals to that of MFR.[19] ART principals focus on muscles, tendons nerves, fascia and add an active component with the participation of the patient in the therapeutic maneuvers. ART employs a shortening as well as stretching of the soft tissues as part of the therapeutic maneuver and its developers believe it to be a comprehensive soft tissue massage technique. ART has been patented, streamlined and offered to practitioners through a course and certification. As with MFR there have been more anecdotal results of improved symptoms and function than large-scale studies on its efficacy. As with MFR, ART is practiced as a supplementary treatment mainly through physical/occupational therapy sessions in the treatment of radiculopathy and myelopathy.

Cervical Traction

Cervical traction is sometimes used for the remediation of pain caused by cervical radiculopathy. Typically, 8–12 lb of traction is applied at an angle of approximately 24° of flexion for 15–20 minute intervals. Traction is best after significant muscular pain has subsided and it is not recommended for patients with signs of myelopathy.[10]

Nonsteroid Anti-inflammatory Drugs

Nonsteroid anti-inflammatory drugs (NSAIDs) are commonly used to reduce pain for patients with cervical myelopathy and radiculopathy. Though there are limited studies on the efficacy of NSAIDs in the cervical spine, there is much evidence about the effectiveness of NSAIDs in the alleviation of lower back pain. In practice, a trial of NSAIDs is usually the first line of treatment for patients with CSM and CR. Safe use of NSAIDs can have low risks but significant benefits in improving CSM and CR related inflammatory pain. However, structural progression may occur in spite of symptomatic reduction.

Oral Steroid Drugs

Pharmacotherapy with oral steroid drugs is indicated in the treatment of cervical myelopathy and radiculopathy acutely or when NSAIDs are not sufficient for significant inflammation. In the presence of significant radiculopathy, early intervention with corticosteroids has been shown to result in a rapid decrease in radicular symptoms.[20] However, excessive or long-term use of steroids may cause a risk of immunosuppression, hyperglycemia (iatrogenic diabetes), osteoporosis, and adrenal insufficiency (Cushing's syndrome).

Cervical Epidural Steroid Injections

When the above treatment options do not relieve pain from cervical myelopathy or radiculopathy, epidural steroid injections (ESIs) may be used for rapid pain relief. Cervical ESIs are often used to treat herniated disks, spinal stenosis, and chronic neck pain. Precise delivery of corticosteroids avoids systemic steroid use and achieves a strong anti-inflammatory effect, which reaches the interneural capillaries of the spinal nerve roots. Thus,

ESIs have been found to rapidly decrease radicular pain. The Task Force for Neck Pain confirmed this short-term relief of radicular symptoms with epidural or selective root injections of corticosteroids.[3] Of note, response to oral steroids does not predict the success of cervical ESIs.

Cervical perineural injections, such as transforaminal ESIs (TFESIs) and interlaminar ESIs, should be used under radiographic guidance and only after confirmation of pathology by MRI.[10] Though ESIs have been shown to successfully reduce pain and decrease the need for surgery, several complications, such as severe neurologic deformity and spinal cord infarction, have been noted. The procedures must be performed by experienced doctors and great care should be taken to ensure that vulnerable structures are not punctured in the injection process.

Transforaminal ESIs

A prospective study by Kolstad et al. found a statistically significant reduction in radicular pain for patients treated with TFESIs.[21] Furthermore, the study found that TFESIs resulted in a reduction in operative treatment required for patients. After receiving TFESIs, 24% of the patients decided to cancel surgery due to the significant reduction in pain from the TFESIs alone.[21]

Interlaminar ESIs

Cervical interlaminar epidural injections significantly reduce chronic cervical pain and provide long-term relief.[22] Anatomically, there is a higher risk of neural and vascular complications of TFESIs over interlaminar ESIs.

Facet Injections

Facet joints are a well-recognized source of pain in the cervical spine. Facet joints are innervated by medial branches of the dorsal rami and can radiate pain to the extremities. Cervical facet joints may be a source of pain for 36–60% of patients with chronic neck pain.[23] Facet joint pain may be managed by intra-articular injections, medial branch blocks, and neurotomies. Facet joint pain may coincide with cervical myelopathy and radiculopathy because facet joint degeneration is directly related to the degeneration of the intervertebral disk, a contributor to both cervical myelopathy and cervical radiculopathy. As a result of aging, the intervertebral disks lose hydration and disk height, which puts greater stress on the posterior facet joints.[24] This degenerative disk process starts as early as the second decade of life. Osteophytic spurs can develop due to the stresses and cause direct compression of the spinal cord, resulting in myelopathy. Facet joint osteophytes have also been found to contribute to nerve root compression, which can induce radiculopathy.[25] Additionally, facet joint inflammation has been found to release inflammatory cytokines that induce nerve root injury and subsequent radiculopathy.[25] Thus, facet injections are important nonoperative considerations as they address the pain and inflammatory processes often at the root of multiple neck pain disorders including cervical myelopathy and radiculopathy.

However, there are conflicting results of the efficacy of facet injections in the cervical spine. According to the Task Force on Neck Pain, facet injections have not proven to be effective in the treatment of cervical myelopathy and radiculopathy.[26] A literature review by Boswell et al. found limited to moderate results in the efficacy of facet injections for the cervical spine.[23] The review examined the short-term (<3 months) and long-term (>3 months) effect of different types of facet injections for the remediation of pain.[23]

Intra-articular Injections

There is limited evidence of the efficacy of cervical intra-articular facet injections and conflicting evidence of the efficacy of lumbar intra-articular facet injections.[23,27,28] Cervical intra-articular facet joint injections have been found to be ineffective at reducing pain for patients with WADs.[29]

Medial Branch Blocks

Therapeutic medial branch blocks have been found to provide significant pain reduction for patients with cervical facet joint pain, diagnosed by local anesthetic agents.[30-33] Although medial branch blocks have been found to be effective in providing pain relief for patients with herniated disks in the cervical spine, patients with myofascial pain, and patients with WAD,[34] they are not typically used for CSM and CR because myelopathy and radiculopathy are not directly associated with facet pathology.

Neurotomy

Percutaneous neurotomy of medial branches is a procedure that offers pain relief by the denervation of the nerves that innervate the painful facet joint. Percutaneous neurotomies have been found to be effective at providing short and long-term pain relief for patients with cervical facet joint pain.[35,36] However, since CSM and CR are not directly related to facet pathology, neurotomies are not often used for patients with CSM and CR. Studies on the efficacy of neurotomies for CSM and CR are limited and further research should be devoted to this topic.[23]

Activity and Sports Modification

Activity and sports modification are important for the restoration of full range of motion. Enhanced muscular strength and increased awareness of proprioception allow the patient to balance the cervical spine.[15] Stretching exercises restore and maintain normal functional movement and are essential to prevent scarring, adhesions, and repetitive microtrauma to the cervical spine.[15,37] Aerobic conditioning is also important for the restoration of full range of motion; however, aerobic capacity may diminish rapidly with the inactivity that often accompanies CR.[15] This may limit a patient's ability to perform strengthening exercises. An exercise program designed to strengthen deconditioned cervical, shoulder, upper trunk, and peripheral musculature is essential for rehabilitation. Activity should be limited to moderate exercise to prevent further damage to the cervical spine. However, it is clear that moderate activity and exercise allows for the restoration of the range of motion of the spine and is a viable option for the conservative treatment of patients with CR and CSM.

Posture and Ergonomics

As individuals age, they develop a kyphotic posture, which includes flexion of the thoracic spine and a compensatory hyperextension of the cervical spine to maintain an effective line of sight. This postural change can result in the new impingement of the cervical spine or progression of previous symptoms. Postural training is an essential nonoperative treatment modality to prevent the progression of the symptoms of cervical myelopathy and radiculopathy. The goal of postural training is to teach the patient to maintain a "neutral spine," while performing activities of everyday life.[15] These proprioceptive skills are applied during rehabilitation and strengthening exercises to teach the patient to keep the cervical spine in a pain-free and stable position during strenuous exercises.[37] Patients should aim to maintain a neutral cervical spine in everyday life by employing ergonomics such as adjusting chair height while sitting at a desk (Fig. 23.3).

OTHER NONOPERATIVE TREATMENT METHODS

Alternative nonoperative treatment procedures include thermal therapy, electrotherapy, massage, and acupuncture. These treatment methods have variable efficacy in reducing pain and are typically used to supplement other nonoperative treatment methods. Additional treatment methods of cervical myelopathy and radiculopathy include adjunct medications, such as opiates, muscle relaxants, and low-dose tricyclic antidepressants.[15] These adjunct medications are effective in reducing the level of pain for the patient.

NONOPERATIVE VERSUS OPERATIVE TREATMENT OF CERVICAL MYELOPATHY

Evaluating the efficacy of treatment options for cervical myelopathy can be difficult. Studies show that as many as 18% of patients with CSM improve spontaneously, 40% stabilize without treatment, and 42% deteriorate without treatment.[38] In order to determine a treatment plan for a patient with cervical myelopathy, the severity of the pathology must be evaluated. For patients with severe myelopathy, surgical procedures designed to decompress the spinal cord and stabilize the spine are utilized. Though often essential for patients with severe myelopathy, surgery has not shown significant results for the treatment of mild to moderate myelopathy. There is currently no evidence indicating decompression with an anterior or posterior approach significantly improves

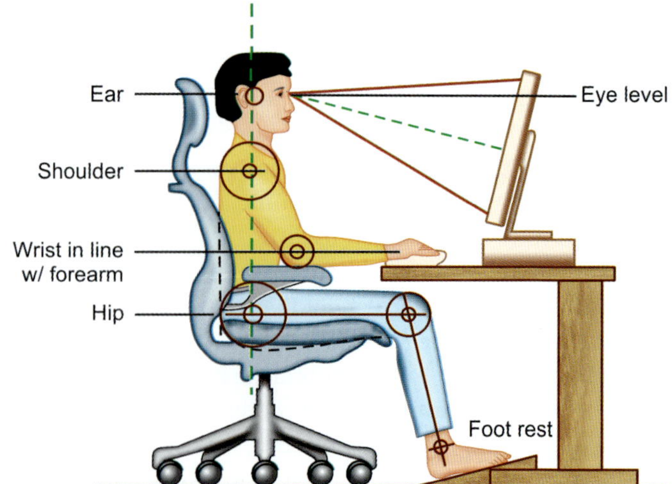

Fig. 23.3: Ergonomics to maintain neutral cervical spine while sitting at a desk.

the outcomes of patients with mild to moderate cervical myelopathy. This may indicate other factors, such as inflammatory reactions, contribute significantly to the symptoms of mild to moderate myelopathy rather than compressive factors. Symptoms may progress to CSM in some patients but not others and it should also be noted that in patients with CSM undergoing surgical intervention, clinical progression may continue.[39] Furthermore, studies have shown that operative procedures do not yield better results than conservative procedures for patients with mild or moderate CSM.[40-43]

It is essential that physicians educate patients about nonoperative treatment options so that surgical techniques can be avoided if not necessary. Nonoperative techniques include cervical immobilization (collar or neck brace), physical therapy, NSAIDs, trigger point injections (TPIs), facet injections, cervical ESIs, and TFESIs. These various nonoperative treatment options will be described in detail later in this chapter.

NONOPERATIVE VERSUS OPERATIVE TREATMENT OF CERVICAL RADICULOPATHY

The treatment of CR also varies according to the extent of cervical spine pathology. Severe cases of CR are commonly treated with surgical techniques, such as laminectomy, discectomy, laminoplasty, anterior and posterior fusion, and/or foraminotomy. However, nonsurgical conservative management has been found to be successful for most patients with CR.[44,45] Thus, surgery is typically deferred until all conservative treatment options have failed. In most cases of cervical spondylotic radiculopathy, the results of conservative management are quite significant. Approximately 80–90% of patients respond to conservative treatment, with improvements in pain, function, and mood in 3–6 months.[17] Nonoperative treatment of CR parallels that of CSM, including cervical immobilization, physical therapy, cervical traction, NSAIDs, TPIs, facet injections, cervical ESIs, and TFESIs. These therapies may be used alone or in combinations. Given these findings, surgical intervention may be deferred unless pain persists or if there is severe neurologic deficit.

CONCLUSION

The severity of the pathology, as well as patient preference and response to treatment, must guide the choice of treatment for the short-term relief of neck pain. Often, taking a "less is more" approach is preferable for patients with cervical myelopathy and radiculopathy. If a patient has mild to moderate cervical myelopathy or radiculopathy, conservative treatment options should be thoroughly considered and utilized before performing surgery. Though conservative treatment options also have risks and associated complications, the risks from conservative procedures are less severe than those associated with surgery and studies have shown that surgical procedures do not yield better results than conservative management.[40-43] Since surgical procedures are much more costly and invasive than nonoperative procedures, surgery should only be performed once conservative treatment has failed to relieve symptoms or neurological progression has been determined.

In most cases, if symptoms can be controlled through nonoperative treatment prior to surgery, the patient's need for surgery can be deferred. However, it is important to keep in mind that multiple visits and treatments without focused goals may make neck pain and disability worse rather than better. Conservative treatment measures, such as injections, should not be administered in excess and clinical judgment is always necessary when balancing between continued short-term interventions versus recommending surgical intervention. On the other hand, delaying surgery could be potentially problematic for the patient and result in worsening of symptoms. Despite the potential drawbacks of using nonoperative treatment options, it is clear that the use of conservative treatment should be the first step in addressing neck pain for patients with mild to moderate cervical myelopathy or radiculopathy. A multidisciplinary approach including multiple nonoperative conservative interventions, with close attention to changing symptoms, is both an excellent treatment plan on its own and as a prerequisite, should surgical intervention be needed.

REFERENCES

1. Young WF. Cervical spondylotic myelopathy: a common cause of spinal cord dysfunction in older persons. Am Fam Physician. 2000;62(5):1064.
2. Galbraith J, Butler J, Dolan A, et al. Operative outcomes for cervical myelopathy and radiculopathy. Adv Orthop. 2012;2012:919153.
3. Haldeman S, Carroll L, Cassidy JD, et al. The bone and joint decade 2000–2010 task force on neck pain and its associated disorders. Eur Spine J. 2008;17:5-7.
4. Boyles R, Toy P, Mellon J, et al. Effectiveness of manual physical therapy in the treatment of cervical radiculopathy: a systematic review. J Man Manip Ther. 2011;19(3):135-42.

5. Stiell IG, Wells GA, Vandemheen KL, et al. The Canadian C-spine rule for radiography in alert and stable trauma patients. JAMA. 2001;286(15):1841-8.
6. Stiell IG, Clement CM, McKnight RD, et al. The Canadian C-spine rule versus the NEXUS low-risk criteria in patients with trauma. N Engl J Med. 2003;349(26):2510-18.
7. Meenen N, Katzer A, Dihlmann S, et al. [Whiplash injury of the cervical spine-on the role of pre-existing degenerative diseases]. Unfallchirurgie. 1994;20(3):138.
8. Ichihara D, Okada E, Chiba K, et al. Longitudinal magnetic resonance imaging study on whiplash injury patients: minimum 10-year follow-up. J Orthop Sci. 2009;14(5):602-10.
9. Roberts A. Myelopathy due to cervical spondylosis treated by collar immobilization. Neurology. 1966;16(9):951.
10. Eubanks JD. Cervical radiculopathy: nonoperative management of neck pain and radicular symptoms. Am Fam Physician. 2010;81(1):33-40.
11. Hurwitz EL, Carragee EJ, Van Der Velde G, et al. Treatment of neck pain: noninvasive interventions: results of the Bone and Joint Decade 2000–2010 Task Force on Neck Pain and Its Associated Disorders. J Manip Physiol Ther. 2009;32(2):S141-S175.
12. Borchgrevink GE, Kaasa A, McDonagh D, et al. Acute treatment of whiplash neck sprain injuries: a randomized trial of treatment during the first 14 days after a car accident. Spine. 1998;23(1):25-31.
13. Gennis P, Miller L, Gallagher EJ, et al. The effect of soft cervical collars on persistent neck pain in patients with whiplash injury. Acad Emerg Med. 1996;3(6):568-73.
14. Persson LCG, Carlsson CA, Carlsson JY. Long-lasting cervical radicular pain managed with surgery, physiotherapy, or a cervical collar: a prospective, randomized study. Spine. 1997;22(7):751.
15. Wolff MW, Levine LA. Cervical radiculopathies: conservative approaches to management. Phys Med Rehab Clin N Am. 2002;13(3):589-608.
16. Atchison J W, Stoll S T, Gilliar W G. Manipulation, traction, and massage. Physical medicine and rehabilitation. Philadelphia: WB Saunders; 1996. pp. 442-6.
17. Kuijper B, Tans JTJ, Schimsheimer R, et al. Degenerative cervical radiculopathy: diagnosis and conservative treatment: a review. Eur J Neurol. 2009;16(1):15-20.
18. DiGiovanna EL, Schiowitz S, Dowling DJ. An osteopathic approach to diagnosis and treatment. Lippincott Philadelphia Williams & Wilkins; 2004.
19. Hammer WI. Functional soft-tissue examination and treatment by manual methods. Sulbury (Mass): Jones & Bartlett Learning; 2007.
20. Saal JS, Saal JA, Yurth EF. Nonoperative management of herniated cervical intervertebral disc with radiculopathy. Spine. 1996;21(16):1877.
21. Kolstad F, Leivseth G, Nygaard O. Transforaminal steroid injections in the treatment of cervical radiculopathy. A prospective outcome study. Acta Neurochir. 2005;147(10):1065-70.
22. Champaign I, Center P, Covington L, et al. Systematic review of the effectiveness of cervical epidurals in the management of chronic neck pain. Pain Physician. 2009;12(1):137-57.
23. Boswell MV, Colson JD, Spillane WF. Therapeutic facet joint interventions in chronic spinal pain: a systematic review of effectiveness and complications. Pain Physician. 2005;8(1):101-14.
24. Varlotta GP, Lefkowitz TR, Schweitzer M, et al. The lumbar facet joint: a review of current knowledge: part 1: anatomy, biomechanics, and grading. Skeletal Radiol. 2011;40(1):13-23.
25. Tachihara H, Kikuchi S, Konno S, et al. Does facet joint inflammation induce radiculopathy?: an investigation using a rat model of lumbar facet joint inflammation. Spine. 2007;32(4):406.
26. Carragee EJ, Hurwitz EL, Cheng I, et al. Treatment of neck pain: injections and surgical interventions: results of the bone and joint decade 2000–2010 task force on neck pain and its associated disorders. J Manipulative Physiol Ther. 2009;32(2):S176-S193.
27. Fuchs S, Erbe T, Fischer HL, et al. Intraarticular hyaluronic acid versus glucocorticoid injections for nonradicular pain in the lumbar spine. J Vascular Int Radiol. 2005;16(11):1493-8.
28. Carette S, Marcoux S, Truchon R, et al. A controlled trial of corticosteroid injections into facet joints for chronic low back pain. N Engl J Med. 1991;325(14):1002-7.
29. Barnsley L, Lord SM, Wallis BJ, et al. Lack of effect of intraarticular corticosteroids for chronic pain in the cervical zygapophyseal joints. N Engl J Med. 1994;330(15):1047-50.
30. Manchikanti L, Manchikanti KN, Damron K, et al. Effectiveness of cervical medial branch blocks in chronic neck pain: a prospective outcome study. Pain Physician. 2004;7(2):195-202.
31. Manchikanti L, Damron K, Cash K, et al. Therapeutic cervical medical branch blocks in managing chronic neck pain: a preliminary report of randomized, double-blind, controlled trial: clinical trial NCT0033272. Pain Physician. 2006;9(346):1533-3159.
32. Niagara W, Manchikanti L. Comparative outcomes of a 2-year follow-up of cervical medial branch blocks in management of chronic neck pain: A randomized, double-blind controlled trial. Pain Physician. 2010;13:437-50.
33. Folman Y, Livshitz A, Shabat S, et al. Relief of chronic cervical pain after selective blockade of zygapophyseal joint. Harefuah. 2004;143(5):339-41.
34. Kim KH, Choi SH, Kim TK, et al. Cervical facet joint injections in the neck and shoulder pain. J Korean Med Sci. 2005;20(4):659-62.
35. Lord SM, Barnsley L, Wallis BJ, et al. Percutaneous radiofrequency neurotomy for chronic cervical zygapophyseal-joint pain. N Engl J Med. 1996;335(23):1721-6.
36. Barnsley L. Percutaneous radiofrequency neurotomy for chronic neck pain: outcomes in a series of consecutive patients. Pain Medicine. 2005;6(4):282-6.
37. Lagattuta F, Falco F. Assessment and treatment of cervical spine disorders. Physical medicine and rehabilitation, 2nd edition. Philadelphia, PA: WB Saunders; 2000. pp. 762-91.
38. Kumar VGR, Rea GL, Mervis LJ, et al. Cervical spondylotic myelopathy: functional and radiographic long-term outcome after laminectomy and posterior fusion. Neurosurgery. 1999;44(4):771.

39. Sampath P, Bendebba M, Davis JD, et al. Outcome in patients with cervical radiculopathy: prospective, multicenter study with independent clinical review. Spine. 1999;24(6):591-7.
40. Kadanka Z, Mareš M, Bednarík J, et al. Approaches to spondylotic cervical myelopathy: conservative versus surgical results in a 3-year follow-up study. Spine. 2002;27(20):2205.
41. Penning L, Wilmink J, Van Woerden H, et al. CT myelographic findings in degenerative disorders of the cervical spine: clinical significance. Am J Roentgenol. 1986;146(4):793-801.
42. Bucciero A, Vizioli L, Tedeschi G. Cord diameters and their significance in prognostication and decisions about management of cervical spondylotic myelopathy. J Neurosurg Sci. 1993;37(4):223.
43. Kadaňka Z, Bednařík J, Voháňka S, et al. Conservative treatment versus surgery in spondylotic cervical myelopathy: a prospective randomised study. Eur Spine J. 2000;9(6):538-44.
44. Swezey RL. Conservative treatment of cervical radiculopathy. Journal of Clinical Rheumatology. 1999;5(2):65.
45. Costello M. Treatment of a patient with cervical radiculopathy using thoracic spine thrust manipulation, soft tissue mobilization, and exercise. J Manual Manipulative Ther. 2008;16(3):129.

CHAPTER

24 Alternative Medicine Treatment in Spinal Disorders: Application of Acupuncture

Alex Moroz, Brian Freed

INTRODUCTION

The National Institutes of Health National Center for Complementary and Alternative Medicine (CAM) defines CAM as a group of diverse medical and healthcare systems, practices, and products that are not generally considered part of conventional medicine. Alternative medicine is the use of CAM instead of conventional medicine. An example of an alternative therapy is using a special diet to treat cancer instead of undergoing surgery, radiation, or chemotherapy that has been recommended by an oncologist. Complementary medicine is used together with convenational medicine. An example of a complementary therapy is using aromatherapy in addition to medication (Table 24.1). Integrative medicine, on the other hand, is a technique that combines treatment modalities from both conventional and CAM, which have high-quality evidence of safety and effectiveness. For example, at New York University Medical Center there is an Integrated Musculoskeletal Program where to provide excellent care for each patient with all available modalities, patients are evaluated medically, a diagnosis is determined, and then a plan is outlined that may combine medical interventions, rehabilitation interventions, and wellness services. Examples of wellness services are the Tai Chi Program and the Mind Body Program.

Table 24.1: Type of complementary and alternative medicine (CAM)

• Medicine systems
– Ayurvedic medicine
– Chinese medicine
– Homeopathy
– Naturopathy
• Biologically based practices
– Vitamins
– Minerals
– Foods and special diets
• Mind and body medicine
– Meditation
– Yoga
– Acupuncture
• Manipulative and body-based practices
– Spinal manipulation
– Massage therapy
– Reflexology

Acupuncture is a complementary modality that has been studied specifically for spinal disorders and is supported in research and literature. Many other complementary modalities have not been as thoroughly studied for spinal disorders. Acupuncture can be viewed from several perspectives. The western point of view has had many theories on its mechanism of action. At the present time there has been no unifying theory to explain all of acupuncture's effects. What is known is that acupuncture releases humoral factors, endorphins being the most commonly known, acting most likely at the spinal cord level. Another theory of acupuncture's mechanism of action is through synaptic inhibition or "gate control". Acupuncture also has impacts on the immune system. Acupuncture releases significant amounts of neurotransmitters and recently has been shown to effect changes in the cerebral cortex. These changes are created using different elements of acupuncture. Needles of various sizes, electrical stimulation, and herbal cigars providing a heat source can all be used throughout a treatment session. Electrical stimulation used with low frequency and high intensity is thought to act on humoral factors, whereas high frequency and low intensity transcutaneous electric nerve stimulation modulates gate control. There is no single theory to date that accounts for the accumulated research data of the past 50 years.[1,2]

The traditional eastern point of view examines acupuncture from a different perspective describing Yin-Yang, Qi, moisture, and blood. This is a logical approach of viewing a disease process as an imbalance. It examines external factors, wind, cold, dampness, heat, and dryness, with internal factors, joy, anger, anxiety, thought, and fear. Acupuncture adjusts imbalance and corrects disharmony. One may ask how a patient's complaints of weight loss and severe neck myofascial pain can be explained from two completely different points of view? It is a question of having different filters, and depending on your filter, or vantage point, you are able to see different aspects of the same three-dimensional problem.

APPLICATIONS OF ACUPUNCTURE

There has been much literature on acupuncture as it pertains to the treatment of spinal disorders, some of which will be discussed here. Many studies have been conducted in eastern cultures, particularly China. Unfortunately, the methodological quality of these studies does not meet acceptable standards. More reliable studies have been performed since the beginning of the 21st century.

The effectiveness of acupuncture for low back pain was examined by a meta-analysis in the Annals of Internal Medicine. Thirty-three randomized controlled trials were included in the analysis. It was found that, to compare the effectiveness of acupuncture on acute low back pain with other therapies, not enough data had been collected to draw any conclusions. However, acupuncture for short-term relief of chronic back pain was significantly more effective than the sham treatment control.[3] Acupuncture for chronic low back pain was further investigated in a large randomized controlled trial studying 638 patients. The patients were divided into four different groups. Three of the groups received acupuncture. The three acupuncture groups were divided to receive either individualized treatments with different combinations of acupuncture points, or a standardized set of acupuncture points, or simulated acupuncture where a sham acupuncture method was used. The fourth was a usual care control group. It was found that each of the acupuncture groups did better than the usual care control group at up to 1 year.[4] This brings up a controversy over the legitimacy of sham acupuncture, how inert it truly is, and whether it can be used. In our scope of discussion, this study is important because it is a large tightly designed study of acupuncture for chronic low back pain.

Another study by the same authors took a subgroup of these same patients and attempted to answer whether the pretreatment expectations and beliefs of acupuncture effectiveness would predict the success of the treatment, i.e. would patients who were fervent believers in acupuncture have better results than acupuncture skeptics? No, they found that neither pretreatment expectations nor preferences for acupuncture were predictive of outcomes. They also found that if a patient's expectations were reassessed after just five treatments, their expectations were predictive of both symptoms and function.[5] This shows that if acupuncture works, patients will know that it is working within five treatment sessions.

To determine if acupuncture is effective in improving patients' quality of life, a review of randomized controlled trials was performed. The ratio of inclusion to exclusion was very low in this study, only 8 of 186 trials were found to be of sufficient quality for inclusion. It was found that there was moderate effect on improvement of physical functioning and pain-related quality of life. However, there was only a very small and delayed effect on improving the mental aspect of quality of life.[6] A smaller study was performed using 69 patients undergoing nucleus pulposus removal and intervertebral fusion. These patients were either assigned to a conventional rehabilitation group or to a conventional rehabilitation group with added acupuncture. It was found that there was a significantly better outcome functionally in the acupuncture group at 3, 6, and 12 months postoperative. It was also found that the group receiving acupuncture recovered more quickly, with 90% of the acupuncture group doing well at only 6 months, significantly different from the conventional group.[7]

Chronic neck pain and acupuncture interventions were recently reviewed, incorporating 10 randomized control trials with varying degrees of control methods. It was found that there was moderate evidence to support the theory that acupuncture relieved pain better than sham treatments. There was also found to be moderate evidence to support acupuncture being better than weightless controls, inactive treatments, or passive treatments.[8] In another small study of 46 patients, a single acupuncture point for cervical radiculopathy from spondylosis was examined. Patients were divided evenly into either an active point group, thought to have an effect on cervical spine symptoms, or into a control point group, not thought to have any effect on cervical spine symptoms. There was improvement in both groups but significantly more improvement in the active point group 78% to 55%, respectively.[9]

Further research and investigation into the effectiveness of CAM modalities like acupuncture is necessary to improve outcome measures in patients with spine disorders.

REFERENCES

1. Moroz A. East-West Medicine: irreconcilably complementary. Am J Acupunct. 1994;22(4):369-74.
2. Moroz A. Issues in acupuncture research: the failure of quantitative methodologies and the possibilities for viable, alternative solutions. Am J Acupunct. 1999;27:95-103.
3. Manheimer E, White A, Berman B, et al. Meta-analysis: acupuncture for low back pain. Ann Intern Med. 2005;142 (8):651-63.
4. Cherkin DC, Sherman KJ, Avins AL, et al. A randomized trial comparing acupuncture, simulated acupuncture, and usual care for chronic low back pain. Arch Intern Med. 2009;169(9):858-66.
5. Sherman KJ, Cherkin DC, Ichikawa L, et al. Treatment expectations and preferences as predictors of outcome of acupuncture for chronic back pain. Spine (Phila Pa 1976). 2010;35(15):1471-7.
6. Lu SC, Zheng Z, Xue CC. Does acupuncture improve quality of life for patients with pain associated with the spine? A systematic review. Evid Based Complement Alternat Med. 2011;2011:301767.
7. Zhao BX, Wang KZ, Zhao JX, et al. Clinical effects of acupuncture after surgical operation in patients with prolapse of the lumbar intervertebral disc. J Tradit Chin Med. 2008;28(4):250-4.
8. Trinh K, Graham N, Gross A, et al. Acupuncture for neck disorders. Spine (Phila Pa 1976). 2007;32(2):236-43.
9. Dong H, Wang X, Meng X, et al. Forty-six cases of the nerve root-involved cervical spondylopathy treated by needling the "Sitian" points. J Tradit Chin Med. 2005;25(3):163-5.

CHAPTER

25

Psychosocial Aspects and Management of Chronic Low Back Pain

Matthew B Smith

INTRODUCTION

Chronic low back pain is a complex matter, a hydra of many heads, reflected in its commonly dramatic and refractory presentation. Treatment calls for recognition and understanding of psychosocial, in addition to physical, contributions. Pain, itself a biopsychosocial phenomenon,[1] rendered more complex by chronicity, then develops an impressive comorbidity with certain psychiatric syndromes.[2] Bidirectional influences of personality and other interpersonal and social factors become symptomatically and therapeutically important.[3] The limited physical component of pain becomes difficult to isolate from global suffering and function. Reductions to "strictly physical", or, alternatively, "volitional", or "psychological", tend to apply only rarely.[4] Even the formulation of "comorbidity", or "overlay", while having merit, is somewhat simplistic.

Understanding the complexity of chronic low back pain, while formidable, is necessary not merely for an empathetic response to the patient, but also in guiding and providing successful treatment. Fully informed intervention calls for a collaborative team approach, providing important perspectives from different vistas, in different dimensions.

It is useful to consider the following psychosocial components: the intrinsic motivational aspect of pain aversion; the neuroplasticity-based psychological changes of central sensitization; the common comorbid psychiatric syndromes; the associated personality features, including early developmental factors; the concurrent interpersonal and social factors; the evolving personal and social role changes; and aspects of the doctor–patient relationship.

AVERSION

Pain involves a localizable sensation that is not merely unpleasant, with negative hedonic valence, but actually aversive, with motivational salience. The associated motivations include cognitive, emotional, behavioral, and social aspects. In chronic pain, as opposed to acute pain, these are maladaptive, contributing to suffering and disability.

Cognitive and executive functions, subordinated to a focus on pain and pain relief, in general are rendered otherwise inefficient. Concentration, for example, becomes challenging.

A number of emotions are involved in aversion.[5] Anxiety is often prominent, though not adaptive in chronic pain. Objects of fear are less identifiable, and anxiety often reaches "catastrophizing"[6] proportions, also becoming generalized or phobic.[7] Autonomic aspects of anxiety may worsen muscular features of low back pain.[1] A vicious circle, involving "anxiety sensitivity" may develop.[8] This facilitates more pain, restricts activities, limits efforts in pain management and treatment, and further reduces quality of life. Fear and anxiety tend to persist, despite clinician reassurances regarding impending injury. This can sometimes take the form of "illness conviction".[9]

Anger spectrum emotions, such as rage, frustration, and irritation, common in chronic pain, while often understandable, are clearly not adaptive. Such emotions are not necessarily imposed on others but certainly tend to be burdensome for the patient, requiring efforts at suppression and control. They can provoke feelings of guilt, and additionally alienate the patient from others. Hate may be directed against the self, with pain now perceived as integral to the self. Violence, however, is rare.[10]

An additional emotion in aversion, disgust, is not commonly expressed, but it is shown at times in patients' visual portrayals of their pain.

Aversion promotes hyperactivity, although in chronic pain it becomes intermittent, alternating with hypoactivity. Pain behaviors such as wincing and moaning offer little in the relief of pain, but they contribute to the reinforcement of the psychological and social role in pain, including the signaling of distress. Such behaviors, over time, tend to worsen the overall pain syndrome.[11]

Chronic aversion tends to seek relief in social soothing, but relief from chronic pain is not thereby found, leaving continued, frustrated social longing, akin to loneliness, even with the presence and comfort of others.[12]

Understanding the aversion involved in chronic pain helps to better understand the patient's subjective experience of helpless frustration and to seek specific interventions to reduce those features that contribute to continuing misery and disability. Psychotherapeutic and psychopharmacologic techniques can specifically address and reduce the maladaptive cognitive, emotional, behavior, and social aspects of the aversiveness of pain.

CENTRAL SENSITIZATION

Central sensitization tends to develop as pain becomes chronic.[13] Neural plasticity processes result in synaptic,[14] neurogenetic,[15] apoptotic,[16] ephaptic,[17] axonal,[18] dendritic,[19] and glial cell[20] changes, with associated neurochemical,[21] endocrine,[22] and immunologic[23] effects. Information processing, both sensory and emotional, is altered, with pain largely augmented.[24] This is a loss of the "stimulus barrier," the psychological function, which manages strong sensory or emotional information input.[25] Clinically, patients develop hyperalgesia or hyperpathia,[26] expanded pain spatial distribution,[27] temporal pain persistence, cross-modality and synesthesia effects, and movement disturbances.[28] Systemically, the "sickness syndrome" is common, associated with steroid release and, clinically, sleepiness and anorexia.[29] It is said that chronic pain becomes an illness unto itself.

Psychologically, pain becomes a more powerful and global force, partly from an amplification of its aversive nature, but also in other ways. Neural plasticity changes, for example, alter the body schema in the parietal lobe.[30] The body image, in turn, is modified but in a conflicted manner.[31] The lower back, experienced as a part of the self, is simultaneously rejected as an unwanted, painful foreign body, intruding itself into the bodily space.[32] The broader self-image also becomes conflicted, illuminated by common metaphoric meanings— "spineless", "no back bone", —with associated disturbances in assertiveness, pride, self-confidence, energy, and sexuality.[33] Such views are often reinforced by other concurrent experiences and losses.

Amplified and extended pain becomes an overwhelming juggernaut of misery and disability. Of particular importance, psychologically, is the lack of predictability, understanding, and control, with associated helplessness, demoralization, mortification, and a reduced sense of subjective agency.[34] Pain becomes pre-eminent, directing moment to moment concerns, daily decisions, and future plans. Everything is seen through its prism. Other experiences and activities are restricted, further limiting quality of life. A psychological regression develops, with egocentricity and primitive modes in relating to others—often with effects on mood and with self-recriminations. Illness behavior may function to channel much of this, but it ultimately reinforces. Pain becomes a central personal reference and developmental force.

Psychotherapeutically, addressing and minimizing helplessness takes priority. Supportive psychotherapy is useful for intense but unavoidable primitive longing, anger, and guilt. Specific efforts to manage cognitive distortions are called for, for example, in the tightrope wherein a painful back is both accepted and hated. It is likely that certain central sensitization effects can be modified pharmacologically, apart from concrete analgesic effects, given plasticity effects of psychiatric medications. Psychotherapeutic and psychopharmacologic interventions reduce the spiraling deteriorations in mind-body interactions, brought on by central sensitization.

PSYCHIATRIC COMORBIDITY

Chronic low back pain is commonly associated with mood and anxiety disorders, odds ratios being significantly increased for both.[35] With respect to depression, the reported prevalence is quite variable, as high as more than 80%;[36] with respect to anxiety disorders, the reported prevalence is consistently 20–27%.[2] Addictive disorders are also associated with chronic pain conditions, with an unclear prevalence, due to varying criteria.[37]

The nature of the relationship between low back pain and psychiatric disorders is complex and variable. A psychiatric disorder may predispose to (diathesis-stress model) or result from the chronic pain condition.[38,39] There may be a common underlying causal contribution, such as a personality factor. A prior psychiatric episode may leave a subclinical residual factor (the "scar" hypothesis).[40] But clinically, since the two syndromes tend to worsen each other, one is often left with a "chicken or egg" determination, complicated by many other factors.

The recognition and treatment of a comorbid psychiatric disorder is necessary for successful pain management. This may call for diagnostic and therapeutic expertise. The diagnosis of a bipolar spectrum disorder, for example, a common but at times challenging and controversial condition, may be especially difficult in the setting of a chronic pain condition.

Addictive disorders deserve special considerations, because opioid medications often play an important role in the management of chronic pain conditions. Although most pain patients treated with opioid medications do not become addicted and reports as high as 50% are probably mistaken, some patients certainly do, posing a clinical challenge.[37] Clinicians need to develop familiarity with certain related phenomena: addiction, pseudo-addiction,[41] physical dependence, psychological dependence, and tachyphylaxis. Opioid medications must be prescribed with attention to their addictive potential, but a preliminary assessment of the addictive potential of the particular patient is also called for.[42] Clinicians must make ongoing efforts to minimize the risks of iatrogenic addiction.[43] Such steps include psychoeducation, close prescription monitoring and control, "contractual" treatment stipulations, compliance determinations, close assessments of aberrant drug taking, and at times, urine and blood assessments.

Because patients with histories of addiction or drug abuse are not immune to chronic pain, and also require treatment, consultation with addiction specialists may be necessary in such cases.

PERSONALITY FACTORS

Some personality features may enable the development of chronic pain. For example, generalized coping difficulties may constitute a risk.[3] But some specific traits have also been considered, including counterdependency,[44] somatoform trends,[45] alexithymia,[46] neuroticism,[47] harm avoidance, and reward dependence.[48] Other maladaptive traits, such as guilt trends,[49] certain narcissistic needs,[50] and histrionic features[51] may find significant partial gratification in a chronic pain syndrome. And traits of impulse or affect dyscontrol, emotional dependency, or masochistic features may also be considered. Personality factors are involved in "secondary gain", considered with the original psychiatric meaning of dependency. The variety of personality traits that may facilitate the development of chronic pain makes it difficult to generalize and difficult to predict. There are apparently many personality problems that can contribute.

Fifteen to fifty percent of chronic pain patients have histories of adversities in childhood,[52] including parental loss and maltreatment (physical, sexual, and emotional). This correlation may be mediated partly through personality features but also through anxiety or mood disorders.

A psychotherapeutic strategy must recognize the influence of early developmental and other personality factors on the development and continuation of chronic lower back pain, as well as its treatment. It will need to specifically inform the general medical and surgical approaches, to maximize a working alliance and minimize resistance.

INTERPERSONAL AND SOCIAL FACTORS

Numerous external factors can influence the suffering and disability of the patient with chronic low back pain.

Interpersonally, pain can be influenced by expectations and responses, with their associated autonomic features, as patients engage and react to other people. Such interactions may be directly about pain and associated changes in function,[53] or may worsen pain less directly in the case of other stress-related muscle or joint usage.[54] Deconditioning from avoidance may also worsen pain.[55] Interactions with others may be supportive, indifferent, or hostile; may be soothing, empowering, enraging, disappointing, or indulging. Pain can be thereby variously influenced in its threshold, intensity, quality, and further effects. In fact, pain itself can be viewed as an interpersonal phenomenon.[56]

Effects on conjugal relationships can be powerful.[57] Other family members and relationships are often influential, either positively or negatively. Role changes in the family can be stressful.[58] With chronicity, family reactions can adapt, or can become obstacles to effective treatment. New family conflicts and alliances may develop around the patient's symptoms or role changes. The patient may take on the role of the "identified patient", now a *nidus* for other family difficulties, making the low back pain an element in a complex dynamic.[59]

Occupational issues can be significant, with work changes, accommodations, and reactions from superiors and coworkers. Insurance matters—often involving worker compensation coverage—and legal issues arise, with direct or indirect psychological aspects. Although financial incentives, in the form of disability or compensation, are commonly viewed as facilitating pain and disability, it is likely that they do so only rarely.[60] The adversarial nature of proceedings may diminish the availability of treatment, or may promote a worsening of pain and the pain role. These may be matters for psychotherapy, in helping the patient to cope more adaptively.

CHRONIC ILLNESS

Illness adaptively calls for the patient's adoption of the sick role, directed toward symptom management, medical maintenance, treatment, restrictions, and social and occupational changes.[61] As chronicity develops, the role becomes a prominent structural element of the self, projecting to the future. Pain, owned and disowned, powerfully inflects primary developmental meaning with pleasure/pain valence. This occurs at an immediate, bodily level, but developing self-image and identity are then constructed unstably and ambivalently, nevertheless with investment and defense.[62] Life revolves around pain and the self of pain.[32] Secondary attachments—people, money, activities, and long-term emotional, and other investments—are affected. Developmental pathways and advantages are pursued through pain and illness. This is clearest in the case of the developing child with a chronic pain syndrome, but it also applies to adults (who are of course also developing).

Treatment is thereby complicated, calling for a modification of role, to limit the effects and the experience of pain. A balance must be struck between realistic accommodation to the illness and its effects, on the one hand, and deliberate reduction in sick role and pain behaviors, with promotion of nonillness related behaviors.

PSYCHIATRIC AND PSYCHOLOGICAL TREATMENT CONSIDERATIONS

Given the refractoriness and complexity of chronic low back pain, treatment is offered from a multidimensional perspective, calling for more than one practitioner, more than one discipline. Chronic pain is a hydra of many heads: dealing with one alone will result in limited, or no, benefit. A specialized biopsychosocial approach must be combined with a more classic pain management approach. A team of practitioners is optimal, and often necessary.[63,64]

Screening for the presence of anxiety syndromes, mood syndromes, and addiction risks can be partially accomplished by questionnaires. Treatments of comorbid conditions, typically mood disorders and anxiety disorders, can proceed with approaches based on their usual treatments, but modified by nuances called for in the setting of pain, and also tend to require psychopharmacologic approaches. Psychotherapy for low back pain is usually offered by a psychotherapist with specialized training and psychopharmacology by a psychiatrist. Conjugal and family matters can often be managed by the psychotherapist or psychiatrist, although in some cases, more specialized practitioners may be called for. Group psychotherapy is an underutilized modality.

Treatment goals need to be explicitly and primarily directed toward improvement in function, rather than pain elimination, for reasons both realistic and heuristic: this implicitly includes elements of pain management and tolerance. Specific therapeutic goals include reduction in pain-associated cognitions, behaviors, and emotions; in self-image disturbances; and in interpersonal avoidances. It includes pursuit of life activities apart from pain.

While specific techniques should favor supportive, cognitive, behavioral, cognitive-behavioral, and psychopharmacological approaches, an overall eclectic, systems point of view is required, including a psychodynamic perspective.[65] Relaxation methods, biofeedback, guided imagery, and hypnosis tend to be useful.[66] Personality features usually are not treated but need to be managed, at first, in conjunction with developmental issues, larger social role and disability matters, and matters related to chronic illness.

Treatments for addictions are not usually offered by orthopedic, neurologic, or pain management specialists. Rather, addiction, when recognized, calls for addictive medications to be appropriately tapered and stopped, usually with the help of an addiction knowledgeable professional. Pain management can proceed with nonaddictive medications. Treatment for addiction itself needs to be placed in the hands of appropriate specialists and grass roots organizations like Alcoholics Anonymous and Narcotics Anonymous. Although some patients with significant addiction problems can still be treated with opioid medications, this usually requires the involvement of an addiction specialist.

COUNTERTRANSFERENCE

Patients with chronic pain syndromes bring challenges to the doctor-patient relationships due to the complexities of pain and its global effects. Such patients have puzzling, refractory, controversial conditions; present subjective complaints that are difficult to objectify; express severe suffering; are often psychologically regressed; often have disability and litigation issues; may have had substance abuse problems; often have had troubles with other providers. There is also the reality of the conflicted expectations that are brought to the relationship by the patient, who has often been a victim of adverse relationships with parental figures, early in his or her life.

Special attention is often necessary to the doctor-patient relationship. Even while remaining objective and professional in manner, providers may develop strong internal emotional reactions—countertransference. Such private reactions may vary from dismissal to fear, suspicion, frustration, and over-identification and can influence premature judgments of victimization, hopelessness, dissimulation, addiction, "secondary gain", or madness. "Blind spots" to psychological factors can develop. While countertransference is universal, with all professionals, a simple private recognition and self-acceptance of strong emotional reaction to a patient often goes a long way to facilitate appropriate objectivity.[67] Consultation may be useful at times.

CONCLUSION

Chronic pain often behaves as a hydra, requiring a simultaneous attack on all heads. Optimal pain management requires recognition of this complexity, including its psychiatric, psychological, and social aspects, and specific interventions for them, in the context of a treatment team, employing psychiatric and psychological methods.

REFERENCES

1. Feuerstein M, Papciak AS, Hoon PE. Biobehavioral mechanisms of chronic low back pain. Clin Psychol Rev. 1987; 7(3):243-73.
2. Wong WS, Chen PP, Yap J, et al. Chronic pain and psychiatric morbidity: a comparison between patients attending specialist orthopedics clinic and multidisciplinary pain clinic. Pain Med. 2011;12(2):246-59.
3. Sivik TM, Rojvall S, Gustafsson E, et al. Relationship between back pain and personality: psychologic vulnerability as risk factor for the development of chronic back pain. Nord J Psychiatry. 1992;46(3):189-93.
4. Sullivan MD. Finding pain between minds and bodies. Clin J Pain. 2001;17(2):146.
5. Wade JB, Price DD, Hamer RM, et al. An emotional component analysis of chronic pain. Pain. 1990;40(3):303-10.
6. Richardson EJ, Ness TJ, Doleys DM, et al. Depressive symptoms and pain evaluations among persons with chronic pain: catastrophizing, but not pain acceptance, shows significant effects. Pain. 2009;147(1-3):147-52.
7. Pfingsten M, Leibing E, Harter W, et al. Fear-avoidance behavior and anticipation of pain in patients with chronic low back pain: a randomized controlled study. Pain Med. 2001;2(4):259-66.
8. Norton PJ, Asmundson GJG. Anxiety sensitivity, fear, and avoidance behavior in headache pain. Pain. 2004;111(1): 218-23.
9. Sullivan MD, Turner JA, Romano J. Chronic pain in primary care. Identification and management of psychosocial factors. J Fam Pract. 1991;32(2):193-9.
10. Bruns D, Disorbio JM, Hanks R. Chronic nonmalignant pain and violent behavior. Curr Pain Headache Rep. 2003;7(2): 127-32.
11. Manchikanti L, Fellows B, Singh V, et al. Correlates of non-physiological behavior in patients with chronic low back pain. Pain Physician. 2003;6(2):159-66.
12. Stein DJ, Van Honk J, Ipser J, et al. Opioids: from physical pain to the pain of social isolation. CNS Spectr. 2007;12(9): 669.
13. Latremoliere A, Woolf CJ. Central sensitization: a generator of pain hypersensitivity by central neural plasticity. J Pain. 2009;10(9):895-926.
14. Ikeda H, Heinke B, Ruscheweyh R, et al. Synaptic plasticity in spinal lamina I projection neurons that mediate hyperalgesia. Science's STKE 2003;299(5610):1237.
15. Duric V, McCarson KE. Persistent pain produces stress-like alterations in hippocampal neurogenesis and gene expression. J Pain. 2006;7(8):544-55.
16. Apkarian AV, Sosa Y, Sonty S, et al. Chronic back pain is associated with decreased prefrontal and thalamic gray matter density. J Neurosci. 2004;24(46):10410-5.
17. Voscopoulos C, Lema M. When does acute pain become chronic? Br J Anaesth. 2010;105(Suppl 1):i69-i85.
18. Howe JF, Loeser JD, Calvin WH. Mechanosensitivity of dorsal root ganglia and chronically injured axons: a physiological basis for the radicular pain of nerve root compression. Pain. 1977;3(1):25-41.
19. Williams SR, Wozny C, Mitchell SJ. The back and forth of dendritic plasticity. Neuron. 2007;56(6):947-53.
20. Gosselin RD, Suter MR, Ji RR, et al. Glial cells and chronic pain. Neuroscientist. 2010;16(5):519-31.
21. Grachev ID, Fredrickson BE, Apkarian AV. Abnormal brain chemistry in chronic back pain: an in vivo proton magnetic resonance spectroscopy study. Pain. 2000;89(1):7-18.
22. Mäntyselkä P, Miettola J, Niskanen L, et al. Glucose regulation and chronic pain at multiple sites. Rheumatology. 2008;47(8):1235-8.
23. Winkelstein BA. Mechanisms of central sensitization, neuroimmunology & injury biomechanics in persistent pain: implications for musculoskeletal disorders. J Electromyogr Kinesiol. 2004;14(1):87-93.

24. Giesecke T, Gracely RH, Grant MAB, et al. Evidence of augmented central pain processing in idiopathic chronic low back pain. Arthritis Rheum. 2004;50(2):613-23.
25. Krystal H. Trauma and the stimulus barrier. Psychoanal Inquiry. 1985;5(1):131-61.
26. O'Neill S, Manniche C, Graven-Nielsen T, et al. Generalized deep-tissue hyperalgesia in patients with chronic low-back pain. Eur J Pain. 2007;11(4):415-20.
27. Forss N, Kirveskari E, Gockel M. Mirror-like spread of chronic pain. Neurology. 2005;65(5):748-50.
28. Schwartzman RJ, Alexander GM, Grothusen J. Pathophysiology of complex regional pain syndrome. Expert Rev Neurother. 2006;6(5):669-81.
29. Saper CB, Romanovsky AA, Scammell TE. Neural circuitry engaged by prostaglandins during the sickness syndrome. Nat Neurosci. 2012;15(8):1088-95.
30. Schmidt-Wilcke T, Leinisch E, Gänssbauer S, et al. Affective components and intensity of pain correlate with structural differences in gray matter in chronic back pain patients. Pain. 2006;125(1):89-97.
31. Moseley GL. I can't find it! Distorted body image and tactile dysfunction in patients with chronic back pain. Pain. 2008;140(1):239-43.
32. Osborn M, Smith JA. Living with a body separate from the self. The experience of the body in chronic benign low back pain: an interpretative phenomenological analysis. Scand J Caring Sci. 2006;20(2):216-22.
33. Kirmayer LJ. Culture and the metaphoric mediation of pain. Transcult Psychiatry. 2008;45(2):318-38.
34. Salomons TV, Johnstone T, Backonja MM, et al. Perceived controllability modulates the neural response to pain. J Neurosci. 2004;24(32):7199-203.
35. Demyttenaere K, Bruffaerts R, Lee S, et al. Mental disorders among persons with chronic back or neck pain: results from the World Mental Health Surveys. Pain. 2007;129(3):332-42.
36. Bair MJ, Robinson RL, Katon W, et al. Depression and pain comorbidity: a literature review. Arch Intern Med. 2003; 163(20):2433.
37. Højsted J, Sjøgren P. Addiction to opioids in chronic pain patients: a literature review. Eur J Pain. 2007;11(5):490-518.
38. Currie SR, Wang J. More data on major depression as an antecedent risk factor for first onset of chronic back pain. Psychol Med. 2005;35(9):1275-82.
39. Linton SJ, Bergbom S. Understanding the link between depression and pain. Scand J Pain. 2011;2(2):47-54.
40. Fishbain DA, Cutler R, Rosomoff HL, et al. Chronic pain-associated depression: antecedent or consequence of chronic pain? A review. Clin J Pain. 1997;13(2):116.
41. Kirsh KL, Whitcomb LA, Donaghy K, et al. Abuse and addiction issues in medically ill patients with pain: attempts at clarification of terms and empirical study. Clin J Pain. 2002;18(4):S52.
42. Wu SM, Compton P, Bolus R, et al. The addiction behaviors checklist: validation of a new clinician-based measure of inappropriate opioid use in chronic pain. J Pain Sympt Manag. 2006;32(4):342-51.
43. Naliboff BD, Wu SM, Pham Q. Clinical considerations in the treatment of chronic pain with opiates. J Clin Psychol. 2006;62(11):1397-408.
44. Gregory R, Manring J, Wade M. Personality traits related to chronic pain location. Ann Clin Psychiatry. 2005;17(2): 59-64.
45. Roberts SJ. Somatization in primary care. The common presentation of psychosocial problems through physical complaints. Nurse Pract. 1994;19(5):47.
46. Lumley MA, Asselin LA, Norman S. Alexithymia in chronic pain patients. Compr Psychiatry. 1997;38(3):160-5.
47. Vossen HGM, van Os J, Hermens H, et al. Evidence that trait-anxiety and trait-depression differentially moderate cortical processing of pain. Clin J Pain. 2006;22(8):725.
48. Pud D, Eisenberg E, Sprecher E, et al. The tridimensional personality theory and pain: harm avoidance and reward dependence traits correlate with pain perception in healthy volunteers. Eur J Pain. 2004;8(1):31-8.
49. Johansson F, Almay BGL, von Knorring L, et al. Personality traits in chronic pain patients related to endorphin levels in cerebrospinal fluid. Psychiatry Res. 1979;1(3):231-9.
50. Arntz A, Peters M. Chronic low back pain and inaccurate predictions of pain: Is being too tough a risk factor for the development and maintenance of chronic pain? Behav Res Ther. 1995;33(1):49-53.
51. Weisberg JN. Personality and personality disorders in chronic pain. Curr Rev Pain. 2000;4(1):60-70.
52. Sachs-Ericsson N, Kendall-Tackett K, Hernandez A. Childhood abuse, chronic pain, and depression in the National Comorbidity Survey. Child Abuse Negl. 2007;31(5):531-47.
53. Harris S, Morley S, Barton SB. Role loss and emotional adjustment in chronic pain. Pain. 2003;105(1):363-70.
54. Hallner D, Hasenbring M. Classification of psychosocial risk factors (yellow flags) for the development of chronic low back and leg pain using artificial neural network. Neurosci Lett. 2004;361(1):151-4.
55. Nachemson A. lumbar intradiscal pressure. The lumbar spine and back pain. Edinburgh, Scotland: Churchill Livingstone, 1987. pp. 191-203.
56. Mikail SF, Henderson PR, Tasca GA. An interpersonally based model of chronic pain: an application of attachment theory. Clin Psychol Rev. 1994;14(1):1-16.
57. Cano A, Gillis M, Heinz W, et al. Marital functioning, chronic pain, and psychological distress. Pain. 2004;107(1-2): 99-106.
58. Walker J, Sofaer B, Holloway I. The experience of chronic back pain: accounts of loss in those seeking help from pain clinics. Eur J Pain. 2006;10(3):199-207.
59. Benton D. Family therapy: problems encountered in defocusing the identified patient. J Psychiatr Nurs Ment Health Serv 1979;17(5):28.
60. Pearce J. Aspects of the failed back syndrome: role of litigation. Spinal Cord. 2000;38(2):63-70.
61. Dantzer R, Kelley KW. Twenty years of research on cytokine-induced sickness behavior. Brain Behav Immun. 2007; 21(2):153-60.
62. Morley S, Davies C, Barton S. Possible selves in chronic pain: self-pain enmeshment, adjustment and acceptance. Pain. 2005;115(1):84-94.

63. Pfingsten M, Hildebrandt J, Leibing E, et al. Effectiveness of a multimodal treatment program for chronic low-back pain. Pain. 1997;73(1):77-85.
64. Stanos S, Houle TT. Multidisciplinary and interdisciplinary management of chronic pain. Phys Med Rehabil Clin N Am. 2006;17(2):435.
65. Molton IR, Graham C, Stoelb BL, et al. Current psychological approaches to the management of chronic pain. Curr Opin Anesthe. 2007;20(5):485.
66. Integration of behavioral and relaxation approaches into the treatment of chronic pain and insomnia. NIH Technology Assessment Panel on Integration of Behavioral and Relaxation Approaches into the Treatment of Chronic Pain and Insomnia. JAMA. 1996;276(4):313-8.
67. Diesfeld K. Interpersonal issues between pain physician and patient: Strategies to reduce conflict. Pain Med. 2008; 9(8):1118-24.

CHAPTER

26 A Conservative Care Approach to the Rehabilitation of Patients with Spine Pain

Angela Lis, Sherri Weiser

INTRODUCTION

Within the past 10 years the global burden of spine pain (SP), as estimated by the World Health Organization, has increased significantly. It has gone from the 115th to the highest ranking condition contributing to years of life living with a disability, making it a world-wide health priority.[1] It is now understood that although most patients with SP recover, recurrences are observed in about 30% of patients who seek care for their pain. It is not known how many people experience SP and do not seek care. However, it is estimated that in North America today, there are about 10 million people living with SP.[1,2] A great majority of individuals with SP are not candidates for surgery and will do poorly if subjected to invasive treatments.[3,4] Most patients suffer from nonspecific SP for which there is no certain cause.[5,6] If pain is prolonged, it can lead to physical, psychological, and social impairments.[7-10] For instance, over time the presence of pain can lead to abnormal dynamic muscle control, which has been found to generate cortical changes in patients with SP.[11,12] In addition, stress hormones that accompany painful conditions have been found to enhance pain transmission.[13] Psychologically, patients with long-term pain often express anxiety about their future and suffer depression from feelings of helplessness and hopelessness. Many develop a fear of movement that restricts social activities including work.[14] The biopsychosocial model of pain and disability proposed by Waddell et al.[15] explains the interactions of the biological, psychological, and social dimensions of pain. For example, catastrophic expectations about pain may lead to fear of movement and avoidance behaviors resulting in changes in muscle patterns. This ultimately leads to muscular atrophy, which is associated with increased pain. Eventually, the individual withdraws from activities and becomes isolated and depressed, making recovery even more unlikely. This model tells us that prolonged back pain is complex and requires multidimensional solutions. Successful interventions require an understanding of the potential impact of all dimensions on the outcome of SP. A flag system has been developed to help identify predictors of poor outcome in different dimensions that may need to be addressed during treatment.[10,16-18] They are as follows:

- Red flags: Biomedical signs and symptoms that indicate a serious spinal pathology and require immediate referral. This includes signs of cauda equina syndrome such as bladder or bowel incontinence, progressive neurological deficit such as drop foot, or worsening of the pain and pain that does not improve with rest.
- Orange flags: Major untreated psychiatric conditions, such as psychosis, mood disorders, and drug or alcohol dependency.
- Yellow flags: Modifiable psychological factors related to SP such as negative outcome expectations, distress, and activity restriction.
- Blue flags: Perceptions of social or work factors such as work stress, low job satisfaction, and poor work/social support.
- Black flags: Economic or socio-organizational contextual factors such workplace or insurance policies and procedures that delay timely treatment or work reintegration and health care systems obstacles.

Ideally, all these factors should be considered. However, patients with complex SP usually receive unimodel treatment to reduce symptoms and improve function. Over the years, empirical studies and systematic reviews of the treatment effectiveness of various conservative interventions for SP have increased exponentially. Unimodel treatments including nonsteroidal anti-inflammatory drugs, exercise, manipulation, acupuncture, and cognitive-behavioral therapy have all been shown to be moderately effective at best in alleviating pain and disability and only in the short term.[17,19,20] There is evidence that multimodel interventions that include exercise programs and psychological treatments are superior to unimodel treatments for patients with prolonged pain.[19-21] However, none of these treatments has been consistently shown to be effective enough in randomized controlled trials to be considered a gold standard treatment.

Is another type of treatment needed to produce better outcomes? Probably not. Instead, we believe that what is needed is the right treatment, for the right patient, at the right time, achieved by triaging for treatment. This approach is implicit in evidence-based guidelines that warn against over treating in the acute stage of SP and encourage multimodal care in later stages.[5,17,18,20,22] However, these guidelines are general and do not take into consideration the specific needs of individual patients. Certainly, there are patients in the acute stage who would benefit from the attention paid to their anxiety about pain that is addressed in the multimodal approach, just as there are patients with chronic SP who need only physical therapy (PT) to reach their functional goals. In addition, guidelines are based on existing empirical findings and do not include information on treatments that have not been well studied, but may be very effective. Therefore, they are never a substitute for clinical judgment. Successful triage requires clinical experience and an appreciation for the complex nature of SP. It is our belief that patients at any stage of SP should be triaged by health care professionals trained to understand the contribution of physical, psychological, and social influences on the patient's pain and disability. In this chapter, we highlight key factors that require consideration when treating patients with SP.

Evidence-based treatment recommendations rooted in the biopsychosocial perspective tell us much about common characteristics of all successful treatment protocols. Most important among these is that a treatment should be responsive to the needs of the patient. It has been shown that active PT, in general, results in much better outcomes than passive care. However, there are numerous active approaches to PT including McKenzie, core stability exercises, and programs based on patient's directional preference. No particular treatment has been shown to be superior to the others.[23] However, the patient's expectation that a treatment will work does predict success.[24,25] This means that the specific type of active treatment is less important than providing a treatment that the patient agrees with or prefers. It also means that if a patient enjoys passive treatments they can be used as an adjunct to an active approach as a mediator of movement but should not be use as substitute for it. Also, implied in a biopsychosocial approach is an emphasis on function rather than on pain. We know that for most patients with chronic problems, pain may improve with treatment, but rarely abates completely. Previous SP, even if acute, is a strong predictor of future episodes, so it is common for those who have experienced back pain to have a recurrence.[26,27] Therefore, a focus on pain can lead to false outcome expectations, disappointments, perceived treatment failures, and ongoing doctor shopping, which reinforces the sick role. A preoccupation with eliminating pain can also lead to unnecessary medical procedures and overuse of medication, which "medicalizes" a more complex problem. A biopsychosocial perspective tells us that pain reduction, although desirable, is not the best indicator of outcome. It is more advantageous to overall well-being to focus on function and returning patients to their former activities that many times includes work.[28,29] Here, the emphases is on learning how to cope better with pain, making pain less bothersome, and alleviating pain-related anxiety and depression by bolstering a sense of control over the pain. Since it is shown that many individuals function quite well with pain, the focus on coping skills seems prudent for patients with SP.[30]

As we have said, best clinical decisions are a function of the clinical state and circumstances of the patient, a good understanding of evidence-based treatments, and a consideration of the needs and preferences of the patient[31] (Fig. 26.1). With this in mind we present our approach to triaging patients with SP for rehabilitation. The purpose of triage is to maximize treatment benefits and minimize costs and suffering to the patient and society.[17,18,20,30] To this end, evidence-based care is a good place to start. By definition, an evidence-based treatment has been proven superior to other treatments. For the majority of patients, evidence-based treatment will have the desired effect. The limitations of relying solely on research evidence

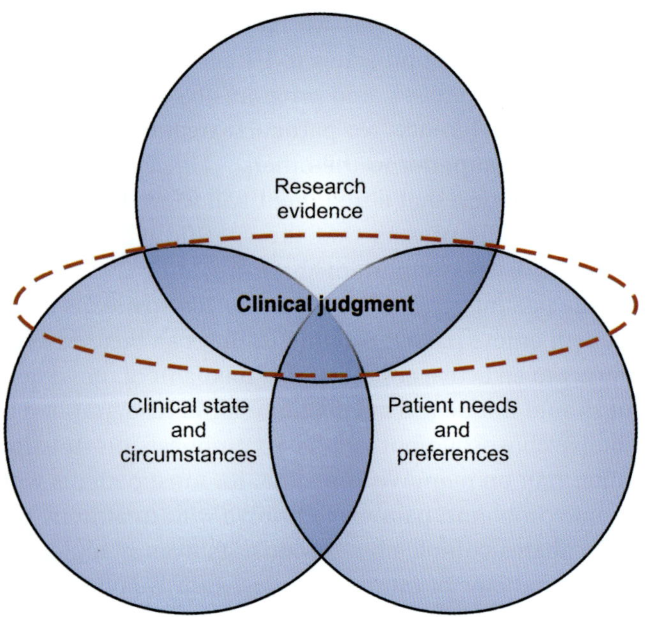

Fig. 26.1: Evidence-based clinical decision model.[31]

to determine treatment has been described earlier. The following triage criteria are, therefore, guideline based and patient preference informed. For SP, where serious medical conditions (red flags) have been ruled out, the first triage criterion is duration of pain.

TRIAGE CRITERION 1: DURATION OF SP

The vast majority of patients with SP get better with no treatment whatsoever in the acute phase (first 4 weeks). This estimate may be extended to up to 6 weeks for patients with sciatica.[32,33] Approximately, 25–30% of patients recover in 1 week, and 60% of patients recover in 7 weeks.[34,35] Therefore, as a rule, do not treat most patients with SP in the acute stage. Instead, self-care such as maintaining activity as tolerated, the application of heat and cold and over-the-counter (OTC) pain relievers should be advised along with strong reassurance about a good outcome to discourage negative thinking. Taking individual differences into account here are some exceptions to the rule:

- Patients with very high pain levels, such that the patient reports unrelenting and intolerable suffering or the pain prevents almost all movement, should be referred to their treating physicians to rule out red flags and provide pain management that may include a short course of opioids.
- In cases of radiating or severe pain when red flags have been ruled out, patients may benefit from a short course of manual therapy.
- Patients who seek PT in the acute phase, who are very physically active, may benefit from instruction on how to maintain current activity levels without exacerbating pain.
- Patients who seek PT in the acute phase and indicate a strong preference for starting therapy, even after they have been reassured, may benefit from a gentle introduction to active PT after 2–3 weeks of pain.
- Patients with recurrent back pain may benefit from an earlier onset of PT.

Patients who have had SP for 4 weeks or longer are good candidates for active PT and should be triaged based on the second criterion.

TRIAGE CRITERION 2: THE PRESENCE OF YELLOW FLAGS

Yellow flags are psychological predictors of poor outcome.[16,28] They include negative beliefs about pain, negative affectivity in response to pain, and pain and avoidance behaviors. Yellow flags are considered maladaptive responses to pain and as such are believed to be modifiable through cognitive-behavioral techniques. Numerous instruments have been developed to assess yellow flags. However, most are cumbersome and not easily administered and interpreted in a clinical setting. Recently, investigators from Keele University in the United Kingdom developed a brief and easily scored instrument called the STarT Back Screening Tool, which includes five of the strongest and consistent yellow flags for SP outcomes.[36–38] These are fear of activity, catastrophizing, pain-related depression, pain-related anxiety, and bothersomeness of pain. An endorsement of at least four of these items has been shown to predict poor outcome in patients with early SP. The STarT Back Screening Tool can be obtained at the following website: http://www.keele.ac.uk/sbst/. Patients who are not at risk for poor outcome should require only evidence-based, active goal oriented PT. It should be noted that some distress is normal in patients with pain and should only be considered a yellow flag if it persists after reassurance of a good outcome by the healthcare provider. Distress in most patients will dissipate after a couple weeks of active PT. Although triage is based on yellow flags, it is helpful screen for other flags and understands their impact on recovery since their presence may require coordinated care.[10,16]

Orange, Blue and Black Flags

It is important to distinguish yellow flags from other possible risk factors of delayed recovery. Some patients may suffer from serious psychiatric conditions, referred to as orange flags. Patients with untreated mood disorders, psychosis, or drug or alcohol dependency may not respond well to treatment. If you suspect that serious psychiatric problems are interfering with treatment, the patient should be referred back to their primary physician to address this issue.

Although there may be little a PT can do to modify the patient's social and work circumstances (blue flags) or economic and organization problems (black flags), understanding potential obstacles posed by these flags can help the PT communicate with the patient about why they may not be getting well and can also be useful in goal setting. For instance, if a patient has a spouse who is encouraging passive care, the PT may suggest that the spouse participate in the patient's education about SP. Similarly, if the patient's insurance will not cover the recommended number of sessions, the PT can introduce a home program earlier for the patient so that the patient can continue with self-care after the end of treatment. In cases where patients are returning to work with residual pain, the healthcare provider may sometimes have the opportunity to speak with a work case manager or supervisor at the patient's workplace and explain any needed modifications so that the patient returns to a more supportive environment.

Patients at risk for poor outcome based on yellow flags require individualized attention and education to modify these beliefs. Hill et al.[36] showed that treatment aimed at yellow flags in this group of patients resulted in better outcomes than PT alone. This treatment can be administered in two ways; by therapists trained in psychologically informed PT or by a psychotherapist trained in cognitive-behavioral pain management (CBPM).

Psychologically Informed PT

Physical therapists who practice psychologically informed PT use evidence-based, active goal-oriented PT while considering the needs of the patient based on demonstrated yellow flags.[28,30,39] To address maladaptive psychological responses to pain, they use cognitive-behavioral principles. This approach modifies false or negative beliefs about pain and replaces them with accurate or more neutral beliefs, thereby reducing related distress. In addition, it incorporates behavioral techniques whereby healthy behaviors are reinforced and illness behaviors are de-emphasized. To achieve this, the physical therapist educates based on the evidence, demonstrates using a behavioral approach, and negotiates to address contextual barriers to recovery. This approach can be very effective in alleviating important yellow flags such as negative affect, negative outcome expectations, and the degree to which a patient allows pain to interfere with daily activities. Education should be rooted in scientific evidence and include direct and clear messages such as:

- The prognosis is good. Most people with SP will get better
- Pain does not mean damage. As time progresses the relationship between pain and physical findings for most patients with SP diminishes, and there is no need to fear further damage
- Normal activity is good for recovery and should not be avoided. It reduces stiffness, increases oxygen and blood flow, and increases feelings of control over pain.
- Modalities and OTCs pain relievers are fine for short-term pain control, but they should not be relied upon for long-term recovery. Instead, a proactive approach to pain reduction that involves progressive increase of activity and avoidance of negative thinking is recommended
- Mind-body techniques such as simple relaxation exercises help increase a sense of coping and reduce pain and discomfort
- Recurrences can be addressed using self-care techniques as described earlier (*see* section Triage criterion 1: duration of spine pain) before seeking care.

Once the patient is educated, a behavioral approach to treatment reinforces what they have been told by demonstrating what they are capable of achieving. A behavioral approach retrains the cortical response to motion that has been altered by the presence of pain by focusing on function rather than on pain. A behavioral approach also emphasizes goal setting as central to recovery. Functional goals should be set up and agreed upon with the patient the day of the evaluation or very soon thereafter. It is advisable to make sure that these goals are realistic to avoid setting the patient up for failure.

Patients who are unable to set goals either because they cannot foresee improvement or because it is not their priority to get better, will not do well unless the physical therapist addresses this early on and makes the patient aware that this may impede progress. A behavioral approach is implemented through the following steps:

- Developing patient-based functional goals that are congruent with the activities the patient hopes and/or needs to pursue to achieve a high quality of life and return to their daily life activities including work
- Using a graded-activity approach starting with small daily achievable goals and larger weekly goals
- Using an exposure approach that specifically targets behaviors that the patient is most anxious to execute in the same manner as above
- Providing oral and written feedback by showing the patient how they have progressed, for example, pounds lifted, or distance walking
- Setting time limits to reinforce the expectation that these goals are realistic and can be met in a reasonable amount of time (usually within 4–6 weeks)
- Incorporating relaxed breathing and a de-emphasis on pain into the exercises.

Sometimes a negotiation with the patient is required for the patients to reach their goals. For instance, a patient may have a preference for a treatment that is not supported in evidence-based guidelines, such as moist heat. To facilitate treatment in this case, the patient could start active treatment in conjunction with the moist heat and use a hot pack while walking on the treadmill. As the patient begins to improve as a result of increased activity, the reliance on heat can be progressively decreased. Alternately if the patient is willing, he or she can be asked to avoid modalities during the first couple of weeks of PT, to give the active approach a chance. Negotiation requires the health care provider to respond to the patient's beliefs and needs and conveys a message of partnership to the patient.

Cognitive-Behavioral Pain Management

Sometimes patients with yellow flags will not improve with psychologically informed PT alone. These patients may benefit from a referral to CBPM in conjunction with PT.[40] CBPM should be administered by a trained psychotherapist; optimally, one who can interact with the PT and provide feedback on a regular basis. The psychotherapist will do a comprehensive evaluation to rule out major psychiatric conditions (orange flags) that require treatment, to identify the patient's strengths and weakness and to identify yellow flags. The therapist will also be able to identify social and contextual barriers to recovery (blue and black flags) that the PT may not be aware of and that require problem solving. CBPM consists of education about the connection between the mind and the body and CBPM techniques that emphasize self-care, such as relaxation, visualization, mindfulness, cognitive restructuring and reinterpretation, and problem solving. This intervention is usually brief; techniques can be taught in four to eight sessions. The goal of treatment is to improve the patient's ability to cope with the pain and to support the functional goals delineated in PT.

If a patient has not made a steady functional progress after combined PT and CBPM, they should be re-evaluated to rule out recently developed red flags and triaged based on criterion 3.

TRIAGE CRITERION 3: IS THE PATIENT A CANDIDATE FOR AN INTENSIVE INTERDISCIPLINARY CONDITIONING PROGRAM?

Patients whose pain has not improved with the combined approach and have no red or orange flags should be sent back to the referring physician/spine specialist to discuss pain management options. In some cases, patients make progress with the combined approach (PT and CBPM) but are still unable to return to their job because of the extreme demands of the job and/or extreme physical deconditioning. These patients, if motivated to go back to work or enroll in vocation training, should be considered for an intensive interdisciplinary conditioning program when available. These programs usually have the goal of returning the patient to work and combine PT, CBPM, and education about SP in an intensive format consisting of several hours of daily treatment for up to 4 weeks.[41] It is crucial to the success of this type of program that the patient forms a partnership with the treating team to develop specific functional goals and timelines for treatment. The patient is treated by a team, including a physical therapist, a psychotherapist, and a physician specializing in rehabilitation, which meets weekly to discuss the patient's progress. This is important because each healthcare provider must give the same message to the patient about what to expect to avoid confusion and doubt on the part of the patient. This type of care is beneficial to patients who want to go back to work because the daily commitment gets them back into a regular routine, and work tasks are simulated to improve ability and self-confidence. Patients who do not improve after a couple of weeks should not continue in the program because the likelihood of success is small. Instead, they should be reassessed and if needed referred to pain management and reconsidered for the program once their pain is controlled.

Table 26.1: Key practice points

• Do not treat most patients in the acute phase of pain
• In the subacute/chronic phase or in cases of recurrent SP, assess for yellow flags
• If the patient has yellow flags, practice PIPT
• If PIPT is unsuccessful, refer to CBPM
• If the patient is having difficulty returning to work in the subacute/chronic phase or in cases of recurrent SP, assess for an intensive conditioning program
• Always refer in cases of red flags, untreated orange flags interfering with PT, severe and unremitting pain interfering with PT; patients who are not reaching agreed upon goals in the expected amount of time

(CBPM: Cognitive-behavioral pain management; PIPT: Psychologically informed physical therapy; PT: Physical therapy; SP: Spine pain).

The authors have used this triaging approach in their clinic with excellent results. Patients show a clinically meaningful decrease in perceived disability and pain from medium to low. In addition, 85% of patients who enrolled in our intensive interdisciplinary conditioning program returned to work, and of those, 75% were still working 1 year later.[41] This is despite the fact that the average time out of work was 8 months, which is well into the chronic phase and has been previously considered difficult to treat.[9,42]

CONCLUSION

Spine pain is complex and requires a biopsychosocial perspective. Patients should be triaged into treatments that have the highest likelihood of success. Empirical data and clinical experience indicate that patients who are triaged according to best clinical practice principles (Table 26.1) have the best outcomes.

REFERENCES

1. Hoy D, Bain C, Williams G, et al. A systematic review of the global prevalence of low back pain. Arthritis Rheum. 2012;64:2068.
2. Loney PL, Stratford PW. The prevalence of low back pain in adults: A methodological review of the literature. Phys Ther. 1999;79:384-96.
3. Deyo RA, Weinstein JN. Low back pain. N Engl J Med. 2001;344:363-70.
4. Carragee EJ, Deyo RA, Kovacs FM, et al. Clinical research: is the spine field a mine field? Spine (Phila Pa 1976). 2009;34:423-30.
5. van Tulder M, Becker A, Bekkering T, et al. European guidelines for the management of acute nonspecific low back pain in primary care. Eur Spine J. 2006;15(Suppl 2):S169.
6. van Tulder M, Koes B, Bombardier C. Low back pain. Best Pract Res Clin Rheumatol. 2002;16:761-75.
7. van Tulder M, Koes B. Chronic low back pain. Am Fam Physician. 2006;74:1577-9.
8. van Tulder M, Becker A, Bekkering T, et al. Chapter 3. European guidelines for the management of acute nonspecific low back pain in primary care. Eur Spine J. 2006;15(Suppl 2):S169-91.
9. Wessels T, van Tulder M, Sigl T, et al. What predicts outcome in non-operative treatments of chronic low back pain? A systematic review. Eur Spine J. 2006;15:1633-44.
10. Shaw WS, van der Windt DA, Main CJ, et al. Early patient screening and intervention to address individual-level occupational factors ("blue flags") in back disability. J Occup Rehabil. 2009;19:64-80.
11. Hodges P, Richardson C. Inefficient muscular stabilization of the lumbar spine associated with low back pain: a motor control evaluation of transversus abdominis. Spine. 1996; 21:2640.
12. Ferreira PH, Ferreira ML, Maher CG, et al. Changes in recruitment of transversus abdominis correlate with disability in people with chronic low back pain. Br J Sports Med. 2009; published online 26 May.
13. Sudhaus S, Möllenberg T, Plaas H, et al. Cortisol awakening response and pain-related fear-avoidance versus endurance in patients six months after lumbar disc surgery. Appl Psychophysiol Biofeedback. 2012;37:121.
14. Dawson A, Schluter P, Hodges P, et al. Fear of movement, passive coping, manual handling, and severe or radiating pain increase the likelihood of sick leave due to low back pain. Pain. 2011;152:1517.
15. Waddell G, Newton M, Henderson I. A fear-avoidance beliefs questionnaire (FABQ) and the role of fear avoidance beliefs in chronic low back pain and disability. Pain. 1993;52:157-68.
16. Nicholas M, Linton S, Watson P, et al. Early identification and management of psychological risk factors ("yellow flags") in patients with low back pain: a reappraisal. Phys Ther. 2011;91:737.
17. Chou R, Qaseem A, Snow V, et al. Diagnosis and treatment of low back pain: A joint clinical practice guideline from the American College of Physicians and the American Pain Society. Ann Intern Med. 2007;147:478.
18. Burton A, Balagué F, Cardon G, et al. European guidelines for prevention in low back pain. Eur Spine J. 2006;15 (Suppl 2):S136.
19. Keller A, Hayden J, Bombardier C, et al. Effect sizes of nonsurgical treatments of non-specific low-back pain. Eur Spine J. 2007;16:1776.
20. Chou R, Loeser JD, Owens DK. Interventional therapies, surgery and interdisciplinary rehabilitation for low back pain: an evidence-based clinical practice guideline from the American Pain Society. Spine. 2009;34:1066.
21. Lamb S, Hansen Z, Lall R, et al. Group cognitive behavioural treatment for low-back pain in primary care: a randomised controlled trial and cost-effectiveness analysis. Lancet. 2010;375:916.

22. Waddell G, Burton AK. Occupational health guidelines for the management of low back pain at work: evidence review. Occup Med (Lond). 2001;51:124-35.
23. Hayden J, van Tulder M, Malmivaara A, et al. Meta-analysis: exercise therapy for nonspecific low back pain. Ann Intern Med. 2005;142:765.
24. Mondloch MV, Cole DC, Frank JW. Does how you do depend on how you think you'll do? A systematic review of the evidence for a relation between patients' recovery expectations and health outcomes. CMAJ 2001;165:174-9. (Erratum in CMAJ 2001 Nov 13;165(10):1303.)
25. Kalauokalani D, Cherkin DC, Sherman KJ, et al. Lessons from a trial of acupuncture and massage for low back pain: patient expectations and treatment effects. Spine. 2001;26:1418-24.
26. Delitto A, George SZ, Van Dillen LR, et al. Low back pain. J Orthop Sports Phys Ther. 2012;42:A1-57.
27. Donelson R, McIntosh G, Hall H. Is it time to rethink the typical course of low back pain? PMR. 2012;4:394-401; quiz 400.
28. Nicholas, M, George, S. Psychologically informed interventions for low back pain: an update for physical therapists. Phys Ther. 2011;91:765.
29. George S, Robinson M. Preference, expectation, and satisfaction in a clinical trial of behavioral interventions for acute and sub-acute low back pain. J Pain. 2010;11:1074.
30. Main C, Foster N, Buchbinder R. How important are back beliefs and expectations for satisfactory recovery from back pain? Best Pract Clin Rheum. 2010;24:205.
31. Haynes B, Devereaux PJ, Guyatt G. Physicians' and patients' choices in evidence based practice: evidence does not make decisions, people do. BMJ. 2002;324:1350.
32. Frymoyer JW. Back pain and sciatica. N Engl J Med. 1988;318:291-300.
33. van Tulder MW, Koes B, Seitsalo S, et al. Outcome of invasive treatment modalities on back pain and sciatica: an evidence-based review. Eur Spine J. 2006;15 (Suppl 1): S82-92.
34. Cherkin D, Deyo R, Street J, et al. Predicting poor outcomes for back pain seen in primary care using patients' own criteria. Spine. 1996;21:2900.
35. Coste J, Delecoeuillerie G, Cohen de Lara A, et al. Clinical course and prognostic factors in acute low back pain: an inception cohort study in primary care practice. BMJ. 1994;308:577.
36. Hill J, Whitehurst D, Lewis M, et al. Comparison of stratified primary care management for low back pain with current best practice (STarT back): a randomised controlled trial. Lancet. 2011;378:1560.
37. Hill J, Dunn K, Main C, et al. Subgrouping low back pain: a comparison of the STarT back tool with the örebro musculoskeletal pain screening questionnaire. Eur J Pain. 2010;14:83.
38. Hay E, Dunn K, Hill J, et al. A randomised clinical trial of subgrouping and targeted treatment for low back pain compared with best current care. the STarT back trial study protocol. BMC Musculoskelet Disord. 2008;9.
39. Foster N, Delitto A. Embedding psychosocial perspectives within clinical management of low back pain: integration of psychosocially informed management principles into physical therapist practice—challenges and opportunities. Phys Ther. 2011;91:790.
40. van Middelkoop M, Rubinstein S, Kuijpers T, et al. A systematic review on the effectiveness of physical and rehabilitation interventions for chronic non-specific low back pain. Eur Spine J. 2011;20:19.
41. Campello MA, Weiser SR, Nordin M, et al. Work retention and nonspecific low back pain. Spine. 2006;31:1850.
42. Spitzer W, LeBlanc F, Dupuis M, et al. Scientific approach to the assessment and management of activity-related spinal disorders: a monograph for clinicians. Report of the Quebec Task Force on spinal disorders. Spine. 1987; 12:S1.

SECTION

3

Spinal Injection

CHAPTER

27

Introduction to Spinal Injections

Jamie R Terran, Rachel N Rattenni, Faruk Razzak, Gerard P Varlotta

INTRODUCTION

Injections have increasingly been utilized in the management of spinal pain. Injections are also useful in diagnosing the cause/s of such pain. Although back pain is a very common ailment—with lower back pain in particular being the leading cause of disability in those less than 45 years old—alleviating it is still quite challenging, as nearly identical symptoms may be caused by varying etiologies. Although injections generally cannot cure the underlying physiological causes of back pain, they can successfully reduce inflammation and pain when used appropriately.[1] The relief in pain may allow a patient to pursue adjunctive therapies, such as physical therapy, with less discomfort and a higher chance of compliance. In addition, for those with early or mild disease, elderly in age, or other contraindications to surgery, injections offer a less invasive treatment option that allows the patient to remain active. Physicians may also use injections of local anesthetics as a diagnostic tool, selectively anesthetizing nerves and/or tissues suspected to be generators of back pain, with relief for the known duration of anesthetic efficacy with return of pain thereafter indicating a successful identification.[2]

HISTORY

The effects of local anesthetics were first recorded in 1884 by the Austrian physician and colleague of Sigmund Freud, Carl Koller, who detailed the numbing effects of cocaine when placed on the tongue.[3] As a result of Koller's discovery, cocaine was widely used as a local anesthetic for a multitude of surgical and nonsurgical invasive procedures by 1885. In 1899, an injected cocaine solution was successfully used to alleviate pain caused by a leg sarcoma, marking the first therapeutic nerve block.[3] Shortly after, Von Gaza used the local anesthetic procaine diagnostically to identify the source of pain as either sympathetic or sensory. Building off of Von Gaza's work, in 1938 Steindler and Luck developed additional diagnostic techniques and highlighted the need for established criteria in determining causal relationships between symptoms and actual nerve compression; they thought this would help increase the accuracy of diagnostic injections. The principles underlying early spine injections still remain in practice among physicians treating pain today.

TRIGGER POINT INJECTIONS

Trigger points are hyperirritable loci of muscle tissue found within taut bands in muscles or fascia that often lead to referred pain in other surrounding areas or structures.[4] The exact factors contributing to the development of trigger points is unknown, but it is presumed that stress, overworking of muscles, and injury are all factors in their formation. Trigger point injections are used to treat patients with myofascial pain symptoms occurring as a result of the hyperirritable loci. While trigger points may occur in patients with osteoarthritis, fibromyalgia, and connective tissue disorders, trigger point injections should not be used on patients with pain due to osteoarthritis or radicular pathology.[4]

The mechanism by which trigger points cause pain is uncertain, but likely stems from inflammation. Increased release of acetylcholine, bradykinin, prostaglandin, serotonin, and substance P—often found in trigger points—can incite an inflammatory response in nearby tissues, causing referred pain.[5] Trigger point injections aim to deactivate trigger points through either mechanical or chemical damage, commonly employing either an injection of 0.5–2 mL of a local anesthetic, botulinum toxin or saline solution, or dry needling. A recent randomized control trial involving trigger point treatment in the upper trapezius muscle with 2 mL of a 1% lidocaine solution versus dry needling revealed significant efficacy for both interventions, with no increased benefit of the lidocaine solution over dry needling.[5] Another study testing only elderly patients had the similar results, with no statistically significant difference between dry needling and 0.5% lidocaine injection.[6]

An earlier meta-analysis of trigger point injections for chronic low back pain found local anesthetic, dry needling, and botulinum toxin injections to be equally as effective in producing statistically significant decreases in pain; all three injection types were also found to be more effective than saline injection. Botulinum toxin is significantly more expensive than dry needling and local anesthetics, but it shows no marked benefit, so its use is not recommended for trigger points. The authors note that these results are questionable, as most saline injections on the market contain 0.9% of the preservative benzyl alcohol, which has local anesthetic properties of its own.[4]

Although the results of studies on trigger point injections have been seemingly contradictory, there are several conclusions that can be recognized in most trials. It is advised that trigger point injections be used only after the failure of several noninvasive techniques, such as physical therapy or the "spray and stretch" technique, to alleviate pain.[4,5] Clinical judgment may be used in cases where acute trigger point pain restricts participation in therapy, perhaps calling for an initial injection. All studies also concluded that an injection was more likely to be effective if a twitch response was generated upon injection. Ultimately, most trigger point injection therapies can offer at least short-term relief of myofascial pain.

SACROILIAC INJECTIONS

The sacroiliac joint (SIJ) has been shown to be the source of approximately 30% of complaints involving chronic low back and buttock pain.[7] However, treatment of SIJ pain has been difficult due, in part, to a lack of any "gold standard" diagnostic test identifying SIJ disease.[8] The most common diagnostic test involves fluoroscopically guided injection of a local anesthetic, but the level of pain improvement required for the test to be considered positive has not been agreed upon.[8] Typically, the treatment of SIJ pain after a positive diagnosis has been corticosteroid injection, although alternative methods are being tested.

A 2006 study aimed to conclude whether or not multiple corticosteroid injections would be more beneficial than a single injection in patients with SIJ spondyloarthropathies. All 31 study participants had persistent and poorly controlled inflammatory back pain. After a single magnetic resonance imaging (MRI) guided injection, patients who did not report marked improvement were given a second injection. Improvement for those who received one injection lasted for about 8.7 months, with a mean visual analog scale (VAS) score of 4.1, whereas the improvement for those who received two injections lasted for 16.1 months, with a mean VAS of 3.5. Thus, there were statistically significant benefits of receiving two injections, with a second injection increasing the likelihood of successful treatment.[9]

Another method of treating SIJ pain is prolotherapy. Prolotherapy injections combine the sugar dextrose with a local anesthetic, a mixture that is believed to initiate dense fibrous tissue formation around the SIJs, thus stabilizing and strengthening fascial structures at their fibro-osseus junctions. The strengthening process is thought to potentially help in the long-term treatment of SIJ pain.[7] Although prolotherapy sounds promising, most experimental evidence has been inconclusive. One study found a clear benefit of prolotherapy over corticosteroid treatment for the SIJ pain. In the double-blind study, patients were diagnosed with SIJ pain after having a 50% decrease in pain symptoms after diagnostic levobupivacaine injection. Patients with positive diagnoses of SIJ pain were then divided and received fluoroscopically guided injections of prolotherapeutic agents (dextrose solution with 0.25% levobupivacaine) or corticosteroids (triamcinolone acetonide in 0.125% levobupivacaine). Although initial 2-week results were identical for pain reduction, a 15-month follow-up favored prolotherapy over steroid injections, with 58.7% of prolotherapy patients sustaining a 50% pain reduction. Comparatively, only 10.2% of steroid patients sustained the same reduction after 15 months. The authors of the study suggested that diagnostic injections to identify appropriate subjects were not utilized in previous tests, with their use in their trial likely contributing to the promising results.[7]

It is not possible to definitively conclude whether prolotherapy is a more efficacious treatment for SIJ pain over steroids, as this has not been repeatedly tested. However, it is clear that both methods offer at least short-term relief.

PERIPHERAL JOINT INJECTIONS

The use of therapeutic peripheral joint injections in patients without inflammatory arthropathies is controversial. Several studies have produced conflicting results as to whether corticosteroids or local anesthetics are more effective in treating peripheral joint pain.[10]

Hyaluronic acid is a naturally occurring component of synovial fluid that has been found at abnormally low levels in the joint spaces of patients with osteoarthritis. Viscosupplementation, which involves the injection of hyaluronic acid, has been shown in a recent meta-analysis to be especially effective for the long-term treatment of patients with osteoarthritis of the knee.[10] More research on viscosupplementation needs to be conducted to assess whether it can eventually be applied to other forms of osteoarthritis.

In the treatment of hip osteoarthritis, local anesthetic and viscosupplementation have not shown to be effective in the very limited research that has been conducted, whereas steroids have been shown to provide short-term relief.

In the upper extremities, corticosteroids can successfully alleviate pain from elbow-lateral epicondylitis in the short-term relief. Although other methods for treating elbow-lateral epicondylitis have shown to have longer lasting effects, the combination of a steroid and local anesthetic provides faster relief for people such as professional athletes who are looking for a quick return to high intensity activity. Use of the peppering injection technique of a steroid and local anesthetic has been statistically favored over other injection methods.[10]

SYMPATHETIC NERVE BLOCKS

The first recorded use of a sympathetic nerve block (SNB) was in 1916 by the French surgeon René Leriche. Leriche used a surgical paravascular sympathetic denervation to treat a soldier with a brachial plexus injury. Leriche was looking for a cure to the soldier's injury, but instead alleviated his pain. Leriche was one of the first physicians to link pain to the sympathetic nervous system.[2]

With the link between pain and the sympathetic nervous system established, SNBs were used as a diagnostic tool for reflex sympathetic dystrophy. However, the diagnostic value of SNBs has since been questioned and is not entirely supported throughout the literature. It was previously believed that an SNB of nerves surrounding particular vertebra could lead to the definitive diagnosis of sympathetically mediated pain. However, choosing which paravertebral location to perform a block on is of utmost importance, as blocking levels unrelated to symptoms can lead to a high incidence of false negative outcomes.[2]

Although SNBs can indicate that pain is somewhat maintained in the sympathetic nervous system, they cannot provide any further etiologic conclusions as once previously thought. The efficacy of SNBs in treating complex regional pain syndromes is about 60%, but it has been shown to decrease with continued use 6 months after diagnosis. SNBs are also different from the previously mentioned spinal injections, in that saline and dry needling techniques have been ineffective beyond a few hours of relief compared with local anesthetics.[2]

The SNBs have also been tested for the treatment of "failed back surgery syndrome", and associated chronic low back pain, with poor results. A study using lidocaine injection followed by bupivacaine versus saline injections twice daily for 4 days produced no significant relief of pain in either group as recorded by VAS and straight leg raises.[11]

EPIDURAL INJECTIONS

The first reported epidural injection took place in 1901 and involved a cocaine solution to treat sciatica.[1] Later, physicians administered procaine, novocaine, and metycaine to patients with sciatica. The injections were often administered in doses exceeding 100 mL of the local anesthetic solution, with the hypothesis being that large volumes of liquid would break adhesions and displace affected nerve roots from herniated disks; the results were mixed. Several patients were declared "cured", yet there were significant adverse effects of such large volumes of injectate. Later, in 1952 Lievre et al. performed the first series of epidural corticosteroid (hydrocortisone) injections in a study of 46 patients with chronic and acute lower back pain. The study of Lievre et al. had decent results: 15 patients had a good response and 8 patients had a mediocre response.[1] Since these early studies, the medications used, the techniques employed, physician skill, and the selectivity of epidural injections have vastly improved.

Epidural steroid injections are designed to treat radicular back pain caused by inflammation. Although a significant amount of empirical evidence suggests that steroid injections are not more beneficial than local anesthetics or other types of injections, it is important to consider that steroids directly address the inflammatory process. Steroid injections are generally intended for the short-term relief of pain; effects start 1 week after the first injection, and relief should last approximately 2 months. A meta-analysis reviewing only studies considering epidural steroid efficacy during the 1-week postinjection to 60-day period found short-term effectiveness to be 75%. Therefore, epidural steroids are clinically beneficial in treating inflammation-mediated back pain in the short-term relief of pain, but they have little evidence supporting their ability to provide long-term relief.[1]

INTRA-ARTICULAR FACET INJECTIONS

Intra-articular facet joint injections are used primarily for diagnosis of facet joint pain, as clinical trials have failed to find any evidence of a therapeutic value or of short- and long-term pain relief in the lumbar spin.[12,13] Computed tomography (CT) and MRI guided local anesthetic injections that include radiopaque contrast dye have proved to be the most effective means of diagnosing facet joint pain.[14] By including a contrast dye into the injectate, clinicians can be sure that only the target structure or nerve has been treated. Other methods, such as unguided injections, have significantly higher false-positive rates and low predictive values.

Guided facet joint injections are also significantly more accurate than CT and MRI imaging findings alone in correctly diagnosing the source of back pain.[12] CT and MRI images alone have been shown to correctly identify the source of chronic back pain in only 15% of patients.

MEDIAN BRANCH BLOCKS AND RHIZOTOMY

Rhizotomy offers an alternative to classic injection therapies in the treatment of chronic back pain. Rhizotomy involves destroying the nerve believed to be causing pain or supplying the area with pain; this destruction thus alleviates symptoms for the patient. Initially, a median branch block is often used to diagnose the source of back pain before rhizotomy. While rhizotomy has shown positive results in the short-term pain relief, the nerve generally grows back in 1 to 2 years, most commonly with a re-emergence of pain.[15,16] Thus, rhizotomy has not been proven as an effective long-term treatment.

A study assessing the efficacy of dorsal ramus medial branch rhizotomy attained by pulsed radiofrequency identified 92 facet joint syndrome patients for inclusion after diagnostic blocks determined the cause of their pain.[15] Only those patients reporting at least a 60% decrease in pain, after the diagnostic anesthetic injection, were offered the procedure. After rhizotomy, patients were assessed at 1, 6, and 12 months, with the intervention only considered successful if pain improved by at least 80%. All patients who underwent complete denervation (confirmed by electromyography) showed successful results to rhizotomy. The excellent results of this study were attributed to strict inclusion criteria and the assessment of denervation by electromyography.[15]

INTRADISCAL ELECTROTHERMAL THERAPY, NUCLEOPLASTY, AND BIACUPLASTY

Intradiscal electrothermal therapy (IDET) procedures are used to treat disk-related chronic low back pain.[17] IDET consists of introducing an intradiscal catheter, with a temperature controlled thermal resistive heating coil, into the inner posterior annulus. This is followed by heating the tip to 90°C over 12.5 minutes and then sustaining the highest temperature for 4 minutes.[17] Although initial trials by the creators of IDET showed promising results, no benefit of IDET over a placebo treatment in 11 subsequent studies was found. The evidence in favor of IDET is inconclusive. In addition, the high cost of IDET—about $8000 per affected disk—makes it an unattainable treatment option for many.[17]

Nucleoplasty is a type of injection therapy designed to treat chronic low back pain caused by herniated disks. Nucleoplasty consists of tissue ablation followed by coagulation. During the ablation phase, injected saline solution and electrodes form a plasma field between the electrodes and tissue, disintegrating the disk nucleus. During coagulation, wand movement leads to thermal coagulation and subsequent collagen shrinkage. The combination of tissue ablation and collagen shrinkage is believed to relieve some of the pressure within the disk, reducing pressure on the compressed nerve.[18]

Nucleoplasty has shown positive results in clinical trials. A 2008 study found 58% of patients reporting a more than 50% decrease in pain symptoms at a 1-year follow-up, whereas a similar study in 2007 found 62% of patients also having pain reduction after 1 year.[18,19]

Intradiscal biacuplasty (IBD) is another nonsurgical treatment for chronic discogenic low back pain. Biacuplasty involves placing two cooled bipolar electrodes in affected disks to lesion the nociceptive fibers of the annulus fibrosus.[20] In one randomized controlled trial, 64 subjects were assigned to either treatment or placebo groups and were tested at 1, 3, and 6 months after treatment. At 6 months, the IBD group exhibited statistically significant improvements in pain, functioning, and disability over the placebo group. Both groups, however, had statistically significant decreases in opioid usage, with no significant difference between the two.[20]

While there has been modest support for the treatment of chronic discogenic low back pain by IDET, nucleoplasty, and biacuplasty, support for the latter two treatments has been the strongest. In addition, nucleoplasty and biacuplasty are significantly easier to administer than the IDET, making them relatively more practical treatment options.

SPINAL CORD STIMULATORS

Although spinal cord stimulation is often successfully used to treat radicular back pain, its application in treating axial low back pain has not been frequently evaluated. However, the few trials testing the use of spinal cord stimulation for chronic low back pain and failed back surgery syndrome have shown promise.[21] One retrospective study, by Van Buyten et al., of 17 patients with failed back surgery syndrome showed statistically significant improvements in back and leg pain for all participants. Another retrospective study, by Ohmeiss and Rashbaum, of 41 patients found 60% of patients improved, whereas 75% of patients would undergo the procedure again for the same result. One prospective study, by Barolat et al., found 68.8% relief in back pain 1 year after treatment, whereas leg pain was relieved by 88.2% during the same time period.[21] While there may not be enough evidence to definitively say whether or not spinal cord stimulation is a valid treatment option for axial low back pain, it has shown to be over 50% effective in alleviating pain symptoms thus far.

COMPLICATIONS AND RISKS

Although injections are not recommended for patients with local infections or who are on antiplatelet or anticoagulant medications, they have been found to be generally safe for healthy patients.[22] A recent meta-analysis revealed the overall complication rate for spinal injections to be 0.8–6%, with cervical injections having the highest risk.[22] In addition, the rate of complications decreases with increasing utilization of high-quality imaging during injection. The most common side effects of injections are mild and short lasting, including headache (typically a result of a dural puncture causing a leak of cerebrospinal fluid and thus intracranial hypotension), temporary pain near injection site, nausea, numbness, and weakness. More rare but very serious complications include epidural hematomas, abscess formation, and brain and/or spinal cord infarctions; even more rarely reported are temporary and permanent paralysis. In an anonymous survey of physicians who administer spinal injections, the 287 responders reported a total of 13 patient deaths from infarctions after injection.[22]

CONCLUSION

There are several nonsurgical treatment options for alleviating back pain that have been shown to be at least moderately effective, most often being injections. Although injections themselves usually do not cure the cause of back pain, they can alleviate its severity enough so that a patient may comfortably undergo a physical therapy program in hopes of attaining more long-term results.

However, when reviewing the results of nonsurgical treatment trials, there are two confounds to keep in mind when assessing the efficacy of any one treatment. First, there is no gold standard for assessing the presence or absence of pain. Unlike many medical maladies that can be definitively detected, pain must be self-reported by a patient and is thus subjective. Second, most studies do not have perfect placebo groups. For instance, dry needles were often treated as placebos in trigger point injection trials, but were later found to cause mechanical damage that may lead to pain alleviation, and thus are not true placebos. In trials that could have a true placebo, it is not ethical to have a placebo group if investigators are knowingly denying helpful treatment.

Any treatment regimen—including the injectable medications and procedures previously discussed—require sound clinical judgment to identify pain generators, performance of an appropriate workup, followed by the forming and administration of a high-quality multidisciplinary plan of care to ensure that patients have the best chance of improvement.

REFERENCES

1. Hession WG, Stanczak JD, Davis KW, et al. Epidural steroid injections. Semin Roentgenol. 2004;39(1):7-23.
2. Boas RA. Sympathetic nerve blocks: in search of a role. Regional Anesthe Pain Med. 1998;23(3):292-305.
3. Manchikanti L, Boswell MV, Raj PP, et al. Evolution of interventional pain management. Pain Physician 2003;6 (4):485-94.
4. Malanga G, Wolff E. Evidence-informed management of chronic low back pain with trigger point injections. Spine J. 2008;8(1):243-52.
5. Ay S, Evcik D, Tur B. Comparison of injection methods in myofascial pain syndrome: a randomized controlled trial. Clin Rheumatol. 2010;29(1):19-23.
6. Ga H, Choi J-H, Park C-H, et al. Acupuncture needling versus lidocaine injection of trigger points in myofascial pain syndrome in elderly patients—a randomised trial. Acupunct Med. 2007;25(4):130-6.
7. Kim WM, Lee HG, Jeong CW, et al. A randomized controlled trial of intra-articular prolotherapy versus steroid injection for sacroiliac joint pain. J Altern Complement Med (New York, NY) 2010;16(12):1285-90.
8. Colonno DV, Harrast MA, Herring SA. Overview of spinal interventions. Clin in Sports Med. 2012;31(3):409-22.
9. Günaydin I, Pereira PL, Fritz J, et al. Magnetic resonance imaging guided corticosteroid injection of sacroiliac joints in patients with spondyloarthropathy. Are multiple injections more beneficial? Rheumatol Int. 2006;26(5):396-400.
10. Peterson C, Hodler J. Evidence-based radiology (part 2): is there sufficient research to support the use of therapeutic injections into the peripheral joints? Skeletal Radiol. 2010;39(1):11-8.
11. Fredman B, Zohar E, Ben Nun M, et al. The effect of repeated epidural sympathetic nerve block on "failed back surgery syndrome" associated chronic low back pain. J Clin Anesth. 1999;11(1):46-51.
12. Peh W. Image-guided facet joint injection. Biomed Imaging Interv J. 2011;7(1):e4.
13. Boswell MV, Colson JD, Sehgal N, et al. A systematic review of therapeutic facet joint interventions in chronic spinal pain. Pain Physician. 2007;10(1):229-53.
14. Sehgal N, Shah RV, McKenzie-Brown AM, et al. Diagnostic utility of facet (zygapophysial) joint injections in chronic spinal pain: a systematic review of evidence. Pain Physician. 2005;8(2):211-24.
15. Masala S, Nano G, Mammucari M, et al. Medial branch neurotomy in low back pain. Neuroradiology. 2012;54(7):737-44.
16. MacVicar J, Borowczyk JM, MacVicar AM, et al. Lumbar medial branch radiofrequency neurotomy in New Zealand. Pain Med. 2013;14(5):639-45.
17. Freeman BC. IDET: a critical appraisal of the evidence. Eur Spine J. 2006;15(3):448-57.
18. Al-Zain F, Lemcke J, Killeen T, et al. Minimally invasive spinal surgery using nucleoplasty: a 1-year follow-up study. Acta Neurochir (Wien). 2008;150(12):1257-62.
19. Masala S, Massari F, Fabiano S, et al. Nucleoplasty in the treatment of lumbar discogenic back pain: one year follow-up. Cardiovasc Intervent Radiol. 2007;30(3):426-32.
20. Kapural L, Vrooman B, Sarwar S, et al. A randomized, placebo-controlled trial of transdiscal radiofrequency, biacuplasty for treatment of discogenic lower back pain. Pain Med. 2013;14(3):362-73.
21. Oakley JC. Spinal cord stimulation in axial low back pain: solving the dilemma. Pain Med. 2006;7:S58-63.
22. Heran MKS, Smith AD, Legiehn GM. Spinal injection procedures: a review of concepts, controversies, and complications. Radiol Clin N Am. 2008;46(3):487-514.

CHAPTER

28

Diagnostic and Therapeutic Value of Spinal Injections

Juan Carlos Robles, Vadim Goz

INTRODUCTION

Spinal injections comprise an increasing popular group of procedures that serve both diagnostic and therapeutic roles in the management of back pain. Various forms of spinal injections are discussed including discography, epidural steroid injections, selective nerve root blocks (SNRBs), facet joint blocks, and median branch nerve blocks.

DISCOGRAMS

As previously described in Chapter 15, discography is a diagnostic test commonly used to identify discogenic back pain at specific vertebral levels. It involves the injection of contrast medium into an intervertebral disk under fluoroscopic guidance. The injection pressure is correlated with pain response of the unsedated patient. The goal of the procedure is to simultaneously evaluate radiographic evidence of disk degeneration and reproduction of concordant pain with injection at a specific level.

Discography has become increasingly useful with the escalating utilization of magnetic resonance imaging (MRI) in patients with chronic back pain. MRI has the potential to demonstrate degenerative findings at multiple levels, but this radiographic evidence fails to connect these findings with clinical symptoms. Further testing is necessary to identify the symptomatic level and direct further management. Discography may offer important information for preoperative planning, directing the surgeon with regards to which and how many levels to fuse. It can also be useful in the postoperative evaluation of a patient who has undergone fusion and returns with recurrent or unresolved back pain. In this case, a discogram can evaluate adjacent levels for discogenic back pain to evaluate for possible extension of fusion.

The diagnostic value of discography is a controversial topic. The significant false positive rate, ranging from < 10% to 50% in the literature, brings the clinical utility of this test into question.[1,2] Some studies demonstrate fairly good sensitivity, with one study showing a positive discogram in 6 out of 7 symptomatic patients.[3] However, a number of other studies suggest that discography is a poor tool for evaluation of the primary cause of lower back pain, raising concerns about its reliability and high false positive rates.[2,4-9] In patients with no history of lower back pain, up to 20% of patients will demonstrate at least one positive level on discography.[7] That proportion increases to 40% in patients who have had prior lumbar fusion but were asymptomatic postoperatively.[8] Abnormal psychogenic testing and long-standing chronic pain are two factors that have been shown to increase the false positive rate of discograms and thus decrease their clinical diagnostic utility.

Another criticism of discography is that the test is largely dependent on the ability of the patient to identify concordant pain, or pain of the same quality as that felt during prior episodes. The ability of patients to reliably identify concordant discogenic pain is a matter of concern. This was emphasized in a study of eight patients with no history of back pain and normal psychometric testing who underwent iliac crest bone grafting for nonspinal reasons. Fifty percent of patients had a positive discogram at 2 to 4 months postoperatively with pain that was concordant with the iliac graft site.[2]

A key question in the evaluation of the utility of discography in clinical management of back pain is the impact that it has on surgical outcomes. However, evidence to this effect remains inconclusive. Some studies indicate that patients who undergo discography have good surgical outcomes, whereas others report no difference.[10,11] There are no major studies providing substantial evidence regarding the impact of discography on surgical decision making. It would be useful to know, for example, how frequently a discogram result translates to fusion of additional levels compared with the original operative plan and the impact of these altered decisions on patient outcomes.

Although the evidence for false positive rates in discography is alarming, it remains the only test with the potential to correlate level-specific radiographic evidence with clinical symptoms by identifying the specific level that produces discogenic back pain. This test should only be considered for patients who are being evaluated for surgical intervention. The risks and discomfort of discography are not justified if identifying the spinal level underlying the patient's symptomatology will not alter management. Specifically, this test is useful in patients with radiographic evidence of multilevel disease, in which case discography may help differentiate symptomatic and asymptomatic levels and avoid unnecessary fusion of asymptomatic levels.

EPIDURAL STEROID INJECTIONS

Epidural steroid injection is one of the most commonly performed interventions in the United States. The number of epidural injections has been increasing precipitously, from 802,735 in 1998 to 1,776,153 in 2005, an increase of 121% over a period of 7 years.[12] Despite this overwhelming trend in use, the evidence for the benefits of epidural spinal injections is mixed at best. The absence of strong evidence for the benefits of these procedures places the astounding increase in utilization in question. Spinal steroid injections are indicated in patients with radiculopathy and should not be used in patients with back pain without radicular symptoms. It is hypothesized that in addition to the mechanical compression of nerve roots, radiculopathy may also be triggered by local pro-inflammatory cytokines and acute phase reactants.[13-16] Although the mechanism of action of steroid injections is poorly understood, it is possible that corticosteroids inhibit pain-inducing inflammatory cytokines.

Current literature has conflicting results regarding the benefits of epidural steroid injections.[17-21] Studies comparing epidural steroid injections with saline or anesthetic epidural injections show less benefit for steroids or no statistically significant difference between the treatment arms in the mid- to long-term time period.[22-26] At 1-year evaluation after epidural spinal injection, pain improvement has been observed in 36–43% of patients.[27,28] It is important to note that this outcome does not significantly differ from the natural history of the disease.[29] These data suggest that epidural spinal steroid injections do not alter the natural trajectory of the disease, but they may lead to transient symptomatic relief while the disease process continues its natural course. While short-term pain relief may be expected from epidural injections, the inability of this intervention to alter the disease entity itself suggests that the long-term outcome is dependent on the course of the underlying disease, the pathophysiology of which is likely unaffected by epidural injections.

A recent randomized controlled trial investigated the efficacy of caudal epidural spinal injections compared with epidural saline injections as well as a sham procedure consisting of subcutaneous saline.[30] A total of 116 patients with radiculopathy of over 12-week duration were randomized to one of the three treatment arms. Outcome measures included the Oswestry disability index, European quality-of-life measure, and visual analog scale for low back pain and leg pain, all measured at baseline, 6 weeks, 12 weeks, and 52 weeks. The results showed no statistical difference between the epidural saline injection, epidural steroid injection, and the sham arms of the study.

In addition to caudal spinal epidural injections, intralaminar lumbar injections can be used to treat lumbar radiculopathy and sciatica. The key difference in these methods is that in the intralaminar approach, the epidural space is accessed by placing the needle between two adjacent laminae. The site of caudal epidural injections, in contrast, is the epidural space at the level of the sacrum/coccyx, making this method more appropriate for patients with sciatica and radiculopathy of the lower limbs. Studies on the efficacy of treatment of lumbar radiculopathy with intralaminar epidural steroid injections report similar outcomes to those on caudal injections.[22,30] An improvement in pain is seen in the short-term period of about 3–4 weeks; however, no benefit is observed during long-term follow-up. Epidural steroid injections have also not been shown to decrease the cumulative probability of surgery in patients with sciatica.[31] The inability of steroids to decrease the rate of surgery at 1-year follow-up is further evidence of the lack of long-term therapeutic value of this treatment.

Epidural steroid injections are also used in the treatment of cervical radiculopathy. Evidence regarding outcomes is poor in both quantity and quality. A limited number of studies available have shown an improvement in both short- and long-term pain.[32,33] However these studies do not include adequate control groups with sham procedures that would account for placebo effect and the natural progression of the disease.

In addition to cervical and lumbar radiculopathy, spinal epidural injections are occasionally used to treat spinal stenosis. However, the evidence for this application is not encouraging. Current literature suggests that epidural injections are associated with mild improvement in pain at 2 weeks when compared with physical therapy and home exercise, after which point the two groups do not show a statistically significant difference.

Given the limited benefit of epidural steroid injections and the possible risks described in Chapter 35, proper selection of patients is of the utmost importance. Since the majority of evidence regarding therapeutic benefit indicates a short-term improvement in pain and function with no long-term benefit, these injections may be suitable for patients with subacute back pain pathology who cannot tolerate, whether financially or otherwise, periods of immobility, and decreased function. In this scenario, the corticosteroid injection may provide short-term pain relief, allowing the patient to function and work while the natural trajectory of the disease leads to resolution of the underlying pathology. An additional benefit of this approach is that with subacute disease, the patient will require a minimum number of injections, which minimizes risks.

The role of epidural steroids injections in the management of chronic back pain is questionable. This is mostly due to the lack of long-term benefits. Long-term pain relief is possible only with recurring injections, which typically show a diminishing duration of effective pain relief and an increase in risk of potential side effects. Furthermore, epidural steroid injections have not been shown to alter the underlying mechanism of disease, change the natural progression of the spinal pathology, or decrease the risk of surgical intervention. However, one possible chronic back pain population for which steroid injections may benefit patients is those with chronic back pain who wish to successfully complete a physical therapy regimen.

SELECTIVE NERVE ROOT BLOCKS, FACET JOINT BLOCKS, AND MEDIAL BRANCH BLOCKS

Selective Nerve Root Blocks

Selective nerve root blocks involve an injection of anesthetic either via the intervertebral foramen or extraforminally to selectively block a specific nerve root.[34] SNRBs theoretically have both therapeutic and diagnostic value. Therapeutic SNRBs are done by injection via the intervertebral foramen, in contrast to diagnostic SNRBs, which are done extraforaminally. To be truly selective these blocks have to be done extraforaminally, distal to the division of the ventral and dorsal rami, to avoid anesthesia of the dorsal ramus and its associated structures.

The SNRBs can be useful in patients who have multilevel radiographic signs of radicular impingement or other pathology. The induction of concordant pain in a specific level with needle placement and pain relief with anesthetic injection in one level over another may suggest that operative intervention at the SNRB positive level will be more beneficial. A number of studies have evaluated the ability of SNRBs to identify various pathologies. Most of the data examining the rate of positive intraoperative findings at levels that are positive on SNRB suggest that pathology will be identified in upward of 90–95% of patients with a positive SNRB at a specific level.[35-40] However, a high false positive rate has been noted in the literature; specifically, blocks that are distal to the pathology will often give a positive result indicating the potential spread of the anesthetic effect and less specificity than anticipated.[41]

The effect of preoperative diagnostic SNRBs on surgical outcomes and decision making has not been extensively studied. A study of 78 surgical patients with preoperative SNRBs found surgical outcomes to be 53% good, 23% fair, and 24% poor as assessed by the surgeon.[42] An interesting note is that patients with prior surgery had 52% more poor surgical outcomes. It is difficult to distinguish whether this is a reflection of worse surgical outcomes in patients requiring multiple surgeries or if the clinical utility of SNRBs and their ability to predict positive postsurgical outcomes is diminished for patients who have had prior surgery. However, some data in postlaminectomy patients with continued sciatica who had a positive diagnostic SNRB and reoperation show that positive surgical outcomes are experienced by the great majority.[36]

Diagnostic SNRBs may be useful in directing preoperative planning in patients with multilevel radicular disease on radiographic studies. A lack of randomized controlled trials comparing surgical outcomes in patients who received or did not receive SNRBs makes it difficult to assess their true value. A number of confounding factors complicate the interpretation of current studies. Injection of anesthetic may spread beyond the intended site, leading to a nonselective block and potentially false positive results. Pain relief due to blockage of a spinal nerve may not distinguish between pathology of the nerve at the site of injection and distal pathology; pain caused by distal pathology will be relieved by proximal anesthesia of the nerve carrying the area's sensory distribution. Previous studies demonstrate that sciatic pain is relieved by blocking the sciatic nerve or contributing collaterals either distally or proximally to the pathology.[43,44] Furthermore, pain produced by proximal pathology can be decreased by anesthetizing the tissue in the area of dermatomal distribution of the affected nerve root.[45] Besides these confounding factors, pain itself is subjective and the reporting of pain is affected by numerous factors external to the underlying pathology including psychological state, socioeconomic status, and legal factors such as ongoing compensation claims.[46,47] The placebo effect may also play a significant role as it does in other interventions. Current studies are not adequately controlled to fully account for these confounders.

In addition to their diagnostic applications, SNRBs are used for the therapeutic treatment of back pain. Therapeutic SNRBs involve the delivery of corticosteroids in addition to an anesthetic into and around the affected nerve root.[36] In essence, this procedure is a selective epidural steroid injection. The advantage of the selective approach is the ability to deliver less volume of a concentrated therapeutic agent into the specific area of pathology, compared with the larger volume required of traditional epidural injections.

The data on effectiveness of therapeutic SNRBs are as inconclusive as that for epidural steroid injections. A number of studies find this intervention to be an effective treatment of radiculopathy not responsive to conservative treatments.[48,49] One study even found SNRBs to be more effective than traditional epidural injections.[48] The duration of effect is limited to short-term improvements, with little to no long-term effect on pain.[50] It is possible that therapeutic SNRBs decrease the need for surgical intervention.[51] Most studies do not have adequate controls to account for placebo effect and other confounding factors. One randomized controlled trial comparing periradicular injections of bupivacaine and methylprednisolone versus saline alone in patients with sciatica found a lack of effectiveness in the bupivacaine and methylprednisolone arm.[24] Recovery was greater in the steroid arm at 2 weeks compared with the saline group, but at 3 and 6 months the saline group had significantly less back pain. The researchers concluded that although there appeared to be an increased effect at 2 weeks post injection with bupivacaine and methylprednisolone, the patients experienced a rebound type phenomenon with increased pain at 3 and 6 months as compared with the control group.

Facet Joint Injections and Medial Branch Nerve Blocks

A significant portion of back pain—up to 40%— is believed to be facet (zygapophyseal) joint mediated.[52-56] Injections of the facet joint capsule itself or blocks of the medial branch nerves that provide sensory innervation to the joint are two diagnostic tools used to differentiate facet joint disease from other back pain etiologies. The critique of diagnostic facet joint injections and medial branch blocks (MBBs) is the same as for other diagnostic spinal injections: the high rate of false positive results.[53,54,57] Indeed, despite their widespread use, facet joint injections have not been rigorously validated as a diagnostic or therapeutic measure.[58]

Although single MBBs are subject to a high rate of false positives, the procedure is considered a reliable tool in the diagnosis of facet-mediated joint pain if the blocks are performed in a controlled manner. Most commonly, control is obtained by performing a comparative block. This procedure involves sequential injection of a short-acting anesthetic and long-acting anesthetic; the long-acting anesthetic is injected once the effect of the short-acting anesthetic has worn off, usually after a period of a few weeks. A positive result is the relief of concordant pain after the injection of a short-acting anesthetic and relief of longer duration after the injection of the long-acting anesthetic. The most common use of MBBs is to evaluate patients for medial branch neurotomy, a procedure that uses a radiofrequency probe to destroy the medial branches of a particular facet joint. A successful neurotomy provides extended pain relief (of 7–9 months duration) to the patient, and the procedure follows logically from a positive MBB. Subsequent neurotomies upon the return of pain are generally successful and are not associated with increased risks.[59]

Although a controlled MBB followed by neurotomy is commonly accepted as the standard of care for suspected facet joint pain, this paradigm is not without flaws and detractors. Although minimal, the risks of MBBs and neurotomy are similar, meaning that unnecessary risk may be introduced by utilizing the diagnostic procedure (MBB) instead of just the definitive treatment (neurotomy). Furthermore, a recent cost analysis of diagnostic MBBs did not reveal favorable results. In this study, the authors concluded that it is more cost-effective to simply perform a neurotomy on patients who are suspected of having facet-mediated pain based on clinical findings alone, although this reduces the success rate of the procedure.[60] However, like any cost-analysis, this analysis is based on reimbursement rates that are subject to change.

CONCLUSION

Spinal injections of various forms are frequently utilized for diagnostic and therapeutic purposes. The current state of the evidence is inconclusive with regard to the effectiveness and value of injections in either role. Discography remains one of the only tests that attempts to correlate clinical and radiographic findings. Various corticosteroid and anesthetic injections may play an important role as part of a multidisciplinary approach to the management of chronic pain and as a temporary pain management measure to preserve function in the management of subacute back pain. Further studies are needed to elucidate the role and effectiveness of spinal injections in both diagnostic and therapeutic settings.

REFERENCES

1. Wolfer LR, Derby R, Lee JE, et al. Systematic review of lumbar provocation discography in asymptomatic subjects with a meta-analysis of false-positive rates. Pain Physician. 2008;11(4):513-38.
2. Carragee EJ, Tanner CM, Yang B, et al. False-positive findings on lumbar discography. Reliability of subjective concordance assessment during provocative disc injection. Spine (Phila Pa 1976). 1999;24(23):2542-7.
3. Walsh TR, Weinstein JN, Spratt KF, et al. Lumbar discography in normal subjects. A controlled, prospective study. J Bone Joint Surg Am. 1990;72(7):1081-8.
4. Carragee EJ, Hannibal M. Diagnostic evaluation of low back pain. Orthop Clin N Am. 2004;35(1):7-16.
5. Carragee EJ, Chen Y, Tanner CM, et al. Provocative discography in patients after limited lumbar discectomy: a controlled, randomized study of pain response in symptomatic and asymptomatic subjects. Spine (Phila Pa 1976). 2000;25(23):3065-71.
6. Carragee EJ, Paragioudakis SJ, Khurana S. 2000 Volvo Award winner in clinical studies: Lumbar high-intensity zone and discography in subjects without low back problems. Spine (Phila Pa 1976). 2000;25(23):2987-92.
7. Carragee EJ, Tanner CM, Khurana S, et al. The rates of false-positive lumbar discography in select patients without low back symptoms. Spine (Phila Pa 1976). 2000;25(11): 1373-80; discussion 1381.
8. Carragee EJ, Tanner CM, Vittum D. Positive provocative discography as a misleading finding in the evaluation of low back pain. In NASS Proceedings 1997, New Orleans, 1997. p. 388.
9. Carragee EJ, Alamin TF, Miller J, et al. Provocative discography in volunteer subjects with mild persistent low back pain. Spine J. 2002;2(1):25-34.
10. Colhoun E, McCall IW, Williams L, et al. Provocation discography as a guide to planning operations on the spine. J Bone Joint Surg Br. 1988;70(2):267-71.
11. Madan S, Gundanna M, Harley JM, et al. Does provocative discography screening of discogenic back pain improve surgical outcome? J Spinal Disord Tech. 2002;15(3):245-51.
12. Manchikanti L. Medicare in interventional pain management: a critical analysis. Pain Physician. 2006;9:171-98.
13. Rydevik B, Brown MD, Lundborg G. Pathoanatomy and pathophysiology of nerve root compression. Spine (Phila Pa 1976). 1984;9(1):7-15.
14. Goupille P, Jayson MI, Valat JP, et al. The role of inflammation in disk herniation-associated radiculopathy. Semin Arthritis Rheum. 1998;28(1):60-71.
15. Autio RA, Karppinen J, Kurunlahti M, et al. Effect of periradicular methylprednisolone on spontaneous resorption of intervertebral disc herniations. Spine (Phila Pa 1976). 2004; 29(15):1601-7.
16. Muramoto T, Atsuta Y, Iwahara T, et al. The action of prostaglandin E2 and triamcinolone acetonide on the firing activity of lumbar nerve roots. Int Orthop. 1997;21(3):172-5.
17. Chou R, Loeser JD, Owens DK, et al. Interventional therapies, surgery, and interdisciplinary rehabilitation for low back pain: an evidence-based clinical practice guideline from the American Pain Society. Spine (Phila Pa 1976). 2009;34(10):1066-77.
18. Koes BW, Scholten RJ, Mens JM, et al. Efficacy of epidural steroid injections for low-back pain and sciatica: a systematic review of randomized clinical trials. Pain. 1995;63(3): 279-88.
19. Watts RW, Silagy CA. A meta-analysis on the efficacy of epidural corticosteroids in the treatment of sciatica. Anaesth Intensive Care. 1995;23(5):564-9.
20. Luijsterburg PA, Verhagen AP, Ostelo RW, et al. Effectiveness of conservative treatments for the lumbosacral radicular syndrome: a systematic review. Eur Spine J. 2007;16(7): 881-99.

21. Conn A, Buenaventura RM, Datta S, et al. Systematic review of caudal epidural injections in the management of chronic low back pain. Pain Physician. 2009;12(1):109-35.
22. Carette S, Leclaire R, Marcoux S, et al. Epidural corticosteroid injections for sciatica due to herniated nucleus pulposus. N Engl J Med. 1997;336(23):1634-40.
23. Ng L, Chaudhary N, Sell P. The efficacy of corticosteroids in periradicular infiltration for chronic radicular pain: a randomized, double-blind, controlled trial. Spine (Phila Pa 1976). 2005;30(8):857-62.
24. Karppinen J, Malmivaara A, Kurunlahti M, et al. Periradicular infiltration for sciatica: a randomized controlled trial. Spine (Phila Pa 1976). 2001;26(9):1059-67.
25. Bush K, Hillier S. A controlled study of caudal epidural injections of triamcinolone plus procaine for the management of intractable sciatica. Spine (Phila Pa 1976). 1991;16(5):572-5.
26. Breivik H, Hesla PE, Molnar I. Treatment of chronic low back pain and sciatica: comparison of caudal epidural injections of bupivacaine and methylprednisolone with bupivacaine followed by saline. Adv Pain Res Ther. 1976;1:927-32.
27. Cuckler JM, Bernini PA, Wiesel SW, et al. The use of epidural steroids in the treatment of lumbar radicular pain. A prospective, randomized, double-blind study. J Bone Joint Surg Am. 1985;67(1):63-6.
28. Buttermann GR. Treatment of lumbar disc herniation: epidural steroid injection compared with discectomy. A prospective, randomized study. J Bone Joint Surg Am. 2004; 86-A(4):670-9.
29. Komori H, Okawa A, Haro H, et al. Factors predicting the prognosis of lumbar radiculopathy due to disc herniation. J Orthop Sci. 2002;7(1):56-61.
30. Iversen T, Solberg TK, Romner B, et al. Effect of caudal epidural steroid or saline injection in chronic lumbar radiculopathy: multicentre, blinded, randomised controlled trial. BMJ. 2011;343:d5278.
31. Wilson-MacDonald J, Burt G, Griffin D, et al. Epidural steroid injection for nerve root compression. A randomised, controlled trial. J Bone Joint Surg Br. 2005;87(3):352-5.
32. Castagnera L, Maurette P, Pointillart V, et al. Long-term results of cervical epidural steroid injection with and without morphine in chronic cervical radicular pain. Pain. 1994;58(2):239-43.
33. Stav A, Ovadia L, Sternberg A, et al. Cervical epidural steroid injection for cervicobrachialgia. Acta Anaesthesiol Scand. 1993;37(6):562-6.
34. Macnab I. Negative disc exploration. An analysis of the causes of nerve-root involvement in sixty-eight patients. J Bone Joint Surg Am. 1971;53(5):891-903.
35. Schutz H, Lougheed WM, Wortzman G, et al. Intervertebral nerve-root in the investigation of chronic lumbar disc disease. Can J Surg. 1973;16(3):217-21.
36. Krempen JF, Smith BS. Nerve-root injection: a method for evaluating the etiology of sciatica. J Bone Joint Surg Am. 1974;56(7):1435-44.
37. Dooley JF, McBroom RJ, Taguchi T, et al. Nerve root infiltration in the diagnosis of radicular pain. Spine (Phila Pa 1976). 1988;13(1):79-83.
38. van Akkerveeken PF. The diagnostic value of nerve root sheath infiltration. Acta Orthop Scand Suppl. 1993;251:61-3.
39. Stanley D, McLaren MI, Euinton HA, et al. A prospective study of nerve root infiltration in the diagnosis of sciatica. A comparison with radiculography, computed tomography, and operative findings. Spine (Phila Pa 1976). 1990;15(6): 540-3.
40. Haueisen DC, Smith BS, Myers SR, et al. The diagnostic accuracy of spinal nerve injection studies. Their role in the evaluation of recurrent sciatica. Clin Orthop Relat Res. 1985(198):179-83.
41. North RB, Kidd DH, Zahurak M, et al. Specificity of diagnostic nerve blocks: a prospective, randomized study of sciatica due to lumbosacral spine disease. Pain. 1996;65(1): 77-85.
42. Herron LD. Selective nerve root block in patient selection for lumbar surgery: surgical results. J Spinal Disord. 1989;2(2):75-9.
43. Xavier AV, Farrell CE, McDanal J, et al. Does antidromic activation of nociceptors play a role in sciatic radicular pain? Pain. 1990;40(1):77-9.
44. Kissin I, Xavier AV, McDanal J. Blockade of sciatic nerve branches relieves sciatic radicular pain. Anesth Analg. 1989;69(2):262-3.
45. Hockaday JM, Whitty CW. Patterns of referred pain in the normal subject. Brain. 1967;90(3):481-96.
46. Beecher HK. The powerful placebo. J Am Med Assoc. 1955;159(17):1602-6.
47. Turner JA, Deyo RA, Loeser JD, et al. The importance of placebo effects in pain treatment and research. JAMA. 1994; 271(20):1609-14.
48. Kraemer J, Ludwig J, Bickert U, et al. Lumbar epidural perineural injection: a new technique. Eur Spine J. 1997;6(5): 357-61.
49. Weiner BK, Fraser RD. Foraminal injection for lateral lumbar disc herniation. J Bone Joint Surg Br. 1997;79(5):804-7.
50. Devulder J, Deene P, De Laat M, et al. Nerve root sleeve injections in patients with failed back surgery syndrome: a comparison of three solutions. Clin J Pain. 1999;15(2): 132-5.
51. Riew KD, Yin Y, Gilula L, et al. The effect of nerve-root injections on the need for operative treatment of lumbar radicular pain. A prospective, randomized, controlled, double-blind study. J Bone Joint Surg Am. 2000;82-A(11):1589-93.
52. Cohen SP, Raja SN. Pathogenesis, diagnosis, and treatment of lumbar zygapophysial (facet) joint pain. Anesthesiology. 2007;106(3):591-614.
53. Schwarzer AC, Aprill CN, Derby R, et al. The false-positive rate of uncontrolled diagnostic blocks of the lumbar zygapophysial joints. Pain. 1994;58(2):195-200.
54. Revel M, Poiraudeau S, Auleley GR, et al. Capacity of the clinical picture to characterize low back pain relieved by facet joint anesthesia. Proposed criteria to identify patients with painful facet joints. Spine (Phila Pa 1976). 1998;23(18): 1972-6; discussion 1977.
55. Schwarzer AC, Aprill CN, Derby R, et al. The relative contributions of the disc and zygapophyseal joint in chronic low back pain. Spine (Phila Pa 1976). 1994;19(7):801-6.

56. Manchikanti L, Boswell MV, Singh V, et al. Prevalence of facet joint pain in chronic spinal pain of cervical, thoracic, and lumbar regions. BMC Musculoskelet Disord. 2004; 5(1):15.
57. Manchikanti L, Pampati V, Fellows B, et al. The diagnostic validity and therapeutic value of lumbar facet joint nerve blocks with or without adjuvant agents. Curr Rev Pain. 2000;4(5):337-44.
58. Varlotta GP, Lefkowitz TR, Schweitzer M, et al. The lumbar facet joint: a review of current knowledge: Part II: diagnosis and management. Skeletal Radiol. 2011;40(2):149-57.
59. Smuck M, Crisostomo RA, Trivedi K, et al. Success of initial and repeated medial branch neurotomy for zygapophysial joint pain: a systematic review. PM&R. 2012;4(9): 686-92.
60. Cohen SP, Williams KA, Kurihara C, et al. Multicenter, randomized, comparative cost-effectiveness study comparing 0, 1, and 2 diagnostic medial branch (facet joint nerve) block treatment paradigms before lumbar facet radiofrequency denervation. Anesthesiology. 2010;113(2): 395-405.

CHAPTER

29

Trigger Point Injections

Benjamin Bieber, Devon Ryan

INTRODUCTION

A trigger point as defined by Travell and Simons is "a hyperirritable spot, usually within a taut band of skeletal muscle or in the muscle fascia, which is painful on compression and can give rise to characteristic referred pain, motor dysfunction, and autonomic phenomena".[1] Trigger points can be classified as either active or latent: active trigger points are spontaneously painful, whereas latent trigger points produce pain only when palpated.[2] Trigger points differ from tender spots, which are not associated with referred pain (Table 29.1). Firm pressure over a trigger point may generate a local twitch response—a transient contraction of the taut band of muscle fibers that contains the trigger point. Affected patients may also present with restricted range of motion and muscle stiffness.[3]

The presence of multiple trigger points is the key characteristic of myofascial pain syndrome, one of the most common causes of musculoskeletal pain. This condition must be differentiated from fibromyalgia, which is associated with pain over various tender spots, although these two disorders may be seen concomitantly.[4]

Trigger points may be caused by repetitive or overuse injuries, sports- and work-related injuries, nerve root compression, disk disease, and arthritis. Muscle tension related to poor posture and stress may be etiological factors. Hormonal disorders such as hypothyroidism and estrogen deficiency, vitamin deficiencies, and metabolic or electrolyte disorders have also been associated with trigger points and tender spots.

The pathophysiology of trigger points is complex and not entirely understood. The most prevalent theory is the Integrated Hypothesis, proposed by Simons.[1,5,6] Briefly, this explanation posits that abnormally high levels of acetylcholine release from motor nerves cause continuous sarcomere shortening, which, in turn, generates a "local energy crisis" characterized by ischemia and increased metabolism. It is this energy crisis that causes the release of substances, which sensitize nociceptors. A 2008 study on the biochemicals present in sites local and distant to trigger points helped solidify the link between the energy crisis and noxious chemical release, providing some evidence for the Integrated Hypothesis.[7]

Table 29.1: Trigger points versus tender points

Trigger points	*Tender points*
• Local tenderness, taut band, local twitch response, jump sign	• Local tenderness
• Singular or multiple	• Multiple
• May occur in any skeletal muscle	• Occur in specific locations that are symmetrically located
• May cause a specific referred pain pattern	• Do not cause referred pain, but often cause a total body increase in pain sensitivity

DIAGNOSIS

There is no gold standard for the diagnosis of trigger points and tender points. Clinicians rely mainly on a detailed history and physical examination, although other diagnostic techniques have been studied. Numerous modalities exist for the treatment of trigger points once they have been successfully identified. Several of these are noninvasive techniques, such as the spray and stretch method, which involves application of a topical anesthetic followed by passive stretching of the affected muscle, and friction massage, which can be performed by a physical therapist.

The specific criteria for diagnosing a trigger point are not standardized and seem to be highly variable across practitioners. The most common factor used is the identification of a tender spot within a taut band of muscle. Often, this finding must coincide with either a reproduction of the patient's referred pain or the generation of a predicted pain referral pattern upon palpation of the tender spot.

The patient should be asked for a detailed account of the course of his or her pain, with an emphasis on characterizing the nature of pain, for example, is it localized or radiating? The patient is asked to point with one finger to the most intense location of pain and give a detailed description of the pattern of referred pain, if present.[8] Then, the examiner can press over the most tender point to verify reproduction of the patient's pain. After localizing the point of maximum tenderness, the entire taut band that contains the trigger point can be palpated. The muscle must be relaxed and palpation should proceed across muscle fibers at a right angle to their length.

Other techniques for the physical identification of trigger points have been outlined, including flat, pincer, and deep palpation.[8] Flat palpation refers to sliding a fingertip across affected muscle fibers with the skin pushed to one side, feeling the firmness of the taut band. Then, the band can be "plucked" to identify the most painful locus—presumably the trigger point. Pincer palpation involves rolling the relevant muscle fibers between the thumb and forefinger to identify the taut band and trigger point. Finally, deep palpation can be used for trigger points that are obscured by superficial tissue. This method involves placing a finger at the point where the affected muscle attaches and looking for symptoms when applying pressure in the appropriate direction.

The ability of the manual physical examination to precisely identify trigger points has been called into question, with a recent review concluding that it is not a reliable test for the condition.[9] In an effort to improve inter-rater reliability in making this diagnosis, Andrew Fischer invented the pressure algometer, a device that allows for quantification of pressure pain thresholds and can be used to supplement the physical examination that was previously described. The algometer measures the minimum pressure or force that causes pain. An abnormal value for this metric is greater than a 2 kg/cm^2 difference relative to a nontender tissue area. The effectiveness of therapeutic measures can also be objectively assessed using the instrument. Some research has described positive results in terms of the reliability and validity of the pressure algometer.[10] However, the device has yet to be adopted broadly in the clinical setting; it is still used more commonly in research than in practice.[11,12]

Other techniques for identifying trigger points have been explored. They have exhibited varying degrees of success, but none has been rigorously validated. Electromyography has also been used to measure abnormal high-frequency potentials at trigger points as compared with normal tissue.[13] Ultrasound has recently proven promising as a method to visualize trigger points,[14] despite the lack of success that was seen in a pilot study.[15] Magnetic resonance elastography, another imaging modality, has also been investigated for use in this setting.[16] Given the lack of evidence for these techniques, however, they cannot be recommended in clinical practice.

Concomitant syndromes, such as spinal segmental sensitization (SSS), that may enhance trigger point pain have also been described.[17] SSS is a state of hyperexcitability of a spinal segment that occurs in reaction to a peripheral irritative focus (trigger point or tender spot). The patient experiences hyperalgesia, or increased sensitivity to pain, along the involved dermatome.

The diagnostic tools used for SSS may aide in locating the trigger point as well as the sensitized spinal segment; they include the skin scratching, pinch and roll, and skin conductance methods. Skin scratching involves dragging an open paper clip across the dermatomal borders, or sensory diagnostic tracks (Fig. 29.1).[18] Patients are asked to indicate when sensation from the paper clip becomes sharper or duller. The pinch and roll method is designed to test the sensitization of the subcutaneous tissue. The technique consists of pinching the skin between the thumb and index finger and making a fold over a nonpainful area. Without releasing the pressure, the skinfold is rolled while the thumb and index finger of the other hand takes over the pinching and continues the rolling. Areas that are sensitized are painful. Finally, a skin conductance meter can be used to quantify increased sympathetic activity, which is characteristic of a sensitized segment.

INDICATIONS

The primary indication for a trigger point injection is a diagnosis of an active trigger point—a spontaneously painful, firm, localized area within a taut band of muscle that is tender and produces referred pain when palpated.

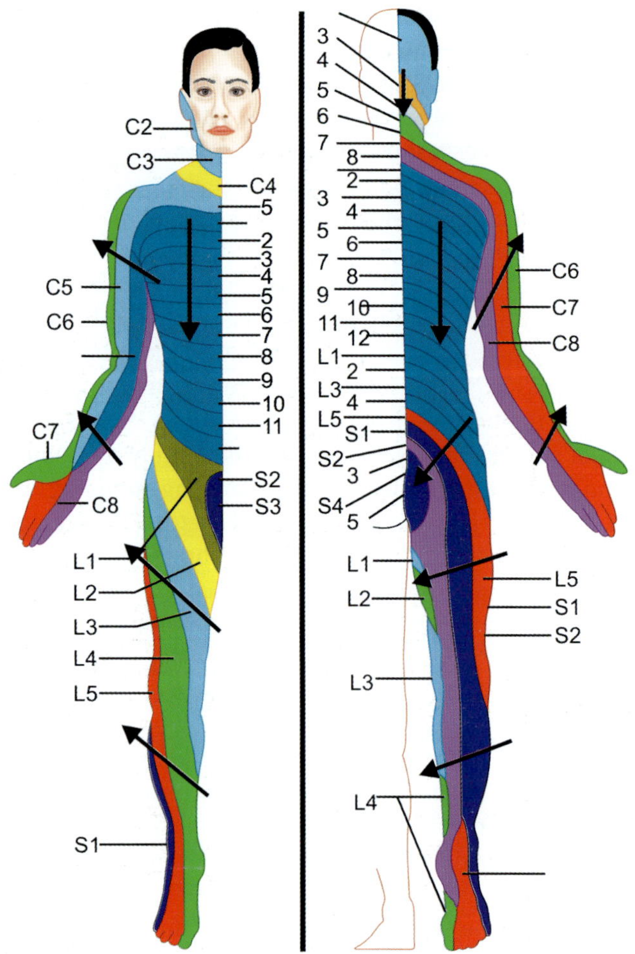

Fig. 29.1: Sensory diagnostic tracks.

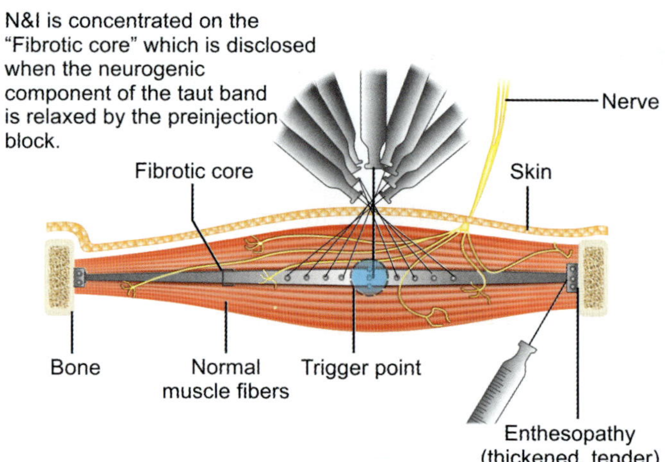

Fig. 29.2: Needling and infiltration of taut band.

In the low back pain population, patients considered for injection should have chronic pain, or pain that fails to resolve itself within the 6 weeks after onset of symptoms.[19] Furthermore, clinicians often recommend injection only for those patients whose pain does not improve with noninvasive manual therapy unless their pain is severe. Such treatment could include deep tissue massage and the spray and stretch method, among other modalities. Pharmacological management is often attempted simultaneously, with medications such as nonsteroidal anti-inflammatory drugs, muscle relaxants, and analgesics.[4] Contraindications for injection include bleeding disorders, anticoagulation, local infection, and fear of needles.[4,19]

TECHNIQUE

Trigger Point Injection

The appropriate needle length for injection depends on the depth of the structure to be injected. It is extremely important to use a needle that will penetrate the entire structure that contains the trigger point or tender spot. For example, a 22-gauge 1.5-inch needle can be used for the upper trapezeii and posterior cervical paraspinal muscles, but for larger muscle groups such as the piriformis and quadratus lumborum, a 22-gauge 3-inch needle is necessary.

Most commonly, the injectate consists of a local anesthetic such as 1% lidocaine or 1% procaine.[4] Dry needling, in which the same procedure is performed without the use of an anesthetic, has also been frequently described. A recent study found no difference between dry needling and anesthetic injection,[20] although previous research has associated the use of an anesthetic with less postinjection soreness.[21] Steroids have also been utilized, but their use is not currently recommended, as no additional benefits have been demonstrated over anesthetic and they are associated with more complications.[2]

The patient should be positioned comfortably, and the trigger points to be injected should be properly identified. The skin at the injection site should then be prepared in a sterile manner.[8] Needling and infiltration is then performed (Fig. 29.2). The needle should be inserted adjacent to the trigger point at an angle to the skin (often 50° to 70°) that directs it toward the trigger point. When the needle is advanced into the trigger point, a small amount of injectate is released. The needle should then be withdrawn to the level of the subcutaneous tissue, redirected slightly, and advanced toward a site adjacent to the trigger point. It is important to withdraw the needle to the subcutaneous tissue so that muscle fibers are not harmed. A similar volume should be injected, and the redirecting procedure should be repeated so that the trigger point, taut band, and associated enthesopathy are mechanically eradicated. At the conclusion of the needling, the tautness of the band should be relieved and no local twitch response should be observed.[4] After removing the needle, the trigger point should be compressed for 2 minutes to allow hemostasis.

The patient should be advised that postinjection soreness is common. Vasovagal syncope during the procedure has been reported. Other complications are rare but include hematoma, abscess development, and pneumothorax.[2]

PREINJECTION BLOCK

Preinjection block refers to a technique in which anesthetic is spread along the normal, non-tender tissue adjacent to the taut band and trigger point on the side where the nerve supply enters the muscle (Fig. 29.3). This practice is meant to anesthetize the painful sensitized area to be infiltrated thus allowing for vigorous needling of the trigger point. The injections should be performed as close to the taut band as possible without actually contacting it.[17]

Paraspinous Block

The paraspinous block is meant to treat SSS by desensitizing the entire affected segment. At the level of the diagnosed sensitized segment, the needle penetrates the skin so that it enters the space between the proximal spinous process and spinalis muscle (Fig. 29.4). The needle proceeds along the spinous process as far as it reaches, injecting small amounts of 1% lidocaine. Without removing the needle from the skin, the needle is redirected to the adjacent spinous process and the same technique is carried out. In the clinical setting, the paraspinous block may be performed first, followed by the preinjection block and subsequently the trigger point injection.[17,18]

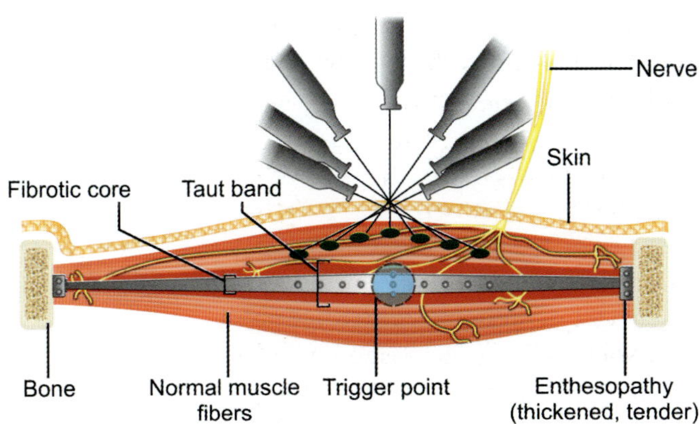

Fig. 29.3: Preinjection block.

EVIDENCE

As with most spinal injections, the evidence for the effectiveness of trigger point injections is inconclusive. They are used commonly in clinical practice, but there are not strong results from placebo-controlled trials to support their use.[22,23] Similarly, some practitioners have reported promising results with preinjection blocks and paraspinous blocks, but the techniques have yet to be rigorously validated.[17]

CONCLUSION

Trigger point injections seem to afford relief to many patients. Their effectiveness is largely dependent on mechanical disruption of muscle fibers, as there is little evidence to support the use of any particular injectate over another.[22] The only way to obtain sustained relief after a trigger point injection is to diagnose the etiological and perpetuating factors that caused the trigger point or tender spot. Otherwise, the pain is likely to recur even after a successful injection procedure.

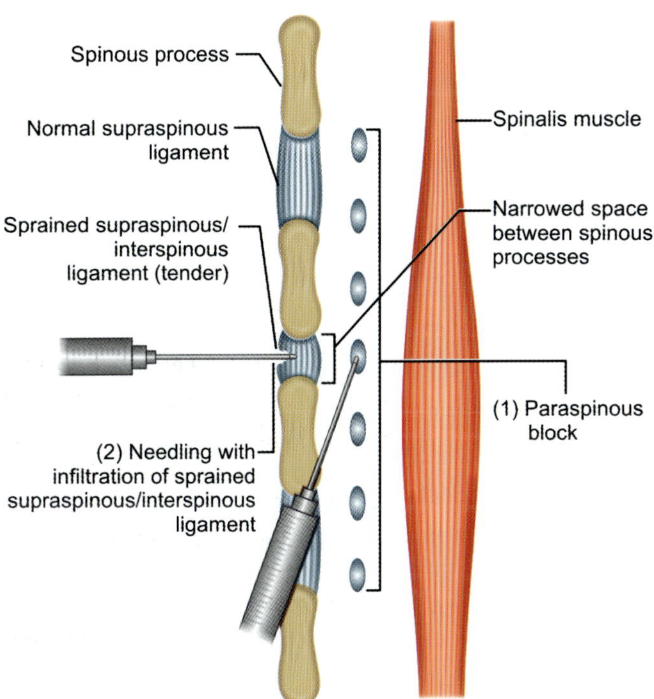

Fig. 29.4: Paraspinous block.

REFERENCES

1. Travell JG, Simons DG, Simons LS. Travell and Simons' myofascial pain and dysfunction: the trigger point manual. Philadelphia, PA: Lippincott Williams & Wilkins; 1999.
2. Malanga G, Wolff E. Evidence-informed management of chronic low back pain with trigger point injections. Spine J. 2008;8(1):243-52.
3. Borg-Stein J, Simons DG. Myofascial pain. Arch Phys Med Rehabil. 2002;83:S40-7.
4. Alvarez DJ, Rockwell PG. Trigger points: diagnosis and management. Am Fam Physician. 2002;65(4):653-62.
5. Simons DG. Review of enigmatic MTrPs as a common cause of enigmatic musculoskeletal pain and dysfunction. J Electromyogr Kinesiol. 2004;14(1):95-107.
6. Simons DG. New views of myofascial trigger points: etiology and diagnosis. Arch Phys Med Rehabil. 2008;89(1):157-9.
7. Shah JP, Danoff JV, Desai MJ, et al. Biochemicals associated with pain and inflammation are elevated in sites near to and remote from active myofascial trigger points. Arch Phys Med Rehabil. 2008;89(1):16-23.
8. Lavelle ED, Lavelle W, Smith HS. Myofascial trigger points. Med Clin N Am. 2007;91(2):229-40.
9. Lucas N, Macaskill P, Irwig L, et al. Reliability of physical examination for diagnosis of myofascial trigger points: a systematic review of the literature. Clin J Pain. 2009;25(1):80-9.
10. Kinser AM, Sands WA, Stone MH. Reliability and validity of a pressure algometer. J Strength Conditioning Res. 2009; 23(1):312.
11. Tough EA, White AR, Richards S, et al. Variability of criteria used to diagnose myofascial trigger point pain syndrome-evidence from a review of the literature. Clin J Pain. 2007; 23(3):278.
12. Wong CSM, Wong SHS. A new look at trigger point injections. Anesthesiol Res Pract. 2011;2012:492452.
13. Hubbard DR, Berkoff GM. Myofascial trigger points show spontaneous needle EMG activity. Spine. 1993;18(13):1803.
14. Sikdar S, Shah JP, Gebreab T, et al. Novel applications of ultrasound technology to visualize and characterize myofascial trigger points and surrounding soft tissue. Arch Phys Med Rehabil. 2009;90(11):1829-38.
15. Lewis J, Tehan P. A blinded pilot study investigating the use of diagnostic ultrasound for detecting active myofascial trigger points. Pain. 1999;79(1):39-44.
16. Chen Q, Bensamoun S, Basford JR, et al. Identification and quantification of myofascial taut bands with magnetic resonance elastography. Arch Phys Med Rehabil. 2007;88 (12):1658-61.
17. Fischer AA. New approaches in treatment of myofascial pain. Phys Med Rehabil Clin North Am. 1997;8:153-69.
18. Fischer AA. Treatment of myofascial pain. J Musculoskelet Pain. 1999;7(1-2):131-42.
19. Malanga GA, Cruz CEJ. Myofascial low back pain: a review. Phys Med Rehabil Clinics N Am. 2010;21(4):711.
20. Ay S, Evcik D, Tur BS. Comparison of injection methods in myofascial pain syndrome: a randomized controlled trial. Clin Rheumatol. 2010;29(1):19-23.
21. Hong CZ, Simons DG. Response to treatment for pectoralis minor myofascial pain syndrome after whiplash. J Musculoskelet Pain. 1993;1(1):89-132.
22. Cummings TM, White AR. Needling therapies in the management of myofascial trigger point pain: a systematic review. Arch Phys Med Rehabil. 2001;82(7):986-92.
23. Scott N, Guo B, Barton PM, et al. Trigger point injections for chronic non-malignant musculoskeletal pain: a systematic review. Pain Med. 2009;10(1):54-69.

CHAPTER

30

Sacroiliac Injections

Jackson Liu, Jeffrey Weinreb, Wayne Stokes

INTRODUCTION

Low back pain (LBP) is the most frequent type of pain reported by adults, the second leading cause of disability, and the leading cause of job-related disability in the United States costing >$50 billion dollars per year. Although LBP is a common complaint in primary and tertiary care, it is often difficult to reach a definitive diagnosis.[1] Identification of the significant pain generator in LBP is challenging to spine specialists.[2,3] The sacroiliac joint (SIJ) has been recognized as a source of LBP and referred pain to the lower limb with a reported prevalence ranging from 7–30%.[1,4–7]

ANATOMY

The SIJ plays an important role in load transfer between the spine, pelvis, and lower extremities. It is auricular in shape, the largest axial joint in the body, and formed by the articulation between the lateral sacrum and the medial surface of the ilium. The sacrum is wedge shaped from posterior to anterior and caudal to cephalad (Fig. 30.1). It is a true synovial (diarthroidal) joint enveloped by a fibrous capsule.[8–10] The sacral surface is covered by hyaline cartilage, whereas the ilial surface has fibrocartilage.[10] Stability of the joint is attributed primarily to the adjacent deep anterior, posterior, and interosseous ligaments and secondarily to its numerous ridges and depressions, suggesting that its function is to minimize movement and enhance stability (Fig. 30.2). Although previously thought to be immobile, studies have shown that there can be motion through the joint mostly from rotation and translation in the sagittal plane, which does not occur in a single axis.[11–14] Important mechanical and myofascial relationships are formed between the joint and other structures, such as the latissimus dorsi via the thoracolumbar fascia, gluteus maximus, piriformis, erector spinae, and iliacus.[9,10] In addition, the sacrotuberous, sacrospinal, and iliolumbar ligaments are intimately related to the SIJ.

The relationship between degenerative changes on imaging and SIJ pain is imprecise.[15] Innervation patterns of the SIJ appear multisegmental, but they are not well defined or agreed upon. Although it is thought to come from the posterior primary rami of L2–S3, a wide number of possibilities have been reported, which may explain how the joint can produce variable unique referral patterns.[1,8,9] Some have suggested ventral rami innervation, whereas others found the innervation to be primarily from dorsal rami.[9,16–19] Histological studies of the richly innervated SIJ have verified the presence of nerve fibers, both myelinated and unmyelinated, as well as mechanoreceptors within the joint capsule and adjoining ligaments.[1,10]

DIAGNOSIS

Distinguishing SIJ pain from other sources, such as the discs, facet joints, or nerve roots, remains a major challenge and is important in targeting treatment strategies.[1,4,5,20] Certain predisposing factors, such as trauma, motor vehicle accident, a direct fall on the buttocks, pregnancy, scoliolis, leg-length discrepancy, and hip osteoarthritis, have been associated with the development of SIJ pain;[8,9] however, no specific finding on clinical history or physical

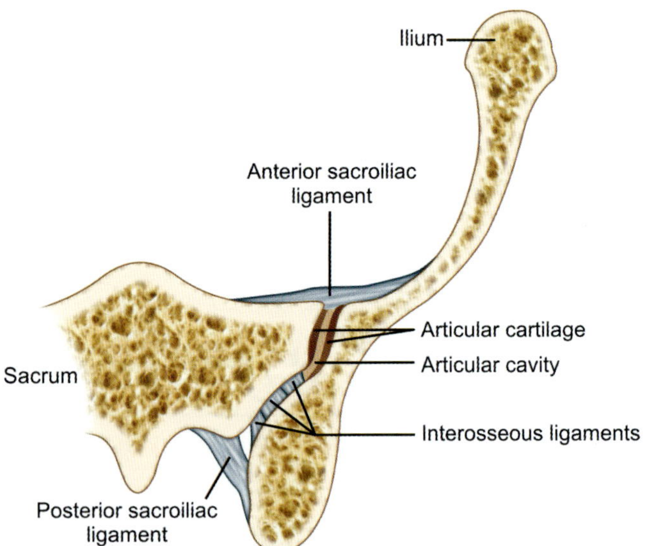

Fig. 30.1: An axial view of the sacroiliac joint demonstrating the orientation of the joint. Note the wedge shape of the joint from posterior to anterior and its articular cavity.

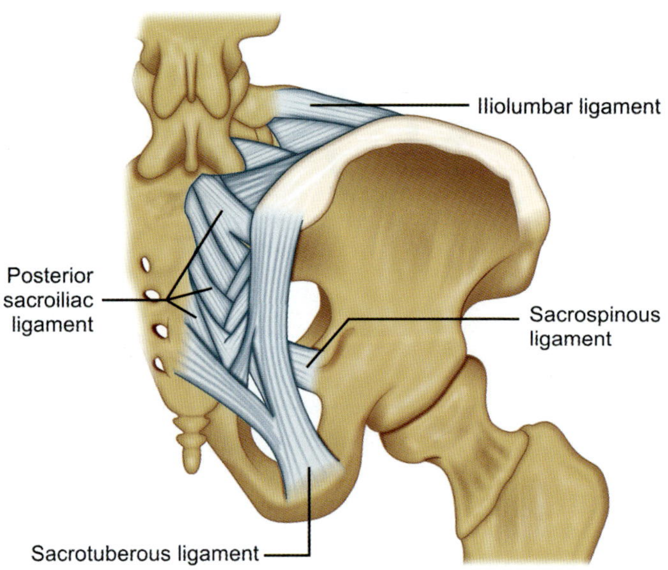

Fig. 30.2: A posterior view of the sacroiliac joint with its associated ligaments and multisegmental innervation pattern.

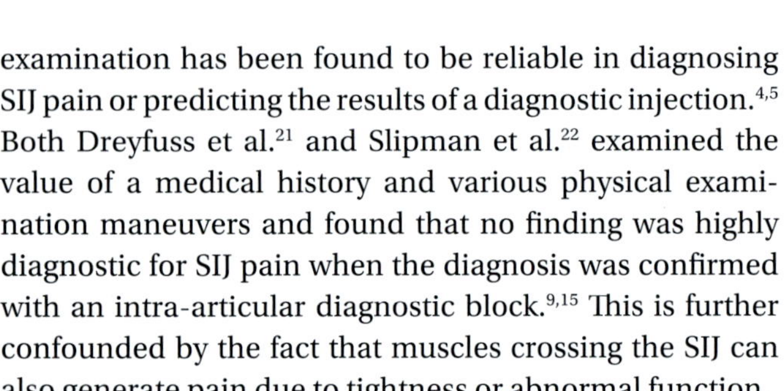

examination has been found to be reliable in diagnosing SIJ pain or predicting the results of a diagnostic injection.[4,5] Both Dreyfuss et al.[21] and Slipman et al.[22] examined the value of a medical history and various physical examination maneuvers and found that no finding was highly diagnostic for SIJ pain when the diagnosis was confirmed with an intra-articular diagnostic block.[9,15] This is further confounded by the fact that muscles crossing the SIJ can also generate pain due to tightness or abnormal function.

The SIJ pain is thought to be located below the L5 level. Dreyfuss et al.[21] and Slipman et al.[22] found that patients having tenderness medial to the posterior superior iliac spine had high predictive value for SIJ pain.[9] A study by Fortin et al.,[20] in which asymptomatic subjects underwent intra-articular injection of contrast medium and local anesthetic, revealed a pain referral pattern with hyperesthesia in the buttocks approximately 10 cm inferiorly and 3 cm laterally from the posterior superior iliac spine. A presumptive diagnosis of SIJ pain on physical examination may correlate with concordant reproduction of the patient's typical or usual pain. Many examination maneuvers are used to this purpose including the thigh thrust, distraction, compression, sacral thrust, stork, Fortin's finger test, Patrick's test, Gaenslen's test, and Gillet's test.[6,9,10,23] These tests, however, fail to target the SIJ independently of other structures.[4,20,23] Increased reliability has been seen when using a multitest regimen and eliciting more positive tests.[4,5,24]

Pain diagrams have been suggested as a good preliminary screening tool for diagnosis and should demonstrate rectangular pattern of pain just inferior to the posterior superior iliac spine. They have been shown to predict patient response to provocative intra-articular injections.[10,20,25] Neurologic examination of the patient is typically normal and any true neurogenic findings, such as deficits in strength, sensory, or reflex testing, should alert the clinician to an alternate diagnosis.[9] Finally, it should be taken into consideration that SIJ can coexist with other conditions like lumbar discogenic or facet pain.[23]

It is important to keep in mind that SIJ pain patterns are diverse and may be dull, sharp, aching, or intense in character. The presence of referred pain, resembling a radiculopathy to the buttocks, thigh, calf, or foot, does not support or discriminate against the diagnosis.[6,21] Computed tomography (CT) arthrography studies in patients with LBP have shown that the joint can communicate with and leak onto nearby neural structures. This was demonstrated as posterior extravasation into the dorsal sacral foramina, superior recess extravasation at the sacral alar level to the fifth lumbar epiradicular sheath, and ventral extravasation onto the lumbosacral plexus (Figs. 30.3A to C). In this model, a traumatized and inflamed joint can extravasate inflammatory mediators such as substance P and possibly explain referral of SIJ pain that resembles sciatica (Figs. 30.4A and B).[10,26,27]

The use of radiologic imaging studies for diagnosis remains controversial, and no specific findings have

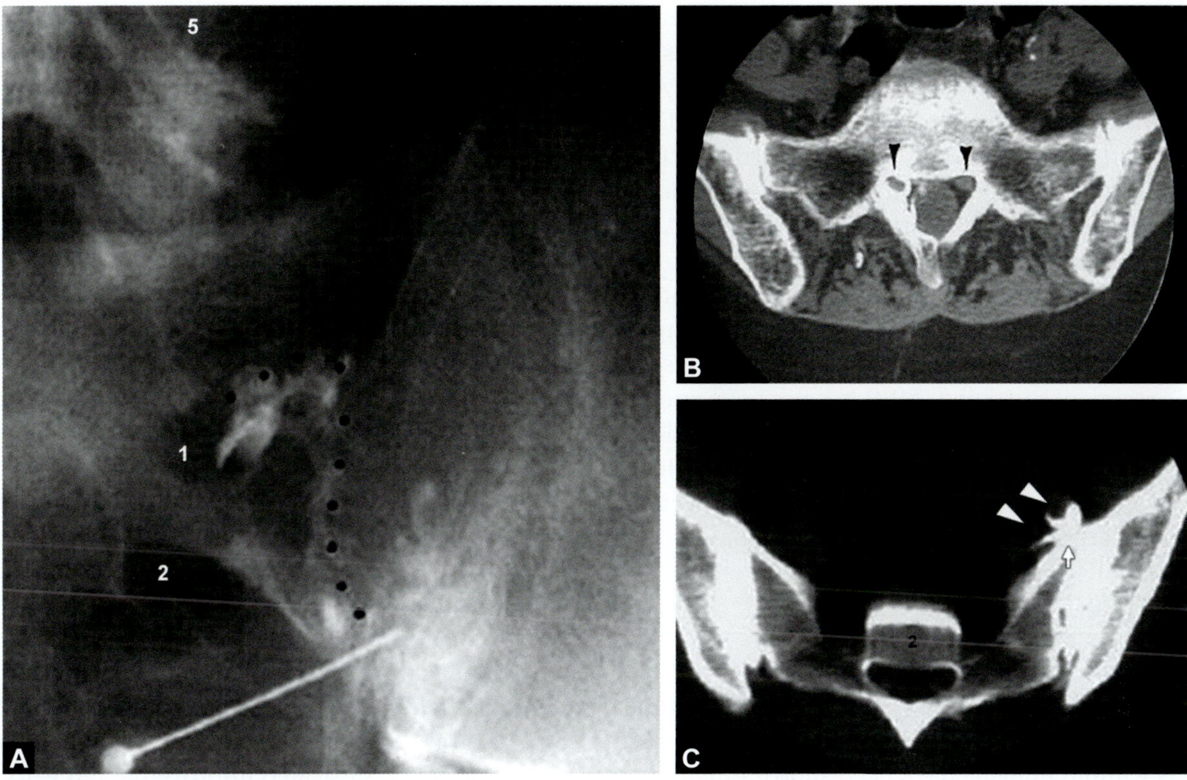

Figs. 30.3A to C: (A) Arthrogram of the anteroposterior view reveals contrast medium extending into the S1 dorsal foramina denoted by the number 1. The S2 dorsal foramina is labeled as 2, and the pedicle of L5 is labeled as 5. (B) Axial computed tomographic (CT) scan post-arthrography at the S1 level with the arrows pointing at the S1 anterior rami bilaterally. Contrast medium has extravasated and encircles the S1 segmental root. (C) Axial CT scan post-arthrography at the S2 level showing contrast medium in both SIJs. A presacral collection of contrast medium is evidence of a left ventral capsular tear (open arrow). Contrast medium contracts the lumbosacral plexus elements (arrowheads). *Source*: With permission from Fortin et al.[26]

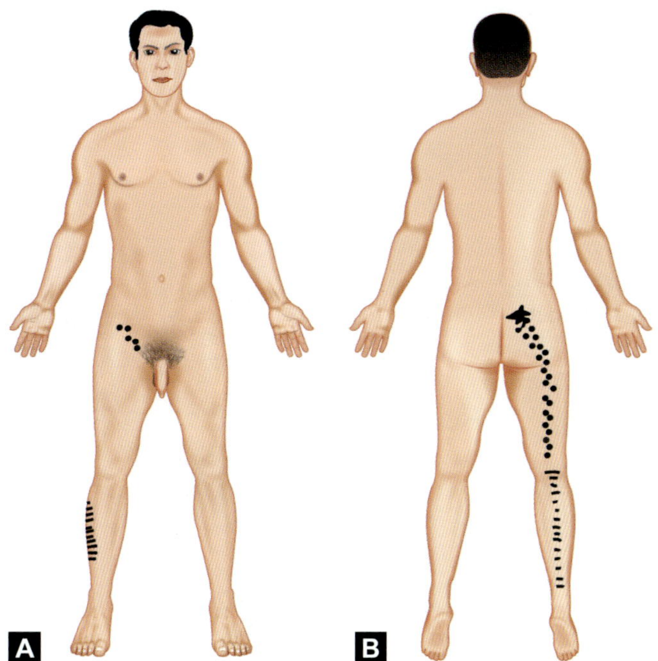

Figs. 30.4A and B: Pain referral diagram of typical sacroiliac joint syndrome.

correlated well with a diagnosis of SIJ pain.[9,28] Cohen et al.[45] found that plain radiographs can be abnormal and show evidence of sacroiliac abnormality in up to 25% of asymptomatic patients above the age of 50. Similarly, CT findings, including joint space narrowing, reactive spurring, sclerosis, or subluxation, have been seen in 77% of asymptomatic subjects < 30 years[29] with a reported sensitivity of 57% and a specificity of 69%.[9,13] Bone scans may reveal enhancement adjacent to the SIJ with inflammatory conditions but have low sensitivity of 12–46% in patients with chronic noninflammatory SIJ disease.[9,30] The diagnostic use of magnetic resonance imaging (MRI) has not been studied for patients with SIJ pain.[31] Laboratory work-up including rheumatologic and inflammatory markers may aid in ruling out spondyloarthropathic, metabolic,or infectious etiologies but are generally nonspecific for SIJ pain.[10]

INJECTION

Fluoroscopically guided SIJ injections are used to both diagnose SIJ pain and provide treatment when other conservative measures fail (Figs. 30.5A and B). Blind injections without imaging have been shown to have low accuracy, being intra-articular in only 22% of subjects.[32] Extravasation of injectant is common and reduces diagnostic specificity, although some studies have indicated that periarticular injections may provide some benefit as well.[29,33] Although there is no accepted gold standard, these injections are considered the best reference test available for diagnosis.[1,8,9,28,31] There is no agreement of what constitutes a positive diagnostic response, but 50–100% pain relief has been reported[9] and 75% has been used in many clinical settings. Comparative or double blocks have been employed to increase the diagnostic value of these injections and decrease false positive findings.[23,28] In such a paradigm, two injections are administered at two separate times, commonly with different anesthetic agents, and pain is accessed pre- and postinjection. A similar response to both injections is considered highly diagnostic.[9]

While intra-articular SIJ injections are used frequently to treat patients with suspected SIJ disease, there is a relative lack of studies on the efficacy of these injections.[33] In patients with seronegative spondyloarthropathies, the efficacy of these injections has been demonstrated both retrospectively and prospectively.[31,34,35] The first study showing efficacy of SIJ corticosteroid injections for treatment in patients with SIJ syndrome was done by Slipman et al.[31] In this retrospective study of 31 patients, patients postinjection demonstrated improvement in work status, reduction in pain scores, and reduction in the Oswestry Disability Index score.[31] There has also been recent research on blocks targeting the lateral branches of the dorsal

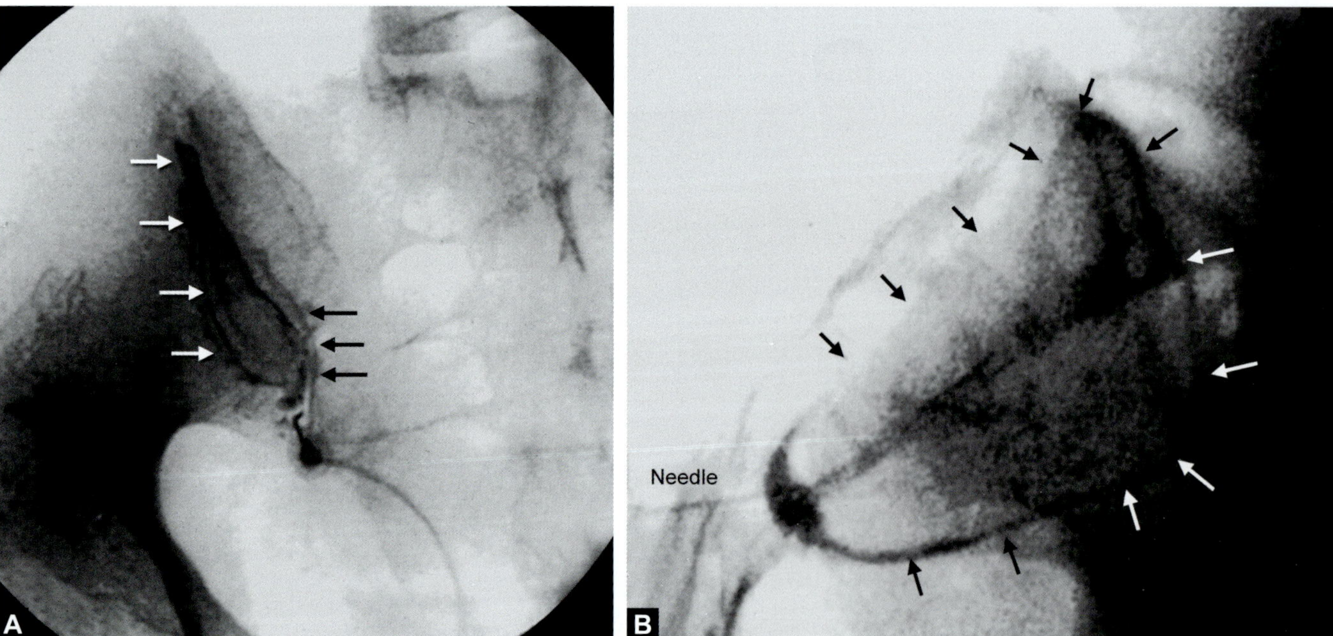

Figs. 30.5A and B: The normal intra-articular contrast pattern of the sacroiliac joint.
Source: Reproduced with permission from Bogduk N (Ed). Practice guidelines for spinal diagnostic and treatment procedures. International Spine Intervention Society, San Francisco, 2004.

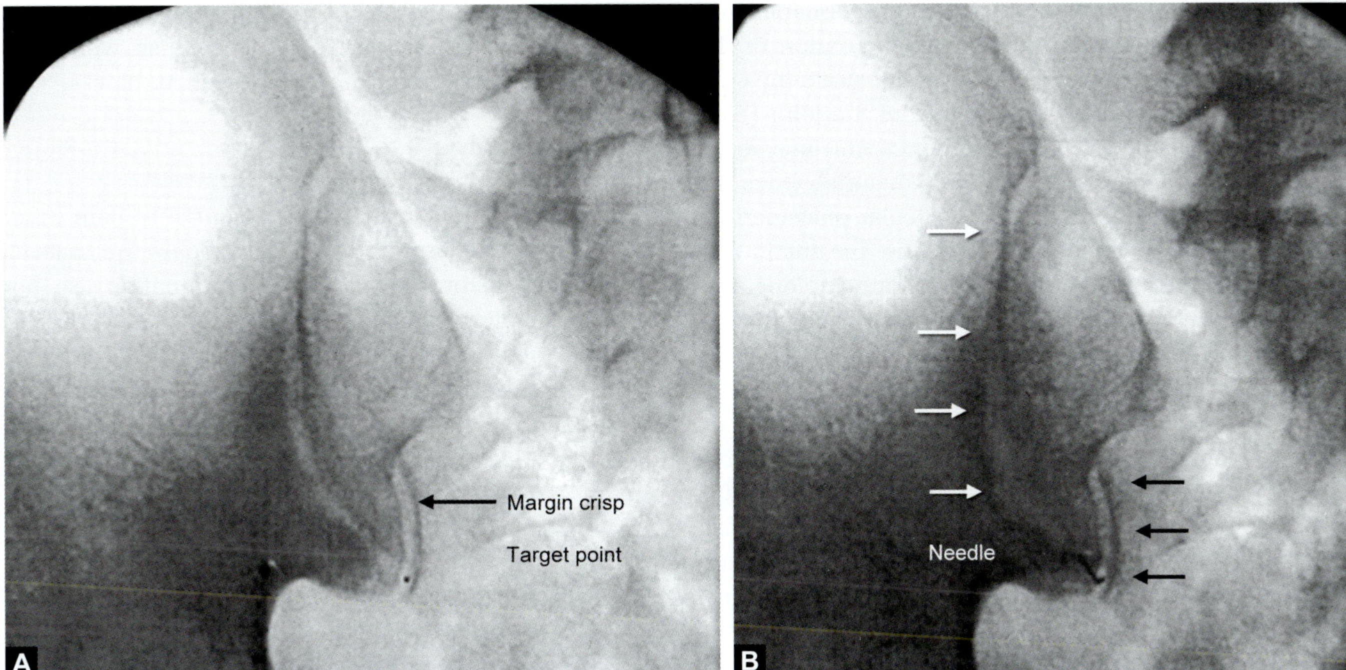

Figs. 30.6A and B: (A) An anteroposterior view of the sacroiliac joint (SIJ) where the posterior margins of the joint are most lucent over the lower 1/3 of the joint. (B) Posterior view of the SIJ where the white arrows delineate the lateral lines marking the ventral joint margin and the black arrows delineate the medial lines marking the dorsal joint margin. The needle is directed toward the inferior aspect of the joint as shown. *Source*: Reproduced with permission from Bogduk N (Ed). Practice guidelines for spinal diagnostic and treatment procedures. International Spine Intervention Society, San Francisco, 2004.

rami at S1–S3 and the medial branches of the L4–5 dorsal rami without actually injecting into the joint, and these have shown some diagnostic value. In addition, there may be a role for radiofrequency (RF) ablation to denervate the sensory fibers transmitting pain from the joint and provide longer lasting pain relief, but further research is needed.[8]

The primary indication for an injection is to rule out the SIJ as a pain generator. This is indicated for patients with chronic LBP that is located at or below the L5 level with or without referred lower extremity pain for whom no other diagnosis is apparent and in whom no other diagnosis is more likely. It includes cases where a diagnosis cannot be made without more invasive options and conservative measures have failed to relieve pain.[36]

INJECTION TECHNIQUE

Proper setup for such an injection requires a fluoroscopy suite including a C-arm and patient monitoring equipment. After obtaining informed consent and explaining the purpose of the injection, the patient is positioned in a prone position on the table with a pillow under the pelvis. Under an anteroposterior (AP) view, the lower margin of the SIJ is identified. The C-arm is rotated until the medial posterior cortical line is most clear and lucent, taking note of the joint projecting medial to lateral while going posterior to anterior. Once a point of entry is targeted, the skin is cleansed with a sterile prep such as an iodine-based solution or chlorhexidine. The injection of a local anesthetic like lidocaine at the site of needle entry and its track is used to decrease the pain of the procedure.

Under image intensifier control, a 22 or 25-gauge 3.5 inch spinal needle is directed toward the inferior aspect of the SIJ from a posterior approach. The most common entry point is in the inferior third of the SIJ, approximately 1–2 cm above the inferior joint margin (Figs. 30.6A and B). The needle is advanced using intermittent screening with the fluoroscope until it engages the dorsal sacroiliac and interosseous ligaments. There may be a slight turn or bend in the needle as it engages the joint and a sense of giving way or change in the tactile feel during penetration.

Injection of a contrast medium is administered into the joint space. This should be a nonionic and hypoallergenic contrast agent such as iopamidol or iohexol. The AP prone view will detail the inferior articular recess and may reveal contrast as a discreet line between the ilium and sacrum.

The end face view (contralateral oblique) is obtained and may highlight a classical auricular configuration of the joint capsule. The lateral view may demonstrate the contrast medium outlining the perimeter of the joint (Figs. 30.5A and B). Disruption of the anterior capsule may result in periarticular spread of the contrast material. Once the clinician is satisfied with an intra-articular placement of the needle, a combination of lidocaine anesthetic and steroid is injected. Betamethasone or triamcinolone acetonide dexamethasone can be used in a 1:1 or 2:1 mixture of anesthetic and steroid. The capacity of most adult SIJs is < 2 cm^3, so care should be taken to use only 0.5 cm^3 of contrast material and 1–1.5 cm^3 of steroid mixture. In 74 patients undergoing sacroiliac injections, the mean volume of the joint was found to be 1.08 mL, with a range from 0.8 to 1.8 mL.[37] A total maximum volume of contrast and local anesthetic of 2.0 mL has been reported.[6] Post procedure care after injections should follow appropriate guidelines.

COMPLICATIONS

Adverse events associated with fluoroscopically guided SIJ injections have been described as rare including transient lower extremity weakness and complete penetration of the joint contacting the sciatic nerve.[38] As with any steroid injection, risks include hematoma, infection, allergic reaction, hyperglycemia, and fluid retention.[33] A large study by Plastaras et al.[38] revealed a 2.6% incidence of adverse events mostly from vagal episodes and a 24.2% of delayed adverse events, including injection site soreness, pain exacerbation, facial flushing, or sweating, possibly related to the effects of the steroid preparations.[38]

NEWER TECHNIQUES

Ultrasound-guided injections of the SIJ are emerging as a new technique that can be done in the office and has the prime advantage of not having to expose patients to harmful radiation. Although one study using MRI and gadolinium revealed only 40% success of an intra-articular SIJ injection,[39] many others have demonstrated success rates of up to 90% when controlled with fluoroscopy.[39-43] This technique is of high interest while research and clinician experience is needed to confirm its efficacy.

Radiofrequency neurotomy is becoming an increasingly popular intervention in the treatment of nonspecific lower back and extremity pain. The procedure utilizes an RF electrode to coagulate suspected painful SIJ nerves. RF lesioning has been used for about 10 years, with generally positive results. Proper patient selection is crucial, and the best candidates are those who have obtained effective but transient relief with SIJ blocks.[44,45]

CONCLUSION

The SIJ should be considered as a source of pain in all patients with LBP, especially when it is below the L5 level. The clinical history and physical examination are not entirely reliable means of diagnosing SIJ pain. Although there has been some controversy regarding the benefits of SIJ pain intervention,[46] an SIJ injection may be both therapeutic and diagnostic in patients with LBP. Obtaining an accurate diagnosis in these patients is a worthwhile pursuit as it can appropriately guide management and direct further care.

REFERENCES

1. Simopoulos T, Manchikanti L, Singh V, et al. A systematic evaluation of prevalence and diagnostic accuracy of sacroiliac joint interventions. Pain Physician. 2012;15(3):E305.
2. Deyo RA, Mirza SK, Martin BI. Back pain prevalence and visit rates: estimates from US national surveys, 2002. Spine. 2006;31(23):2724-7.
3. Sembrano JN, Polly DW Jr. How often is low back pain not coming from the back? Spine. 2009;34(1):E27-E32.
4. Laslett M, Aprill CN, McDonald B, et al. Diagnosis of sacroiliac joint pain: validity of individual provocation tests and composites of tests. Man Ther. 2005;10(3):207-18.
5. van der Wurff P, Buijs EJ, Groen GJ. A multitest regimen of pain provocation tests as an aid to reduce unnecessary minimally invasive sacroiliac joint procedures. Arch Phys Med Rehabil. 2006;87(1):10-14.
6. Schwarzer AC, Aprill CN, Bogduk N. The sacroiliac joint in chronic low back pain. Spine. 1995;20(1):31.
7. Migliore A, Bizzi E, Massafra U, et al. A new technical contribution for ultrasound-guided injections of sacro-iliac joints. Eur Rev Med Pharmacol Sci. 2010;14(5):465-9.
8. Aydin SM, Gharibo CG, Mehnert M, et al. The role of radiofrequency ablation for sacroiliac joint pain: a meta-analysis. PM&R. 2010;2(9):842-51.
9. Sembrano JN, Reiley MA, Polly DW, Jr, Garfin SR. Diagnosis and treatment of sacroiliac joint pain. Curr Orthop Pract. 2011;22(4):344-50.
10. Forst S, Wheeler M, Fortin J, et al. The sacroiliac joint: anatomy, physiology and clinical significance. Pain Physician. 2006;9(1):61.
11. Vleeming A, Schuenke M, Masi A, et al. The sacroiliac joint: an overview of its anatomy, function and potential clinical implications. J Anat. 2012;221(6):537-67.
12. Vleeming A, Van Wingerden J, Dijkstra P, et al. Mobility in the sacroiliac joints in the elderly: a kinematic and radiological study. Clin Biomech. 1992;7(3):170-6.

13. Greenman PE. Principles of manual medicine. Baltimore, MD: Lippincott Williams & Wilkins, 1989.
14. Harrison DE, Harrison DD, Troyanovich SJ. The sacroiliac joint: a review of anatomy and biomechanics with clinical implications. J Manipulative Physiol Ther. 1997; 20(9): 607-17.
15. Bernard T, Cassidy J. The sacroiliac joint syndrome: pathophysiology, diagnosis, and management. In: The adult spine: principles and practice. New York, NY: Raven Press Ltd, 1991:2107-30.
16. Solonen KA. The sacroiliac joint in the light of anatomical, roentgenological and clinical studies. Acta Orthop Scand Suppl. 1957;27:1.
17. Nakagawa T. Study on the distribution of nerve filaments over the iliosacral joint and its adjacent region in the Japanese. Nihon Seikeigeka Gakkai zasshi. 1966;40(4):419.
18. Grob K, Neuhuber W, Kissling R. Die innervation des sacroiliacalgelenkes beim menschen. Zeitschrift für Rheumatologie. 1995;54(2):117-22.
19. Fortin J, Kissling R, O'Connor B, et al. Sacroiliac joint innervation and pain. Am J Orthop (Belle Mead, NJ). 1999;28(12): 687.
20. Fortin JD, Dwyer AP, West S, et al. Sacroiliac joint: pain referral maps upon applying a new injection/arthrography technique. Part I: Asymptomatic volunteers. Spine (Phila Pa 1976). 1994;19(13):1475-82.
21. Dreyfuss P, Michaelsen M, Pauza K, et al. The value of medical history and physical examination in diagnosing sacroiliac joint pain. Spine. 1996;21(22):2594.
22. Slipman CW, Sterenfeld EB, Chou LH, et al. The predictive value of provocative sacroiliac joint stress maneuvers in the diagnosis of sacroiliac joint syndrome. Arch Phys Med Rehabil. 1998;79(3):288.
23. Maigne JY, Aivaliklis A, Pfefer F. Results of sacroiliac joint double block and value of sacroiliac pain provocation tests in 54 patients with low back pain. Spine. 1996;21(16):1889-92.
24. Kokmeyer DJ, van der Wurff P, Aufdemkampe G, et al. The reliability of multitest regimens with sacroiliac pain provocation tests. J Manipulative Physiol Ther. 2002;25(1):42-8.
25. Fortin JD, Aprill CN, Ponthieux B, et al. Sacroiliac joint: pain referral maps upon applying a new injection/arthrography technique. Part II: Clinical evaluation. Spine. 1994;19(13): 1483.
26. Fortin JD, Washington WJ, Falco FJE. Three pathways between the sacroiliac joint and neural structures. Am J Neuroradiol. 1999;20(8):1429-34.
27. Fortin JD, Vilensky JA, Merkel GJ. Can the sacroiliac joint cause sciatica? Pain Physician. 2003;6(3):269-72.
28. Slipman CW, Whyte W, Chow DW, et al. Sacroiliac joint syndrome. Pain Physician. 2001;4(2):143-52.
29. Vogler J, Brown W, Helms C, Genant H. The normal sacroiliac joint: a CT study of asymptomatic patients. Radiology. 1984;151(2):433-7.
30. Slipman CW, Sterenfeld EB, Chou LH, et al. The value of radionuclide imaging in the diagnosis of sacroiliac joint syndrome. Spine. 1996;21(19):2251-4.
31. Slipman CW, Lipetz JS, Plastaras CT, et al. Fluoroscopically guided therapeutic sacroiliac joint injections for sacroiliac joint syndrome. Am J Phys Med Rehabil. 2001;80(6):425-32.
32. Rosenberg JM, Quint DJ, de Rosayro AM. Computerized tomographic localization of clinically-guided sacroiliac joint injections. Clin J Pain. 2000;16(1):18-21.
33. Colonno DV, Harrast MA, Herring SA. Overview of spinal interventions. Clin Sports Med. 2012;31(3):409.
34. Maugars Y, Mathis C, Berthelot JM, Charlier C, Prost A. Assessment of the efficacy of sacroiliac corticosteroid injections in spondyloarthropathies: a double-blind study. Rheumatology. 1996;35(8):767-70.
35. Maugars Y, Mathis C, Vilon P, et al. Corticosteroid injection of the sacroiliac joint in patients with seronegative spondyloarthropathy. Arthritis Rheum. 1992;35(5):564-8.
36. Manchikanti L, Boswell MV, Singh V, et al. Comprehensive evidence-based guidelines for interventional techniques in the management of chronic spinal pain. Pain Physician. 2009;12(4):699-802.
37. Fortin JD, Tolchin RB. Sacroiliac arthrograms and post-arthrography computerized tomography. Pain Physician. 2003;6(3):287-90.
38. Plastaras CT, Joshi AB, Garvan C, et al. Adverse events associated with fluoroscopically guided sacroiliac joint injections. PM&R. 2012;4(7):473-8.
39. Hartung W, Ross CJ, Straub R, et al. Ultrasound-guided sacroiliac joint injection in patients with established sacroiliitis: precise IA injection verified by MRI scanning does not predict clinical outcome. Rheumatology. 2010;49(8): 1479-82.
40. Chen CPC, Lew HL, Tsai WC, et al. Ultrasound-guided injection techniques for the low back and hip joint. Am J Phys Med Rehabil. 2011;90(10):860-7.
41. Klauser A, De Zordo T, Feuchtner G, et al. Feasibility of ultrasound-guided sacroiliac joint injection considering sonoanatomic landmarks at two different levels in cadavers and patients. Arthritis Care Res. 2008;59(11):1618-24.
42. Pekkafalı MZ, Kıralp MZ, Başekim CÇ, et al. Sacroiliac joint injections performed with sonographic guidance. J Ultrasound Med. 2003;22(6):553-9.
43. Harmon D, O'Sullivan M. Ultrasound-guided sacroiliac joint injection technique. Pain Physician. 2008;11(4):543-7.
44. Burnham RS, Yasui Y. An alternate method of radiofrequency neurotomy of the sacroiliac joint: a pilot study of the effect on pain, function, and satisfaction. Reg Anesth Pain Med. 2007;32(1):12-9.
45. Cohen SP, Chen Y, Neufeld NJ. Sacroiliac joint pain: a comprehensive review of epidemiology, diagnosis and treatment. Expert Rev Neurother. 2013;13(1):99-116.
46. Conover N. A systematic evaluation of the therapeutic effectiveness of sacroiliac joint interventions. Pain Physician. 2012; 15:E247-78.

CHAPTER

31

Peripheral Joint and Soft Tissue Injections

Warren Young

INTRODUCTION

Musculoskeletal aspiration and injection of the peripheral joints and soft tissues can have diagnostic and therapeutic purpose. Corticosteroids injections were first performed by Thorn in 1940, but it was Hollander in 1951 who established the use of it in practice for placement at intra-articular joints, bursa, and tendon sheaths.[1] Over the past seven decades, the efficacy and safety of corticosteroid injections have been debated, and recent studies have sought to answer questions regarding side effects, cartilage injury, and risk versus benefits. As new medications and injectates such as viscosupplementation, platelet-rich plasma (PRP), sclerosing agents for prolotherapy, and stem cells are utilized, more studies are needed to determine their safety and efficacy.

Peripheral injections used for diagnostic means can help differentiate between intra-articular versus extra-articular sources of pain in areas such as the shoulder, hip, and knee. Therapeutic injections of corticosteroids in the joints and soft tissues can help alleviate pain in musculoskeletal and rheumatologic conditions and allow continuation and completion of necessary physical therapy. Newer therapies such as PRP and stem cell injections may prove to be useful for various conditions, but continued research is needed.

Overall, injections and aspirations of the peripheral joints and soft tissues can be done safely and effectively with the proper training of injection techniques, understanding of the risks and benefits of the medications used, and utilization for appropriate diagnoses. Discussion of specific technique for every injection location is beyond the scope of this chapter.

INJECTABLES

Corticosteroids

Corticosteroids are one of the most common medications injected into peripheral joints and soft tissues. They are used to treat an extensive list of musculoskeletal diagnoses, including osteoarthritis, rheumatoid arthritis, bursitis, tenosynovitis, systemic lupus erythematosus, and gout. The most common corticosteroids used in musculoskeletal injections are synthetic derivatives of prednisolone such as methylprednisolone, betamethasone, dexamethasone, and triamcinolone. These corticosteroids have predominantly glucocorticoid and anti-inflammatory effects. Their primary mechanism of action is to increase lipocortin-1 synthesis, suppressing phospholipase A2, thereby inhibiting prostaglandin and leukotriene production, as well as suppressing cyclooxygenase expression.[2]

Corticosteroids preparations are described by their potency, solubility, and crystalline composition. Most preparations are insoluble and contain corticosteroid esters, which form microcrystalline suspension. The advantage of crystalline formation is that they require hydrolysis in the tissues to become active and therefore have a longer duration of effect than nonester preparations.[3] Insoluble steroids such as methylprednisolone, triamcinolone hexacetonide will have a longer duration of action, whereas more soluble steroids such as betamethasone acetate will have a shorter duration of action. Preparations with higher solubility will have higher chance of systemic effects, whereas insoluble solution have higher incidence of cutaneous side effects such as tissue atrophy. Table 31.1 lists the commonly used corticosteroids in musculoskeletal injections.

Table 31.1: Common corticosteroid preparations

Corticosteroid	*Commercial name*	*Approximate duration of action (days)*	*Solubility*	*Dose equivalent (mg)*	*Dose for large joints (knee/ shoulder) (mg)*
Betamethasone sodium phosphate/ betamethasone acetate	Celestone Soluspan	7	Soluble/slightly soluble	0.75	12
Triamcinolone acetonide	Kenalog	14	Insoluble	4	40–80
Triamcinolone hexacetonide	Aristospan	21	Insoluble	4	40–80
Dexamethasone sodium phosphate	Decadron	6	Relatively insoluble	0.75	4
Methylprednisolone acetate	Depo Medrol	28	Relatively insoluble	4	40–80

Data combined from multiple sources: Official drug labels of respective medications, Saunders 2002 "The Clinics Atlas of Office Procedures", Saunders 2008, The Sports Medicine Resource Manual.

Indications

Corticosteroid injection is commonly indicated for intra-articular, periarticular, and soft tissue conditions. They can be used as definitive treatment, adjuvant treatment of pain to promote more effective rehabilitation, or temporary pain relief for chronic pain syndromes. (Table 31.2)

Adverse Effects

The potential adverse effects of cortisone injection into joint or soft tissue are listed in Table 31.3. Most common local effects are postinjection pain flare, subcutaneous fat atrophy, and skin atrophy and depigmentation. Facial flushing is a common systemic effect. Systemic effects associated with prolong oral steroids are rare after a one-time injection. The risk of adverse events is increased with increased frequency and dose of corticosteroids.

Cartilage injury is of particular interest. One randomized controlled trial showed no radiographic changes of joint deterioration over a 2-year period consisting of triamcinolone injections every 3 months compared with saline injections.[4] Animal studies of intra-articular hydrocortisone and methylprednisolone injections have shown cartilage injury.[5,6] More recently, in vitro studies of human chondrocytes have shown significant decrease in viability from a single-injection dose of betamethasone.[7] A synergistic increase in chondrotoxicity may also exist when a mixture of betamethasone and a local anesthetic such as lidocaine or bupivacaine is injected into joints.[8]

Increased rates of tendon rupture in weight-bearing locations such as the Achilles tendon and plantar fascia are associated with peritendinous injections of cortisone.[9,10] While the exact incidence is not known, one retrospective

Table 31.2: Potential indications for corticosteroid injection

Inflammatory arthritides
- Rheumatoid arthritis
- Seronegative spondyloarthropathies
  - Ankylosing spondylitis
  - Psoriatic arthritis
  - Reiter's syndrome
- Crystal-induced arthropathies
  - Gout/pseudogout

Noninflammatory arthritides
- Osteoarthritis

Periarticular/soft tissue injection
- Adhesive capsulitis
- Bursitis
  - Pes anserine
  - Prepatella
  - Olecranon
  - Trochanteric
  - Subacromial
- Tenosynovitis/tendonitis
  - Proximal biceps tendonitis
  - De Quervain's tenosynovitis
  - Stenosing tenosynovitis (trigger finger)
  - Lateral and medial epicondylitis
  - Plantar fasciitis
- Entrapments neuropathies
  - Carpal tunnel syndrome
  - Tarsal tunnel syndrome
  - Cubital tunnel syndrome
- Other conditions
  - Trigger points
  - Ganglion cysts

Adapted from The clinics Atlas of Office Procedures: Joint Injection Techniques, vol 5, Number 4. Philadelphia, PA: WB Saunders, 2002.

study reported an annual incidence of total Achilles ruptures to be 2.4 and 0.2%, respectively, for patients with and without prior corticosteroid injection.[11]

Absolute and relative contraindications for the use of corticosteroids are listed in Table 31.4.

Local Anesthetics

Anesthetics can be injected alone or with corticosteroids into joints and soft tissue. The most commonly used anesthetics are lidocaine, bupivacaine, and ropivacaine (Table 31.5). They can aid for diagnostic and therapeutic purposes of the procedure. Anesthetics with epinephrine are typically not used in peripheral musculoskeletal aspiration and injections.

Table 31.3: Potential adverse outcomes from corticosteroid injections

Complication
Local
• Postinjection pain flare
• Joint or soft tissue infection
• Skin atrophy/depigmentation
• Subcutaneous fat atrophy
• Tendon rupture
• Steroid arthropathy
Systemic
• Facial flushing
• Syncope or temporary dizziness
• Transient paresis
• Hypersensitivity reaction
• Addisons
• Psychiatric changes
• Hyperphagia
• Hyperglycemia
• Immunosuppression
• Acne
• Weight gain
• Hypertension
• Osteoporosis
• Cataracts

Local anesthetics can also facilitate steroid spread and serve to dilute the preservatives contained in the corticosteroid.

Preservative free local anesthetics are preferred injectate of choice. Parabens are present in multiuse vials as a preservative and may cause allergic reactions. Parabens can precipitate corticosteroids and can potentially lead to a post injection flare. Single-use vials of anesthetics are therefore preferred when mixing with corticosteroids.

Nole et al.[12] were the first to publish the chondrotoxic effects of bupivacaine on porcine and canine articular cartilage. Multiple studies since have shown that lidocaine, bupivacaine, and ropivacaine all have cytotoxic effects on chondrocytes, which are increased with longer duration of exposure and higher concentrations of the anesthetic.[13] Ropivacaine may have less chondrotoxic effects than lidocaine and bupivacaine.[14] It is recommended that for intra-articular injections, only the minimum dose of anesthetic necessary for diagnosis and therapy be used.

Viscosupplementation

Hyaluronan is an anionic, nonsulfated, high molecular weight glycosaminoglycan that is present in joints as well as other locations in the human body. It is also referred to as hyaluronate and hyaluronic acid. The properties of hyaluronan were first described by Karl Meyer in

Table 31.4: Absolute and relative contraindications for corticosteroid injection

Absolute
• Acute systemic infection
• Overlying skin or soft tissue infection
• Septic effusion
• Intra-articular fracture
• Hypersensitivity reaction to the medication
• Prosthetic joint
• Unstable joint
Relative
• Coagulopathy or anticoagulated
• Poorly controlled diabetes
• Immunosuppressed
• Uncooperative patient

Table 31.5: Local anesthetics

Anesthetic	*Strengths*	*Onset of action (minutes)*	*Duration of action t½ (hours)*
Lidocaine (Xylocaine)	1%, 2%	1–2	1
Bupivacaine (Marcaine)	0.25%, 0.5%, 0.75%	3–5	2–4
Ropivacaine (Naropin)	0.5%, 0.75%	10–30	2–6

Data obtained from official drug labels of respective medications.

the 1930s. It is a polymer of disaccharides composed of repeating sequences of D-glucuronic acid and D-N-acetyl-glucosamine.[15] There are on average about 2500 repeating disaccharide units in hyaluronan with a molecular weight of 4000 Daltons (Da), but the number of repeating disaccharides varies. Polymers of hyaluronan can vary in size from 5,000 to 20,000,000 Da. In joints, it is produced by fibroblasts in the synovial membrane.[16]

In the healthy human knee, the average molecular weight of hyaluronan in human synovial fluid is 6–7 million Da, with a concentration of 2.5–4.0 mg/mL. In injured and diseased knees, the concentration and molecular weight of hyaluronan is decreased. For osteoarthritis of the knee, the concentration of hyaluronic acid is reduced to one half to one third of the normal value.[17,18]

The full spectrum of function of hyaluronan is not entirely known. In the human joint, hyaluronan functions as a lubricant, shock absorber, and an anti-inflammatory. It may also have anabolic effects, analgesic, and chondroprotective activity.[18] Hyaluronan is viscoelastic, meaning that it has both viscous and elastic properties, acting as a lubricant during slow activity, and as a shock absorber during fast movements. It has been shown in vivo and in vitro to have effects on leukocyte function including inhibition of phagocytosis, adherence,[19] and mitogen-induced stimulation.[20]

In patients with arthritis, intra-articular injection of hyaluronan has been reported to decrease the levels of prostaglandin and cyclic adenosine phosphate in synovial fluid.[21] Animal studies of intra-articular hyaluronic acid have shown that it suppresses production of inflammatory cytokines and other inflammatory mediators.[22] It may act to stimulate endogenous hyaluronic acid production in patients with osteoarthritis.[23] Its chondroprotective effects may include functioning as a scavenger of free radicals,[15] inhibiting degenerative changes within chondrocytes and the cartilage matrix, enhancing cartilage proteoglycan content, inhibiting apoptosis, and improving cartilage metabolism adjacent to cartilage injury.[24]

Formulations of hyaluronan available in the United States are listed in Table 31.6.

Indications

Hyaluronan injections are currently only Food and Drug Administration approved for use in the osteoarthritis of the knee. A Cochran Review in 2006 of viscosupplementation for the treatment of osteoarthritis of the knee concluded from 76 studies that viscosupplementation was an effective treatment for osteoarthritis of the knee as compared with placebo, with more prolonged effects than intra-articular corticosteroids, and comparable efficacy to nonsteroidal anti-inflammatory drugs.[25]

In addition to osteoarthritis of the knee, intra-articular hyaluronan injections may be useful after partial meniscectomy[26] and microfracture surgery.[27] Studies have also suggested possible benefits in osteoarthritis of the ankle,[28,29] shoulder,[30-33] and hip.[34,35] but further studies are necessary.

Adverse Effects

Intra-articular hyaluronan injections of the knee are associated with low rates of adverse effects. The most common adverse reactions consist of localized pain or effusion and resolved within 1 to 3 days. No systemic effects have been linked to hyaluronan. No long-term side effects have been

Table 31.6: Types of hyaluronan (available in the United States)

Brand	*Molecular weight x 10^6 Da*	*Dose/vial*	*Manufacturer*	*Treatment regimen*
Synvisc	6.0	16-mg hylan polymer/2-mL vial	Genzyme Biosurgery (Ridgefield, NJ)	1 vial/week x 3 weeks
Synvisc-One	6.0	48-mg hylan polymer/6-mL vial	Genzyme Biosurgery (Ridgefield, NJ)	1 vial only
Supartz	0.62–1.17	25-mg sodium hyaluronate/2.5-mL vial	Seikagaku Corporation (Tokyo, Japan)	1 vial/week x 5 weeks
Hyalgan	0.5–0.73	20-mg sodium hyaluronate/2-mL vial	Fidia Pharma USA Inc. (Parsippany, NJ)	1 vial/week x 5 weeks
Euflexxa	2.4–3.6	20-mg sodium hyaluronate/2-mL vial	Bio-Technology General, Ltd (Israel)	1 vial/week x 3 weeks
Orthovisc	1.0–2.9	30-mg sodium hyaluronate/2-mL vial	Anika Therapeutics (Woburn, MA)	1 vial/week x 3–4 weeks

Data obtained from official drug labels of respective medications.

reported. Hyaluronan is contraindicated in those who have had hypersensitivity reactions to the medication, or with current knee infection or overlying skin and soft tissue infection. Synvisc and Orthovisc are contraindicated for those with hypersensitivity to avian products.

Platelet-rich Plasma

Platelet-rich plasma is autologous plasma with higher concentration of platelets than normal. It contains seven known growth factors (Table 31.7) that facilitate healing of soft tissue and bone. Normal platelet concentration in whole blood ranges between 150,000/μL to 350,000/μL with an average of 200,000/μL. PRP generally contains at least four times the normal concentration. The ideal platelet concentration for healing potential is not known. The optimal platelet concentration has been recommended to be at least 1,000,000/μL in a 5-mL volume,[36] whereas others suggest four to six times the normal serum levels.[37] However, the efficacy of PRP therapy has been demonstrated at lower levels.[38]

The PRP is prepared first by drawing a sample of autologous, anticoagulated blood from the patient. It is then centrifuged or filtered to separate platelet-poor and platelet-rich plasma. An activating agent such as calcium chloride, thrombin, or tendon-derived collagen is added, and the preparation is injected into the treatment site. The concentration of platelets and growth factors in a PRP preparation can vary depending on the patient's blood concentrations, the process, and the PRP system used (Table 31.8).

Indications

The PRP has been studied, with mixed results, for use in joints and soft tissue injuries, such as osteoarthritis, tendonitis, tendinopathy, epicondylitis, partial tendon tears, ligament tears, and muscle tears.

In studies of PRP for Achilles tendon injuries, the recent literature has shown no significant benefit of PRP injections for midsubstance Achilles tendinopathy.[39] Results of two trials conflict on whether it may shorten recovery times when used in surgical repair of Achilles ruptures.[40,41]

There have been positive results of PRP therapy for Achilles tendinosis in the literature.[42] In prospective studies, it has shown benefits for treatment of chronic patellar tendinopathy.[43,44] PRP may have more benefits for lateral epicondylitis than corticosteroids.[45-47] Early results for treatment of plantar fasciitis have shown improved safety and improvement of pain of PRP therapy when compared with corticosteroid injections.[48,49]

PRP may be beneficial for knee osteoarthritis by having anabolic effects on chondrocytes and inhibiting inflammatory effects of IL-1β and inhibiting NFkβ activation.[50] Clinical trials evaluating PRP for knee osteoarthritis suggest that it is safe and effective[51] and may be comparable with hyaluronan injections.[52]

Although it is considered safe, many questions still remain regarding the proper application and the efficacy of PRP therapy. Table 31.9 lists diagnoses for which PRP therapy is potentially indicated.

Adverse Effects

When autologous blood is used for the PRP therapy, the adverse effects are minimal. Side effects in human PRP trials have ranged from a rate of 1.3 to 5%. Local pain is the most common side effect and can last in some cases for 3–4 weeks post injection.[53]

INJECTION TECHNIQUES

The majority of peripheral joint and soft tissue injections are performed by palpation and are based on anatomic

Table 31.7: Growth factors in platelet-rich plasma

Growth factor	*Source*	*Function*
Platelet-derived growth factor	Platelets	Stimulates cell replication, angiogenesis, mitogenesis of fibroblasts
Vascular endothelial growth factor	Platelets	Angiogenesis
Transforming growth factor-β1	Platelets	Key regulator between fibrosis and myocyte regeneration
Fibroblast growth factor	Platelets	Stimulates proliferation of myoblasts, angiogenesis
Epidermal growth factor	Platelets	Proliferation of mesenchymal and epithelial cells, potentiation of growth factors
Hepatocyte growth factor	Plasma	Angiogenesis, mitogenesis of endothelial cells, antifibrotic
Insulin-like growth factor-1	Plasma	Stimulates myoblasts and fibroblasts, mediates growth and repair of skeletal muscle

Reproduced from Creaney and Hamilton. Growth factor delivery methods in the management of sports injuries: the state of play. Br J Sports Med. 2008;42;314-20.

Table 31.8: Commercial platelet-rich plasma systems (PRP)

System	*Volume of blood (mL)*	*Centrifuge time/ speed*	*Final PRP volume (mL)*	*Final platelet concentration (compared with average whole blood)*	*Activator*	*Level of growth factors (compared with average)*
Autologous Conditioned Plasma (Arthrex, Naples, FL)†	9	5 min/1500 rpm	3–5	2–3x	None	PDGF (25x) EGF (5x) VEGF (11x) TGF- β1 (4x) IGF-1 (1x)
Cascade (Musculoskeletal tissue foundation, Edison, NJ)‡	9 or 18	6 min/1100 g; 15 min/1450 g	2 or 4	N/A	Calcium	PDGF (N/A) EGF (5–10x) VEGF (5–10x) TGF- β1 (5–10x) IGF-1 (5–10x)
GPS III (Biomet, Warsaw, IN)§	27 or 54	15 min/1100 g	3 or 6	4–8x	Calcium chloride/ thrombin	PDGF (N/A) EGF (3.9x) VEGF (6.2x) TGF-β1 (3.6x) IGF-1 (1x)
SmartPREP (Harvest, Plymouth, MA)	20 or 60	14 min/1000 g	3 or 7	4.4–7.6x	Thrombin	PDGF (4.4x) EGF (4.4x) VEGF (4.4x) TGF-β1 (4.4x) IGF-1 (N/A)

Reproduced from Hall et al. Platelet-rich plasma: current concepts and application in sports medicine. J Am Acad Orthop Surg. 2009;17:602-8.
† Arthrex: https://www.arthrex.com/innovations/index.cfm?adid=28&CFID=2168033&CFTOKEN=63754575
‡ Musculoskeletal Tissue Foundation: http://plateletttherapy.com/
§ Biomet: http://www.biomet.com/biologics/information/pdf/BBI0003.0.pdf

Table 31.9: Potential indications for platelet-rich plasma therapy

• Intra-articular joint
• Knee osteoarthritis
• Periarticular/soft tissue
• Rotator cuff tendinopathy
• Patellar tendinopathy
• Achilles tendinopathy
• Lateral and medial epicondylitis
• Plantar fasciitis

landmarks and identifying the point of maximal tenderness. Imaging with fluoroscopy and ultrasound can be helpful in needle guidance and placement and may increase accuracy of injections depending on the treated location. Fluoroscopy-guided joint injections are generally considered reliable, but subject the patient and the clinician to radiation. Therefore, ultrasound-guided joint injections may sometimes be preferred. For soft tissue injections, ultrasound guidance has been shown to be superior in most instances to palpation (Table 31.10).

CONCLUSION

Peripheral joint and soft tissue injections can be very useful and effective in diagnosis and treatment. An understanding of the side effects and limitations of corticosteroids and local anesthetics can allow the safe and efficacious use of these medications. Newer injectables such as hyaluronan and PRP can be used in certain diagnoses in conjunction with corticosteroids and may even be preferred. Stem cells therapy, not discussed in this text, can also prove to be useful in the future.

Table 31.10: Accuracy of peripheral joint and soft tissue injections

Location	*Approach technique*	*Palpation accuracy (%)*	*Ultrasound accuracy (%)*
Intra-articular			
Acromioclavicular	N/A	40–70%[54–57]	90–100%[54,56]
Glenohumeral	Anterior, posterior	27–85%[58–62]	92.5–100%[59,63]
Hip	N/A	80%[64]	97–100%[65,66]
Knee	Anterolateral, anteromedial, patellofemoral, medial, midlateral, superolateral	55–93%[67–71]	96–100%[68,69,71]
Tibiotalar joint	N/A	85%[72]	100%[72,73]
PIP and MCP joints	N/A	59%[74]	96%[74]
Soft tissue			
Biceps tendon sheath	N/A	66.7%[75]	100%[75]
Peroneal tendon sheath	N/A	60%[76]	100%[76]
Subacromial-subdeltoid bursa	Anterior, posterior, lateral	30–100%[55,58,77,78]	100%[78]
Pes anserine bursa	N/A	17%[79]	92%[79]
Trigger finger	N/A	15%[80]	70%[80]
Sinus tarsi	N/A	35%[72]	90%[72]

(MCP: Metacarpophalangeal; N/A: Not available; PIP: Proximal interphalangeal).

REFERENCES

1. Hollander JL, Brown EM Jr, Jessar RA, et al. Hydrocortisone and cortisone injected into arthritic joints; comparative effects of and use of hydrocortisone as a local antiarthritic agent. J Am Med Assoc. 1951;147(17):1629-35.
2. Goppelt-Struebe M, Wolter D, Resch K. Glucocorticoids inhibit prostaglandin synthesis not only at the level of phospholipase A2 but also at the level of cyclo-oxygenase/PGE isomerase. Br J Pharmacol. 1989;98(4):1287-95.
3. Wright JM, Cowper JJ, Page Thomas DP, et al. The hydrolysis of cortisol 21-esters by a homogenate of inflamed rabbit synovium and by rheumatoid synovial fluid. Clin Exp Rheumatol. 1983;1(2):137-41.
4. Godwin M, Dawes M. Intra-articular steroid injections for painful knees. Systematic review with meta-analysis. Can Fam Physician. 2004;50:241-8.
5. Shoemaker RS, Bertone AL, Martin GS, et al. Effects of intra-articular administration of methylprednisolone acetate on normal articular cartilage and on healing of experimentally induced osteochondral defects in horses. Am J Vet Res. 1992;53(8):1446-53.
6. Papacrhistou G, Anagnostou S, Katsorhis T. The effect of intraarticular hydrocortisone injection on the articular cartilage of rabbits. Acta Orthop Scand Suppl. 1997;275:132-4.
7. Dragoo JL, Danial CM, Braun HJ, et al. The chondrotoxicity of single-dose corticosteroids. Knee Surg Sports Traumatol Arthrosc. 2012;20(9):1809-14.
8. Braun HJ, Wilcox-Fogel N, Kim HJ, et al. The effect of local anesthetic and corticosteroid combinations on chondrocyte viability. Knee Surg Sports Traumatol Arthrosc. 2012;20(9):1689-95.
9. Paavola M, Kannus P, Jarvinen TA, et al. Treatment of tendon disorders. Is there a role for corticosteroid injection? Foot Ankle Clin. 2002;7(3):501-13.
10. Sellman JR. Plantar fascia rupture associated with corticosteroid injection. Foot Ankle Int. 1994;15(7):376-81.
11. Moller M, Movin T, Granhed H, et al. Acute rupture of tendon Achillis. A prospective randomised study of comparison between surgical and non-surgical treatment. J Bone Joint Surg Br. 2001;83(6):843-8.
12. Nole R, Munson NM, Fulkerson JP. Bupivacaine and saline effects on articular cartilage. Arthroscopy. 1985;1(2):123-7.
13. Piper SL, Kramer JD, Kim HT, et al. Effects of local anesthetics on articular cartilage. Am J Sports Med. 2011; 39(10): 2245-53.
14. Piper SL, Kim HT. Comparison of ropivacaine and bupivacaine toxicity in human articular chondrocytes. J Bone Joint Surg Am. 2008;90(5):986-91.
15. Laurent TC, Laurent UB, Fraser JR. The structure and function of hyaluronan: an overview. Immunol Cell Biol. 1996; 74(2):A1-7.
16. Edwards JC, Wilkinson LS, Jones HM, et al. The formation of human synovial joint cavities: a possible role for hyaluronan and CD44 in altered interzone cohesion. J Anat. 1994;185 (Pt 2):355-67.
17. Dahl LB, Dahl IM, Engstrom-Laurent A, Granath K. Concentration and molecular weight of sodium hyaluronate in synovial fluid from patients with rheumatoid arthritis and other arthropathies. Ann Rheum Dis. 1985;44(12):817-22.
18. Watterson JR, Esdaile JM. Viscosupplementation: therapeutic mechanisms and clinical potential in osteoarthritis of the knee. J Am Acad Orthop Surg. 2000;8(5):277-84.
19. Forrester JV, Balazs EA. Inhibition of phagocytosis by high molecular weight hyaluronate. Immunology. 1980;40(3): 435-46.

20. Hakansson L, Hallgren R, Venge P. Regulation of granulocyte function by hyaluronic acid. In vitro and in vivo effects on phagocytosis, locomotion, and metabolism. J Clin Invest. 1980;66(2):298-305.
21. Punzi L, Schiavon F, Cavasin F, et al. The influence of intra-articular hyaluronic acid on PGE2 and cAMP of synovial fluid. Clin Exp Rheumatol. 1989;7(3):247-50.
22. Miyakoshi N, Kobayashi M, Nozaka K, et al. Effects of intraarticular administration of basic fibroblast growth factor with hyaluronic acid on osteochondral defects of the knee in rabbits. Arch Orthop Trauma Surg. 2005;125(10):683-92.
23. Smith MM, Ghosh P. The synthesis of hyaluronic acid by human synovial fibroblasts is influenced by the nature of the hyaluronate in the extracellular environment. Rheumatol Int. 1987;7(3):113-22.
24. Jansen EJ, Emans PJ, Douw CM, et al. One intra-articular injection of hyaluronan prevents cell death and improves cell metabolism in a model of injured articular cartilage in the rabbit. J Orthop Res. 2008;26(5):624-30.
25. Bellamy N, Campbell J, Robinson V, et al. Viscosupplementation for the treatment of osteoarthritis of the knee. Cochrane Database Syst Rev. 2006;(2):CD005321.
26. Sonoda M, Harwood FL, Wada Y, et al. The effects of hyaluronan on the meniscus and on the articular cartilage after partial meniscectomy. Am J Sports Med. 1997;25(6):755-62.
27. Strauss E, Schachter A, Frenkel S, et al. The efficacy of intra-articular hyaluronan injection after the microfracture technique for the treatment of articular cartilage lesions. Am J Sports Med. 2009;37(4):720-6.
28. Salk RS, Chang TJ, D'Costa WF, et al. Sodium hyaluronate in the treatment of osteoarthritis of the ankle: a controlled, randomized, double-blind pilot study. J Bone Joint Surg Am. 2006;88(2):295-302.
29. Mei-Dan O, Kish B, Shabat S, et al. Treatment of osteoarthritis of the ankle by intra-articular injections of hyaluronic acid: a prospective study. J Am Podiatr Med Assoc. 2010;100(2):93-100.
30. Blaine T, Moskowitz R, Udell J, et al. Treatment of persistent shoulder pain with sodium hyaluronate: a randomized, controlled trial. A multicenter study. J Bone Joint Surg Am. 2008;90(5):970-9.
31. Noel E, Hardy P, Hagena FW, et al. Efficacy and safety of Hylan G-F 20 in shoulder osteoarthritis with an intact rotator cuff. Open-label prospective multicenter study. Joint Bone Spine. 2009;76(6):670-3.
32. Weil AJ. High molecular weight hyaluronan for treatment of chronic shoulder pain associated with glenohumeral arthritis. Med Devices (Auckl). 2011;4:99-105.
33. Brander VA, Gomberawalla A, Chambers M, et al. Efficacy and safety of hylan G-F 20 for symptomatic glenohumeral osteoarthritis: a prospective, pilot study. PMR. 2010;2(4):259-67.
34. Migliore A, Massafra U, Bizzi E, et al. Intra-articular injection of hyaluronic acid (MW 1,500-2,000 kDa; HyalOne) in symptomatic osteoarthritis of the hip: a prospective cohort study. Arch Orthop Trauma Surg. 2011;131(12):1677-85.
35. Migliore A, Granata M, Tormenta S, et al. Hip viscosupplementation under ultrasound guidance reduces NSAID consumption in symptomatic hip osteoarthritis patients in a long follow-up. Data from Italian registry. Eur Rev Med Pharmacol Sci. 2011;15(1):25-34.
36. Marx RE. Platelet-rich plasma (PRP): what is PRP and what is not PRP? Implant Dent. 2001;10(4):225-8.
37. Weibrich G, Hansen T, Kleis W, et al. Effect of platelet concentration in platelet-rich plasma on peri-implant bone regeneration. Bone. 2004;34(4):665-71.
38. Creaney L, Hamilton B. Growth factor delivery methods in the management of sports injuries: the state of play. Br J Sports Med. 2008;42(5):314-20.
39. de Vos RJ, Weir A, van Schie HT, et al. Platelet-rich plasma injection for chronic Achilles tendinopathy: a randomized controlled trial. JAMA. 2010;303(2):144-9.
40. Schepull T, Kvist J, Norrman H, et al. Autologous platelets have no effect on the healing of human Achilles tendon ruptures: a randomized single-blind study. Am J Sports Med. 2011;39(1):38-47.
41. Sanchez M, Anitua E, Azofra J, et al. Comparison of surgically repaired Achilles tendon tears using platelet-rich fibrin matrices. Am J Sports Med. 2007;35(2):245-51.
42. Gaweda K, Tarczynska M, Krzyzanowski W. Treatment of Achilles tendinopathy with platelet-rich plasma. Int J Sports Med. 2010;31(8):577-83.
43. Filardo G, Kon E, Della Villa S, et al. Use of platelet-rich plasma for the treatment of refractory jumper's knee. Int Orthop. 2010;34(6):909-15.
44. Kon E, Filardo G, Delcogliano M, et al. Platelet-rich plasma: new clinical application: a pilot study for treatment of jumper's knee. Injury. 2009;40(6):598-603.
45. Edwards SG, Calandruccio JH. Autologous blood injections for refractory lateral epicondylitis. J Hand Surg Am. 2003;28(2):272-8.
46. Peerbooms JC, Sluimer J, Bruijn DJ, et al. Positive effect of an autologous platelet concentrate in lateral epicondylitis in a double-blind randomized controlled trial: platelet-rich plasma versus corticosteroid injection with a 1-year follow-up. Am J Sports Med. 2010;38(2):255-62.
47. Mishra A, Pavelko T. Treatment of chronic elbow tendinosis with buffered platelet-rich plasma. Am J Sports Med. 2006;34(11):1774-8.
48. Martinelli N, Marinozzi A, Carni S, et al. Platelet-rich plasma injections for chronic plantar fasciitis. Int Orthop. 2013;37(5):839-42
49. Ragab EM, Othman AM. Platelets rich plasma for treatment of chronic plantar fasciitis. Arch Orthop Trauma Surg. 2012;132(8):1065-70.
50. van Buul GM, Koevoet WL, Kops N, et al. Platelet-rich plasma releasate inhibits inflammatory processes in osteoarthritic chondrocytes. Am J Sports Med. 2011;39(11): 2362-70.
51. Patel S, Dhillon MS, Aggarwal S, Marwaha N, Jain A. Treatment with platelet-rich plasma is more effective than placebo for knee osteoarthritis: a prospective, double-blind, randomized trial. Am J Sports Med. 2013;41(2):356-64.

52. Spakova T, Rosocha J, Lacko M, et al. Treatment of knee joint osteoarthritis with autologous platelet-rich plasma in comparison with hyaluronic acid. Am J Phys Med Rehabil. 2012;91(5):411-7.
53. Paoloni J, De Vos RJ, Hamilton B, et al. Platelet-rich plasma treatment for ligament and tendon injuries. Clin J Sport Med. 2011;21(1):37-45.
54. Borbas P, Kraus T, Clement H, et al. The influence of ultrasound guidance in the rate of success of acromioclavicular joint injection: an experimental study on human cadavers. J Shoulder Elbow Surg. 2012;21(12):1694-7.
55. Partington PF, Broome GH. Diagnostic injection around the shoulder: hit and miss? A cadaveric study of injection accuracy. J Shoulder Elbow Surg. 1998;7(2):147-50.
56. Peck E, Lai JK, Pawlina W, et al. Accuracy of ultrasound-guided versus palpation-guided acromioclavicular joint injections: a cadaveric study. PM R. 2010;2(9):817-21.
57. Pichler W, Weinberg AM, Grechenig S, et al. Intra-articular injection of the acromioclavicular joint. J Bone Joint Surg Br. 2009;91(12):1638-40.
58. Eustace JA, Brophy DP, Gibney RP, et al. Comparison of the accuracy of steroid placement with clinical outcome in patients with shoulder symptoms. Ann Rheum Dis. 1997; 56(1):59-63.
59. Patel DN, Nayyar S, Hasan S, et al. Comparison of ultrasound-guided versus blind glenohumeral injections: a cadaveric study. J Shoulder Elbow Surg. 2012;21(12):1664-8.
60. Porat S, Leupold JA, Burnett KR, et al. Reliability of non-imaging-guided glenohumeral joint injection through rotator interval approach in patients undergoing diagnostic MR arthrography. AJR Am J Roentgenol. 2008;191(3): W96-9.
61. Sethi PM, Kingston S, Elattrache N. Accuracy of anterior intra-articular injection of the glenohumeral joint. Arthroscopy. 2005;21(1):77-80.
62. Catalano OA, Manfredi R, Vanzulli A, et al. MR arthrography of the glenohumeral joint: modified posterior approach without imaging guidance. Radiology. 2007;242(2):550-4.
63. Rutten MJ, Collins JM, Maresch BJ, et al. Glenohumeral joint injection: a comparative study of ultrasound and fluoroscopically guided techniques before MR arthrography. Eur Radiol. 2009;19(3):722-30.
64. Leopold SS, Battista V, Oliverio JA. Safety and efficacy of intraarticular hip injection using anatomic landmarks. Clin Orthop Relat Res. 2001(391):192-7.
65. Pourbagher MA, Ozalay M, Pourbagher A. Accuracy and outcome of sonographically guided intra-articular sodium hyaluronate injections in patients with osteoarthritis of the hip. J Ultrasound Med. 2005;24(10):1391-5.
66. Smith J, Hurdle MF, Weingarten TN. Accuracy of sonographically guided intra-articular injections in the native adult hip. J Ultrasound Med. 2009;28(3):329-35.
67. Bliddal H. Placement of intra-articular injections verified by mini air-arthrography. Ann Rheum Dis. 1999;58(10): 641-3.
68. Bum Park Y, Ah Choi W, Kim YK, et al. Accuracy of blind versus ultrasound-guided suprapatellar bursal injection. J Clin Ultrasound. 2012;40(1):20-5.
69. Curtiss HM, Finnoff JT, Peck E, et al. Accuracy of ultrasound-guided and palpation-guided knee injections by an experienced and less-experienced injector using a superolateral approach: a cadaveric study. PM R. 2011;3(6): 507-15.
70. Jackson DW, Evans NA, Thomas BM. Accuracy of needle placement into the intra-articular space of the knee. J Bone Joint Surg Am. 2002;84-A(9):1522-7.
71. Park Y, Lee SC, Nam HS, et al. Comparison of sonographically guided intra-articular injections at 3 different sites of the knee. J Ultrasound Med. 2011;30(12):1669-76.
72. Wisniewski SJ, Smith J, Patterson DG, et al. Ultrasound-guided versus nonguided tibiotalar joint and sinus tarsi injections: a cadaveric study. PM R. 2010;2(4):277-81.
73. Reach JS, Easley ME, Chuckpaiwong B, et al. Accuracy of ultrasound guided injections in the foot and ankle. Foot Ankle Int. 2009;30(3):239-42.
74. Raza K, Lee CY, Pilling D, et al. Ultrasound guidance allows accurate needle placement and aspiration from small joints in patients with early inflammatory arthritis. Rheumatology (Oxford). 2003;42(8):976-9.
75. Hashiuchi T, Sakurai G, Morimoto M, et al. Accuracy of the biceps tendon sheath injection: ultrasound-guided or unguided injection? A randomized controlled trial. J Shoulder Elbow Surg. 2011;20(7):1069-73.
76. Muir JJ, Curtiss HM, Hollman J, et al. The accuracy of ultrasound-guided and palpation-guided peroneal tendon sheath injections. Am J Phys Med Rehabil. 2011;90(7): 564-71.
77. Henkus HE, Cobben LP, Coerkamp EG, et al. The accuracy of subacromial injections: a prospective randomized magnetic resonance imaging study. Arthroscopy. 2006;22(3): 277-82.
78. Rutten MJ, Maresch BJ, Jager GJ, et al. Injection of the subacromial-subdeltoid bursa: blind or ultrasound-guided? Acta Orthop. 2007;78(2):254-7.
79. Finnoff JT, Henning PT, Cederholm SK, et al. Accuracy of medial foot compartment pressure testing: a comparison of two techniques. Foot Ankle Int. 2010;31(11): 1001-5.
80. Lee DH, Han SB, Park JW, et al. Sonographically guided tendon sheath injections are more accurate than blind injections: implications for trigger finger treatment. J Ultrasound Med. 2011;30(2):197-203.

CHAPTER 32

Sympathetic Blocks: Utility in Complex Regional Pain Syndrome

Kseniya Slobodyanyuk, Christopher Gharibo

NOCICEPTIVE AND NEUROPATHIC PAIN

The rationale behind the indications of sympathetic blocks relies on understanding the differences between normal and abnormal pain responses. Nociceptive pain is often due to an expected inflammatory response such as due to a herniated nucleus pulposus or degenerative spine disease. Nociceptive pain is transmitted via distinct pathways: the lateral spinothalamic tracts, which may modulate the area and intensity of the pain, and the medial spinothalamic tracts, which control autonomic and emotional reactions to pain.

In contrast, neuropathic pain is an abnormal, enhanced response to a stimulus related to peripheral or central nerve irritation or excitability from nerve damage such as from trauma, inflammation, or chronic pain. Several mechanisms are thought to contribute to neuropathic pain. Central sensitization involves a lowered activation threshold of A-δ and C fibers, leading to enhanced release of neurotransmitters and modulators from peripheral afferent terminals, creating an algesic environment of cytokines, prostaglandins, bradykinins, nitric oxide, interleukins, substance P, and others. This altered environment is conducive to depolarization of pain pathways and amplification of the pain signal, with the result being an ongoing level of transmission even with the removal of the original noxious stimulus. Other mechanisms of neuropathic pain are peripheral sensitization due to upregulation and activation of select sodium channels, and α-receptor upregulation on nociceptors.[2]

COMPLEX REGIONAL PAIN SYNDROME

The peripheral and central neuropathic pain mechanisms are thought to contribute to what is now referred to as complex regional pain syndrome (CRPS), an abnormal prolongation of responses to noxious events such as trauma or surgery, which include heightened pain response, changes in temperature perception, local structural degeneration, autonomic dysfunction, and functional impairment.[3] Originally known as causalgia, this disorder was initially described during the American Civil War by Silas Weir Mitchell when observing soldiers with traumatic nerve injury who developed chronic pain.[4] Decades later, the term reflex sympathetic dystrophy (RSD) was coined for those syndromes characterized by continuous and excessive pain after injury, which is responsive to sympathetic blocks. The two related observations were combined in 1994 by the International Association for the Study of Pain, yielding two types of CRPS: type I, formerly RSD, which occurs without a definable nerve lesion, and type II, formerly causalgia, which occurs in the presence of a defined nerve lesion.[5]

Epidemiology

Studies monitoring the incidence of CRPS have yielded an estimated range of 5.6–26.2 per 100,000 person-years.[4] After peripheral nerve injury, CRPS II incidence rate is estimated at 2–14%, with a mean around 4%.[6] Females develop CRPS more frequently than males at a rate of 4:1. Mean age at diagnosis is 53 years; thus, the typical CRPS patient is a postmenopausal woman. However, the disease has been known to occur in children, particularly after a sports injury, with mean onset at 13 years of age.[4]

Pathophysiology

Although CRPS occurs largely in the extremities, it can occur anywhere in the body. Evidence suggests that it is largely a central nervous system phenomenon. Symptoms of CRPS can be exacerbated by a variety of stimuli, including touch, range of motion, changes in temperature, visual or auditory stimuli, or emotional disturbances. Furthermore, the disorder occurs even in phantom limbs, where peripheral innervation or nociception may be missing. Pain is often described as burning, shooting, pricking, tearing, crushing, and gnawing while being nonpositional and nonmechanical, qualities which are not as common with peripheral sensory fiber damage. In addition, if the pain were to involve purely peripheral innervations, it would be cured by both rhizotomy and sympathectomy. However, while sympathectomy is widely used in the treatment of CRPS, peripheral rhizotomy does not appear to have efficacy in CRPS.

A possible mechanism leading to central manifestations in CRPS after peripheral damage involves injury-induced changes, which result in scarring and neuroma formation, distorting conduction along peripheral sensory fibers, and contributing to development of secondary central sensitization. Subsequently, altered conduction of sensory neurons can affect all of its branches, and central involvement can lead to regionalization of the pain seen in CRPS.[7]

Clinical Presentation

The clinical presentation of CRPS includes a variety of original injuries such as sprains, strains, minor or major trauma, fractures (particularly of the wrist), and cast immobilization.[4] The necessary clinical manifestation is pain that may be described as burning, shooting, or pricking. Additional pain manifestations are allodynia, hyperalgesia (particularly in response to mechanical stimuli), joint movement, and altered sensation, including hypoesthesia. The behavior patterns of activity avoidance, guarding of the involved area, and secondary pain often develop within months of disease onset. Autonomic changes are also observed, including swelling, vasomotor changes (color change to blue or pale, temperature change, and asymmetry), sweating abnormalities (sudomotor changes), and osteoporosis. Motor changes involve weakness, tremor, dystonia, and myoclonus, as well as early and late restricted range of motion from joint effusions and contractures, respectively. Other manifestations are dystrophic, including changes in hair and nail growth, hyperkeratosis, and thin, glossy skin. Myofascial dysfunction is also common in CRPS.[3,8] In the majority of cases, CRPS spontaneously improves. In long-standing CRPS, manifestations of peripheral and central sensitization such as mechanical and tactile allodynia and behavioral patterns of activity avoidance and guarding result in persistent atrophy, dystrophy, contractions, and orthopedic impairment (Fig. 32.1).

While symptoms are initially localized to the site of injury, they can spread. In cases of spontaneous spread (i.e. without additional trauma), proximal spread pattern is most common, followed by symmetric contralateral or ipsilateral spread. Several mechanisms have been offered to explain the observed patterns of spread. Genetic involvement is supported by the younger age of onset and increased frequency of movement disorders in patients with multiple affected limbs, as well as the supposed association between CRPS and human leukocyte antigens. The pattern of spread can also be explained by immobilization; cortical or spinal rather than systemic involvement, including altered spinal processing with glial modulation in the spinal cord rather than just at the affected level; alterations in the thalamus; and an interhemispheric spread of cortical sensitization, thought to involve the somatosensory and the motor cortices.[9]

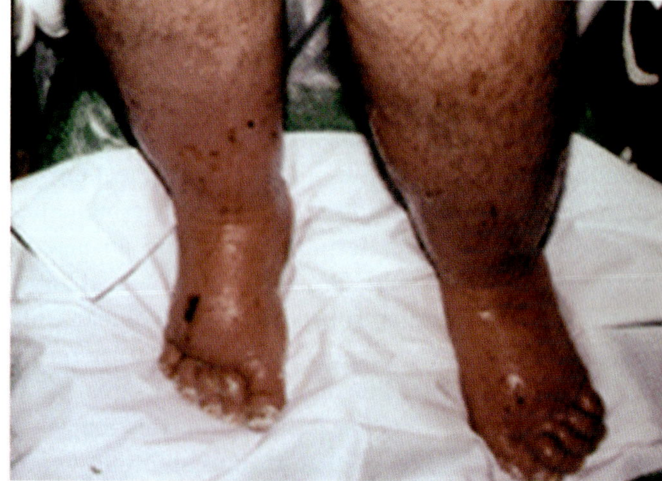

Fig. 32.1: Advanced complex regional pain syndrome of the right lower extremities.
Source: (RSDSA.org).

Diagnosis

Diagnosis of CRPS is based on history and physical examination. There are no diagnostic tests. The most recent clinical diagnostic criteria were defined at a convention held in Budapest in 2007 based on the four major diagnostic clusters of CRPS, with separate categories for clinical and research purposes (Table 32.1). Because there is a wide range of symptoms, CRPS carries a wide differential diagnosis, including peripheral vascular disease, infection, rheumatoid arthritis, osteomyelitis, lymphedema, tenosynovitis, osteoporosis, and others.[10] Furthermore, in select cases, the clinical presentation of acute radiculopathy with pathophysiology involving edema and inflammation of the nerve roots may be hard to distinguish from that of CRPS.

Prognosis

Despite the well-published potentially devastating effects, CRPS generally carries a good prognosis, with 80% of those treated within 1 year of injury improving considerably and 50% of those treated after 1 year also demonstrating substantial improvement.[3]

Table 32.1: Budapest criteria for diagnosis of complex regional pain syndrome (CRPS)[11]

Clinical criteria
1. Continuing pain, which is out of proportion to any inciting event
2. Must report at least one symptom in three of the four categories:
*Sensory: Hyperesthesia/allodynia
*Vasomotor: Temperature asymmetry/skin color changes/skin color asymmetry
*Sudomotor/edema: Reports of edema and/or sweating changes and/or sweating asymmetry
*Motor/trophic: Reports of decreased range of motion and/or motor dysfunction (weakness, tremor, dystonia) and/or trophic changes (hair, nail, skin)
3. Must display at least one *sign* at the time of evaluation in two or more categories:
*Sensory: Evidence of hyperalgesia (pinprick) and/or allodynia
*Vasomotor: Evidence of temperature asymmetry (>1°C)/skin color changes/color asymmetry
*Sudomotor/edema: Evidence of edema/sweating changes/ sweating asymmetry
*Motor/trophic: Evidence of decreased range of motion/motor dysfunction (weakness, tremor, dystonia)/trophic changes (hair, nail, skin)
4. There is no other diagnosis that better explains the signs and symptoms

*For research criteria, patient must report at least one symptom in all four symptom categories and at least one observed sign in two or more sign categories.

CRPS MANAGEMENT

Optimal management of CRPS requires the cooperation of an interdisciplinary treatment team. Treatment priorities include physical rehabilitation, pain control, functional restoration, and psychological support. A wide range of pharmacologic agents have been studied: antiepileptics; local anesthetics; antidepressants, including tricyclic antidepressants (TCAs), serotonin-norepinephrine reuptake inhibitors (SNRIs), and selective serotonin reuptake inhibitors (SSRIs); systemic corticosteroids; bisphosphonates; topical agents, such as casaicin and clonidine; intrathecal baclofen; and opioids. Recently, benefits of ketamine have been investigated on the basis of its supposed mitigation of central sensitization.

More invasive options are available to patients with refractory CRPS. Efficacy of intravenous (IV) regional anesthesia has been supported by multiple studies including randomized controlled trials.[12,13] Evidence also supports efficacy of spinal cord stimulators; however, literature supporting use of peripheral nerve stimulators for causalgia is limited.[6,14] Treatments targeting enhanced sympathetic response, including sympathetic nerve blocks and sympathectomies, are discussed below.[6]

Sympathetic Block

There are several anatomic targets for sympathetic blocks such as stellate ganglion block or lumbar sympathetic block (Figs. 32.2A and B). A sympathetic block is not required for diagnosis of CRPS but is widely used to classify CRPS into sympathetically mediated and sympathetically independent pain. Other sympathetic blocks include brachial plexus block and epidural blocks. Figures 32.3A and B demonstrated placement of stellate ganglion block under fluoroscopy. In the lower extremity, the sympathetic nervous system may be blocked at the peripheral nerves, lumbar plexus, or the lumbar epidural space.[15]

The theoretical benefit of sympathetic blocks is quite broad. Sympathetic nerve blocks may not only be utilized for prolonged pain control but may also provide diagnostic information (for example, is the pain sympathetically mediated or independent?). They may improve limb functionality, enhancing its engagement in activities of daily living and improving participation in physical

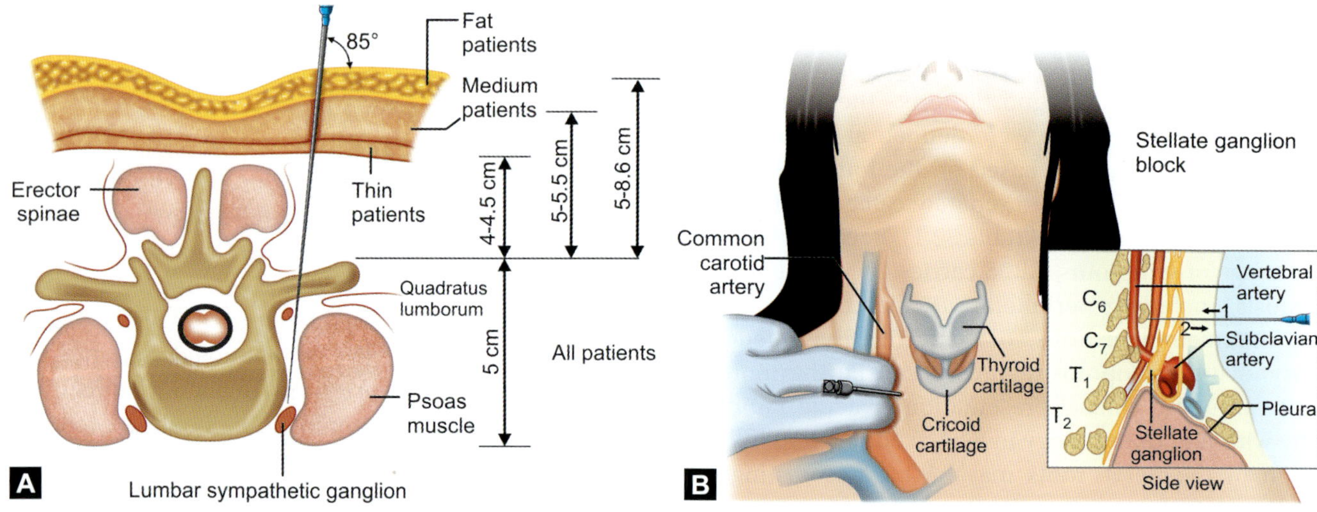

Figs. 32.2A and B: (A) Lumbar sympathetic block. (B) Stellate ganglion block.

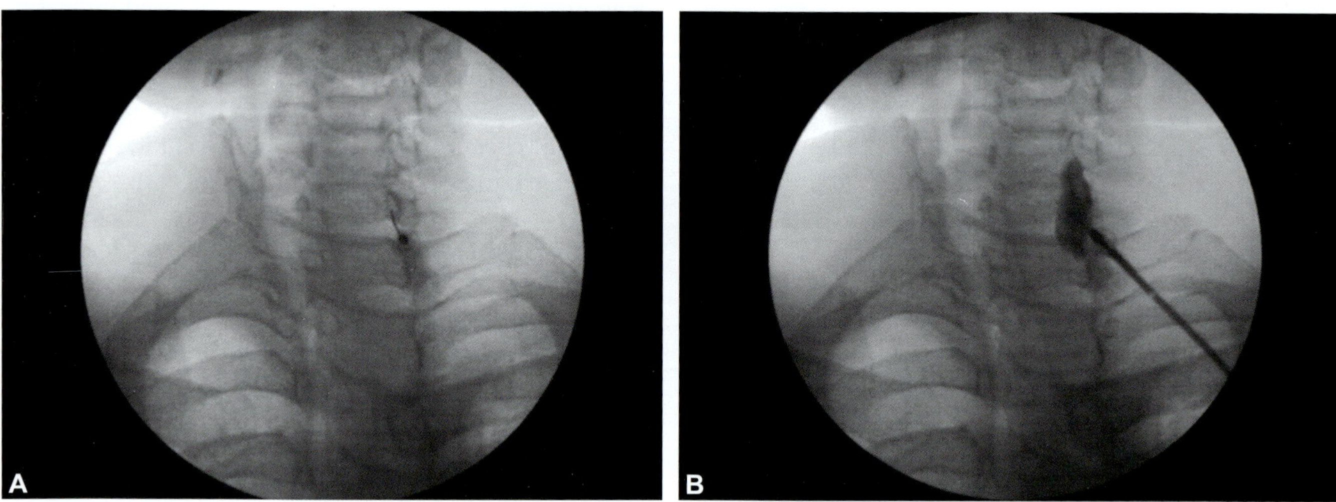

Figs. 32.3A and B: Stellate ganglion block fluoroscopy.[1]

therapy. A study by Reuben et al.[16] evaluated preoperative sympathetic blocks in an alternative role, as a postoperative prophylactic measure against CRPS recurrence in previously diagnosed and successfully treated patients. A comparison of 50 patients with postoperative stellate ganglion block to 50 patients without intervention concluded that stellate ganglion blocks significantly decreased CRPS recurrence rate, from 72% to 10%, compared with no intervention.[16] Use of sympathetic blocks is not limited solely to CRPS but potentially has diagnostic, prognostic, and therapeutic utility in peripheral vascular disease, cold-induced injuries, chronic vasospasticity, postherpectic neuralgia, and vascular headaches.

Sympathetic Block in CRPS Type I (RSD)

Evidence that sympathetic involvement contributes to CRPS type I is based on the improvement after sympathetic block.[17] Aberrant sympathetic activity has been offered as a possible mechanism: although there is normally no connection between C-fibers and sympathetic activity, sympathetic stimulation may excite cutaneous C-fibers after nerve damage, leading to allodynia and hyperalgesia.[18] However, recent findings suggest that it is initial sympathetic hypoactivity and increased arterial flow, which lead to CRPS-I, progressing to sympathetic hyperactivity and vasoconstriction over time.[19]

Nonsympathetic block-related mechanisms of relief have also been attributed to sympathetic blocks. Given the conductive block of local anesthetics, there is a possible reduction of the abnormal nerve impulse generators leading to reduction of nociceptive and neuropathic pain. Clinically, studies of sympathetic block efficacy have yielded mixed results. This has been attributed to the overpreponderance of case series that fail to reach controlled research standards such as an adequately powered sample and consistent methodology of diagnosis, treatment methods, and outcomes.[18] Overall, it is estimated that one-third of patients with CRPS respond well to sympathetic block, one-third only have a partial response, and the remaining third have no response.[15,17,18,20] A study by Wang et al.[21] comparing long-term efficacy of sympathetic block to conservative medical management found that 65% of patients reported improvement at 3 years, compared with 41% of those treated only medically. However, some investigators believe that any relief afforded by the sympathetic block is either due to temporary local anesthetic effect or placebo.[17,10] A 2001 review of randomized controlled trials concluded that analgesic effectiveness of sympathetic blocks was low, and just one of the studies reached a significant clinical effect size.[22] Price et al.[23] showed peak effect between saline and lidocaine block was not statistically different and concluded that improvement in pain could be the result of either placebo or other systemic effects of the block unrelated to sympathetic mechanisms. Ackerman and Zhang[20] addressed the potential effect of the local anesthetic.

A possible explanation for the paucity of high-quality studies investigating efficacy of sympathetic blocks is the lack of evidence-based information about number of blocks, their timing, frequency, and indications for CRPS diagnosis and treatment.[8] Several studies have demonstrated a significantly higher proportion of patients showing improvement if treated within 6 months of symptom onset.[17,21] One such study suggested that increased efficacy is seen when there is increased vasomotor activity, with efficacy decreasing with the onset of sustained vasoconstriction.[20]

In attempting to enhance efficacy and avoid unnecessary expenditure on interventional pain techniques, studies have evaluated predictors of response to sympathetic block. Although it is seemingly intuitive that the most "sympathetic-seeming" presentation would respond best to sympathetic block, there is currently no consensus regarding the presence of these symptoms and increased sympathetic nerve block efficacy. While Merritt[17] reported that these symptoms, including abnormal skin color, temperature, and sweat, predict efficacy, Van Eijs et al.[15] found that temperature alterations had no correlation with rate of response. Price concluded that signs of sympathetic change, including Horner's syndrome and surface temperature differences were not predictive of pain relief but were positively correlated with prolonged relief duration.[15,17,23]

Surprisingly, a search for negative predictors of effect pointed to allodynia and hyperesthesia.[15] The explanation offered was one involving central versus peripherally mediated pain: while sympathetic blocks are mainly a peripheral intervention, both allodynia and hyperesthesia reflect the alterations to central processing described above that may not respond to sympathetic blocks.[15,17]

Pharmacological Infusions

In attempting to develop alternatives to sympathetic blocks, numerous studies have investigated IV guanethidine. In theory, guanethidine should have a longer duration of response than stellate ganglion blocks.[17] However, numerous studies, including double-blind randomized controlled trials, have failed to show a difference in effect between IV guanethidine and placebo.[8,17,22,24] Other pharmacological infusions include reserpine and phentolamine, which are not currently approved in the United States, along with bretylium tosylate, usually used with steroids.[17]

Sympathetic Block in CRPS Type II

Similar to CRPS type I, there is a paucity of research investigating efficacy of sympathetic blocks and sympathectomies in CRPS type II. Nevertheless, several studies have upheld the efficacy of sympathetic blocks in CRPS type II, including one meta-analysis, which showed that 88% of 822 patients treated with sympathetic block demonstrated a beneficial response.[17,25] Reasons offered for the lack of efficacy in nonresponders include presence of a sympathetically mediated pain condition distinct from causalgia and failure of the injections to anesthetize the appropriate part of the sympathetic chain.[25]

Once a patient with causalgia has demonstrated consistent temporary relief after sympathetic block, the possibility of sympathectomy may be considered.

Post Discectomy Causalgia

In the civilian setting, causalgia can manifest in patients who have undergone previous surgery, particularly involving nerve decompression in the spine. Notably, Mockus et al.[26] performed a 15-year retrospective review of 34 sympathectomies for causalgic pain, investigating the predisposing factors of causalgia, its complications, and response to sympathectomy. He found that in his series, only 8 patients (26%) had known trauma as the precipitating event, whereas 15 (48%) had previous surgery with inadequate relief of nerve compression. The authors suggested residual nerve damage occurring prior to decompression as a possible etiology. They noted that in this subgroup of patients, sympathectomy was an equally effective treatment method.[26]

AbuRahma et al.[27] reviewed 12 patients who underwent lumbar sympathectomies for causalgia after lumbar laminectomy. The authors categorized their patients according to Drucker et al.[10] stages of causalgia (Table 32.2).

They noted that these distinct categories were important for their differential response to treatment: whereas for stage I or II patients there is possibility of permanent relief, possibly even without sympathectomy, for those in stage III the prognosis is relatively poor. Thus, the authors stressed prompt treatment as the key to effective relief, noting that in their own patients, the time between lumbar laminectomy and sympathectomy was significantly shorter in patients who had satisfactory treatment outcomes. Furthermore, the authors suggested a treatment algorithm involving prompt use of sympathetic blocks if conservative measures fail or if there is progression of symptoms over several days.[27]

More recently, Lee et al.[29] confirmed AbuRahma's findings in a retrospective review, investigating the outcomes of computed tomography-guided chemical sympathectomy for patients presenting with post discectomy causalgia, endorsing the relief of sympathetic vasoconstriction and subsequent improvement in perfusion as a possible mechanism.[28] Noted complications of the sympathectomy included injury to the ureter or lumbar vein and neuralgia or paresthesia, with an estimated 5–10% incidence of genitofemoral neuralgia.[29]

Table 32.2: Drucker's stages of causalgia

Stage I	Most immediate manifestation of causalgia, which can begin immediately or not until a few weeks after injury. This stage is characterized by hyperthermia, hyperalgesia, burning, increased hair and nail growth, and muscle atrophy
Stage II	Dystrophic stage, develops about 3 months after initial manifestations. In this stage, skin is pale and cyanotic, there is hair loss with brittle nails, persistent pain, and evidence of osteoporosis on X-ray
Stage III	Atrophic stage, generally considered to be irreversible. There is decreased dermal blood flow, atrophic skin, and marked loss of bone mineral. Pain is spreading and intractable. Sweating and growth of hair and nails may have resumed its normal pattern

CONCLUSION

Much is still unknown regarding the pathophysiology and treatment of CRPS. Studies of sympathetic blocks and sympathectomy have been limited by poor research design and inconclusive results. Nevertheless, these treatments continue to be widely supported by clinicians and have been known to provide relief, particularly when utilized early in treatment. They are relatively safe procedures, which are a reasonable option to improve quality of life for even a fraction of patients with this debilitating disease.

REFERENCES

1. Jadon A. Revalidation of a modified and safe approach of stellate ganglion block. Indian J Anaesth. 2011;55(1):52-6.
2. Azari P, Lindsay DR, Briones D, et al. Efficacy and safety of ketamine in patients with complex regional pain syndrome: a systematic review. CNS Drugs. 2012;26(3):215-28.
3. Patterson RW, Li Z, Smith BP, et al. Complex regional pain syndrome of the upper extremity. J Hand Surg Am. 2011;36(9):1553-62.
4. Veizi IE, Chelimsky TC, Janata JW. Chronic regional pain syndrome: what specialized rehabilitation services do patients require? Curr Pain Headache Rep. 2012;16(2):139-46.
5. Galer BS, Bruehl S, Harden RN. IASP diagnostic criteria for complex regional pain syndrome: a preliminary empirical validation study. International Association for the Study of Pain. Clin J Pain. 1998;14(1):48-54.
6. Hsu ES. Practical management of complex regional pain syndrome. Am J Ther. 2009;16(2):147-54.
7. Sunderland S. Pain mechanisms in causalgia. J Neurol Neurosurg Psychiatry. 1976;39(5):471-80.
8. Ghai B, Dureja GP. Complex regional pain syndrome: a review. J Postgrad Med. 2004;50(4):300-7.
9. van Rijn MA, Marinus J, Putter H, et al. Spreading of complex regional pain syndrome: not a random process. J Neural Transm. 2011;118(9):1301-9.
10. Drucker WR, Hubay CA, Holden WD, et al. Pathogenesis of post-traumatic sympathetic dystrophy. Am J Surg. 1959;97(4):454-65.
11. Harden RN, Bruehl S, Stanton-Hicks M, et al. Proposed new diagnostic criteria for complex regional pain syndrome. Pain Med. 2007;8(4):326-31.
12. Reuben SS, Pristas R, Dixon D, et al. The incidence of complex regional pain syndrome after fasciectomy for Dupuytren's contracture: a prospective observational study of four anesthetic techniques. Anesth Analg. 2006;102(2):499-503.

13. Reuben SS, Rosenthal EA, Steinberg RB, et al. Surgery on the affected upper extremity of patients with a history of complex regional pain syndrome: the use of intravenous regional anesthesia with clonidine. J Clin Anesth. 2004;16(7):517-22.
14. Kemler MA, Barendse GA, van Kleef M, et al. Spinal cord stimulation in patients with chronic reflex sympathetic dystrophy. N Engl J Med. 2000;343(9):618-24.
15. van Eijs F, Geurts J, van Kleef M, et al. Predictors of pain relieving response to sympathetic blockade in complex regional pain syndrome type 1. Anesthesiology. 2012;116(1):113-21.
16. Reuben SS, Rosenthal EA, Steinberg RB. Surgery on the affected upper extremity of patients with a history of complex regional pain syndrome: a retrospective study of 100 patients. J Hand Surg Am. 2000;25(6):1147-51.
17. Merritt WH. The challenge to manage reflex sympathetic dystrophy/complex regional pain syndrome. Clin Plast Surg. 2005;32(4):575-604, vii-viii.
18. Cepeda MS, Lau J, Carr DB. Defining the therapeutic role of local anesthetic sympathetic blockade in complex regional pain syndrome: a narrative and systematic review. Clin J Pain. 2002;18(4):216-33.
19. Fishman S, Ballantyne J, Rathmell JP, Bonica JJ. Bonica's Management of Pain, 4th edition. Baltimore, MD: Lippincott Williams & Wilkins; 2010.
20. Ackerman WE, Zhang JM. Efficacy of stellate ganglion blockade for the management of type 1 complex regional pain syndrome. South Med J. 2006;99(10):1084-8.
21. Wang JK, Johnson KA, Ilstrup DM. Sympathetic blocks for reflex sympathetic dystrophy. Pain. 1985;23(1):13-7.
22. Perez RS, Kwakkel G, Zuurmond WW, et al. Treatment of reflex sympathetic dystrophy (CRPS type 1): a research synthesis of 21 randomized clinical trials. J Pain Symptom Manage. 2001;21(6):511-26.
23. Price DD, Long S, Wilsey B, et al. Analysis of peak magnitude and duration of analgesia produced by local anesthetics injected into sympathetic ganglia of complex regional pain syndrome patients. Clin J Pain. 1998;14(3):216-26.
24. Schott GD. Interrupting the sympathetic outflow in causalgia and reflex sympathetic dystrophy. BMJ. 1998;316(7134): 792-3.
25. Hassantash SA, Afrakhteh M, Maier RV. Causalgia: a meta-analysis of the literature. Arch Surg. 2003;138(11):1226-31.
26. Mockus MB, Rutherford RB, Rosales C, et al. Sympathectomy for causalgia. Patient selection and long-term results. Arch Surg. 1987;122(6):668-72.
27. AbuRahma AF, Thaxton L, Robinson PA. Lumbar sympathectomy for causalgia secondary to lumbar laminectomy. Am J Surg. 1996;171(4):423-6.
28. Lindenauer SM, Cronenwett JL. What is the place of lumbar sympathectomy? Br J Surg. 1982;69(Suppl):S32-3.
29. Lee KS, Su YF, Lieu AS, et al. The outcome of percutaneous computed tomography-guided chemical lumbar sympathectomy for patients with causalgia after lumbar discectomy. Surg Neurol. 2008;69(3):274-9; discussion 279-80.

CHAPTER

33

Epidural Steroid Injections

Kseniya Slobodyanyuk, Christopher Gharibo

INTRODUCTION

The first use of neural blockade for low back pain was described in 1901, and epidural steroid injections (ESIs) for treatment of low back pain and radiculopathy were introduced in 1952.[1] However, in the past 20 years, ESIs have been more widely used than ever, with Medicare rates showing a 271% increase over a recent 7-year period. ESIs are now considered to be the most commonly performed interventional pain procedures in the world.[2] At the same time, their efficacy has been the subject of extensive debate. Data show that disability rates and other objective functional measures have remained unchanged despite the increased ESI use, whereas social, psychological, and functional consequences of chronic back pain have worsened over the past 15 years.[3]

EPIDURAL STEROID INJECTIONS

Structural changes of the spine can trigger an inflammatory response in the epidural space and tears or herniations of the intervertebral disk can lead to leakage of the nucleus pulposus, provoking an inflammatory reaction at the dura and surrounding regions including posterior longitudinal ligament and nerve roots. Indeed, one of the rationales behind the use of ESIs is based on their anti-inflammatory action: steroids inhibit aggregation of leukocytes, prevent inflammatory mediator release, and reduce synthesis and release of proinflammatory factors. Other ESI mechanisms contributing to pain relief include irrigation of the inflamed area, prolonged sodium channel blockade, C-fiber neurolysis, lysis of adhesions, relief of muscle spasms, sympathetic block, and central and peripheral desensitization.

Evidence-based utility of ESIs is primarily in relief of radicular pain, particularly from a herniated disk. Patients with spinal stenosis may also benefit, although in this population, a lesser effect and shorter duration have been observed. Lately, ESIs have been used for axial back pain but evidence for this indication is lacking.[2]

ESI Efficacy

Even for the most appropriate indications, studies of ESI efficacy have been inconclusive. Meta-analyses have been difficult to perform owing to wide variations in study methodology.[2,4] Half of 12 randomized controlled trials performed between 1952 and 1997 have concluded that ESIs are effective, whereas the other half have shown them to be no more effective than placebo.[5] In one study, from 1997, ESIs were administered to 78 patients with sciatica due to herniated nucleus pulposus, whereas another 80 patients were given placebo. At 3-week follow-up, significant differences were only seen in finger-to-floor distance and sensory deficits. At 6 weeks, only improvement in leg pain was significant. At 3 months, no significant differences were seen between groups. The authors concluded that the benefits of ESIs in sciatica, if any, are only short term.[5]

More recently, Benoist et al.[6] performed a systematic review, which separated studies into two categories to account for variability in design: Cochrane reviews and US Preventive Services Task Force (USPSTF) reviews. Cochrane reviews presented nonconclusive results, mainly attributed to small sample sizes and study heterogeneity.

On the other hand, the USPSTF reviews were more conclusive, suggesting that ESIs have moderate short-term efficacy. Suggestions for improvement of future study design included stratifying studies by pathology, imaging guidance of needle placement, extent of long-term evaluation, and changing placebo administration technique, perhaps to nonepidural, to account for wash-out effect. Despite the lack of definitive evidence, expert clinical opinions generally endorse ESIs, suggesting that the possibility of substituting a more costly and risky spine surgery for even a small proportion of patients makes ESIs an option worth considering.[6]

One explanation for the variability in study outcomes is the lack of consistency of ESI technique and injectate administration.[7,8] Regarding the optimal amount of injections, one study concluded that while some patients improve after one injection, some patients will need as many as three.[4] Regarding appropriate volume of injectate, a 2008 systematic review found that although there was a positive overall correlation between volume of fluid injected and immediate positive outcome, any conclusions are limited because the reviewed studies were heterogeneous and of limited quality. One of the few technical aspects of ESIs, which is generally agreed upon, however, is the use of imaging to guide needle placement. Evidence shows that one quarter to one third of "blind" injections without imaging guidance are not epidural.[6,9] Furthermore, the altered anatomy in spinal disorders and postsurgical backs increases the likelihood that medication is not reaching the target nerve. Using imaging guidance, confirming placement, level, laterality, optimizing nerve root coverage, placing the injectate anterolaterally, and covering the exiting and descending nerve root are all strategies that pain specialists can use to potentially enhance ESI efficacy.

INTERLAMINAR, TRANSFORAMINAL, AND CAUDAL ESIs

The difference between interlaminar (IL) and transforaminal (TF) injections lies in the location of needle placement and subsequent spread of injectate. TF ESIs, by spreading transforaminally into the epidural space, generally may cover a greater area of nerve root inflammation than can be achieved by IL (Figs. 33.1 and 33.2). Furthermore, TF ESIs have additional diagnostic utility in foraminal stenosis and may be useful in predicting foraminotomy outcomes. A study by Rho and Tang[4] concluded that there is "strong evidence to support the use of lumbar TF ESIs in patients with acute to subacute unilateral radicular pain caused by herniated nucleus pulposus or spinal stenosis", with greatest pain relief in the leg. On the other hand, IL ESIs provide multilevel and potential bilateral spread of injectate and may be the more reasonable approach for patients with multilevel or bilateral symptoms (Figs. 33.3A and B).

An alternative approach to epidural steroids is caudal. When caudal ESIs were first implemented, they were widely used owing to their low risk of serious complications and easier technique. Although caudal use declined over time due to heterogeneous anatomy, lack of consensus regarding technique, and a high rate of inaccurate

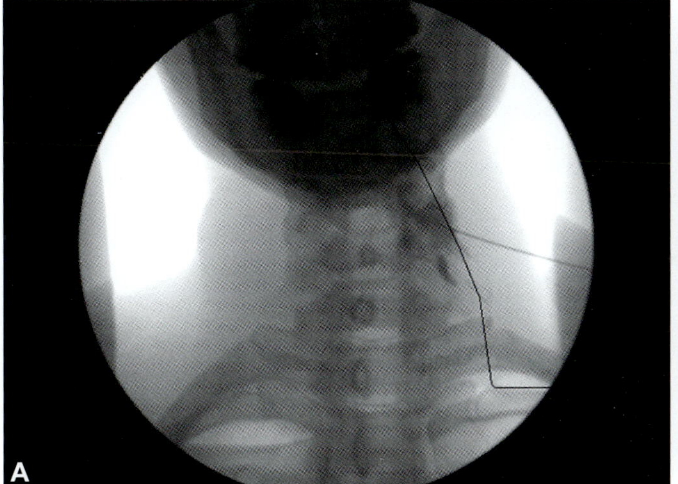

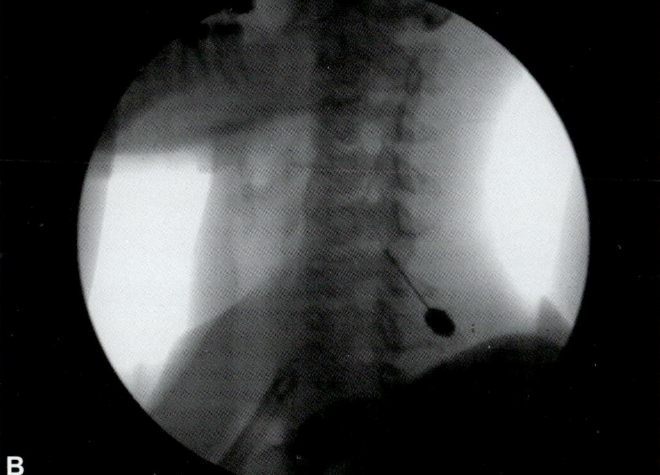

Figs. 33.1A and B: Transforaminal cervical epidural injection, anteroposterior and lateral.

needle placement, there has recently been an increase in interest in the caudal approach with fluoroscopic guidance. Indications for caudal epidural steroids include annular tears, herniated nucleus pulposus, chemical neuritis of the cauda equina, internal disk disruption, spondylolisthesis, scoliosis, and spinal stenosis.[10]

Interlaminar Procedure

When performing an IL ESI, the patient is placed in a prone position with a pillow under the abdomen. Anteroposterior (AP) imaging identifies the target IL space. The skin overlying the superior border of the ipsilateral lower lamina is marked and injected with local anesthetic. A needle is then advanced paramedian under fluoroscopic guidance until there is loss of resistance. Contrast medium may be injected to confirm placement in the epidural space. Once placement is confirmed, a mix of steroid and local anesthetic or saline is injected.

Transforaminal Procedure

The patient is positioned prone and AP and oblique imaging is performed. Six o'clock pedicle position is marked under oblique ipsilateral imaging angle. The skin overlying the 6 o'clock position of the pedicle is injected. A needle is advanced toward the upper one-third of the foramen under fluoroscopic guidance such that the tip rests within the triangle composed of the nerve root medially, bony pedicle superiorly, and lateral edge of

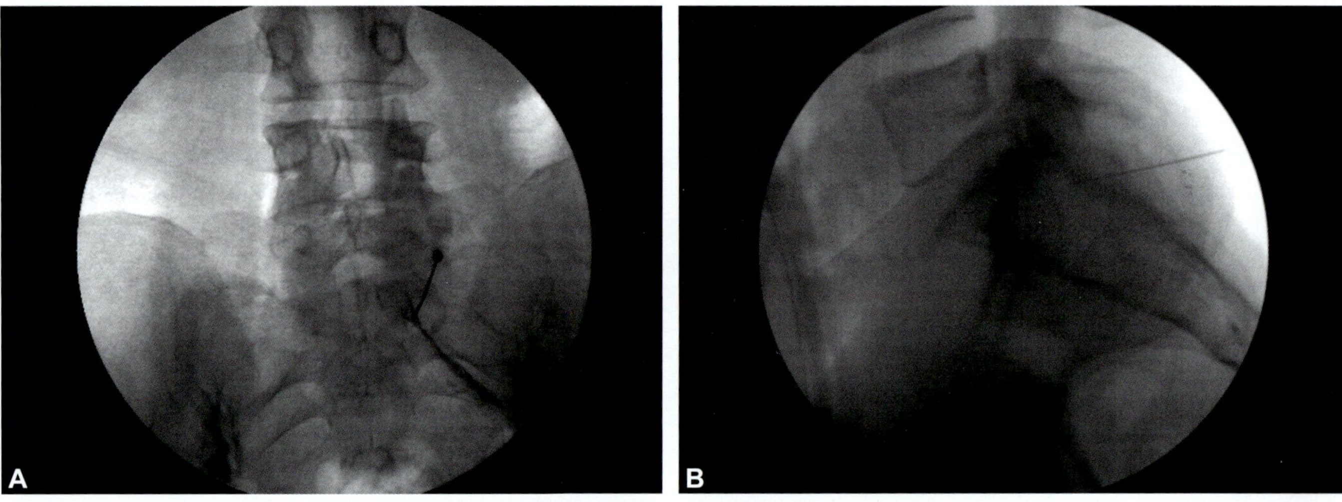

Figs. 33.2A and B: Transforaminal lumbar epidural injection, anteroposterior and lateral.

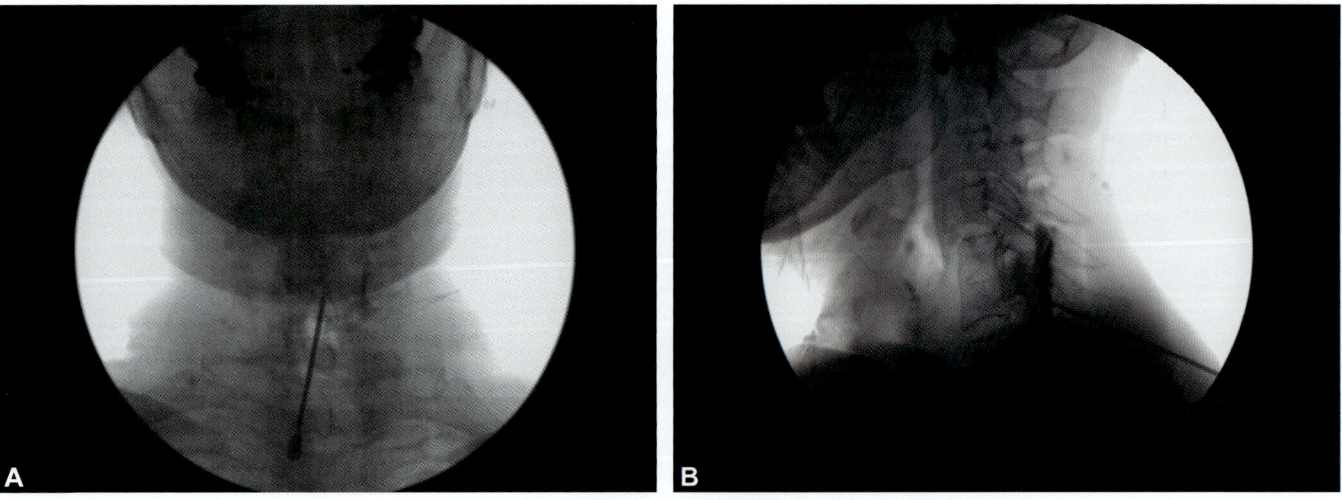

Figs. 33.3A and B: Interlaminar cervical epidural injection, anteroposterior and lateral.

the foramen laterally. Contrast confirmation is followed by an injection of a mixture of steroid and local anesthetic.

Caudal Procedure

The patient is placed in a prone position, and the skin below the sacral hiatus is injected with local anesthetic. The epidural needle is inserted at a 45° angle, and the approach is confirmed with AP and lateral imaging. The needle is then advanced until there is a loss of resistance, indicating passage through the sacrococcygeal ligament. After the ligament is penetrated, the needle is advanced into the epidural space and placement is confirmed using AP and lateral imaging. The needle is aspirated for blood and cerebrospinal fluid, and a mixture of steroid and local anesthetic is then injected.

COMPLICATIONS

Dural puncture and subarachnoid or epiarachnoid injections can lead to postdural puncture headache, aseptic meningitis, arachnoiditis, and conus medullaris syndrome. Direct trauma to the cord can occur depending on the level of the injection. In addition, as with all steroid use, especially with repeat administrations, one must consider potential systemic effects, including Cushing's syndrome, adrenal suppression, insulin resistance, psychosis, osteoporosis, congestive heart failure, gastrointestinal bleeding, and others. There are also inherent differences in complications between the IL and TF techniques.[8]

Disruption of the radiculomedullary or anterior spinal artery, which can traverse the length of the intervertebral foramen medially, can lead to paralysis, a risk that holds especial weight when considering TF injections. The exact cause of vascular injury may be compression of the arterial supply by the injectate, producing neural ischemia, compression of the venous side leading to back-pressure ischemia, mechanical needle injury to vasculature, increased irritability of arterial vasculature leading to vasospasm, distal embolization of the particulate steroid, alteration of spinal anatomy, air embolization, arterial dissection and neovascularization due to previous spine surgery.[8] It is suggested that particulate steroids are more effective and require lesser number of injections to desired therapeutic effect when compared with nonparticulate steroids. It has also been suggested that larger particles have longer half-lives and thus provide greater therapeutic effect. There is a lack of robust outcome data that compare particulate and nonparticulate steroid outcomes although the available literature and the body of experience favors nonparticulate steroids in terms of extent and duration of efficacy as well as minimizing the number of injections to desired effect.[2,8]

Relative Efficacy of TF vs IL ESIs

The subject of TF and IL complications is balanced by the question of their relative efficacy, which has been evaluated in a number of recent studies. A 2007 randomized controlled trial by Ackerman and Ahmad[11] performed IL, TF, or caudal ESIs on 90 patients every 2 weeks for a total three injections. Although all patients reported relief, by the 12- and 24-week evaluation periods, significantly more TF patients were reporting complete or partial pain relief. The authors hypothesized that the "V" spread of injectate of the TF approach allows for better steroid exposure to the affected area.[11] Another randomized controlled trial by Lee separated results by pathology, randomizing 100 herniated disk patients and 102 spinal stenosis patients to receive IL or TF injections, with a 4-month follow-up. They found that while patients with herniated disks demonstrated equal improvement with both IL and TF injections, patients with spinal stenosis randomized to TF reported significantly greater pain score improvement between 2 weeks and 4 months.[12] Most recently, efficacy was compared in a narrative review, which included level I, II, and III data. They concluded that the greatest pain relief and the lowest average number of injections were achieved with TF ESIs, an approach which "demonstrates more ventral epidural flow, which is where most of the pathologic changes occur".[4]

In 2011, a prospective, randomized, double-blind crossover cohort evaluating short-term benefits of IL versus TF ESIs for subacute lumbar radicular pain was done by the author. Forty-two patients with low back and radicular pain, all of whom failed conservative therapy, were randomly assigned to TF or IL ESIs. Overall, the study authors reported above-average results with both injection types, with a collective 90% of patients achieving 75% or greater relief after just one ESI, regardless of the type, and only four patients requiring repeat injection. When comparing results of the two arms, both IL and TF produced similar clinically significant improvements in pain, function, and depression assays. While the TF group reported statistically significant superior pain reduction in Numeric Rating Scale, other scores, including Oswestry Disability Index (ODI), were similar for both groups. The authors concluded that considering the equal functional benefit of both IL and TF ESIs, as reflected by ODI, and the superior safety and comfort of IL, the former is the recommended initial technique, with TF as a reasonable option for cases of inadequate relief after 2 weeks.[13]

Caudal ESI Efficacy

Efficacy of caudal ESIs has been the subject of numerous studies since the 1970s.[14] In 2012, a systematic review of 11 randomized trials and 5 nonrandomized trials of at least moderate quality supported the efficacy of caudal ESIs. The authors concluded that there is good evidence for caudal ESIs in managing disk herniation-induced radiculopathy leading to chronic low back and lower extremity pain. Fair evidence was found to support "spinal stenosis, axial pain, and post surgery syndrome". Furthermore, the results of the current review were found to correspond with those of previous reviews.[14]

CONCLUSION

The evaluation of ESI efficacy and comparison of TF and IL approaches are limited by the paucity of comparative short- and long-term research. Suggestions for improving future studies include standardization of technique and well-powered research to produce more systematic conclusions; stratification of results by pathology; and increased long-term follow-up. ESIs, regardless of the approach, are relatively safe and are virtually a default option to consider in those patients who have failed non-interventional treatment, prior to undergoing surgery.

REFERENCES

1. Manchikanti L. Role of neuraxial steroids in interventional pain management. Pain Physician. 2002;5:182-99.
2. Wilkinson IM, Cohen SP. Epidural steroid injections. Curr Pain Headache Rep. 2012;16:50-9.
3. Deyo RA, Mirza SK, Turner JA, et al. Overtreating chronic back pain: time to back off? J Am Board Fam Med. 2009;22:62-8.
4. Rho ME, Tang CT. The efficacy of lumbar epidural steroid injections: transforaminal, interlaminar, and caudal approaches. Phys Med Rehabil Clin N Am. 2011;22:139-48.
5. Carette S, Leclaire R, Marcoux S, et al. Epidural corticosteroid injections for sciatica due to herniated nucleus pulposus. N Engl J Med. 1997;336:1634-40.
6. Benoist M, Boulu P, Hayem G. Epidural steroid injections in the management of low-back pain with radiculopathy: an update of their efficacy and safety. Eur Spine J. 2012;21:204-13.
7. Fishman S, Ballantyne J, Rathmell JP, Bonica JJ. Bonica's Management of Pain, 4th edition. Baltimore, MD: Lippincott Williams & Wilkins; 2010.
8. Gharibo C, Koo C, Chung J, et al. Epidural steroid injections: an update on mechanisms of injury and safety. Techn Reg Anesth Pain Manage. 2009;13:266-71.
9. Bartynski WS, Grahovac SZ, Rothfus WE. Incorrect needle-position during lumbar epidural steroid administration: inaccuracy of loss of air pressure resistance and requirement of fluoroscopy and epidurography during needle insertion. AJNR Am J Neuroradiol. 2005;26:502-5.
10. Ogoke BA. Caudal epidural steroid injections. Pain Physician. 2000;3:305-12.
11. Ackerman WE, 3rd, Ahmad M. The efficacy of lumbar epidural steroid injections in patients with lumbar disc herniations. Anesth Analg. 2007;104:1217-22.
12. Lee CW, Park DW, Lee SH, et al. Comparison of the efficacy and safety of zotarolimus-, sirolimus-, and paclitaxel-eluting stents in patients with ST-elevation myocardial infarction. Am J Cardiol. 2009;104:1370-6.
13. Gharibo CG, Varlotta GP, Rhame EE, et al. Interlaminar versus transforaminal epidural steroids for the treatment of subacute lumbar radicular pain: a randomized, blinded, prospective outcome study. Pain Physician. 2011;14: 499-511.
14. Parr AT, Manchikanti L, Hameed H, et al. Caudal epidural injections in the management of chronic low back pain: a systematic appraisal of the literature. Pain Physician. 2012;15:E159-98.

CHAPTER

34

Intra-articular Facet Injections

Kristina L Bianco, Jeffrey H Weinreb, Gerard P Varlotta

INTRODUCTION

Spinal degeneration is among the most common causes of low back pain and often results in segmental incompetence of the spinal elements. In each spinal segment, an anterior intervertebral disk (IVD) and two posterior zygapophyseal (facet) joints comprise a "three-joint complex", as discussed in Chapter 1.[1] While the flexible consistency of the IVD allows for motion in all planes, facet joints are synovial joints that are restricted in movement. Degenerative disk disease results in the dehydration of the IVD and loss of disk height. This results in increased facet joint motion, which leads to facet arthropathy and inflammation. Consequently, the joint may become painful, as the inflammatory response can lead to nerve irritation or compression. Facet cysts can also arise due to microtrauma of the facet joints, leading to inflammation and pain. Anti-inflammatory injections are common treatment techniques to reduce inflammation caused by degenerative facet joints or facet cysts. Intra-articular injections alleviate facet-mediated pain and might limit the need for costly and high-risk surgical procedures. This chapter provides an overview of the evaluation and identification of facet joint pathologies and describes various intra-articular injections.

FACET JOINT ANATOMY

The facet joints are paired diarthrodial joints on the posterior side of the vertebral bodies.[2] Facet joints limit excessive joint motion and contribute to the stability of the spine.[3] In addition, they play a crucial role in both the transmission of intervertebral loads and rotational kinematics.[4] On axial imaging, the lumbar facet joint is parallel to the intervertebral disk space and has been described to resemble a "C" or "J" shape (Fig. 34.1).[1]

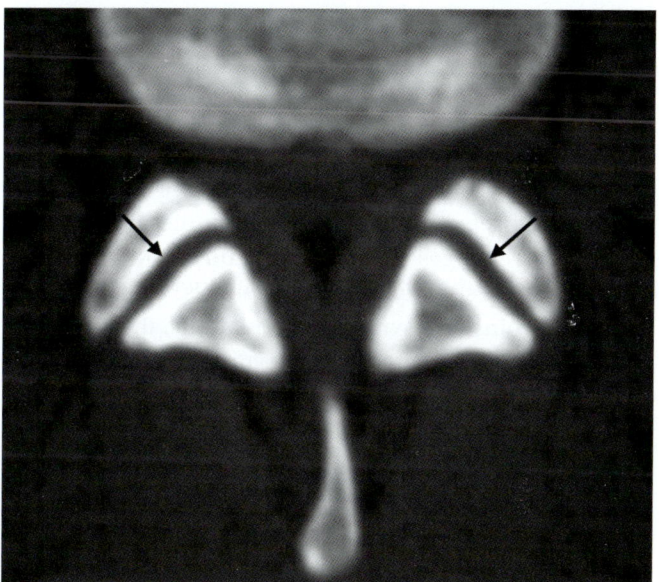

Fig. 34.1: An axial computed tomographic image of a lumbar facet joint (arrows), approximating a "C" or "J" shape.

Facet joint capsules have low-threshold nociceptors, making them a potential source of pain.[5,6] Due to a robust nerve supply, they reproduce pain similar to that of peripheral joints.[2] Not only do facet joint injections, such as intra-articular injections, have a therapeutic role, but they also aid in the diagnosis of facet-mediated pain.

ETIOLOGY AND PATHOPHYSIOLOGY

Degenerative changes to the spine usually start in one joint but eventually affect all components of the three-joint

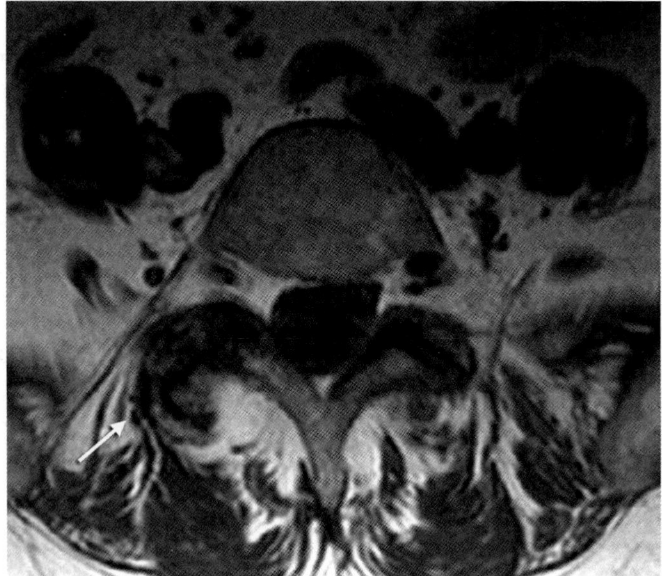

Fig. 34.2: Axial T1 weighted image of the lumbar spine. Severe degeneration of the right facet joint results in a "wraparound bumper" configuration (arrow).

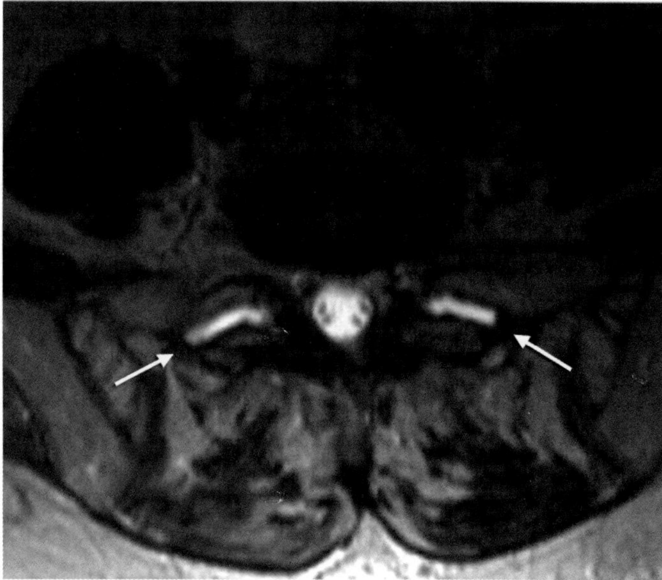

Fig. 34.3: An axial computed tomographic image of the lumbar spine illustrating bilateral facet joint effusions (arrow).

complex. For example, degeneration of the anterior IVD leads to subsequent deterioration of the facet joints. These joint changes may subsequently lead to pathologies such as spondylosis and stenosis.[7] Furthermore, since facet joints are synovial articulations, they undergo degenerative changes typical of synovial joints, such as osteoarthritis (OA).[3]

As described in Chapter 1, disk degeneration is a multifactorial process that begins in the nucleus pulposus of the IVD. In a degenerative disk, the nucleus pulposus is unable to dissipate compressive loads equally, resulting in an uneven distribution of the load and subsequent bulges in the annulus fibrosus (AF).[8,9] As disk degeneration progresses, the outer fibers of the AF begin to fragment and weight is shifted posteriorly to the facet joints. This results in increased mechanical loading and movement of the facet joints. While a healthy facet joint serves to limit joint motion, a degenerating facet joint undergoes excessive motion, resulting in both morphological and physical changes.[1] As progression of the IVD occurs, up to 47% increased pressure is placed on the posterior facet joints, resulting in facet joint degeneration (Fig. 34.2).[10] As a result of severe degeneration of the facet joints and the IVD, osteophytes form and movement is drastically reduced.

Osteophyte formation, facet hypertrophy, and apophyseal malalignment may lead to central or lateral stenosis. In degenerative spondylolisthesis, disk narrowing and osteophyte formation in the posterior joints result in a loss of articular cartilage, allowing upper vertebra to slip forward.[7] The sagittal orientation of the lumbar facet joint is identified as a risk factor in developing degenerative spondylolisthesis, and significantly greater sagittal orientations of the L4-5 facet joints have been found for patients with degenerative spondylolisthesis.[11] The measurement of facet joint angles is increasingly being used to evaluate degenerative spondylolisthesis.[1] Studies have found that patients with narrow facet joint angles have a 2.5 times greater risk of developing degenerative spondylolisthesis than patients with larger facet joint angles.[12]

Facet cysts are extradural membranous sacs that arise near the facet joints (Fig. 34.3). The formation of a facet cyst often occurs from microtrauma of the facet joints.[13] On the basis of the histopathological and radiographic findings, Kusakabe et al.[14] proposed a pathogenesis for the development of facet cysts (Fig. 34.4). In the first step of facet cyst formation, increased motion in the lumbar spine and degenerative arthritic changes results in degeneration of the ligamentum flavum. Spinal instability then causes rupture and fissure in the ligamentum flavum, which creates a fluid-filled cavity. These stages of cyst formation correspond with Type 1 and Type 2 cysts. In the second stage of facet cyst formation, growth of the cyst wall leads to increased damage of the ligamentum flavum. This results in an inflammatory reaction that consequently leads to growth of the cell wall. These stages of cyst formation correspond to Type 2 and 3a cysts. In the third step of facet cyst formation, the cyst grows within the cyst wall. The shape of the cyst is dependent on the elasticity and intensity of the cyst wall. As the cyst becomes larger, the cystic wall becomes thinner and the contents of the cystic cavity show myxoid degeneration. These stages of cyst formation correspond to cyst Types 3b, 4a, and 4b.

Synovial cysts, ganglion cysts, and juxtafacet cysts have all been used to describe cysts located near the facet joints. These are differentiated on the basis of the presence or absence of a synovial lining; while synovial cysts have a synovial lining, the other types of cysts do not.[1,13-15] Synovial cysts extrude into the spinal canal and are in direct contact with facet joints and the articular cavity. They represent synovial exvaginations that arise secondary to recurrent joint effusions. In contrast, ganglion cysts, also known as pseudosynovial cysts, lack a synovial membrane and have no communication with the articular cavity. Juxtafacet cysts are not conventionally associated with a facet joint and do not have a synovial membrane. Because intra-articular, synovial cysts have been defined as cysts that exhibit communication with the facet joints, they are the only type of cysts that can be classified as facet cysts. Facet cysts exhibit three distinct shapes: a small protrusion, a semicircular cyst, or a round cyst. Cysts associated with facet joint OA and degenerative spondylolisthesis are potential causes of low back pain. Intra-articular injections can be used for the therapeutic management of pain caused by facet cysts and are preferred over invasive surgical procedures.

Facet cysts are most commonly found in the L4-5 segment of the lumbar spine (Figs. 34.5A and B) and typically arise from arthritic facet joints, may contribute to, or indicate the development of, degenerative spondylolisthesis.[16] A retrospective study found that lumbar synovial cysts were accompanied by degenerative spondylolisthesis in 54% of cases.[13] Furthermore, patients with degenerative spondylolisthesis are more likely to have a higher grade of facet joint OA and synovial cysts with larger effusion sizes.[17] Although most facet cysts form after facet hypertrophy, cysts can also arise after surgical procedures such as decompressive laminectomies or instrument-augmented fusion.

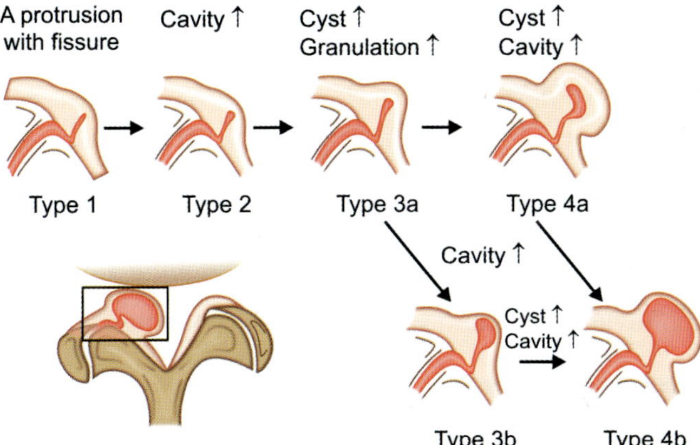

Fig. 34.4: Development of facet cysts in the lumbar spine.[14]

GRADING SCALES FOR FACET JOINT ARTHROPATHY

Grading systems can be used for the classification of facet joint arthropathy.[18] The Pathria grading scale, developed in 1983, has become the research standard for grading facet joint arthropathy. According to the Pathria's grading scale, radiographically normal facets are classified as grade 0. Facets with joint space narrowing are classified as grade 1. Facets with joint space narrowing as well as sclerosis or hypertrophy are classified as grade 2. Finally, facets with severe degenerative disease with sclerosis, narrowing, and osteophyte formation are classified as grade 3 (Table 34.1).[19] However, the authors regard radiographic imaging to be only a screening tool for facet disease as it is relatively insensitive for early- or mid-stage degenerative changes. Weishaupt's grading system also uses a 0–3 grading scale.[20] It is based on the idea that magnetic resonance imaging (MRI) and computed tomography (CT) are clinically equivalent and statistically relevant in the classification of lumbar facet OA.[1] However, MRI tends to underestimate the severity of facet OA in comparison with CT.[21]

DIAGNOSIS

Early studies injected hypertonic saline directly into the lumbar intra-articular facet joints to better understand where facet mediated pain manifests itself. These studies

Table 34.1: Pathria's grading scale for facet joint pathology[19]

Grade	*Description*
0	Radiographically normal facets.
1	Facets with joint space narrowing.
2	Facets with joint space narrowing, as well as sclerosis or hypertrophy.
3	Facets with severe degenerative diseases, as well as sclerosis, narrowing, and osteophyte formation.

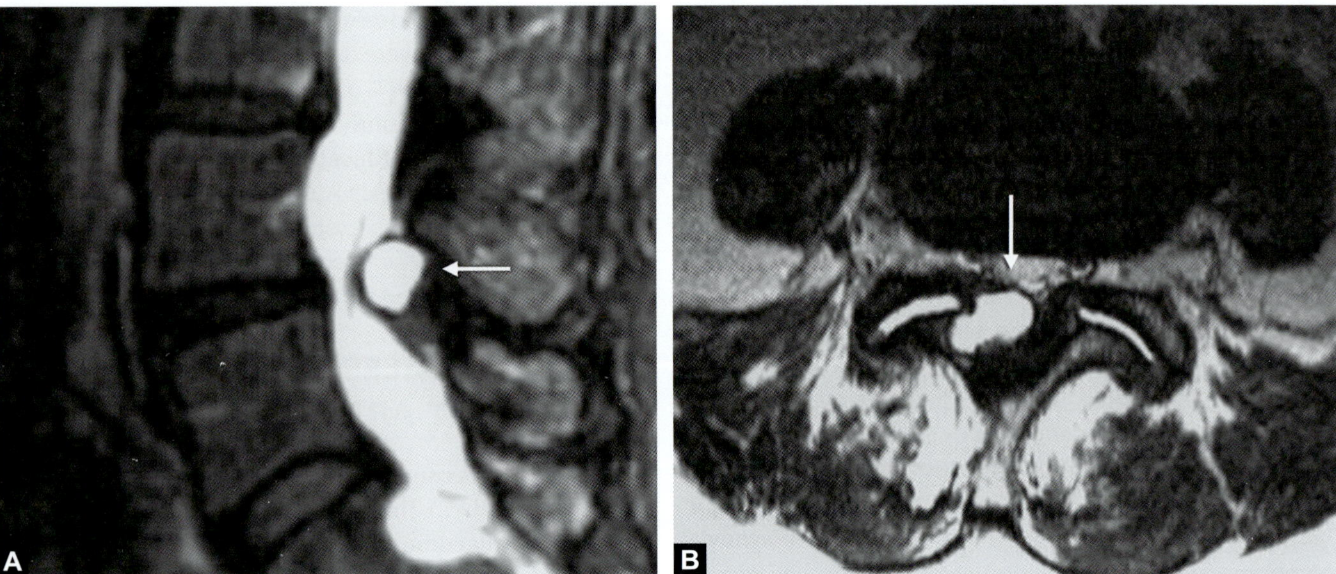

Figs. 34.5A and B: (A) Sagittal and (B) axial T2-weighted MR images of the lumbar spine. A facet cyst (arrow) is located in the L4-5 segment, causing compression of the thecal sac.

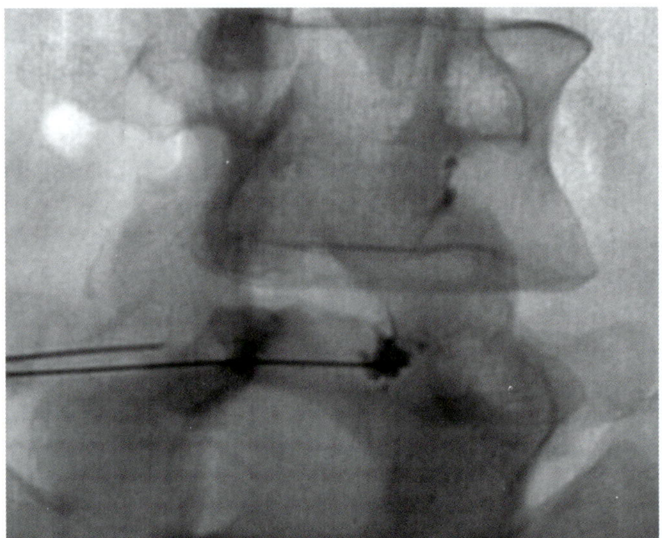

Fig. 34.6: A fluoroscopic oblique image of the lumbar spine during a facet injection demonstrating an arthrogram with contrast outlining the joint.

demonstrated that asymptomatic subjects report pain in the back, buttocks, and proximal thigh.[22] Utilizing the knowledge of where intra-articular facet-mediated joint pain radiates, controlled diagnostic blocks can be used to definitively determine the source of zygapophyseal joint pain. History, physical examination, and current imaging techniques are inadequate for diagnosis.[23-25] Pain reduction is the primary goal, but pain source identification is crucial for effective treatment.

To diagnose the source of zygapophyseal joint pain, an anesthetic agent injection with a known half-life can be used to determine pain origin, along with an arthrogram to confirm the targeted joint (Fig. 34.6).[24] However, despite initial promising results, this method has not been tested as a diagnostic tool.[23] A medial branch block (MBB) can also be used to locate the origin of pain. In this technique, the medial branches from the dorsal primary ramus of one level and the above level are anesthetized. Less than a complete pain reduction may indicate alternate pain origins. For additional information on MBB, *see* Chapter 36.

IMAGING

MRI is typically utilized for the evaluation of disk degeneration; however, there is currently no standard radiographic technique to evaluate facet joint arthrosis.[1] MRI tends to underestimate the severity of facet joint OA in comparison with CT.[21] Although CT is better at diagnosing lumbar stenosis and ossification of the ligamentum flavum, MRI is preferred for the evaluation of facet joint cysts and effusions. Increased fluid in the facet joints, as identified by MRI, is highly correlated with degenerative spondylolisthesis and synovial cyst degeneration.[13,14]

TREATMENT

Prior to undergoing facet joint injections, patients with facet-mediated pain are often recommended to try other types of conservative management techniques, such as physical therapy, manual therapy, or oral medications. However, none of these forms of conservative management has been evaluated for efficacy in facet joint pain relief.[23]

INDICATIONS FOR INJECTIONS

Indications for intra-articular facet joint injection include nonspecific and intractable low back and extremity pain. Injection intervention usually follows a course of activity modification, pharmacologic therapy, and exercise treatment. Bracing has been shown to be effective for low back pain, but long-term use may cause muscular atrophy and further pain when an exercise program is not maintained. Pharmacologic intervention, such as nonsteroidal anti-inflammatory drugs (NSAIDs), may reduce pain associated with facet joint arthrosis. Analgesics have been found to have no significant benefit compared with NSAIDs when treating low back pain.[26] Exercise treatment, including aerobic and core strength training, is also effective and should be used in conjunction with any treatment.[27] If these treatments do not alleviate pain, injection intervention is recommended. Intra-articular facet joint injections are indicated in varied pathologies including rheumatoid arthritis, ankylosing spondylitis, facet joint arthritis, paravertebral spasm, and the presence of intra-articular cysts. These diseases generally present with symptoms such as low back pain, unilateral radicular pain, and neurogenic claudication.[28] Contraindications of facet injections include signs of cellulitis, bacteremia, blood thinning or clotting disorder, and uncontrolled diabetes.[29]

INTRA-ARTICULAR FACET JOINT INJECTIONS

Pain reduction is a primary objective with an intra-articular facet joint injection. Corticosteroids are commonly utilized in intra-articular facet injections. Because inflammation is thought to contribute to pain, corticosteroids may reduce facet-mediated pain by reducing inflammation around the facet joints.

When the presence of an intra-articular facet cyst is radiographically confirmed, an intra-articular injection is a potential therapy (Fig. 34.7). Injections may be preferable to a surgical approach as they are associated with fewer complications than invasive surgery. Complications from cyst treatment surgery include dural tear, spinal nerve injury, epidural hematoma, seroma, cyst recurrence, and deep venous thrombosis.[30]

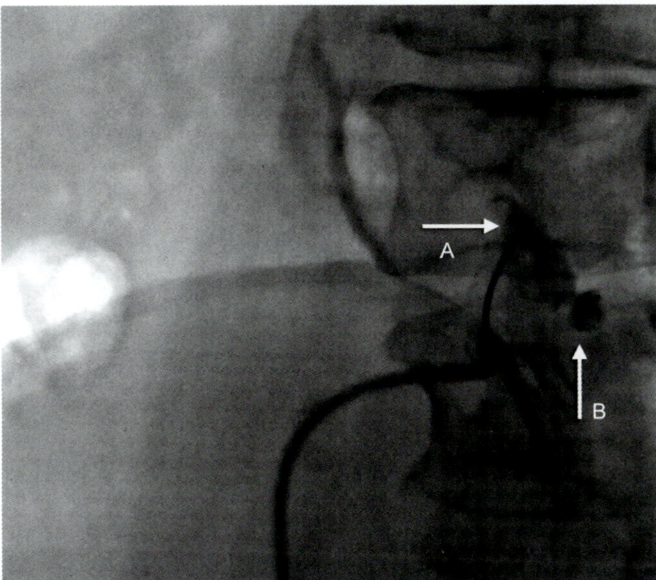

Fig. 34.7: (A) Percutaneous injection of corticosteroids into the extracystic space, surrounding the (B) facet cyst.

Percutaneous Injection

The cyst is first radiographically located. The area is anesthetized and contrast material is injected to confirm the intra-articular needle tip position. Then, corticosteroids are injected into the extracystic space or epidural space by an interlaminar, caudal, or transforaminal approach. The mechanism by which the corticosteroids reduce cyst size is still unclear.[30,31]

Fluoroscopic Aspiration

After locating the cyst radiographically, the area is then anesthetized and a needle and syringe are fluoroscopically guided into the facet joint. The syringe is then used to aspirate the cyst fluid.[32] It should be noted that cyst morphology varies and the viscosity of the cyst fluid or the extent of cyst calcification may impair aspiration attempts. Corticosteroids may then be injected into the extracystic or epidural space.[30]

Percutaneous Injection (Intracyst Distention and Drainage)

The cyst is located using either fluoroscopic or CT imaging, and a needle is inserted with local anesthetic. Then, contrast is introduced to ensure needle placement in the facet joint. The needle is used to penetrate the cyst, and a combination of equal parts long-acting corticosteroid and anesthetic is injected into the cyst. This injection is followed by normal saline with the intention of distending and rupturing the cyst.[33]

CYST INTERVENTION RESULTS

Although injections do not remove facet cysts in the way that surgery would, injections are preferred because they limit the potential complications caused by the surgical removal of facet cysts. Intra-articular injections for facet cysts reduce their size and severity and thereby reduce pain caused by the cysts.

However, percutaneous cyst intervention has been limited to low-quality research studies and has had mixed results. In one study, five patients underwent cyst aspiration followed by steroid instillation and five others underwent cyst aspiration followed by transforaminal epidural steroid injection. Of these 10 patients, only one experienced sustained pain reduction. Eight went on to receive surgical intervention with complete pain relief.[34] In another study, 9 of 12 patients who underwent a cyst distention and rupture had excellent pain relief.[33] Even in cyst rupture, one study reported a 38% cyst reoccurrence, and those who underwent a second rupture had a 50% chance of recovery.[30] In addition, when spondylostenosis or spondylolisthesis is found to be concurrent with intra-articular facet joint cysts, surgical intervention is indicated.[16]

COMPLICATIONS

The complication rate associated with injections are very low. However, severe complications such as infection, subcutaneous fat atrophy, fistulous tract formation, exacerbation of diabetes, and neurologic injury have been reported. Potential complications of facet cyst drainage include incomplete penetration of the facet joint with extravasation of contrast and failure to pressurize the cyst, resulting in incomplete cyst drainage.

DIFFERENTIAL DIAGNOSIS

Possible alternative etiologies may include tabes dorsalis, syringomyelia, diabetes mellitus, and infection. Although the spread of pyogenic bacteria is uncommon in the lumbar spine, it is crucial to consider infection in a differential diagnosis.[1] Septic arthropathy can be a differential diagnosis of facet cysts. Patients present with severe low back pain, stiffness, fever, and asthenia. Inflammatory markers including erythrocyte sedimentation rate and C-reactive protein level may be elevated, with or without leukocytes. To differentiate a simple facet cyst from a septic arthropathy, an MRI with contrast and a radionuclide bone scan can be used.

CONCLUSION

Intra-articular injection is a commonly used technique for the reduction of facet-mediated pain; however, it does not address the fundamental problem of degeneration of the three-joint complex and does not typically result in long-term pain reduction. Thus, intra-articular injections are not a sustainable singular treatment method, and multiple injections might be necessary for meaningful therapeutic management of facet joint pain. Although Chou et al. concluded that there has been little evidence to support the effectiveness of facet joint injections and MBBs, this review has been critiqued for the lack of methodological rigor, leading to misleading results.[36]

Intra-articular injections are most effective when used in conjunction with other pain-management techniques, such as medications, physical therapy, and manual therapy. When used as continuous care techniques in conjunction with other pain management techniques, intra-articular injections for facet joint pain and facet cysts might provide effective therapeutic management of facet-mediated pain.

REFERENCES

1. Varlotta GP, Lefkowitz TR, Schweitzer M, et al. The lumbar facet joint: a review of current knowledge: part 1: anatomy, biomechanics, and grading. Skeletal Radiol. 2011;40:13-23.
2. Benzel EC. Spine surgery: techniques, complication avoidance, and management, vol 2. Houston, TX: Gulf Professional Publishing, 2005.
3. Fujiwara A, Lim TH, An HS, et al. The effect of disc degeneration and facet joint osteoarthritis on the segmental flexibility of the lumbar spine. Spine. 2000;25:3036.
4. Tischer T, Aktas T, Milz S, et al. Detailed pathological changes of human lumbar facet joints L1–L5 in elderly individuals. Eur Spine J. 2006;15:308-15.
5. McLain RF, Pickar JG. Mechanoreceptor endings in human thoracic and lumbar facet joints. Spine. 1998;23:168.
6. Giles L, Taylor J. Human zygapophyseal joint capsule and synovial fold innervation. Rheumatology. 1987;26:93-8.
7. Yong-Hing K, Kirkaldy-Willis W. The pathophysiology of degenerative disease of the lumbar spine. Orthop Clin North Am. 1983;14:491.
8. Haefeli M, Kalberer F, Saegesser D, et al. The course of macroscopic degeneration in the human lumbar intervertebral disc. Spine. 2006;31:1522.

9. Horst M, Brinckmann P. 1980 Volvo award in biomechanics. Measurement of the distribution of axial stress on the end-plate of the vertebral body. Spine. 1981;6:217.
10. Yang KH, King A. Mechanism of facet load transmission as a hypothesis for low-back pain. Spine. 1984;9:557.
11. Grobler LJ, Robertson PA, Novotny JE, et al. Etiology of spondylolisthesis. Assessment of the role played by lumbar facet joint morphology. Spine. 1993;18:80.
12. Kim N, Lee J. The relationship between isthmic and degenerative spondylolisthesis and the configuration of the lamina and facet joints. Eur Spine J. 1995;4:139-44.
13. Pirotte B, Gabrovsky N, Massager N, et al. Synovial cysts of the lumbar spine: surgery-related results and outcome. J Neurosurg Spine. 2003;99:14-9.
14. Kusakabe T, Kasama F, Aizawa T, et al. Facet cyst in the lumbar spine: radiological and histopathological findings and possible pathogenesis. J Neurosurg Spine. 2006;5:398-403.
15. Epstein N, Baisden J. The diagnosis and management of synovial cysts: efficacy of surgery versus cyst aspiration. Surg Neurol Int. 2012;3:157.
16. Epstein NE. Lumbar synovial cysts: a review of diagnosis, surgical management, and outcome assessment. J Spinal Disord Tech. 2004;17:321.
17. Chaput C, Padon D, Rush J, et al. The significance of increased fluid signal on magnetic resonance imaging in lumbar facets in relationship to degenerative spondylolisthesis. Spine. 2007;32:1883.
18. Kettler A, Wilke HJ. Review of existing grading systems for cervical or lumbar disc and facet joint degeneration. Eur Spine J. 2006;15:705-18.
19. Pathria M, Sartoris D, Resnick D. Osteoarthritis of the facet joints: accuracy of oblique radiographic measurement. Radiology. 1987:227-30.
20. Weishaupt D, Zanetti M, Boos N, et al. MR imaging and CT in osteoarthritis of the lumbar facet joints. Skeletal Radiol. 1999;28:215-9.
21. Fujiwara A, Tamai K, Yamato M, et al. The relationship between facet joint osteoarthritis and disc degeneration of the lumbar spine: an MRI study. Eur Spine J. 1999;8:396-401.
22. Mccall I, Park WM, O'brien JP. Induced pain referral from posterior lumbar elements in normal subjects. Spine. 1979;4:441.
23. Bogduk N. Evidence-informed management of chronic low back pain with facet injections and radiofrequency neurotomy. Spine J. 2008;8:56-64.
24. Varlotta GP, Lefkowitz TR, Schweitzer M, et al. The lumbar facet joint: a review of current knowledge: Part II: diagnosis and management. Skeletal Radiol. 2011;40:149-57.
25. Bogduk N. A narrative review of intra-articular corticosteroid injections for low back pain. Pain Med. 2005;6:287-96.
26. van Tulder MW, Scholten RJ, Koes BW, et al. Non-steroidal anti-inflammatory drugs for low back pain. Cochrane Database Syst Rev. 2000;(2):CD000396.
27. Benzel EC, Henwood AM. Spine Surgery: Techniques, Complication Avoidance, and Management, vol 2, 3rd edition. Houston, TX: Gulf Professional Publishing; 2005. pp. 1807-13.
28. Benzel EC, Ahmed M, Modic MT. Spine Surgery: Techniques, Complication Avoidance, and Management, vol 2. Houston, TX: Gulf Professional Publishing; 2005. pp. 1623-46.
29. Rifat SF, Moeller JL. Basics of joint injection. General techniques and tips for safe, effective use. Postgrad Med. 2001; 109:157.
30. Allen TL, Tatli Y, Lutz GE. Fluoroscopic percutaneous lumbar zygapophyseal joint cyst rupture: a clinical outcome study. Spine J: official journal of the North American Spine Society. 2009;9:387-95.
31. Bjorkengren A, Kurz L, Resnick D, et al. Symptomatic intraspinal synovial cysts: opacification and treatment by percutaneous injection. Am J Roentgenol. 1987;149:105-7.
32. Lutz GE, Shen TC. Fluoroscopically guided aspiration of a symptomatic lumbar zygapophyseal joint cyst: a case report. Arch Phys Med Rehabil. 2002;83:1789-91.
33. Bureau NJ, Kaplan PA, Dussault RG. Lumbar facet joint synovial cyst: percutaneous treatment with steroid injections and distention–clinical and imaging follow-up in 12 patients. Radiology. 2001;221:179-85.
34. Shah RV, Lutz GE. Lumbar intraspinal synovial cysts: conservative management and review of the world's literature. Spine J. 2003;3:479-88.
35. Chou R, Atlas SJ, Stanos SP, et al. Nonsurgical interventional therapies for low back pain: a review of the evidence for an American Pain Society clinical practice guideline. Spine. 2009;34(10):1078-93.
36. Manchikanti L, Datta S, Gupta S, et al. A critical review of the American Pain Society clinical practice guidelines for interventional techniques: part 2. Therapeutic interventions. Pain Physician. 2010;13:E215.

CHAPTER

35

Complications of Spinal Injections

Brian Forzani, Stephen P Maier II, Kseniya Slobodyanyuk, Thomas J Errico, Thomas Cheriyan, Christopher Gharibo

INTRODUCTION

Spinal injections, while relatively safe, are associated with potential complications. These complications may be of mechanical, vascular or chemical origin. Spinal injections include epidural, facet joint, injections as well as nerve root, selective nerve root, and sympathetic blocks (Table 35.1). Epidural steroid injections (ESIs) are now among the most commonly performed interventional pain procedures in the United States.[1] Generally, they are considered safe, with complication rates ranging from 1:10,000 to 100,000 and side effect rates ranging 0.5–21.3% in prospective and retrospective analyses.[2,3] The majority of these side effects are deemed minor, including facial flushing, fever, vasovagal reactions, skin rashes, dizziness, nausea, and vomiting. Available epidural approaches include caudal, interlaminar, and more recently, transforaminal. By definition, an interlaminar injection passes between the upper and lower lamina of the vertebrae to reach the epidural space, whereas a transforaminal injection is directed via the intervertebral foramen to where the spinal nerves exit. As these injections have grown in popularity, there has been mounting evidence of more serious adverse events, including brain and spinal cord strokes resulting in hemiplegia, paraplegia, quadriplegia, or death. Mechanisms of ESI-related injury can broadly be classified into three major categories: mechanical, vascular, and chemical. Complications may also arise due to side effect profiles of the commonly administered drugs, including steroids, anesthetics, and myelographic contrast (Table 35.2). Injected medications might elicit allergic reactions, dizziness, headache, insomnia, mood swings, suppression of the hypothalamic-pituitary-adrenal axis, transient weight gain due to fluid retention, menstrual irregularities, facial erythema, transient hypertension or hypotension, gastritis, and pruritus. Furthermore, diabetics may experience elevations in blood sugar levels. This chapter will elaborate upon the relevant anatomy, pathophysiology, and specific examples of potential complications within each topic.

Table 35.1: Types of spinal injections and their associated functions and complications

Types of injection	*Description*
Epidural steroid injections	Relieves axial and radicular pain by reducing inflammation of spinal nerves
Nerve root blocks	Relieves radicular pain by reducing inflammation of spinal nerves
Facet joint injections	Diagnostic and therapeutic injection of steroids and local anesthetic into the facet joint
Sacroiliac joint injections	Used to diagnose and relieve causes of chronic low back pain
Stellate ganglion blocks	Injection of anesthetic to block sympathetic nerves and increase mobility
Trigger point injections	Deactivate trigger points, hyperirritable sites from which pain emanates, to relieve pain
Selective nerve root blocks	Nerve root blocked performed solely for diagnostic purposes

REGIONAL/MECHANICAL INJURY

Mechanical damage to neural tissue can occur from many sources. These include, but are not limited to, direct trauma from medical instruments, alterations in local pressure

Table 35.2: Types of injected drugs and their associated purposes and complications

Types of injected drug	*Purpose*	*Complications*
Steroid	anti-inflammation and neuromodulatory effects	Dizziness, headache, insomnia, mood swings, menstrual irregularities, facial erythema, transient hypertension or hypotension, gastritis, and pruritus
Anesthetic (e.g. lidocaine, bupivacaine)	Neural blockade	Allergic reaction
Dye (nonionic radiocontrast agents)	May be used for confirmatory diagnostic purposes	Allergic reactions [immunoglobulin (IgE) mediated] Pseudoallergic reactions (non-IgE mediated)

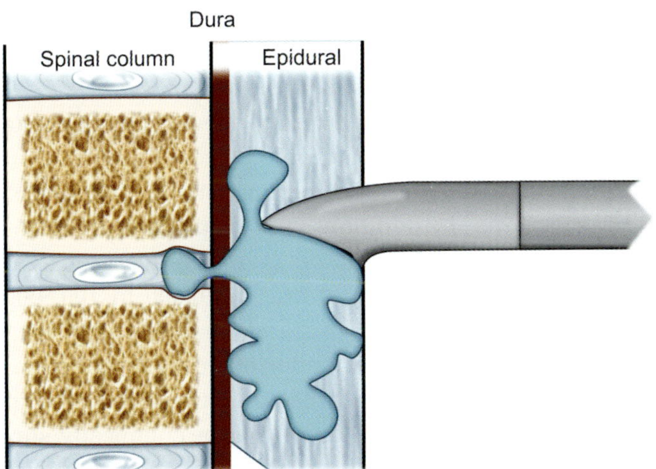

Fig. 35.1: Schema of an inadvertent dural puncture, in which cerebrospinal fluid leaks from the spinal canal/subarachnoid space into the epidural space.

during injection, and compression of nervous or vascular structures from volume buildup or resulting hematomas or abscesses.

NEEDLE/INJECTATE-RELATED INJURIES

Dural Puncture

Inadvertent dural puncture, also referred to as a dural tap, is the most common complication of epidural injections, with reported incidence ranging from 0.25–2.65% to 5–17% in the cervical and lumbar regions, respectively.[4,5] However, the consequences are often relatively minor and symptoms usually resolve spontaneously. An estimated 0.9–1.1% of patients develop post dural puncture headache (PDPH) due to cerebrospinal fluid (CSF) leakage from the subarachnoid into the epidural space from traction on cerebral tissue, which consequently lowers CSF pressure on intracranial tissues (Fig. 35.1).[4,6] The headache is presumed to persists until the defect in the dura heals and the CSF pressure returns to baseline. Symptoms generally appear immediately or within 2–3 days after puncture and last 3–4 days.[7] Failure of dural closure can result in adhesions, continuing CSF leak, and the risk of infection. A persistent spinal fluid leak after a dural tear may be surgically closed either directly or by using synthetic or biological graft material. Rarely, decreased intracranial pressure from a CSF leak has been reported to induce downward displacement of the brain and subsequent tearing of bridging veins, resulting in a subdural hematoma.[8]

Pneumocephalus

In addition to PDPH, pneumocephalus is another cause of headache after spinal injection. Pneumocephalus is the presence of air or gas in the intracranial cavity and may be epidural, subdural, subarachnoid, spinal, parenchymal, or intraventricular, causing pressure alterations within the intracranial or intraspinal tissues and leading to headache. Pneumocephalus has been associated with both cervical and lumbar interlaminar ESIs (ILESIs), often occurring when physicians utilize the loss of resistance technique, which allows for introduction of air into the meninges.[9,10] Symptoms include an headache, lethargy, confusion, and slow arousal. Headaches from pneumocephalus manifest on the day of the injection, worsen with movement, and do not abate with lying supine, as opposed to dural puncture headaches, which manifest up to 3 days post procedure and are relieved with lying supine. The diagnosis can be confirmed by subarachnoid air on brain computed tomography (CT) or magnetic resonance imaging (MRI) scan. Most symptoms resolve within 2–7 days.[9]

Intradiskal Injections

Aberrant injections can also enter intervertebral disks, depending on approach and anatomic pathology. Two groups performed retrospective studies to calculate the incidence of inadvertent disk injection.[11,12] The incidence of intradiscal entry with lumbar transforaminal ESIs (TFESI) is infinitely higher than with other epidural approaches. This may be associated with degenerative disc disease and ipsilateral posterolateral disc herniations as well as higher incidence of discitis and related infection approaching that of discograms. Two other incidences of disk injection were reported and both were associated with large foraminal disk herniations.[12]

Direct Nerve or Spinal Cord Trauma

In all spinal injections, there is a possibility of nerve damage that can lead to temporary or permanent deficits. The magnitude of neurological damage is dependent upon the nerve or group of nerves that are affected by the injection; hence larger groups of nerves that are damaged produce greater consequential deficits than independent or smaller nerves. Neurological damage may range from paresthesia and anesthesia to paralysis.

Inappropriate needle placement can lead to direct neural tissue damage. Nerve root or spinal cord injury will often be signaled by acute radicular pain during needle positioning, at which point needle position and advancement should be reassessed. Needle or injectate-related trauma can lead to multiple complications including severe neuropathic pain, complex regional pain syndrome, and/or paresthesias, which may be transient, prolonged, or permanent.[4] More severe consequences can occur after injection of material into spinal cord parenchyma. Lee et al.[13] reported the case of a 55-year-old man who developed quadriparesis during a C6–C7 TFESI. Radiologic findings revealed air bubbles and contrast medium within the cord substance, indicating needle penetration and intracord injection (Fig. 35.1). Repeat imaging demonstrated contrast absorption, which correlated with motor recovery. However, 1 year after the event, the patient still suffered from a left claw hand deformity.[13] The risk of spinal cord trauma may be heightened when performing injections at the level of stenotic thoracic or cervical spine where the epidural space is minimal. Large disk protrusions may actually push the cord posteriorly and obliterate the already small epidural space.[14]

Spinal cord injury from direct needle and injectate trauma is a serious form of neurological damage. Complications may likely result including paresis, paraparesis, or arachnoiditis. In addition, spinal epidural injections may cause epidural hematomas or epidural abscess formation at an incidence of one in 10,000 to 100, 000 injections, which may result in paraparesis or paraplegia.

Arachnoiditis, the inflammation of the arachnoid membrane that provides one of three protective layers around the central nervous system (CNS), may be chemically, surgically, or infectiously induced. Regardless of its origin, however, the thickened arachnoid may then adhere to its adjacent meninges and/or nerve roots, thereby reducing the available subarachnoid space and potentially introducing nerve root tension or ischemia (Figs. 35.2A and B).[15] This meningeal reaction may manifest as painful

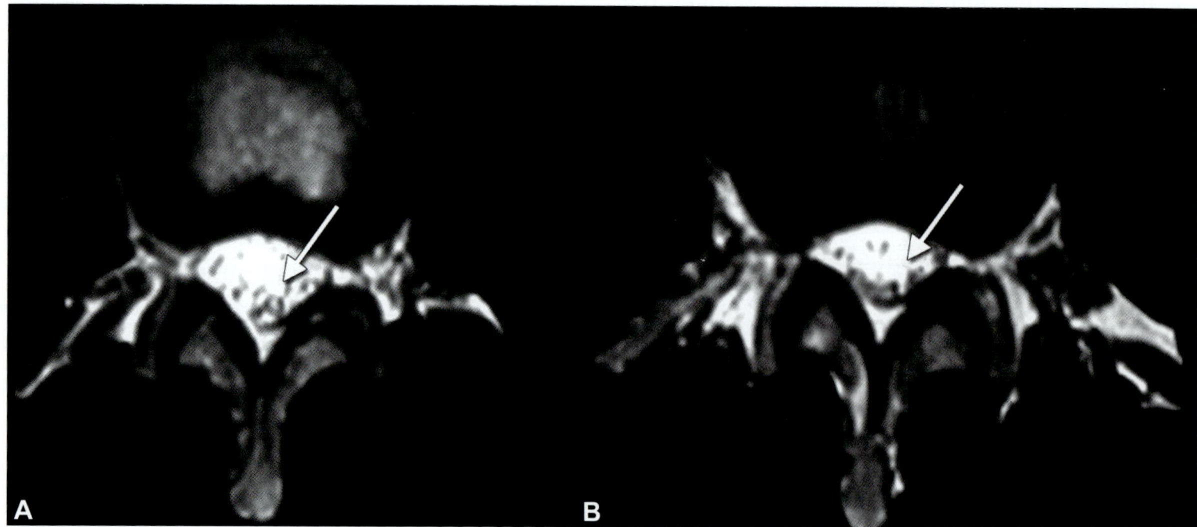

Figs. 35.2A and B: Magnetic resonance imaging adhesion of spinal roots to each other in lumbar subarachnoid space (arrow) suggestive of arachnoiditis.

Source: With permission from Paliwal VK, Kumar A, Rahi SK, Pradhan S. Charcot foot in post-tubercular spinal arachnoiditis may indicate emerging dorsal cord syringomyelia. Neurol India. 2011;59(2):299-301.

and debilitating symptoms, including muscle weakness, paraparesis, headache, urinary incontinence, or itching, burning/throbbing/sharp pain, and back pain with leg radiation. The incidence of persistent postoperative symptomatic arachnoiditis ranges from 3.5 to 16% of spine surgeries.[16,17]

Awareness of relative injection and cavity pressures is critical to minimizing complications. If sustained injectate pressure is greater than venous pressure, backpressure ischemia may result. If injectate pressure is greater than perfusion pressure, arterial ischemia may result. Nerve injury may also be caused by high-velocity injectate trauma, also called jetting.

PRESSURE-RELATED INJURIES

Practitioners must also be aware that indirect injuries can cause significant morbidity. Depositing or encroachment of space occupying materials into the small spaces surrounding the spinal cord can result in critical pressure changes and compromise neural structures.

Hematomas

Spinal epidural hematoma (SEH) is a localized accumulation of blood that forms a pocket in the spinal epidural space, increasing the CSF pressure (Figs. 35.3A and B).[18] If not treated promptly, the resulting acute, progressive spinal compression may lead to permanent neurologic deficits. While the incidence and prevalence of SEH due to spinal injections are not known, the incidence of hematomas after general epidural anesthesia has been estimated to range from 1/150,000 to 1/190,000.[19] Although the risk of SEH is very low, its consequences a resevere. Underlying coagulation dysfunction should also be considered as a possible etiology for SEH formation.

Piercing of blood vessels is an inherent risk of spinal injections and can lead to hematoma formation, with increased potential of bleeding complications especially in patients taking anticoagulants or with undiagnosed coagulopathies. In a review of 61 reports of epidural or subdural hematomas after neuraxial procedures, a clotting anomaly or use of anticoagulant medication was present in 68% of the cases.[20] Generally, presenting symptoms are the onset of radicular pain followed by progressive neurologic deterioration arising from compression of neural tissue.

Epidural hematomas are the most common form of bleeding in the spinal canal (Figs. 35.3A and B), with a reported incidence of 1 per 150,000–190,000 epidural procedures.[21] Classically, the venous plexus surrounding the epidural space is implicated as the likely source of bleeding. Subdural or parenchymal hematomas are felt to be less common but can still result in severe neurological consequences.[22]

Injectate Associated

Space-occupying and pressure-applying fluids are primarily introduced with injection of medication or contrast during procedures. Onset of acute monoplegia has been reported after injection of L5 nerve roots and lysis of

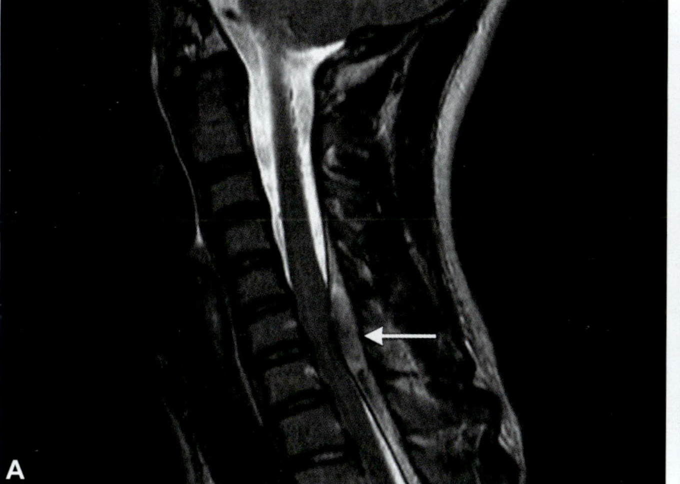

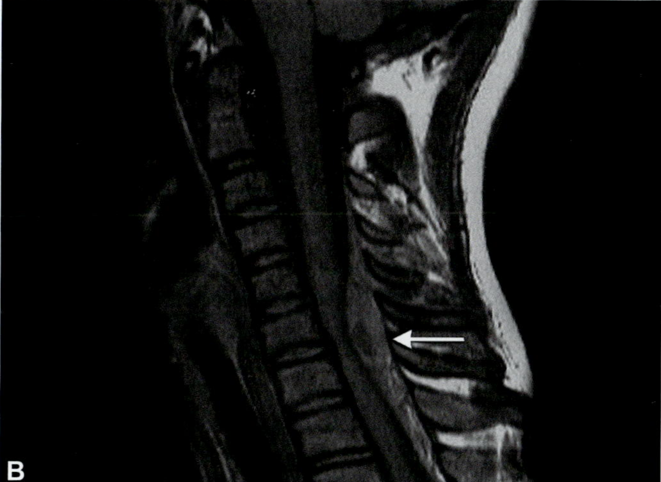

Figs. 35.3A and B: Magnetic resonance imaging showing a spinal epidural hematoma in the cervical spine as indicated by the arrows. *Source*: With permission from Al-Mutair A, Bednar DA. Spinal epidural hematoma. J Am Acad Orthop Surg. 2010;18(8):494-502. With permission from Department of Surgery, McMaster University, Hamilton, Ontario, Canada.

adhesions with both small and large injectate volumes.[23] Transient blindness is another rare complication. The mechanism involves a rise in CSF pressure as high as 85 cm H_2O after an epidural injection of 20 mL of fluid. The magnitude of the pressure rise is proportional to the speed and volume of injection. A rapid elevation of intracranial pressure can lead to an increase in retinal venous pressure and ensuing retinal hemorrhages. Of the 10 reported cases of transient blindness, 9 occurred in female patients.[24] Other risk factors include diabetes mellitus, obesity, and hypertension, all of which may alter ophthalmic vasculature. Visual acuity returns to baseline in most patients.[24]

Epidural Abscess

Abscess formation can result in severe morbidity and generally requires urgent treatment. Cervical epidural abscesses have been reported to occur after cervical ILESI, leading to central cord syndrome with subsequent resolution after surgical decompression.[25] In a 2004 review of epidural abscesses by Hooten et al.[26] clinical outcomes were documented in 13 of the 14 cases and were highly variable. Four patients experienced a full recovery, two of whom did not undergo surgery. Two patients died of perioperative complications, one patient became paraplegic, and one became quadriplegic. The remaining patients had memory impairment or focal neurologic deficits involving the extremities or bladder.[26]

Granuloma Related

Granuloma formation can also cause neurologic compromise as the thickening dura encroaches upon nervous structures. This inflammatory response often occurs after neural irritation. The risk is potentiated by multiple injections as outlined in the case of a 39-year-old woman who was treated with a series of three ESIs, over a 6-week period, for the treatment of a C6–C7 herniated disk. She experienced headaches, upper neck pain, and lower extremity paresthesias. Subsequent MRI revealed a gadolinium-enhancing mass consistent with an epidural granuloma.[27]

INFECTIONS

Infections are a risk of any invasive procedure and have been reported to occur in 0.1–0.01% of spinal injections.[28] Depending on the site of inoculation, they can result in osteomyelitis, discitis, meningitis, or an epidural abscess (Figs. 35.4A to D), all of which may lead to neurologic deficits and death (Figs. 35.5A to D). Common bacteria include *Staphylococcus aureus*, followed by *Streptococcus* species and *Staphylococcus epidermidis*. Organisms may be introduced deep via instrumentation from skin flora, unsterile needles, or contaminated medications. Alternatively, they may migrate to the injection site with localized bleeding. Individuals with compromised immune systems, such as diabetics, are more likely to become infected. Furthermore, administration of steroids can hinder the local inflammatory response by interfering with cytokine production and suppressing the hypothalamic–pituitary–adrenocortical axis, which may lead to a systemic immune suppression.

Osteomyelitis/Diskitis

Osteomyelitis and diskitis usually occurs simultaneously with epidural abscesses secondary to local spread. Adjacent disk infection also develop with concomitant osteomyelitis. Diagnosis is challenging and often delayed. Often, patients do not manifest symptoms and signs of infection. A 73-year-old woman underwent an L3/4 epidural injection for mechanical low back pain with neurogenic claudication. One month later she returned with increased back pain and MRI revealed L4/5 and L2/3 diskitis with osteomyelitis. Biopsy culture grew *Pseudomonas aeruginosa*. She was successfully treated with intravenous ciprofloxacin and gentamicin.[29]

Meningitis

The risk of contracting CNS infections after spinal injection is estimated at 1/1,000.[30] A recent meta-analysis studied patients admitted to a neurological care unit for the treatment of meningitis between 1992 and 2000. A total of 128 patients were treated during this time interval, eight of whom previously received corticosteroid injections. The probability of developing meningitis is believed to be higher in cases of accidental dural puncture.[30]

VASCULAR INJURY

The incidence of intravascular injection differs depending on approach and spinal location, estimated at 19.4% in cervical TFESIs and 11.2% in lumbar TFESIs.[31] Cervical and lumbar ILESIs are thought to be safer from a vascular perspective, with rates of 4.2% and 0.5%, respectively.[32] Caudal ESIs fall in between at 9.2%.[33] Despite these statistics, the transforaminal approach has gained

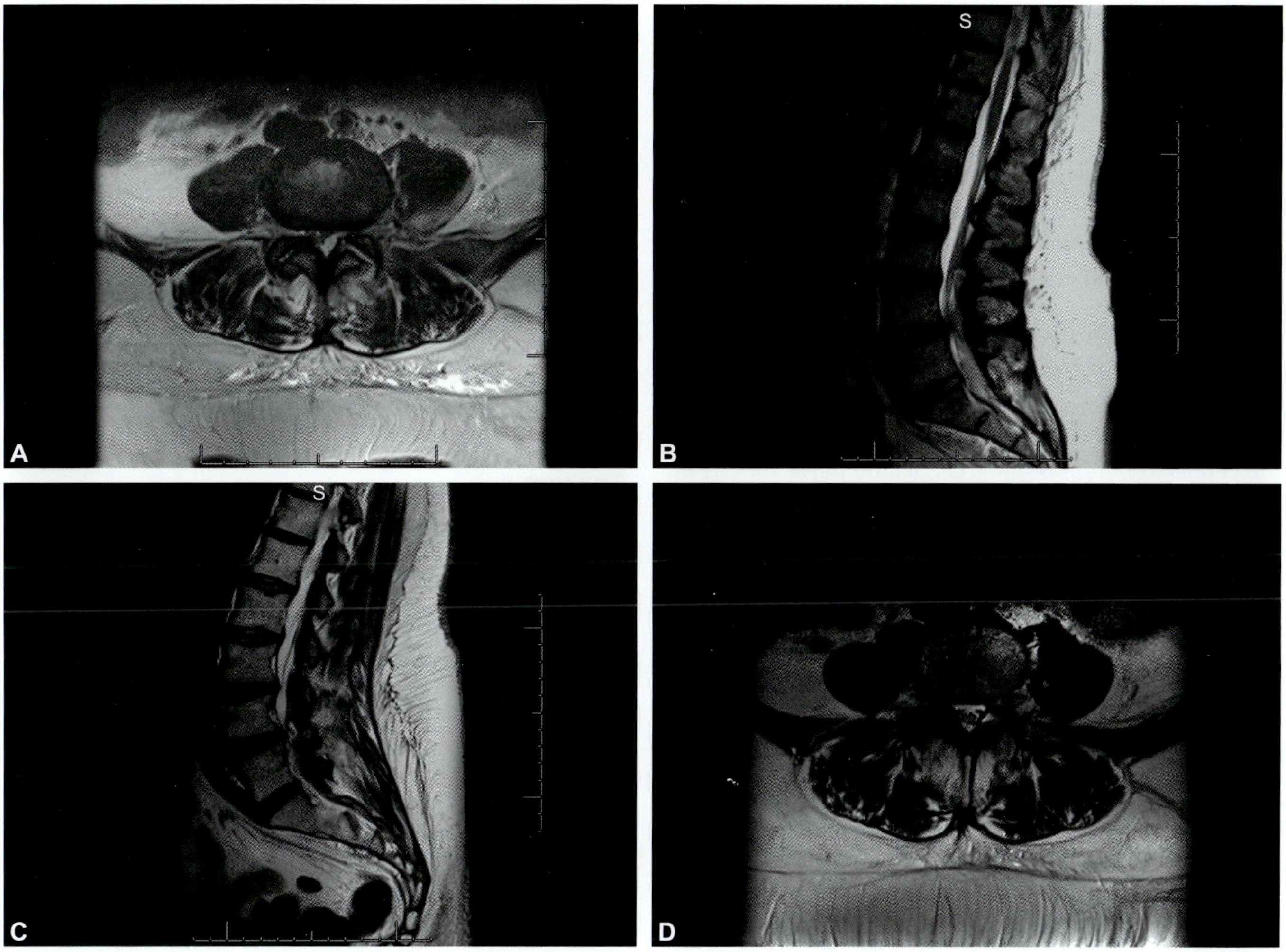

Figs. 35.4A to D: (A) Septic epidural abscess, leakage of pus into spinal canal due to infected facet joint. (B) Sagittal view of a septic epidural abscess. (C) An epidural injection healed the abscess. (D) Upon further investigation, a synovial cyst was discovered (arrow). An additional injection was administered and the patient fully recovered.

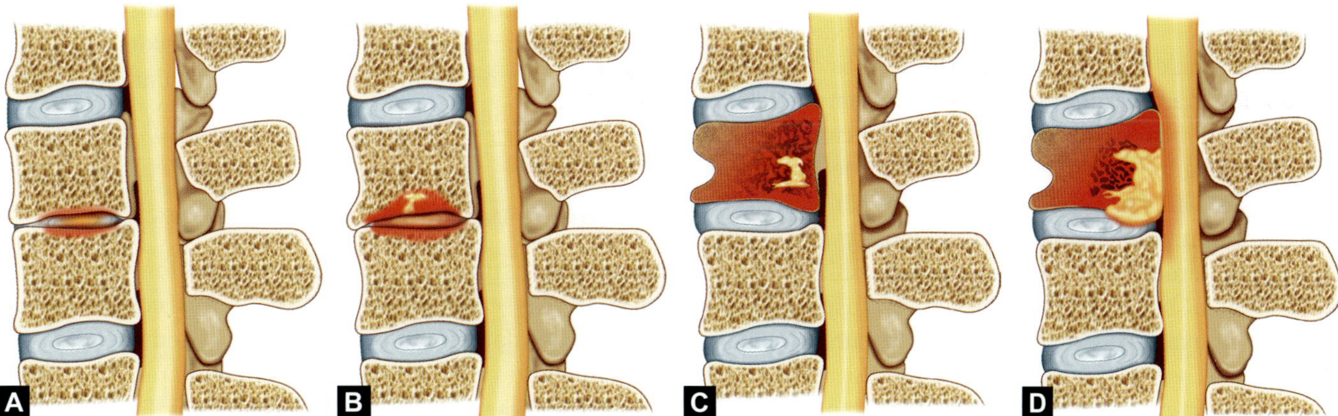

Figs. 35.5A to D: The progression of spinal infection (clockwise from top left) from the initial inflammation to vertebral body penetration and compression of the spinal cord.

popularity in recent years for a number of reasons. Theoretically, it allows for direct access to the dorsal root ganglion pathologically involved in causing a patient's radicular pain. Comparatively, in studies of interlaminar cervical epidural injections, medication spreads ventrally toward the nerve root only 28% of the time.[34] Multiple articles have corroborated these sentiments clinically. In head-to-head comparisons of ILESI and TFESI for the treatment of lumbar radicular back pain, two independent trials reported a 44 versus 74% and 35 versus 82% reduction in pain scores, respectively.[35,36]

The classically recommended approach of needle placement is defined by the "safe triangle". When viewed from posterior to anterior, it consists of the pedicle as the cephalad border of the triangle, the nerve root as the tangential base, and a side wall overlying the lateral edge of the vertebral body. Approaching the safe triangle is thought to provide the best balance of risk and benefit for patients. Avoids the nerve root. However, notably absent from the traditional depiction of the "safe triangle" is the vascular anatomy. Some proponents urge practitioners to perform TFESI at the caudal aspect of the foramen underneath the nerve root. This region is known as Kambin's triangle, whose hypotenuse is the exiting nerve, base is the caudal vertebral body, and height is the traversing nerve root. This method is hypothetically proposed to be more efficacious as steroids are instilled directly at the nerve-disk interface in contrast to the standard technique, which delivers the injectate further cephalad.[37] However, the approach to the Kambin's places the nerve at the path of the needle as well as exposing to the patient to disproportionate risk of infection due to intradiskal entry.

Vascular damage can result in catastrophic damage, including spinal cord or brain infarction. Therefore, safety practices are constantly created to decrease the probability of complications. Aspiration or "flashback" within the spinal needle is generally felt to indicate vascular penetration; however, recent papers have reported that detecting blood within the needle conferred a sensitivity of 44.7–45.9%.[33] This low value may, in part, be due to a combination of factors. If the venous system is punctured, pressure is often inadequate to result in spontaneous flow of blood into the syringe, and aspiration may actually generate sufficient negative pressure to collapse small caliber vessels. Accordingly, administration of contrast in conjunction with live fluoroscopic imaging is used to confirm instrument position and prevent intravascular medication delivery. Unfortunately, studies of lumbosacral transforaminal ESIs still indicate a simultaneous epidural and vessel injection incidence of 8.9%.[38] Digital subtraction angiography may enhances visualization of contrast diffusion by removing background structures identified on an initial scout film from subsequent images after contrast administration. However, many practitioners do not accept it as a genuinely useful tool. Finally, modified needles have been implemented to minimize the rate of arterial cannulation. A single preliminary trial of the needle-catheter hybrid delivery system reported vascular trespass rates, which were one third of those standard spinal needles during cervical TFESIs.[39]

Anatomy

To appreciate the complications that can arise due to vascular injury, one must understand the intricate anatomy of the spinal cord vasculature. Blood is delivered to the spinal cord through a single anterior artery and paired posterior spinal arteries, which send penetrating branches. The cervical level is supplied by the vertebral, ascending cervical, and deep cervical arteries that originate from the subclavian artery. The vertebral artery travels up the spinal column within each cervical transverse process, lying anterior and adjacent to the cervical neural foramen, which makes unintended penetration possible during cervical transforaminal blockade. At the thoracic and lumbar levels, local spinal branches arise from tributaries of the aorta and iliac vessels. The spinal branches traverse the intervertebral foramina adjacent to the spinal nerves at multiple levels and continue as radicular arteries. In turn, the radicular arteries penetrate the dura and divide to follow the ventral and dorsal nerve roots, where they eventually join the anterior and posterior spinal arteries. The artery of Adamkiewicz is an enlargement of a lumbar anterior radicular artery and contributes the majority of the blood supply to the lower two thirds of the spinal cord.

Anatomic Variation

Anomalous structures such as arteriovenous malformations (AVMs) can increase the likelihood of complications. Often, vascular anomalies are not visualized on soft tissue imaging and cannot be anticipated. The artery of Adamkiewicz enters the spine at varying locations. Eighty percent of the time the artery enters on the left side, as high as T7 or as low as S1. Photographic evidence has confirmed the presence of a cervical radicular artery at the C6 level, which anastomoses with the anterior spinal artery, providing a direct route for spinal cord infarction.[40] Radicular arteries have been found to fluctuate in both connections and local path. Typically, they follow a tortuous path along the spinal-nerve roots in the anterior-inferior aspect of the foramina. However, in cadaveric studies, Huntoon[41] recorded a branch that was located in the posterior-inferior aspect of the foramen, which could readily be pierced during injection. Previous publications have correlated history of spine operations with negative outcomes after ESIs.[42] Anomalous vasculature is postulated to be the root cause for several reasons. First, post surgical lumbar tissue has been shown to undergo neoangiogenesis.[43] Newly created vessels may form aberrant connections with the spinal blood supply and serve as unintended targets. Alternately, surrounding scar tissue may displace or fix a previously established radiculomedullary artery and make its penetration more probable.[42]

Vascular Compromise

Venous Injection

Although the consequences of arterial injections are more deleterious than their venous counterparts, all unwarranted intravascular injections should be avoided when possible. Venous injections can produce an air embolism. Furthermore, they can misplace medication to a nontarget site, reducing its diagnostic and therapeutic benefits.[38]

Perfusion Disruption

The pathogenesis of arterial compromise is decidedly complex and several mechanisms can impair vascular perfusion. One factor that increases the risk of spinal cord ischemia is delivery of large volumes of anesthetic solution into the epidural space, which can promote hypotension and watershed infarction. Furthermore, two situations may arise causing vascular stasis. When the sustained compressive effect of the injectate produces pressures that surpass the local arterial pressure, neural ischemia can take place. Second, a so-called backpressure ischemia may result if sustained venous compression occurs.

Anatomic Predisposition (AVM, AVF)

Unforeseen abnormalities, namely AVMs or arteriovenous fistulas (AVFs), are susceptible to vascular injury. The majority of AVMs are congenital and located intradurally, on the surface or within the parenchyma of the spinal cord. AVFs are a direct connection between arterial and venous pathways without the benefit of intervening capillaries. AVM and AVFs, elevated venous pressure, and fragile vessel walls predispose to ischemia or hemorrhage.

Arterial Puncture and Vasospasm

Another proposed mechanism of ischemia involves a mechanically induced arterial vasospasm. Studies of the cerebral circulation catalogued the response of the basilar artery when touched with a fine glass needle. An annular contraction was exhibited at the site of stimulation and lasted between 5 seconds and 10 minutes. When the vessel was punctured, it contracted at the point of rupture as well as a considerable distance on either side.[44] A study of the internal carotid, middle cerebral, and anterior cerebral arteries of Rhesus monkeys corroborated these findings. Puncture with a 30-gauge needle produced immediate intense vasospasm. Serial angiograms proved that distal perfusion was typically compromised for 4 hours and in one case was still evident up to 4 days later.[45] Moreover, mechanical insult may lead to arterial compression or vasospasm, which can precipitate intravascular thrombosis.[42]

There has been speculation that the size and sharpness of the needle tip may be modified to reduce risk. Although the idea lacks supporting evidence, it has been proposed that a blunt needle may eliminate intravascular entry or prevent vasospasm or vessel injury.[46] The potential consequences of arterial puncture are life threatening. An intra-articular injection might result in embolus formation and brain or spinal cord infarction. Arterial gas embolus has been reported to be a potentially fatal complication of ESI.[47]

Vasospasm might occur due to hemorrhage from an arterial puncture (Fig. 35.4) or cervical transforaminal epidural injection and may cause spinal cord infarction.

Embolization

Brain or spinal cord infarction due to arterial occlusion from air or particulate steroids. This theory has been substantiated in animal models and has been proposed as another mechanism of injury.[41,48-54] The prevailing model assumes this occurs via antegrade flow of material through direct cannulation of a vertebral or radiculomedullary artery. Nevertheless, one study also raises the possibility of retrograde flow into a common arterial trunk with subsequent antegrade flow into vulnerable structures. Once again, this emphasizes the crucial role anatomic variability plays in neurologic complications.

Particulate steroid embolization to the cerebral vasculature can pose multiple dangers. It has been listed as a differential cause of posterior hemisphere reversible leukoencephalopathy.[55] This disease is characterized clinically by reversible symptoms, including headache, decreased alertness, altered mental status, seizures, and visual loss and radiologically by white matter edema in the posterior hemispheres. Some publications have called attention to sedation, particularly before cervical injections, as the patient is unable to relay critical information although the ASA Closed Claims database contains an abundant number of injections into the spinal cord in a wake patients.[54] Particulate embolization may also have fatal outcomes. Edlow et al.[53] reported the case of a 64-year-old man with chronic cervical pain who consented to a C1–C2 intra-articular facet steroid injection. Of note, the procedure was executed without fluoroscopic assistance. He lost and never regained consciousness directly after infusion of 2 mL of triamcinolone. Given the poor prognosis, the family withdrew life support and the patient died shortly thereafter. Postmortem studies were consistent with left vertebral artery puncture. Brain dissection was consistent with a showering of infarcts throughout the posterior circulation territory, including the pons, inferomedial left temporal lobe, left occipital lobe, cerebellar hemispheres, and bilateral thalami, which confirmed an embolic etiology.[53]

A representative example of the dangers posed by local spread of injectate within the spinal cord vasculature is anterior spinal artery syndrome. It is classically categorized by abrupt motor loss, sphincter disturbance, and nonconcordant sensory examination with preservation of sensation to light touch but loss of pain and temperature.[41] When it occurs during ESI, the patient may have sudden back or abdominal pain soon after injection. MRI is the early test of choice and will demonstrate T2 signal change consistent with cord ischemia/infarct.[41] Permanent neurologic deterioration, including varying levels of paraplegia, have been acknowledged with spinal cord infarcts.[48] At lower levels, progression of conus medullaris syndrome may also take place.

Pre-existing Medical Disease

Concurrent medical conditions such as atherosclerosis or other comorbidities that would predispose one to develop arterial disease, including diabetes and vasculitides, potentiate the risk of impaired perfusion. Disruption of the muscular arterial wall with the sharp bevel of the needle can displace plaque and form an intimal flap. Furthermore, plaque disruption can initiate the coagulation cascade causing clot production or result in distal embolization.

Mechanical Vascular Disruption

A report of arterial dissection was published with grave consequences. The case involved a 44-year-old woman who suffered from migraine headaches and neck pain with radiculopathy. A transforaminal ESI via the left C6–C7 neural foramen was performed. After initial positioning under fluoroscopic guidance, aspiration of blood was positive and the needle was relocated. Repeat aspiration was negative, followed by contrast and medication instillation. The patient became immediately unresponsive and died later the ensuing day. The cause of death was clarified by autopsy. Vertebral artery puncture catalyzed intimal wall dissection and thrombosis creation with subsequent massive cerebral edema and cerebellar herniation. The authors believe this terrible outcome may be averted in the future with the use of CT guidance for cervical TFESIs.[56]

NEURAL COMPLICATIONS

Exacerbation of Pain

The most common complication of spinal injections is worsening of the pain being treated. The complication rate is dependent upon injection type. For example, in the administration of ESIs, roughly 1 in every 100 injections results in greater pain and 1 in 300 results in increased pain at the injection site.[57] However, in lumbosacral selective nerve root blocks (SNRBs), roughly 17% of injections result in increased pain at the injection site and 5% in increased spinal pain; in cervical SNRBs, pain increases at the injection site and spine by 23% and 9 %, respectively.[58]

Vasovagal Syncope

Sudden loss of consciousness from cerebral ischemia related to altered vagus activity has a significantly higher reported incidence in cervical (8%) than in lumbar injections (1–2%).[59] This condition is secondary to decreased cardiac output, peripheral vasodilation, and bradycardia. Upon removal of the needle and with supportive care, symptoms are self-limiting.

CHEMICAL INJURY

A multitude of substances are employed during ESIs including therapeutic medications, chemical preservatives, and contrast dyes, all of which have toxic profiles. This section will expand upon the properties and potential hazards of these commonly utilized compounds.

Steroid-Related Complications

Synthetic corticosteroids frequently selected for spinal injection procedures are derivatives of prednisolone, an analog of cortisol, and have long half-lives ranging from 36–72 hours. They exist in several forms including dexamethasone, betamethasone, methylprednisolone, and triamcinolone. The latter two are hydrophobic and form particulate suspensions. Theoretically, their tissue depot of large, slowly absorbing particles results in a longer duration of action. Of note, both methylprednisolone and triamcinolone have been found to regularly form crystal aggregates >10 μm in solution (Table 35.1). At this size, they are larger than the diameter of an average red blood cell, which makes it possible for them to cause CNS infarctions during unintended intravascular injections. Examples of these devastating consequences were discussed earlier in the chapter. Furthermore, simple occlusion of blood vessels may not be the only mechanism of CNS damage. An in vivo analysis of Depo Medrol, Solu Medrol, and Depo Medrol carrier groups was performed by Dawley et al.[60] After direct vascular inoculation, microscopic evaluation revealed erythrocyte extravasation into the parenchyma and cortex of the brain. It is theorized that the steroid solution produces direct endothelial toxicity, causing blood-brain barrier degradation and subsequent hemorrhagic injury.[60]

Neurotoxicity

The dura and arachnoid serve as barriers against chemical injury to intraspinal structures. Neural irritation can be a consequence of inadvertent intrathecal injection, in particular, arachnoiditis or aseptic meningitis. Arachnoiditis is defined as inflammation of the leptomeninges triggering production of fibrin exudates that cause nerve roots to adhere to each other and to the dural sac. The most common symptoms include burning pain in the lower back and lower extremities, variable motor impairment, numbness not after the dermatomal distribution, and bladder dysfunction. Latham et al.[61] demonstrated that high doses of betamethasone injected into the intrathecal spaces of sheep can precipitate arachnoiditis. Furthermore, drug vehicles, such as polyethylene glycol, within the steroid preparation were implicated in two cases of adhesive arachnoiditis among a series of 23 patients who received a total of 83 injections of methylprednisolone acetate.[62]

Aseptic meningitis is a generally benign condition accompanied by fever, nausea, headaches, meningismus, and in severe cases, seizures. The CSF examination reveals pleocytosis, elevated protein, and decreased glucose. Researchers documented the occurrence of this syndrome after intrathecal injections of 40 to 200 mg of methylprednisolone, with a dose-related polymorphonuclear pleocytosis that lasted up to 6 days.[14] Animal studies have also confirmed histological changes of feline nerve tissue after epidural injections of triamcinolone and lidocaine mixtures. Mild inflammatory changes were noted 30 days after injection with complete resolution in 120 days.[63]

Systemic Effects

Spinal corticosteroids may have systemic endocrine, renal, or cardiovascular side effects. Increased blood pressure may occur due to renal mineralocorticoid effects, which promote water and sodium retention. Mild peripheral edema may ensue; however, significant fluid shifts have been reported, resulting in congestive heart failure exacerbation after a single ESI.[64] Steroids may lead to an elevation in blood glucose, particularly in the postprandial diabetic population. These effects may last up to 2 weeks after administration. Additional finger stick monitoring and diabetic medication adjustment may be warranted during this period. Cushing's syndrome is a well-known complication of prolonged steroid use. It is defined by the presence of facial edema, a buffalo hump, skin bruising, and scaly skin lesions. Another lesser-known sequela is epidural lipomatosis, or enlargement of epidural fatty tissue. It is hypothesized that glucocorticoids induce certain fat deposits in the body to undergo selective hypertrophy. Excessive expansion can cause symptomatic spinal stenosis and direct compression of neural structures.

Local Anesthetics

Administration of local anesthetics, such as lidocaine or bupivacaine, in combination with steroids is commonplace in ESIs. Depending upon the area being injected, effects of local anesthetics range from benign to life threatening.

CNS Effects

Swift onset of transient paresthesias and motor weakness can occur after inadvertent subarachnoid administration causing spinal anesthesia. It is important to differentiate between the presentations of subdural and intrathecal blocks. In the former, slow progression (5–30 minutes) of respiratory depression with moderate hypotension should be distinguished from more prompt onset (2–3 minutes) of acute cardiovascular collapse, seen with the latter.[4]

Systemic Toxicity

This is likely to occur after excessive dosage, excessive accidental vascular injection, or anesthetic test dose application. The concept of a test dose was designed to detect any temporary and reversible neurologic signs of intravascular instillation of a short-duration local anesthetic agent so that subsequent steroid injection, which may potentially result in permanent neurologic complications, can be withheld. Positive symptoms elicited by test dose can include metallic taste, dizziness, full body paresthesias, auditory changes, and slurred speech. At larger systemic local anesthetic doses, detrimental cardiac effects may occur and include a widened PR* interval, widened QRS** duration, atrioventricular dissociation, sinus arrest, and sinus tachycardia. In addition, occurrence of a grand mal seizure has been reported after administration of 2 mL of 1% lidocaine.[65]

Contrast Dye

In more recent decades, nonionic water-soluble contrast has been developed with lesser neurotoxicity than previous ionic or oil-based agents. Controlled studies verified the safety of intrathecal delivery of 10–15 mL of nonionic compounds. The most common adverse reactions, in descending order of frequency, included headache (18%), nausea (7.3%), muscular pain (3.7%), and hypotension (1.1%).[66] However, hypersensitivity reactions remain the most worrisome complication as they can cause cardiovascular collapse and airway compromise. Rare but severe anaphylactic responses involve immunoglobulin E-mediated release of vasoactive substances after re-exposure to an antigen after initial sensitization. More commonly encountered and just as complicating are anaphylactoid reactions, nonimmune-guided pseudoallergic reactions initiated by the direct release of histamine and other mediators from basophils and mast cells. Allergic encephalomyelitis can be produced after the introduction of an antigenic substance into the body, causing simultaneous inflammation of both the brain and spinal cord. If an allergy is suspected, some authors have recommended and confirmed the utility of alternative products, such as gadolinium, when performing ESIs.[67]

CONCLUSION

Although infrequent, spinal injections are associated with inherent and unavoidable risks. Depending on the patient profile, the probability of severe complications such as hematoma and infection are 1:10,000 to 1:100,000. Mild side effects are common and are part of the routine recovery of these patients. The risk of PDPH is about 1%, although in most fluoroscopic series this drops to about 1:500.[6] In conclusion, although absolute safety in medicine is challenging, further investigation of spinal injection practices is needed to mitigate the mechanisms of injury described in this chapter.

REFERENCES

1. Carrino JA, Morrison WB, Parker L, et al. Spinal injection procedures: volume, provider distribution, and reimbursement in the U.S. medicare population from 1993 to 1999. Radiology. 2002;225(3):723-9.
2. Botwin KP, Baskin M, Rao S. Adverse effects of fluoroscopically guided interlaminar thoracic epidural steroid injections. Am J Phys Med Rehabil. 2006;85(1):14-23.
3. Scanlon GC, Moeller-Bertram T, Romanowsky SM, et al. Cervical transforaminal epidural steroid injections: more dangerous than we think? Spine (Phila Pa 1976). 2007;32(11):1249-56.
4. Abbasi A, Malhotra G, Malanga G, et al. Complications of interlaminar cervical epidural steroid injections: a review of the literature. Spine (Phila Pa 1976). 2007;32(19):2144-51.
5. Dilke TF, Burry HC, Grahame R. Extradural corticosteroid injection in management of lumbar nerve root compression. Br Med J. 1973;2(5867):635-7.
6. Sprigge JS, Harper SJ. Accidental dural puncture and post dural puncture headache in obstetric anaesthesia: presentation and management: a 23-year survey in a district general hospital. Anaesthesia. 2008;63(1):36-43.
7. Crawford JS. The prevention of headache consequent upon dural puncture. Br J Anaesth. 1972;44(6):598-600.
8. Ozdemir O, Calisaneller T, Yildirim E, et al. Acute intracranial subdural hematoma after epidural steroid injection: a case report. J Manipulative Physiol Ther. 2007; 30(7):536-8.

* The PR interval represents the time between initial contraction of the atria and initial contraction of the ventricles.

** The QRS duration reflects the time of initial depolarization to final repolarization during ventricle contraction.

9. Simopoulos T, Peeters-Asdourian C. Pneumocephalus after cervical epidural steroid injection. Anesth Analg. 2001;92(6):1576-7.
10. Guarino AH, Wright NM. Pneumocephalus after a lumbar epidural steroid injection. Pain Physician. 2005;8(2):239-41.
11. Candido KD, Katz JA, Chinthagada M, et al. Incidence of intradiscal injection during lumbar fluoroscopically guided transforaminal and interlaminar epidural steroid injections. Anesth Analg. 2010; 110(5):1464-7.
12. Plastaras CT, Casey E, Goodman BS, et al. Inadvertent intradiscal contrast flow during lumbar transforaminal epidural steroid injections: a case series examining the prevalence of intradiscal injection as well as potential associated factors and adverse events. Pain Med. 2010;11(12):1765-73.
13. Lee JY, Nassr A, Ponnappan RK. Epidural hematoma causing paraplegia after a fluoroscopically guided cervical nerve-root injection. A case report. J Bone Joint Surg Am. 2007;89(9):2037-9.
14. Moore RJ. Handbook of pain and palliative care: biobehavioral approaches for the life course. New York, London: Springer; 2012.
15. Chronic spinal arachnoiditis. Br Med J. 1978;2(6136):518-9.
16. Ribeiro C. [Adhesive lumbar arachnoiditis]. Acta Med Port. 1998;11(1):59-65.
17. Ozgen S, Naderi S, Ozek MM, et al. Findings and outcome of revision lumbar disc surgery. J Spinal Disord. 1999;12(4):287-92.
18. Pear BL. Spinal epidural hematoma. Am J Roentgenol Radium Ther Nucl Med. 1972;115(1):155-64.
19. Xu R, Bydon M, Gokaslan ZL, et al. Epidural steroid injection resulting in epidural hematoma in a patient despite strict adherence to anticoagulation guidelines. J Neurosurg Spine. 2009;11(3):358-64.
20. Vandermeulen EP, Van Aken H, Vermylen J. Anticoagulants and spinal-epidural anesthesia. Anesth Analg. 1994;79(6):1165-77.
21. Horlocker TT, Wedel DJ. Infectious complications of regional anesthesia. Best Pract Res Clin Anaesthesiol. 2008;22(3):451-75.
22. Reitman CA, Watters W, 3rd. Subdural hematoma after cervical epidural steroid injection. Spine (Phila Pa 1976). 2002;27(6):E174-6.
23. Ho KY, Manghnani P. Acute monoplegia after lysis of epidural adhesions: a case report. Pain Pract. 2008;8(5):404-7.
24. Young WF. Transient blindness after lumbar epidural steroid injection: a case report and literature review. Spine (Phila Pa 1976). 2002;27(21):E476-7.
25. Waldman SD. Cervical epidural abscess after cervical epidural nerve block with steroids. Anesth Analg. 1991;72(5):717-8.
26. Hooten WM, Kinney MO, Huntoon MA. Epidural abscess and meningitis after epidural corticosteroid injection. Mayo Clin Proc. 2004;79(5):682-6.
27. Dietrich CL, Smith CE. Epidural granuloma and intracranial hypotension resulting from cervical epidural steroid injection. Anesthesiology. 2004;100(2):445-7.
28. Goodman BS, Posecion LW, Mallempati S, et al. Complications and pitfalls of lumbar interlaminar and transforaminal epidural injections. Curr Rev Musculoskelet Med. 2008;1(3-4):212-22.
29. Yue WM, Tan SB. Distant skip level discitis and vertebral osteomyelitis after caudal epidural injection: a case report of a rare complication of epidural injections. Spine (Phila Pa 1976). 2003;28(11):E209-11.
30. Gaul C, Neundorfer B, Winterholler M. Iatrogenic (para-) spinal abscesses and meningitis following injection therapy for low back pain. Pain. 2005;116(3):407-10.
31. Furman MB, Giovanniello MT, O'Brien EM. Incidence of intravascular penetration in transforaminal cervical epidural steroid injections. Spine (Phila Pa 1976). 2003;28(1):21-5.
32. Manchikanti L, Malla Y, Wargo BW, et al. A prospective evaluation of complications of 10,000 fluoroscopically directed epidural injections. Pain Physician. 2012;15(2): 131-40.
33. Renfrew DL, Moore TE, Kathol MH, et al. Correct placement of epidural steroid injections: fluoroscopic guidance and contrast administration. AJNR Am J Neuroradiol. 1991;12(5):1003-7.
34. Stojanovic MP, Vu TN, Caneris O, et al. The role of fluoroscopy in cervical epidural steroid injections: an analysis of contrast dispersal patterns. Spine (Phila Pa 1976). 2002;27(5):509-14.
35. Ackerman WE, 3rd, Ahmad M. The efficacy of lumbar epidural steroid injections in patients with lumbar disc herniations. Anesth Analg. 2007;104(5):1217-22.
36. Gharibo CG, Varlotta GP, Rhame EE, et al. Interlaminar versus transforaminal epidural steroids for the treatment of subacute lumbar radicular pain: a randomized, blinded, prospective outcome study. Pain Physician. 2011;14(6):499-511.
37. Glaser SE, Shah RV. Root cause analysis of paraplegia following transforaminal epidural steroid injections: the 'unsafe' triangle. Pain Physician. 2010;13(3):237-44.
38. Smuck M, Fuller BJ, Yoder B, et al. Incidence of simultaneous epidural and vascular injection during lumbosacral transforaminal epidural injections. Spine J. 2007;7(1):79-82.
39. Kloth DS, Calodney AK, Derby R, et al. Improving the safety of transforaminal epidural steroid injections in the treatment of cervical radiculopathy. Pain Physician. 2011;14(3):285-93.
40. Verrills P, Nowesenitz G, Barnard A. Penetration of a cervical radicular artery during a transforaminal epidural injection. Pain Med. 2010;11(2):229-31.
41. Huntoon MA. Anatomy of the cervical intervertebral foramina: vulnerable arteries and ischemic neurologic injuries after transforaminal epidural injections. Pain. 2005;117(1-2):104-11.
42. Wybier M, Gaudart S, Petrover D, et al. Paraplegia complicating selective steroid injections of the lumbar spine. Report of five cases and review of the literature. Eur Radiol. 2010;20(1):181-9.
43. Van Goethem JW, Parizel PM, Jinkins JR. Review article: MRI of the postoperative lumbar spine. Neuroradiology. 2002;44(9):723-39.

44. Florey H. Microscopical observations on the circulation of the blood in the cerebral cortex. Brain. 1925;48:43-64.
45. Simeone FA, Ryan KG, Cotter JR. Prolonged experimental cerebral vasospasm. J Neurosurg. 1968;29(4):357-66.
46. Gharibo C. Epidural steroid injections: an update on mechanisms of injury and safety. Techn Regl Anesth Pain Manage. 2009;13(4):266-71.
47. MacLean CA, Bachman DT. Documented arterial gas embolism after spinal epidural injection. Ann Emerg Med. 2001; 38(5):592-5.
48. Houten JK, Errico TJ. Paraplegia after lumbosacral nerve root block: report of three cases. Spine J. 2002;2(1):70-5.
49. Chan LL, Kumar AJ, Leeds NE, et al. Post-epidural analgesia spinal cord infarction: MRI correlation. Acta Neurol Scand. 2002;105(4):344-8.
50. Ludwig MA, Burns SP. Spinal cord infarction following cervical transforaminal epidural injection: a case report. Spine (Phila Pa 1976). 2005;30(10):E266-8.
51. Muro K, O'Shaughnessy B, Ganju A. Infarction of the cervical spinal cord following multilevel transforaminal epidural steroid injection: case report and review of the literature. J Spinal Cord Med. 2007;30(4):385-8.
52. Kennedy DJ, Dreyfuss P, Aprill CN, et al. Paraplegia following image-guided transforaminal lumbar spine epidural steroid injection: two case reports. Pain Med. 2009;10(8):1389-94.
53. Edlow BL, Wainger BJ, Frosch MP, et al. Posterior circulation stroke after C1-C2 intra-articular facet steroid injection: evidence for diffuse microvascular injury. Anesthesiology. 2010;112(6):1532-5.
54. Beckman WA, Mendez RJ, Paine GF, et al. Cerebellar herniation after cervical transforaminal epidural injection. Reg Anesth Pain Med. 2006;31(3):282-5.
55. Kim W, Kim JS, Lim SC, et al. Reversible posterior leukoencephalopathy syndrome after cervical transforaminal epidural steroid injection presenting as transient blindness. Anesth Analg. 2011;112(4):967-70.
56. Rozin L, Rozin R, Koehler SA, et al. Death during transforaminal epidural steroid nerve root block (C7) due to perforation of the left vertebral artery. Am J Forensic Med Pathol. 2003;24(4):351-5.
57. McGrath JM, Schaefer MP, Malkamaki DM. Incidence and characteristics of complications from epidural steroid injections. Pain Med. 2011;12(5):726-31.
58. Huston CW, Slipman CW, Garvin C. Complications and side effects of cervical and lumbosacral selective nerve root injections. Arch Phys Med Rehabil. 2005;86(2):277-83.
59. Friedrich JM, Harrast MA. Lumbar epidural steroid injections: indications, contraindications, risks, and benefits. Curr Sports Med Rep. 2010;9(1):43-9.
60. Dawley JD, Moeller-Bertram T, Wallace MS, et al. Intra-arterial injection in the rat brain: evaluation of steroids used for transforaminal epidurals. Spine (Phila Pa 1976). 2009;34(16):1638-43.
61. Latham JM, Fraser RD, Moore RJ, et al. The pathologic effects of intrathecal betamethasone. Spine (Phila Pa 1976). 1997;22(14):1558-62.
62. Nelson DA, Vates TS, Jr, Thomas RB, Jr. Complications from intrathecal steroid therapy in patients wsith multiple sclerosis. Acta Neurol Scand. 1973;49(2):176-88.
63. Delaney TJ, Rowlingson JC, Carron H, et al. Epidural steroid effects on nerves and meninges. Anesth Analg. 1980;59(8): 610-4.
64. Goebert HW, Jr, Jallo SJ, Gardner WJ, et al. Painful radiculopathy treated with epidural injections of procaine and hydrocortisone acetate: results in 113 patients. Anesth Analg. 1961;40:130-4.
65. Chung SG. Convulsion caused by a lidocaine test in cervical transforaminal epidural steroid injection. PM R. 2011;3 (7):674-7.
66. Drayer BP, Vassallo C, Sudilovsky A, et al. A double-blind clinical trial of iopamidol versus metrizamide for lumbosacral myelography. J Neurosurg. 1983;58(4):531-7.
67. Safriel Y, Ali M, Hayt M, et al. Gadolinium use in spine procedures for patients with allergy to iodinated contrast-experience of 127 procedures. AJNR Am J Neuroradiol. 2006;27(6):1194-7.

CHAPTER

36

Medial Branch Block and Rhizotomy

Devon Ryan, Jamie Terran, Mohammed Khan

INTRODUCTION

Back pain is a common medical problem, with a lifetime prevalence reported between 54% and 80%.[1] It is a leading reason for physician visits and hospitalizations and has become very costly due to both health care utilization and lost productivity.[2] Spinal pain is responsible for the majority of cases of chronic, unresolved pain, and treatment failures.[1] Patients may, of course, present with pain in any region of the spine; however, cervical and lumbar pain are much more common than thoracic pain.[3] Techniques that may diagnose the cause of a patient's back pain are of great interest to the physician, who then may offer targeted treatment to resolve the pain.

A significant portion of back pain patients have symptoms originating from the facet (zygapophyseal) joint. For those with pain in the lumbar spine, 31% are estimated to have facet-mediated joint pain, with that value increasing to 42% and 55% for thoracic and cervical pain, respectively.[4] The anatomy of the facet joint is best explained in the context of the spinal motion segment, which consists of two adjacent vertebrae and the intervening disk. In each segment, the disk and a pair of facet joints comprise a three-joint complex, with the disk within the anterior column and the facet joints as part of the posterior elements. Each facet joint itself consists of an articulation of the superior articular process of the inferior vertebra and the inferior articular process of the superior vertebra (Fig. 36.1). The facet joint is synovial, with the two processes surrounded by a fluid-filled capsule. The orientation of the processes varies throughout the spine, guiding and limiting motion appropriately for each region.[5]

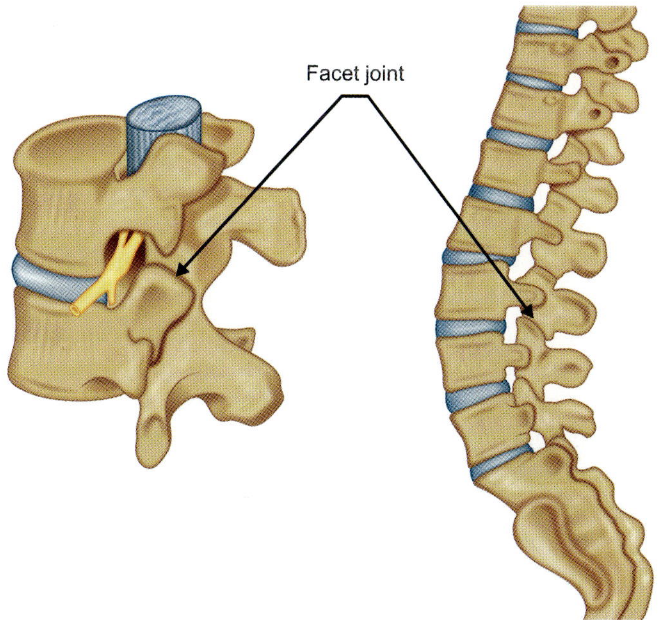

Fig. 36.1: The facet joint, in a spinal segment and the entire spine.

Degeneration of the joints within each spinal segment is a normal process of aging. Typically, the disk breaks down first, which exerts axial pressure on the facet joints. As the facet joints carry more of the load, the degeneration of the joint cartilage, capsule, and synovium may be accelerated, leading to increased friction and stress at the joint.[6] This, in turn, can cause osteophytic overgrowth and osteoarthritis. Ultimately, it is osteoarthritis of the joint complex that causes facet joint pain in the majority of cases.

There is no specific sign or symptom for the identification of facet joint pain from patient history or physical examination. Typically, patients are older and present with nonspecific back pain greater on one side (in any region) that fails to resolve itself over a period of weeks or months. Segmental examination that reveals tenderness over the relevant joint is often used as a signal,[11] although there is some evidence that this is not a reliable indicator for facet joint pain.[12] Symptoms may mimic those of herniated disk or nerve root impingement, as patients can present with "pseudoradicular" referred pain in one or more extremities. Typically, this pain will not be accompanied by a neurological deficit, which may help rule out peripheral neuralgia or radiculopathy.[13] In addition, in the lower back, facet joint pain has been shown to be more common in patients whose symptoms are relieved by recumbence and not exacerbated by coughing, forward flexion, rising from forward flexion, hyperextension, or extension rotation.[14] In general, facet joint pain should be suspected in an older patient with chronic back pain that cannot be ascribed to any other common etiologies.

Osteoarthritis can usually be visualized on X-rays, magnetic resonance imaging, or computed tomography (CT) imaging; however, many patients with objective evidence of facet degeneration in their scans are asymptomatic and do not have facet joint pain.[7] Bone scintigraphy (bone scanning) with single photon emission computed tomography, a more advanced imaging modality that enables the physician to identify areas of active bone remodeling, has shown promise in identifying those patients who will benefit from facet joint interventions.[8] More research on this technique is necessary, however, as it has only proven superior to ordinary CT imaging, an unreliable diagnostic method.

Indeed, identification of true facet joint pain is not straightforward. General consensus is that controlled diagnostic blocks are the most reliable method for detecting facet joint pain. Such techniques include intra-articular injections and medial branch blocks. Intra-articular injections, in which a small amount of a local anesthetic, with or without steroids, is injected into the facet joint capsule, have enjoyed widespread use as both a diagnostic tool and therapeutic treatment for decades.[9] It is perhaps surprising, then, that these injections have never been validated for use as a diagnostic tool. Medial branch blocks are the most reliable tests to conclusively identify facet joint pain.[10] In this technique, the target of the anesthetic injection is the pair of nerves that innervate superior and inferior poles of each facet joint.

A few studies have shown medial branch blocks to have some therapeutic effectiveness, indicating a potential use for them beyond diagnosis.[7] The more proven technique for treatment of confirmed facet joint pain, however, is rhizotomy (also known as medial branch neurotomy or radiofrequency neurotomy). This procedure targets the same nerves as the medial branch block, but instead of an injection, a radiofrequency electrode is inserted to coagulate the nerves and denervate the facet joint.[10] The overall goal of this chapter is to present the salient aspects of medial branch blocks and rhizotomy, thus providing an introduction to the most widely verified techniques for the identification and treatment of facet joint pain.

MEDIAL BRANCH BLOCK

Medial branch block is a well-studied technique for confirming facet joint pain in the presence of a clinical suspicion. Facet joints are innervated by two medial branches that emanate from the dorsal ramus at the same level and the level above the joint. For example, the L3–L4 facet joint is innervated by the medial branches of the L2 and L3 dorsal rami (Fig. 36.2). Each nerve is typically targeted for injection as it crosses the superior articular process of the appropriate vertebra.[15] Before the procedure, a small amount of local anesthetic should be applied over the planned needle insertion point to numb the skin. It is important that the quantity of the anesthetic at the skin and as part of the nerve block is minimized since using too much could local anesthetic can relieve pain caused by structures other than the facet joints, such as ligaments, muscles, or the nerve root, and thereby produce false positive results. A 22-gauge needle is often utilized, and even smaller instruments have been employed to further reduce procedure-related pain that can confound the outcome.

Fluoroscopy is utilized to guide accurate needle placement and help rule out potential intravascular needle placement by allowing the clinician to visualize appropriate contrast flow pattern after injection of a small amount of contrast dye. Recent literature has suggested that ultrasound may also be useful for ensuring accurate administration of the injectate, but this technique has yet to be validated.[16] Furthermore, ultrasound does not allow for the detection of intravascular needle placement, meaning that fluoroscopy should continue to prove useful. The necessary injection volume is just 0.25–0.30 mL of

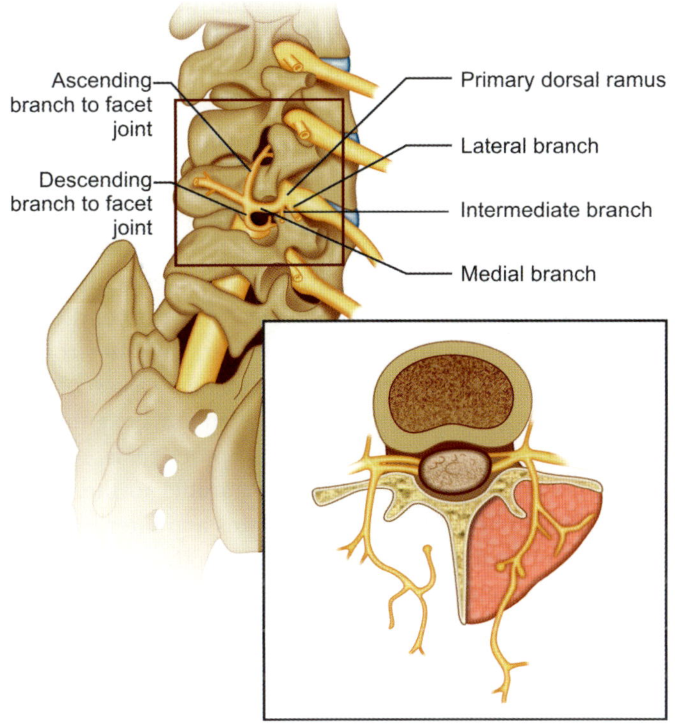

Fig. 36.2: Innervation of the facet joint.

anesthetic solution. This amount is sufficient to block the medial branch and makes it unlikely that the anesthetic will spread to and act upon nearby structures such as the epidural space or the nerve root, which can generate a false-positive result.[17] Major side effects are unlikely, although local tenderness and oozing at the injection site are relatively common.[18]

After the injection, the patient can be re-examined and his or her pain level is monitored. The pain level can be assessed before, immediately after the procedure and subsequent to discharge using a standardized metric such as the numeric rating scale. An optimal result is, of course, complete cessation of pain; however, this seems to be an unrealistic standard in clinical practice. As such, an 80% reduction in pain is a commonly accepted threshold for a "positive" test, with 50% relief typically viewed as too relaxed a standard. More ideally, the temporary pain relief should also be accompanied by an ability to perform previously painful activities, such as extension, rotation, and prolonged sitting.[10]

Medial branch blocks, even when performed properly, are prone to false-positive results. Such an outcome could be due to some manifestation of the placebo effect or spread of the anesthetic agent to nearby structures that are pain generators. Specifically, the false-positive rate for single medial branch blocks in the cervical spine has been estimated as 45%, with similar values of 42% and 45% found for the thoracic and lumbar regions, respectively.[11]

A number of multiple-procedure paradigms that aim to minimize the chance of a false-positive result have been specified, but the risk, expense, and patient inconvenience of additional, multilevel medial branch blocks must be acknowledged. One method, placebo control, involves a series of three injections. The initial block uses an active anesthetic, and if the result is positive, second and third blocks are performed on later dates—one with an active anesthetic and one with a placebo. These two are administered in random order and, ideally, under double-blind conditions. The result of the entire procedure is positive if pain relief occurs when anesthetic is used but does not occur when placebo is injected.

Another commonly implemented protocol, called comparative control, involves only two procedures. Two anesthetics that confer different durations of relief, such as lidocaine and bupivacaine, are administered on separate occasions. The result is positive only if both blocks relieve pain and the longer lasting agent (bupivacaine, in the preceding example) provides a longer period of relief. In this paradigm, the relative duration of relief is the only important consideration. It may be argued that comparative control, given that it involves two injections instead of three, is more easily utilized and cost-effective than placebo control. However, it also seems somewhat less reliable.[19] Other practical paradigms suggest that even single-administration local anesthetic blockade of the medial branch nerve can serve to provide relief for much longer than the duration of local anesthetic effect due to a termination of the cycle of pre-existing pain. This would seem to evaluating the comparative control method, which also depends crucially on eliciting an accurate patient history.

If a medial branch block is performed correctly under controlled conditions, the clinician should take a positive result to mean that the source of the patient's pain is the tested facet joint(s). Correspondingly, in the event of a negative result, the physician should continue to look for other causes of the patient's chronic back pain. Following a positive result, the practitioner is in a position to deliver longer term therapeutic care. Two treatment options in response to this scenario have been studied.

The first is to deliver another medial branch block using essentially the same procedure as outlined above.

This therapeutic approach has been tested in a series of three studies: one on the lumbar spine, one on the thoracic spine, and one on the cervical spine.[20-22] In all three trials, the investigators used diagnostic medial branch blocks to establish the presence of facet joint pain in subjects and then performed a subsequent injection using either local anesthetic or local anesthetic mixed with steroids. Across the studies, they found long-term pain relief (on average, 17–20 weeks before regression to 50% of original pain level)—a much longer duration of relief than would be expected given the characteristics of the anesthetic. Patients also experienced decreased disability and continued to obtain relief with additional injections. There was no difference in outcomes between the groups with and without steroids in the injectate. The mechanism for this longer duration of relief is not well understood but may be secondary to neuromodulatory effect of the steroid on the C fibers. Furthermore, the investigators decided against including a placebo group, citing difficulties with identifying a true spinal injection placebo and ethical considerations.[20-22] Given these shortcomings, more research is needed on the use of medial branch block as a long-term treatment.

RHIZOTOMY (MEDIAL BRANCH NEUROTOMY, RADIOFREQUENCY NEUROTOMY)

The second and better-studied therapeutic option is rhizotomy. Rhizotomy involves targeted insertion of an electrode with the goal of coagulating the medial branches that innervate painful facet joints. The procedure follows logically from a positive medial branch block: if certain nerves are shown to be transmitting pain signals, ablating them for a prolonged period should provide extended relief. A positive, diagnostic medial branch block can be considered an appropriate indication threshold for rhizotomy.

Procedurally, rhizotomy bears resemblance to a medial branch block. The patient may receive a sedative for relaxation and a local anesthetic to numb the electrode insertion site. The relevant medial branches (two for each joint) are similarly targeted as they wrap around the superior articular process of the relevant vertebra. There is some variation across physicians in the size of electrode utilized. A 22-gauge cannula with a 5 mm active tip is the most commonly used,[23] but some physicians have advocated for a larger instrument such as an 18-gauge electrode with a 10-mm tip.[24] The reasoning behind this suggestion is that the bigger electrode has a larger radius of action, endowing the physician with a more substantial margin of error in positioning the device. In any case, fluoroscopic guidance is utilized to ensure accurate placement of the electrode.

The orientation of the electrode relative to the target nerve has proven to be an important consideration. In the past, physicians have often attempted to coagulate the medial branch by positioning the electrode perpendicular to the nerve.[10] This technique, however, only destroys a small segment of the nerve even in the best case scenario and may result in incomplete or even no coagulation. Current consensus is that the best practice is instead to position the tip of the electrode parallel to the target nerve (Fig. 36.3).[25] This method ablates a greater number of nodes of Ranvier to provide an effective conduction block and prevent jumping of the impulse due to too short a segment of ablation.[25] Parallel positioning thus makes a successful procedure more likely and results in a longer duration of relief. Sixty to one hundred twenty seconds of radiofrequency treatment at a temperature of 80°C should be sufficient to coagulate all types of fibers in the target nerve.[23,26]

The effectiveness of medial branch neurotomy has been examined to varying degrees in the different regions of the spine. In the cervical segment, the procedure is generally accepted as effective provided that the proper

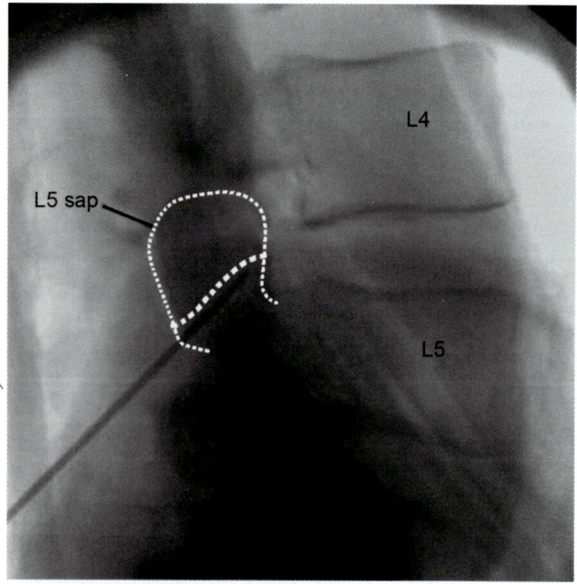

Fig. 36.3: Lateral radiograph showing accurate electrode placement for neurotomy.

diagnostic criteria and procedure are implemented.[27,28] The average duration of pain relief in rigorous studies has been found to be between 7 and 9 months.[29] The consensus regarding rhizotomy in the lumbar spine is comparable,[7,10,23,30] with an average period of relief of about 9 months.[29] In both the cervical and lumbar regions, repeat neurotomies have proven to be effective, particularly in those patients for whom the original ablation was effective. Furthermore, no harms or reduction in relief have been associated with subsequent procedures.[29] As for the thoracic region, evidence supporting medial branch neurotomy is much more limited.[31] This is likely due to the dearth of studies on the topic, a situation not surprising given the low prevalence of thoracic back pain in comparison to cervical or lumbar pain. Nevertheless, research on rhizotomy in the thoracic spine is needed, and the procedure may prove useful given the similarities in facet joint anatomy throughout the spine.

CONCLUSION

Most adults in the United States will, at some point in their lives, experience back pain, making it a very relevant medical condition. However, it is often difficult to pinpoint the source of such pain conclusively. Any techniques that allow the physician to do so are useful and allow for more effective, specific, and lasting treatment. Patients with facet-mediated joint pain comprise a significant portion of the back pain population at large, so identification and therapeutic mechanisms for such pain are important. Medial branch blocks are an established diagnostic method for identifying facet joint pain. Following a positive result, the best-studied treatment option is medial branch neurotomy. With such a course, patients have a good chance of alleviating their pain for up to 9 months after each therapeutic radiofrequency neurotomy.

REFERENCES

1. Manchikanti L, Singh V, Datta S, et al. Comprehensive review of epidemiology, scope, and impact of spinal pain. Pain Physician. 2009;12(4):E35-70.
2. Luo X, Pietrobon R, Sun SX, et al. Estimates and patterns of direct health care expenditures among individuals with back pain in the United States. Spine. 2004;29(1):79-86.
3. Leboeuf-Yde C, Nielsen J, Kyvik K, et al. Pain in the lumbar, thoracic or cervical regions: do age and gender matter? A population-based study of 34,902 Danish twins 20–71 years of age. BMC Musculoskelet Disord. 2009;10(1):39.
4. Manchikanti L, Boswell MV, Singh V, et al. Prevalence of facet joint pain in chronic spinal pain of cervical, thoracic, and lumbar regions. BMC Musculoskelet Disord. 2004; 5(1):15.
5. Varlotta GP, Lefkowitz TR, Schweitzer M, et al. The lumbar facet joint: a review of current knowledge: part 1: anatomy, biomechanics, and grading. Skeletal Radiol. 2011;40 (1):13-23.
6. Butler D, Trafimow J, Andersson G, et al. Discs degenerate before facets. Spine. 1990;15(2):111.
7. Varlotta GP, Lefkowitz TR, Schweitzer M, et al. The lumbar facet joint: a review of current knowledge: part II: diagnosis and management. Skeletal Radiol. 2011;40(2):149-57.
8. Pneumaticos SG, Chatziioannou SN, Hipp JA, et al. Low back pain: prediction of short-term outcome of facet joint injection with bone scintigraphy. Radiology. 2006; 238(2): 693-8.
9. Lynch M, Taylor J. Facet joint injection for low back pain. A clinical study. J Bone Joint Surg Br. 1986;68(1):138-41.
10. Bogduk N. Evidence-informed management of chronic low back pain with facet injections and radiofrequency neurotomy. Spine J. 2008;8(1):56-64.
11. Manchukonda R, Manchikanti KN, Cash KA, et al. Facet joint pain in chronic spinal pain: an evaluation of prevalence and false-positive rate of diagnostic blocks. J Spinal Disord Techn. 2007;20(7):539-45.
12. Siegenthaler A, Eichenberger U, Schmidlin K, et al. What does local tenderness say about the origin of pain? An investigation of cervical zygapophysial joint pain. Anesth Analg. 2010;110(3):923-7.
13. Kalichman L, Hunter DJ. Lumbar facet joint osteoarthritis: a review. Semin Arthritis Rheum. 2007;37(2):60-82.
14. Revel M, Poiraudeau S, Auleley GR, et al. Capacity of the clinical picture to characterize low back pain relieved by facet joint anesthesia: Proposed criteria to identify patients with painful facet joints. Spine. 1998;23(18):1972-6.
15. Cohen SP, Raja SN. Pathogenesis, diagnosis, and treatment of lumbar zygapophysial (facet) joint pain. Anesthesiology. 2007;106(3):591.
16. Siegenthaler A, Mlekusch S, Trelle S, et al. Accuracy of ultrasound-guided nerve blocks of the cervical zygapophysial joints. Anesthesiology. 2012;117:347-52.
17. Cohen SP, Strassels SA, Kurihara C, et al. Randomized study assessing the accuracy of cervical facet joint nerve (medial branch) blocks using different injectate volumes. Anesthesiology. 2010;112(1):144.
18. Manchikanti L, Malla Y, Wargo BW, et al. Complications of fluoroscopically directed facet joint nerve blocks: a prospective evaluation of 7,500 episodes with 43,000 nerve blocks. Pain Physician. 2012;15:E143-50.
19. Bogduk N. Diagnostic nerve blocks in chronic pain. Best Pract Res Clin Anaesthesiol. 2002;16(4):565-78.
20. Manchikanti L, Singh V, Falco FJE, et al. Comparative outcomes of a 2-year follow-up of cervical medial branch blocks in management of chronic neck pain: a randomized, double-blind controlled trial. Pain Physician. 2010;13:437-50.

21. Manchikanti L, Singh V, Falco FJE, et al. Evaluation of lumbar facet joint nerve blocks in managing chronic low back pain: a randomized, double-blind, controlled trial with a 2-year follow-up. Int J Med Sci. 2010;7(3):124.
22. Manchikanti L, Singh V, Falco FJE, et al. The role of thoracic medial branch blocks in managing chronic mid and upper back pain: a randomized, double-blind, active-control trial with a 2-year follow up. Anesthesiol Res Pract. 2012;2012:585806.
23. Gofeld M, Faclier G. Radiofrequency denervation of the lumbar zygapophysial joints—targeting the best practice. Pain Med. 2008;9(2):204-11.
24. Hooten WM, Martin DP, Huntoon MA. Radiofrequency neurotomy for low back pain: evidence-based procedural guidelines. Pain Med. 2005;6(2):129-38.
25. Lau P, Mercer S, Govind J, et al. The surgical anatomy of lumbar medial branch neurotomy (facet denervation). Pain Med. 2004;5(3):289-98.
26. Fröhling M, Schlote W, Wolburg-Buchholz K. Nonselective nerve fibre damage in peripheral nerves after experimental thermocoagulation. Acta Neurochir. 1998;140(12): 1297-302.
27. Falco F, Erhart S, Wargo B, et al. Systematic review of diagnostic utility and therapeutic effectiveness of cervical facet joint interventions. Pain Physician. 2009;12(2):323.
28. Lord SM, Barnsley L, Wallis BJ, et al. Percutaneous radiofrequency neurotomy for chronic cervical zygapophyseal-joint pain. N Engl J Med. 1996;335 (23):1721-6.
29. Smuck M, Crisostomo RA, Trivedi K, et al. Success of initial and repeated medial branch neurotomy for zygapophysial joint pain: a systematic review. PM R. 2012;4(9):686-92.
30. Dreyfuss P, Halbrook B, Pauza K, et al. Efficacy and validity of radiofrequency neurotomy for chronic lumbar zygapophysial joint pain. Spine. 2000;25(10):1270-7.
31. Manchikanti KN, Atluri S, Singh V, et al. An update of evaluation of therapeutic thoracic facet joint interventions. Pain Physician. 2012;15:E463-81.

CHAPTER

37 Intradiscal Electrothermal Therapy, Nucleoplasty and Biacuplasty

Steven Calvino, Rohan Bannis, Sachin Shah

INTRODUCTION

Discogenic pain and associated internal disk disruption (IDD) has been reported to account for 30–50% of chronic low back pain.[1] IDD is defined as biochemical, biophysical, and morphological disruption of the disk.[1] The intervertebral disks have a major role in the function and stability of spine. Disk degeneration is a frequent cause of pain and disability, and herniated disks appear to be the most common reason for back surgery in the United States.[2]

Each disk is composed of the nucleus pulposus and the annulus fibrosus that is surrounded by the vertebral end plates. The nucleus pulposus is located in the center of the disk. It contains collagen and elastin fibers, which are embedded in a highly hydrated aggrecan-containing gel. The annulus fibrosus is made up of a series of 15 to 25 concentric rings called lamellae, with the collagen fibers lying in parallel within each lamella.[3] The structure of each end plate is a thin horizontal layer, usually <1-mm thick, of hyaline cartilage. The disk has blood vessels and some nerves, mainly restricted to the outer lamellae. With advanced age and degeneration, the disk changes in morphology, becoming more disorganized. Cleft formation and fissures may appear within the disk.[4]

Mechanical forces can be distributed evenly as long as the inner nucleus pulposus and outer annulus fibrosus remain intact. If cleft formation and fissuring develop, then mechanical stresses on the disk may become disproportionate in areas leading to the potential for tears of the annulus fibrosus. In addition to the development of tears, it has been shown that the nerve ending typically present in the outer one third of the annulus fibrosus may grow inward toward the center of the disk in the normal degenerative process. In the presence of annular tears and nerve ingrowth into the disk it has been postulated that there is a "chemical" irritation, pain mediators called cytokines can then enter through these defects and "sensitize" the disk.[5] Discogenic pain is primarily axial. The quality of discogenic pain is usually described as deep and aching and is exacerbated with axial loading activities such as sitting or standing.[6]

While the disk itself may become painful through mechanical and chemical changes, the presence of annular tears also allows for disk material to extend beyond the limits of the intervertebral disk space resulting in what is called a disk herniation.[7] According to the American Journal of Neuro-Radiology (AJNR) guidelines, disk herniations may be classified as "focal", which equates to <25% of the disk circumference or "broad-based", which is between 25% and 50% of the disk circumference. Herniations may be further classified as protrusions or extrusions. When the disk material beyond the disk space boundaries in any plane is less than the distance between the edges of the base of the herniation in the same plane, the herniation is characterized as a protrusion. For a herniation to be considered an extrusion the disk material beyond the disk space boundaries in any plane must be greater than the distance between the edges of the base of the herniation in the same plane. It is only possible to make the distinction between the two types of herniation with sagittal images.[7] The pain associated with a disk herniation differs from that of primary discogenic pain in that it is often radicular in nature due to compression of nerve roots by the disk material. The quality of radicular pain is most often described as sharp, lancinating, electric in character, and travels in a specific band that corresponds to the nerve root dermatome.[6,8]

Discogenic pain due to IDD is most often diagnosed by a procedure called provocative discography with optional follow-up computed tomographic (CT) discogram. First, the physician attempts to reproduce the patient's usual pain by pressurizing the disk with an injection of contrast material. Then the physician examines the spread of the contrast medium using a CT scan. This procedure may be repeated on adjacent disks that are suspected to be symptomatic. The exact mechanisms of discogenic pain are still controversial. One of the most popular theories is the development of a full thickness radial annular tear that leaks nuclear material (cytokines) into posterior annulus where discal innervations reside. This annular disk leak theory has been supported by numerous high-quality peer-reviewed investigations.[9]

INTRADISCAL ELECTROTHERMAL THERAPY

Intradiscal electrothermal therapy (IDET) is a minimally invasive procedure that involves the thermal heating of the posterior and posteriolateral disk annulus within a painful intervertebral disk (diagnosed using discography). The technique was developed by Jeffrey Saal and Joel Saal as an alternative to fusion for patients with chronic discogenic low back pain. IDET received US regulatory clearance in 1998. The exact mechanism which results in the proposed reduction of discogenic pain remains unclear even today, but it has been postulated that thermal heating results in collagen fiber modification (shrinkage), potential segmental stabilization, and/or ablation of nociceptors.[10]

A 17-gauge needle is inserted posterolaterally into the affected disk. A 30-cm catheter with a flexible 5–6 cm heating tip is then threaded circumferentially into the disk through the nucleus pulposus to the pathologic area of the annulus. After fluoroscopic confirmation, the catheter tip is heated to 90°C over a 13-minute period. Once at 90°C, the temperature is maintained for an additional 4 minutes. The catheter and needle are then withdrawn (Figs. 37.1A to D).

Evidence for the efficacy of IDET in the treatment of chronic lower back pain is conflicting. One prospective study looked at 18 month Oswestry Disability Index (ODI) scores for 39 patients with chronic discogenic low back pain who failed to improve after conservative treatment. These patients had 1- or 2-level symptomatic disk degeneration without evidence of nerve root compression, symptoms of degenerative disk disease >6 months, failure to improve with a minimum of 6 weeks of conservative treatment and a normal neurological examination. Individuals who had severe disk degeneration with (>50% loss of disk height), previous spinal surgery, and other spinal conditions that can mimic lower back pain were excluded from the study. There was a significant difference between mean ODI scores after treatment as compared with before treatment. The study concluded that nearly four out of five patients clearly benefited from IDET.[11] However, a systematic review of the effectiveness of thermal annular procedures in treating discogenic lower back pain has also been published and reached a more moderate conclusion. The primary outcome examined was pain relief of at least 6 months with a secondary outcome of improvement in functional status. Forty-three studies were identified; three randomized controlled trials and one observational study met the inclusion criteria. The evidence for IDET was only fair.[12]

Nonetheless, IDET may be an effective treatment for chronic lower back pain in carefully selected patients with functional limitations, normal neurological examination, absence of neural compressive lesion on magnetic resonance imaging or CT, and no history of prior back surgery where other axial pain generators have been ruled out. Evidence suggests that patients with severe disk space narrowing, disk extrusion >5 mm, or previous back surgery are not likely to benefit from the procedure.[12]

NUCLEOPLASTY

Nucleoplasty is another minimally invasive procedure used in the treatment of chronic lower back pain and associated radiculopathy. Nucleoplasty combines coagulation and tissue ablation to form channels in the nucleus and decompress the herniated disk. Patented "Coblation" (controlled ablation) technology uses radiofrequency energy, which is applied to a conductive medium, creating a highly focused plasma field around the energized electrodes. This is then used to remove some of the nucleus pulposus and form channels within the disk.[13] Temperatures between 40° and 70° are used. Removal of the nucleus pulposus in contained disks has been shown to decompress herniated disks and relieve pressure on nerve roots (Fig. 37.2).[14]

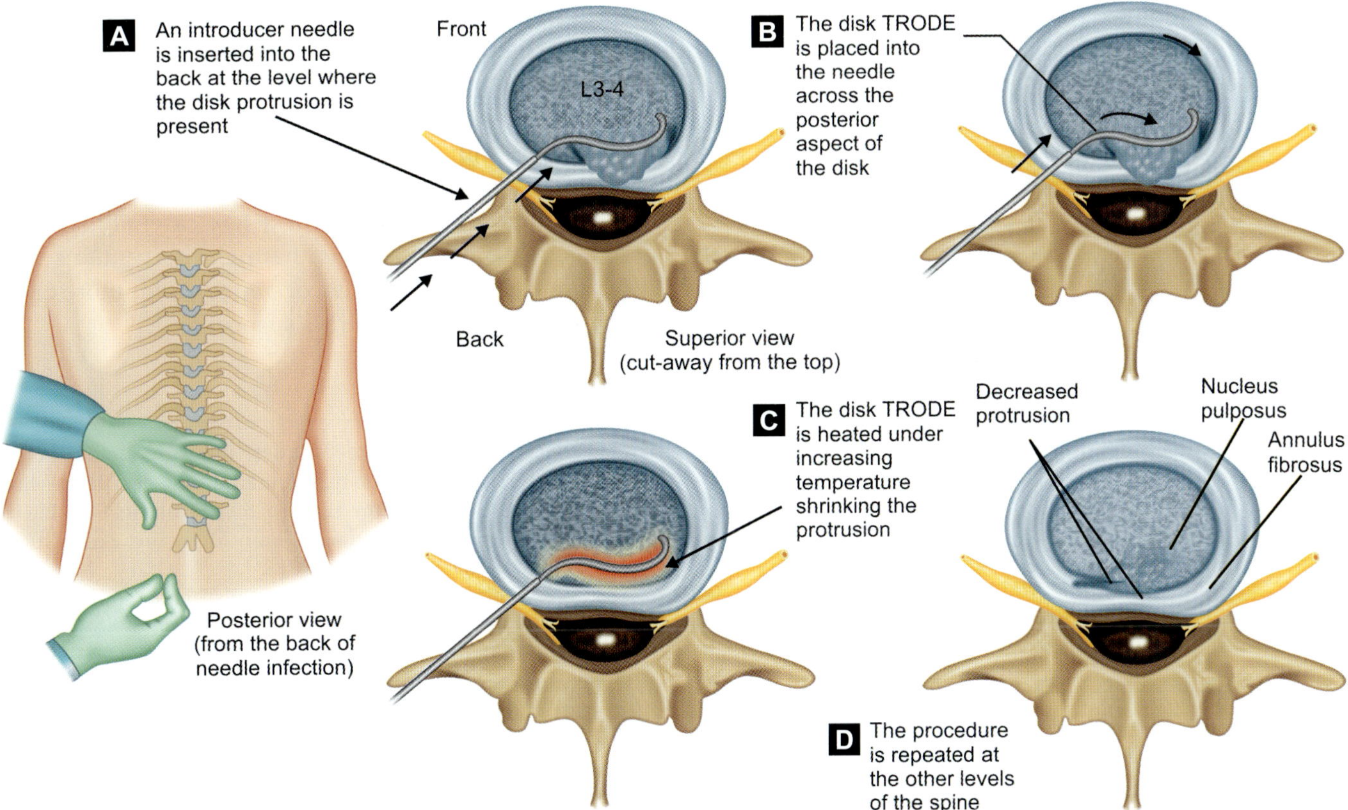

Figs. 37.1A to D: Intradiscal electrothermal therapy technique. (A) A 17-gauge needle is first inserted posterolaterally into the affected disk. (B) A 30-cm catheter with a flexible 5 to 6 cm heating tip is then threaded circumferentially into the disk through the nucleus pulposus to the pathologic area of the annulus. (C) After fluoroscopic confirmation, the catheter tip is heated to 90°C over a 13-minute period. Once at 90°C, the temperature is maintained for an additional 4 minutes. The catheter and needle are then withdrawn. (D) The procedure is repeated at disk levels necessary.

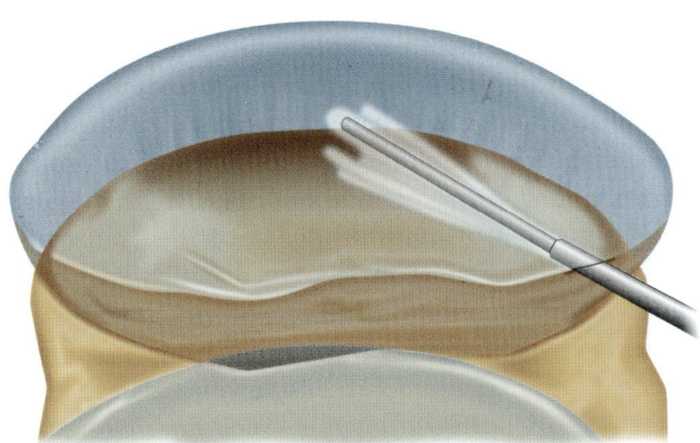

Fig. 37.2: Nucleoplasty combines coagulation and tissue ablation to form channels in the nucleus and decompresses the herniated disk.

As with IDET, the efficacy of nucleoplasty is not well established. One prospective study looked at 50 patients who all underwent percutaneous disk decompression with nucleoplasty. The inclusion criteria included: disk protrusion or contained herniated disk <6 mm at a single level, disk heigh >50%, and radicular pain resistant to previous medical treatment and physical therapy for >3 months. The exclusion criteria included: previous lumbar spine surgery, significant spinal stenosis, and two or more symptomatic levels. Patients were assessed using the visual analog scale (VAS) and the ODI scale after 2 weeks, 3 months, 6 months, and 1 year. VAS scores improved and analgesic consumption was reduced or stopped in 90% of cases after 1 year. There was complete resolution of symptoms in 38 patients at 6 months and in 40 patients after 1 year.[15] Although there was significant improvement in the patients' perceived pain, it is evident that strict criteria must be adhered to for the selection of patients who will undergo nucleoplasty.

BIACUPLASTY

Like nucleoplasty, biacuplasty is a minimally invasive thermal annular treatment modality. In this procedure,

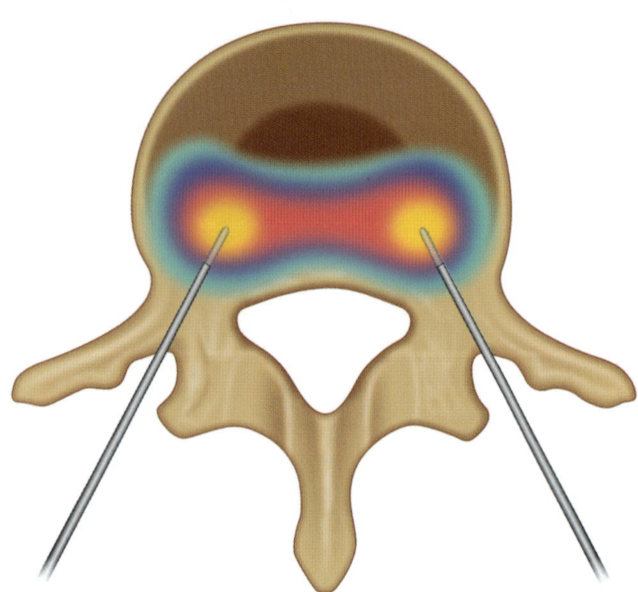

Fig. 37.3: Biacuplasty technique involves introducing two electrodes percutaneously into the disk in a bipolar arrangement, allowing radiofrequency energy to be concentrated in the disk.

two electrodes are introduced percutaneously into the disk in a bipolar arrangement, allowing radiofrequency energy to be concentrated in the disk. Water circulating in the electrodes gently cools the electrode surfaces, which allows the temperature of tissue across the posterior aspect of the disk to be elevated while preventing overheating of tissue local to the electrodes (Fig. 37.3).[16]

A prospective, observational study of transdiscal biacuplasty of patients with discogenic low back pain showed a statistically significant improvement in the VAS and ODI score. A total of 14 patients (of the 15 patients enrolled) completed the study with 1-, 3-, and 6-month follow-ups. More than 50% of the patients reported a decrease in their pain at 6 months post-treatment.[17] However, the study was limited by its small sample size and very restrictive inclusion criteria.

Patients who may benefit from biacuplasty are generally those who are young, have not had previous back surgeries, show very little pathology on neuroradiographic images, and do not have neurological symptoms or deficits in the physical examination. However, further research is needed to validate the utility of this technique.

CONCLUSION

Chronic low back pain is a challenge to treat even for the most astute physician. Although minimally invasive procedures are attractive forms of therapy, given their quick recovery time and low risk, the questionable efficacy of these procedures and strict selection criteria limits their clinical usefulness. A recent systematic review of the literature for three procedures discussed above showed that the evidence with regards to the treatment of lower back pain was fair for IDET and limited or poor for nucleoplasty and biacuplasty.[14] However, for a few carefully selected patients, these percutaneous thermal interventions may serve as a viable option in lieu of surgery or for those cases where the surgical indication is suspect.

REFERENCES

1. Walega D. Intradiscal techniques: intradiscal electrothermal therapy, biacuplasty, percutaneous decompression techniques. In: Benzon H, Raja SN, Fishman SM, Liu S, Cohen SP (Eds). Essentials of Pain Medicine, 3rd edition. Philadelphia, PA: Saunders; 2011.
2. Luo X, Pietrobon R, Sun SX, et al. Estimates and patterns of direct health care expenditures among individuals with back pain in the United States. Spine. 2004;29(1):79-86.
3. Bogduk N. Clinical anatomy of the lumbar spine and sacrum. London, UK: Churchill Livingstone, 2005.
4. Roberts S, Menage J, Urban J. Biochemical and structural properties of the cartilage end-plate and its relation to the intervertebral disc. Spine. 1989;14(2):166.
5. Cohen SP, Larkin TM, Barna SA, et al. Lumbar discography: a comprehensive review of outcome studies, diagnostic accuracy, and principles. Reg Anesth Pain Med. 2005;30(2):163-83.
6. Maus TP, Aprill CN. Lumbar discogenci pain, provocation discography, and imaging correlates. Radiol Clin N Am. 2012;50:681-704.
7. Bailey WM. A practical guide to the application of AJNR guidelines for nomenclature and classification of lumbar disc pathology in magnetic resonance imaging (MRI). Radiography. 2006;12:175-82.
8. Benzon HT, Rathmell JP, Wu CL. Low back pain. In: Raj's Practical Managemet of Pain, 4th edition. Philadelphia, Pa: Mosby, Inc; 2008. pp. 367-87.
9. Marshall LL, Trethewie E, Curtain C. Chemical radiculitis: a clinical, physiological and immunological study. Clini Orthop Relat Res. 1977;129:61-7.
10. Hurri H, Karppinen J. Discogenic pain. Pain. 2004;112(3): 225-8.
11. Ergun R, Sekerci Z, Bulut H, et al. Intradiscal electrothermal treatment for chronic discogenic low back pain: a prospective outcome study of 39 patients with the Oswestry disability index at 18 month follow-up. Neurol Res. May 2008; 30(4):411-6.
12. Helm II S, Deer TR, Manchikanti L, et al. Effectiveness of thermal annular procedures in treating discogenic low back pain. Pain Physician. 2012;15(3):E279-304.
13. Chen YC, Lee S, Chen D. Intradiscal pressure study of percutaneous disc decompression with nucleoplasty in human cadavers. Spine. 2003;28(7):661-5.

14. Hirsch JA, Singh V, Falco FJ, et al. Automated percutaneous lumbar discectomy for the contained herniated lumbar disc: a systematic assessment of evidence. Pain Physician. 2009;12(3):601-20.
15. Azzazi A, AlMekawi S, Zein M. Lumbar disc nucleoplasty using coblation technology: clinical outcome. J Neurointerv Surg. 2011;3(3):288-92.
16. Petersohn JD, Conquergood LR, Leung M. Acute histologic effects and thermal distribution profile of disc biacuplasty using a novel water-cooled bipolar electrode system in an in vivo porcine model. Pain Med. 2007;9(1):26-32.
17. Karaman H, Tüfek A, Kavak GÖ, et al. 6-Month results of transdiscal biacuplasty on patients with discogenic low back pain: preliminary findings. Int J Med Sci. 2011;8(1):1.

CHAPTER

38

Spinal Cord Stimulators

Brian Park, Yong H Kim

INTRODUCTION

According to the Institute of Medicine, 116 million Americans, 30% of the population, suffer from chronic pain. Chronic pain affects physical and mental functioning, quality of life, and productivity. This affliction costs the nation US $635 billion in medical treatment and lost productivity.[1]

Two types of pain exist: nociceptic and neuropathic. Both types are completely disparate in etiology and mechanism. Nociceptic pain is caused by stimulation of peripheral nerve fibers in response to harmful stimuli. It is a warning sign to one's body that something is wrong. Examples include acute sciatica, pain from fractured bones, postoperative pain, and headaches from an intracranial mass.

On the other hand, neuropathic pain stems from damage to the sensory nervous system. Chronic pain is often neuropathic in nature. The mechanism of neuropathic pain is not clearly elucidated, but it is categorized into peripheral nerve damage and central nervous system alterations. Peripheral nerve damage may result in the formation of a neuroma and proliferation of unmyelinated C fibers. These C fibers have been shown to have upregulation of sodium channel expression and become hyperexcitable. This phenomenon is called peripheral sensitization.[2,3] Animal studies have also revealed that peripheral sensitization may, in turn, result in an increase in background activity of the spinothalamic tracts, the primary ascending nociceptive pathway. This is thought to enlarge the receptive field and increase response to all afferent impulses.[2,3]

A multimodal approach to pain management is most effective. Options include oral medications, psychotherapy, desensitization physical therapy, injections, intrathecal pumps, and neuromodulation. Spinal cord stimulators are one type of neuromodulation, which have attained success and popularity.

WHAT ARE SPINAL CORD STIMULATORS?

Spinal cord stimulators have been in use for chronic pain since first being described by Shealy et al. in 1967.[4] Spinal cord stimulators are implantable devices, which provide low-voltage electrical stimulation to the spinal cord and ultimately block the sensation of pain. These devices are implanted over the dorsal columns/spinal cord and produce an electric field. This electric field provides a neuromodulating milieu and presumably blocks afferent pain signals.

Prior to the advent of spinal cord stimulators, physicians observed that patients with tabes dorsalis would suffer from intractable paroxysms of pain. This was thought to be related to the degeneration of the dorsal columns, and some theorized that the dorsal columns played a role in pain modulation. In 1965, Melzack and Wall proposed the gate control theory on pain.[5] In this theory, he described that large diameter afferent nerve fibers and small diameter nerve fibers synapse on the substantia gelatinosa in the dorsal columns of the spinal cord. Activation of the large diameter afferent fibers would "close the gate" and prevent transmission of the small diameter afferent fibers up to the central nervous system and thereby block certain pain signals.

Spinal cord stimulators were developed on the basis of this theory. Originally termed dorsal column stimulators, they were thought to provide stimulation to large afferent dorsal column fibers and close the gate to the smaller afferent fibers. However, some theorized that stimulation extends to other tracts of the spinal cord, such as the spinothalamictracts.[6,7] The observation that spinal cord stimulators reduced certain types of pain (such as neuropathic and ischemic pain) better than others (namely, nociceptive pain) further complicates the issue and clouds our understanding of the mechanism of action of these devices.[8] Current understanding of the physiology of spinal cord stimulators suggests that there are several different mechanisms of action when treating various pain conditions. In neuropathic pain, stimulation of large afferent dorsal column fiber and suppression of dorsal horn neurons may play important roles. Relief of ischemic pain appears to be secondary to re-establishment of oxygen supply and demand either by decreased tissue demand or increased flow mediated by inhibition of sympathetic activity.

INDICATIONS

In their first decade of use in the 1970s, spinal cord stimulators were used widely and injudiciously to a myriad of pain diagnoses of various etiologies. Therefore, early results were poor and spinal cord stimulators fell out of favor quickly. However, in recent times, spinal cord stimulators have achieved a resurgence and have been successful in treating selective diagnoses. Despite a poor understanding of the mechanism of action of spinal cord stimulators, relatively clear indications exist. Certain types of pain are stimulator resistant. Typical axial back and neck pain and nociceptive type pain are historically poor indications for spinal cord stimulation.[9,10] Indicated types of pain can be categorized into ischemic/visceral pain, neuropathic pain, and mixed type pain syndromes.[11]

ISCHEMIC/VISCERAL PAIN

Spinal cord stimulator implantation may be indicated in cases of inoperable ischemic limb pain or angina pectoris. In fact, the most common indication for spinal cord stimulators in Europe is peripheral ischemic pain.[11] Several studies have demonstrated decreased pain and higher limb survival rates in in-operable peripheral ischemic disease.[12–14] Refractory angina pectoris has also been successfully treated with neuromodulation. Spinal cord stimulation has shown to have equivalent survival rates, rates of angina attacks, and quality-of-life measures in some studies.[15–18]

Recently, the dorsal columns have been thought to play a role in visceral pain pathways. In addition to angina pectoris, other types of visceral pain may also be treated with spinal cord stimulation. Although good clinical data are lacking, chronic visceral abdominal and pelvic pain due to various conditions, such as irritable bowel syndrome, chronic pancreatitis, diffuse abdominal adhesions, Mediterranean fever, and endometriosis have been successfully treated with spinal cord stimulation.[19–21]

NEUROGENIC PAIN

Examples of neurogenic type pain that have successfully responded to spinal cord stimulation include lower extremity pain due to multiple sclerosis, post herpetic neuralgia, and other polyneuropathies,[22,23] including diabetic neuropathy.[24] Amputation stump pain and phantom limb pain has responded poorly to spinal cord stimulation.[22,23] Furthermore, spinal cord stimulators are often used in the treatment of mixed type pain syndromes, which have both neuropathic and nociceptive elements. The two most prominent mixed type pain syndromes treated with neuromodulation are chronic regional pain syndrome (CRPS) and failed back surgery syndrome (FBSS).

The CRPS is a poorly understood pain disorder, which affects 1 in 2,000 cases of extremity trauma.[25] CRPS, previously known as reflex sympathetic dystrophy, is a debilitating ailment, which results in severe pain and disability with few known treatments. Spinal cord stimulators are one of the few options, which have achieved success in treating patients afflicted with CRPS. In a randomized control trial, spinal cord stimulators used in combination with physical therapy produced greater pain relief and higher health-related quality-of-life scores than did physical therapy alone.[26–28]

SPINE-RELATED CONDITIONS

While spine surgery has progressed a great deal, unfortunately not all spine operations result in success. Possible etiologies of incomplete relief of back or radicular pain after spine surgery include pseudarthrosis, inadequate decompression, hardware failure, iatrogenic neurologic injury, arachnoiditis, and epidural scarring. When these diagnoses have been ruled out, some patients still have unexplained pain. This had led to the description of FBSS.

FBSS is defined as persistent or recurrent pain, mainly in the region of the lower back and legs, after lumbosacral spine surgeries that are technically and anatomically successful.

Treatment of FBSS falls into two categories: reoperation or pain management. While some may benefit from reoperations, for many, this is ineffective. FBSS is the most common indication for spinal cord stimulators in the United States.[11] Long-term studies have shown successful use of spinal cord stimulators for FBSS with improved pain, higher functionality, and higher quality-of-life scores.[22,23,29-32] In 1995, Turner et al. performed a meta-analysis of 39 studies on the effectiveness of spinal cord stimulators in FBSS. They concluded that approximately 50–60% of patients treated with spinal cord stimulators had at least 50% pain relief; however, this systematic review did not include any randomized control trials.[33]

In response, two large randomized control trials were performed. North et al. conducted a prospective trial of 50 subjects randomized to repeated lumbar spine surgery or spinal cord stimulator placement. Forty-seven percent of subjects receiving spinal cord stimulators versus only 12% of reoperation subjects achieved success.[32] Kumar et al. performed a multicenter randomized control trial of 100 subjects with FBSS randomized to spinal cord stimulator plus conventional medical management or conventional medical management alone. At 1-year and 2-year intervals, subjects receiving spinal cord stimulators had significantly improved leg pain, quality of life, and functional capacity; however, back pain was not significantly improved.[29,30] In another meta-analysis, Taylor et al. reviewed 74 studies comprising > 3,000 subjects. Of those receiving spinal cord stimulation, 62% of patients had > 50% reduction in pain and 53% no longer required analgesic medications. In addition, 40% were able to return to work, and there was an overall 70% satisfaction rate with spinal cord stimulator implantation.

In addition, spinal cord stimulators are now being used for spine-related conditions prior to any previous surgical intervention. Lumbar spinal stenosis is the most common and fastest growing indication for spine surgery in those > 65 years old.[34] However, many patients may not be good candidates for a large open procedure often required to treat spinal stenosis. Implantation of a spinal cord stimulator provides a minimally invasive and reversible alternative. In one study, all 69 patients in the study population had significant improvement in pain relief. In addition, there was a reduction in analgesic medication use and improvement in functional outcomes.[35]

Spinal cord stimulators have historically been poor at treating low back pain, because balancing pain relief with uncomfortable, stimulator-induced paresthesia is difficult. However, new studies question this belief. Although their superiority is still unproven,[36] newer multicontact electrodes and computer-assisted multichannel programming has allowed for finer adjustments in treating axial back pain. Rigoard et al. reported that 9 of 11 patients implanted with tripolar spinal cord stimulators for primarily low back pain achieved successful paresthesia coverage and had significant pain relief compared with preimplantation.[37] In a prospective cohort study, Van Buyten et al. investigated the effects of newer high-frequency spinal cord stimulators on 83 subjects with low back pain. Specifically, low back pain was the end point studied. Eighty-eight percent of patients had successful trials of spinal cord stimulation and underwent permanent implantation. Of these, 74% of subjects reported > 50% back pain relief at 6-month follow-up. Eighty-one percent of the study population was being treated for FBSS; however, of the 16 subjects who were treated for low back pain without history of prior spine surgery, 15 had successful trial implantation.[38] Although data are limited at this time, development of newer techniques and programming may allow us to successfully treat low back pain with neuromodulation.

TECHNIQUE

One of the most appealing aspects of spinal cord stimulator is being able to trial the potential benefit of the procedure before deciding to proceed with the permanent procedure. There is trial/screening part of the procedure followed by permanent implantation when the trial is successful.

TRIAL/SCREENING

Patient is positioned on a radiolucent table. The entire procedure is performed percutaneously with local anesthesia (Fig. 38.1). Typical entry point for the epidural needle is T12–L1. After the skin is prepped and draped, the local anesthetic is injected. Using the paramedian approach, a 14-gauge Touhy needle is introduced into epidural space. This is done under fluoroscopic guidance and utilizing the loss of resistance technique. Once the needle is in the midline of the epidural space, the percutaneous lead is inserted through the needle and advanced in the epidural space to the initial empirical position based on the patient's typical pain distribution.

Percutaneous Implantation of trial spinal cord stimulator

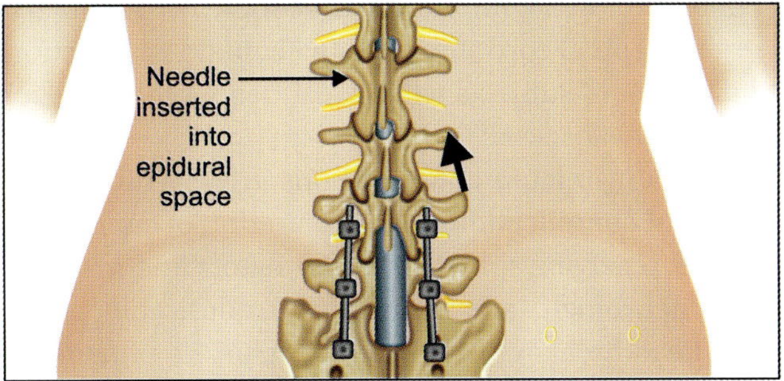

Placement of needle

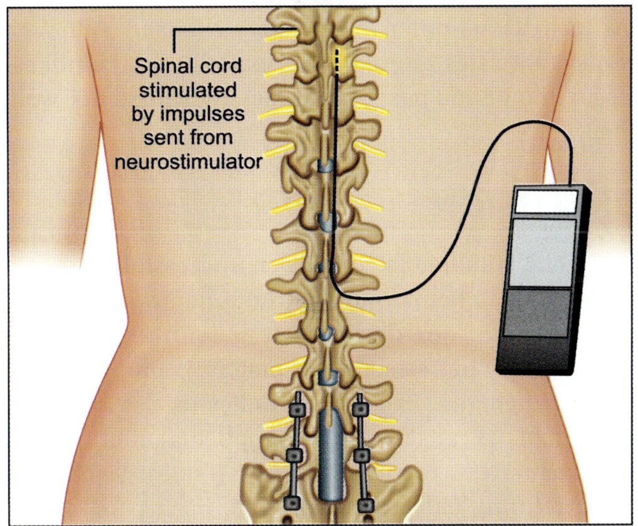

Lead connected to neurostimulator

Midsagittal view of spine

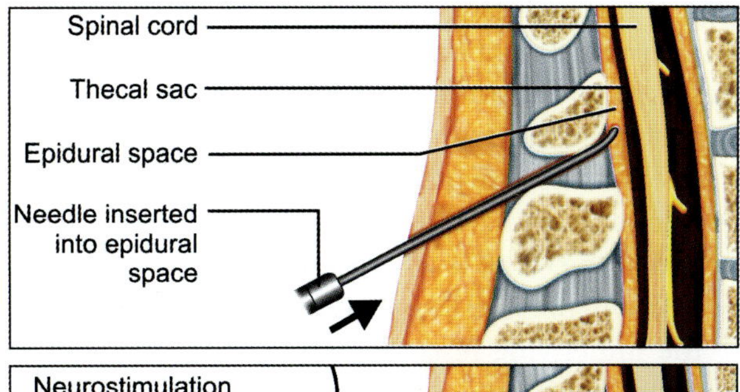

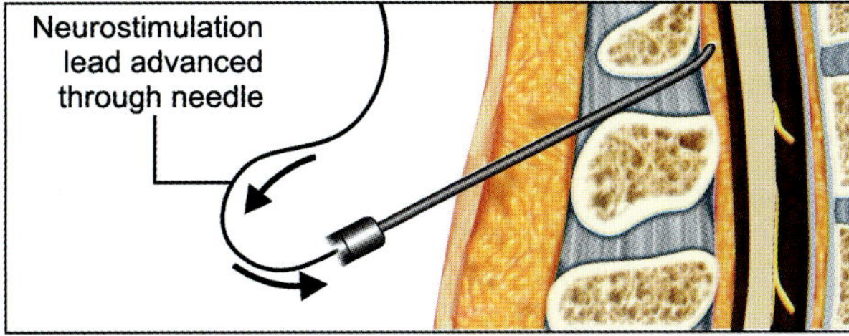

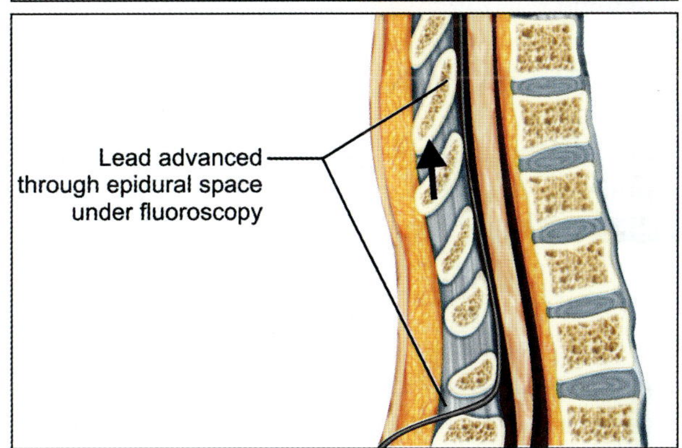

Fig. 38.1: Schematic diagram of percutaneous implantation of trial spinal cord stimulator.

Typically, low back pain is T8–9, buttock and leg is T9–10, but it can vary individually. It is crucial that the position of the lead is as midline as possible favoring slightly toward the side of the pain. Two leads are used when trying to cover bilateral symptoms or mostly low back pain. The lead placed too laterally will result in unpleasant "visceral" stimulation. Once the lead is positioned correctly and confirmed with fluoroscopy, the lead is then stimulated and the patient is asked whether the stimulation covers all the areas of pain. The position of the lead is then adjusted by advancing or pulling back the lead to optimize the area of coverage. Initially, the middle electrodes are stimulated to allow for the possible migration of the lead. The lead is then secured to the skin either with sutures looped around the lead or with tape. Once the patient is transferred to the postanesthesia care unit, the stimulator is programmed and the patient is given instructions on the uses of the device. Patient is also instructed to avoid excessive bending, twisting or reaching overhead to prevent the possible lead migration. Typical trial period lasts 3 to 7 days. During this period, it is crucial that the coverage is closely monitored and if it is inadequate, then it should be reprogrammed immediately. At the end of the trial period, the lead is removed in the office and the patient is assessed. It is important that the pain relief and the improvement in the quality of life are significant, typically >50%, to justify proceeding with the permanent implantation.

PERMANENT IMPLANTATION

Once the trial lead is removed and the decision is made to proceed with the permanent implantation, the patient is typically given a choice between percutaneous lead versus surgical paddle lead. The advantage of the percutaneous lead is that it avoids an open laminotomy that required for the insertion of the paddle lead. However, the paddle lead is inherently more stable against the lead migration. Percutaneous permanent lead is placed by making a small incision at the previous needle insertion site. The Touhy needle is introduced, and the lead is inserted and positioned at the same level as the trial lead. Once the lead is positioned, the needle is removed and the lead is secured to the underlying fascia via an anchor. The lead is then tunneled subcutaneously to the pocket that has been created to hold the battery. The typical location for the battery is upper buttock area. If the paddle lead is chosen, then a small laminotomy is performed, typically, a level below the location of the lead determined during the trial. The lead is then secured along the dorsal fascia and then tunneled subcutaneously to the battery site (Figs. 38.2A and B).

COMPLICATIONS

Although recent data support the use of spinal cord stimulators in carefully selected patients, no surgical procedure is without complications. Turner described a high complication rate of 42%. [33] Complications include superficial or deep infections, dural tear, lead migration, lead breakage, equipment failure, and pain about stimulator components. Complications could be classified into two categories: surgical/biologic or equipment related.

Surgical or biologic complications include infection, dural tears, cerebrospinal fluid leak, spinal headache, hematoma/seroma formtion, and rarely neural injury. Overall rate of surgical/biologic complications is approximately 14%. Nine percent of patients sustain noninfectious biologic complications. About 5% of subjects undergoing spinal cord stimulator will obtain an infection, but only 0.1% of subjects will have a deep infection such as an epidural abscess.[33,39]

Equipment-related complications are the most common type of complications. Lead migration occurs in 24% of patients receiving spinal cord stimulators and may lead adverse neurologic affects such as undesirable paresthesias. Lead breakage or failure occurs in 7% of patients. Pulse generator failure occurs in 2%.[33,39]

Overall, 23% of stimulators require unplanned revisions for reasons other than battery change.[39] Although complication rates are high, the majorities of complications are minor and pose little threat to the patients' well-being.

CONCLUSION

Spinal cord stimulators have been successfully used in patients with ischemic pain, chronic neuropathic pain, CRPS, and FBSS for decades. As is with any medical procedures, proper selection of patient is paramount in achieving high rate of success. Judicious use of spinal cord stimulators can effectively aid patients suffering from chronic pain. New reports with uses of latest technology may be refuting old belief that axial, back pain cannot be successfully treated. The future of neuromodulation holds promise. Its indications may go beyond the scope of treating chronic pain syndrome. Early reports and animal studies have shown great improvement in motor function with spinal cord stimulation in Parkinson's

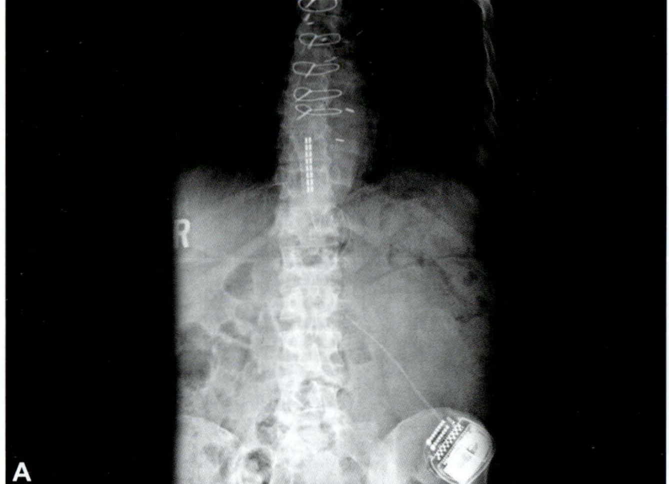

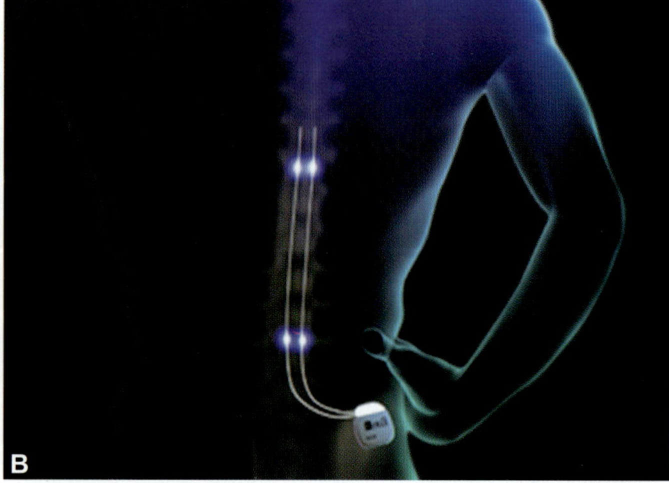

Figs. 38.2A and B: (A) Plain radiograph and (B) schematic diagram of a permanently placed spinal cord stimulator.

disease.[40-42] Spinal cord stimulators have proven and potent utility in managing chronic pain, and further awareness of these devices may help develop and expand their uses.

REFERENCES

1. Institute of Medicine (US) Committee on Advancing Pain Research, Care, and Education. Relieving pain in America: a blueprint for transforming prevention, care, education, and research. Washington, DC: National Academies Press (US);2011.
2. Truini A, Cruccu G. Pathophysiological mechanisms of neuropathic pain. Neurol Sci: official journal of the Italian Neurological Society and of the Italian Society of Clinical Neurophysiology. 2006;27(Suppl 2):S179-82.
3. Campbell JN, Meyer RA. Mechanisms of neuropathic pain. Neuron. 2006;52(1):77-92.
4. Shealy CN, Mortimer JT, Reswick JB. Electrical inhibition of pain by stimulation of the dorsal columns: preliminary clinical report. Anesth Analg. 1967;46(4):489-91.
5. Melzack R, Wall PD. Pain mechanisms: a new theory. Science. 1965;150(3699):971-9.
6. North RB, Ewend MG, Lawton MT, et al. Failed back surgery syndrome: 5-year follow-up after spinal cord stimulator implantation. Neurosurgery. 1991;28(5):692-9.
7. Larson SJ, Sances A, Jr, Riegel DH, et al. Neurophysiological effects of dorsal column stimulation in man and monkey. J Neurosurg. 1974;41(2):217-23.
8. Linderoth B, Foreman RD. Physiology of spinal cord stimulation: review and update. Neuromodulation. 1999;2 (3):150-64.
9. Meyerson BA, Linderoth B. Mechanisms of spinal cord stimulation in neuropathic pain. Neurol Res. 2000;22(3):285-92.
10. Stojanovic MP, Abdi S. Spinal cord stimulation. Pain Physician. 2002;5(2):156-66.
11. Kunnumpurath S, Srinivasagopalan R, Vadivelu N. Spinal cord stimulation: principles of past, present and future practice: a review. J Clin Monit Comput. 2009;23(5):333-9.
12. Amann W, Berg P, Gersbach P, et al. Spinal cord stimulation in the treatment of non-reconstructable stable critical leg ischaemia: results of the European Peripheral Vascular Disease Outcome Study (SCS-EPOS). Eur J Vasc Endovasc Surg: the official journal of the European Society for Vascular Surgery. 2003;26(3):280-6.
13. Augustinsson LE, Carlsson CA, Holm J, et al. Epidural electrical stimulation in severe limb ischemia. Pain relief, increased blood flow, and a possible limb-saving effect. Ann Surg. 1985;202(1):104-10.
14. Ubbink DT, Vermeulen H. Spinal cord stimulation for non-reconstructable chronic critical leg ischaemia. Cochrane Database Syst Rev. 2005(3):CD004001.
15. Taylor RS, De Vries J, Buchser E, et al. Spinal cord stimulation in the treatment of refractory angina: systematic review and meta-analysis of randomised controlled trials. BMC Cardiovasc Disord. 2009;9:13.
16. Ekre O, Eliasson T, Norrsell H, et al. Long-term effects of spinal cord stimulation and coronary artery bypass grafting on quality of life and survival in the ESBY study. Eur Heart J. 2002;23(24):1938-45.
17. Borjesson M, Andrell P, Lundberg D, et al. Spinal cord stimulation in severe angina pectoris—a systematic review based on the Swedish Council on Technology assessment in health care report on long-standing pain. Pain. 2008; 140(3):501-8.
18. Lapenna E, Rapati D, Cardano P, et al. Spinal cord stimulation for patients with refractory angina and previous coronary surgery. Ann Thorac Surg. 2006;82(5):1704-8.
19. Kapural L, Narouze SN, Janicki TI, et al. Spinal cord stimulation is an effective treatment for the chronic intractable visceral pelvic pain. Pain Med. 2006;7(5):440-3.
20. Kapural L, Nagem H, Tlucek H, et al. Spinal cord stimulation for chronic visceral abdominal pain. Pain Med. 2010;11 (3):347-55.
21. Kapural L, Deer T, Yakovlev A, et al. Technical aspects of spinal cord stimulation for managing chronic visceral abdominal pain: the results from the national survey. Pain Med. 2010;11(5):685-91.
22. Kumar K, Toth C, Nath RK, Laing P. Epidural spinal cord stimulation for treatment of chronic pain—some predictors of success. A 15-year experience. Surg Neurol. 1998;50 (2):110-20; discussion 120-1.
23. Kumar K, Hunter G, Demeria D. Spinal cord stimulation in treatment of chronic benign pain: challenges in treatment planning and present status, a 22-year experience. Neurosurgery. 2006;58(3):481-96; discussion 481-96.
24. Tesfaye S, Watt J, Benbow SJ, et al. Electrical spinal-cord stimulation for painful diabetic peripheral neuropathy. Lancet. 1996;348(9043):1698-701.
25. Sandroni P, Benrud-Larson LM, McClelland RL, et al. Complex regional pain syndrome type I: incidence and prevalence in Olmsted county, a population-based study. Pain. 2003;103(1-2):199-207.
26. Kemler MA, De Vet HC, Barendse GA, et al. The effect of spinal cord stimulation in patients with chronic reflex sympathetic dystrophy: two years' follow-up of the randomized controlled trial. Annals of neurology 2004;55(1):13-8.
27. Kemler MA, de Vet HC, Barendse GA, et al. Effect of spinal cord stimulation for chronic complex regional pain syndrome Type I: five-year final follow-up of patients in a randomized controlled trial. J Neurosurg. 2008;108(2):292-8.
28. Kemler MA, Barendse GA, van Kleef M, et al. Spinal cord stimulation in patients with chronic reflex sympathetic dystrophy. New England J Med. 2000;343(9):618-24.
29. Kumar K, Taylor RS, Jacques L, et al. Spinal cord stimulation versus conventional medical management for neuropathic pain: a multicentre randomised controlled trial in patients with failed back surgery syndrome. Pain. 2007;132(1-2): 179-88.
30. Kumar K, Taylor RS, Jacques L, et al. The effects of spinal cord stimulation in neuropathic pain are sustained: a 24-month follow-up of the prospective randomized controlled multicenter trial of the effectiveness of spinal cord stimulation. Neurosurgery. 2008;63(4):762-70; discussion 770.

31. Manca A, Kumar K, Taylor RS, et al. Quality of life, resource consumption and costs of spinal cord stimulation versus conventional medical management in neuropathic pain patients with failed back surgery syndrome (PROCESS trial). Eur J Pain. 2008;12(8):1047-58.
32. North RB, Kidd DH, Farrokhi F, et al. Spinal cord stimulation versus repeated lumbosacral spine surgery for chronic pain: a randomized, controlled trial. Neurosurgery. 2005;56(1):98-106; discussion 106-7.
33. Turner JA, Loeser JD, Bell KG. Spinal cord stimulation for chronic low back pain: a systematic literature synthesis. Neurosurgery. 1995;37(6):1088-95; discussion 1095-6.
34. Ciol MA, Deyo RA, Howell E, et al. An assessment of surgery for spinal stenosis: time trends, geographic variations, complications, and reoperations. J Am Geriatr Soc. 1996;44(3):285-90.
35. Costantini A, Buchser E, Van Buyten JP. Spinal cord stimulation for the treatment of chronic pain in patients with lumbar spinal stenosis. Neuromodulation. 2010;13(4):275-9; discussion 279-80.
36. North RB, Kidd DH, Olin J, et al. Spinal cord stimulation for axial low back pain: a prospective controlled trial comparing 16-contact insulated electrodes with 4-contact percutaneous electrodes. Neuromodulation. 2006;9(1):56-67.
37. Rigoard P, Delmotte A, D'Houtaud S, et al. Back pain: a real target for spinal cord stimulation? Neurosurgery. 2012;70(3):574-84; discussion 584-5.
38. Van Buyten JP, Al-Kaisy A, Smet I, et al. High-frequency spinal cord stimulation for the treatment of chronic back pain patients: results of a prospective multicenter European clinical study. Neuromodulation. 2013;16(1):59-66.
39. Turner JA, Loeser JD, Deyo RA, et al. Spinal cord stimulation for patients with failed back surgery syndrome or complex regional pain syndrome: a systematic review of effectiveness and complications. Pain. 2004;108(1-2):137-47.
40. Fuentes R, Petersson P, Siesser WB, et al. Spinal cord stimulation restores locomotion in animal models of Parkinson's disease. Science. 2009;323(5921):1578-82.
41. Fuentes R, Petersson P, Nicolelis MA. Restoration of locomotive function in Parkinson's disease by spinal cord stimulation: mechanistic approach. Eur J Neurosci. 2010; 32(7):1100-8.
42. Fenelon G, Goujon C, Gurruchaga JM, et al. Spinal cord stimulation for chronic pain improved motor function in a patient with Parkinson's disease. Parkinsonism Relat Disord. 2012;18(2):213-4.

SECTION

4

Surgical Management

CHAPTER

39

History of Surgical Management of Spinal Disorders

Justin Paul, Thomas Cheriyan, Thomas J Errico

INTRODUCTION

Treatment of spinal deformity has found mention in the ancient Indian Hindu epic Srimad Bhagwat Mahapuranam (3500–1800 BCE). The epic describes Lord Krishna applying axial traction to correct the hunchback of one of his devotees, Kubja, by pressing her feet down and pulling her chin upward. Cases of vertebral subluxation and dislocation resulting in traumatic quadriplegia and paraplegia have also been recorded in the Edwin Smith papyrus (2600–2200 BCE).

In the fourth century BCE, Hippocrates invented two devices—the hippocratic ladder and hippocratic board— designed to treat disorders, such as scoliosis and kyphosis, through applied physical force (Figs. 39.1A and B).[1] The earliest account of surgical treatment for a spine disorder comes from the seventh century CE, when the first laminectomy was performed by the Byzantine Greek physician, Paulus of Aegina for a spinal fracture with cord compression.[1-4]

Spine disorders can manifest with disability and sometimes crippling pain even without obvious deformity or

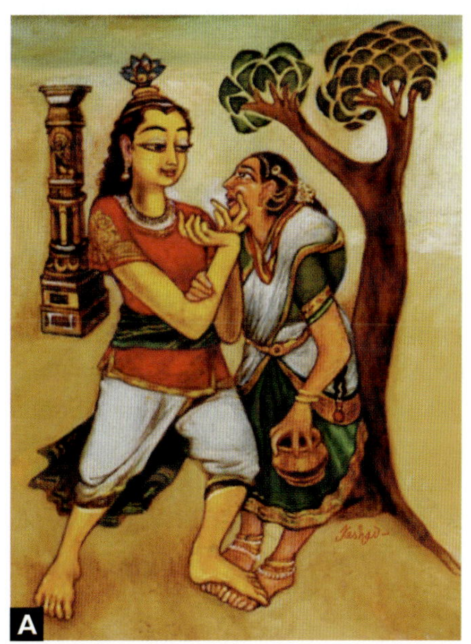

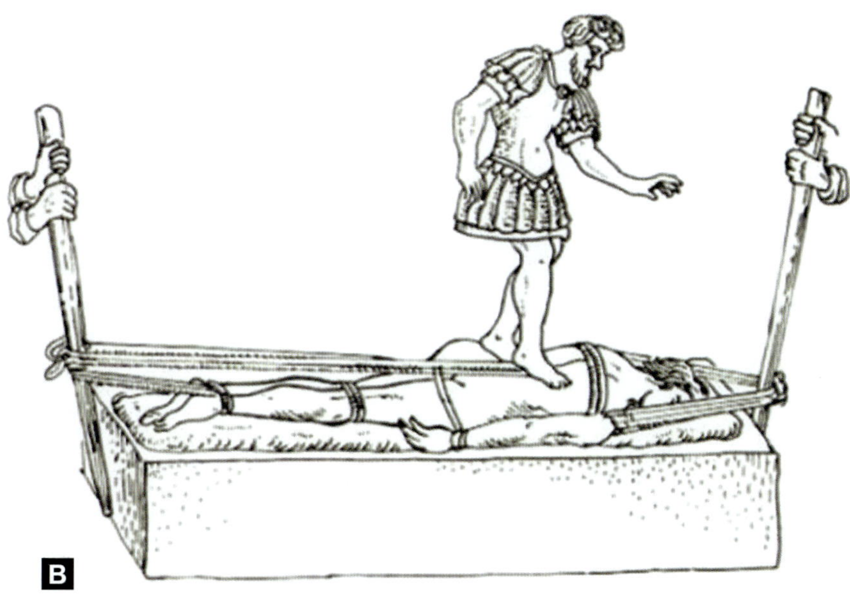

Figs. 39.1A and B: (A) Krishna straightened the spine of Kubja, one of his devotees. (B) An illustration of Galen's method of spinal deformity correction using a device similar to the Hippocratic traction board with pressure applied to the patient's back.

trauma. Both acute and chronic spine disorders can be treated today with a multitude of operative procedures that can be grouped conceptually around three surgical aims: decompression (relief of neural compression), stabilization, and correction of a spinal deformity (Fig. 39.2).

DECOMPRESSION OF SPINAL ELEMENTS

Laminectomy

In the infancy of spine surgery during the 19th century, decompression of the neural elements was the single most common indication to undertake the risks of spinal surgery. The risks of surgery were high as antibiotics were unavailable, and deep bone infection could have disastrous consequences. Laminectomy was the most commonly used technique to achieve decompression. Initial attempts at the surgery were controversial opponents of laminectomy often referenced the failed multilevel procedure on a 26-year-old male patient who had sustained a thoracic fracture-dislocation from a fall that resulted in paraplegia.[5] Surgical reduction of the fracture was unsuccessful, complete decompression of the neural elements was not achieved, and the patient died on postoperative day 4. While the patient's outcome was untoward, it cannot necessarily be attributed to an inefficiency of laminectomy, as inadequate anesthesia the frequent septic complications of the era likely contributed to the failure.

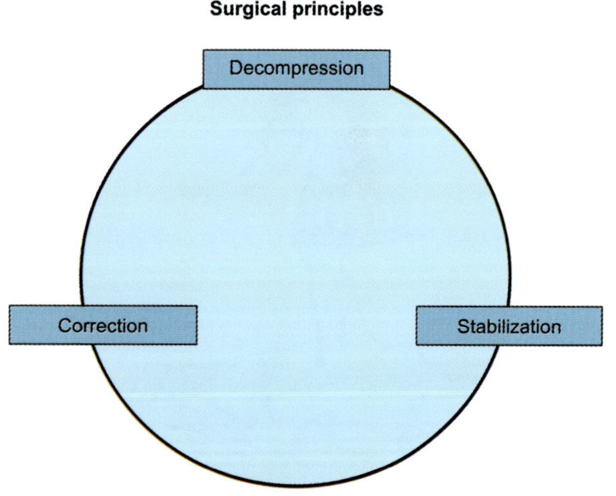

Fig. 39.2: Spinal surgery revolves around three basic surgical goals: decompression, surgical stabilization, and deformity correction. In the 19th century, spinal surgery was almost exclusively reserved for neural element decompression in cases of tumor, trauma, and infection. By the 20th century, the field had evolved to achieve surgical stabilization and deformity correction.

Restored faith in the usefulness of laminectomy came after repeated attempts demonstrating survival and even partial neurologic recovery for traumatic paraplegia, thus affirming trauma as an indication for spine surgery. By the end of the 19th century, indications for surgical decompression included neural compression resulting from trauma, tumors, and infection.[6] The later discovery that degenerative diseases might result in neural compression led to an important expansion of surgical indications for the spine.

Decompression in Sciatica

"Thou cold sciatica, cripple our senators, that their limbs may halt as lamely as their manners"—William Shakespeare (Timon of Athens: IV, i)

Sciatica is one of the most ill-famed yet poorly understood neural compression syndromes. Greek and Roman physicians attributed the pain of sciatica (deep lower back and shooting leg pain) to the hip joint. Hippocrates referred to pain in the pelvis and leg "sciatica", derived from *ischios*, the Greek word for hip.[7] It was the Italian physician Domencio Cotugno's experiments in 1764 that led to the realization that pain of nerve origin, such as sciatica, can be distinguished from pain of arthritic origin.[8]

Understanding that sciatica arises from spinal compression did not immediately clarify the causes of such compression. In 1932, a patient with sciatica that was thought to result from a chondroma was referred to the surgeon William Mixter at Massachusetts General Hospital. After removal of the suspected chondroma, histology revealed that it was actually the nucleus pulposus, therefore representing a ruptured intervertebral disk. Upon further review, Mixter and Barr found that all of the misdiagnosed chondromas at Massachusetts General Hospital were ruptured intervertebral disks as well, thus an important cause of neural compression and irritation (Figs. 39.3A and B).[9] Currently, sciatica is considered more as a symptom than a diagnosis as it can be caused by compression from various structures. The disorder is most often caused by age-related degeneration of the spinal column, which occurs more frequently in the cervical and lumbar spine than in the thoracic as these regions have increased motion.

Cord and nerve compression are not limited to the lumbar spine. The increased motion in both the cervical

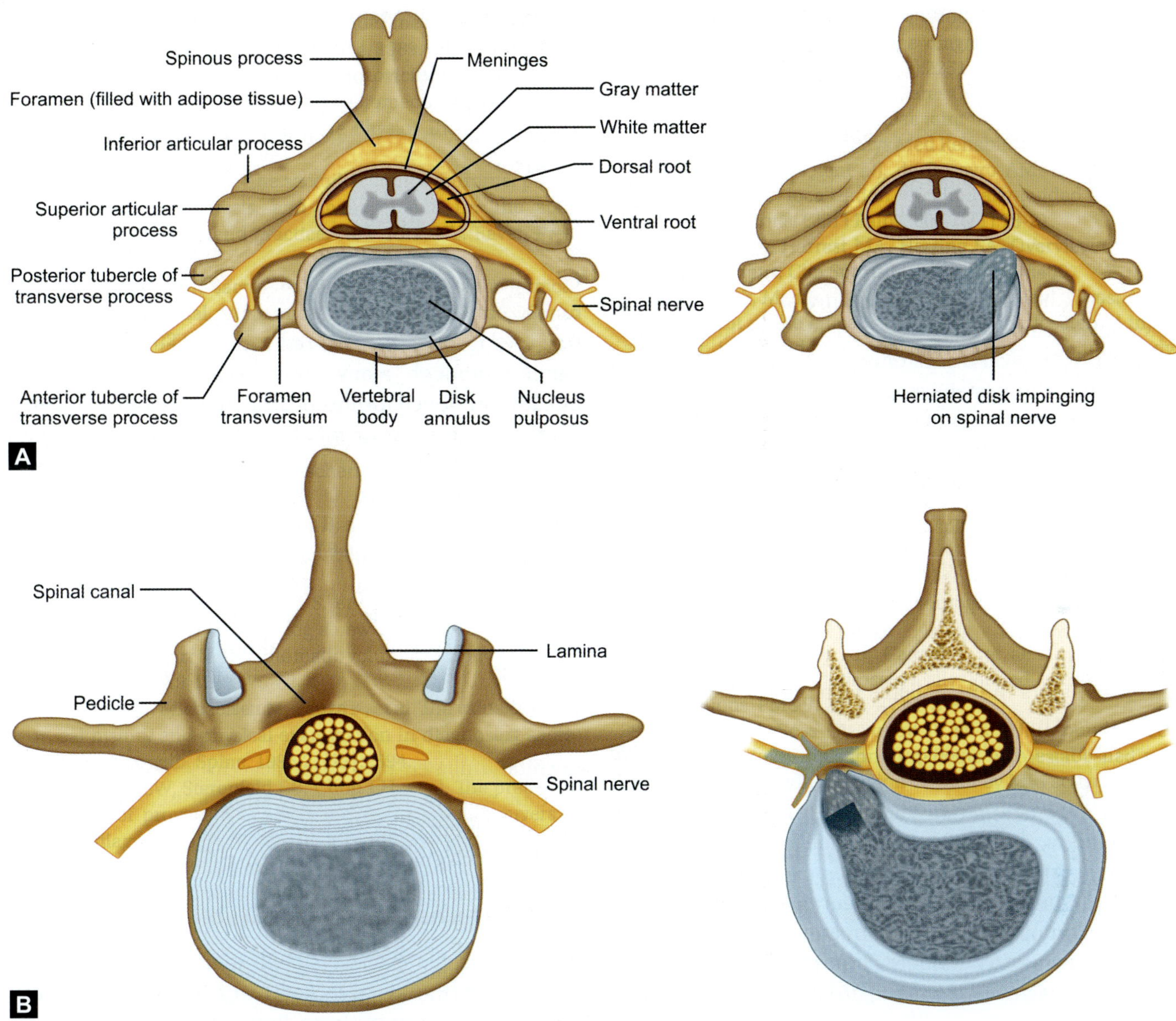

Figs. 39.3A and B: (A) Herniation of nucleus pulposus compresses and irritates nerve root at the cord level and (B) lumbar level where cord is no longer present.

and lumbar regions can lead to degenerative conditions that cause axial pain (neck or back pain) and/or radicular pain (arm pain-brachalgia or leg pain-sciatica). As in most orthopedic disorders, surgical intervention for compression is typically regarded as the last resort, an option only to be used once all other forms of conservative treatment have been exhausted.

Cervical Spine Decompression

In the cervical spine, a vertebral stress fracture, known as spondylosis, that causes nerve root compression (radiculopathy) can result in severe pain, paresthesias, and motor deficits. Spondylosis that results in spinal cord compression is one etiology of myelopathy, which can be identified by symptoms of clumsiness and gait disturbance. Anterior cord or radicular compression is frequently treated with anterior cervical discectomy and fusion (ACDF), frequently performed for 1-, 2-, or even 3-level disease. When a more extensive decompression is warranted, posterior techniques may be employed.

Laminoplasty is a method of decompression that preserves the posterior lamina but expands the spinal canal over multiple levels. In cases with greater instability, decompression is obtained by removal of the mid-line posterior elements (laminectomy), with or without stabilization and fusion.

Lumbar Spine Decompression

As in the cervical spine, decompression surgery of the lumbar spine should be appropriate for the cause of the axial back pain, radicular pain, or both. When nonsurgical options have failed to relieve nerve or cord impingement due to disk herniation, a discectomy may provide relief. Although decompression was initially thought to be best achieved by radical discectomy, surgeons soon began to understand the destabilizing nature of this procedure. Thus, simply removing the protruding portion of the herniated disk has shown to provide satisfactory decompression, preserving stability.

Familiar with the advantages of using the operating microscope, Williams popularized microdiscectomy technique (Fig. 39.4). The popularity could be associated with the minimal surgical scar noted on his patients, many of whom happened to include Las Vegas show girls where the size of the scar was quite important. The small scars in his patients were supplemented by a faster return to work.[10]

Although disk herniation is part of a degenerative process, degeneration of the lumbar spine can also result in disk degeneration (axial loss of disk height), facet degeneration, instability (spondylolisthesis, retrolisthesis, lateral listhesis, and/or degenerative scoliosis), spinal stenosis (compression of the neural elements), or any combination of these. Surgical treatment of degenerative disorders is most commonly performed through a posterior approach, involving partial laminotomy and discectomy, laminectomy, partial facetectomy, or other techniques of decompression based on pathoanatomy. When instability is found preoperatively (usually from spondylolisthesis or degenerative scoliosis) or created iatrogenically from surgical decompression, the spine is fused for stabilization.

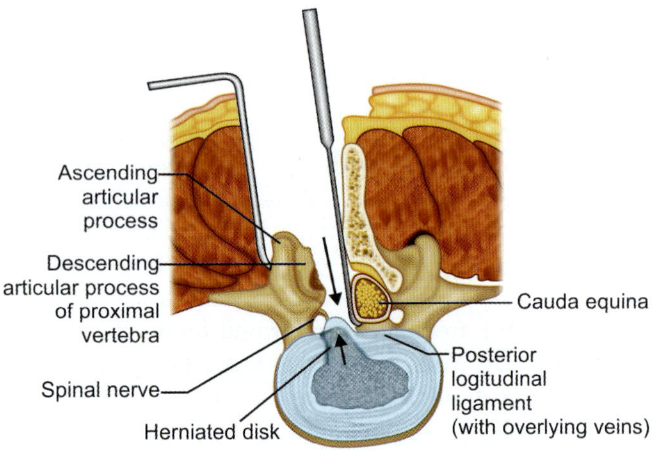

Fig. 39.4: Surgical approach to the microdiscectomy.

STABILIZATION OF THE SPINE

Orthopedists during the Civil War were considered primarily cast and brace makers who provided stability to fractures through indirect reduction and external stabilization. Although many other medical specialties had already developed forums of academic discourse, the first North American Academic Department of Orthopaedics was not established until 1853, at the Bellevue Medical College in Manhattan. Dr Lewis Albert Sayre served as the first professor of orthopedics at Bellevue (Figs. 39.5A and B).[11] However, clinical instruction of orthopedics at New York University (NYU) began as early as 1819. In 1898, the Bellevue Hospital Medical College merged with NYU Medical College, although the NYU School of Medicine did not assume complete responsibility for Bellevue's clinical services until 1968.

Bellevue Hospital Medical College was the first hospital-affiliated medical college in New York State. In treating orthopedics as a professional discipline, meticulous documentation, sketches, and photographs were all used to teach guiding principles to trainees.

From External to Internal Stabilization

Sayre advocated external stabilization of the spine using plaster vests (the "Sayre jacket"), which could theoretically reduce the deformity from Pott's disease (tuberculosis of the spine resulting in destruction of vertebral bodies) (Fig. 39.6). But the Sayre jacket and other common external measures of stabilization proved unsuccessful, providing the impetus for more invasive techniques. The first report of a surgical means of internal fixation to stabilize the deformity of Pott's disease made use of simple loops of silver wire around the spinous processes as documented by Hadra in 1891.[12]

The idea of stabilizing the spine with a "bony ridge" used to achieve fusion was proposed in 1911. Russell A Hibbs, a surgeon working at the New York Orthopaedic Hospital, used a cantilever support for the bony fusion in the lumbar spine to prevent kyphosis.[13] Also working in New York City, Fred H Albee used autologous tibial

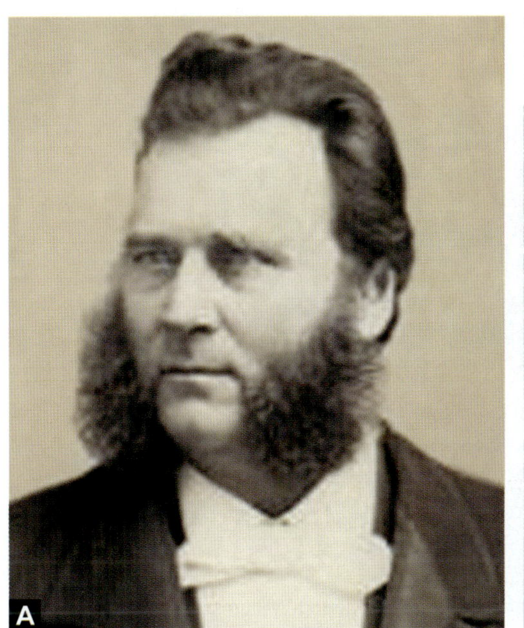

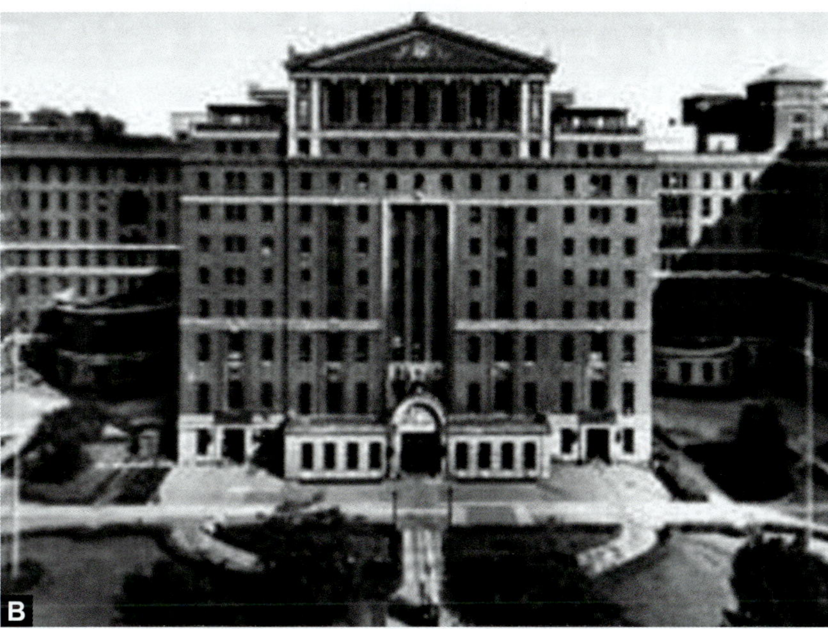

Figs. 39.5A and B: Lewis Albert Sayre began the first Academic Department of Orthopaedics at Bellevue Medical College.

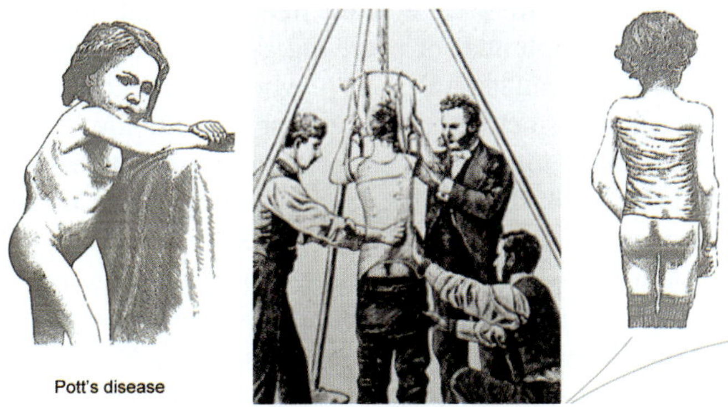

Fig. 39.6: Sayre advocated use of plaster vests "Sayre jacket" to reduce spine deformity from Pott's disease.

bone grafts between spinal processes instead of metal to fuse Pott's disease.[14] Together, Hibbs and Albee developed what is now known as a posterior fusion. When decompression (laminectomy) was initially performed, there was no bed for a posterior fusion so the bone graft was placed laterally in the gutters over the transverse processes. This became known as a posterolateral fusion and was initially popularized at NYU by George Truckley and Walter Thompson, the former chair of orthopedic surgery at NYU Hospital for Joint Diseases (Fig. 39.7).[15]

Fusion techniques were employed in the cervical spine with early procedures using posterior wiring and grafting methods. Posterior wiring was first described by Rogers in 1942 for cervical trauma.[16] However, wiring techniques for the posterior elements of the spine were initially limited by inadequate stiffness and poor resistance to rotation and extension forces. In addition, removing spinous processes for grafting made wiring impossible.

ANTIBIOTICS AND ORTHOPEDIC INSTRUMENTATION

The advent of antibiotics and antisepsis during the World War II era improved surgical safety across all medical disciplines. In orthopedic surgeries, the risk of developing osteomyelitis was reduced to the point where orthopedic surgeons were comfortable leaving plates and screws—which are prone to harboring infection—inside of the body after operative reduction and internal fixation. Advances in caring for trauma to the appendicular skeleton had a strong influence on fusion techniques in the axial skeleton. An organization dedicated to improving musculoskeletal patient care called Arbeitsgemeinschaft für Osteosynthesefragen (AO) was founded in Switzerland in 1958 and taught principles of internal fracture fixation to physicians. The principles taught in Sweden were later adapted to the spine for stabilization, and although concepts of rigid fixation were developed, spine surgeons adhered to the maxim that "internal fixation is a race between bony fusion and hardware failure". As Boucher noted in 1959, adequate bony fusion is essential to his proposed lumbosacral screw fixation technique.[17]

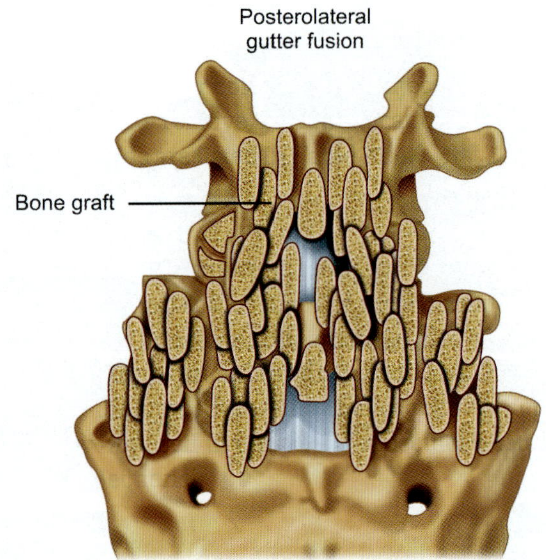

Fig. 39.7: Spinal fusion, also known as "spondylodesis", uses supplementary bone tissue to join two or more vertebrae. In a posterolateral fusion, bone graft (from patient or donor) placed over the transverse processes in the back of the spine is used in conjunction with the body's natural bone growth processes to fuse the vertebrae.

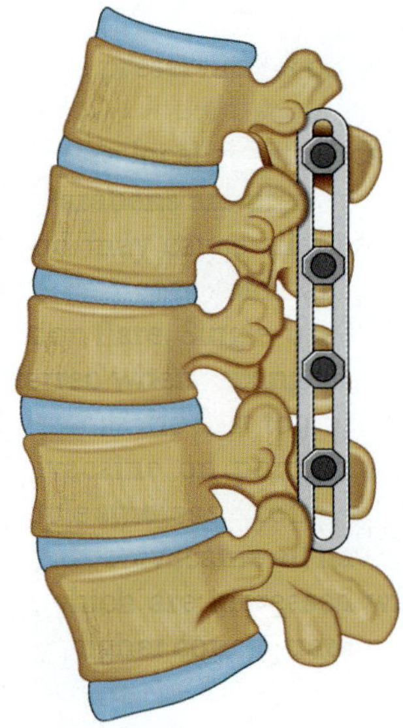

Fig. 39.8: Posterior plating with Meurig-Williams plate.

POSTERIOR THORACOLUMBAR INSTRUMENTATION

The use of facet screws in the lumbosacral spine was reported by King in 1948, who placed them internally through the spine's lateral articulations for stabilization, thus avoiding external casting in plaster.[18] However, surgeons using stainless steel machine screws across facet articulations have noted that pseudarthrosis was a common complication, despite King's initially low rates.[19]

As screws alone seemed inadequate when fractures in the extremities were being treated with plate-screw constructs, innovators such as Philip D Wilson in New York started using plates for spine fixation in the 1940s to provide more rigid fixation than screws alone. The Wilson plate, the Meurig-Williams plating system (Fig. 39.8), and other early plate-screw designs provided greater strength in resisting motion and allowing fusion, although they attached to the spinous processes.[20] Holdsworth and Hardy proposed a similar design of plates secured with screws, but additionally proposed a model for stability and a classification scheme for disruption of this stability by mechanism and fracture morphology.[21]

The attachment sites for the screws in these plate-screw constructs involved the facets, lamina, or spinous processes, which could be damaged or needed for bone graft. While the plates were more stabilizing than screws alone, they were often too superficial, limiting the healing potential of overlying skin and soft tissues. It was Roy-Camille et al. in 1970 who first integrated the orthopedic principles of plate fixation with the spine-specific technique of screws inserted through pedicles.[22] Exploitation of the pedicle as an attachment site is credited to this influential report (Fig. 39.9).

After Roy-Camille et al. invented the plate-screw construct using pedicle screws, Arthur Steffee popularized the use of pedicle screws in the United States. Steffe used a contoured plate as opposed to the screw-rod devices developed in Europe. Proponents of screw-plate and screw-rod constructs debated the strength advantages of the plates versus the flexibility and added space for fusion mass of the rods.[23] Ultimately, dual-rod constructs attached to lumbar pedicle screws proved superior in correcting deformity.

ANTERIOR THORACOLUMBAR INSTRUMENTATION

In 1969, Dwyer et al. introduced a technique for instrumenting the convex side of curvature with titanium screws inserted into vertebral bodies securing a titanium plate hooked over the end plates.[24] A cable threaded through the screw heads could be tensioned to provide correction of deformity. With a ventral approach, the intervertebral disks were easily removed, resulting in increased mobility

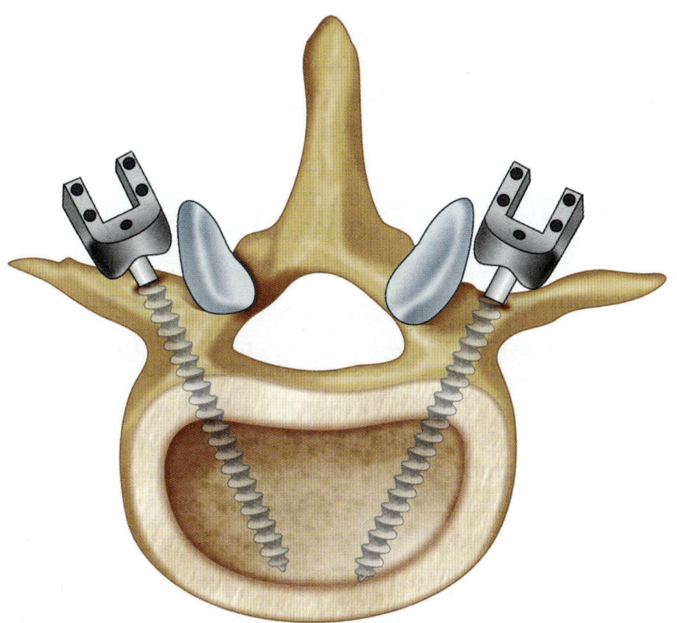

Fig. 39.9: Roy-Camille is credited with the use of the pedicle as an attachment site for screws, commonly used today for posterior thoracolumbar instrumentation.

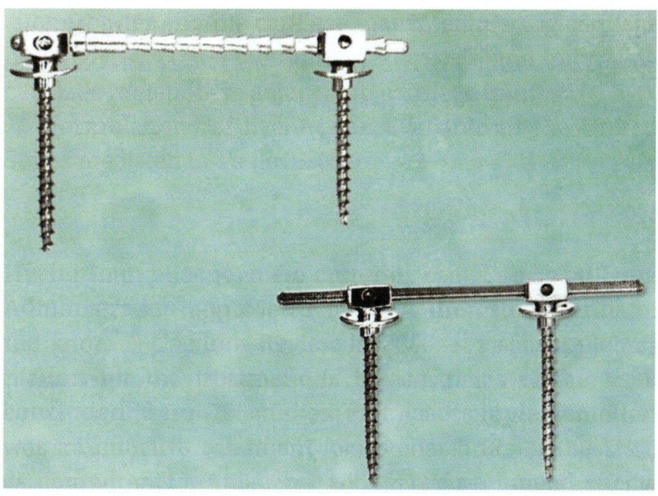

Fig. 39.10: Top, the Kostuik-Harrington system with round-ended Harrington distraction rod used with ratchet end screws, collar-ended screws, and washers. On the bottom, a heavy compression Harrington rod.

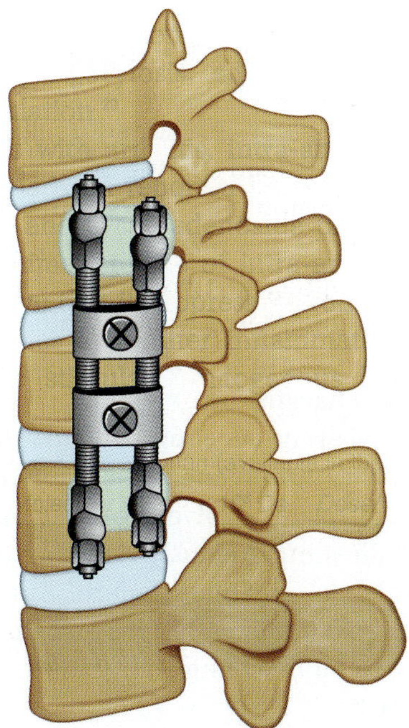

Fig. 39.11: Anterior thoracolumbar instrumentation with Kaneda's two threaded rods secured by staples and vertebral body screws.

of the spine to achieve greater amounts of correction than posterior techniques; this proved especially useful in adult scoliosis patients who did not tolerate bracing and were at high risk for pseudarthrosis.[25]

The Zielke system modified Dwyer et al.'s instruments with a compression rod with nuts to allow more rigid fixation and derotation. This system showed best results when combined with dorsal fixation, but it could still produce kyphosis. Systems later evolved with rods rigidly linked by "vertebral body bridges": a ventrolateral staple into the vertebral body and a dorsolateral intervertebral body screw; unfortunately, this system went too far anterior under the vessels, and after a few complications ceased being used.[26]

Using the ventrolateral vertebral body screw attachment site, the Kostuik-Harrington instrumentation (Fig. 39.10) introduced an innovative method of short-segment fixation with the ability to correct the kyphotic deformity associated with burst fractures. The added cross-fixators over the rods enhanced stability, as they were the biomechanical equivalent of a plate. Bolt-plate systems continued to develop, but the single bolt design was less resistant to rotation.[27]

A meeting between the innovators Kostuik and Kaneda led to another important adaptation in spinal stabilization. Kaneda introduced vertebral body staples with threaded longitudinal rods that provided reduction of kyphosis with the simultaneous compression of intervertebral bone graft for fusion (Fig. 39.11).[28] The concept was adapted to a system using rigid bolt-plate interfaces with semirigid screw-plate interfaces. The bolts provided distraction for kyphotic deformities, but slots on the plate achieved compression for the bone graft.[29] Newer generations of plates retained the ability to both compress graft and distract kyphotic deformity while providing lower profile titanium alloy designs.

POSTERIOR CERVICAL INSTRUMENTATION

As surgeons noticed the inadequacies of wiring techniques, screw fixation alternatives emerged. The stainless-steel Daab plate, shaped like an H, could be compressed to fit and fix with screws to the spinous processes, but it did not show significant improvement over wiring. Later cervical fusion techniques included instrumentation with a stainless steel interlaminar Halifax clamp, consisting of two sublaminar hooks tightened together with a screw.[30,31] The hooks in the spinal canal proved hazardous, and usefulness was limited when multiple segments required fixation.

Roy-Camille introduced the technique of using the lateral mass as an attachment site for the screws, allowing for strong fixation when spinous processes or lamina are unavailable due to trauma or procedure.[32,33] Initially, lateral mass fixation required accommodation from plates with proper hole positions and ability to contour, which can be better achieved with screw-rod constructs.

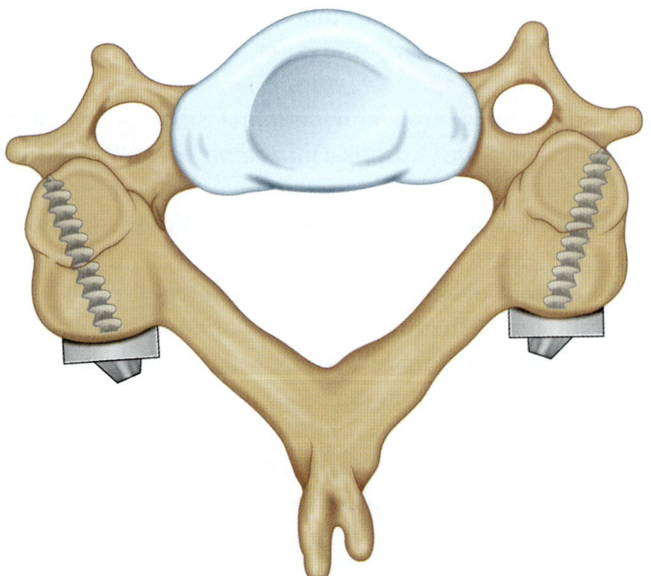

Fig. 39.12: Lateral mass screws are often used for the subaxial cervical spine.

Lateral mass screws are often used for the subaxial cervical spine as they are considered safer than pedicle screws, despite the higher pullout strength of pedicle screws (Fig. 39.12).

ANTERIOR CERVICAL INSTRUMENTATION

The technique of enhancing cervical fusion by introducing a horseshoe-shaped bone graft was introduced by Robinson and Smith. With another spine surgeon at Johns Hopkins, Lee Riley, Robinson and Smith pioneered the ACDF with the use of intervertebral graft to promote the biologic process. Cloward followed, introducing intervertebral fusion using bone grafted from the iliac crests in 1953.[34] However, Cloward's use of allograft and sometimes xenograft would often result in extreme cases of graft-host immunogenicity. Disk removal and replacement with bone graft is one of the most common cervical spine procedures performed today, but it is now usually stabilized with an anterior plate; the plate functions as a tension band during neck extension and as a buttress in flexion.

The use of plate implants to stabilize fusion was pioneered by Bohler in the 1960s, which became a popular supplement to the operation.[35] Anterior plate-screw constructs were to provide load sharing between the graft and plate while bony fusion took place. However, the vital structures anterior to the plate are at an increased risk of tracheal or esophageal erosion from screw backout or breakage. Technique was thus essential and care was taken to obtain bicortical purchase and to angle the screws to prevent backing out.

Plate material eventually improved to mostly titanium alloy, and in light of problems with overly rigid designs, dynamic cervical plates evolved to limit intersegmental movement while simultaneously reducing the incidence of graft subsidence and plate failure. Anterior cervical plates are available in many designs and can be categorized according to biomechanical or graft-loading properties (Fig. 39.13).[36]

INTERBODY FUSION

The idea of an intervertebral implant with biologic properties to enhance fusion inspired the design of the hollow stainless steel implant known as an intervertebral cage. The use of a biological implant was first explored in horses with wobbler-neck syndrome, a type of cervical

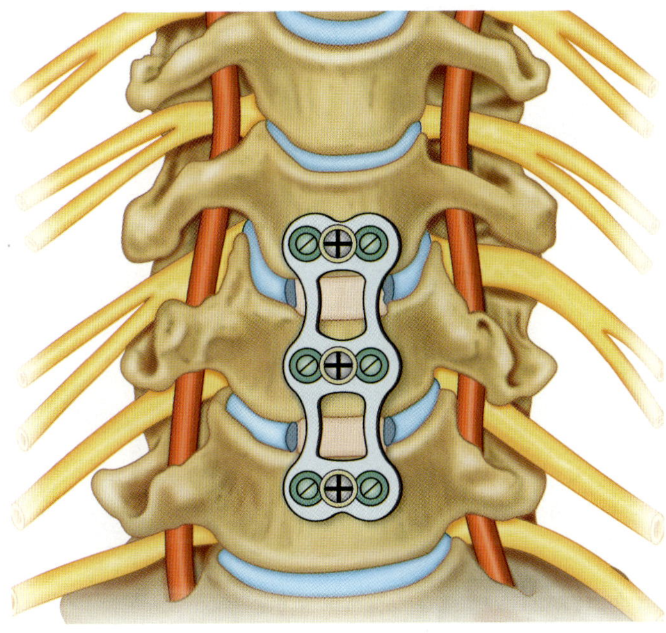

Fig. 39.13: Example of an anterior cervical plate-screw construct.

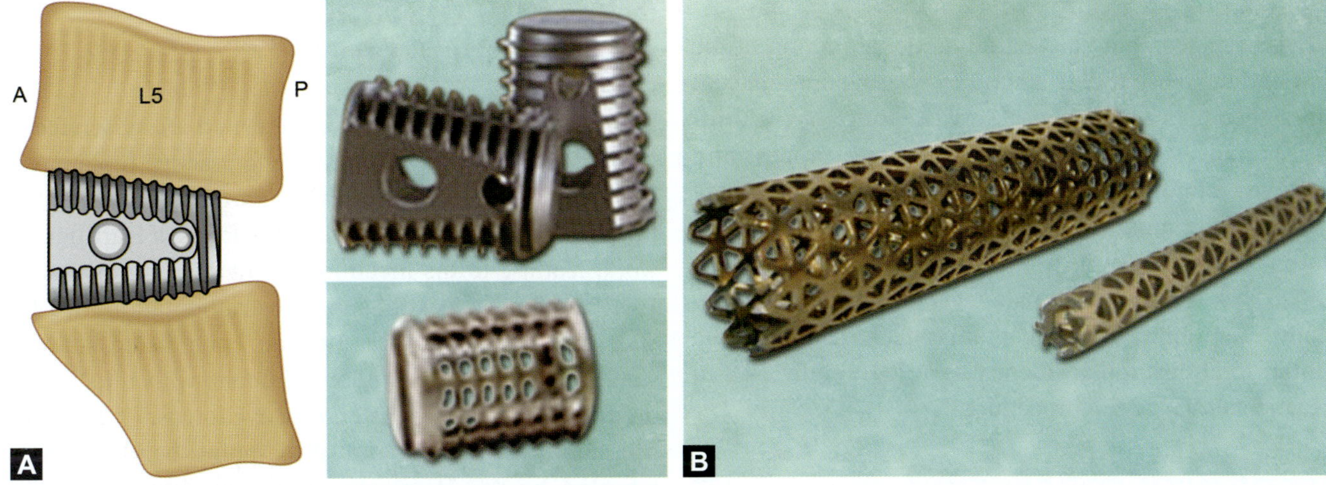

Figs. 39.14A and B: (A) Intervertebral cages. (B) Long-titanium mesh cages.

spondylomyelopathy. The cage was designed to function as a spacer and a "basket", containing bone graft and any other augment for the interbody fusion (Figs. 39.14A and B).[37] Success of the cage in treating horses with wobbler-neck syndrome led to its quick adaptation for surgical in humans with cervical spine disorders.[38,39]

Despite implant's initial development for the cervical spine, the cage became widely used in the lumbar spine as well, leading to the "cage rage" of the 1990s. The cage allowed for ventral or dorsal approaches to lumbar interbody fusions, termed anterior lumbar interbody fusion (ALIF) and posterior lumbar interbody fusion (PLIF), respectively.[40] Considered a more direct approach with less retraction than PLIF, the transforaminal lumbar interbody fusion (TLIF) was also popularized in the 1990s. However, an anterior approach was necessary when the space to be filled extended beyond an intervertebral level, such as with bone destruction from metastatic disease or trauma. For special cases necessitating an anterior approach, Harms developed a long titanium mesh cage for vertebral body height replacement that is packed with bone and seated between remaining end plates (Figs. 39.14A and B).[41]

ALTERNATIVES TO FUSION—TOTAL DISK REPLACEMENT

Fusion of the knee and hip joints were common pain-relieving procedures before the advent and success total joint arthroplasty in the 1960s. Although the spine involves more complex intersegmental motion than either the hip or knee, there is potential benefit in replacing a degenerated intervertebral disk rather than fusing the two surrounding vertebrae. Despite the successes of fusion in ACDF, the loss of mobility and potential to develop adjacent segment disease—wearing out of the levels above and below the fusion—can eventually necessitate revision surgery.[42] Posterior fusions for scoliosis similarly present a risk, as skeletally immature children can develop crankshaft phenomenon, which occurs when anterior growth around a posterior fusion worsens the deformity. Motion preservation has also become an important consideration, furthering the debate on the long-term success of vertebral fusion.

Disk replacement can spare functional motion at the joint and decrease the likelihood of wearing out adjacent joints seen in rigid fusions. Cervical total disk arthroplasty removes any compressive pathologic process and preserves motion with satisfactory 2-year follow-up data available.[43] Lumbar total disk arthroplasty is another motion-preserving surgical option for patients with degenerative disk disease at a single level (Fig. 39.15). A prospective, randomized, multicenter clinical trial evaluating lumbar total disk replacement was at least equivalent to the gold standard ALIF procedure.[44]

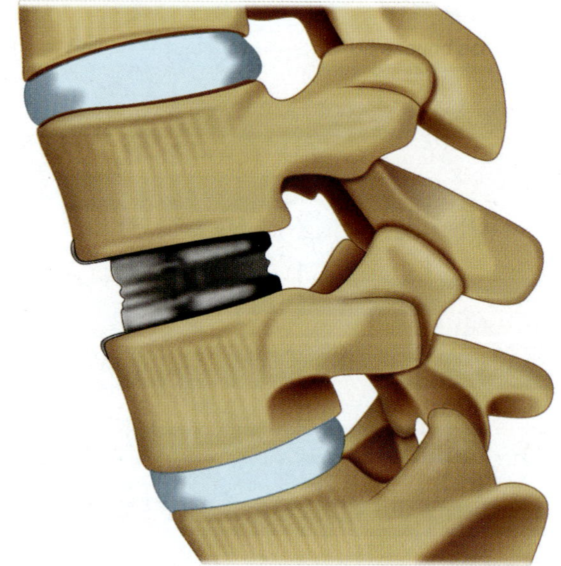

Fig. 39.15: Artificial disk replacement in the lumbar spine.

DEFORMITY CORRECTION

Deformity or loss of normal spinal alignment can develop after trauma (acute), as a result of a gradual process of imbalance among dynamic stabilizers such as muscles and static stabilizers such as ligaments and joint capsules, or after a failure of osseous support from destructive lesions. But scoliosis, the most common spine deformity, has no clear etiology and is thus termed adolescent idiopathic scoliosis. Although some early advances in stabilization devices were able to achieve short-segment correction of the deformity, the means to surgically reduce large curves spanning many segments was not available until the 1940s.

RODS FOR DISTRACTION AND COMPRESSION

In 1945, Dr Paul Harrington returned from service in World War II to find his orthopedic practice replete with scoliotic spinal deformity resulting from the polio epidemic. Scoliosis deformity became the focus of Harrington's work, leading to his invention of the Harrington Rod in 1953, the first successful spinal instrumentation. In 1973, Harrington reported that he had been using stainless steel hooks on the posterior elements, with nuts placed on threaded rods to adjust corrective forces.[45,46] The compression, distraction, and three-point bending forces afforded by the Harrington Rod were able to achieve both stability and correction of the deformity.

The important underlying principles of orthopedics resounded as they emerged from Harrington's and others' early successes and failures. In reviewing records of early surgical treatments for scoliosis, it was reported that implantation without fusion resulted in complete loss of correction, re-emphasizing the importance of promoting solid biological fusion, and how the implant is only a temporary measure.[47] Still, even with solid fusion there were frequent implant-related complications, and surgeons soon learned that distraction of the spine often decreases normal lumbar lordosis, resulting in flat back deformity (Figs. 39.16A to C).

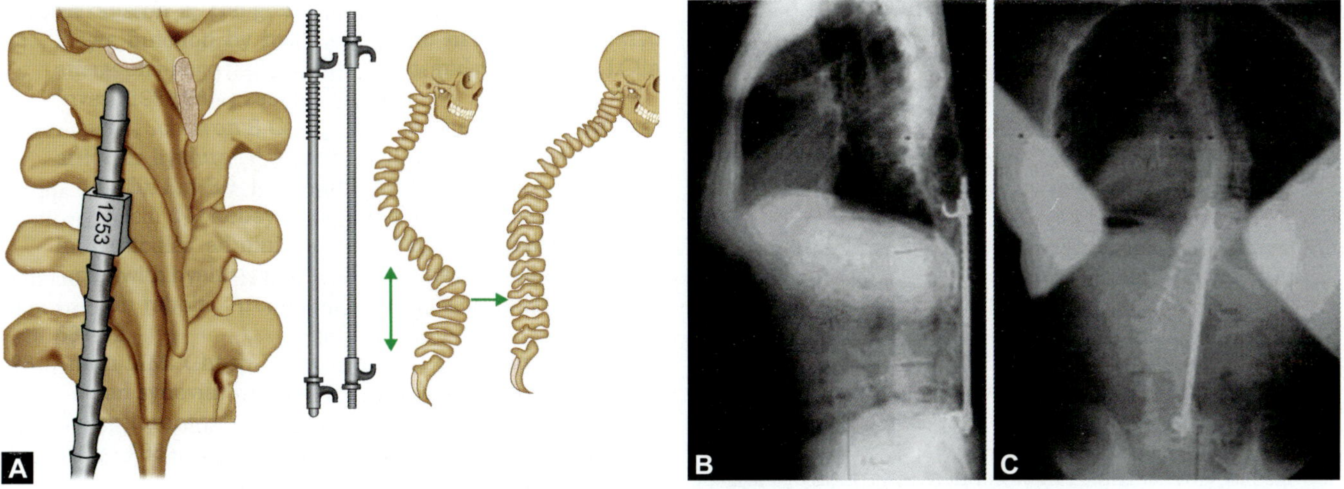

Figs. 39.16A to C: Harrington rod instrumentation resulting in flat back syndrome with loss of normal lumbar lordosis.

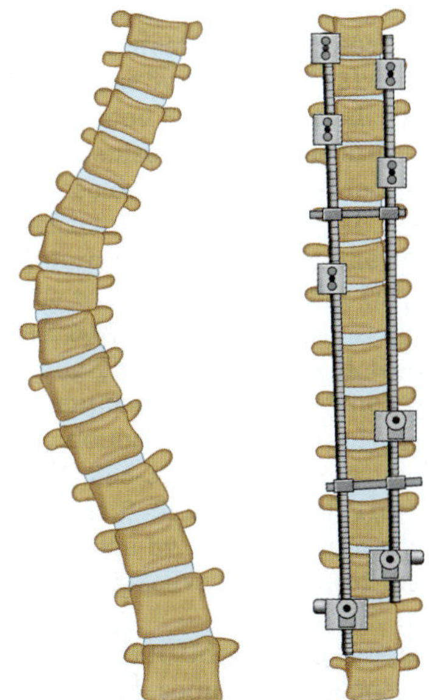

Fig. 39.17: Cotrel and Dubousset instrumentation for correction of scoliosis attaching rods to the spine with hooks and/or screws.

SEGMENTAL FIXATION FOR INCREASED RIGIDITY

As difficulties with the Harrington system manifested, Dr Luque from Mexico introduced what he termed segmental spinal instrumentation (SSI) for fixation and correction of scoliosis.[48] SSI involves sublaminar wire loops that secure prebent stainless steel rods in place. By increasing the points of fixation, SSI increased the corrective power of previous scoliosis instrumentation and obviated the need for postoperative immobilization from a brace.

MULTIPLE HOOK ROD FOR ROTATION

Cotrel and Dubousset introduced rods for scoliosis correction with hooks used superiorly and pedicle screws in the lumbosacral region in 1984 (Fig. 39.17).[49] The instrument's multiple hooks allowed spinal surgeons to apply compression and distraction over different areas within the same rod and applied the principles of segmental fixation without the need for sublaminar wires, which require passage encroaching on the spinal canal. The compression-distraction system also provided rod rotation, a powerful force in the correction of scoliosis, with further stability provided by cross-linking the two parallel rods together.

Various anchoring and rod construct combinations are also frequently used, resulting in segmental pedicle screw-rod fixation.[50] Combined anchoring and rod constructs provide fixation of all three columns of stability and correction in three planes.[51] The current all-transpedicle screw and rod constructs are also able to manipulate and potentially derotate the caudal-most end of the construct. The caudal levels horizontally neutral position can spare the need for more distal levels.

SUMMARY

Decompression, stabilization, and correction form the core principles of surgical management for spine disorders. Advances in instrumentation have dramatically improved the surgeon's ability to provide stabilization, correction, and reduction while minimizing the need for postoperative external bracing.

REFERENCES

1. Goodrich JT. History of spine surgery in the ancient and medieval worlds. Neurosurg Focus. 2004;16(1):E2.
2. Deshaies EM, DiRisio D, Popp AJ. Medieval management of spinal injuries: parallels between Theodoric of Bologna and contemporary spine surgeons. Neurosurg Focus. 2004; 16(1):E3.
3. Singh H, Rahimi SY, Yeh DJ, et al. History of posterior thoracic instrumentation. Neurosurg Focus. 2004;16(1):E11.
4. Omeis I, DeMattia JA, Hillard VH, et al. History of instrumentation for stabilization of the subaxial cervical spine. Neurosurg Focus. 2004;16(1):E10.
5. Hayward G. An account of a case of fracture and dislocation of the spine. N Engl J Med Surg Collateral Branches Sci. 1815;4(1):1-3.
6. Elsberg CA. Diagnosis and treatment of surgical diseases of the spinal cord and its membranes. St Louis, MO: WB Saunders Company; 1916.
7. Adams F, Kelly EC. The Genuine Works of Hippocrates. Whitefish, MT: Kessinger Pub; 2006.
8. Brunori A, De Caro GM, Giuffre R. [Surgery of lumbar disk hernia: historical perspective]. Annali italiani di chirurgia. 1998;69(3):285-93.
9. Mixter WJ, Barr JS. Rupture of the intervertebral disc with involvement of the spinal canal. N Engl J Med. 1934; 211(5):210-5.
10. Williams RW. Microlumbar discectomy: a conservative surgical approach to the virgin herniated lumbar disc. Spine. 1978;3(2):175-82.
11. Zampini JM, Sherk HH. Lewis A. Sayre: the first Professor of Orthopaedic Surgery in America. Clin Orthop Relat Res. 2008;466(9):2263-7.
12. Keller T, Holland MC. Some notable American spine surgeons of the 19th century. Spine. 1997;22(12):1413-7.
13. Hibbs RA. An operation for progressive spinal deformities: a preliminary report of three cases from the service of the orthopaedic hospital. 1911. Clin Orthop Relat Res. 2007;460:17-20.
14. Albee FH. Transplantation of a portion of the tibia into the spine for Pott's disease: a preliminary report 1911. Clin Orthop Relat Res. 2007;460:14-6.
15. Truchly G, Thompson WA. Posterolateral fusion of the lumbosacral spine. J Bone Joint Surg Am Vol. 1962;44-A:505-12.
16. Rogers WA. Treatment of fracture-dislocation of the cervical spine. J Bone Joint Surg. 1942;24(2):245-58.
17. Boucher HH. A method of spinal fusion. J Bone Joint Surg Br Vol. 1959;41-B(2):248-59.
18. King D. Internal fixation for lumbosacral fusion. J Bone Joint Surg Am Vol. 1948;30A(3):560-5.
19. Thompson WA, Ralston EL. Pseudarthrosis following spine fusion. J Bone Joint Surg Am Vol. 1949;31A(2):400-5.
20. Wilson PD, Straub LR. Spine fusion with internal plate fixation. New York State J Med. 1952;52(24):3003-4.
21. Holdsworth FW, Hardy A. Early treatment of paraplegia from fractures of the thoraco-lumbar spine. J Bone Joint Surg Br Vol. 1953;35-B(4):540-50.
22. Roy-Camille R, Roy-Camille M, Demeulenaere C. [Osteosynthesis of dorsal, lumbar, and lumbosacral spine with metallic plates screwed into vertebral pedicles and articular apophyses]. La Presse medicale. 1970;78(32):1447-8.
23. Esses SI, Bednar DA. The spinal pedicle screw: techniques and systems. Orthop Rev. 1989;18(6):676-82.
24. Dwyer AF, Newton NC, Sherwood AA. An anterior approach to scoliosis. A preliminary report. Clin Orthop Relat Res. 1969;62:192-202.
25. Winter RB. Combined Dwyer and Harrington instrumentation and fusion in the treatment of selected patients with painful adult idiopathic scoliosis. Spine. 1978;3(2):135-41.
26. Dunn HK. Anterior stabilization of thoracolumbar injuries. Clin Orthop Relat Research. 1984(189):116-24.
27. Ryan MD, Taylor TK, Sherwood AA. Bolt-plate fixation for anterior spinal fusion. Clin Orthop Relat Res. 1986(203): 196-202.
28. Bridwell KH. Spinal instrumentation in the management of adolescent scoliosis. Clin Orthop Relat Res. 1997(335): 64-72.
29. McDonough PW, Davis R, Tribus C, et al. The management of acute thoracolumbar burst fractures with anterior corpectomy and Z-plate fixation. Spine. 2004;29(17):1901-8; discussion 1909.
30. Bostman O, Myllynen P, Riska EB. Posterior spinal fusion using internal fixation with the Daab plate. Acta Orthop Scandinavica. 1984;55(3):310-4.
31. Holness RO, Huestis WS, Howes WJ, et al. Posterior stabilization with an interlaminar clamp in cervical injuries: technical note and review of the long term experience with the method. Neurosurg. 1984;14(3):318-22.
32. Ebraheim NA, Rupp RE, Savolaine ER, et al. Posterior plating of the cervical spine. J Spinal Disord. 1995;8(2):111-5.
33. An HS, Gordin R, Renner K. Anatomic considerations for plate-screw fixation of the cervical spine. Spine. 1991;16 (10 Suppl):S548-51.
34. Cloward RB. The treatment of ruptured lumbar intervertebral discs by vertebral body fusion. I. Indications, operative technique, after care. J Neurosurg. 1953;10(2):154-68.
35. Vaccaro AR, Balderston RA. Anterior plate instrumentation for disorders of the subaxial cervical spine. Clinic Orthop Relat Res. 1997(335):112-21.
36. Haid RW, Foley KT, Rodts GE, et al. The Cervical Spine Study Group anterior cervical plate nomenclature. Neurosurg Focus. 2002;12(1):E15.
37. DeBowes RM, Grant BD, Bagby GW, et al. Cervical vertebral interbody fusion in the horse: a comparative study of bovine xenografts and autografts supported by stainless steel baskets. Am J Vet Res. 1984;45(1):191-9.
38. Bagby GW. Arthrodesis by the distraction-compression method using a stainless steel implant. Orthopedics. 1988; 11(6):931-4.
39. Kuslich SD, Ulstrom CL, Griffith SL, et al. The Bagby and Kuslich method of lumbar interbody fusion. History, techniques, and 2-year follow-up results of a United States prospective, multicenter trial. Spine. 1998;23(11):1267-78; discussion 1279.

40. Burns BH. An operation for spondylolisthesis. Lancet. 1933;221(5728):1233.
41. Togawa D, Bauer TW, Brantigan JW, et al. Bone graft incorporation in radiographically successful human intervertebral body fusion cages. Spine. 2001;26(24):2744-50.
42. Hilibrand AS, Carlson GD, Palumbo MA, et al. Radiculopathy and myelopathy at segments adjacent to the site of a previous anterior cervical arthrodesis. J Bone Joint Surg Am Vol. 1999;81(4):519-28.
43. Boselie TF, Willems PC, van Mameren H, et al. Arthroplasty versus fusion in single-level cervical degenerative disc disease. Cochrane Database Syst Reviews (Online) 2012;9: CD009173.
44. Blumenthal S, McAfee PC, Guyer RD, et al. A prospective, randomized, multicenter Food and Drug Administration investigational device exemptions study of lumbar total disc replacement with the CHARITE artificial disc versus lumbar fusion: part I: evaluation of clinical outcomes. Spine. 2005;30(14):1565-75; discussion E387-91.
45. Harrington PR. Treatment of Scoliosis: correction and internal fixation by spine instrumentation. J Bone Joint Surg. 2002;84(2):316.
46. Harrington PR. 1973 Nicoals Andry Award Contribution: the history and development of Harrington instrumentation. Clin Orthop Relat Res. 1973;93:110-2.
47. Vaccaro AR, Garfin SR. Pedicle-screw fixation in the lumbar spine. J Am Acad Orthop Surgeons. 1995;3(5):263-74.
48. Luque ER. Segmental spinal instrumentation of the lumbar spine. Clin Orthop Relat Res. 1986(203):126-34.
49. Cotrel Y, Dubousset J. [A new technic for segmental spinal osteosynthesis using the posterior approach]. Revue de chirurgie orthopedique et reparatrice de l'appareil moteur. 1984;70(6):489-94.
50. Suk SI, Lee CK, Kim WJ, et al. Segmental pedicle screw fixation in the treatment of thoracic idiopathic scoliosis. Spine. 1995;20(12):1399-405.
51. Denis F. The three column spine and its significance in the classification of acute thoracolumbar spinal injuries. Spine. 1983;8(8):817-31.

CHAPTER

40 Surgical Management of Lumbar Degenerative Spondylolisthesis

Qasim M Husain, Robert P Norton, Jeffrey M Spivak

INTRODUCTION

Degenerative spondylolisthesis refers to a sagittal translational malalignment of two vertebrae due to progressive degenerative changes of the disk and accompanying facet joints. Typically, this is a forward slippage of the cephalad vertebra relative to the caudal vertebra (anterolisthesis), although backward slippage (retrolisthesis) can be seen as well (more commonly at the L5–S1 level. As the posterior bony arch is intact with this condition, degenerative spondylolisthesis is commonly accompanied by stenosis of the spinal canal. The condition predominantly affects individuals > 40 years of age and has an increasing incidence as the general population is aging. The condition was first described by Junghanns[1] in 1930 which he termed "pseudospondylolisthesis", and over 20 years later, Newman[2] coined the ubiquitously used term degenerative spondylolisthesis. The translation of one vertebral body with respect to another in the setting of a degenerated disk and facet arthrosis is found most commonly at the L4–5 level, followed by the L3–4 level, and rarely at L5–S1 level.[3] Several etiologic factors have been linked to this condition.

PATHOGENESIS

The pathogenesis of degenerative spondylolisthesis is thought to be related to arthrosis and loss of stability of the facet joints, with or without accompanying degeneration of the intervertebral disk. The facet joints may become lax and commonly enlarge and remodel with osteophyte formation. Disk degeneration leads to an increase in stress borne by the posterior elements, which can accelerate and worsen the facet arthrosis.[4]

The L3–4 and L4–5 facets have a more sagittal orientation compared with the coronal alignment of the L5–S1 joint. This anatomic variation decreases the ability of the facets at L3–4 and L4–5 to resist the forces of forward flexion, thereby contributing to olisthesis and facet arthritis. Also, while the L3–4 disk level is commonly parallel to the ground, the L4–5 disk is commonly angled down anteriorly, placing more shear forces on the facets at this level with any weight bearing in the upright position. Transitional lumbosacral junctions, with limited mobility due to partial or complete sacralization at L5–S1 may also predispose to increased forces and more likely development of degenerative spondylolisthesis at L4–5.[5] Degenerative spondylolisthesis does not progress beyond grade 2. As a result of the intact posterior arch, forward progression of the cephalad vertebrae is halted as the inferior articular processes contact the posterior aspect of the caudal vertebral body.

INCIDENCE

The overall incidence of degenerative spondylolisthesis in adults is between 4 and 9%.[6] This condition is five times more common in women, which is thought to be related to an increased ligamentous laxity compared with men. Recent studies have shown there to be a higher expression of estrogen receptors in the articular cartilage of facet joints, which is likely related to degenerative spondylolisthesis in postmenopausal women.[7] Also, women typically have a more open pelvis with a less deep-seated L4–5 level, which may result in higher forces at that level and may predispose to the development of olisthesis. Degenerative spondylolisthesis is also three times more common in people of African descent. This is believed to be due to anatomic features, including decreased lumbosacral lordosis and an increased prevalence of L5 sacralization.[3]

PRESENTATION

The clinical presentation of degenerative spondylolisthesis overlaps significantly with that of spinal stenosis. Complaints consistent with neurogenic claudication, radicular symptoms (usually the L5 nerve root if the olisthesis is at L4–5), and a history of waxing and waning low back pain are typical. Bowel and bladder complaints, although less common, can also be present.

NONOPERATIVE MEASURES

According to many authors, up to 90% of patients presenting with degenerative spondylolisthesis will have their symptoms controlled with nonoperative measures.[8] These treatment modalities include formal physical therapy, home exercise programs with an emphasis on lumbar flexion, nonsteroidal anti-inflammatory medications, narcotic medications, adaptive changes in activity and lifestyle, and epidural steroid injections.

Surgical Indications and Goals

Surgical intervention is most commonly indicated for those patients with persistent symptoms and functional deficits despite an adequate attempt of nonsurgical treatment. Much literature, including the ongoing landmark SPORT study,[9] have demonstrated the sustainable benefit of surgical treatment for spinal stenosis with degenerative spondylolisthesis. Herkowitz and Kurz[10] recommend the following surgical indications:

- Persistent or recurrent leg pain despite a minimum of 3 months of nonoperative treatment or
- Progressive or functionally significant neurologic deficit

The clinical symptoms and signs should be resulting in a significant reduction in quality of life, and they should also be consistent with the imaging studies.

Anatomic goals of surgery include decompression of compressed neurologic elements, stabilizing any unstable motion segments, and correction of significant spinal deformity. Decompression can be direct via laminectomy, or indirect by interspinous distraction or spinal realignment and disk height restoration. Fusion for stabilization may be required for a preoperatively unstable motion segment, or one made unstable at surgery as a consequence of the needed decompression. Newer interbody stabilization devices are also available, which do not require fusion. Correction of spinal deformity requires instrumentation to achieve the correction and fusion to maintain it over time.

Once the surgeon and patient together have made the decision to embark upon surgery, the specific surgical plan depends on the specific anatomic goals, choosing among various options when more than one surgical plan can be used to achieve all of the goals. Most of the surgical treatment options are supported by a significant amount of validated research and ongoing trials. Surgical procedures range from simple outpatient interspinous process device application to laminectomy alone to decompression and interbody fusion with instrumentation. There are various surgical approach options for obtaining an interbody fusion, which can be considered when desired.

SURGICAL OPTIONS

Interspinous Process Devices

There are several Food and Drug Administration approved interspinous devices (ISDs) currently available for use (e.g. X-Stop and Coflex). Although they vary in design and composition, the common goal of these devices is to distract between adjacent spinous processes, thereby increasing the spinal canal diameter and blocking segmental extension. Certain ISDs have been approved for up to a grade 1 slip, and others have been indicated to be used alone, or in conjunction with direct decompression via laminotomies.

Kabir et al.[11] performed a systematic review of the clinical and biomechanical research that has been performed on these devices. They found biomechanical evidence to support the notion of a potential beneficial effect of ISDs on the kinematics of the degenerative spine; however, clinical studies are not as conclusive.

Anderson et al.[12] conducted a prospective, randomized trial on 75 patients with neurogenic claudication and grade 1 degenerative spondylolisthesis. Forty-two patients underwent implantation of an ISD and 33 patients were treated nonoperatively. Significant improvements were observed in ZCQ (Zurich Claudication Questionnaire) score, patient satisfaction, and SF-36 outcome measures in the ISD group compared with control group. They reported overall clinical success in 63% in the implant group compared with 13% in the nonsurgical group at 2 years. Other noncomparative studies on the same ISD have reported varying degrees of satisfactory outcomes, whereas some have reported high rates of failure and complications requiring revision surgery. Moreover, comparative studies of this implant and other surgical interventions are lacking.

Richter et al.[13] recently reported their experience with a different ISD. They performed a prospective controlled study on 62 patients comparing decompression alone versus decompression with implantation of the ISD. Improvements in Oswestry Disability Index (ODI), visual analog scales (VAS), and Roland-Morris score clinical outcome measures were significant in both groups compared with baseline without any significant intergroup differences in all parameters evaluated. They concluded that at 2-year follow-up, the addition of an ISD does not improve the already good clinical outcome made after decompression alone.

Lumbar ISD may have a beneficial effect in a select group of patients. However, many studies show only marginal degrees of clinical success. More high-quality studies are needed to fully elucidate the proper indications for ISD use and the long-term outcomes of such devices.

Direct Decompression Alone

Decompression of the neural elements is the key component to surgical management of degenerative spondylolisthesis. The goal is to relieve pressure on the involved neural structures thereby relieving pain and other neurologic symptoms. This is achieved by an entire spectrum of techniques, including uni/bilateral laminotomy (Fig. 40.1) or laminectomy (Fig. 40.2), depending on the anatomy of the patient's compression and symptoms. Laminotomy refers to a removal of a portion of the lamina. When this is done, the lateral recess can be directly decompressed. Central stenosis can also be decompressed with a laminotomy by undercutting the central lamina. Furthermore, a contralateral lateral recess decompression can also be performed through a unilateral laminotomy by adjusting the patient position and the surgical retractors to gain access to the contralateral side. Depending on the patient's anatomy and compression, as well as surgeon's preference, this technique can also be performed using bilateral incisions. Laminotomy has the benefit of preserving the posterior elements that contribute to continued stability. Removal of the entire lamina, or laminectomy, can also be performed. This can be done unilaterally or bilaterally, depending on the patient's stenosis and symptoms. Performing a laminectomy that extends between the pedicles, referred to as a ''pedicle-to-pedicle'' decompression, is often done to achieve a thorough bilateral decompression. This technique, however, does have the drawback of sacrificing more bone (decreased potential fusion bed) as well as the posterior ligamentous complex. Inadequate decompressions, which leave residual areas of neural compression, are associated with poor clinical outcome. In contrast, appropriate decompressions have demonstrated up to 80% good or excellent outcomes.[10] The surgeon must carefully consider the patient's symptoms and anatomic points of compression when choosing a decompression technique.

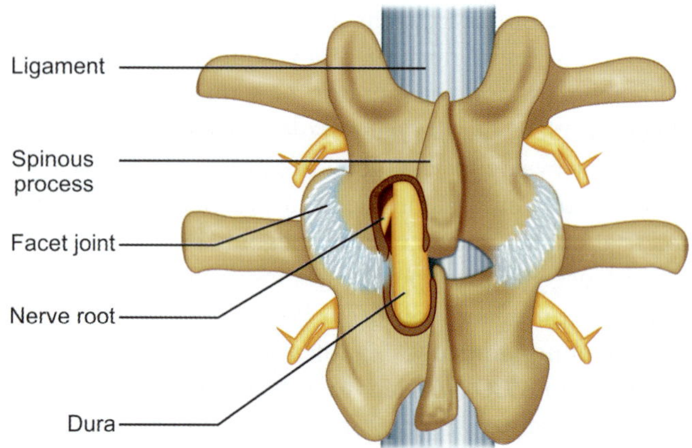

Fig. 40.1: Laminotomy.

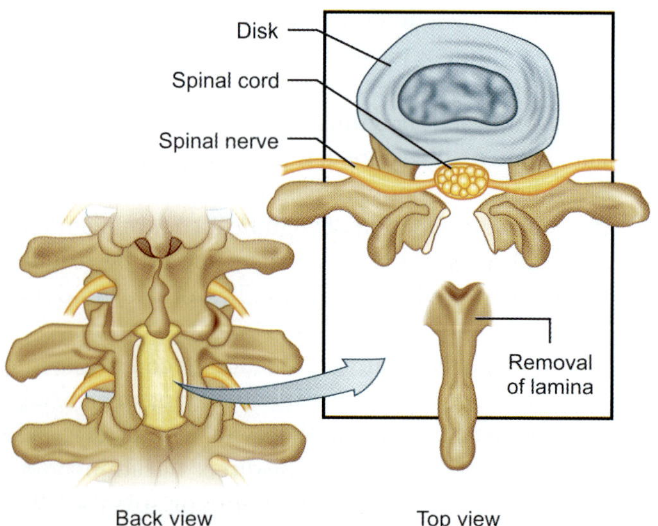

Fig. 40.2: Laminectomy.

Lombardi et al.[14] showed good to excellent results in 33% of patients after decompression with total facetectomy, 80% of patients after decompression with facet preservation, and 90% of patients with concomitant posterolateral intertransverse fusion. The authors thus recommended a facet-sparing decompression and noted that fusion further improved results. It is important to note that while inadequate decompression may lead to residual symptoms, overzealous removal of the posterior elements may lead to iatrogenic further destabilization at an already unstable motion segment, olisthesis progression, and an unsatisfactory clinical result.

Decompression and Posterolateral Fusion ± Instrumentation

In 1991, a prospective randomized study comparing decompression versus decompression and fusion for the treatment of degenerative spondylolisthesis was published by Herkowitz and Kurz.[10] About 50 patients were studied and assigned alternately either to decompression alone or decompression with noninstrumented bilateral posterolateral arthrodesis. Patients were followed for an average of 36 months, and clinical outcome was significantly improved in the cohort that had undergone decompression with concomitant fusion.

This result was supported by Ghogawala et al.'s [15] prospective study evaluating the outcomes of patients to determine whether or not fusion had an effect on functional outcome 12 months after surgery. All of the patients had the diagnosis of Meyerding grade I degenerative spondylolisthesis. None of the patient's had gross instability (i.e. >3 mm of motion at the involved level). Twenty patients received a decompression alone, and 14 underwent decompression in addition to posterolateral arthrodesis, with instrumentation being used at the discretion of the surgeon. Baseline roentgenographic findings, demographics, ODI, and SF-36 forms were matched between the two groups. Both groups showed independent improvement in ODI and SF-36 compared with baseline. Overall, 93% of the patients undergoing arthrodesis achieved successful fusion, and this was associated with greater functional improvement.

The adjunct use of spinal instrumentation to support arthrodesis has been evaluated and reviewed in several studies. Zdeblick[16] performed a study in which 124 patients (56 of whom were diagnosed with spondylolisthesis), which compared noninstrumented fusion with semirigid and rigid instrumented fusion. The rigidly instrumented group had improved fusion rates and superior clinical outcome compared with the noninstrumented group. Bridwell et al.[17] found similar results in a study of 44 patients. The patients either underwent laminectomy without fusion, noninstrumented posterolateral fusion, or instrumented posterolateral fusion with the use of pedicle screws. The use of instrumentation had a significant positive effect on fusion rates, sagittal alignment, and functional outcome.

In 1994, Mardjetko et al.[18] presented a meta-analysis of the literature dealing with degenerative spondylolisthesis. The study critically reviewed the effects of fusion as well as the adjunct use of instrumentation. Satisfactory outcomes were reported in 69% of patients who underwent decompression alone. Progression of olisthesis was noted in a significant number of cases. Concomitant arthrodesis increased the satisfactory outcome rate to 90%, with 86% of patients achieving evidence of a solid fusion. At the time, the authors found five studies appropriate for reviewing the relative value of the use of spinal instrumentation. A strong trend showing increased fusion rates with the use of segmental instrumentation was found, but the difference in clinical outcomes was negligible.

In 1997, Fischgrund et al.[5] reported on a prospective randomized study comparing the results of decompression and fusion with and without instrumentation. Overall, 67 patients were randomly assigned to one of the treatment groups and followed, on average, for 24 months. The use of spinal instrumentation improved the rate of arthrodesis, 82% compared with 45%. However, no difference was found in terms of clinical outcome between the two groups. Short-term results did not appear to indicate that successful fusion influenced clinical outcomes in patients.

Interestingly, in a long-term (between 5 and 14 years) study following up the patients initially studied by Herkowitz and Kurz[10], Fischgrund et al.[5] and Kornblum et al.[19] were able to show that patients who developed a pseudarthrosis did not do as well clinically as those who achieved a solid arthrodesis. On the basis of this finding, the authors remarked that solid fusion was of benefit to long-term patient outcomes and that surgeons should certainly consider the use of spinal instrumentation when performing a decompression and fusion to surgically treat degenerative spondylolisthesis.

Interbody Fusion

Patients presenting with degenerative spondylolisthesis will often have a concomitant degenerated intervertebral disk, although this is not always the case. There is likely to be desiccation, loss of height, and potentially disk displacement. The degenerated disk itself may be a source of back pain, the loss of disk height can lead to foraminal stenosis, and disk displacement can lead to direct compression of neural elements. As a result, the performance of a discectomy and interbody fusion, in conjunction with decompression and posterolateral fusion, is becoming an increasingly utilized option.

Placement of an interbody graft provides an indirect decompression of the nerve roots by increasing foraminal height. By elevating the vertebral body anteriorly, interbody devices can additionally be used to restore lumbar lordosis and prevent kyphotic deformity progression. Bridwell et al.[17] recommended the use of an interbody fusion if the patient demonstrates frank kyphosis at the involved level.

In theory, performance of an interbody fusion increases the area available for potential arthrodesis, thereby increasing fusion rates, and thus, patient outcomes. In addition, the interbody fusion heals under compressive forces, as compared with a posterolateral fusion, which must heal under tension forces. The increased surface area of interbody fusions may be especially useful when performing revision surgery secondary to pseudarthrosis in which prior procedures will have likely decreased the size of the potential fusion bed. Furthermore, interbody graft or cage placement in addition to posterolateral fusion has been shown to have significantly increased mechanical strength when compared with the posterolateral fusion alone.

Interbody fusion can be accomplished through many approaches, including anterior [anterior lumbar interbody fusion, (ALIF)], lateral [extreme lumbar interbody fusion, (XLIF); direct lateral interbody fusion, (DLIF)], posterior [posterior lumbar interbody fusion (PLIF)], and transforaminal [transforaminal lumbar interbody fusion (TLIF)] (Figs. 40.3 to 40.6). ALIF is performed through an anterior skin incision. The spine can then be approached either trans or retroperitoneally. The lateral approach to the lumbar intervertebral disk (e.g. XLIF, DLIF) is performed from a laterally based incision and carried out through the psoas muscle. Anterior and lateral approaches when combined with posterior surgery increase surgery duration are less cost-effective than a posterior-only approach and may increase patient morbidity. On the other hand, the anterior approach provides superior access to the disk space for discectomy and allows for the placement of a cage with a larger footprint, thereby increasing fusion potential. Restoration of lumbar lordosis is also better achieved anteriorly with the insertion of a cage with lordotic angulation.

Also in 2005, Sears[20] published the results of a prospective, single-cohort, observational study of 34 patients with degenerative spondylolisthesis treated with decompressive laminectomy and PLIF with lordotic spacers. Patients were followed on average for 21 months, and 91% considered their outcome to be good or excellent. Mean focal lordosis increased from 13.1 to 16.1°, and there were no device-related complications. The authors concluded that the use of PLIF for degenerative spondylolisthesis can yield high levels of patient satisfaction with an increase in lumbar lordosis with low levels of complications, all from a single posterior approach.

Lateral transpsoas interbody fusion (e.g. XLIF, DLIF) was introduced in 2006 as a less invasive alternative to conventional anterior or posterior approaches to interbody fusion. This surgical approach mitigates the risks of vascular and visceral injury associated with an anterior approach as well as the neural complications and posterior element disruption associated with a posterior approach, albeit with an increased risk of injury to the lumbar plexus during dissection through the psoas muscle. Lateral interbody fusion appears to have short-term clinical and radiographic success comparable with traditional anterior or posterior approach procedures with the added benefit of minimal invasiveness; however, intermediate and long-term studies are lacking.

Marchi et al.[21] recently published their prospective nonrandomized observational study on 52 consecutive patients undergoing stand-alone lateral interbody fusion for the treatment of low-grade degenerative spondylolisthesis. The fusion rate was 86.5%, ODI improved 54%, VAS improved 60%, and the mean listhesis was reduced from 15.1 to 7.1% at a minimum 24-month follow-up. However, cage subsidence occurred in 17% and pseudarthrosis was found in 13.5% of cases. Overall, 13% of cases required a revision surgery secondary to subsidence with instability/recurrent stenosis or due to inadequate indirect decompression.

Preliminary studies have demonstrated TLIF to be effective, with decreased expense and patient morbidity when compared with a combined anterior/posterior approach. In 2005, McAfee et al.[22] reported on a series of 58 patients with degenerative spondylolisthesis treated by TLIF. Successful circumferential fusion was demonstrated in >90% of patients. There were no reported failures of

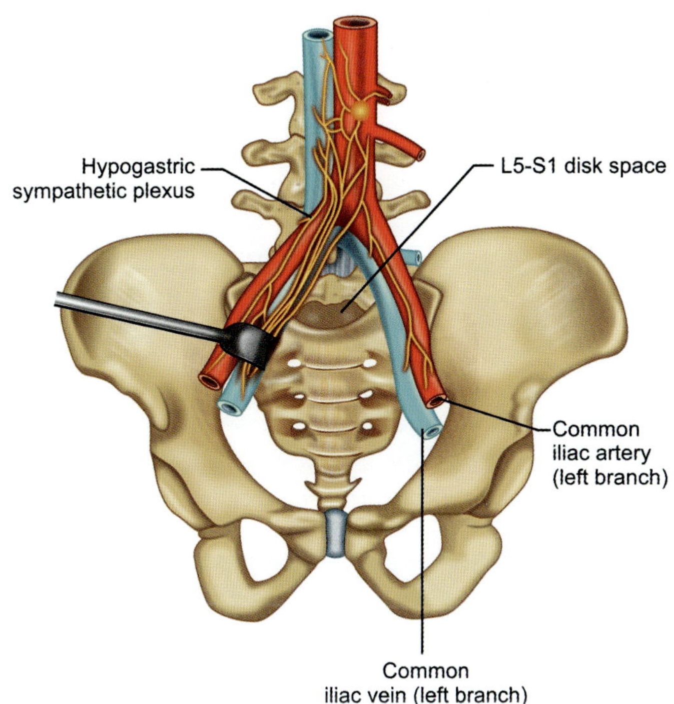

Fig. 40.3: Anterior lumbar interbody fusion approach.

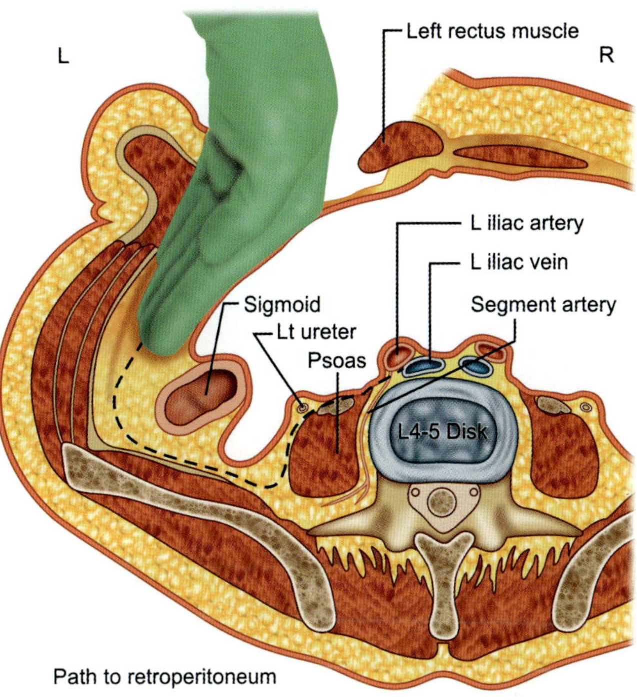

Fig. 40.4: Axial view of anterior lumbar interbody fusion approach.

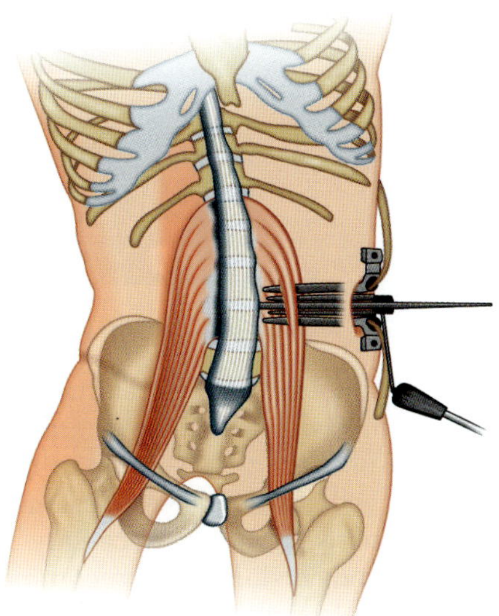

Fig. 40.5: Lateral transpsoas approach.

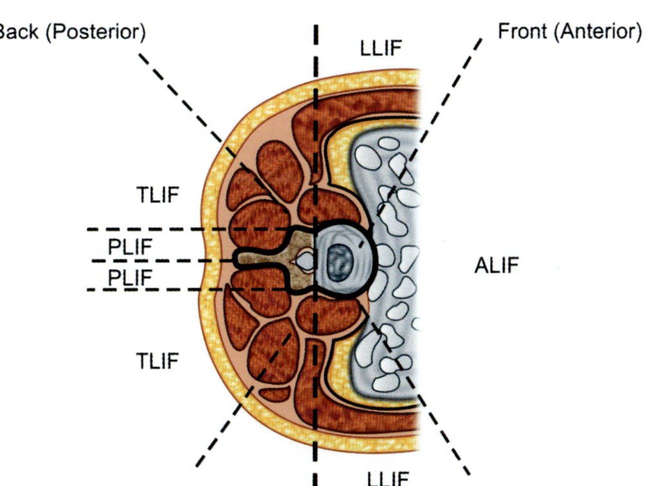

Fig. 40.6: Lumbar interbody fusion (LIF) can be accomplished through many surgical approaches, including anterior (ALIF), lateral (LLIF; company named examples include XLIF and DLIF), posterior (PLIF), and transforaminal (TLIF) (Figs. 40.3 to 40.6).

posterior instrumentation or instances of cage subsidence. There was one case of posterior cage migration secondary to a traumatic event sustained by a patient. The authors concluded that interbody cages increase foraminal height and improve chances of achieving a circumferential fusion when treating degenerative spondylolisthesis. This increased chance of fusion may lead to improved patient outcomes.

The transforaminal, lateral transpsoas, and anteroposterior combined approach each have their own benefits, risks, and morbidities. The decision on which to pursue is heavily based on surgeon's preference and patient factors (e.g. avoidance of an anterior approach secondary to prior abdominal surgery).

The concomitant use of interbody fusion with decompression and posterolateral fusion, regardless of technique,

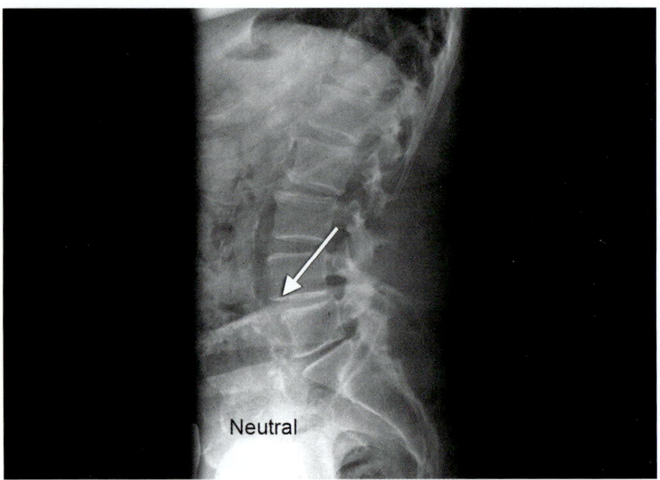

Fig. 40.7: Lateral radiograph demonstration L4–5 degenerative spondylolisthesis.

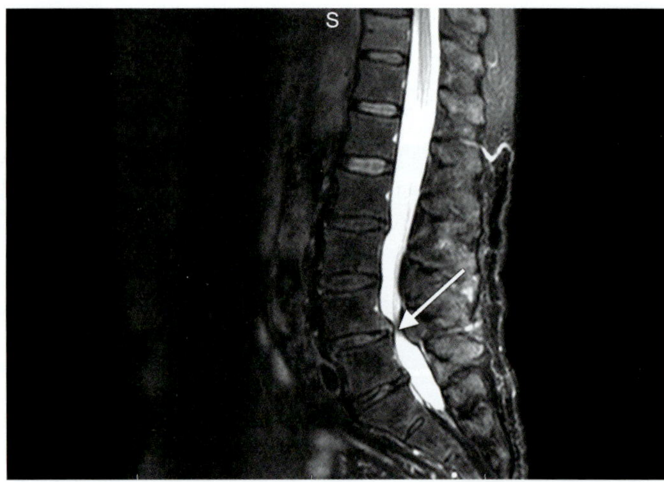

Fig. 40.8: Mid-sagittal T2 magnetic resonance imaging demonstrating severe spinal stenosis at the L4–5 level.

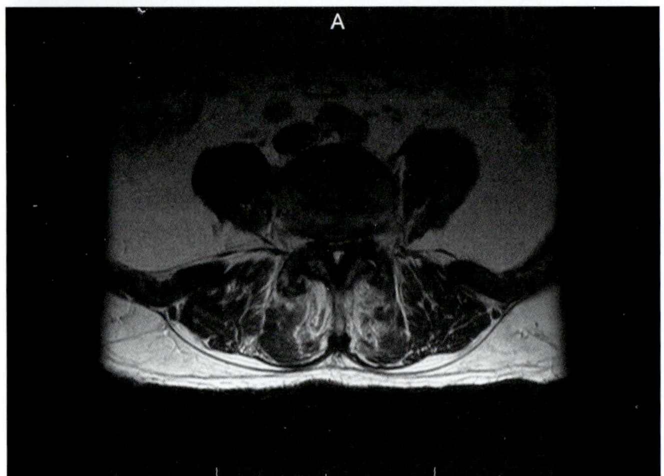

Fig. 40.9: Axial T2 magnetic resonance imaging demonstrating severe spinal stenosis at the L4–5 level.

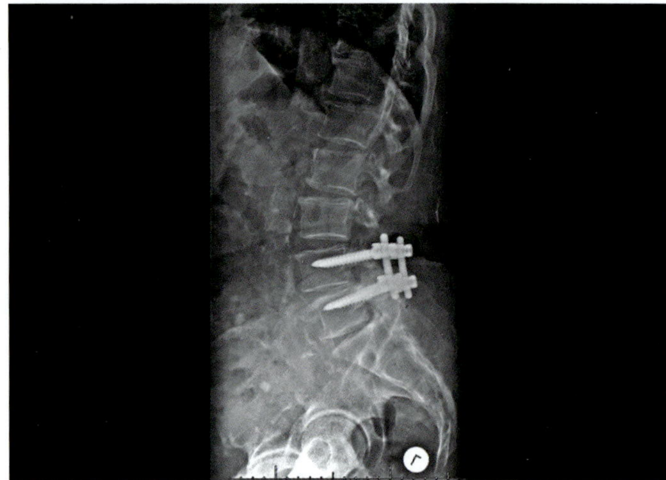

Fig. 40.10: Lateral postoperative X-ray.

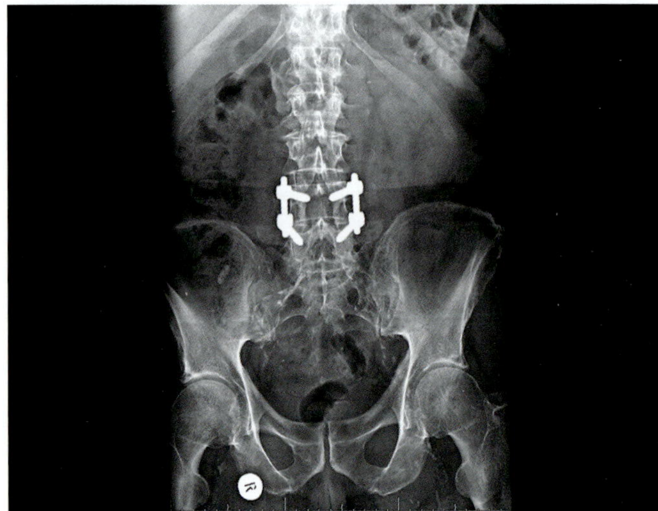

Fig. 40.11: Anterior/posterior postoperative X-ray.

shows significant potential in the treatment of degenerative spondylolisthesis. Further long-term evaluation, in addition to prospective studies comparing the results of decompression with posterolateral fusion versus circumferential fusion, is certainly necessary before the routine use of interbody fusion can be recommended. The early results, nevertheless, appear to be promising.

CASE EXAMPLE

A 75-year-old man with significant complaints of back and leg pain consistent with neurogenic claudication secondary to spinal stenosis in the setting of an L4-5 degenerative spondylolisthesis, refractory to nonoperative measures. The patient underwent an L4-5 decompressive laminectomy with concomitant instrumented posterior spinal fusion. The patient had near-complete resolution of his preoperative symptoms (Figs. 40.7 to 40.11).

SUMMARY

Degenerative spondylolisthesis is a common pathology with symptoms similar to that of spinal stenosis. Most patients can be managed nonoperatively, although a subset of patients will have symptoms recalcitrant to nonsurgical measures and will require surgical intervention. Procedures utilized to address degenerative spondylolisthesis range from isolated decompression to decompression and circumferential fusion with instrumentation. There is ample evidence to support the use of decompression with an instrumented posterolateral fusion. Although early results of interbody fusion are promising, further studies to evaluate the long-term results are necessary.

REFERENCES

1. Junghanns H. Spondylolisthesen ohne Spaltim Zwischergelenkstulcz (Pseudospondylisthen). Arch Orthop Unfallchir. 1931;29:118-27.
2. Newman PH. Spondylolisthesis, its cause and effect. Ann R Coll Surg Engl. 1955;16(5):305-23.
3. Rosenberg NJ. Degenerative spondylolisthesis. Predisposing factors. J Bone Joint Surg Am. 1975;57(4):467-74.
4. Love TW, Fagan AB, Fraser RD. Degenerative spondylolisthesis. Developmental or acquired? J Bone Joint Surg Br. 1999;81(4):670-4.
5. Fischgrund JS. The argument for instrumented decompressive posterolateral fusion for patients with degenerative spondylolisthesis and spinal stenosis. Spine (Phila Pa 1976). 2004;29(2):173-4.
6. Iguchi T, Wakami T, Kurihara A, et al. Lumbar multilevel degenerative spondylolisthesis: radiological evaluation and factors related to anterolisthesis and retrolisthesis. J Spinal Disord Tech. 2002;15(2):93-9.
7. Ha KY, Chang CH, Kim KW, et al. Expression of estrogen receptor of the facet joints in degenerative spondylolisthesis. Spine (Phila Pa 1976). 2005;30(5):562-6.
8. O'Rourke MR, Grobler LJ. L4-L5 degenerative spondylolisthesis: indications and technique for operative management. Iowa Orthop J. 1998;18:76-86.
9. Weinstein JN, Lurie JD, Tosteson TD, et al. Surgical versus nonsurgical treatment for lumbar degenerative spondylolisthesis. N Engl J Med. 2007;356(22):2257-70.
10. Herkowitz HN, Kurz LT. Degenerative lumbar spondylolisthesis with spinal stenosis. A prospective study comparing decompression with decompression and intertransverse process arthrodesis. J Bone Joint Surg Am. 1991;73(6):802-8.
11. Kabir SM, Gupta SR, Casey AT. Lumbar interspinous spacers: a systematic review of clinical and biomechanical evidence. Spine (Phila Pa 1976). 2010;35(25):E1499-506.
12. Anderson PA, Tribus CB, Kitchel SH. Treatment of neurogenic claudication by interspinous decompression: application of the X STOP device in patients with lumbar degenerative spondylolisthesis. J Neurosurg Spine. 2006;4(6):463-71.
13. Richter A, Halm HF, Hauck M, et al. 2-year follow-up after decompressive surgery with and without implantation of an interspinous device for lumbar spinal stenosis: a prospective controlled study. J Spinal Disord Tech. [published online ahead of print 24 May 2012.
14. Lombardi JS, Wiltse LL, Reynolds J, et al. Treatment of degenerative spondylolisthesis. Spine (Phila Pa 1976). 1985;10 (9):821-7.
15. Ghogawala Z, Benzel EC, Amin-Hanjani S, et al. Prospective outcomes evaluation after decompression with or without instrumented fusion for lumbar stenosis and degenerative grade I spondylolisthesis. J Neurosurg Spine. 2004;1(3):267-72.
16. Zdeblick TA. A prospective, randomized study of lumbar fusion. Preliminary results. Spine (Phila Pa 1976). 1993;1 8(8):983-91.
17. Bridwell KH, Sedgewick TA, O'Brien MF, et al. The role of fusion and instrumentation in the treatment of degenerative spondylolisthesis with spinal stenosis. J Spinal Disord. 1993;6(6):461-72.
18. Mardjetko SM, Connolly PJ, Shott S. Degenerative lumbar spondylolisthesis. A meta-analysis of literature 1970-1993. Spine (Phila Pa 1976). 1994;19(20 Suppl):2256S-65S.
19. Kornblum MB, Fischgrund JS, Herkowitz HN, et al. Degenerative lumbar spondylolisthesis with spinal stenosis: a prospective long-term study comparing fusion and pseudarthrosis. Spine (Phila Pa 1976). 2004;29(7):726-33; discussion 733-4.
20. Sears W. Posterior lumbar interbody fusion for degenerative spondylolisthesis: restoration of sagittal balance using insert-and-rotate interbody spacers. Spine J. 2005;5(2):170-9.
21. Marchi L, Abdala N, Oliveira L, et al. Stand-alone lateral interbody fusion for the treatment of low-grade degenerative spondylolisthesis. ScientificWorldJournal. 2012;2012:456346.
22. McAfee PC, DeVine JG, Chaput CD, et al. The indications for interbody fusion cages in the treatment of spondylolisthesis: analysis of 120 cases. Spine (Phila Pa 1976). 2005;30(6 Suppl):S60-5.

CHAPTER

41 Differentiating Cervical Radiculopathy and Peripheral Compressive Neuropathy

Themistocles S Protopsaltis, John A Bendo

INTRODUCTION

Cervical radiculopathy and peripheral compressive neuropathies can present with similar constellations of symptoms, creating a challenge in diagnosis. Cervical radiculopathy usually presents as pain, sensory disturbance, or motor weakness in a distribution subserved by a particular cervical nerve root, resulting from a soft disk herniation or a disk-osteophyte complex. A radiculopathy can be accompanied by axial neck pain, but this is not always the case.[1,2] Alternatively, peripheral nerve compressive syndromes such as carpal tunnel and cubital tunnel are other common causes of pain, sensory disturbance, and weakness in the upper extremities. Between the cervical spine and the hand, there are several sites where nerve compression commonly occurs, leading to a familiar set of nerve entrapment syndromes. Common peripheral entrapment neuropathies include carpal tunnel syndrome (CTS); cubital tunnel syndrome; posterior interosseous nerve (PIN) syndrome; and radial tunnel syndrome (RTS), ulnar tunnel syndrome, and pronator syndrome.

EPIDEMIOLOGY

The annual incidence of cervical radiculopathy was estimated to be 83.2/100,000 with a male preponderance (107 for males and 64 for females) in an epidemiologic study from Mayo Clinic, Rochester, MN.[3] The most common of peripheral entrapment neuropathy is CTS. The annual age-adjusted incidence of carpal tunnel was found to be 106/100,000 with a female preponderance (166 in women and 44 in men).[4] In another study, the age-adjusted annual incidence of CTS was found to be 149/100,000 for women and 105/100,000 for men.[5] In a broad study of common compressive neuropathies, the annual age-standardized rates per 100,000 were 87.8 men and 192.8 women for carpal tunnel, 25.3 men and 18.9 women for ulnar neuropathy, 2.97 men and 1.42 women for radial neuropathy.[6]

CLINICAL PRESENTATION AND RELEVANT ANATOMY

Cervical radiculopathies and peripheral neuropathies can be differentiated by the location of symptoms in the upper extremities. In general, cervical radiculopathies will have radiating symptoms in a dermatomal distribution. In contrast, peripheral compressive neuropathies will cause symptoms in more than one nerve root distribution.

In cervical radiculopathies, the distinctive pain and sensory pattern and the muscle group affected are referred to as the "root signature". In general, paresthesias and sensory disturbances have been found to fit more reliably to a dermatomal distribution, whereas, pain is less predictably limited to a particular dermatome.[3]

The key to differentiating cervical radiculopathy and peripheral neuropathies lies in understanding the anatomy of the brachial plexus. Brachial plexus anatomy (Fig. 41.1) can serve as a road map to hone down a diagnosis to a particular nerve root or to a specific peripheral nerve entrapment. Certain radiculopathies can masquerade as peripheral entrapments, and vice versa, particularly if the constellation of symptoms has an incomplete expression. The following are peripheral compressive neuropathies and the corresponding cervical radiculopathies that commonly cloud the differential diagnosis.

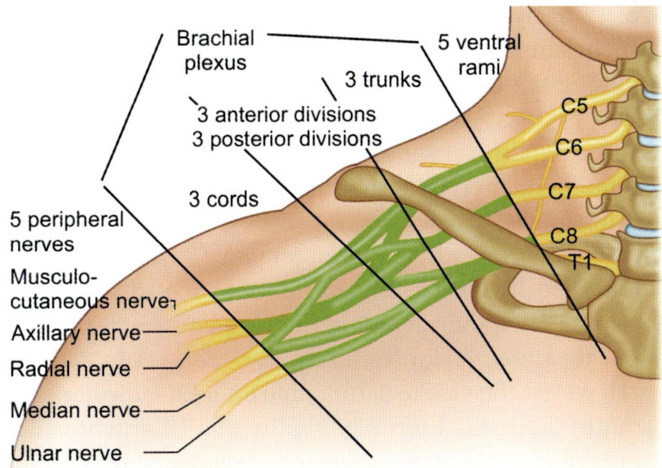

Fig. 41.1: Schematic representation of anatomy of the brachial plexus.

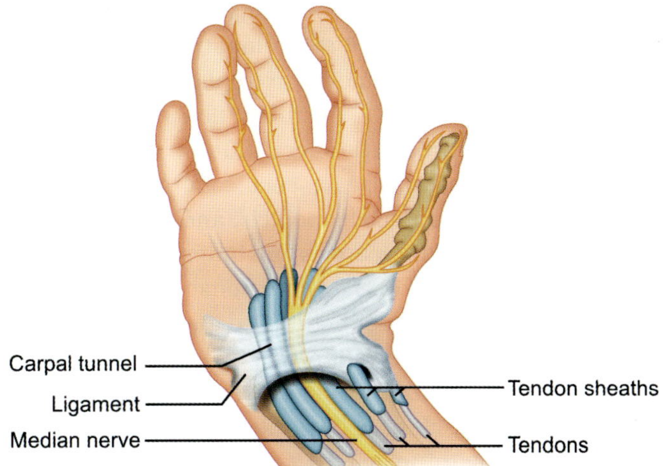

Fig. 41.2: Schematic representation of the distribution of the median nerve in the hand.

There is considerable variation in neural anatomy. Published diagrams, figures, and tables project concepts of uniformity that do not correlate with the practical reality of a population of individuals, each with variable anatomical differences. The classic myotome patterns can vary to a great extent from one patient to another. In a study correlating intraoperative pathology and preoperative electromyography (EMG), Levin et al. showed that there is considerable variability between patients regarding the muscles innervated by specific nerve roots.[6] C6 demonstrated the greatest variability. Anatomic studies of the brachial plexus have shown that between one third and two thirds of plexuses are "prefixed" where C4 contributes to muscle innervation. The incidence of "postfixed" plexuses in which there are contributions from T2 can occur ranges from 16% to 73%.[7]

Carpal Tunnel Syndrome and C6 Radiculopathy

Common presenting symptoms for CTS include paresthesias, numbness, and pain, particularly at night. However, the distribution of the pain is not always reliable. Any or all of the three and half fingers in the median nerve distribution (Fig. 41.2) can be involved. Some have reported that the pain of CTS can radiate or refer proximally along the course of the median nerve to the volar forearm or anterior brachium. Numbness is another common presenting symptom, one that is more reliably present in a dermatomal distribution corresponding to regions of the hand and finger subserved by the median nerve fibers that pass beneath the transverse carpal ligament. An early finding in CTS is a loss of sensation detectable with a threshold test such as the Semmes-Weinstein monofilament test.[8] A later finding is an increase in two-point discrimination (normal is 4–6 mm).[8] However, these tests or the subjective sensations of numbness are not necessarily uniform across the entire classic distribution of CTS. The sensory innervation of the median nerve includes contributions from the C6 and C7 nerve roots, whereas the motor contribution to the median nerve innervated musculature of the hand distal to the carpal tunnel is primarily via C8.

In contrast, the volar sensory distribution of the C6 nerve root includes contributions from three major nerve branches: innervating the radial forearm, the lateral antebrachial cutaneous nerve, a continuation of the musculocutaneous nerve, which is a branch of the lateral cord; the palmar cutaneous branch of the median nerve, which branches from the median nerve proximal to the carpal tunnel in the distal forearm between the tendons of the flexor carpi radialis and the palmaris longus, and the portion of the median nerve that passes within the carpal tunnel giving rise to the digital branches of the index and long fingers. Thus, only the latter group of nerves will be involved in CTS, whereas any or all of the former two groups can be affected by a C6 radiculopathy. Also of note, a C6 radiculopathy can involve the radial and dorsal aspect of the hand via the superficial branch of the radial nerve. However, it is important to emphasize, again, that radiculopathies can have an incomplete expression whereby only a portion of the classic dermatome is involved in the presenting symptomatology.

Another important differentiating factor can be the motor examination. In a C6 radiculopathy, elbow flexion and wrist extension weakness are implicated classically. In contrast, in chronic CTS, the motor fibers to the thumb intrinsic musculature can be affected. These median nerve innervated thenar muscles, specifically the abductor pollicis brevis, the opponens pollicis, and the superficial head of the flexor pollicis brevis, are innervated by the C8 nerve root. The patient may exhibit thenar muscle wasting and weakness of thumb abduction and the thenar muscles will show signs of denervation by EMG. However, in an isolated chronic CTS, one would expect no deficits in other C8 innervated muscles, such as the flexor pollicis longus and the flexor digitorum longus to fingers II through V.

However, it is important to understand that there is considerable variation within the population with regard to myotomes and their corresponding nerve roots.[6] Moreover, if a radiculopathy is acute or if the dorsal portion of the root is more affected than the volar (a primarily sensory radiculopathy), then motor weakness may not be present at all.

The reflex examination may show an absent or diminished brachioradialis in a C6 radiculopathy, whereas this reflex would not be affected in an isolated CTS.

C8 RADICULOPATHY VS CUBITAL TUNNEL SYNDROME VS T1 RADICULOPATHY

Cubital tunnel syndrome is the second most common compressive mononeuropathy in the upper extremity. It can be confused with a C8 radiculopathy. In cubital tunnel syndrome, the ulnar nerve is compressed at the level of the elbow. The most likely site of compression is Osborne's ligament, which is the fibrous band that forms the roof of the cubital tunnel. However, other compression points have been described and a complete release should address all the following structures: the intramuscular septum medial to the triceps, a fascial band between the intermuscular septum and the triceps (the Arcade of Struthers), the retinaculum of the cubital tunnel (Osborne's ligament), and the proximal fascial edge of the flexor carpi ulnaris.

Sensory portions of the ulnar nerve, which branch distal to the cubital tunnel, include the dorsal and volar sensory branches, which divide from the main trunk of the nerve proximal to Guyon's canal and the wrist. The palmar cutaneous branch of the ulnar nerve innervates the area over the hypothenar eminence. The dorsal sensory branches innervate the dorsal-medial aspect of the hand, including the dorsal small finger and frequently the ring finger. Distal to Guyon's canal, the ulnar nerve divides into the superficial sensory branch that gives rise to the palmar digital nerves of the small finger and ulnar half of the ring finger.

Similar to an ulnar neuropathy, a C8 radiculopathy would also involve a sensory disturbance in the ulnar aspect of the hand including the ring and small fingers, hence the potential for confusion.

However, the classic dermatome for a C8 radiculopathy includes the medial forearm via the medial antebrachial cutaneous nerve that branches directly from medial cord. An ulnar neuropathy should not involve the medial forearm, and symptoms would not extend proximally to the elbow as they could in a C8 radiculopathy. This is often true for numbness and paresthesias. As discussed earlier, pain is less reliably limited to a dermatomal distribution, and patients with cubital tunnel syndrome frequently complain of pain about the site of compression near the medial elbow and more distally in the forearm.

The motor examination is helpful in differentiating these neuropathies. In an advanced ulnar neuropathy, the flexor digitorum profundus (FDP) tendons to the ring and small fingers may be weak. The FDP to a finger is isolated by blocking the proximal interphalangeal (PIP) and metacarpophalangeal flexion of a finger and asking the patient to flex the tip of the finger. The FDP to the index and long fingers are innervated by the anterior interosseous nerve, a branch of the median nerve, thus they should not exhibit any weakness.

In contrast, a C8 radiculopathy would involve all the long finger flexors, including the FDP to all four of these fingers. Moreover, weakness could be detected in the thenar muscles, which are C8 innervated via the median nerve.

In differentiating between a T1 radiculopathy and ulnar nerve compression, knowledge of the myotomes, dermatomes, and ulnar nerve innervations is essential. Like an ulnar neuropathy, a T1 radiculopathy could affect the intrinsic muscles of the hand. However, the FDP to the ring and small finger should not be affected in a T1 radiculopathy as they would be in cubital tunnel syndrome. The T1 dermatome includes the medial brachium via the medial brachial cutaneous nerve, a branch of the medial cord. Numbness, tingling and pain should not be present in the medial brachium in a patient with an ulnar neuropathy.

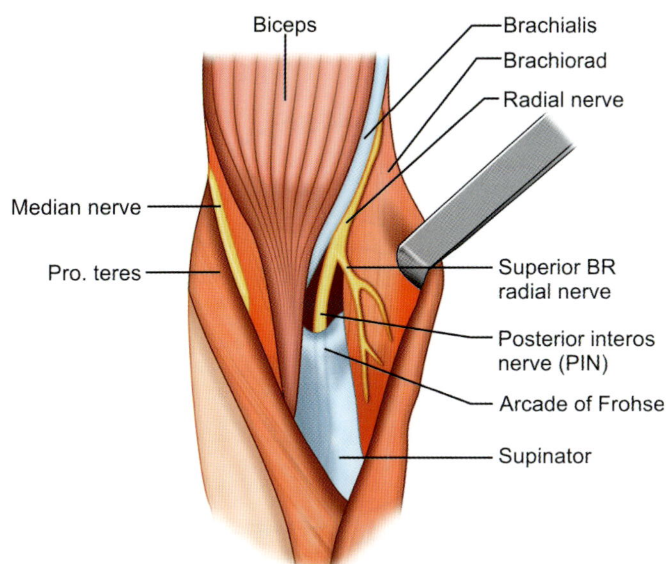

Fig. 41.3: Posterior interosseous nerve supplies all the muscles on the radial side and dorsal surface of the forearm, except the anconeus, brachioradialis and extensor carpi radialis longus.

C7 Radiculopathy vs RTS vs PIN Syndrome

The PIN syndrome is the loss of motor function of one of the muscles innervated by the PIN. It supplies all the muscles on the radial side and dorsal surface of the forearm, except the anconeus, brachioradialis, and extensor carpi radialis longus. It is classically defined as a motor palsy without a sensory disturbance. Anatomic sites of compression in PIN syndrome include the fibrous bands adjacent to the radiocapitellar joint, the tendinous edge of the extensor carpi radialis brevis, the radial recurrent artery (the Leash of Henry), the tendinous edge of the supinator (the Arcade of Frohse), and the distal edge of the supinator (Fig. 41.3).

In contrast, RTS is a pain syndrome. Pain in RTS localizes to the proximal radial forearm and so this syndrome must be differentiated from lateral epicondylitis or "tennis elbow", which occurs approximately 5 cm proximal to the RTS site of pain. The pain can be exacerbated by activity, and it can awaken the patient at night. If motor weakness is present it is usually due to pain causing the patient to guard. Electrodiagnostic abnormalities are usually absent.

A C7 radiculopathy may present with pain in a distribution similar to RTS: along the radial forearm, but it may also include the dorsum of the hand to the long finger, possibly the fingers adjacent. Numbness or paresthesias may be present in this dermatome. However, a C7 radiculopathy can be differentiated by the motor examination. In addition to weakness of metacarpophalangeal extension, triceps weakness can be present as this muscle reliably belongs to the C7 myotome. Wrist extension is usually controlled by C6 and finger PIP and distal interphalangeal joint extension are controlled by the hand intrinsic, which are mostly T1 innervated via the ulnar nerve. A C7 radiculopathy may cause weakness of pronation and wrist flexion as the pronator teres and flexor carpi radialis muscles can be affected.

The reflex examination may show an absent or diminished triceps in a C7 radiculopathy, whereas this reflex would not be affected in RTS or PIN syndrome.

Double Crush Phenomenon

The double crush hypothesis contends that two sites of compression along a peripheral nerve can summate to create a more severe neuropathy by an underlying mechanism of impaired axoplasmic flow. The hypothesis was first described by Upton and McComas in 1973, following their clinical observation that many of their patients with median and ulnar neuropathy had associated cervical radiculopathy as well.[9] Several basic science studies have corroborated the double crush hypothesis. Dellon and Mackinnon demonstrated significantly worse nerve function in the presence of two concurrent sites of nerve compression or an additional delayed site of compression using a rat model of sciatic nerve banding. A patient with a C6 or C7 radiculopathy with concurrent CTS would be a clinical example of a double crush phenomenon. Such patients may suffer persistent symptoms if only one of the two nerve compressions is addressed therapeutically.

PHYSICAL EXAMINATION

When differentiating cervical radiculopathy and peripheral entrapment neuropathies, complete spine and peripheral nerve examinations are indicated. A complete examination of the cervical spine includes testing neck range of motion, motor strength, sensation, reflexes, and provocative maneuvers.

Motor strength testing is performed on muscle groups innervated by each nerve root from C5 to T1 (Fig. 41.4). Major muscle groups representing each of these nerve roots include the deltoid, biceps, triceps, wrist flexors, wrist extensors, thumb abductors, and dorsal interossei.

In a patient in whom a rotator cuff tear or shoulder pathology is suspected, the supraspinatus can be isolated

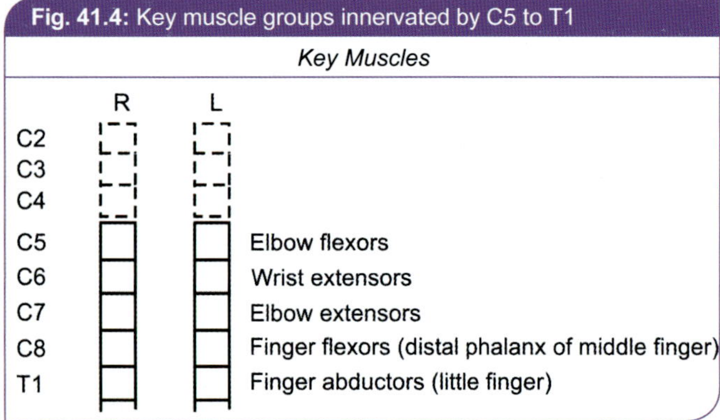

Fig. 41.4: Key muscle groups innervated by C5 to T1

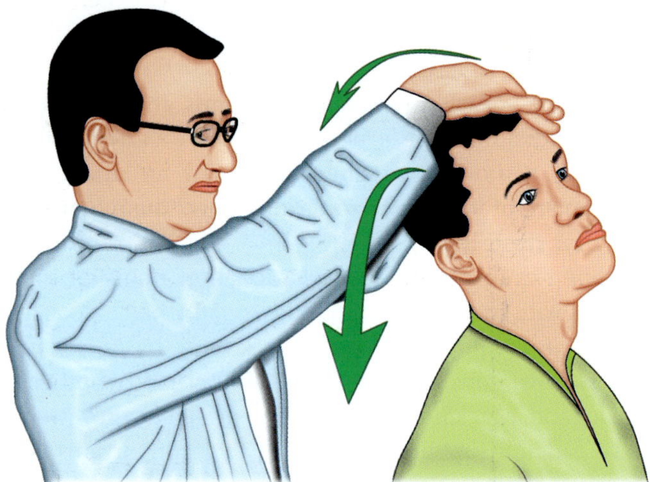

Fig. 41.6: Spurling's test is a provocative maneuver where the patient's head is positioned with the neck extended slightly and laterally flexed, which will close down the neural foramina. An axial compressive force is then applied, which further compresses the nerve root in a tight foramen. Spurling's test is positive if it reproduces the radicular pain that shoots down the arm.

from the deltoid by internally rotating the arm while actively resisting shoulder abduction. The supraspinatus, infraspinatus, and the deltoid are all innervated by C5. Shoulder external rotation should be tested as the major shoulder external rotators, the infraspinatus, teres minor, and supraspinatus are all C5 innervated. Testing for impingement signs such as the Neer and Hawkin's tests can rule out subacromial impingement/bursitis.

If an ulnar neuropathy is suspected versus a C8 radiculopathy, FDP testing should be compared between the index and long fingers (median nerve innervated) and the ring and small fingers (ulnar nerve innervated). When testing FDP to a finger, resisted DIP flexion is performed with the PIP maintained extended. The other fingers should be extended and prevented from flexing at the DIP to prevent the assisting action of adjacent FDP

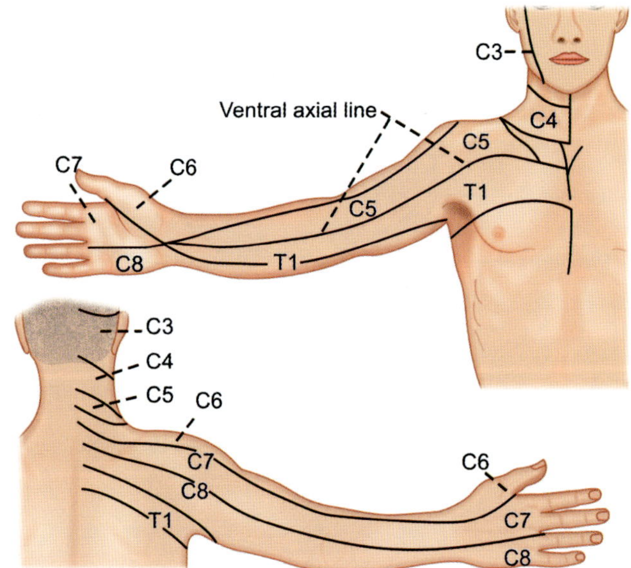

Fig. 41.5: Dermatomal distribution of C3 to T1.

muscle bellies. Upon inspection of patients with intrinsic muscle weakness, Wartenberg's sign may be present. The small finger will abduct due to weakness of the small finger adductor resulting from ulnar neuropathy or chronic T1 radiculopathy. If Wartenberg's sign is present, patients often will complain of difficulty placing their hand in the pocket of their pants. This sign would not be present in a C8 radiculopathy.

Sensory testing can be performed to light touch and pain (anterior spinothalamic tracts) or vibration and proprioception (dorsal column). Dermatomes from C3 to T1 should be tested (Fig. 41.5).

Reflex testing should include the biceps (C5), brachioradialis (C6), and the triceps (C7). Reflexes are graded 0 to 3+, where grade 1 or 2 is within the normal range. Hoffman's test, the inverted radial reflex and hand clench-release tests are positive in upper motor neuron dysfunction.

Spurling's test is a provocative maneuver whereby the patient's head is positioned with the neck extended slightly and laterally flexed, which will close down the neural foramina. An axial compressive force is then applied, which further compresses the nerve root in a tight foramen. Spurling's test is positive if it reproduces the radicular pain that shoots down the arm (Fig. 41.6).

The shoulder abduction relief sign is useful after a positive Spurling's test or in a patient with acute radicular pain. For this test, the arm is abducted at the shoulder and the hand is placed over the top of the patient's head.

This maneuver decreases tension along the course of the nerve roots exiting the cervical spine, relieving acute radiculopathic pain. The cervical distraction test is another relief sign where manual axial distraction is performed on the patient to widen the cervical foramen and relieve acute radicular pain.

For examination of the peripheral nervous system, testing with a Semmes-Weinstein monofilament or two-point discrimination (normal is 4–6 mm in the fingers) provides an objective assessment of sensation. A Tinel's test should be performed at common sites of compression such as the carpal tunnel and the cubital tunnel.[10] Phalen's and Durkan's compression tests are important to perform when CTS is suspected. In a systematic review of common diagnostic examinations, the sensitivity and specificity of combining the Phalen's test and Durkan's compression test was found to be highest among 14 different physical examination maneuvers.[11]

Active compression of the ulnar nerve at the cubital tunnel with the elbow flexed will elicit paresthesias or numbness in the ulnar nerve distribution in a patient with cubital tunnel. The elbow should be flexed and extended while palpating the ulnar nerve in the cubital tunnel to identify a subluxing ulnar nerve or a snapping triceps tendon.

ELECTRODIAGNOSTIC STUDIES

Cervical Radiculopathies and EMG

Electrodiagnostic studies can be helpful in differentiating between radiculopathy and peripheral neuropathies. They are a valuable adjunct but not a substitute for astute clinical diagnostic findings. When cervical radiculopathy is suspected, EMG is utilized. Increased insertional activity, fibrillations, fasciculations, and diminished motor unit recruitment are indicative of denervation. The diagnosis of a radiculopathy is made when there are abnormal EMG findings in two muscles belonging to the same myotome but they are innervated by different peripheral nerves. Early studies demonstrated a limited role for EMG as a primary diagnostic modality due to a low reported sensitivity. The more muscle groups tested, the more confident a diagnosis of radiculopathy can be made or excluded. However, EMG needle examination can be very painful for patients, and therefore, a balance must be struck by testing an optimal number of muscle groups to minimize discomfort while increasing diagnostic sensitivity and specificity. Dillingham et al. showed that the addition of paraspinal muscles to the needle examination diagnosed 94–99% of radiculopathies when six upper limb muscles were tested.[12] However, some radiculopathies cannot be confirmed by EMG. Radiculopathies that predominantly cause sensory root involvements will not show abnormal findings since the EMG is exclusively a test of the motor units. Moreover, a mild radiculopathy, an early radiculopathy, or one in which the rate of denervation is balanced by reinnervation is less likely to yield abnormal EMG findings.

The EMG and nerve conduction studies (NCS) should be performed at least 3–4 weeks after the onset of radicular symptoms to allow for the delay in Wallerian degeneration. Fibrillation potentials, increased insertional activity, and other signs of denervation changes on the EMG will be seen in proximal muscles as early as 10–14 days, but they may take 3–6 weeks to be seen in more distal muscles.

PERIPHERAL ENTRAPMENT NEUROPATHIES AND NCS

The NCS are quite useful in the evaluation of peripheral neuropathies. Decreased amplitude, decreased velocity, and increased latency are the hallmarks of abnormal neuroelectrodiagnostics across a nerve segment where compression is suspected. In general, abnormal findings in CTS are sensory nerve action potential (SNAP) latencies above 3.5 ms and compound muscle action potentials (CMAP) latencies above 4.5 ms, SNAP amplitudes <20 μV and CMAP amplitudes <4.5 mV when measured across the wrist. Abnormal EMG testing is a late finding in the natural history of a peripheral nerve entrapment, and thus, it is indicative of a chronic compression; patients usually will present with sensory complaints well before the onset of motor findings.

Negative NCS/EMG studies do not exclude a peripheral neuropathy especially if the clinical picture is consistent with one. There are several studies demonstrating excellent results from surgical release of clinically apparent but electrodiagnostically negative peripheral neuropathies.[8] Thus, the specificity of neuroelectrodiagnostic testing is better than its sensitivity.

TREATMENT

Nonoperative management of cervical radiculopathy includes rest, activity modification, physical therapy, nonsteroidal anti-inflammatory drugs (NSAIDs), and epidural steroid injections. The natural history of cervical radiculopathy has been described to be very favorable. The majority of patients will improve without treatment or with the aforementioned nonoperative measures. Level-1 randomized controlled trials comparing nonoperative treatment, and no treatment is available.

Nonoperative treatment of CTS includes wrist splinting, NSAIDS, activity modification, and steroid injections. The aim of splinting is to brace the wrist in neutral to avoid wrist flexion and extension, positions that increase carpal tunnel pressures and exacerbate symptoms. Steroid injections have been shown to be effective in patients with mild and some with moderate CTS, especially when the duration of symptoms is short.

Bracing and activity modification can also be effective for mild cubital tunnel syndrome. A brace that maintains the elbow is approximately 50° of elbow flexion will decrease pressure within the cubital tunnel. Such braces are effective when worn at night or in the workplace when permitting. Patients should avoiding positions and activities that exacerbate symptoms, particularly those involving maximal elbow flexion.

SURGICAL RESULTS

The results of surgical management of cervical radiculopathy are very favorable. Henderson et al. demonstrated 91.4% good or excellent results for posterior laminoforamenotomy for the treatment of cervical radiculopathy regardless of the underlying etiology: herniated soft disk versus spondylotic disk-osteophyte complex.[1] Relief of arm pain and recovery of motor function have been shown in multiple studies with anterior and posterior approaches with successful results in the 80–90% range.[9,13-15]

The surgical results of CTS have been shown to be very favorable regardless of the technique utilized: open, endoscopic, or miniopen.[16,17] Operative results of cubital tunnel syndrome also have been shown to be favorable regardless of the technique utilized: in situ release, subcutaneous transposition, or submuscular transposition.[18]

There is a paucity of studies addressing operative results of patients with double crush phenomenon. Using unvalidated outcome measures, Osterman et al. showed that patients with double crush phenomenon had poorer postoperative clinical results when compared with those with isolated CTS.[19]

REFERENCES

1. Henderson CM, Hennessy RG, Shuey HM, et al. Posterior-lateral foraminotomy as an exclusive operative technique for cervical radiculopathy: a review of 846 consecutively operated cases. Neurosurgery. 1983;12(5):505-12.
2. Cote P, Cassidy JD, Carroll LJ, et al. The annual incidence and course of neck pain in the general population: a population-based cohort study. Pain. 2004;112:267-73.
3. Radhakrishnan K, Litchy WJ, O'Fallon WM, et al. Epidemiology of cervical radiculopathy. Brain. 1994;117: 325-35.
4. Stevens JC, Sun S, Beard CM. Carpal tunnel syndrome in Rochester, Minnesota, 1961 to 1980. Neurology. 1988;38: 134-8.
5. Latinovic R, Gulliford MC, Hughes RA. Incidence of common compressive neuropathies in primary care. J Neurol Neurosurg Psychiatry. 2006;77:263-5.
6. Levin KH, Maggiano HJ, Wilbourn AJ. Cervical radiculopathies: comparison of surgical and EMG localization of single-root lesions. Neurology. 1996;46:1022-5.
7. Kerr AT. The brachial plexus of nerves in man, the variations in its formation and branches. Am J Anat. 1918;23:285-395.
8. Szabo RM, Gelberman RH, Dimick MP. Sensibility testing in patients with carpal tunnel syndrome. J Bone Joint Surg Am. 1984;66:60-4.
9. Upton AR, McComas AJ. The double crush in nerve entrapment syndromes. Lancet. 1973;2:359-62.
10. Grunderg AB. Carpal tunnel decompression in spite of normal electromyography. J Hand Surg Am. 1983;8:348-9.
11. Kuhlman KA, Hennessey WJ. Sensitivity and specificity of carpal tunnel syndrome signs. Am J Phys Med Rehabil. 1997;76:451-7.
12. Dillingham TR, Lauder TD, Andary M, et al. Identification of cervical radiculopathies: optimizing the electromyographic screen. Am J Phys Med Rehab. 2001;80:(2)84-91
13. Bohlman HH, Emery SE, Goodfellow DB, et al. Robinson anterior cervical discectomy and arthrodesis for cervical radiculopathy. Long-term follow-up of one hundred and twenty-two patients. J Bone Joint Surg. 1993;75:1298-307.
14. Herkowitz HN, Kurz LT, Overholt DP. Surgical management of cervical disc herniation. A comparison between the anterior and posterior approach. Spine. 1990;15:1026-30.
15. Sasso RC, Smucker JD, Hacker RJ, et al. Clinical outcomes for BRYAN cervical disc arthroplasty: a prospective, randomized, controlled, multicenter trial with 24-month follow-up. J Spinal Disord Tech. 2007;20:481-91.
16. Murrey D, Janssen M, Delamarter R, et al. Results of the prospective, randomized, controlled multicenter Food and Drug Administration investigational device exemption study of the ProDisc-C total disc replacement versus anterior discectomy and fusion for the treatment of 1-level symptomatic cervical disc disease. Spine J. 2009;9:275-86.
17. Burke FD, Wilgis EF, Dubin NH, et al. Relationship between the duration and severity of symptoms and the outcome of carpal tunnel syndrome. J Hand Surg Am. 2006;31:1478-82.
18. Hui AC, Wong S, Leung CH, et al. A randomized controlled trial of surgery vs. steroid injection for carpal tunnel syndrome. Neurology. 2006;64:2074-978.
19. Osterman AL. The double crush syndrome. Orthop Clin North Am. 1988;19(1): 147-55.

CHAPTER

42

Surgical Management of Cervical Disk Herniation

Kseniya Slobodyanyuk, Jonathan Stieber

INTRODUCTION

In 1934, Mixter and Barr's landmark publication correlated intervertebral disk herniation with neurologic symptomatology and underlined the vital role of surgery in the management of herniations.[1] Since then, much has been elucidated about the structure of a healthy intervertebral disk and the consequences of its herniation. A healthy disk consists of an outer annulus fibrosus: a tough, fibrous, ring, which encases a gel-like nucleus pulposus. Degenerative disk changes seen with aging have been described in detail in Chapter 1. Briefly, disk water content decreases due to decreased quantity and size of proteoglycans, the water-binding matrix proteins, consequently making the disks less elastic, promoting rupture and herniation.[2] Chronic degenerative changes often related to aging may result in a hard disk herniation involving osteophytosis and irreversible damage. Such a disk herniation may be partially calcified or may be associated with uncovertebral joint osteophytes. Chronic changes and spondylosis may lead to decreased disk height with subsequent loss of neuroforaminal space. In contrast, soft herniation can also occur, often associated with acute trauma. This herniation type may resolve spontaneously and is usually treated conservatively.[3] Due to the anatomic proximity of the neural elements in the cervical spine to the intervertebral disk, both types of disk herniation have the potential to result in neurologic symptomatology. Impingement upon the spinal cord can result in cervical myelopathy and associated upper motor neuron symptoms, whereas compression of an exiting nerve root can result in radiculopathy with associated lower motor neuron deficits.

EPIDEMIOLOGY

Herniation of the cervical intervertebral disk has an estimated incidence of 107/100,000 men and 64/100,000 women. Incidence peaks at 50–54 years, with only 15% of cases associated with trauma or physical exertion.[4] Risk factors include tobacco, occupation, and aging.[5–7] Although less common than lumbar disk herniation, cervical disk disease has been identified as the most common cause of acquired disability in adults >50 years of age and is thus important to recognize and treat.[8]

SIGNS AND SYMPTOMS

Common signs and symptoms associated with cervical disk herniation can be divided into neurologic symptomatology and axial or referred paraxial pain. Paracentral or foraminal cervical disk herniation will frequently compress the exiting nerve root resulting in radiculopathy. Radiculopathy manifests as radiating pain, paresthesias, and/or numbness in a dermatomal distribution (Fig. 42.1). Disruption of the motor fibers may result in weakness of the muscle groups supplied by the affected nerve root. A large central disk herniation can cause cervical stenosis with compression of the spinal cord and consequent myelopathy. Upper motor neuron symptoms secondary to myelopathy may include loss of manual dexterity, gait disturbance, clumsiness, and bowel or bladder incontinence. Not uncommonly, myelopathy can present as isolated weakness with the absence of pain.[9]

Cervical disk herniation commonly causes axial or paraxial neck pain. Pain is also frequently referred to the

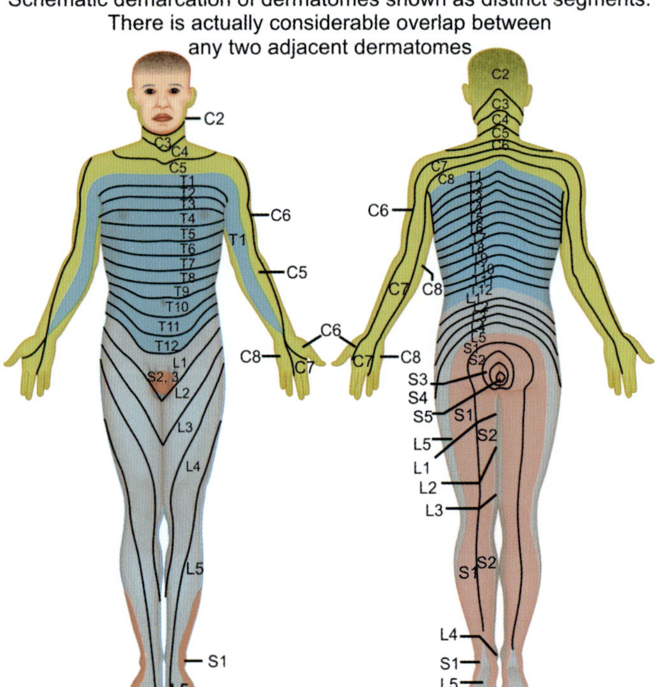

Levels of principal dermatomes

C5	Clavicles	L1–L4	Anterior and inner surfaces of lower limbs
C5–C7	Lateral parts of upper limbs		
C8, T1	Medial sides of upper limbs		
C6	Thumb	L4, 5, S1	Foot
C6–C8	Hand	L4	Medial sides of great toe
C8	Ring and little fingers		
C4	Level of nipple	S1, 2, L5	Posterior and outer surfaces of lower limbs
C10	Level of umbilicus		
C12	Inguinal or groin regions	S1	Lateral margin of foot and little toe
		S2–S4	Perineum

Fig. 42.1: Schematic diagram of dermatomal distribution.

medial periscapular region. These pain symptoms are often coupled with neurologic symptoms.

TREATMENT

There is no consensus regarding optimal nonoperative treatment; it is usually individualized, depending upon patient needs and preferences. Many cases resolve spontaneously within 4-6 months with nonoperative treatment, and more rapid regression is often seen with larger herniations than those, which are smaller and more confined.[10] In the absence of profound or progressive neurologic deficit, initial nonoperative treatment is always warranted.

Surgical indications for cervical disk herniation include profound or progressive myelopathy, herniation resulting in severe stenosis, or magnetic resonance imaging evidence of myelomalacia. Surgery is also indicated in patients presenting with radiculopathy manifesting in profound or progressive weakness or numbness, or in those who have had unrelenting and intractable symptoms that are unresponsive to thorough and comprehensive nonoperative treatment. The primary goal of surgical treatment is decompression of the neural elements. An effective procedure will also preserve or restore cervical lordosis and spinal stability. There is evidence to suggest that for patients who ultimately require surgical treatment, an optimal outcome is more likely if intervention occurs within 6 months of symptom onset.[11] A number of surgical treatment options are available, none of which has conclusively demonstrated superiority over the others.[12,13] Consequently, the choice of surgical approach is determined on an individualized basis.

SURGICAL OPTIONS

Cervical disk herniation may be treated surgically with both anterior and posterior approaches. Surgical treatment of the spine initially gained recognition as safe and effective soon after AG Smith performed the first successful laminectomy in 1829.[14] Posterior laminectomy and foraminotomy became the most frequently performed procedures owing to their direct access to the neural elements. However, the anatomic limitations of the posterior approach with its limited access to more anterior structures resulted in a shift toward anterior discectomy, developed independently by Smith and Robinson in 1955 and Cloward in 1958.[15] Currently, anterior discectomy and its variations are the most commonly performed spine surgeries.[16] Other anterior approaches include cervical arthroplasty and anterior cervical foraminotomy.

ANTERIOR APPROACH

Anterior Cervical Discectomy and Fusion

The most frequently performed anterior surgery, and one of the most common spine surgeries overall, is an anterior cervical discectomy and fusion (ACDF).[17] This option involves removal of the pathologic disk and osteophytes, if present, to decompress the spinal cord and/or the exiting nerve root(s). Decompression is then followed by fusion and stabilization.

The ACDF is accomplished utilizing a standard Smith-Robinson approach. A small transverse skin incision is performed anteriorly over the affected level from the

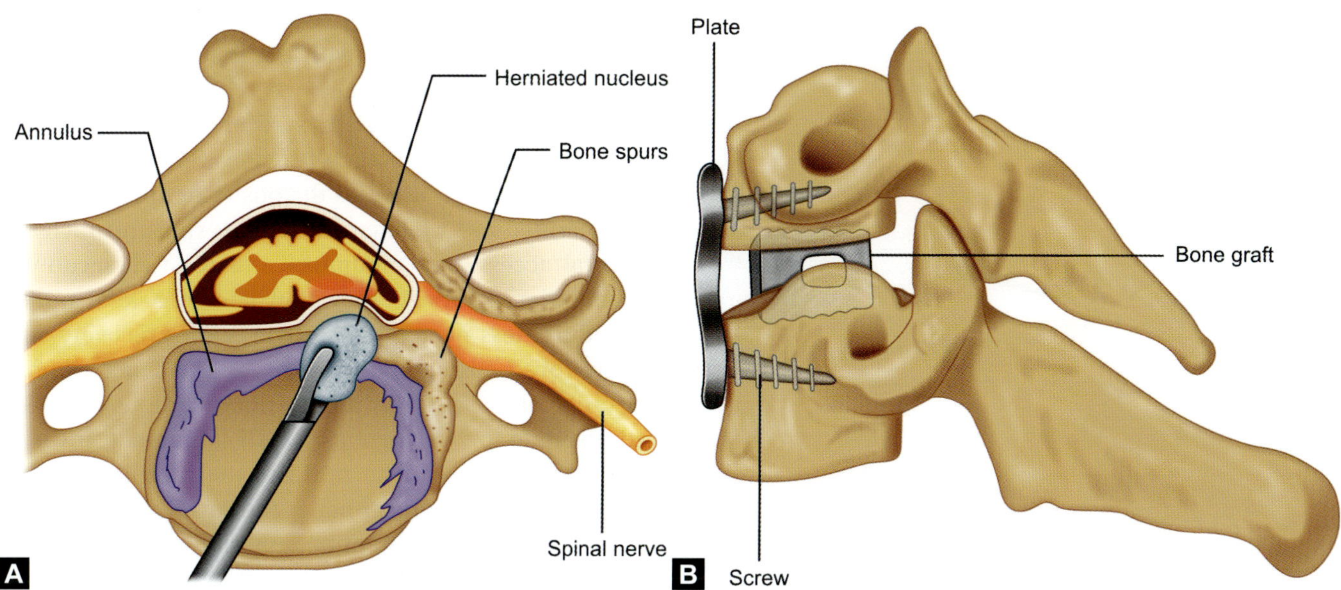

Figs. 42.2A and B: Basic anterior technique: (A) Dissection is performed through an anterior skin incision to reach the herniated disk that is then excised down to the posterior ligament, removing all disk material and the cartilaginous endplates. Decompression is then performed with removal of any extruded disk fragments and compressive osteophytes. (B) Fusion is achieved by replacing disk materials with a bone graft, a spacer, or osteobiologics. Instrumentation with a plate and screws facilitates biologic fusion and maintains spinal alignment.

medial border of the sternocleidomastoid toward midline. The surgeon incises the platysma, retracting the sternocleidomastoid and carotid sheath laterally and the strap muscles and esophagus medially. The longus colli muscles are elevated to expose the lateral aspect of the disk and uncovertebral joints. The herniated disk is then excised down to the posterior longitudinal ligament, removing all disk material as well as the cartilaginous end plates. The neural elements are then decompressed with removal of any extruded disk fragments and compressive osteophytes. If necessary, the posterior longitudinal ligament is resected to achieve full exposure of the spinal cord and neural foramen. Fusion is achieved by replacing the disk with structural bone allograft, an intervertebral spacer device (e.g. synthetic or metal cage) filled with osteobiologics, and/or autologous bone graft (usually harvested from the iliac crest). Instrumentation is commonly performed with a plate and screws to facilitate biologic fusion and maintain spinal alignment (Figs. 42.2A and B and Fig. 42.5).

Because ACDF involves fusion, which necessarily limits motion of the spine, a number of alternative anterior procedures have been designed taking motion preservation into account. One of these procedures, cervical arthroplasty or total disk replacement, is nearly identical to ACDF. Rather than using a graft and plating, however, the intervertebral disk is replaced with a mechanic disk replacement with the potential to allow segmental motion. Another procedure, anterior cervical foraminotomy, described by Jho in 1996, may also preserve motion but has not gained widespread popularity.[18] Since both of these techniques employ similar surgical approaches to ACDF, they have largely similar characteristics. These have been briefly mentioned, but a comprehensive discussion is beyond the scope of this chapter.

POSTERIOR APPROACH

Laminoforaminotomy

The most frequent posterior surgery for the treatment of cervical disk herniation is the laminoforaminotomy (keyhole foraminotomy), described by Spurling and Scoville 10 years prior to the advent of the ACDF (Figs. 42.3A to F).[19] A laminoforaminotomy usually involves a midline posterior surgical incision with unilateral muscular exposure. The paraspinal musculature is then reflected off the spinous process and lamina. This procedure entails removing part of the lamina of the medial facet joint to uncover the neural foramen, indirectly decompressing the affected exiting nerve root. After foraminotomy, a soft disk herniation may also be amenable to removal. This approach does not involve instrumentation or fusion as it serves to preserve both stability and motion. Minimally invasive approaches with tubular retractors have also been advanced.

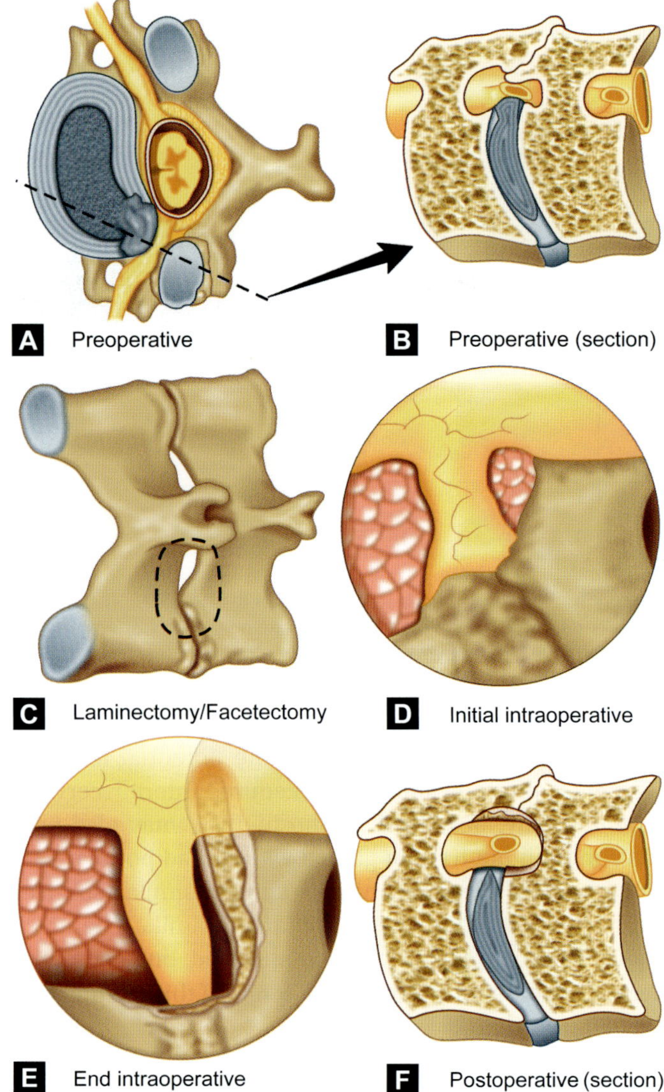

Figs. 42.3A to F: Basic posterior technique: A portion of the lamina of the medial facet joint is removed through a midline posterior incision to expose the neural foramen, indirectly decompressing the affected exiting nerve root.
Source: Adapted from Jagannathan et al. J Neurosurg Spine. 2009;10 (4):347-56.

SELECTION OF APPROACH

The choice of surgical approach is primarily dictated by the anatomic location of the compressive pathology (Figs. 42.4A and B). While the anterior approach provides access to central, paracentral, and foraminal pathology, the posterior laminoforaminotomy allows safe access to foraminal pathology alone. A posterior approach, even when incorporating a wide laminectomy, does not allow direct exposure to central or paracentral pathology as the spinal cord interferes with access and cannot be safely retracted as can be done with the thecal sac and cauda equina in the lumbar spine.

The anterior approach has several advantages over the posterior. This approach provides facile exposure to bilateral pathology, whereas the posterior approach must be performed with a bilateral muscular exposure to achieve bilateral access. The minimized muscular dissection of the anterior approach may translate to a less morbid procedure, less postoperative pain, easier recovery, and an improved cosmetic outcome. The incidence of postoperative neck pain after a posterior technique has been estimated to be as high as 22%.[20] Minimally invasive techniques may serve to mitigate the morbidity of the posterior approach and enhance the cosmesis.

In cases of hard herniation, anterior access allows for excision of calcified disk and/or osteophytes that may emanate from the end plates or uncovertebral joints. Although the laminoforaminotomy often allows removal of a soft disk fragment that may be free or extruded, it does not allow for removal of calcified or bony compressive pathology. Instead, posterior decompression relies upon indirect means, allowing the neurologic elements to shift dorsally. This type of indirect decompression may not be sufficiently effective in all cases of neurologic compression.

Use of a bone graft or cage in ACDF also serves to restore the height of the intervertebral space and neural foramen, providing indirect vertical foraminal decompression. Subsequent fusion prevents recurrent neural compression over time, which is an issue seen in posterior surgery where recurrent disk herniation or further loss of foraminal height may lead to recurrent symptomatology. An additional benefit of fusion is the potential treatment of pain generators in those patients who experience axial neck pain concomitant with their neurologic symptoms due to cervical disk herniation, spondylosis, or facet joint arthrosis.

The posterior laminoforaminotomy is an excellent surgical option, particularly in those patients with foraminal disk herniation, absent/limited neck pain, and unilateral pathology (Figs. 42.6A and B). There are potential advantages offered by this approach. Posterior surgery avoids exposure of the anterior neck anatomy and complications potentially associated with the Smith-Robinson approach. Avoidance of fusion allows preservation of motion, which is sacrificed with ACDF—approximately 10% of motion per level in the absence of spondylosis.[21] As attempted fusion is not among the surgical goals, the risk of pseudarthrosis

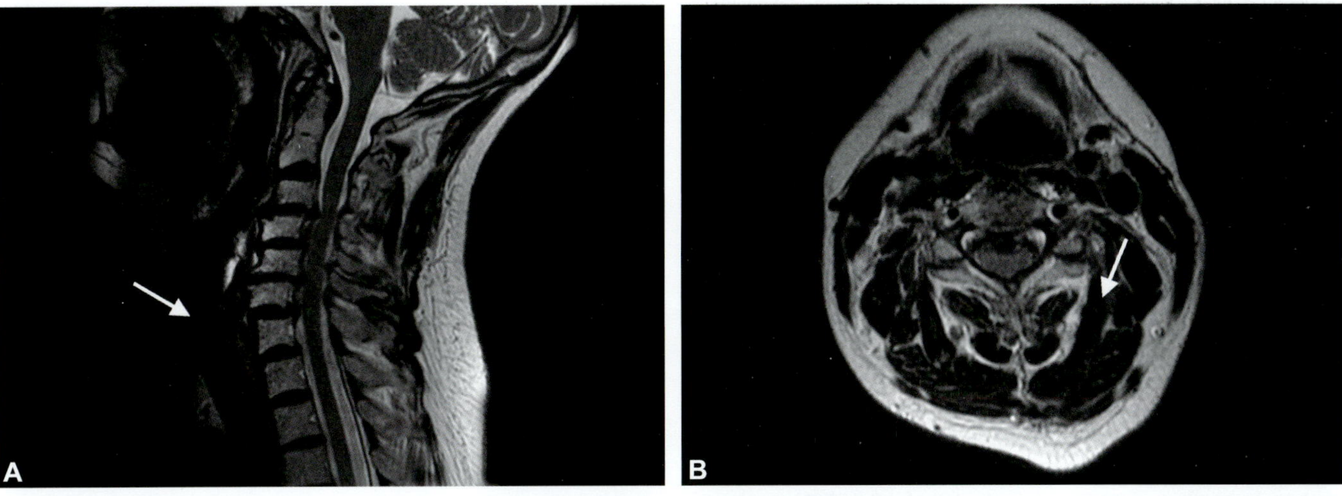

Figs. 42.4A and B: Large central C3–C4 disk herniation resulting in spinal cord compression and myelopathy. This central disk herniation requires ACDF for safe and effective decompression.

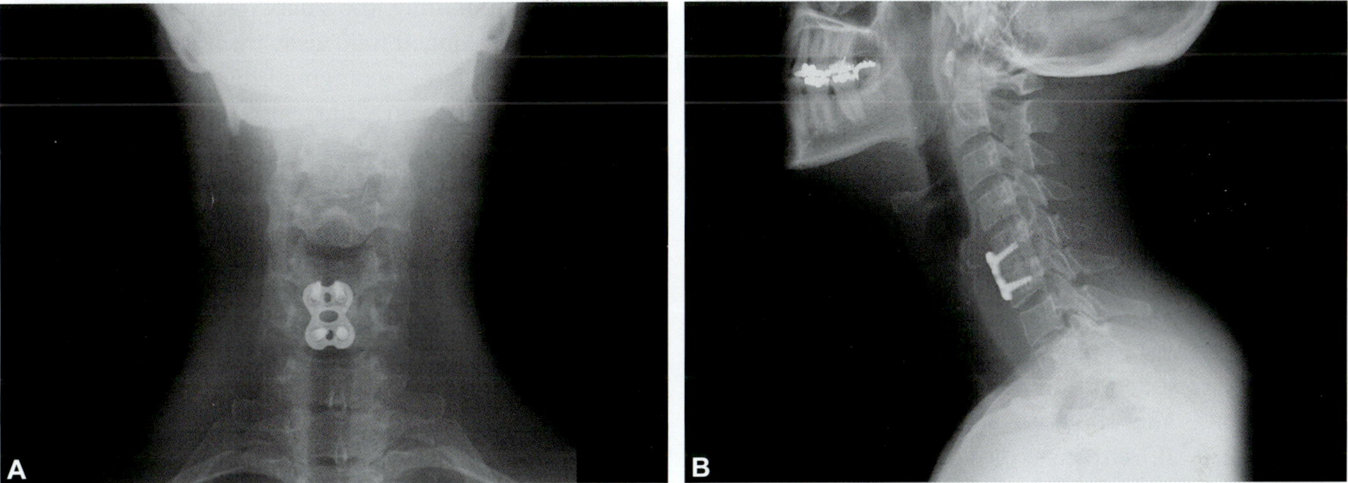

Figs. 42.5A and B: Anteroposterior and lateral postoperative plain radiographs following C5–C6 ACDF.

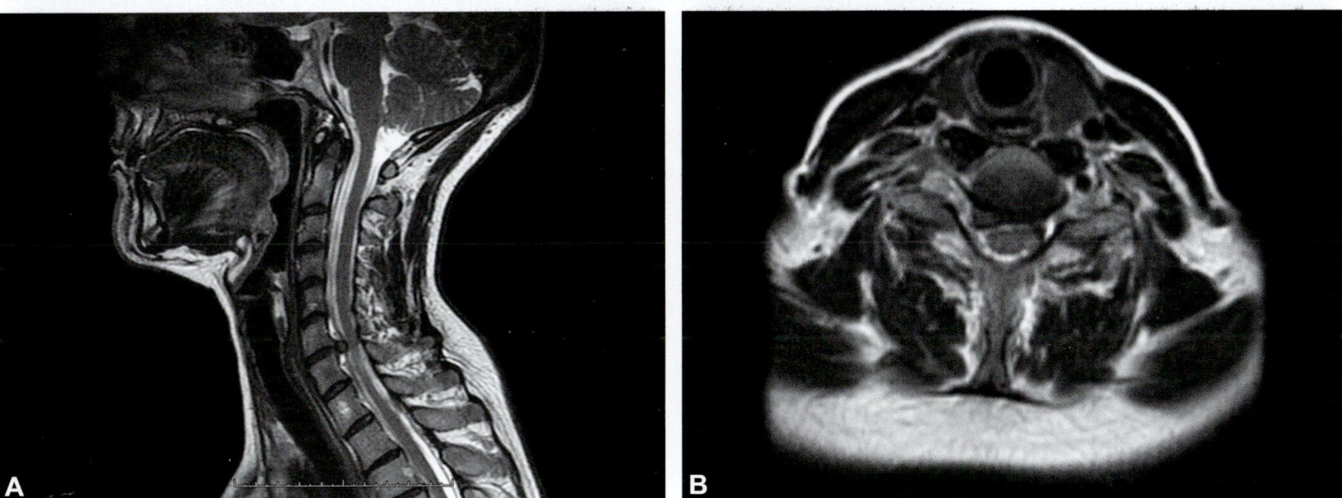

Figs. 42.6A and B: Right paracentral C6–C7 disk herniation: T2 sagittal and axial views. This type of disk herniation is amenable to surgical treatment with foraminotomy and discectomy.

is eliminated along with any associated pain or need for revision fusion surgery. Because laminoforaminotomy does not require implants or allograft, this procedure may be more cost-effective and long-term device-related issues are not a factor.

Few studies have directly compared the efficacies of anterior and posterior approaches. Conclusive results have been limited by small, heterogeneous sample sizes, and lack of long-term follow-up. A prospective study by Herkowitz et al. compared anterior fusion to laminoforaminotomy for single-level anterolateral herniation manifesting with signs and symptoms of radiculopathy. At the end of a mean 4.2-year follow-up, 16 of 17 (94%) patients in the anterior fusion group reported excellent or good results, compared with 12 of 16 (75%) patients who underwent laminoforaminotomy. These results, however, were not statistically significant. Complications were minor in both groups and were not considered when comparing outcomes.[12]

A similar study by Onimus et al. retrospectively compared two groups of 14 patients who underwent anterior discectomy and fusion versus partial lateral laminectomy for treatment of myelopathy or radiculopathy secondary to chronic spondylosis. Mean follow-up was 36 months. Although more patients complained of cervical pain in the posterior group at 3 months, on late follow-up, both groups reported 13 patients with excellent/good results with one fair result. Furthermore, both groups returned to work 3 months after surgery.[13]

Korinth et al. retrospectively compared 168 patients who underwent posterior foraminotomy to 124 patients after ventral microdiscectomy and polymethyl methacrylate interbody stabilization. All patients presented with cervical monoradiculopathy secondary to soft disk disease. Mean follow-up was 72 months. Outcomes were measured on the basis of the Odom's criteria and included morphologic findings, neurologic findings, duration of symptoms, operative technique, age, sex, and cervical levels. Other studied outcomes included length of operation and postoperative complications. The overall success rate was found to be significantly higher after the anterior surgery (93.6%) than after the posterior foraminotomy (85.1%, $p < 0.05$). At the same time, posterior foraminotomy offered significantly lower mean operating time and postoperative complication rates. On the basis of these findings, the author suggested that both approaches are equally valuable when making clinical decisions on a case-by-case basis.[22]

More recently, a retrospective review by Tumialán investigated cost-effectiveness of the anterior and posterior approaches in military personnel. Nineteen active-duty military patients with cervical disk herniation treated with ACDF were matched to a second group of 19 who received posterior foraminotomy. Matching was based on age, treatment level, and surgery, between July 2007 and August 2009. Study outcomes included difference in time to return to active duty, as well as direct and indirect costs associated with each surgery. There were no statistically significant differences in operating room time, estimated blood loss, or narcotic refills between the two groups. Average time to return to duty was 4.8 weeks for foraminotomy versus 19.6 weeks for ACDF, a statistically significant difference of 14.8 weeks. Furthermore, while there was a difference of > $6,000 in direct costs of surgery favoring foraminotomy, the salary lost by ACDF patients during their prolonged time away from work contributed to a total cost difference ranging from $20,094 to $30,553 in favor of foraminotomy. The results of this study suggest that in those military patients eligible for posterior cervical foraminotomy (PCF), there is an advantage in terms of immediate and long-term direct and indirect costs.[23] It should be noted that these military personnel are involved in particularly demanding duties and, in the author's experience, return to work is fairly similar among patients undergoing either foraminotomy or ACDF at approximately 2 weeks.

COMPLICATIONS

Although an anterior approach offers many advantages, it brings with it risk of injury to anterior structures of the neck. Incidence of damage to the recurrent laryngeal nerve, resulting in hoarseness, has been estimated at 0.2–16.7%.[24] This is an important complication to consider especially for those patients with a career or valued avocation that is reliant upon their voice. Other structures at risk include the esophagus and the carotid artery.[25] Risk of damage to the vertebral artery occurs in up to 0.3% of cases and, while uncommon, carries serious consequences, including hemorrhage, cerebrovascular accident, and the potential for long-term neurologic sequelae.[24] Dysphagia is among the most common complications of anterior surgery and is usually transient, generally resolving spontaneously within a month of surgery. The incidence is widely estimated at 2–67%, depending upon the sensitivity of the study and severity of dysphagia described.[24,26] Respiratory distress is a

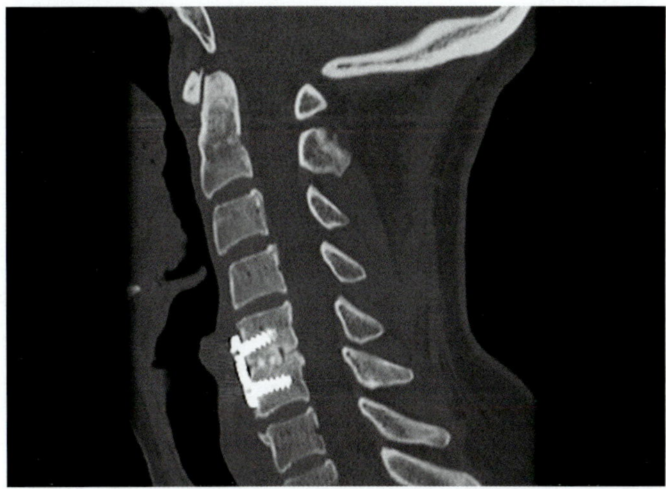

Fig. 42.7: Postoperative CT scan at 1 year demonstrates solid fusion.

rare, but potentially life-threatening, complication seen in more complex procedures and those involving the upper cervical spine.[26] The estimated incidence of pseudarthrosis ranges from 0% to 50%, depending on the number of levels fused, risk factors present, and complexity of the case.[27-33] The fusion rate for more straightforward one- or two-level ACDF with plating has been demonstrated to range from 91% to 100% (Fig. 42.7).[32,34] The risk of pseudarthrosis can be minimized with the use of modern techniques, instrumentation, autologous bone graft, and preoperative smoking cessation. It should be noted that solid fusion or pseudarthrosis does not necessarily correlate completely with clinical outcome.

Although fusion is avoided in posterior techniques, the maintenance of motion allows a risk of progressive spinal instability and/or kyphosis. In a series by Jagannathan et al., 8 of 162 patients (4.9%) developed postoperative instability after undergoing foraminotomy, with one of these patients requiring fusion. Another 30 patients developed postoperative loss of cervical lordosis, of which 9 were symptomatic.[35] Other uncommon complications, estimated to occur at a rate <10%, include intraoperative air emboli, dural tears, and transient nerve root palsy (especially C5).[14]

Adjacent Segment Disease

Another frequently studied adverse effect of spine surgery, traditionally associated with the anterior approach, is adjacent segment disease (ASD), with an estimated risk ranging from 1.6% to 4.2% per year.[36-38] ASD has an annual estimated reoperation rate of 0.8–2.9% in cervical fusion patients, with a cumulative 10-year rate of 25.6%.[39] Factors associated with increased cervical ASD risk include age more than 60 years, fusion adjacent to C5–6 or C6–7, and pre-existing compression of the spinal cord, with a diameter of 13 mm or smaller.[37]

It has been postulated that the limitation of motion resulting from fusion increases degeneration of adjacent disks. Another possibility, however, is that ASD is a combined result of limited motion, natural history and surgical manipulation, regardless of approach. In fact, a similar rate of ASD has been observed when ACDF has been compared with both posterior surgery and motion preserving techniques.[40,41] A retrospective study by Acikbas et al. found no significant difference between ASD development in patients who underwent anterior versus posterior surgery, concluding that factors other than fusion contribute to disease.[40] Furthermore, a 2012 systematic review found no significant difference between total disk replacement and ACDF in the development of ASD. No conclusions could be made, however, regarding the various nonarthroplasty motion-sparing techniques or different fusion techniques.[41,39]

CONCLUSION

The surgical treatment of cervical disk herniation can be highly effective, with among the highest outcomes not just in spinal surgery, but in all of orthopedic surgery. Studies comparing anterior and posterior approaches have been limited and have yet to provide conclusive evidence in favor of a specific approach. Thus, choice of approach should be tailored to the individual patient and pathology to achieve optimal outcome.

REFERENCES

1. Parisien RC, Ball PA. William Jason Mixter (1880-1958). Ushering in the "dynasty of the disc." Spine (Phila Pa 1976). 1998;23(21):2363-6.
2. Hubert MG, Vadala G, Sowa G, et al. Gene therapy for the treatment of degenerative disk disease. J Am Acad Orthop Surg. 2008;16(6):312-9.
3. Zmurko MG, Tannoury TY, Tannoury CA, et al. Cervical sprains, disc herniations, minor fractures, and other cervical injuries in the athlete. Clin Sports Med. 2003;22(3): 513-21.
4. Benzel EC. The Cervical Spine, 5th edition. Philadelphia, PA: Wolters Kluwer Health/Lippincott Williams & Wilkins; 2013.
5. Gore DR. Roentgenographic findings in the cervical spine in asymptomatic persons: a ten-year follow-up. Spine (Phila Pa 1976). 2001;26(22):2463-6.

6. An HS, Silveri CP, Simpson JM, et al. Comparison of smoking habits between patients with surgically confirmed herniated lumbar and cervical disc disease and controls. J Spinal Disord. 1994;7(5):369-73.
7. Hagberg M, Wegman DH. Prevalence rates and odds ratios of shoulder-neck diseases in different occupational groups. Br J Ind Med. 1987;44(9):602-10.
8. Fehlings MG, Arvin B. Surgical management of cervical degenerative disease: the evidence related to indications, impact, and outcome. J Neurosurg Spine. 2009;11(2):97-100.
9. Ropper AH, Adams RD, Victor M, et al. Adams and Victor's principles of neurology, 9th edition. New York: McGraw-Hill Medical; 2009.
10. Mochida K, Komori H, Okawa A, et al. Regression of cervical disc herniation observed on magnetic resonance images. Spine (Phila Pa 1976). 1998;23(9):990-5; discussion 996-7.
11. Bertalanffy H, Eggert HR. Clinical long-term results of anterior discectomy without fusion for treatment of cervical radiculopathy and myelopathy. A follow-up of 164 cases. Acta Neurochir (Wien). 1988;90(3-4):127-35.
12. Herkowitz HN, Kurz LT, Overholt DP. Surgical management of cervical soft disc herniation. A comparison between the anterior and posterior approach. Spine (Phila Pa 1976). 1990;15(10):1026-30.
13. Onimus M, Destrumelle N, Gangloff S. [Surgical treatment of cervical disk displacement. Anterior or posterior approach?]. Rev Chir Orthop Reparatrice Appar Mot. 1995; 81(4):296-301.
14. Benzel EC, Francis TB. Spine surgery: techniques, complication avoidance, and management, 3rd edition. Philadelphia, PA, Elsevier/Saunders; 2012.
15. Denaro V, Di Martino A. Cervical spine surgery: an historical perspective. Clin Orthop Relat Res. 2011;469(3):639-48.
16. Decker RC. Surgical treatment and outcomes of cervical radiculopathy. Phys Med Rehabil Clin N Am. 2011;22(1): 179-91.
17. Patil PG, Turner DA, Pietrobon R. National trends in surgical procedures for degenerative cervical spine disease: 1990-2000. Neurosurgery. 2005;57(4):753-8; discussion 753-8.
18. Jho HD. Microsurgical anterior cervical foraminotomy for radiculopathy: a new approach to cervical disc herniation. J Neurosurg. 1996;84(2):155-60.
19. American Chemical Society. Meeting (228th: 2004 : Philadelphia Pa.), Fishman ML, Qi PX, Wicker L, American Chemical Society. Division of Agricultural and Food Chemistry. Advances in biopolymers: molecules, clusters, networks, and interactions. Washington, DC: American Chemical Society: Distributed by Oxford University Press, 2006.
20. Grieve JP, Kitchen ND, Moore AJ, et al. Results of posterior cervical foraminotomy for treatment of cervical spondylitic radiculopathy. Br J Neurosurg. 2000;14(1):40-3.
21. Lin HL, Cho DY, Liu YF, et al. Change of cervical balance following single to multi-level interbody fusion with cage. Br J Neurosurg. 2008;22(6):758-63.
22. Korinth MC, Kruger A, Oertel MF, et al. Posterior foraminotomy or anterior discectomy with polymethyl methacrylate interbody stabilization for cervical soft disc disease: results in 292 patients with monoradiculopathy. Spine (Phila Pa 1976). 2006;31(11):1207-14; discussion 1215-6.
23. Tumialan LM, Ponton RP, Gluf WM. Management of unilateral cervical radiculopathy in the military: the cost effectiveness of posterior cervical foraminotomy compared with anterior cervical discectomy and fusion. Neurosurg Focus. 2010;28(5):E17.
24. Fountas KN, Kapsalaki EZ, Nikolakakos LG, et al. Anterior cervical discectomy and fusion associated complications. Spine (Phila Pa 1976). 2007;32(21):2310-7.
25. Vrouenraets BC, Been HD, Brouwer-Mladin R, et al. Esophageal perforation associated with cervical spine surgery: report of two cases and review of the literature. Dig Surg. 2004;21(3):246-9.
26. Stieber JR, Brown K, Donald GD, et al. Anterior cervical decompression and fusion with plate fixation as an outpatient procedure. Spine J. 2005;5(5):503-7.
27. Pradhan BB, Nassar JA, Delamarter RB, et al. Single-level lumbar spine fusion: a comparison of anterior and posterior approaches. J Spinal Disord Tech. 2002;15(5):355-61.
28. Christensen FB. Lumbar spinal fusion. Outcome in relation to surgical methods, choice of implant and postoperative rehabilitation. Acta Orthop Scand Suppl. 2004;75(313):2-43.
29. Phillips FM, Carlson G, Emery SE, et al. Anterior cervical pseudarthrosis. Natural history and treatment. Spine (Phila Pa 1976). 1997;22(14):1585-9.
30. Fourney DR, Skelly AC, Devine JG. Treatment of cervical adjacent segment pathology: a systematic review. Spine (Phila Pa 1976). 2012;37(22 Suppl):S113-22.
31. Gause PR, Davis RA, Smith PN, et al. Success of junctional anterior cervical discectomy and fusion. Spine J. 2008;8(5): 723-8.
32. Wang JC, McDonough PW, Endow KK, et al. Increased fusion rates with cervical plating for two-level anterior cervical discectomy and fusion. Spine (Phila Pa 1976). 2000;25(1):41-5.
33. Wang JC, McDonough PW, Endow KK, et al. A comparison of fusion rates between single-level cervical corpectomy and two-level discectomy and fusion. J Spinal Disord. 2001;14(3):222-5.
34. Kaiser MG, Haid RW, Jr, Subach BR, et al. Anterior cervical plating enhances arthrodesis after discectomy and fusion with cortical allograft. Neurosurgery. 2002;50(2):229-36; discussion 236-8.
35. Jagannathan J, Sherman JH, Szabo T, et al. The posterior cervical foraminotomy in the treatment of cervical disc/ osteophyte disease: a single-surgeon experience with a minimum of 5 years' clinical and radiographic follow-up. J Neurosurg Spine. 2009;10(4):347-56.
36. Kepler CK, Hilibrand AS. Management of adjacent segment disease after cervical spinal fusion. Orthop Clin North Am. 2012;43(1):53-62, viii.
37. Lawrence BD, Hilibrand A, Brodt E, et al. Predicting the risk of adjacent segment pathology in the cervical spine: a systematic review. Spine (Phila Pa 1976). 2012;37(22 Suppl): S52-64.
38. Lawrence BD, Wang J, Arnold PM, et al. Predicting the risk of adjacent segment pathology after lumbar fusion: a systematic review. Spine (Phila Pa 1976). 2012;37(22 Suppl):S123-32.

39. Hilibrand AS, Carlson GD, Palumbo MA, et al. Radiculopathy and myelopathy at segments adjacent to the site of a previous anterior cervical arthrodesis. J Bone Joint Surg Am. 1999;81(4):519-28.
40. Acikbas SC, Ermol C, Akyuz M, et al. Assessment of adjacent segment degeneration in and between patients treated with anterior or posterior cervical simple discectomy. Turk Neurosurg. 2010;20(3):334-40.
41. Harrod CC, Hilibrand AS, Fischer DJ, et al. Adjacent segment pathology following cervical motion sparing procedures or devices compared to fusion surgery: a systematic review. Spine (Phila Pa 1976). 2012;37(22 Suppl): S96-S112.

CHAPTER

43

Surgical Treatment of Cervical Stenosis

Jane S Hoashi, Stephen P Maier II, Jeffrey D Klein

INTRODUCTION

Cervical stenosis refers to the narrowing of the cervical spinal canal, generally as a result of degenerative changes that often begin in the cervical disk. As the disk degenerates, the nucleus pulposus and disk annulus progressively lose their viscoelastic properties; there is a loss of disk height, with bulging of the disk posteriorly. This leads to retraction and hypertrophy of the ligamentum flavum and soft tissues, as well as osteophyte development.[1] These degenerative, or spondylotic, changes are commonly found after the age of 50 years.[2-4] Between ages 60 and 65 years, at least one radiographic degenerative change can be seen in 95% of asymptomatic men and 70% of asymptomatic women.[5] These radiographic changes include disk space narrowing, osteophyte formation, loss of lordosis, subluxation, and ankylosis[6] and can lead to narrowing of the spinal canal as well as the neuroforamen. Cervical spondylosis can be asymptomatic, or present as neck stiffness or pain radiating to the shoulders or the occiput. Although the presence of stenosis does not necessarily cause symptoms, nerve root compression typically presents as upper extremity radiculopathy while spinal cord compression may present with the clinical features of myelopathy. Clinical findings, however, do not always correlate with radiographic images; many asymptomatic individuals are noted to have significant radiographic changes with marked narrowing of the spinal canal.[7] A thorough history and physical examination are needed to appropriately diagnose and manage these patients.

Although cervical spondylotic radiculopathy is often a self-limiting condition,[8] myelopathy is considered a progressive and irreversible disorder characterized by stable periods punctuated by stepwise deterioration. Clinical resolution of myelopathy is rare without surgical treatment, especially for moderate to severe cases.[9,10] A range of treatment options exist on the basis of the severity of the clinical presentation.

CERVICAL SPONDYLOTIC RADICULOPATHY

Cervical spondylotic radiculopathy occurs as a result of nerve root compression from uncovertebral osteophytes, disk herniations, and spondylotic bars. These degenerative features are seen in association with loss of disk height. Soft disk herniation refers to a relatively acute displacement of the nucleus pulposus causing compression of the nerve root. Hard disks refer to osteophyte formation as an adaptive response to the greater loads placed on the facet and uncovertebral bodies. These spondylotic findings, especially in the presence of decreased disk height, can cause nerve root compression with or without an associated soft disk herniation.

Patients with cervical spondylotic radiculopathy may complain of arm pain or weakness in a dermatomal distribution, but it is not uncommon for classic radiculopathic symptoms of radiating pain down the arm to be absent. Patients may also present with overlapping radiculopathic symptoms from multiple levels. Neck pain may be unilateral or bilateral, often associated with pain in the trapezial and periscapular areas.[11] The diagnosis of the exact level or levels affected is, therefore, often a challenge.

Diagnosis involves a detailed physical examination, in which provocative tests consisting of cervical compression and distraction can help diagnose the radiculopathy. The Spurling maneuver may also be positive; by rotating and extending the neck to the side of the pathology, tension is placed on an entrapped nerve root and can reproduce symptoms of radiculopathy. In the shoulder abduction test, the nerve roots experience decrease in tension, and relief of radicular pain is observed. Plain X-rays in anteroposterior (AP), lateral, and oblique views are useful for identifying osteophytes or even an ossified posterior longitudinal ligament, another cause of cervical stenosis. Magnetic resonance imaging (MRI) is most useful for identifying disk herniations, but a computerized tomography (CT) with myelogram can best differentiate whether nerve root compression is due to an osteophyte or a disk herniation. Electromyography and nerve conduction studies can also help differentiate peripheral nerve compression, such as carpal tunnel syndrome, from nerve root compression in the cervical spine.

Disorders unrelated to the spine may mimic cervical radiculopathy and should be ruled out when examining the patient. Tumors such as schwannoma and meningioma, peripheral nerve entrapment syndrome, brachial neuritis, thoracic outlet syndrome, infection, and shoulder impingement can all lead to symptoms similar to those of cervical radiculopathy. Shoulder impingement can present as shoulder pain that is aggravated by shoulder abduction. Periscapular pain may be a sign of radiculopathy from the lower cervical nerve roots or referred cervical facet pain. Pain in the superomedial scapula, however, may be a sign of occult shoulder pathology.[12]

The prognosis of cervical spondylotic radiculopathy is generally favorable. Conservative treatment includes nonsteroidal anti-inflammatory medication, oral steroids, physical therapy, and targeted steroid injections.[11] Improvement or resolution of symptoms has been reported in 45–90% of patients with nonoperative treatment of acute cervical radiculopathy.[13,14] Surgery is indicated when there is severe pain and weakness despite prolonged conservative treatment and certainly in the setting of a progressive neurologic deficit. The goal of surgery is to decompress the compromised neural elements.

CERVICAL SPONDYLOTIC MYELOPATHY

Cervical spondylotic myelopathy (CSM) refers to the clinical condition caused by spinal cord compression in the setting of cervical spondylosis. Unlike cervical spondylotic radiculopathy, which is commonly a more benign and self-limiting condition,[11] CSM is a progressive disorder characterized by stepwise deterioration and intermittent stable periods.[9,10] CSM is the most common cause of myelopathy in patients over the age of 55 years.[15] Symptoms are variable, and sometimes can be confused with the normal aging process. Patients with early signs of myelopathy may report decreased manual dexterity, such as clumsiness when handling keys, frequent dropping of items, or the inability to button their shirts. This may progress to weakness or loss of balance when walking, which can also mimic symptoms caused by other conditions related to aging such as osteoarthritis in the lower extremities. Loss of bowel and bladder control is rare but can exist in severe and later stages of cervical myelopathy. Although the symptoms generally reflect the degree of spinal cord compression, this is not always the case. Significant cord compression on imaging studies can be found in relatively asymptomatic patients with normal neurological examinations. Therefore, it is important to maintain a high level of suspicion when evaluating for myelopathy, with close attention to a detailed history and physical examination.

PATHOGENESIS

In addition to the degenerative processes causing mechanical compression of the spinal cord, other factors contribute to the pathogenesis of cervical myelopathy. These include canal diameter, dynamic compression of the cord, and ischemia. A normal cervical spinal canal in the sagittal plane (between the posterior aspect of the vertebral body and the spinolaminar line) measures 17–18 mm.[16] A congenitally narrow cervical canal defined as < 13 mm, or having a Pavlov ratio—the AP diameter of the canal divided by the AP diameter of the vertebral body—of < 0.8, is a predisposing factor for developing CSM;[17,18] the reduced space available for the cord creates a decreased tolerance for symptoms of spinal cord compression. While a normal sized canal can often accommodate space occupying degenerative changes, a degenerative disk herniation or osteophyte formation can induce radicular or myelopathic symptoms earlier in patients with congenital cervical stenosis. Ossification of the posterior longitudinal ligament (OPLL) is another cause of cervical stenosis (Fig. 43.1) and may coexist with spondylotic changes.

Dynamic factors also play a role in the pathogenesis of cervical myelopathy. Neck flexion and extension can change the diameter of the spinal canal by 2–3 mm.[19]

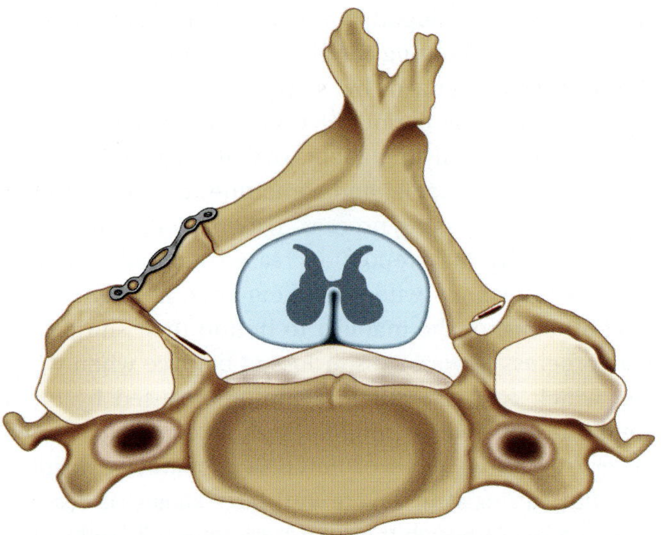

Fig. 43.1: Ossification of the posterior longitudinal ligament further constricts the spinal canal impinging upon the cord, leading to myelopathy in the cervical spine.

In extension, the shingling of the laminae can cause the ligamentum flavum to buckle ventrally into the canal and thereby reduce the cross-sectional area of the canal by 24%.[20] In flexion, the cord stretches and, if compressed against an anterior protruding disk or spondylotic ridge, can result in ongoing compression that can lead to ischemia and axonal injury.

Decreased vascular flow to the spinal cord from the mechanical compression has been hypothesized as a key factor in the development of myelopathy.[21,22] Oligodendrocytes, whose role is to insulate axons with myelin sheath, are affected most from these ischemic changes and suffer apoptosis. Histopathologic evidence shows irreversible changes such as demyelination, gliosis, and cystic cavitation in central gray matter and lateral columns.[23-25] This may explain why decompressive surgery does not improve the neurologic symptoms in some patients.

Physical Examination

A thorough neurological examination should be performed in both the upper and lower extremities, keeping in mind that a normal neurological examination does not exclude the diagnosis of myelopathy. Patients with mild CSM may report pain and limited motion in the neck, with or without radicular symptoms in the upper extremities, depending on the presence or absence of coexisting nerve root compression. L'hermitte's phenomenon (electric sensations radiating down the spine and extremities) can be elicited with neck flexion. The motor examination may reveal weakness in upper and lower extremities. Sensory examination may be abnormal to touch or pinprick and may not follow a dermatomal pattern. There may also be signs of early, decreased vibration, and proprioception; it is important to examine the patient's gait for the overall balance, including heel-to-toe tandem walking. Nurick classified incapacity due to CSM into five grades, from no gait impairment (Grade I) to bed or chair-bound (Grade V).[10] Posterior column dysfunction should be evaluated with vibratory testing and the Romberg's test.

Sometimes, patients present with localized wasting and weakness of the extrinsic and intrinsic hand muscles. They may also complain of diffuse numbness of the hands, which can be confused with carpal tunnel syndrome or peripheral neuropathy. These symptoms are referred to as myelopathy hand,[26] for which two specific signs have been described. In the finger-escape sign, the patient holds the fingers in extension and adduction. The myelopathic patient will be unable to maintain this position for 30 seconds, and the two ulnar digits will start to drift into flexion and abduction. With the grip-and-release test, in which the patient is asked to repetitively make a fist and release, a patient with myelopathic hand will be unable to perform 20 of these movements in 10 seconds.

Patients with CSM often show signs of upper motor neuron dysfunction. Hyper-reflexia is often found in patients with CSM in both upper and lower extremities, along with sustained or >3 beats of clonus. Pathological reflexes, including Babinski's, Hoffman's, and inverted radial reflexes, may be present. The inverted radial reflex is positive if finger flexion is seen along with a hypoactive brachioradialis. This is indicative of cord compression at the C6 level. Other pathological reflexes for higher cervical levels include a hyperactive scapulohumeral reflex. Brisk elevation of the scapula or humerus is observed with tapping of the acromion, which is suggestive of cord compression cephalad to C3. Lastly, the jaw jerk test, in which upward jerking of the mandible is present when tapping on the lower jaw, is suggestive of upper motor dysfunction originating from the brain, as opposed to the cervical spinal cord.

Differential Diagnosis

Differential diagnoses are broad and include many spinal and nonspinal conditions. Spinal pathologies other than spondylosis causing cord compression include OPLL, trauma, tumor, epidural abscess, osteomyelitis, and discitis. Nonspinal conditions that mimic cervical myelopathy include neurological disorders such as multiple sclerosis, peripheral polyneuropathy, motor neuron disease like amyotrophic lateral sclerosis (ALS), syringomyelia, stroke, and vitamin B12 deficiency.[27] In an elderly patient with gait instability and urinary incontinence, it is important to rule out normal pressure hydrocephalus due to the similarities in presentation to myelopathy.

Diagnostic Studies

Imaging studies include plain AP and lateral radiographs. The size of the canal and the overall sagittal alignment of the cervical spine can be seen in the lateral projection. Oblique films can reveal uncovertebral joint spurring causing foraminal narrowing. Flexion and extension lateral films are necessary to identify instability and ankylosed vertebral segments.

The MRI is used to evaluate spinal cord and nerve root compression. A recent systematic review showed a correlation between cord signal changes on the MRI and overall prognosis, with multisegmental high-intensity signal changes on T2 and low-intensity T1 changes predictors of poor prognosis for neurologic recovery after surgical decompression.[28] CT scans are used to visualize osteophyte formation, foraminal stenosis, and OPLL. CT myelography, although an invasive procedure, is useful for patients with metal implants or those with spinal deformities, because it outlines the exact degree of cord compression. It also provides the best evaluation of nerve root compression in the neuroforamen.[29]

Electromyography and nerve conduction studies can be useful when differentiating cervical radiculopathy from peripheral neuropathy or root entrapment syndromes such as carpal tunnel or cubital tunnel syndrome. These tests may also help distinguish peripheral disorders from central processes such as ALS.[29] However, its use is limited by its low sensitivity, high false negative rate,[30] and low concordance with MRI findings.[31]

TREATMENT OPTIONS

The Role of Conservative Treatment in CSM

The treatment options for CSM include nonoperative and surgical treatments. Given the natural history of CSM, with the majority of patients suffering a stepwise neurological deterioration, most surgeons have favored surgical decompression in an effort to stop or at least slow the progression of the disease. Several large retrospective studies using different outcome measures have shown the benefits of surgical decompression on neurologic function.[32-34] A more recent prospective study comparing conservatively and surgically treated patients demonstrated improved neurologic symptoms and functional status and less overall pain in the surgically treated group; the conservatively treated group showed worsening of neurologic symptoms.[35] Other prospective randomized studies comparing conservative to surgical treatment in patients with mild to moderate CSM found that both groups had similar Japanese Orthopaedic Association (JOA) scores and functional status at 3 and 10 years, respectively.[36,37] Although the optimal management for mild to moderate CSM is not clear, there is a role for conservative treatment. Indications for conservative treatment include mild cervical myelopathy (mild hyper-reflexia without motor deficit or weakness) or myelopathic patients in a plateau period who have not suffered a recent exacerbation of symptoms.

Conservative treatment includes nonsteroidal anti-inflammatory medication, soft collar immobilization, and physical therapy (active only motion) for neck strengthening. The patient should be re-evaluated within 3–6 months to assess for neurological deterioration.

Surgical Treatment

Surgery is indicated in patients with moderate-to-severe myelopathy or in those who show progressive neurologic dysfunction or increasing pain or disability. The goals of surgery are to decompress the neural elements, alleviate the pain, and correct and prevent cervical deformity. Surgical approaches for cervical stenosis and spondylosis can be anterior, posterior, or a combination of both. The decision to use any of these approaches is made on the basis of a number of factors. These include the sagittal profile of the cervical spine, anatomic location and severity of the stenosis, the number of pathological levels, the presence of neck versus arm pain, and a history of previous surgery on the neck.[38]

As spondylosis progresses, there is a general loss of lordosis in the cervical spine.[39] When there is cervical kyphosis, the spinal cord is draped over the vertebral bodies and compressive elements anteriorly (Fig. 43.2). If a posterior decompressive procedure is performed in a kyphotic spine, there is minimal posterior drift of the spinal cord, and the cord remains draped over the compressive anterior structures. Improvement of symptoms

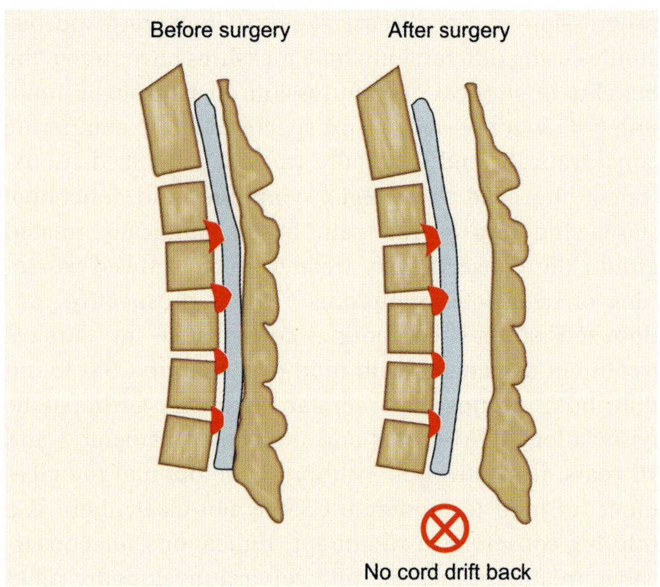

Fig. 43.2: A posterior surgical approach in a kyphotic cervical spine. The spinal cord continues to drape over the compressive structures anteriorly thus preventing any relief.

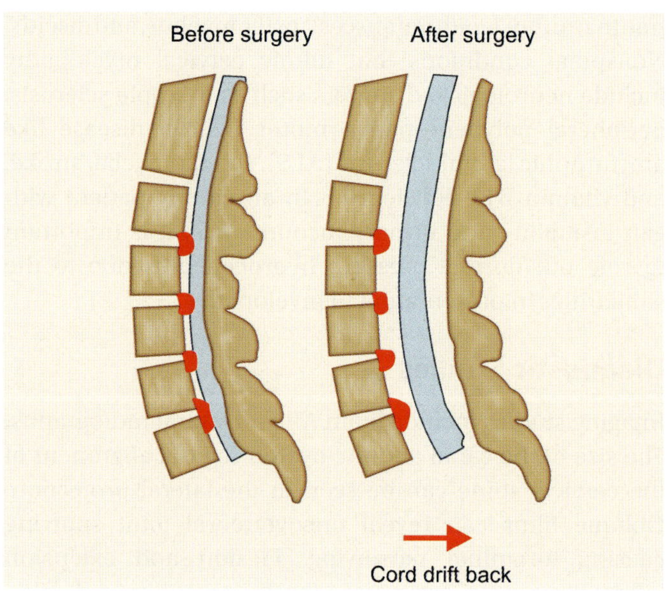

Fig. 43.3: A posterior surgical approach to a lordotic cervical spine yields superior results to the same approach in a kyphotic cervical spine due to the allowance for cord drift back.

is suboptimal compared with the results commonly achieved in a lordotic cervical spine, where a similar posterior decompression permits posterior drifting of the cord (Fig. 43.3).[40,41] A kyphotic cervical alignment, then, is considered a relative contraindication for the posterior approach.

Congenital stenosis is typically multilevel, and the posterior approach is often chosen as a way to increase the diameter of the canal and allow for the spinal cord to drift posteriorly after decompression. An anterior approach is usually contraindicated in these four- to five-level surgical decompressions.[38]

The extent and location of the stenosis must also be considered in determining the surgical approach. The anterior approach is typically favored in one- or two-level presentations,[38] whereas four levels or more are usually treated posteriorly.[42] Three-level cases can be treated from either approach as dictated by other factors. The nonunion rate of anterior cervical interbody fusions increases with increasing number of levels.[42-45] Also, risk of soft tissue injury increases with multiple levels. Dysphagia due to esophageal retraction is a frequent postoperative complaint from the anterior approach and has been associated with multiple level involvement.[46,47] Cervical radiculopathy resulting from narrowing of the lateral recess from cervical spondylosis or disk herniation can be treated using either the anterior or posterior approach.[48]

Finally, when the symptoms include significant axial neck pain, an anterior approach should be considered because a posterior approach will often exacerbate the neck pain. However, if there is previous anterior surgery to the neck, a posterior approach might be preferred to avoid issues related to a difficult revision exposure.

ANTERIOR APPROACH

Anterior Cervical Discectomy and Fusion (ACDF)

Anterior cervical discectomy and fusion is currently considered the gold standard for surgical treatment in cervical degenerative disease. It involves direct decompression by removing the entire disk including the herniated portion along with any offending osteophytes that may be compressing centrally on the spinal cord or laterally on the nerve roots. Indirect decompression of the foramen and canal is also achieved by placing bone graft in the distracted disk space for fusion to take place. The technique was initially described using autogenous iliac crest bone graft[43,49] without instrumentation, but today, allograft with plate instrumentation is commonly used (Figs. 43.4A to D).

In this approach, the patient is positioned supine, sometimes with head halter traction. Slight cervical lordosis is applied by placing a roll in between the scapulae.

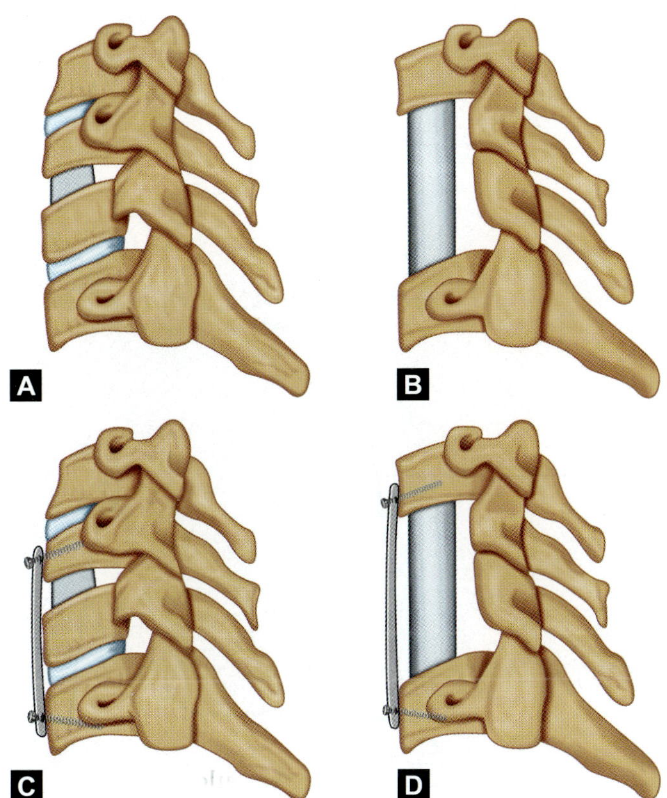

Figs. 43.4A to D: Visual representation of (A and C) anterior cervical discectomy and fusion (ACDF) and (B and D) anterior cervical corpectomy and fusion (ACCF) procedures used to treat cervical myelopathy. ACDF and ACCF procedures use bone spacers (A and C) and bone strut-grafting (B and D), respectively, to fuse the vertebral bodies after the removal of the cervical elements; however, occasionally cervical anterior plating (C and D) supplements the grafting.

Care must be taken not to hyperextend the neck in cases with stenosis and cord compression. The incision is made in the anterolateral aspect of the neck at the level of vertebral involvement.[49] The main anatomic landmarks are the hyoid for C3, thyroid cartilage for C4–C5 intervertebral disk space, and the cricoid cartilage for C6.[50] A left-sided approach is recommended to minimize injury to the recurrent laryngeal nerve. The left recurrent laryngeal nerve descends into the thorax and loops around the aortic arch before ascending in between the esophagus and the trachea. The left-sided approach is considered safer than the right-sided approach due to the longer and anatomically protected nature of the left recurrent laryngeal nerve.[51] However, in lower cervical levels, one must be aware of the thoracic duct, which lies behind the carotid sheath, ending at the junction of the subclavian and left internal jugular veins. A horizontal incision is made in the anterolateral aspect of the neck in line with the natural skin creases. After dividing the platysma, the spine is approached via a blunt dissection medial to the sternocleidomastoid muscle and through the natural fascial planes between the carotid sheaths laterally and the esophagus and trachea medially (Figs. 43.5A and B). The disk is removed using curettes and Kerrison rongeurs. The cartilaginous end plates are carefully removed with curettes and the burr, whereas the bony end plates are left intact, but abraded. The allograft is placed and then secured with an anterior plate.

Anterior Cervical Corpectomy and Fusion (ACCF)

If the stenosis is not confined to the disk space and extends behind the posterior vertebral body, then a corpectomy is indicated. Neurological deterioration in myelopathy has been reported with large osteophyte removal of the posterior aspect of the vertebral end plates with ACDF procedures due to the relatively limited space and visualization rendered by this procedure.[52] ACCF is a good surgical option in CSM or when large osteophyte removal from multiple segments is expected. Using the same approach as an ACDF, the ACCF consists of removing a portion of the vertebral body, along with the adjacent caudal and cephalad disks.[38] A central trough is created anteriorly down to the posterior longitudinal ligament or dura, expanding the vertebral canal and allowing easier and safer access for removing osteophytes than with an ACDF.[38,52] It is important to stay within the uncinate processes, with a safety margin of 5 mm to the uncovertebral joint, to avoid injury to the vertebral artery that runs within the foramen transversarium (Fig. 43.6). The defect is then reconstructed with iliac crest autograft, fibular strut allograft, or metallic cages with anterior plating for fixation (Figs. 43.4 and 43.7).

Advantages and Complications of the Anterior Approach

An advantage to using this approach is that natural fascial planes are used, thus avoiding retraction of neural elements. Postoperative pain is usually quite tolerable and infectious complications are rare.[11] Anterior cervical surgery is associated, however, with complications related to speech and swallowing due to esophageal and recurrent laryngeal nerve compression, with reports of dysphagia ranging from 28% to 57% and dysphonia from 2% to 30%.[46,47,53,54] Other disadvantages include loss of a motion segment and possible disk degeneration of

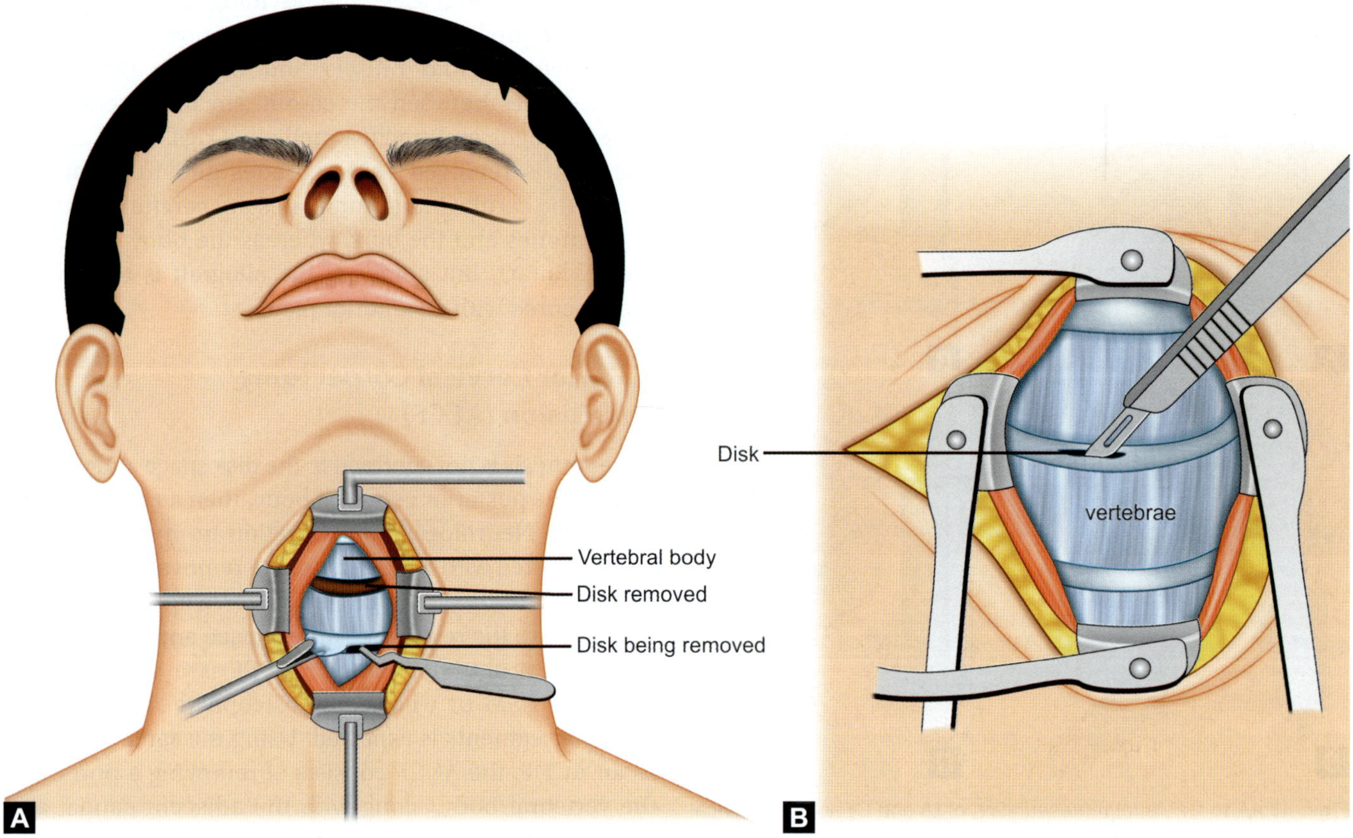

Vertebral body
Disk removed
Disk being removed
Disk
vertebrae

Figs. 43.5A and B: The anatomical approach of an anterior cervical discectomy and fusion showing the incision made anteriorly and the subsequent removal of the appropriate disk(s). Replacement of the disk(s) with autologous bone grafts follows and instrumentation is inserted to fuse the vertebrae.

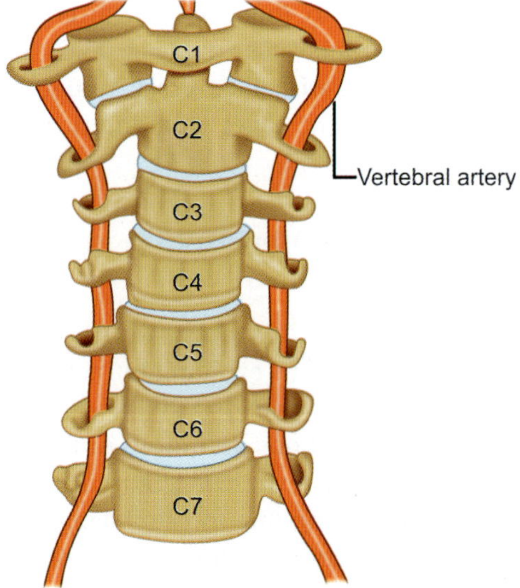

Fig. 43.6: It is critical to avoid injury to the vertebral arteries, the blood vessels that run bilaterally within the foramen transversarium.

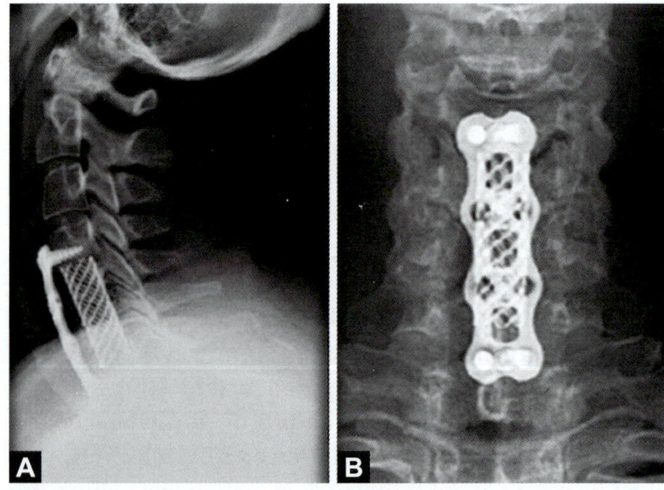

Figs. 43.7A and B: Plain radiographs, (A) lateral and (B) anteroposterior of a patient after undergoing corpectomy of C5 and C6 with insertion of a strut graft and titanium mesh cage. Autologous bone is packed inside the cage to promote fusion.

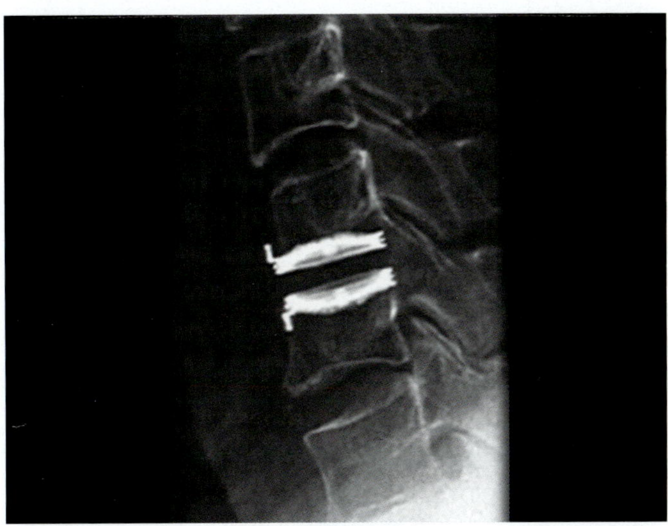

Fig. 43.8: Lateral X-ray after C5/C6 cervical disk arthroplasty with Bryan system instrumentation.

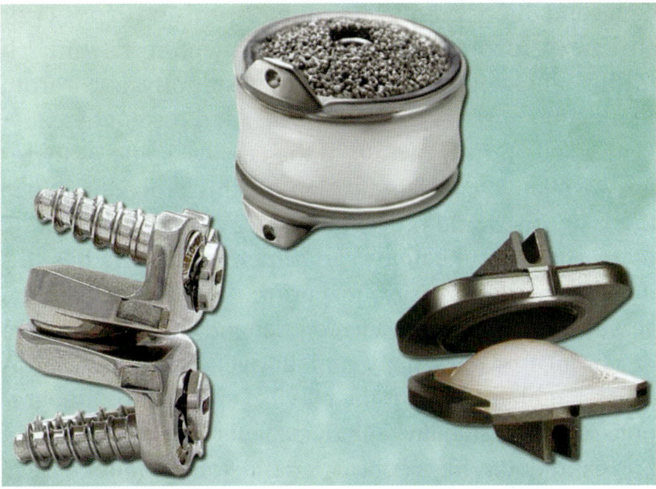

Fig. 43.9: The instrumentation used in cervical arthroplasty may vary. Images shown above are the Food and Drug Administration certified instruments: (l to r) Prestige ST, Bryan system, Pro-disk C.

adjacent levels.[11,55] Hilibrand et al. found a 25% risk of developing adjacent segment disease, mostly occurring at C5–C6 and C6–C7 levels.[55] Risk of pseudarthrosis exists with the anterior approach, with rates reported between 5–10% for a single level,[56-59] although plate fixation has been shown to have higher fusion rates when compared with bone graft or cages alone.[59] C5 palsy, typically associated with posterior approaches, is also a possible complication of the anterior approach. It is thought to be due to a possible traction injury to the spinal cord and C5 nerve root. A recent study on 750 consecutive anterior approach cases found a greater risk of nerve palsy as the number of levels corpectomized increased.[60]

For patients with CSM, a long-term study found high rates of neurological improvement and pain relief after anterior cervical procedures including anterior discectomy, partial corpectomy, or subtotal corpectomy (*see* ACCF). Improvement in the average Nurick's score from 2.4 preoperatively to 1.2 postoperatively was reported.[61] For cervical radiculopathy, a recent systematic review showed ACDF to provide more rapid relief of neck and arm pain or weakness, as well as longer term (12 months) maintenance of arm function as compared with nonoperative treatment including physical therapy or cervical collar immobilization.[62]

Cervical Arthroplasty

Arthroplasty has gained momentum as an alternative to fusion in an effort to address concerns of possible adjacent level disk degeneration associated with fusion procedures (ACDF and ACCF). Its use has primarily been for cervical radiculopathy. The same anterior approach is used to access the intervertebral space, and the entire disk space is replaced with an artificial disk (Figs. 43.8 and 43.9). With arthroplasty, it is hoped that preservation of mobility in the affected cervical level results in less stress placed on the adjacent levels than is thought to occur in a fusion. A recent systematic review of arthroplasty compared with fusion for single-level cervical degenerative disk disease[63] found low to moderate quality evidence showing a small difference favoring arthroplasty in alleviating arm pain and improving neck-related functional status at 1–2 years. However, the systematic review could not confirm that adjacent level disk degeneration occurred less in arthroplasty than in fusion cases at 2 years. The authors concluded that longer term studies are needed to observe whether arthroplasty indeed has a protective effect against adjacent degenerative disk disease.

For cervical myelopathy, arthroplasty has been described, but concerns have been raised regarding preserving motion in a cervical spine with a compromised cord. The contraindications for arthroplasty are severe osteoporosis, cervical kyphosis, segmental instability, lack of motion at the involved segment, severe facet arthrosis, and OPLL.

POSTERIOR APPROACH

Laminectomy

Laminectomy involves a posterior decompression of the spinal cord by enlarging the dimensions of the cervical canal and directly removing compression due to posterior structures such as a redundant ligamentum flavum.[64] It further allows the cord to shift posteriorly away from impinging anterior bulging disks and osteophytes. A kyphotic deformity of > 10° in the cervical spine is, therefore, a relative contraindication for this procedure since the kyphosis would prevent an effective posterior drifting of the cord. Laminectomy can be performed with or without fusion. The decision to perform laminectomy alone versus laminectomy and fusion depends on the presence or absence of neck pain, patient age, existing comorbidities, sagittal profile of the cervical spine, and radiographic signs of instability. Elderly patients with comorbidities are candidates for cervical laminectomy alone if they preserve cervical lordosis of at least 10° without signs of instability.[38,65,66] The removal of the posterior elements, however, can disrupt normal biomechanics, leading to destabilization of the spine, and postlaminectomy kyphosis in 11–47% of patients.[67] Delayed neurological deterioration, including recurrence of myelopathy, is also a potential complication due to exuberant scar tissue affecting the cord.[64] Adding instrumentation and fusion can help avoid postlaminectomy instability and kyphosis.[68,69] Fusion should be considered when there is loss of cervical lordosis, signs of instability are present, or in younger patients whose complaints include significant neck pain.[65] In addition to providing immediate stabilization, instrumentation and fusion promotes early mobilization and can eliminate the need for a brace.

The patient is positioned prone with the patient's head fixed in a Mayfield tong. Through a midline cervical incision, the cervical muscles are dissected to expose the spinous processes and laminae. In laminectomy alone, the dissection is carried out laterally just beyond the medial aspect of the facet joint. Care must be taken to not compromise the facet capsules. During decompression, 50% of the facet joints should be preserved to avoid iatrogenic instability.[65,70] If instrumentation is to be added, the dissection is carried out to the lateral margin of the facet for lateral mass screw placement. Lateral mass screws are inserted before laminectomies are performed. The laminectomy is performed at the lamina-facet junction bilaterally (Fig. 43.10).[71]

Short-term postoperative results from a systematic review have shown successful outcomes of cervical laminectomy.[66] However, longer term results show increased risk of postlaminectomy kyphosis and neurological deterioration as compared with other posterior techniques

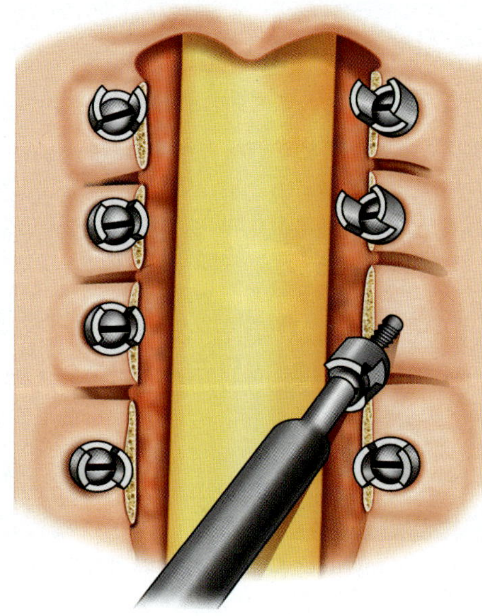

Fig. 43.10: The lateral masses are implanted prior to the osteotomy and the screws are inserted after the removal of the laminae.

such as laminectomy and fusion or laminoplasty. Studies report neurological deterioration, as measured by the Nurick's scale or JOA score, in 10 to 39.4% of patients.[33,52,72-75] Although the development of postlaminectomy kyphosis was not found to diminish outcome,[66] there are other concerns such as scar tissue invasion from the laminectomy site into the spinal canal, with consequent worsening of neurologic symptoms. Such complications have led to the development and use of techniques that preserve the posterior structural elements such as laminoplasty.

LAMINOPLASTY

Recognizing the potential iatrogenic instability and long-term neurological complications associated with laminectomy, laminoplasty was developed as a way to preserve the posterior bony structures of the cervical spine while allowing for decompression of the spinal cord. Oyama et al. performed the first laminoplasty in 1973, consisting of a Z-plasty of the laminae and reconstruction of the posterior arch.[76,77] Since then, several modifications of the technique have been described.

Laminoplasty is a technique in which the laminae are dorsally "lifted" but preserved, thereby enlarging the diameter of the spinal canal and allowing for the posterior drift of the cord.[78] Laminoplasty is indicated in C3–C7 levels in neutral to lordotic cervical spines with multisegmental stenosis. Because the laminae and ligamentum flavum are preserved, risk for iatrogenic instability is minimized.[79-81] Fusion is not routinely required in laminoplasty, although instrumentation and fusion can be performed with the procedure if necessary.

Common laminoplasty techniques to achieve decompression are the single-door (or open-door) technique and the double-door (or French-door) technique. In the single-door technique, the lamina on one side is detached by an osteotomy at the junction of the lateral masses and lamina. On the contralateral side, a trough is created until reaching the ventral cortex of the lamina causing a greenstick fracture. This creates a bone hinge at this site to posteriorly shift the lamina (Figs. 43.11A to D).[82,83] In the original technique described by Hirabayashi et al. stay sutures were used to secure the spinous processes to the facet capsule to maintain the open position of lamina. However, it did not completely avoid the closing down of the hinge, or "spring back" phenomenon. Modern techniques have incorporated different materials to maintain a patent canal, such as bone graft, spacers, or titanium plates (Figs. 43.11 A to D). An advantage to the single-door technique is the relative ease of the procedure in creating the bilateral troughs at the laminofacet junctions in which one becomes the hinge door.[84] Foraminotomies are easily performed on the "open-door" side of the construct.

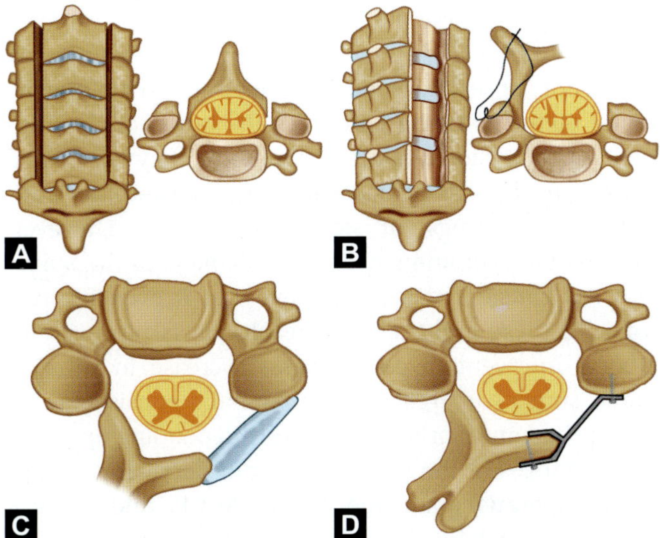

Figs. 43.11A to D: Single-door, or open-door laminoplasty, (A) utilizes multiples osteotomies, one in each of the laminae, (B to D) to create a bone hinge and expand the cervical spinal canal to decompress the neural elements. Multiple techniques for the single-door laminoplasty are currently employed including (B) sutures, (C) bone grafts/spacers, and (D) plates.

Fixation of a spacer, however, by threading it through the lamina, and the medial border of the facet joint is technically challenging. Another disadvantage is that the posterior elements of the spine shift to an asymmetric position as the hinge door opens.[84]

The double-door technique by Kurokawa et al.[85] involves splitting of the spinous processes at the midline. Bilateral troughs are made at the junction of the laminae and the lateral masses, and the two laminar halves are separated laterally. The space between the split spinous processes is maintained by a spacer or graft material (Figs. 43.12A and B). Unlike the single-door technique, this procedure results in a symmetric spine.

Several complications are characteristic of laminoplasty, the most common being postoperative neck pain.[86] Reports of postoperative neck pain from laminoplasty are up to 60%,[87] most of them resolving within a year. Although the etiology is unclear, it is believed to be due to posterior muscle dissection or facet joint disruption. A 30–70% loss of range of motion in the neck has also been described from laminoplasty. Recent data have shown that by preserving the semispinalis cervicis from the C2 spinous process, less cervical brace wear (limited to 2 weeks postoperatively) and early postoperative neck exercises can help preserve range of motion in the neck.[88]

C5 nerve root palsy is another complication associated with laminoplasty with an incidence ranging between 5% and 8%.[89-94] Patients complain of deltoid and bicep weakness, which typically resolves over a few months.[64] It is believed that the palsy is caused by traction on the relatively short C5 nerve root as the decompressed spinal cord shifts posteriorly.[64] Uematsu et al. reported that elevation of the laminae >60° during laminoplasty was associated with a higher risk for C5 palsy.[94] Prophylactic C5 foraminotomy with limited opening of the laminoplasty has been suggested by some authors as a method that may avoid excessive posterior shifting of the spinal cord and subsequent traction on the C5 nerve root.[95,96] However, the clinical usefulness of this procedure has not yet been proven.[97]

In a recent review, outcomes for laminoplasty for CSM showed a 55–60% neurologic recovery rate (as measured by the JOA scale).[97] Laminoplasty has been shown to have a lower complication rate with lower implant costs than laminectomy and fusion.[98] However, outcomes with laminoplasty have not demonstrated superiority over laminectomy and fusion with regard to Nurick's scores,

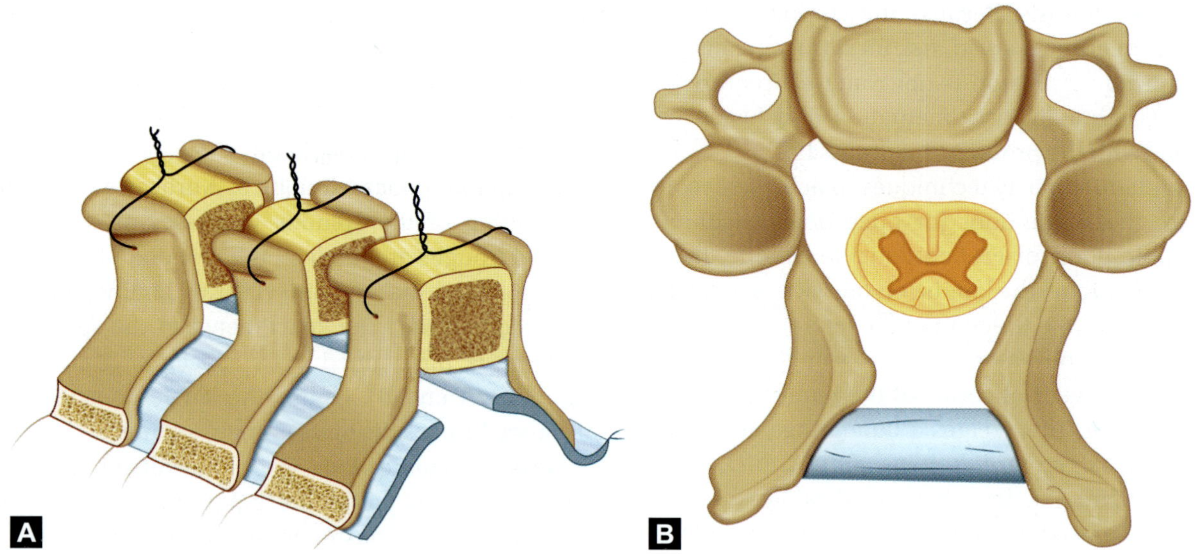

Figs. 43.12A and B: The double-door (or French door), technique uses bone graft to fill the space left by the splitting of the spinous processes, allowing neural elements room to migrate posteriorly reducing compression.

JOA scores, and Odom outcome criteria.[97,98] Also, laminoplasty may not be appropriate for patients with significant neck pain, as laminectomy and fusion appears to be more effective in pain reduction.[98]

POSTERIOR LAMINOFORAMINOTOMY

For single-level cervical radiculopathy resulting from narrowing of the lateral recess from cervical spondylosis or disk herniation, the posterior approach is a viable alternative to an ACDF. A patient with a "reverse Spurling's sign" (where relief of pain is experienced when the neck is flexed and rotated away from the symptomatic side) is considered a good candidate for posterior foraminal decompression because the maneuver enlarges the foramen, thus theoretically reproducing the potential result from a foraminal decompression.[11] There are multiple advantages to this technique—it avoids fusion of a motion segment and also avoids the tracheoesophageal morbidity associated with the anterior approach. However, because this procedure is rather limited in its exposure, there is the possibility for incomplete decompression and recurrence of symptoms. A recent systematic review on cervical laminoforaminotomy for the treatment of cervical degenerative radiculopathy found the treatment to have good to excellent outcomes for arm pain and neurologic deficit as well as for return to baseline activities and employment.[48] In terms of choosing between the anterior and posterior approaches for cervical radiculopathy, current literature does not provide clear answers as to which approach yields better long-term outcomes. The surgeon must always consider the risks and benefits to each approach and procedure, and discuss this thoroughly with the patient.

CONCLUSION

The severity of cervical stenosis depends upon the specific neural elements being compressed. Nerve root entrapment causing radiculopathic symptoms may be treated conservatively with physical therapy, nonsteroidal anti-inflammatory drugs, or steroid medication. However, myelopathic symptoms caused by damage to the spinal cord are considered a progressive and irreversible disorder. In these cases, clinical resolution is rare without surgical intervention as the cases increase in severity. Spinal surgery to treat cervical spinal stenosis may be approached anteriorly or posteriorly depending upon the circumstances of the patient. Anterior cervical decompressive operations include ACDF, ACCF, and cervical arthroplasty, whereas posterior cervical decompressive operations include laminectomy, laminoplasty, and laminoforaminotomy. The literature cites advantages and disadvantages of each, although all of the aforementioned procedures are well established in contemporary spine surgery.

REFERENCES

1. Kumaresan S, Yoganandan N, Pintar FA, et al. Contribution of disc degeneration to osteophyte formation in the cervical spine: a biomechanical investigation. J Orthop Res. 2006;19(5):977-84.
2. Adams CB, Logue V. Studies in cervical spondylotic myelopathy. II. The movement and contour of the spine in relation to the neural complications of cervical spondylosis. Brain. 1971;94(3):568-86.
3. Law MD, Jr, Bernhardt M, White AA, 3rd. Evaluation and management of cervical spondylotic myelopathy. Instr Course Lect. 1995;44:99-110.
4. Kellgren JH, Lawrence JS. Osteo-arthrosis and disk degeneration in an urban population. Ann Rheum Dis. 1958; 17(4):388-97.
5. Gore DR, Sepic SB, Gardner GM. Roentgenographic findings of the cervical spine in asymptomatic people. Spine (Phila Pa 1976). 1986;11(6):521-4.
6. Edwards CC, Riew KD, Anderson PA, et al. Cervical myelopathy: current diagnostic and treatment strategies. Spine J. 2003;3(1):68-81.
7. Boden SD, Davis DO, Dina TS, et al. Abnormal magnetic-resonance scans of the lumbar spine in asymptomatic subjects. A prospective investigation. J Bone Joint Surg Am. 1990;72(3):403-8.
8. Lees F, Turner JW. Natural history and prognosis of cervical spondylosis. Br Med J. 1963;2(5373):1607-10.
9. Clarke E, Robinson PK. Cervical myelopathy: a complication of cervical spondylosis. Brain. 1956;79(3):483-510.
10. Nurick S. The pathogenesis of the spinal cord disorder associated with cervical spondylosis. Brain. 1972;95(1):87-100.
11. Rhee JM, Riew KD. Cervical degenerative disease. In: Flynn J (Ed). Orthopaedic Knowledge Update 10: Spine. Rosemont, IL: American Academy of Orthopaedic Surgeons; 2011. pp. 611-22.
12. Aprill C, Dwyer A, Bogduk N. Cervical zygapophyseal joint pain patterns. II: a clinical evaluation. Spine (Phila Pa 1976). 1990;15(6):458-61.
13. DePalma A, Rothman R, Lewinnek G, et al. Anterior interbody fusion for severe cervical disc degeneration. Surg Gynecol Obstet. 1972;134(5):755.
14. Murphy DR, Hurwitz EL, Gregory A, et al. A nonsurgical approach to the management of patients with cervical radiculopathy: a prospective observational cohort study. J Manipulative Physiol Ther. 2006;29(4):279-87.
15. McCormick WE, Steinmetz MP, Benzel EC. Cervical spondylotic myelopathy: make the difficult diagnosis, then refer for surgery. Cleve Clin J Med. 2003;70(10):899-904.
16. Lebl DR, Hughes A, Cammisa FP, Jr, et al. Cervical spondylotic myelopathy: pathophysiology, clinical presentation, and treatment. HSS J. 2011;7(2):170-8.
17. Edwards WC, LaRocca H. The developmental segmental sagittal diameter of the cervical spinal canal in patients with cervical spondylosis. Spine (Phila Pa 1976). 1983; 8(1):20-7.
18. Morishita Y, Naito M, Hymanson H, et al. The relationship between the cervical spinal canal diameter and the pathological changes in the cervical spine. Eur Spine J. 2009;18(6):877-83.
19. Hochman M, Tuli S. Cervical spondylotic myelopathy: a review. Internet Journal of Urology. 2005;2(2):14-33.
20. Chen IH, Vasavada A, Panjabi MM. Kinematics of the cervical spine canal: changes with sagittal plane loads. J Spinal Disord. 1994;7(2):93-101.
21. Barre JA. Troubles pyramidaux et arthrite vertebrale chronique. Medecine. 1924;3:58-60.
22. Breig A, Turnbull I, Hassler O. Effects of mechanical stresses on the spinal cord in cervical spondylosis. A study on fresh cadaver material. J Neurosurg. 1966;25(1):45-56.
23. Ito T, Oyanagi K, Takahashi H, et al. Cervical spondylotic myelopathy. Clinicopathologic study on the progression pattern and thin myelinated fibers of the lesions of seven patients examined during complete autopsy. Spine (Phila Pa 1976). 1996;21(7):827-33.
24. Ogino H, Tada K, Okada K, et al. Canal diameter, anteroposterior compression ratio, and spondylotic myelopathy of the cervical spine. Spine (Phila Pa 1976). 1983;8(1):1-15.
25. Ono K, Ota H, Tada K, et al. Ossified posterior longitudinal ligament: a clinicopathologic study. Spine. 1977;2:126-38.
26. Ono K, Ebara S, Fuji T, et al. Myelopathy hand. New clinical signs of cervical cord damage. J Bone Joint Surg Br. 1987;69(2):215-9.
27. Rao R. Neck pain, cervical radiculopathy, and cervical myelopathy: pathophysiology, natural history, and clinical evaluation. J Bone Joint Surg Am. 2002;84-A(10):1872-81.
28. Mummaneni PV, Kaiser MG, Matz PG, et al. Preoperative patient selection with magnetic resonance imaging, computed tomography, and electroencephalography: does the test predict outcome after cervical surgery? J Neurosurg Spine. 2009;11(2):119-29.
29. Rao RD, Currier BL, Albert TJ, et al. Degenerative cervical spondylosis: clinical syndromes, pathogenesis, and management. J Bone Joint Surg. 2007;89-A(6):1360-78.
30. Bednarik J, Kadanka Z, Vohanka S, et al. The value of somatosensory and motor evoked evoked potentials in preclinical spondylotic cervical cord compression. Eur Spine J. 1998;7 (6):493-500.
31. Nardin RA, Patel MR, Gudas TF, et al. Electromyography and magnetic resonance imaging in the evaluation of radiculopathy. Muscle Nerve. 1999;22(2):151-5.
32. Hukuda S, Mochizuki T, Ogata M, et al. Operations for cervical spondylotic myelopathy. A comparison of the results of anterior and posterior procedures. J Bone Joint Surg Br. 1985;67(4):609-15.
33. Ebersold MJ, Pare MC, Quast LM. Surgical treatment for cervical spondylotic myelopathy. J Neurosurg. 1995;82(5): 745-51.
34. Chiles BW, 3rd, Leonard MA, Choudhri HF, et al. Cervical spondylotic myelopathy: patterns of neurological deficit and recovery after anterior cervical decompression. Neurosurgery. 1999;44(4):762-9; discussion 769-70.

35. Sampath P, Bendebba M, Davis JD, et al. Outcome of patients treated for cervical myelopathy. A prospective, multicenter study with independent clinical review. Spine (Phila Pa 1976). 2000;25(6):670-6.
36. Kadanka Z, Mares M, Bednanik J, et al. Approaches to spondylotic cervical myelopathy: conservative versus surgical results in a 3-year follow-up study. Spine (Phila Pa 1976). 2002;27(20):2205-10; discussion 2210-1.
37. Kadanka Z, Bednarik J, Novotny O, et al. Cervical spondylotic myelopathy: conservative versus surgical treatment after 10 years. Eur Spine J. 2011;20(9):1533-8.
38. Rao RD, Gourab K, David KS. Operative treatment of cervical spondylotic myelopathy. J Bone Joint Surg Am. 2006;88(7):1619-40.
39. Baba H, Maezawa Y, Furusawa N, et al. Flexibility and alignment of the cervical spine after laminoplasty for spondylotic myelopathy. A radiographic study. Int Orthop. 1995;19 (2):116-21.
40. Suda K, Abumi K, Ito M, et al. Local kyphosis reduces surgical outcomes of expansive open-door laminoplasty for cervical spondylotic myelopathy. Spine (Phila Pa 1976). 2003;28(12):1258-62.
41. Satomi K, Nishu Y, Kohno T, et al. Long-term follow-up studies of open-door expansive laminoplasty for cervical stenotic myelopathy. Spine (Phila Pa 1976). 1994;19(5):507-10.
42. Lunsford LD, Bissonette DJ, Jannetta PJ, et al. Anterior surgery for cervical disc disease. Part 1: treatment of lateral cervical disc herniation in 253 cases. J Neurosurg. 1980; 53(1):1-11.
43. Robinson RA, Walker AE, Ferlic DC, et al. The results of anterior interbody fusion of the cervical spine. J Bone Joint Surg (American). 1962;44(8):1569-87.
44. Boni M, Cherubino P, Denaro V, et al. Multiple subtotal somatectomy. Technique and evaluation of a series of 39 cases. Spine (Phila Pa 1976). 1984;9(4):358-62.
45. Brigham CD, Tsahakis PJ. Anterior cervical foraminotomy and fusion. Surgical technique and results. Spine (Phila Pa 1976). 1995;20(7):766-70.
46. Riley LH, 3rd, Vaccaro AR, Dettori JR, et al. Postoperative dysphagia in anterior cervical spine surgery. Spine (Phila Pa 1976). 2010;35(9 Suppl):S76-85.
47. Bazaz R, Lee MJ, Yoo JU. Incidence of dysphagia after anterior cervical spine surgery: a prospective study. Spine (Phila Pa 1976). 2002;27(22):2453-8.
48. Heary RF, Ryken TC, Matz PG, et al. Cervical laminoforaminotomy for the treatment of cervical degenerative radiculopathy. J Neurosurg Spine. 2009;11(2):198-202.
49. Robinson RA. Anterolateral cervical disc removal and interbody fusion for the cervical disc syndrome. Bull John Hopkins Hosp. 1955;96:223-4.
50. Hoppenfeld S, Hutton R, Thomas H. Physical examination of the spine and extremities. East Norwalk, CT: Appleton-Century-Crofts; 1976.
51. Tew JM, Jr, Mayfield FH. Complications of surgery of the anterior cervical spine. Clin Neurosurg. 1976;23:424-34.
52. Yonenobu K, Okada K, Fuji T, et al. Causes of neurologic deterioration following surgical treatment of cervical myelopathy. Spine (Phila Pa 1976). 1986;11(8):818-23.
53. Daniels AH, Riew KD, Yoo JU, et al. Adverse events associated with anterior cervical spine surgery. J Am Acad Orthop Surg. 2008;16(12):729-38.
54. Winslow CP, Winslow TJ, Wax MK. Dysphonia and dysphagia following the anterior approach to the cervical spine. Arch Otolaryngol Head Neck Surg. 2001;127(1):51-5.
55. Hilibrand AS, Carlson GD, Palumbo MA, et al. Radiculopathy and myelopathy at segments adjacent to the site of a previous anterior cervical arthrodesis. J Bone Joint Surg Am. 1999;81(4):519-28.
56. Wang JC, McDonough PW, Endow K, et al. The effect of cervical plating on single-level anterior cervical discectomy and fusion. J Spinal Disord. 1999;12(6):467-71.
57. Martin GJ, Jr, Haid RW, Jr, MacMilan M, et al. Anterior cervical discectomy with freeze-dried fibula allograft. Overview of 317 cases and literature review. Spine (Phila Pa 1976). 1999;24(9):852-8; discussion 858-9.
58. Samartzis D, Shen FH, Goldberg EJ, et al. Is autograft the gold standard in achieving radiographic fusion in one-level anterior cervical discectomy and fusion with rigid anterior plate fixation? Spine (Phila Pa 1976). 2005;30(15):1756-61.
59. Song KJ, Taghavi CE, Lee KB, et al. The efficacy of plate construct augmentation versus cage alone in anterior cervical fusion. Spine (Phila Pa 1976). 2009;34(26):2886-92.
60. Nassr A, Eck JC, Ponnappan RK, et al. The incidence of C5 palsy after multilevel cervical decompression procedures: a review of 750 consecutive cases. Spine (Phila Pa 1976). 2012;37(3):174-8.
61. Emery SE, Bohlman HH, Bolesta MJ, et al. Anterior cervical decompression and arthrodesis for the treatment of cervical spondylotic myelopathy. Two to seventeen-year follow-up. J Bone Joint Surg Am. 1998;80(7):941-51.
62. Matz PG, Holly LT, Groff MW, et al. Indications for anterior cervical decompression for the treatment of cervical degenerative radiculopathy. J Neurosurg Spine. 2009;11(2): 174-82.
63. Boselie TF, Willems PC, van Mameren H, et al. Arthroplasty versus fusion in single-level cervical degenerative disc disease. Cochrane Database Syst Rev. 2012;9:CD009173.
64. Rhee JM, Riew KD. Cervical spondylotic myelopathy: including ossification of the posterior longitudinal ligament. In: Spivak JM, Connolly PJ (Eds). Orthopaedic Knowledge Update: Spine 3. Rosemont, IL: American Academy of Orthopaedic Surgeons; 2006. pp. 235-49.
65. McAllister BD, Rebholz BJ, Wang JC. Is posterior fusion necessary with laminectomy in the cervical spine? Surg Neurol Int. 2012;3(Suppl 3):S225-31.
66. Ryken TC, Heary RF, Matz PG, et al. Cervical laminectomy for the treatment of cervical degenerative myelopathy. J Neurosurg Spine. 2009;11(2):142-9.
67. Techy F, Bell GR. Laminectomy. In: Mandell BF (Ed). Perioperative Management of Patients with Rheumatic Disease. New York: Springer; 2013. p. 301.
68. Huang RC, Girardi FP, Poynton AR, et al. Treatment of multilevel cervical spondylotic myeloradiculopathy with posterior decompression and fusion with lateral mass plate fixation and local bone graft. J Spinal Disord Tech. 2003;16(2):123-9.

69. Sekhon LH. Posterior cervical decompression and fusion for circumferential spondylotic cervical stenosis: review of 50 consecutive cases. J Clin Neurosci. 2006;13(1):23-30.
70. Zdeblick TA, Zou D, Warden KE, et al. Cervical stability after foraminotomy. A biomechanical in vitro analysis. J Bone Joint Surg Am. 1992;74(1):22-7.
71. Komotar RJ, Mocco J, Kaiser MG. Surgical management of cervical myelopathy: indications and techniques for laminectomy and fusion. Spine J. 2006;6(6 Suppl):252S-67S.
72. Arnold H, Feldmann U, Missler U. Chronic spondylogenic cervical myelopathy. A critical evaluation of surgical treatment after early and long-term follow-up. Neurosurg Rev. 1993;16(2):105-9.
73. Kato Y, Iwasaki M, Fuji T, et al. Long-term follow-up results of laminectomy for cervical myelopathy caused by ossification of the posterior longitudinal ligament. J Neurosurg. 1998;89(2):217-23.
74. Snow RB, Weiner H. Cervical laminectomy and foraminotomy as surgical treatment of cervical spondylosis: a follow-up study with analysis of failures. J Spinal Disord. 1993;6(3):245-50; discussion 250-1.
75. Yonenobu K, Fuji T, Ono K, et al. Choice of surgical treatment for multisegmental cervical spondylotic myelopathy. Spine. 1985;10(8):710.
76. Oyama M, Hattori S, Moriwaki N, et al. A new method of cervical laminectomy. Chubu Nippon Seikeigeka Gakkai Zasshi. 1973;16:792-94.
77. Kawai S, Sunago K, Doi K, et al. Cervical laminoplasty (Hattori's method). Procedure and follow-up results. Spine (Phila Pa 1976). 1988;13(11):1245-50.
78. Aita I, Hayashi K, Wadano Y, et al. Posterior movement and enlargement of the spinal cord after cervical laminoplasty. J Bone Joint Surg Br. 1998;80(1):33-7.
79. Shaffrey CI, Wiggins GC, Piccirilli CB, et al. Modified open-door laminoplasty for treatment of neurological deficits in younger patients with congenital spinal stenosis: analysis of clinical and radiographic data. J Neurosurg. 1999;90 (2 Suppl):170-7.
80. Mikawa Y, Shikata J, Yamamuro T. Spinal deformity and instability after multilevel cervical laminectomy. Spine (Phila Pa 1976). 1987;12(1):6-11.
81. Ishida Y, Suzuki K, Ohmori K, et al. Critical analysis of extensive cervical laminectomy. Neurosurgery. 1989;24 (2):215-22.
82. Hirabayashi K, Watanabe K, Wakano K, et al. Expansive open-door laminoplasty for cervical spinal stenotic myelopathy. Spine (Phila Pa 1976). 1983;8(7):693-9.
83. Hirabayashi K, Satomi K. Operative procedure and results of expansive open-door laminoplasty. Spine (Phila Pa 1976). 1988;13(7):870-6.
84. Hirabayashi S, Yamada H, Motosuneya T, et al. Comparison of enlargement of the spinal canal after cervical laminoplasty: open-door type and double-door type. Euro Spine J. 2010;19(10):1690-4.
85. Kurokawa T, Tsuyama N, Tanaka H. Enlargement of spinal canal by the sagittal splitting of the spinous process. Bessatsu Seikeigeka. 1982;2(2):234-40.
86. Hosono N, Yonenobu K, Ono K. Neck and shoulder pain after laminoplasty. A noticeable complication. Spine (Phila Pa 1976). 1996;21(17):1969-73.
87. Ratliff JK, Cooper PR. Cervical laminoplasty: a critical review. J Neurosurg. 2003;98(3 Suppl):230-8.
88. Machino M, Yukawa Y, Hida T, et al. Cervical alignment and range of motion after laminoplasty: radiographical data from more than 500 cases with cervical spondylotic myelopathy and a review of the literature. Spine (Phila Pa 1976). 2012;37(20):E1243-50.
89. Iwasaki M, Kawaguchi Y, Kimura T, et al. Long-term results of expansive laminoplasty for ossification of the posterior longitudinal ligament of the cervical spine: more than 10 years follow up. J Neurosurg. 2002;96(2 Suppl):180-9.
90. Ogawa Y, Toyama Y, Chiba K, et al. Long-term results of expansive open-door laminoplasty for ossification of the posterior longitudinal ligament of the cervical spine. J Neurosurg Spine. 2004;1(2):168-74.
91. Satomi K, Ogawa J, Ishii Y, et al. Short-term complications and long-term results of expansive open-door laminoplasty for cervical stenotic myelopathy. Spine J. 2001;1(1):26-30.
92. Wada E, Suzuki S, Kanazawa A, et al. Subtotal corpectomy versus laminoplasty for multilevel cervical spondylotic myelopathy: a long-term follow-up study over 10 years. Spine (Phila Pa 1976). 2001;26(13):1443-7; discussion 1448.
93. Yonenobu K, Hosono N, Iwasaki M, et al. Laminoplasty versus subtotal corpectomy. A comparative study of results in multisegmental cervical spondylotic myelopathy. Spine (Phila Pa 1976). 1992;17(11):1281-4.
94. Uematsu Y, Tokuhashi Y, Matsuzaki H. Radiculopathy after laminoplasty of the cervical spine. Spine (Phila Pa 1976). 1998;23(19):2057-62.
95. Sasai K, Saito T, Akagi S, et al. Preventing C5 palsy after laminoplasty. Spine (Phila Pa 1976). 2003;28(17):1972-7.
96. Komagata M, Nishiyama M, Endo K, et al. Prophylaxis of C5 palsy after cervical expansive laminoplasty by bilateral partial foraminotomy. Spine J. 2004;4(6):650-5.
97. Matz PG, Anderson PA, Groff MW, et al. Cervical laminoplasty for the treatment of cervical degenerative myelopathy. J Neurosurg Spine. 2009;11(2):157-69.
98. Highsmith JM, Dhall SS, Haid RW, Jr, et al. Treatment of cervical stenotic myelopathy: a cost and outcome comparison of laminoplasty versus laminectomy and lateral mass fusion. J Neurosurg Spine. 2011;14(5):619-25.

CHAPTER

44 Operative Management of Degenerative Cervical Disorders

Hiroyuki Yoshihara, John A Bendo

INTRODUCTION

Cervical spondylosis, also referred to as cervical degenerative disease, is among the most common spinal ailments encountered in elderly people. The pathophysiology of cervical degenerative disk disease includes imbalance in the proteoglycan composition leading to intervertebral disk dehydration and subsequent desiccation and cracking. The pathophysiology of degenerative changes has been described in detail in Chapter 1. As intervertebral disk degeneration progresses, the disks become less capable of load bearing and as a consequence exert additional mechanical load stress on adjacent structures, including the facet joints and vertebral bodies. At levels of advanced degeneration, imbalanced strain forces between contacting surfaces of adjacent bony structures result in new bone formation and development of osteophytes, bony ridges, and spurs. In addition, the ligamentum flavum hypertrophies posterior to the spinal cord, narrowing the spinal canal, and this might cause impingement of nerve roots and/or the spinal cord.

Depending on phase of disease progression, cervical spondylosis may cause symptoms of neck pain, radiculopathy, and/or myelopathy. Mechanical neck pain is the most common symptom. However, there is poor correlation between radiologically defined spondylosis and neck pain. For example, some patients can have severe spondylosis on imaging studies without having any symptoms at all. Pain due to cervical spondylosis might come from a variety of sources like new bone formation in the facets or vertebral bodies, or the degenerating disk (discogenic pain). Compression of the nerve roots or the spinal cord might result in manifestation of symptoms of radiculopathy and myelopathy, respectively.

Ossification of the posterior longitudinal ligament (OPLL) is a hyperostotic spinal condition associated with neurological deficit. The pathogenesis of OPLL is not clearly understood. OPLL generally is seen in patients > 40 years of age and is not common before the third decade of life. In Asian countries, the prevalence of OPLL has been 1.9 to 4.3% among individuals > 30 years of age.[1-3] In North American populations, it appears that the disease prevalence is much lower. The rate of classic disease in Caucasian individuals from North America is 0.12%.[4]

As the disease progresses, narrowing of spinal cord causes compression of the spinal cord and symptoms of myelopathy. It has been estimated that up to 25% of Caucasian patients presenting with cervical myelopathy have OPLL.[5] The investigation committee on the ossification of the spinal ligaments of the Japanese Ministry of Public Health and Welfare classified OPLL into four major groups: continuous type, segmental type, mixed type, and other type (Figs. 44.1A to D).[6]

SURGICAL INDICATIONS

Surgery is indicated in patients with radicular pain and demonstrated root compression on imaging studies, where the pain and/or neurological deficit reduce the quality of life and nonsurgical treatments have not been beneficial.

The primary indication for surgery in patients with OPLL is progressive myelopathy, which usually is manifested by

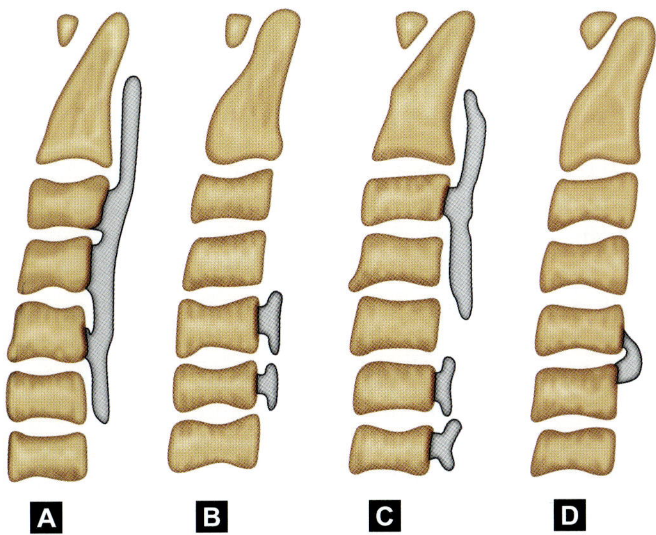

Figs. 44.1A to D: Classification of ossification of the posterior longitudinal ligament by the Investigation Committee on the Ossification of the Spinal Ligaments, Japanese Ministry of Public Health and Welfare. (A) Continuous type; continuous ossification over several vertebral bodies. (B) Segmental type; segmental ossification of one or more vertebral bodies. (C) Mixed type; continuous type ossification associated with segmental type. (D) Other type; ossification of intervertebral disk level. *Source*: Reprinted with permission from Matsunaga et al.[6]

considerable numbness, weakness of the upper extremity, and a spastic gait. Without surgical decompression, symptomatic OPLL tends to progress with time. In a long-term follow-up study, Matsunaga et al.[7] demonstrated that 38% of patients presenting with baseline myelopathy had progressive worsening of their symptoms. Preventative surgery for OPLL in asymptomatic patients is controversial because of the inherent risks, although asymptomatic patients with significant canal stenosis caused by OPLL can develop severe acute neurological deficits in association with relatively minor cervical injury.

In a systematic review, it has been recommended that operative therapy be offered to cervical spondylotic myelopathy (CSM) patients with severe and/or long lasting symptoms, because the likelihood of improvement with nonoperative measures is low (Class III).[8]

Patients with axial pain, who have a one- or two-level disease on imaging studies and have exhausted nonsurgical treatment options, quite often respond well to surgery. These patients should have a confirmatory test, usually a positive response to facet injections, to be sure the abnormalities on the imaging studies are the source of the pain. Satisfactory pain relief can be expected in a moderate number of well-selected patients.

SURGICAL OPTIONS

The surgical options include cervical decompression and fusion, cervical corpectomy and fusion, total disk replacement (TDR), cervical laminoforaminotomy, laminectomy with/without fusion, or laminoplasty. The surgical approach can be anterior, posterior, or a combination of both, depending on the site of pathology. Frequently, patients have a combination of pain and neurologic deficit, and the surgical plan should take these factors into consideration, in addition to the condition of the bone, spinal alignment, and adjacent segments.

Anterior Cervical Decompression and Fusion (ACDF)

Anterior cervical decompression and fusion is indicated when a spondylotic bony spur is causing radiculopathy, myelopathy, or intolerable intractable neck pain. This procedure is rarely indicated for OPLL due to risk of potential complications like dural atresia and cerebrospinal fluid (CSF) leakage.

A standard Smith-Robinson approach[9] via the carotid triangle is used, which allows access C2–T1 spinal segments. The incision may be made transversely or obliquely, depending on the target levels. Anatomical landmarks include the hyoid bone overlying C3, thyroid cartilage overlying C4–5 interspace, and cricothyroid membrane for the C5–6 level. The platysma is incised either longitudinally or transversely. Blunt dissection is done along the medial border of sternocleidomastoid muscle, and both sides of the longus colli muscle are identified. The carotid sheath and associated vessels are gently retracted laterally. The midline structures, such as esophagus, trachea, and thyroid gland, are retracted medially with care. Excessive retraction might result in esophageal and recurrent laryngeal nerve injury resulting in hoarseness. Verification of the level is done through fluoroscopy, and the retractor blades are carefully inserted under the longus colli muscle. Discectomies are performed through the anterior longitudinal ligament and anterior annulus, and the intervertebral disk is completely removed. Along the posterior aspect, a small curette or 1-mm Kerrison rongeur may be used to remove the disk and bony spur. After decompression is achieved, the end plates are prepared for fusion. Appropriately, sized bone graft or cage and then plate fixation are applied.

Anterior Cervical Corpectomy and Fusion (ACCF)

Anterior cervical corpectomy and fusion is indicated when spondylotic bony compression-causing myelopathy is located posterior to the vertebral body necessitating partial or complete corpectomy, i.e. removal of vertebral body (Fig. 44.2). The majority of patients with OPLL present with multilevel cervical disease that often requires extensive decompression with ACCF.

As in ACDF, a standard Smith-Robinson approach is utilized. Once adequate exposure is achieved, discectomies are performed above and below each intended corpectomy level. Corpectomy is performed using a small rongeur or high-speed drill to create a trough in the center of the vertebral body and is extended posteriorly to the posterior cortex. The lateral walls of the vertebral body are left intact to protect the vertebral artery. Bone wax on a Penfield may be used to stop bleeding. As the posterior cortex is thinned, a small curette or 1-mm Kerrison rongeur may be used to carefully remove the cortex. In cases of OPLL with severe dural ossification, the "anterior floating method"[10] can be used, where central areas of densely ossified ligament, and dura are detached laterally and superoinferiorly from the surrounding posterior longitudinal ligament. This results in a "floating" ossified island of bone that will move freely and does not compress the cord. With the decompression complete, end-plate cartilage is removed with a curette to achieve adequate fusion. The intended strut graft is measured with the disk space distracted. Various grafts and cage devices can be used for corpectomy defects. Plate fixation is then applied.

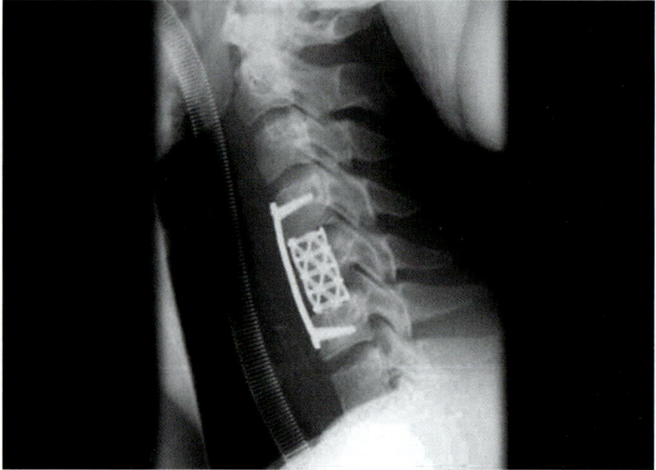

Fig. 44.2: Cervical lateral X-ray shows C5 corpectomy.
Source: Reprinted with permission from Nakase H, Park YS, Kimura H, Sakaki T, Morimoto T. Complications and long-term follow-up results in titanium mesh cage reconstruction after cervical corpectomy. J Spinal Disord Tech. 2006;19(5):353-7.

Total Disk Replacement

Total disk replacement may be advantageous in avoiding complications like dysphagia from anterior plate fixation and adjacent spinal segment disease after cervical fusion. TDR has been approved by the Food and Drug Administration (FDA) for single-level cervical disease causing either radiculopathy or myelopathy. Usually, TDR has favorable outcomes when the facet joints are relatively well preserved, and the spinal alignment is relatively normal. The artificial disk, therefore, has limited utility in patients with advanced spondylosis. In addition, cervical instability and OPLL are contraindications to TDR.

Similar to ACDF and ACCF, a standard Smith-Robinson approach is used. Once adequate exposure is achieved, the intervertebral disk is removed and the cartilaginous end plates of the vertebral bodies are prepared. No part of the vertebral body is removed so as to prevent postoperative implant subsidence. However, posterior impinging osteophytes are removed. It is vital to adequately releasing the posterior annulus fibrosus to allow correct positioning and functioning of the prosthesis. The proper size and lordotic angle are determined with anteroposterior or lateral fluoroscopy and ensure proper spinal implant placement.

Posterior Cervical Laminoforaminotomy

Laminoforaminotomy is primarily indicated for patients with radiculopathy without significant neck pain due to foraminal stenosis and/or herniated disk(s). However, this procedure is not indicated for OPLL. The advantage of this procedure is that dissection is minimal and segmental motion is preserved.

After the appropriate interspace is identified and exposed, a 1-mm Kerrison rongeur is used to create a small laminotomy. Half of this laminotomy is made on the superior lamina, and the other half is on the inferior lamina, forming the circular portion of a keyhole. The exiting nerve root is then palpated with a fine dental probe, which allows the surgeon to identify the pathway for the foraminotomy. A high-speed drill with a 3-mm tip is used to thin the bone over the nerve root. Because the nerve root exits between the laminae, the drilling straddles the facet joint. Superior and inferior extension of the drilling process is done from pedicle to pedicle. The majority of the facet joint should be preserved to maintain stability.

Once the bone is thinned adequately, a fine-angled curette or a 1-mm Kerrison rongeur is used to remove the layer of the remaining bone over the nerve root.

Laminectomy

Laminectomy is done to indirectly decompress the most severe area of cervical spinal stenosis. This allows the cord to migrate dorsally away from areas of anterior compression. Laminectomy is indicated to treat patients with multilevel spinal stenosis due to spondylotic disease and OPLL. Good outcomes are obtained in lordotic cervical spine.

Laminectomy is done through a midline posterior cervical incision. A subperiosteal dissection of the underlying ligaments and paracervical muscles exposes the spinous processes as well as laminae of the subaxial cervical spine. Laminectomy is performed by creating two bony troughs through the lateral lamina at the junction of the lamina and bony lateral mass using a high-speed drill and removing the lamina using a 1-mm Kerrison rongeur.

Laminectomy with Fusion

Laminectomy with fusion (Figs. 44.3A and B) is indicated for multilevel spinal stenosis due to spondylotic disease and OPLL with instability or loss of cervical alignment.

There are multiple fusion techniques that can be used, including facet wiring, lateral mass screws, and pedicles screws. Placement of screw trajectories prior to decompression maintains familiar landmarks, eases attainment of correct trajectories, and is safer. Satisfactory placement of the screws is confirmed using intraoperative fluoroscopy. Both lateral mass screws and pedicle screws have demonstrated to have sufficient stability and high fusion rates. Pedicle screw placement in the mid-cervical spine (C3–6) is not approved by FDA due to the inherent risk, although it is a common procedure in some Asian countries.

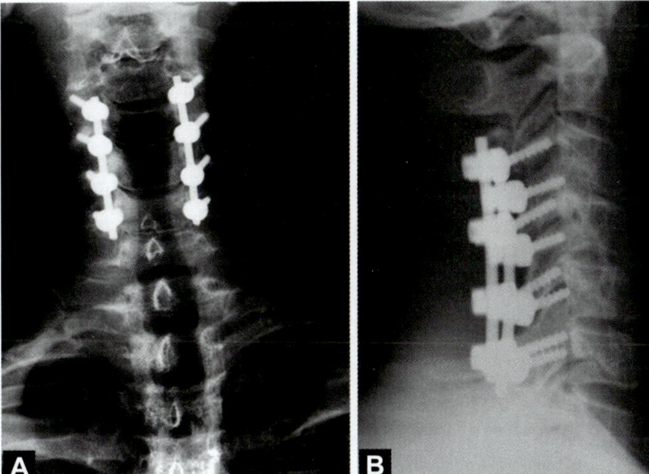

Figs. 44.3A and B: (A) Anteroposterior and (B) lateral postoperative C-spine radiographs of a patient who underwent decompression with laminectomy and C3 to C6 lateral mass fixation.
Source: Reprinted with permission Katonis P, Papadakis SA, Galanakos S, Paskou D, Bano A, Sapkas G, Hadjipavlou AG. Lateral mass screw complications: analysis of 1662 screws. J Spinal Disord Tech. 2011;24(7):415-20.

Laminoplasty

Hirabayashi and Satomi[11] first reported cervical laminoplasty as an alternative to laminectomy in patients with myelopathy. Laminoplasty (Figs. 44.4 and 44.5) is best

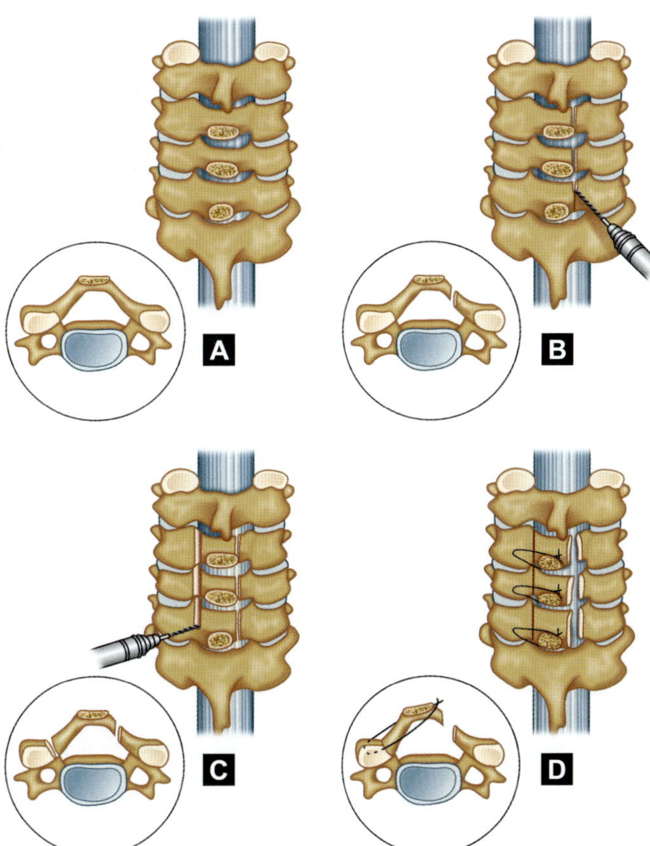

Figs. 44.4A to D: The Hirabayashi-type "open-door" laminoplasty technique. (A) After the spinous processes are removed, (B) bone troughs are created at both laminae–lateral mass junctions using a high-speed drill. (C) The trough is left incomplete on the contralateral side. (D) The hemilamina is elevated and fixed to the ipsilateral facet or surrounding musculature with sutures, maintaining patency of the canal.
Source: Reprinted with permission from Ratliff and Cooper[14] and from Hale JJ, Gruson KI, Spivak JM. Laminoplasty: a review of its role in compressive cervical myelopathy. Spine J. 2006;6(6 Suppl):289S-98S.

used to treat patients with multilevel spinal stenosis due to spondylotic disease and OPLL. It offers dorsal decompression of the cervical spine without decreasing stability. Another theoretical advantage of the technique is that laminoplasty avoids the development of the post-laminectomy membrane and delays the onset of recurrent stenosis.[12] Laminoplasty for CSM is best indicated for patients with local kyphosis <13°.[13] Multiple different approaches have been developed for cervical laminoplasty. These include the "open-door" hinge, the midline "French-door", and the Z-plasty techniques.[11,14] Each technique is aimed to allow expansion of the cervical canal with simultaneous preservation of a dorsal laminar cover.

"Open-door" laminoplasty technique was originally described by Hirabayashi and Satomi.[11] This involves a standard dorsal exposure that includes the lamina and extends out to the facets bilaterally. A high-speed drill is used to make a unilateral bony trough on one side through the lateral lamina at the junction of the lamina and bony lateral mass. This is the "open door" side of the laminoplasty, which conveniently allows for nerve root decompression. On the contralateral side, the drill is used to create a "greenstick" fracture and the "hinge" side of the trough is only developed to partial depth. Gentle tension is then applied with a Kocher or similar instrument and allows the spinous process and laminar complex to be hinged dorsally, away from the thecal sac. This effectively increases the volume of the cervical canal. The decompression is then maintained with the application of titanium miniplates in the modified technique.

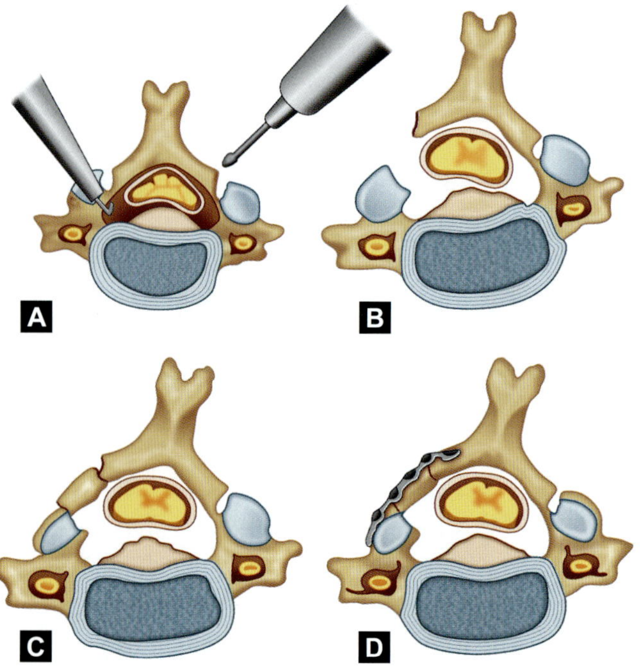

Figs. 44.5A to D: The use of titanium miniplates in maintaining canal patency after laminoplasty. (A and B) The technique follows that described for the "open-door" laminoplasty, except for the final steps. (C) Typically, a piece of allograft is notched at both ends to allow for more secure fit to the hinged hemilaminae. (D) A miniplate is contoured to the lateral mass and hinged posterior elements and secured with screws to maintain canal patency.

Source: Reprinted with permission from Shaffrey CI, Wiggins GC, Piccirilli CB, et al. Modified open-door laminoplasty for treatment of neurological deficits in younger patients with congenital spinal stenosis: analysis of clinical and radiographic data. J Neurosurg Spine. 1999;90:170–7.

Modified from O'Brien MF, Peterson D, Casey ATH, Crockard HA. A novel technique for laminoplasty augmentation of spinal canal area using titanium miniplate stabilization: a computerized morphometric analysis. Spine. 1996;21:474–83.

SURGICAL OUTCOMES

Cervical Spondylosis

Surgical intervention for intractable radiculopathy and progressive myelopathy have shown good to excellent results.[15,16] Cervical myelopathy secondary to a large central disk herniation with acute neurologic deterioration responds exceptionally well to urgent decompressive surgery. In the case of long-standing (>1 year) symptoms secondary to CSM, surgery serves to halt the progression of the disease, although there may be minimal clinical improvement in this situation. However, a recent Cochrane review[17] suggested that there was not sufficient evidence from controlled trials to support surgical treatment of patients with spondylotic radiculopathy or myelopathy. There is low-quality evidence from one trial[18] comprising 81 patients that surgery appears to provide pain relief faster in patients who suffer from cervical radiculopathy, compared with physiotherapy or hard collar immobilization. There is very low quality evidence from one trial[19] (68 patients) that patients with mild myelopathy feel subjectively better after surgery, but there was no evidence of benefit for up to 3 years, objectively. It is not clear whether the short-term risks of surgery are offset by any long-term benefits.[17]

A variety of techniques have improved functional outcome after surgical treatment for CSM, including ACDF, ACCF, laminoplasty, laminectomy, and laminectomy with fusion (Class III).[20] Cervical laminoplasty is recommended in the treatment of myelopathy in the setting of CSM or OPLL. Using the Japanese Orthopaedic Association (JOA) scale, 55–60% recovery rate is anticipated

(Class III).[21] However, laminectomy for CSM is associated with late deterioration compared with the other types of anterior and posterior surgeries (Class III).[20] Multilevel T2 hyperintensity, T1 focal hypointensity combined with T2 focal hyperintensity, and spinal cord atrophy convey poor prognosis (Class III).[22]

OPLL

The long-term outcomes of laminoplasty seem to be favorable, although late neurological deterioration has been noted in some patients. In studies of open-door laminoplasty for OPLL with a long-term follow-up period (>5 years), the recovery rates varied from 47.9% to 63.1% in JOA scores.[23-27] Neurological improvement rates in anterior approaches for cervical OPLL varied from 51% to 71.7%.[28-30] Although progression of OPLL after posterior decompression is of concern, symptomatic recurrence of OPLL is rare, and the frequency of symptomatic progression is <1%.[31,32]

COMPLICATIONS

Approach-related Injuries

Anterior approach-related injuries to the soft tissue structures of the neck are well known. The most common complications include dysphagia and odynophagia. Uncommon complications include temporary or permanent, recurrent laryngeal or superior laryngeal nerve injury, vertebral artery injury, esophageal perforation, and soft tissue swelling that constricts the airway, which necessitates prolonged intubation or tracheostomy.[33]

With regard to posterior approach-related complications, significant postoperative muscular spasm and pain is not uncommon. In a meta-analysis evaluating the outcomes after laminoplasty, the overall incidence of neck pain ranged from 6% to 60% without apparent dependence on the specific variations of laminoplasty.[34] However, meticulous realignment of muscles and early range of motion exercise can decrease the pain.[35,36]

Dural Injury

In cases of OPLL, the anterior approach presents a significant risk of dural injury and subsequent CSF leak. Epstein[37] reported that this can occur in up to 35% of patients treated with anterior corpectomy for advanced OPLL. In the systematic analysis, Li and Dai[38] reported that the incidence of CSF leak in OPLL patients treated surgically was approximately 5.1%. The "anterior floating method"[10] described above might help prevent this complication. However, if a CSF leak is encountered, a lumbar drain may be placed and drainage maintained for 5–7 days for sealing of the dura.[39]

C5 Palsy

Postoperative upper extremity paresis is a well-known and troubling complication after cervical decompression surgery. There are several potential pathophysiologies, which include tethering of nerve root and localized reperfusion spinal cord injury.[40] Paresis of not only the C5 nerve but also of the other cervical nerves (C6–8) can occur in isolation or combination. Some patients with postoperative C5 palsy present primarily with sensory deficits and/or severe pain. In an analysis of multiple reports, Sakaura et al.[41] found the average incidence of postoperative C5 palsy to be 4.6% (range 0–30%). The frequency of this complication did not appear to correlate with the direction (anterior vs posterior) or exact type of approach. The average incidence was 4.3% for anterior decompressive techniques, and there was a similar rate, 4.7%, for laminoplasty. However, patients with postoperative C5 palsy generally have a good prognosis for functional recovery.

Postlaminectomy Kyphosis

The incidence of kyphotic change after multilevel laminectomy has been reported to be between 21% and 47% in larger retrospective series.[42,43] Facet injury is the most important contributor to postoperative kyphosis. When the degree of facetectomy approaches 50%, significant kyphosis and resultant instability may ensue.[44]

Other Complications

Similar to other spine surgeries, iatrogenic neurological injuries, hematoma, infection, hardware complications, and pseudarthrosis can occur, although the incidence is not high.

REFERENCES

1. Matsuoka T, Yamaura I, Kurosa Y, et al. Long-term results of the anterior floating method for cervical myelopathy caused by ossification of the posterior longitudinal ligament. Spine (Phila Pa 1976). 2001;26(3):241-8.

2. Sakou T, Matsunaga S, Koga H. Recent progress in the study of pathogenesis of ossification of the posterior longitudinal ligament. J Orthop Sci. 2000;5(3):310-5.
3. Wang PN, Chen SS, Liu HC, et al. Ossification of the posterior longitudinal ligament of the spine. A case-control risk factor study. Spine (Phila Pa 1976). 1999;24(2):142-4; discussion 145.
4. Resnick D, Niwayama G (Eds). Diagnosis of bone and joint disorders: with emphasis on articular abnormalities. London: WB Saunders; 1994.
5. Epstein N. Ossification of the cervical posterior longitudinal ligament: a review. Neurosurg Focus. 2002;13(2):ECP1.
6. Matsunaga S, Sakou T, Taketomi E, et al. The natural course of myelopathy caused by ossification of the posterior longitudinal ligament in the cervical spine. Clin Orthop Relat Res. 1994;(305):168-77.
7. Matsunaga S, Sakou T, Taketomi E, et al. Clinical course of patients with ossification of the posterior longitudinal ligament: a minimum 10-year cohort study. J Neurosurg. 2004;100(3 Suppl Spine):245-8.
8. Matz PG, Anderson PA, Holly LT, et al. The natural history of cervical spondylotic myelopathy. J Neurosurg Spine. 2009;11(2):104-11.
9. Robinson RA, Smith G. Anterolateral cervical disk removal and interbody fusion for cervical disk syndrome. Bull Johns Hopkins Hosp. 1955;96:223-4.
10. Yamaura I, Kurosa Y, Matuoka T, et al. Anterior floating method for cervical myelopathy caused by ossification of the posterior longitudinal ligament. Clin Orthop Relat Res. 1999;(359):27-34.
11. Hirabayashi K, Satomi K. Operative procedure and results of expansive open-door laminoplasty. Spine. 1988;13:870-6.
12. Hirabayashi K, Bohlman HH. Multilevel cervical spondylosis. Laminoplasty versus anterior decompression. Spine. 1995;20:1732-4.
13. Suda K, Abumi K, Ito M, et al. Local kyphosis reduces surgical outcomes of expansive open-door laminoplasty for cervical spondylotic myelopathy. Spine (Phila Pa 1976). 2003;28(12):1258-62.
14. Ratliff JK, Cooper PR. Cervical laminoplasty: a critical review. J Neurosurg. 2003;98(3 Suppl):230-8.
15. Hilibrand AS, Fye MA, Emery SE, et al. Increased rate of arthrodesis with strut grafting after multilevel anterior cervical decompression. Spine. 2002;27:146-51.
16. Yonenobu K, Hosono N, Iwasaki M, et al. Laminoplasty versus subtotal corpectomy. A comparative study of results in multisegmental cervical spondylotic myelopathy. Spine. 1992;17:1281-4.
17. Nikolaidis I, Fouyas IP, Sandercock PA, et al. Surgery for cervical radiculopathy or myelopathy. Cochrane Database Syst Rev. 2010;(1):CD001466.
18. Persson LC, Moritz U, Brandt L, et al. Cervical radiculopathy: pain, muscle weakness and sensory loss in patients with cervical radiculopathy treated with surgery, physiotherapy or cervical collar. A prospective, controlled study. Eur Spine J. 1997;6(4):256-66.
19. Kadanka Z, Mares M, Bednaník J, et al. Approaches to spondylotic cervical myelopathy: conservative versus surgical results in a 3-year follow-up study. Spine (Phila Pa 1976). 2002;27(20):2205-10; discussion 2210-1.
20. Mummaneni PV, Kaiser MG, Matz PG, et al. Cervical surgical techniques for the treatment of cervical spondylotic myelopathy. J Neurosurg Spine. 2009;11(2):130-41.
21. Matz PG, Anderson PA, Groff MW, et al. Cervical laminoplasty for the treatment of cervical degenerative myelopathy. J Neurosurg Spine. 2009;11(2):157-69.
22. Mummaneni PV, Kaiser MG, Matz PG, et al. Preoperative patient selection with magnetic resonance imaging, computed tomography, and electroencephalography: does the test predict outcome after cervical surgery? J Neurosurg Spine. 2009;11(2):119-29.
23. Chiba K, Ogawa Y, Ishii K, et al. Long-term results of expansive open-door laminoplasty for cervical myelopathy-average 14-year follow-up study. Spine (Phila Pa 1976). 2006;31 (26):2998-3005.
24. Fujimura Y, Nishi Y, Chiba K, et al. Multiple regression analysis of the factors influencing the results of expansive open-door laminoplasty for cervical myelopathy due to ossification of the posterior longitudinal ligament. Arch Orthop Trauma Surg. 1998;117(8):471-4.
25. Iwasaki M, Kawaguchi Y, Kimura T, et al. Long-term results of expansive laminoplasty for ossification of the posterior longitudinal ligament of the cervical spine: more than 10 years follow up. J Neurosurg. 2002;96(2 Suppl):180-9.
26. Iwasaki M, Okuda S, Miyauchi A, et al. Surgical strategy for cervical myelopathy due to ossification of the posterior longitudinal ligament: Part 1: Clinical results and limitations of laminoplasty. Spine (Phila Pa 1976). 2007;32(6):647-53.
27. Ogawa Y, Toyama Y, Chiba K, et al. Long-term results of expansive open-door laminoplasty for ossification of the posterior longitudinal ligament of the cervical spine. J Neurosurg Spine. 2004;1(2):168-74.
28. Iwasaki M, Okuda S, Miyauchi A, et al. Surgical strategy for cervical myelopathy due to ossification of the posterior longitudinal ligament: Part 2: advantages of anterior decompression and fusion over laminoplasty. Spine (Phila Pa 1976). 2007;32(6):654-60.
29. Chen Y, Chen D, Wang X, et al. Anterior corpectomy and fusion for severe ossification of posterior longitudinal ligament in the cervical spine. Int Orthop. 2009;33(2):477-82.
30. Kim K, Isu T, Sugawara A. Treatment of cervical OPLL by cervical anterior fusion using autologous vertebral bone grafts. Acta Neurochir (Wien). 2009;151(11):1549-55.
31. Kato Y, Iwasaki M, Yonenobu K. Long-term results of posterior decompressive surgery for cervical myelopathy due to OPLL. In: Terayama K (Ed). Investigation committee report of 1995 on the ossification of the spinal ligaments. Tokyo: Japanese Ministry of Public Health and Welfare, 1995:209-13. (In Japanese).
32. Tomita T, Harada M, Ueyama K, et al. Radiological follow-up evaluation of the progression of ossification of the posterior longitudinal ligament. In: Terayama K (Ed). Investigation committee report of 1995 on the ossification of the spinal ligaments. Tokyo: Japanese Ministry of Public Health and Welfare, 1995:241-4. (In Japanese).

33. Bilbao G, Duart M, Aurrecoechea JJ, et al. Surgical results and complications in a series of 71 consecutive cervical spondylotic corpectomies. Acta Neurochir (Wien). 2010; 152:1155-63.
34. Sani S, Ratliff JK, Cooper PR. A critical review of cervical laminoplasty. Neurosurg Quart. 2004;14:5-16.
35. Okada M, Minamide A, Endo T, et al. A prospective randomized study of clinical outcomes in patients with cervical compressive myelopathy treated with open-door or French-door laminoplasty. Spine. 2009;34:1119-26.
36. Kotani Y, Abumi K, Ito M, et al. Minimum 2-year outcome of cervical laminoplasty with deep extensor muscle-preserving approach: impact on cervical spine function and quality of life. Eur Spine J. 2009;18:663-71.
37. Epstein NE. Ossification of the yellow ligament and spondylosis and/or ossification of the posterior longitudinal ligament of the thoracic and lumbar spine. J Spinal Disord. 1999:12:250-6.
38. Li H, Dai LY. A systematic review of complications in cervical spine surgery for ossification of the posterior longitudinal ligament. Spine J. 2011;11(11):1049-57.
39. Smith ZA, Buchanan CC, Raphael D, et al. Ossification of the posterior longitudinal ligament: pathogenesis, management, and current surgical approaches. A review. Neurosurg Focus. 2011;30(3):E10.
40. Yoshihara H. Letter to the Editor concerning "C5 palsy following anterior decompression and spinal fusion for cervical degenerative diseases" by Hashimoto M et al. (2010) Eur Spine J. 19:1702-10. Eur Spine J. 2011 Jul;20(7):1188-9; author reply 1190-1.
41. Sakaura H, Hosono N, Mukai Y, et al. C5 palsy after decompression surgery for cervical myelopathy: review of the literature. Spine (Phila Pa 1976). 2003;28(21):2447-51.
42. Kaptain GJ, Simmons NE, Replogle RE, et al. Incidence and outcome of kyphotic deformity following laminectomy for cervical spondylotic myelopathy. J Neurosurg. 2000;93(2 Suppl):199-204.
43. Kato Y, Iwasaki M, Fuji T, et al. Long-term follow-up results of laminectomy for cervical myelopathy caused by ossification of the posterior longitudinal ligament. J Neurosurg. 1998;89:217-23.
44. Zdeblick TA, Abitbol JJ, Kunz DN, et al. Cervical stability after sequential capsule resection. Spine. 1993;18:2005-8.

CHAPTER

45

Newer Motion Preservation Technologies

Kseniya Slobodyanyuk, Rachel N Rattenni, Thomas Cheriyan, Thomas J Errico

INTRODUCTION

Over the past 50 years, clinical outcomes attained with vertebral arthrodesis have been excellent. However, with an improved understanding of spine biomechanics, there has been growing concern about the altered kinematics of regions adjacent to fused levels. Studies have demonstrated that arthrodesis causes increased stress due to increased motion and intradiscal pressure on adjacent levels that may lead to progression of adjacent segment degeneration. In addition, while single-level fusion does not significantly affect global motion, multilevel fusion can affect range of motion.

Recent efforts to preserve motion have centered on disk arthroplasty, a promising technique that addresses concerns about arthrodesis to some extent. Disk replacement has been discussed in detail in Chapters 47 and 48; this chapter will review other potential developments in motion preservation technology.

NUCLEUS REPLACEMENT

Nucleus replacement has become an area of interest for mild and moderate degenerative disease. Ideally, nucleus replacement would be used when existing changes to the lumbar spine, including disruption of the annulus, end plates, and facet joints, are minimal.[1] The goal of nucleus replacement surgery is to approximate the physiologic function of the nucleus pulposus, thus protecting the annulus and facet joints of the involved disk. The damaged nucleus can be substituted with a synthetic replacement or autologous cartilage implantation. Methods of regrowing and replanting the nucleus include autologous chondrocyte transplantation, which involves harvesting, culturing, and reimplanting nucleus pulposus cells through a minimally invasive percutaneous route, injection of growth factors, and genetic manipulation.

SYNTHETIC NUCLEUS REPLACEMENT

Numerous synthetic nucleus prosthesis replacement technologies that function as an alternative to regrowing the nucleus are currently being investigated. Nucleus replacement may slow the aging process by increasing disk height and restoring stability. The nuclear implants can be made of a variety of materials, including metals, ceramics, injectable fluids, hydrogels, inflatables, and elastic coils. Some of the more common materials utilized in replacement are hydrogels.

Hydrogels function like the natural disk, exuding fluid when under pressure and imbibing it when pressure is removed. Hydrogel-based nucleus replacement devices have been in development for > 25 years; both constrained and unconstrained implants have been described. Constrained implants undergo controlled deformation when loaded and are thus designed to minimize creep under load. Unconstrained hydrogel implants are designed to swell and fill maximally, preventing migration from the disk space. Although it is intuitive to think that ideal hydrogel implants would approximate the physiologic disk structure, the best implants are actually firmer than a natural disk. Firmer implants are effective because patients with disk disease often have a damaged annulus, thus increasing the likelihood that a natural nucleus would again be extruded. The hydrogel core is typically contained in a polyethylene jacket. Thus far, two types of hydrogel devices have made headway, though neither has been used in a clinical setting: the Raymedica nucleus has been undergoing trials outside the United States, whereas the prosthetic disk nucleus device calle the PDN-SOLO device has been undergoing prospective clinical trials in the United States. Efficacies of the two devices were analyzed in a 2011 retrospective analysis of a non-randomized, single-center clinical series by Pimenta et al.[1] One hundred twenty-five patients presented with moderate disk degeneration, of whom 80 received the Raymedica prosthesis, 26 the percutaneous nucleus replacement, and 19 the NUBAC articulating nucleus disk prosthesis device. NUBAC is another mechanical nucleus replacement device with a large surface area to distribute stress and theoretically, reduce subsidence. Follow-up extended up to 9 years after initial recruitment. Incidence of device retrieval was 48.8%, most frequently with percutaneous nucleus replacement. Study authors attributed the high failure rate of all prosthetic disks to their reliance on the central region of the vertebral end plates, the weakest portion of the vertebral bone, which may fail with load bearing.

Other nucleus replacement devices include DASCOR, NeuDisc Artificial Lumbar Nucleus Replacement, NuCore Injectable Nucleus, Aquarelle Hydrogel Disk Nucleus, BioDisk Nucleus Polposus Replacement, TranS1 Percutaneous Nucleus Replacement, and the Satellite Spherical Partial Disk.[2] The NeuDisc is currently undergoing a two-arm pilot study in Europe, with early outcomes indicating a fast resolution of symptoms that is maintained at a 12-month follow-up. The NuCore Injectable Nucleus utilizes a minimally invasive, in situ technique, and is currently being tested in Switzerland, with early clinical outcomes indicating improvements as measured by leg and back pain visual analog scale (VAS) and Oswestry Disability Index (ODI) scales; radiographic analysis concurrently shows up to 100% maintenance of restored disk height at 12 months postoperatively. The Aquarelle device, another hydrogel implant, has yet to be clinically tested in humans. The BioDisk Nucleus Polposus Replacement is also a hydrogel and has so far been tested in 11 patients with sciatica, who all experienced relief immediately after surgery; the results of this study have not yet been published. The TranS1 device has shown improvements on VAS and ODI scales at a 3-week follow-up in an initial investigation. Clinical trials of the Satellite Spherical Partial Disk have not yet been initiated, but the device aims to treat low back pain secondary to disk degeneration.[2]

Cell Therapy

Cell-based therapies are based on the premise that diseased disks are deficient in matrix components, including collagen and proteoglycan, which help retain the strength and hydration of the disk; supplementing cells may significantly increase rates of matrix synthesis. Target cells include growth factors such as platelet derived growth factor and insulin-like growth factor, matrix components such as type II collagen, transcription factors including SOX6 and SOX9, signal transduction molecules, regulators such as Sonic Hedgehog, anti-inflammatory mediators such as anti-IL1 and anti-TNF α, inhibitors of apoptosis such as Bcl-2, and mesenchymal stem cells, which are either adult or embryonic and could be multipotent or specific.[1]

Although cell therapy has many potential advantages, there are several limitations to this approach. First, injecting growth factors into cells of reduced viability may limit their function in restoring disk structure. Growth factor injection into diseased cells may also increase metabolic demand and lead to further damage; thus, healthy cells may also need to be transplanted. Second, structural modification would not necessarily result in symptom relief. Finally, direct injection of cytokines or growth factors has had short-lived effects.[2]

Gene Therapy

The goal of gene therapy is to promote proteoglycan synthesis in degenerative disk disease (DDD), which would result in increased water content, restoring disk height and properties.[2] Proteoglycan synthesis can be achieved by transducing the cells of the NP with a target gene. Introduction of desired genes is achieved through either a viral or a nonviral vector. Nonviral vectors include liposomes and DNA-ligand complexes.

However, the efficacy of gene therapy is somewhat limited. The current gold standard employs bone marrow stimulation to grow fibrocartilage, a material that has a relatively poorly organized structure with significant amounts of type I collagen and is thus more susceptible to injury and premature osteoarthritis.[3] A second limitation is the limited utility of gene therapy in partial thickness lesions. In treating partial thickness lesions, the defect remains completely contained within the avascular articular cartilage—there is no way for growth factors to reach the damaged regions. This is in contrast to full-thickness lesions, in which there is rupture of the blood vessels and thus repair of the defect.[3]

INTERSPINOUS DISTRACTION

Distraction utilizes a posterior device to restrict lumbar extension, thus potentially limiting compression on the existing nerve roots. Interspinous distraction devices may be implanted under a mild sedative or local anesthesia, often as a same-day surgical procedure. One such device is the X-STOP (Fig. 45.1). Indicated for lumbar stenosis, this is the first device that was shown to be superior to nonoperative management in this patient population at 1- and 2-year follow-up. One major benefit of the X-STOP device is its ability to limit extension only at affected levels while sparing other types of motion. In addition, the X-STOP boasts a reduced complication rate, avoids pseudarthrosis, and does not contribute to adult spinal deformity.[4] In a 2006 4-year follow-up of 18 patients, 78% had successful outcomes, with all but 1 patient reporting some improvement.[4] However, a 2008 retrospective review of 12 patients with spondylolisthesis-related symptomatic lumbar stenosis noted an extremely high failure rate, suggesting that spondylolisthesis may be a contraindication to use of the X-STOP.[5]

The Coflex interspinous implant (Fig. 45.2) was approved by the Food and Drug Administration (FDA) in 2012 for used in one- or two-level lumbar stenosis from L1–L5, after decompression of affected levels. Two-year results from the noninferiority FDA Investigational Device Exemption (IDE) trials that compared decompression and Coflex interlaminar stabilization to decompression and instrumented fusion for spinal stenosis and low-grade spondylolisthesis, demonstrated similar clinical outcomes with greater improvements in SF-12 health outcomes, Zurich Claudication questionnaire, physical function, and patient satisfaction in the Coflex group.[6,7] The Coflex system seems to have a low complication and reoperation rate. However, spinal process fracture, device loosening, wing breakage, and dura mater tear have been reported.[8]

Other interspinous distraction systems include the DIAM Spinal Stabilization System, Wallis Dynamic Stabilization, and the Coflex Interspinous Implant for Stabilization of the Lumbar Spine. The DIAM system was shown to produce satisfactory or very satisfactory results in 87% of patients undergoing surgery for extruded disk herniations, stenosis, and topping off, as measured by the VAS. The Wallis device has shown similar promise in clinical trials, with an improvement in postoperative VAS scores of at least 50% in 93% of patients at a 1-year follow-up.

DYNAMIC STABILIZATION

A second option for reconstructing the posterior column is dynamic stabilization. The idea of this technique is to alter abnormal loads on the degenerated disk, facilitating regeneration by inserting flexible rods to connect one or multiple spinal segments to provide stability while avoiding complete fusion.[9] This technique of "semirigid" fixation has already achieved success in other parts of the body.[10] The goal of the posterior dynamic stabilization is to function like an internal brace of the spine. It allows for controlled movement in such a way as to achieve more normal spinal motion. These devices are typically used to treat patients with spondylolisthesis and DDD. To date, they have been approved for use with fusion but not for independent use as dynamic stabilizers. Advantages include stabilization of a segment (which can be potentially unstable or intrinsically unstable) without fusion of the segment and reduction of adjacent

Fig. 45.1: Schematic representation of the X-STOP interspinous device.

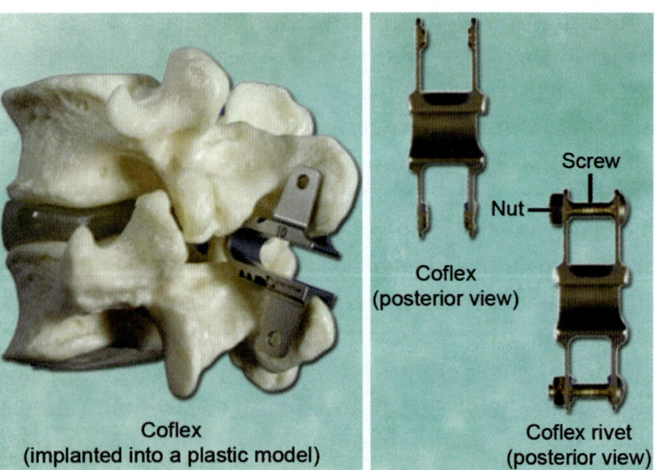

Fig. 45.2: Schematic representation of the Coflex device.

segment disease. Potential disadvantages include loosening at the bone-implant interface, mechanical failures, insufficient stabilization, and autofusion. In general, although short-term studies have supported noninferiority of posterior dynamic stabilization compared with fusion, the approach is of unclear clinical value and lacks long-term studies.[9,10]

There are a variety of devices available for posterior dynamic stabilization, many of which are already used in conjunction with fusion. The two most extensively studied devices are the Graf ligamentoplasty and the Dynesys. The Graf ligamentoplasty, created in 1992, is one of the earliest pedicle screw-based systems. The Graf system consists of polyester bands wrapped around screws. After insertion of the screws, bands are connected under applied compressive force to stabilize the segment in extension. The major disadvantage of the Graf system is that although it eases the load on the anterior annulus, it increases the load on the posterior annulus. There is also a lack of empirical support for the effectiveness of the Graf system in relieving symptoms of low back pain.[9]

The Dynesys device resembles the Graf and was designed to resist excessive compression force.[10] Currently, this device is FDA-approved as an adjunct to fusion and is undergoing study in the United States for nonfusion use.

Other methods of dynamic stabilization include the Stablimax Neutral Zone Posterior Lumbar Dynamic Stabilization System, Scient'x IsoBar TTL Dynamic Rod Stabilization, the Cosmic device, the Innovative Spinal Technologies Dynamic Stabilization Device, the Nflex, and the coflex. The Stablimax device is currently undergoing an IDE clinical trial approved by the FDA. The Scient'x IsoBar has shown 45% absolute improvement when combined with fusion and 83% improvement when used alone at an 18-month follow-up in an initial clinical trial. The Cosmic device has shown improvements over fusion in postoperative VAS and ODI scales. The Innovative Spinal Technologies Dynamic Stabilization Device has yet to undergo clinical testing, as has the Nflex. The coflex, however, has shown an 88% patient satisfaction rating at a 2-year follow-up of 68 surgery patients in a retrospective analysis.[2]

FACET REPLACEMENT

Some facet replacement designs involve replacement with a metal articulation, whereas others involve redesigning a posterior joint dissimilar to a natural facet joint. A number of joint implants have already been designed and patented. As joint implants undergo mechanical testing and clinical trials, a major criticism that has surfaced is that replacement of only the facet joint does not solve the problem of the damaged disk. The total disk replacement options that are currently available may result in nonphysiologic motion and thus place increased strain on the joint implants.[2] Three facet replacement systems currently under investigation include the Total Facet Arthroplasty System (TFAS), the Anatomic Facet Replacement System (AFRS), and the Total Posterior Arthroplasty System (TOPS).

Total Facet Arthroplasty System

The TFAS is similar in design to hip and knee replacement devices, using metal-on-metal joint prostheses.[9] Indicated for patients with moderate to severe lumbar stenosis, the TFAS can stabilize the affected segment and maintain, or even restore, motion and sagittal balance.[2] Currently, the TFAS is undergoing randomized comparison studies with fusion.

Anatomic Facet Replacement System

The AFRS, composed of superior and inferior facet implants with pedicle screw fixation, is indicated for patients with osteoarthritis of the facet joints resulting in subarticular, lateral, and central canal stenosis or stenosis with spondylolisthesis. Patients without stenosis or degeneration that present with isolated facet-joint pain or traumatic facet fractures may also benefit from this system.[2] Advantages of the AFRS include its design, which preserves physiologic lumbar motion and thus minimizes adjacent-level degeneration; its ease of use; and its use of pedicle screw fixation, a technique already well known to spine surgeons.

Total Posterior Arthroplasty System

Another pedicle screw-based system, TOPS, is indicated for patients with coexisting spinal stenosis and facet joint arthritis. Like the other facet systems, TOPS aims to maximize physiologic spinal motion and to minimize loads at adjacent levels. It is composed of titanium plates that permit flexion, extension, rotation, and lateral movement while limiting anterior and posterior sagittal motion.[2] Currently, a prospective, multicenter study is underway that compares TOPS to fusion, with a 2- to 3-year follow-up.

Other facet joint treatment modalities include the Zyre Facet Replacement Device, the FENIX Facet Resurfacing

Implant, and dynamic pedicle-screw stabilization with nucleus replacement. The Zyre implant is an interpositional arthroplasty device that does not require bony resection and has yet to be clinically tested. The FENIX facet resurfacing implant has also not yet undergone clinical testing, but it is designed as an alternative to more extensive facet joint replacements. Dynamic pedicle-screw stabilization with nucleus replacement is a hybrid surgical technique that has yet to be clinically tested as the procedure is theoretically beneficial; the combination of pedicle-screw stabilization and nucleus replacement may have greater complication rates than either procedure alone.

ANNULUS REPAIR

The Inclose Surgical Mesh System and the Barricaid devices are both used for annulus repair and are designed to supplement disk repair by containing intradiscal contents and reducing rates of reherniation. Both devices have shown benefit in reducing reherniation rates in initial clinical testing. The Inclose Surgical Mesh system is a complete nuclear implant, whereas the Barricaid device acts as an internal patch between the annulus and the nucleus that covers that posterior annulus.

CONCLUSION

Many of the options described above are still in the early stages of testing, and it is not expected that motion preservation or tissue engineering techniques will be widely used in the near future. Nevertheless, a greater understanding of spine mechanics will lead to the creation of more sophisticated approaches that will provide lifelong relief and mitigate the adverse effects of current systems.

REFERENCES

1. Pimenta L, Marchi L, Coutinho E, et al. Lessons learned after 9 years' clinical experience with 3 different nucleus replacement devices. In: Seminars in spine surgery. Elsevier; 2012. pp. 43-7
2. Yue JJ, Bertagnoli R, McAfee PC, An HS. Motion Preservation Surgery of the Spine: Advanced Techniques and Controversies: Elsevier Health Sciences; 2008.
3. Longo UG, Petrillo S, Franceschetti E, et al. Stem cells and gene therapy for cartilage repair. Stem Cells Int. 2012;2012: 168385.
4. Kondrashov DG, Hannibal M, Hsu KY, et al. Interspinous process decompression with the X-STOP device for lumbar spinal stenosis: a 4-year follow-up study. J Spinal Disord Tech. 2006;19(5):323-7.
5. Verhoof OJ, Bron JL, Wapstra FH, et al. High failure rate of the interspinous distraction device (X-Stop) for the treatment of lumbar spinal stenosis caused by degenerative spondylolisthesis. Eur Spine J. 2008;17(2):188-92.
6. Davis RJ, Errico TJ, Bae H, et al. Decompression and Coflex interlaminar stabilization compared with decompression and instrumented spinal fusion for spinal stenosis and low-grade degenerative spondylolisthesis: two-year results from the prospective, randomized, multicenter, Food and Drug Administration Investigational Device Exemption trial. Spine (Phila Pa 1976). 2013;38(18):1529-39.
7. Davis R, Auerbach JD, Bae H, et al. Can low-grade spondylolisthesis be effectively treated by either Coflex interlaminar stabilization or laminectomy and posterior spinal fusion? Two-year clinical and radiographic results from the randomized, prospective, multicenter US investigational device exemption trial: clinical article. J Neurosurg Spine. 2013;19(2):174-84.
8. Xu C, Ni WF, Tian NF, et al. Complications in degenerative lumbar disease treated with a dynamic interspinous spacer (Coflex). Int Orthop. 2013 Nov;37(11):2199-204. doi: 10.1007/s00264-013-2006-2. Epub 2013 Jul 27.
9. Bono CM, Kadaba M, Vaccaro AR. Posterior pedicle fixation-based dynamic stabilization devices for the treatment of degenerative diseases of the lumbar spine. J Spinal Disord Tech. 2009;22(5):376-83.
10. Lee MJ, Lindsey JD, Bransford RJ. Pedicle screw-based posterior dynamic stabilization in the lumbar spine. J Am Acad Orthop Surg. 2010;18(10):581-8.

CHAPTER

46

Minimally Invasive Lumbar Spine Fusion

Noel I Perin

INTRODUCTION

Minimally invasive and minimal access procedures are gaining wider acceptance within the spine community and the general population. Minimally invasive techniques reduce access-related tissue trauma, reduce surgical pain in the early postoperative period and allow for faster recovery and return to normal activities. Patients have smaller, cosmetically pleasing incisions and they experience a reduction in muscle ischemia and scarring, as noted on long-term magnetic resonance imaging (MRI). More importantly, patients achieve fusion rates similar to those experienced by patients undergoing open procedures.

INDICATIONS

The indications for minimally invasive lumbar interbody fusion are essentially similar to the indications for open lumbar interbody fusion.[1] In most cases, lumbar spine fusion operations are indicated when there is clinical and radiological evidence of segmental instability, recurrent disk herniation, herniation that requires wide decompression that may lead to instability, and patients who risk progression of pre-existing deformity if decompressed.[1-3] Spondylolisthesis with movement on flexion/extension X-rays is a classic indication for fusion surgery. Patients having MRI evidence of type 1 modic changes, such as black disk with disk desiccation is a relative indication, if the patient responds positively to facet blocks and provocative discography.

Minimally invasive and minimal access lumbar fusions can be performed using anterior, posterior, lateral, and para-axial approaches, or using a combination of these approaches (Figs. 46.1A and B).

ANTERIOR APPROACHES (ALIF)

Anterior lumbar interbody fusion (ALIF) has produced good clinical results with open and minimally invasive techniques.[4,5] ALIF provides direct visualization and access to the disk space, thus allowing a more complete discectomy and preparation of the end plates leading to better fusion. ALIF is also advantageous over transforaminal lumbar interbody fusion (TLIF) in that the posterior anatomy is preserved. However, the anterior approach does pose risks to the great vessels, inferior hypogastric plexus, and other intra-abdominal structures.

Transperitoneal and Retroperitoneal Approaches for ALIF

Endoscopic transperitoneal approaches, once a popular technique for ALIFs at L4–5 and L5–S1, are no longer performed. The predominant reason for their falling out of favor was the high incidence of major (11%) and minor complications (24%), especially retrograde ejaculation and loss of sexual function in male patients.[6]

However, minimal access retroperitoneal anterior approaches performed for ALIF in male patients carry a reduced incidence of sexual complications when working with experienced general and vascular surgeons (4%).

After the anterior interbody cage/bone fusion, these patients are turned prone and have percutaneous pedicle screws placed at the respective levels, thus limiting posterior muscle dissection. However, patients requiring decompression for canal stenosis can have a tubular retractor guided procedure prior to placement of percutaneous screws.

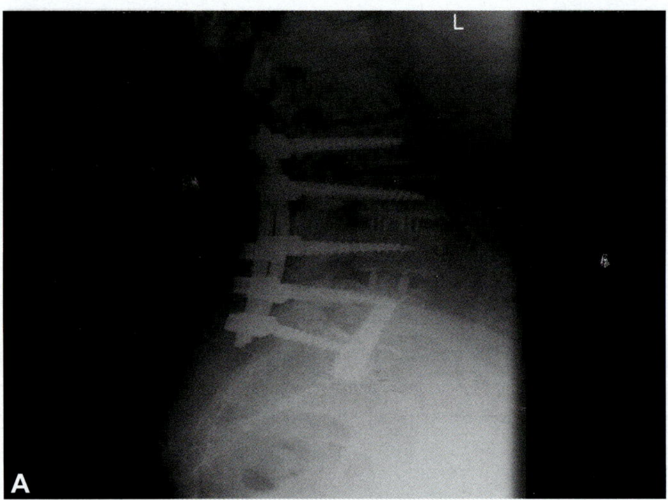

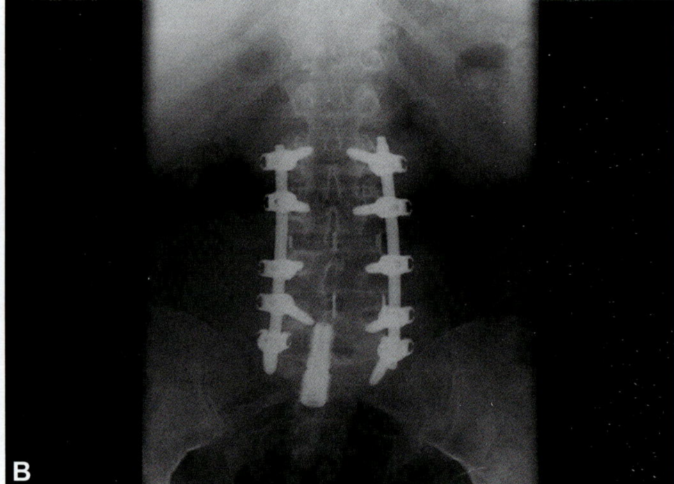

Figs. 46.1A and B: (A) Lateral and (B) anteroposterior (AP) radiographs showing stabilization/fusion at L2–S1; eXtreme Lateral Interbody Fusion (XLIF) at L3–4, L4–5 ; Axial Lumbar Interbody Fusion (AxiaLIF) at L5–S1; and onlay at L2–L3.

Minimal Access Retroperitoneal Interbody Fusion

Patient is positioned supine on the operating table, which is placed in a reverse Trendelenberg position, with pillows under the knees to relax the psoas muscles. A blanket may be placed below the buttocks to rotate the pelvis. A 5-7 cm paramedian vertical or Pfannenstiel incision is made, and the abdominal wall muscles are opened in the direction of the fibers. As the transversalis fascia is opened, care is taken to protect the peritoneum, working retroperitoneally the peritoneal contents are pushed to the right and upward. The aorta, inferior vena-cava and their branches are identified and protected. With blunt and sharp dissection the vessels and the hypogastric plexus are protected and retractor blades placed to protect and hold them out of the disk space. After discectomy and preparation of the end plates, a lordotic femoral ring allograft or cage is placed in the interspace. A screw and washer are placed into the adjacent body to hold the graft in place. The wound is closed in routine fashion.

Anterior Trans-Sacral Interbody Fusion (AxiaLIF)

This technique utilizes a novel corridor via a small paracoccygeal incision through the presacral space to access the L5-S1 disk space. The technique preserves the integrity of the muscles, ligaments, and the annulus of the disk. The technique entails developing the presacral plane to the junction of S1-2. Using biplaner fluoroscopy a working tube is docked at the junction of S1-2 and a reamer is used to drill through the S1, L5-S1 disk and L5 bodies. Using cutting loops and wire-brush type capture devices the discectomy is performed, and allograft bone and bone fusion enhancers are packed into the disk space. The titanium prosthetic device is then threaded after drilling and tapping across the disk space into the L5 body. This technique still requires posterior stabilization, which can be performed percutaneously either with facet screws or pedicle screws. The technique has been used to incorporate the L4-5 disk space using a longer titanium screw bridging both L5-S1 and L4-5 (Figs. 46.1A and B). This approach, however, has not gained wide acceptance due in part to the technical difficulties involved with the approach itself, as well as the incidence of bowel injuries and relatively high pseudarthrosis rates.

Lateral Transpsoas Approaches

The minimally invasive lateral transpsoas interbody fusion differs from the traditional lateral lumbar approaches in that it involves a retroperitoneal access followed by the use of a tubular retractor directly through the psoas muscle. Utilization of the transpsoas surgical approach has undergone tremendous growth after the development of novel instrumentation that has allowed increasingly sophisticated and pathology-specific lumbar interbody fusion techniques. Only recently have outcome studies begun to provide details regarding the efficacy of these procedures, including the benefit of minimally invasive versus traditionally open techniques.

Patient Selection

This approach is applicable in the lumbar spine from L1–2 through L4–5. L5–S1 is not accessible because of the iliac crest. Accessibility to L4–5 should be determined preoperatively with standing anteroposterior (AP) X-rays that show the relationship of the L4–5 disk space to the iliac crest. Standing AP X-rays, lateral flexion X-rays and MRI of the lumbar spine are essential for planning purposes. Once the determination of the need for an interbody fusion and the levels to be fused has been made, the suitability of the lateral approach to these levels has to be determined. If the standing AP X-rays shows the L4–5 disk space to be at or above the crest, then the level can be accessed laterally. In a patient with scoliosis, it is easier to access the disk spaces from the concave side, whereas in patients with greater than grade 1 spondylolisthesis as noted on the flexion/extension films, this level is not suitable for lateral access surgery. MRI should be evaluated for any abnormal anatomy along the access routes (i.e., anomalous vessels). Also in cases where indirect decompression of the foramina and spinal canal (mild to moderate stenosis) is to be achieved, an assessment of the height of the disk space is critical. If the disk space is not collapsed, it is not possible to achieve good decompression with lateral access surgery.

Procedure

The patient under general anesthesia is positioned on a standard operating room table that has its base reversed. Patient is placed in the lateral decubitus position with the greater trochanter at the break in the table, with the iliac crest about 3–4 inches above the break. All pressure points are padded and the patient is taped to the table, as shown in Figure 46.2. AP X-rays are obtained before final taping to maintain the spinous processes midway between the pedicles by adjusting the patient on the table before taping and, to have sharp end plates by moving the fluoro machine. The optimal position of the fluoro machine is marked on the floor.

The table is flexed to open the interspace between the ribs and the crest as needed. However, care must be taken not to overdo the flexion and to limit overstretching the psoas muscle. With lateral fluoroscopy the incision site is marked in the flank—a horizontal incision if a single level is to be fused or a vertical incision if more than one level. After routine preparation and draping, the incision is carried through the subcutaneous fat to the dorsolumbar

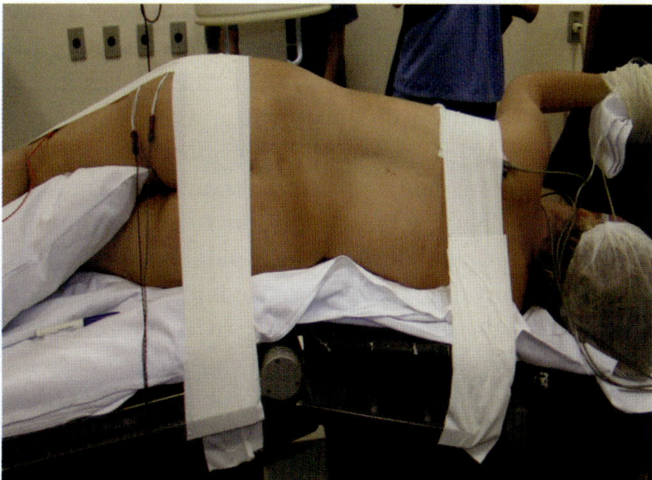

Fig. 46.2: Lateral decubitus position with appropriate taping and table flexion for lateral transpsoas approach.

fascia. The fascia is opened sharply and thereafter a tonsil clamp is used to open the external oblique, internal oblique, and the transversus abdominis muscles in the direction of the fibers. Once the transversalis fascia is reached, a finger is used to bluntly push through the fascia. Once in the retroperitoneal space, the finger is directed posteriorly and sweeps the retroperitoneal fat anteriorly to palpate the transverse process posteriorly and the psoas muscle. Care should be exercised not to break any bands in the retroperitoneal space as the ilioinguinal and iliohypogastric nerves may be disrupted.

With lateral fluoroscopy, the initial dilator/stimulation probe is carried to the surface of the psoas muscle, with continuous electromyography stimulation. It is carried through the psoas muscle and docked on the disk space, docking at the junction of the anterior two thirds and the posterior one third of the space (safe zone) from L1–2 to L3–4 and more anteriorly at the L4-5 disk space to avoid the femoral nerve. A Kirschner (K) wire is then placed into the disk space and confirm appropriate placement with AP and lateral fluoroscopy. At this stage, the working tubular retractor is placed and docked on the surface of the psoas muscle, and a light source is introduced. The genitofemoral nerve is identified and protected. The muscle is then teased open in the direction of the fibers with a "freer" elevator to identify anterior nerves within the muscle and protect them. The working tube is then collapsed and carried down under direct vision to dock on the disk space before opening the blades. This technique has significantly reduced the incidence of injury to the sensory nerves and in many cases, the femoral nerve as well. AP and lateral fluoroscopy are used to confirm that the retractor is docked in the middle of the body before proceeding with surgery (Fig. 46.3). The discectomy is performed removing disk material and the end plates prepared for fusion. Using Cobb elevators and curettes, the end plates are prepared, and the contralateral annulus is opened using the Cobb elevator. It is important to make sure that the anterior longitudinal ligament is not breached at any time so as to prevent injury to abdominal contents. Trials are used, followed by the appropriate-sized polyetheretherketone (PEEK) cage, to increase the disk height to match the adjacent normal disk height. The cage is packed with allograft and bone fusion enhancers. If more than one level is to be fused the procedure is repeated, placing the tubular retractor through a separate fascial opening (Figs. 46.4A and B).

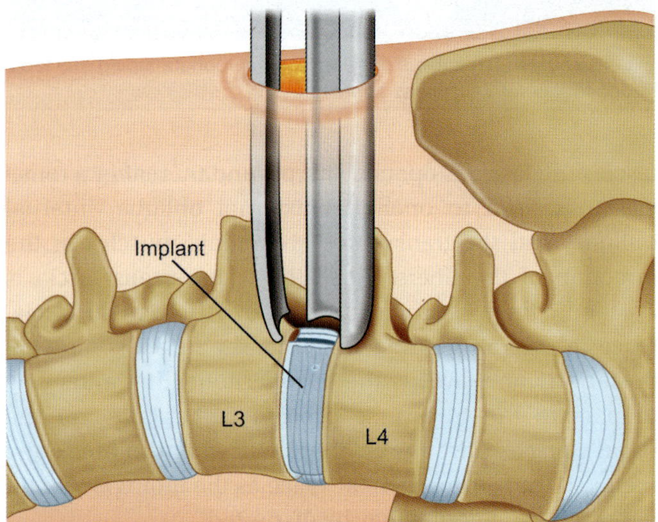

Fig. 46.3: Retractor in place straddling the disk for lateral transpsoas discectomy/fusion.

POSTERIOR APPROACHES

PLIF Approach

It is not utilized with the minimally invasive techniques due to the significant thecal sac retraction and incidence of nerve root injuries.

TLIF Approach

Most complications due to posterior lumbar interbody fusion (PLIF) are related to the approach; TLIF was developed by Harms and Rollinger in an attempt to minimize approach-related morbidity. This procedure is associated with many of the advantages of PLIF (for example, single approach, no need for an access surgeon, and limited risk to peritoneal structures) while avoiding many of the drawbacks of the traditional PLIF procedure. The unilateral TLIF procedure allows access to the disk space via a far-lateral approach, after removal of the facet, which requires less mobilization of the thecal sac and preservation of the contralateral anatomy.

Surgical Technique

After appropriate preoperative evaluation, the patient's general anesthesia is induced in the operating room. The

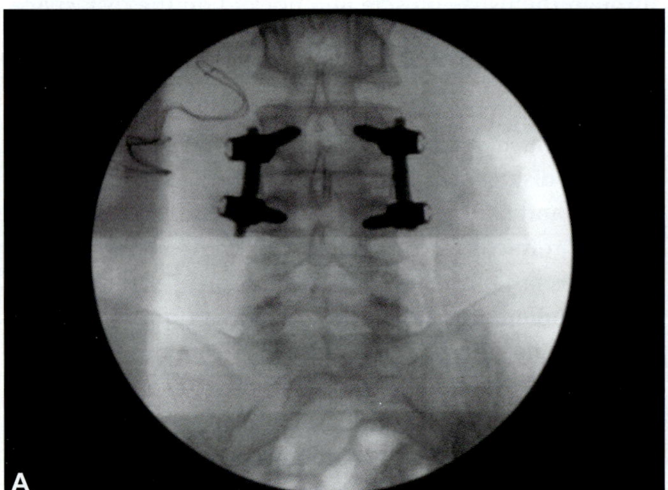

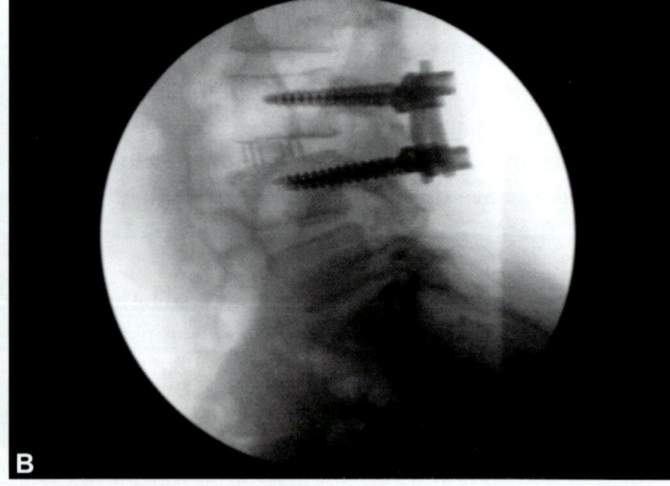

Figs. 46.4A and B: (A) Anteroposterior and (B) lateral fluoroscopic images after interbody cage placement via transpsoas approach with pedicle fixation at L3–4.

more symptomatic side determines the surgical approach. When symptoms are bilaterally identical, a left-sided approach is preferred. All other equipment—support for the working channel, the base and monitor for the fluoroscopy, and the video monitor—are typically placed on the contralateral side.

The patient is positioned prone on the "Jackson table" (Fig. 46.5), and the operative level is confirmed using AP and lateral fluoroscopy. Using AP fluoroscopy, the transverse pedicular lines are drawn through the pedicles on the AP view. A vertical pedicular line is drawn along the lateral borders of the facets. The fluoroscope is then rotated 15° to either side, and the oblique pedicular line is drawn. The incision is then marked between the transverse pedicular lines along the oblique pedicular line (3–4 cm from midline) (Fig. 46.6).

After routine preparation and draping, a stab wound is made with a 15 blade and the smallest dilator tube is carried down through the fascia and muscle and docked on the facet joint under lateral fluoroscopic guidance (Figs. 46.7A and B). The incision is extended to 25 mm and the sequential soft tissue dilators are then inserted until the final working tube can be placed and affixed to the table mounted holder (Quadrant; Medtronic Sofamor Danek, Memphis, TN) (Fig. 46.8). The soft tissue overlying the laminae and facets are taken down.

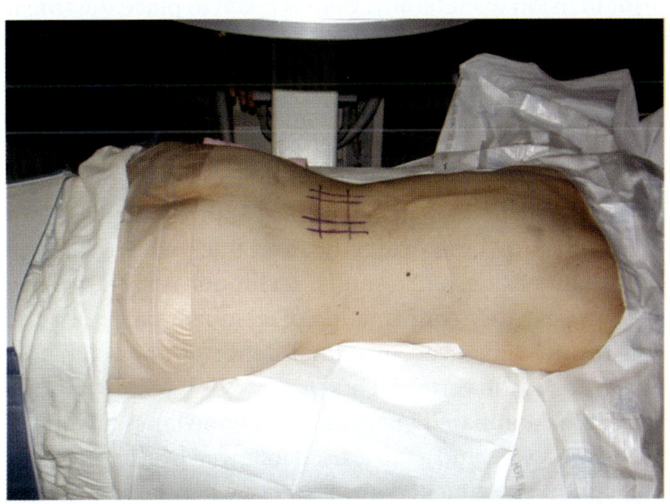

Fig. 46.5: Patient positioning and incision site at intersection of transverse pedicular lines with the lateral most oblique pedicular line.

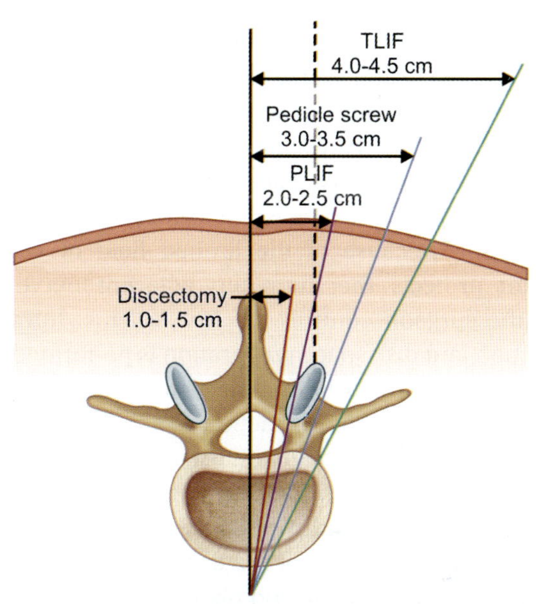

Fig. 46.6: Guidelines of measurements for locating incision site in MISS.

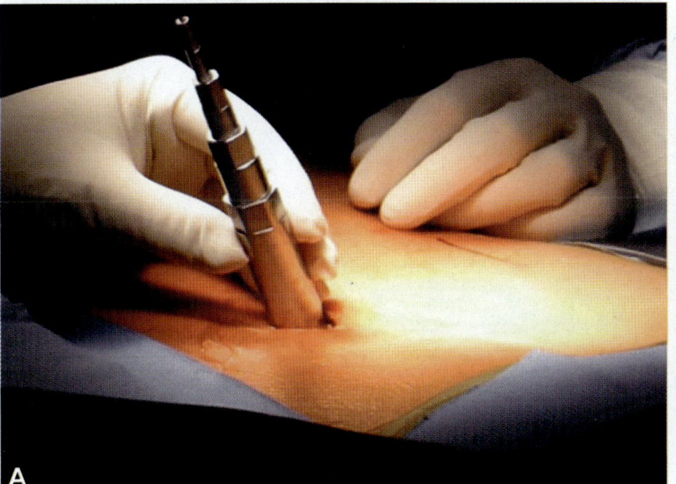

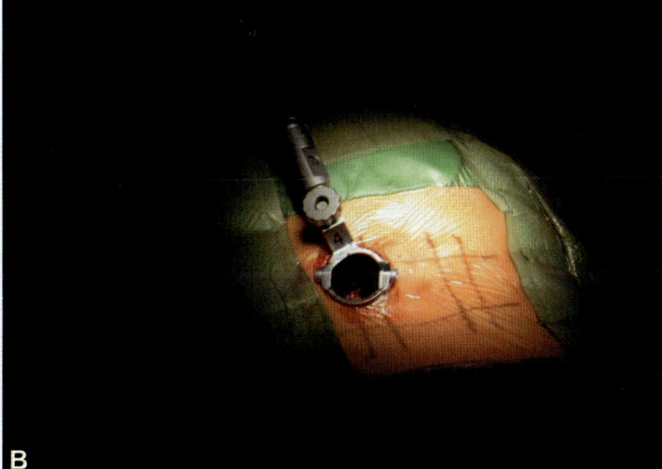

Figs. 46.7A and B: Sequential muscle dilation placement of working tube.

Using the operating microscope, the lower half of the superior lamina, the superior one third of the inferior lamina and the facet joint are drilled. The bone removal is completed by removing the inferior facet of the superior segment and the pars interarticularis, identifying the traversing root and exiting roots at the level. The ligamentum flavum is removed piecemeal in order to decompress the canal and foramen on the ipsilateral side. Next, the tubular retractor is angled medially, the under surface of the spinous processes is drilled, and the ligamentum is removed in order to decompress the contralateral lateral recess and foramen. Bone obtained from the laminotomy and facetectomy is saved for the fusion.

Both nerve roots must be clearly visualized to perform the interbody fusion safely. After visualization of both nerve roots, it is safe to perform the discectomy. The disk material is removed using standard techniques in conjunction with a disk space reamer and an end plate scraper. This prepares the disk space to accept placement of the graft. Because of the limited field of view, an assistant protects the dura and adjacent nerve roots while the surgeon controls the instruments. Intradiscal distraction and disk space preparation is performed using standard interbody fusion instruments. After performing facetectomy and serial distraction in the disk space, we find that we are able to maintain reasonable disk height to allow implantation of the bone grafts. During placement of the grafts, fluoroscopic guidance allows the surgeon to gauge safely the depth of the instruments while in the disk space. After adequate end plate preparation, some of the bone graft material is packed ahead of the cage in the interspace. A single-bullet-shaped PEEK cage is placed obliquely from one side. Under fluoroscopic guidance, the interbody age is hammered into place (Fig. 46.9). Care is taken to ensure that the exiting nerve roots and lateral aspect of the dura mater are protected. Endoscopic visualization and intraoperative neuromonitoring help in the safe placement of the cage.

Attention is then turned to implantation of the instrumentation. The working channel is removed and the fluoroscope is brought into the AP position (i.e., the fluoroscope is angled into the owl's-eye position with respect to the pedicle, such that the X-ray beam is directly in line with the axis of the pedicle). On the side of the decompression, a Jamshidi needle is placed through the prior incision ipsilaterally. Care is taken to place the trocar in the center of the pedicle in line with the long axis of the pedicle. A lateral fluoroscopic image is used to confirm the trocar location when advancing the Jamshidi into the vertebral body. The Jamshidi trocar, once directed along this path, serves as a conduit for safe passage of a K-wire into the pedicle. Two stab incisions, approximately 1.5 cm in length, are made directly over the pedicles on the contralateral side, and a similar technique is used to place the K-wires. After confirmation of adequate trajectory, the K-wires are advanced to a final depth of approximately two thirds of the vertebral body.

Using cannulated instruments, a bone tap is advanced over the K-wire, and a tap is used followed by a cannulated pedicle screw attached to a screw extender (''Mantis'' Stryker) is placed over the wire (Figs. 46.10A and B).

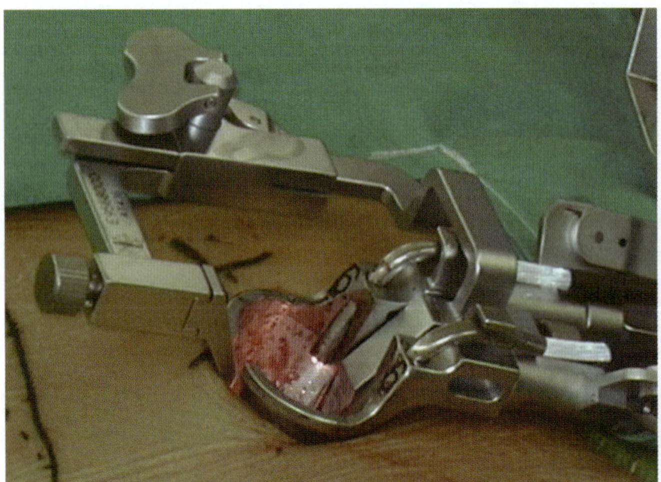

Fig. 46.8: Final working tube in place with rostrocaudal and mediolateral retractors.

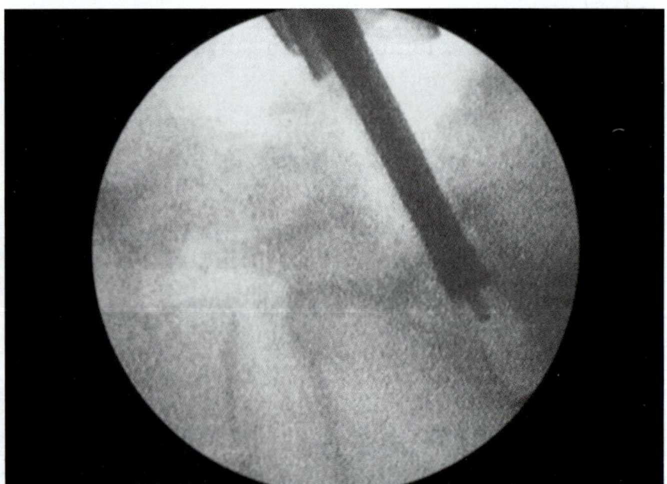

Fig. 46.9: Transforaminal lumbar interbody fusion—interbody polyetheretherketone cage placed through the working tube.

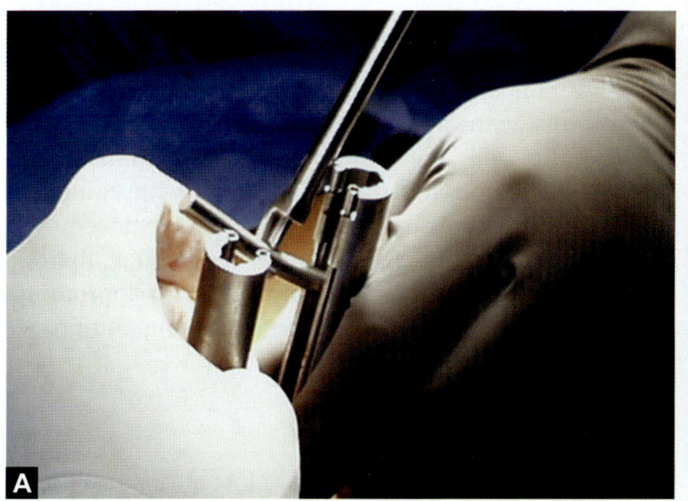

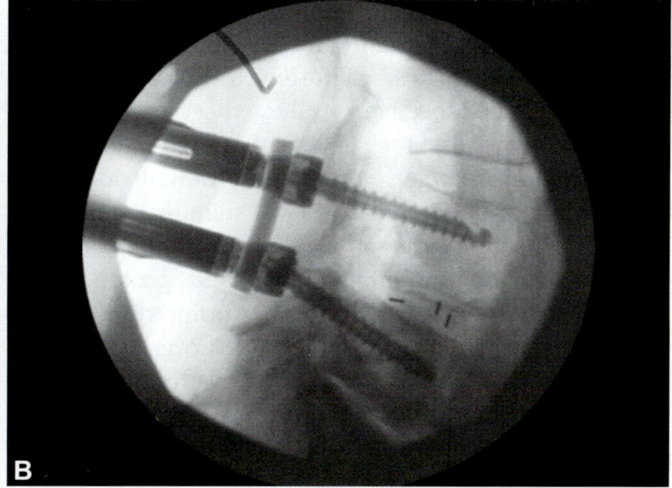

Figs. 46.10A and B: Minimally invasive spine surgery—transforaminal lumbar interbody fusion and percutaneous pedicle fixation.

Fluoroscopy is used to ensure that the Steinmann pin did not advance as the tap and screw are advanced over the K-wire. The screw is advanced until it almost abuts the facet joint. The second screw on the ipsilateral side is also placed in a similar fashion. Attention is then shifted to the contralateral side, and the process is repeated. The rod size is measured, and the rod is introduced down the screw extenders and guided into the head of the screw. Locking caps are then placed. Compression can be applied across the screw extenders. The screw extenders are detached and the wounds are closed.

DISCUSSION

The goal of spinal fusion surgery is to afford maximum benefit to the patient while minimizing associated morbidity. Conventional lumbar fusion surgery is associated with approach-related iatrogenic soft-tissue injury that can have deleterious short- and long-term effects on patient outcomes. Numerous studies have demonstrated that irreversible ischemic muscle injury occurs as a result of muscle stripping and retraction and can be associated with poor clinical results. This muscle injury can lead to muscle scarring and long-term back pain. Advances in fiberoptic technology and spinal instrumentation have played a pivotal role in the advancement of this field. Despite these advancements, however, the surgery related objective and techniques underlying minimally invasive spinal surgery compared with the traditional open surgery remain the same.

Currently accepted interbody fusion techniques include ALIF, PLIF, lateral transpsoas approach and the trans-sacral approach to L5–S1. Interbody techniques afford good results with fusion by placing bone dowels and cages under compression. The ALIF approach that is currently practiced is performed in conjunction with the miniopen technique and carries with it the risk of retrograde ejaculation. The thoracoscopic transperitoneal approach was abandoned because of the high incidence of retrograde ejaculation; in addition, stand-alone ALIF procedures were associated with a high incidence of nonunion. The TLIF approach has significantly reduced the risk of nerve root injury and dural lacerations by accessing the disk far laterally. The percutaneous minimally invasive tubular retractor guided unilateral approach lends itself well to minimize approach-related tissue trauma when followed by the placement of percutaneous screws. In addition, patients experience reduced blood loss and shorter hospital stays, as well as immediately reduced postoperative pain.

The lateral transpsoas approach offers the unique ability to place an anterior interbody cage from L4–5 through L1–2 without an anterior retroperitoneal or transperitoneal approach or the attendant risks with such approaches. This technique also allows access to the upper lumbar spine and the ability to correct deformity in both the coronal and sagittal planes. In selected cases with moderate lumbar stenosis allows, it allowed for indirect decompression of the spinal canal and foramina without posterior decompression. In selected older patients, this can be performed as a stand-alone procedure without posterior instrumentation. However, there are some complications uniquely related to this approach—transient postoperative groin numbness and iliopsoas weakness.

Significant femoral nerve weakness, as well as groin and inner thigh numbness, can occur and grows increasingly likely when procedures are performed at the L4-5 level.

Gejo et al. prospectively evaluated serial changes in trunk muscle performance in 20 patients who underwent posterior lumbar surgery. The patients were divided into short (<80 minutes) and long (>80 minutes) retraction time groups. The degree of back muscle injury was estimated by comparing preoperative and postoperative MRI. Muscle strength was evaluated during trunk flexion and extension by using a kinetic measuring device and dynamometer. The authors determined that damage to the multifidus muscle was more severe, and the recovery of extensor muscle strength was delayed in the long retraction-time group.

Sihvonen et al.[7] studied a group of patients with severe postoperative failed-back surgery syndrome, using radiological and neurophysiological studies as well as muscle biopsy procedures. They concluded that disrupted back-muscle innervation and loss of muscular support could be an important factor in the development of failed-back surgery syndrome. They suggested the potential role of developing surgical methods that preserve back muscle innervation better than conventional techniques.

A meta-analysis and review by Cizik et al. concluded that most outcomes between open TLIF and minimally invasive TLIF were comparable.[8] However, the minimally invasive technique was associated with less blood loss and longer surgical times. Another meta-analysis by Tian et al. similarly showed that minimally invasive TLIF procedures were associated with less blood loss and shorter hospital stays. In addition, they were associated with better functional outcomes as compared to open TLIF. There was no difference in operative time, reoperation rate or complication rates. However, there was increased intraoperative X-ray exposure when using the minimally invasive technique.[9] Currently, there is a paucity of high-level evidence with regard to the efficacy and outcomes of minimally invasive spine surgery. However, present evidence indicates that minimally invasive procedures might be at least as effective as open procedures. Complication rates are low and compare favorably to open procedures.[10] Minimally invasive surgery also appears to be cost-saving advancement.[11]

SUMMARY

The goal of any minimally invasive procedure is to achieve the same surgical objectives as the corresponding open procedure with reduced access-related tissue damage. These less invasive approaches result in decreased intraoperative blood loss, less immediate postoperative pain and shorter hospital stay. Furthermore, they do so without compromising the efficiency of the procedure.

The minimally invasive approaches for spinal fusion can be safely and effectively performed with complication rates and clinical outcomes similar to those of the open techniques. As with all novel techniques, there is a learning curve that can be overcome with appropriate attention to detail, sufficient clinical training and proper cadaver work.

REFERENCES

1. Shen FH, Samartzis D, Khanna AJ, et al. Minimally invasive techniques for lumbar interbody fusions. Orthop Clin North Am. 2007;38(3):373-86.
2. Satoh I, Yonenobu K, Hosono N, et al. Indication of posterior lumbar interbody fusion for lumbar disc herniation. J Spinal Disord Tech. 2006;19(2):104-8.
3. Wang JC, Mummaneni PV, Haid RW. Current treatment strategies for the painful lumbar motion segment: posterolateral fusion versus interbody fusion. Spine (Phila Pa 1976). 2005;30(16 Suppl):S33-43.
4. McAfee PC, Regan JJ, Geis WP, et al. Minimally invasive anterior retroperitoneal approach to the lumbar spine. Emphasis on the lateral BAK. Spine (Phila Pa 1976). 1998;23(13):1476-84.
5. Mummaneni PV, Haid RW, Rodts GE. Lumbar interbody fusion: state-of-the-art technical advances. Invited submission from the Joint Section Meeting on Disorders of the Spine and Peripheral Nerves, March 2004. J Neurosurg Spine. 2004;1(1):24-30.
6. McDonnell MF, Glassman SD, Dimar JR, 2nd, et al. Perioperative complications of anterior procedures on the spine. J Bone Joint Surg Am. 1996;78(6):839-47.
7. Sihvonen T, Herno A, Paljarvi, et al. Local denervation atrophy of paraspinal muscles in postoperative failed back syndrome. Spine (Phila Pa 1976). 1993;18(5)575 -81.
8. Cizik AM, Devine EB, Wolf FM, et al. Systematic review and meta-analysis of open spine fusion versus minimally invasive spine fusion for the diagnosis and treatment of lumbar spine conditions. Value Health. 2013;16(3):A217.
9. Tian NF, Wu YS, Zhang XL, et al. Minimally invasive versus open transforaminal lumbar interbody fusion: a meta-analysis based on the current evidence. Eur Spine J. 2013;22 (8):1741-9.
10. Tsahtsarlis A, Efendy JL, Mannion RJ, et al. Complications from minimally invasive lumbar interbody fusion: experience from 100 patients. J Clin Neurosci. 2013; 20(6): 813-7.
11. Parker SL, Mendenhall SK, Shau DN, et al. Minimally invasive versus open transforaminal lumbar interbody fusion (TLIF) for degenerative spondylolisthesis: comparative effectiveness and cost-utility analysis. World Neurosurg. [published online ahead of print 12 Jan 2013].

CHAPTER

47

Cervical Total Disk Replacement

Robert P Norton, Jeffrey A Goldstein

INTRODUCTION

Cervical spondylosis with associated radiculopathy and/or myelopathy is a common cause of disability and loss of work. Fortunately, it can often be treated with nonoperative measures, such as physical therapy, soft collar use, modalities, or steroid injections. However, if a patient fails a trial of nonsurgical management, operative intervention may be warranted. Both surgical and nonsurgical management aim to restore function and reduce pain with minimized risk. With this in mind, the operative management of symptomatic cervical disk disease has evolved and continues to be fine tuned in an effort to improve outcomes, patient satisfaction, and safety. Currently, the Food and Drug Administration (FDA) has approved multiple cervical devices with ongoing investigational device exemption (IDE) trials underway.

EVOLUTION OF IMPLANTS

Anterior cervical discectomy and fusion (ACDF) has been widely accepted as the gold standard surgical procedure for anterior cervical degenerative disk disease. Originally described by Robinson and Smith in the 1950s, this procedure has, indeed, withstood the test of time. Numerous studies have documented its effectiveness with excellent results and relatively low complication rates. Furthermore, increased use of allograft has reduced the complications associated with iliac crest bone graft harvesting, and widespread use of supplemental instrumentation has reduced the incidence of pseudarthrosis. However, complications such as instrumentation failure or dislodgement, dysphagia, pseudarthrosis, and adjacent segment disease (ASD) do occur, and the opportunity for improvement does exist. Indeed, a major impetus for the development of cervical total disk replacement (TDR) was to reduce the incidence of ASD after spinal fusion. ACDF has been shown to alter adjacent-segment kinematics by increasing adjacent segment motion, shear strains, and intradiscal pressures,[1,2] which may thereby predispose to hastening of degeneration. Hilibrand et al.[3] in 1999 reported an annual incidence of 2.9% per year and prevalence of 25.6% over 10 years of symptomatic ASD requiring surgical management after ACDF. As it turns out, they found that the risk of ASD was higher with single-level fusion compared with multilevel fusions, suggesting that ASD is the result of natural progression of cervical spondylosis rather than changes in kinematics from the fusion itself. The progression of spondylosis has been supported in the literature to be both secondary to fusion[4] as well as hereditary predisposition.[5] Goffin et al.[6] reported a 92% incidence of ASD after ACDF at a mean of 100 months. They attributed their findings to both natural progression and the biomechanical impact of the interbody fusion. A study by Garrido et al.[7] analyzed the prospectively collected data on the Bryan TDR versus ACDF. They reported a significantly lower incidence of adjacent-level ossification development at 2- and 4-year follow-up with arthroplasty compared with ACDF. Nunley et al.[8] recently studied the incidence of clinically symptomatic ASD after cervical TDR. They established an annual incidence of symptomatic ASD to be 3.1% with a median follow-up of 51 months, regardless of age, sex, smoking status, number of levels operated, or design of TDR device. In short, the literature on the subject is bountiful but inconclusive, with higher rates of degeneration and instability adjacent to fusion levels being both supported[9] and refuted.[10] In reality, the pathology of ASD can likely be attributed to both the natural progression of the disease process and postsurgical biomechanical alterations.

Pseudarthrosis is another complication associated with ACDF that has been studied extensively. Fusion rates for single-level ACDF have varied in the literature depending on study design, instrumentation use, surgeon experience, patient comorbidities, and risk factors. Brodke and Zdeblick[11] reported 97% fusion rate, whereas Bohlman et al.[12] reported a 89% fusion rate with single-level ACDF. More recently, Fraser and Hartl[13] performed a meta-analysis and found an average fusion rate of 97.1% with single-level ACDF and plating. However, most of these articles were retrospective small series without universal standards of identifying fusion. Therefore, the fusion rate results may not be as predictable as would seem. Interestingly, perhaps the most accurate determination of fusion rate after single-level ACDF came from the results of the FDA IDE study of the ProDisc-C TDR versus ACDF by Murrey et al.[14] This trial may have been the largest prospective series of ACDF with plating with the highest patient accountability ever reported and showed a fusion rate of 90.2%. Regardless of the exact rate of pseudarthrosis, the fact remains that nonunion is a serious complication that can be improved upon.

Because of the aforementioned limitations specific to ACDF, investigators sought ways to address these biomechanical and kinematic concerns related to fusion and ASD. This led to the development of cervical disk arthroplasty. The goal of this procedure is to avoid the limitations of a fusion mass by preserving motion while decompressing neural elements, restoring disk height, and restoring cervical alignment. Secondary goals are to preserve normal motion at adjacent segments thereby attempting to retard ASD, eliminate the risk of pseudarthrosis, and remove the morbidity associated with graft donor site.

Cervical TDR acts as an interbody spacer that is mobile, allowing for motion at the diseased level. It is a reconstruction of the anterior column, and therefore, this procedure is not suitable if there is significant facet degeneration or instability. The implant acts as a motion preservation device and not a motion creation device. After appropriate exposure with the anterior Smith-Robinson approach, a discectomy and decompression of the neural elements is performed via foraminotomies, resection of osteophytes, and/or the posterior longitudinal ligament. Once all neural elements are adequately decompressed and the vertebral body end plates are prepared, the artificial disk is placed with careful attention to place the prosthesis within the center of rotation (COR) of the disk space. When properly placed, sagittal balance and stability is improved while segmental height is restored. Furthermore, because a fusion is not required and the implant is inherently stable, patients do not require postsurgical immobilization.

TECHNICAL CONSIDERATIONS

Many designs exist with various permutations of evolving cervical disk implants. They all take into consideration the various axes of movement (rotation, translation, and axial compression), which occur around a COR. The COR represents a point, which varies with each vertebral segment, in which the vertebral body can rotate without translating. Beyond this point rotation is coupled with translation to create what is known as the instantaneous axis of rotation. Arthroplasty designs have been created to take advantage of mobility with varying degrees of freedom. A constrained implant is one in which the implant itself has a limit on the amount of motion allowed within the normal range of motion (ROM) of a vertebral segment. This type of implant may protect the facet joints from excessive shear force with time. A semiconstrained implant stops motion outside of the normal physiologic ROM of a vertebral segment. An unconstrained implant has no internal restriction on motion and relies upon the anatomic restrictions placed on it by the anatomy of the patient. Advocates of this design argue that facet joints are able to glide more naturally compared with limited facet motion of a constrained implant. Furthermore, in a constrained design, much like the design of a constrained hip, as motion occurs further from the neutral position the implant-bone interface is subjected to greater stress. It should be noted that in any design, constraint is not synonymous with stability. All types of implants strive for maximal stability. Poorly placed implants may accelerate index level facet joint degeneration.

Similar to total joint arthroplasty, cervical arthroplasty has been designed with various bearing surfaces and bearing surface geometry. The two most common types of bearing surface materials used are metal-on-polyethylene or metal-on-metal design. Both metal-on-metal and ultrahigh molecular weight polyethylene coupled to cobalt-chromium alloy implants have shown to possess low wear rates. Furthermore, the cervical spine is not subjected to the degree of mechanical loading seen in a total hip arthroplasty or total knee arthroplasty. Subsequently, the clinical significance of articular bearing surface wear remains unclear but has not been shown to be a problem.

The geometry of the bearing surface is most commonly a ball and socket or trough with a semiconstrained design. Finally, the implant fixation techniques vary with manufacturer and implant design. A more constrained implant requires more rigid fixation in the form of a keel or screw; however, a less constrained implant may use serrations or teeth to resist implant extrusion. Again, there are many designs that are either currently FDA approved or under investigation.

INDICATIONS AND CONTRAINDICATIONS

Cervical TDR is indicated for degenerative disk disease at 1 level between C3 and C7. The ideal candidate is a patient with a single-level disk herniation, minimal spondylosis, and concordant radiculopathy that has failed a trial of nonoperative management for at least 6 weeks or has a severe or progressive neurological deficit.

Contraindications to cervical arthroplasty based upon present FDA criteria include severe spondylosis with more than a single-level involvement, bridging osteophytes or ossification of the posterior longitudinal ligament, spondylosis involving levels other than C3–C7, disk height loss of > 50%, significant facet joint arthrosis, significant kyphosis or focal deformity, instability, tumor, infection, metabolic bone disease, morbid obesity, metal allergy, or revision surgery.

Indications and contraindications to cervical TDR have been established by the FDA trials and are the criteria used in the IDE studies. Therefore, any cervical TDR performed with differing criteria may be subject to differing outcomes or device failures. In addition, results of outcomes will vary with the inevitable evolution of inclusion and exclusion criteria when performing cervical arthroplasty.

ANALYSIS OF THE FDA IDE TRIALS

The US FDA performed multiple separate large, multicenter, noninferiority, prospective, randomized IDE studies comparing cervical arthroplasty to ACDF for the operative management of symptomatic single-level cervical disk disease from C3 to C7.[14-18] The objective of these trials was to determine the safety and efficacy of cervical TDR. These FDA studies had similar inclusion and exclusion criteria, and all had similar outcome measures. Overall success of the cervical arthroplasty was defined as having achieved a ≥15-point improvement in neck disability index (NDI) score from baseline, maintenance or improvement in neurologic status, no major complication related to the implant/surgical procedure, and no subsequent surgery or intervention.[19] The overall success rate of each trial was defined as the percentage of patients who achieved success in all four composite end points. All initial FDA IDE trails from the ProDisc-C, Bryan, Prestige-ST, Kineflex-C, PCM, and Secure-C (Figs. 47.1A to F) arthroplasty systems with 24-month follow-up reported primary outcome measures to be slightly superior or equivalent to ACDF.[14-18]

Longer follow-up from these initial trials is now becoming available. Zigler et al. recently published their 5-year results on the FDA study of the ProDisc-C implant versus ACDF.[20] They found that at 5 years, ProDisc-C patients had significantly less neck pain than patients who underwent ACDF. Both groups found significant improvement in NDI score, arm pain, visual analog scale (VAS) satisfaction score, and SF-36 outcome summary measures maintained at 5 years. No device failures or implant migration was noted with the ProDisc-C. Furthermore, the ProDisc-C patients maintained motion at their index level and had significantly lower reoperation rates compared with ACDF (2.9 vs 11.3%).

Similarly, the 4-year results on the Bryan cervical disk FDA IDE trial by Sasso et al.[21] have been published. They concluded that at 48 months, cervical arthroplasty continued to show consistent, sustained significant superior outcomes compared with cervical fusion. The 5-year outcomes of the Prestige disk by Burkus et al.[22] have also demonstrated maintenance of improved clinical outcomes after arthroplasty versus fusion.

Furthermore, two of the studies[21,22] found significantly higher number of patients returned to work earlier in the arthroplasty group compared with the fusion group, and all three trials[20-22] found physiological segmental motion to be maintained.

FURTHER LITERATURE ANALYSIS

In an interesting article by Coric et al.[23] three separate IDE studies from a single investigation site with a

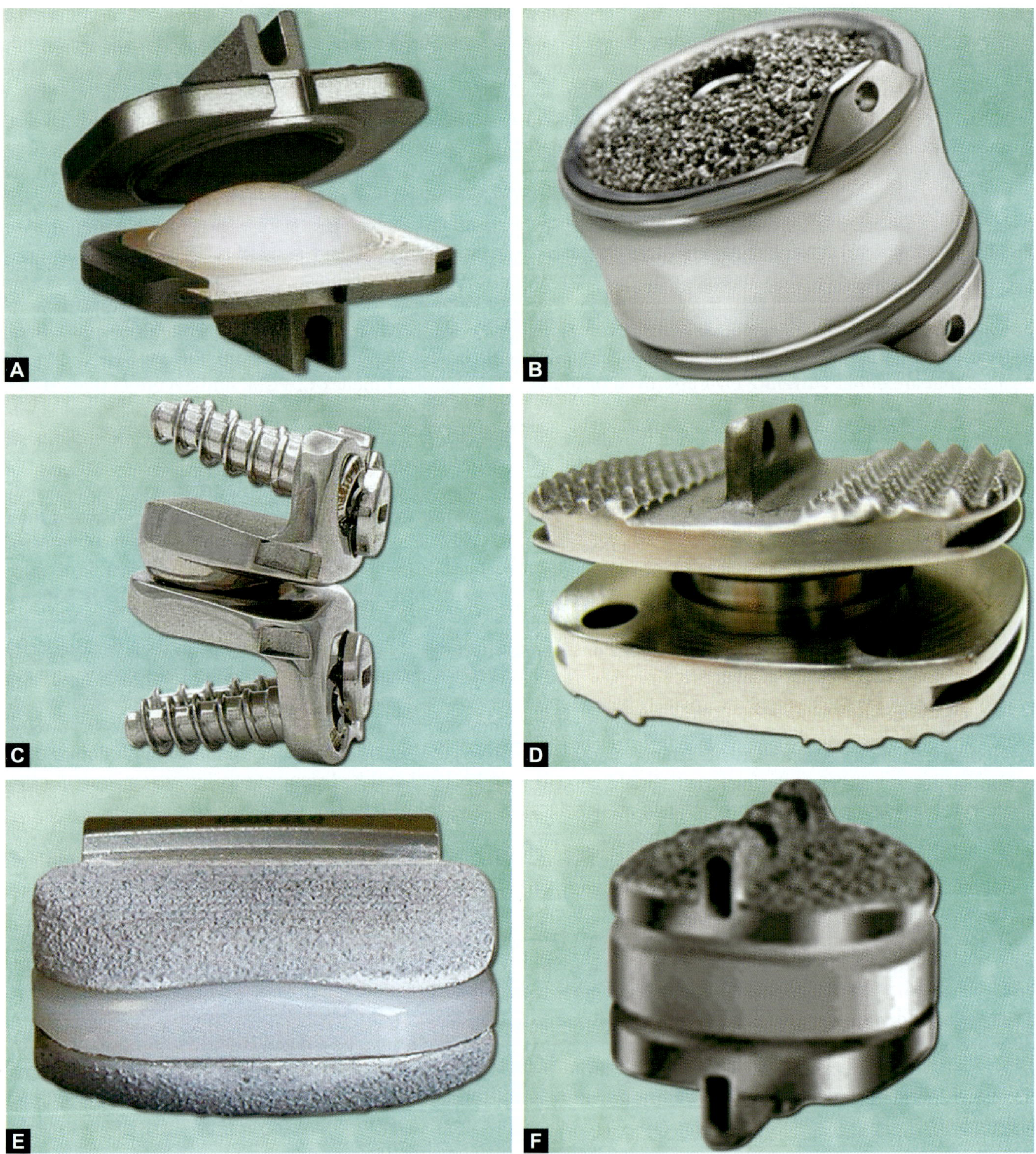

Figs. 47.1A to F: Various cervical total disk replacement devices. (A) Prodisc-C, (B) Bryan, (C) Prestige-ST, (D) Kineflex-C, (E) PCM and (F) Secure-C.

minimum of 2-year follow-up were analyzed. Despite the substantial design differences of the three implants, there was no significant difference in clinical outcome between arthroplasty groups. As a group, the arthroplasty patient's outcomes were statistically superior to the ACDF patients. Moreover, patients treated with an artificial disk maintained their motion and had a rate of ASD of 1.7% compared with 8.1% in the ACDF group.

Lastly, in a review of the journal articles pertaining to cervical arthroplasty, three separate literature review analyses have been published to date.[19,24,25] After filtering all articles in the English language that held the highest standard of only randomized, prospective, controlled trials, they all concluded that total disk replacement proves to be noninferior to ACDF and, in fact, superior on many outcome measures.

COMPLICATIONS

As with any surgical procedure complications do exist with cervical TDR. Because cervical arthroplasty has the same surgical approach to ACDF, both have similar intraoperative and postoperative approach-related complications. These complications include neurovascular injury, esophageal injury, dural tear, infection, dysphagia and dysphonia, and postoperative airway compromise from edema or hematoma formation. Pickett et al. reported on surgical complications related to cervical TDR[26] and found an overall perioperative complication rate of 6.2% per treated level.

It appears that dysphagia and dysphonia occurrence reported in the literature is lower after arthroplasty compared with traditional ACDF. Riley at al.[27] found a 29.8% incidence of dysphagia after ACDF with plating. McAfee et al.[28] performed a prospective randomized clinical study comparing both procedures and found a significantly reduced rate of dysphagia with cervical TDR compared with ACDF. Tortolani et al.[29] set out to investigate potential reasons why this is the case since both procedures have the same approach and surgical exposure. They determined that cervical TDR requires less esophageal retraction and therefore reduced intraesophageal pressure compared with ACDF.

Heterotopic ossification (HO) is a complication of particular concern since its occurrence may negate a major theoretical benefit ascribed to TDR, specifically, maintaining motion. A recent meta-analysis[30] found a prevalence of HO in 58.2% at 24 months of patients undergoing cervical TDR. Furthermore, advanced HO as defined by McAfee et al.[31] was found in 16.7% of patients at 24 months. Fortunately, the majority of these are clinically asymptomatic in as much that a fused cervical TDR patient behaves like an ACDF patient. In an effort to reduce the risk of HO, some authors[32] required patients to receive a 2-week postoperative course of nonsteroidal anti-inflammatory drugs (NSAIDs). Variations in cervical technique focusing on reduced soft tissue and periosteum dissection and improved hemostasis are also recommended.

Wear debris and its associated osteolysis is a well-known complication of total joint arthroplasty; however, data are limited on this topic in relation to disk arthroplasty. Complications associated with wear debris include pain, osteolysis, implant loosening, metal hypersensitivity, and pseudotumor.[33] The few studies that do exist that evaluate this topic have shown minimal foreign body debris production and inflammatory response. This may be secondary to limited motion and altered mechanics within the functional unit of the spine undergoing TDR compared with other joint replacements and the subsequent reduced volumetric wear rates. Long-term studies may bear out complications similar to the total joint literature.

Implant failures, including polyethylene fractures, dislocations, bearing surface wear, and implant breakage are uncommon complications but never the less, have been reported.[34] Furthermore, implant migration and loosening can occur with poor intraoperative implant sizing, poor bony ingrowth, subsidence, and end plate resorption.

Postoperative segmental kyphosis and/or poor implant positioning has also been reported in the literature, and the risk appears to increase with multilevel TDR.[35] This may be caused by both segmental misalignment of the functional spinal unit and or the prosthesis itself.[36] Overall, alignment and balance of the cervical spine is dictated by the implant positioning. Abnormal stress may be placed on the facet joints and paraspinal muscles resulting in patient discomfort. Furthermore, improper placement of the prosthesis with overdistraction or underdistraction of the disk space may result in worsening facet joint disease with altered biomechanics of the posterior elements or persistent radiculopathy/myelopathy from poor recreation of vertical disk and foraminal height.

Finally, adjacent segment degeneration is being observed after patients undergo cervical arthroplasty. As previously mentioned, at present time, insufficient data exist to determine conclusively if TDR results in less ASD than the current gold standard ACDF.

However, the rate of reoperations in many studies appears to be significantly lower than a comparative

ACDF.[37,38] Delamarter and Zigler[39] sought out to determine the reasons for and rates of secondary surgery at both index and adjacent levels after undergoing cervical TDR with the ProDisc-C versus an ACDF. They found ACDF patients had five times higher rate of reoperations than TDR patients. Others have reported that both ACDF and TDR have similar reoperation rates for ASD and, in fact, reoperation rates within ACDF patients may actually be lower than reported in the FDA trials secondary to study design.[40]

SUMMARY

The development of cervical TDR has stemmed from the desire to improve upon existing technology. Although ACDF has proved to be a successful surgery, it is not perfect. Cervical TDR allows for direct decompression and removal of the pathologic process as in ACDF with the added benefit of potentially maintaining spinal kinematics thereby avoiding the complications and limitations associated with anterior cervical fusion.

CASE EXAMPLE

A 30-year-old male patient presented with persistent neck pain and radicular right arm pain within the C6 dermatome that impaired his ability to work. On physical examination, he was found to have a global decrease in neck ROM, normal motor and sensory examination, and normal reflexes. His main complaint was unrelenting pain with a neck VAS score of 5/10 and right arm VAS score of 9/10. His NDI score measured 30/50. He failed a trial of nonoperative management, which included physical therapy, NSAIDS, narcotics, and epidural steroid injections.

Radiographic imaging of the cervical spine (Figs. 47. 2A and B) demonstrated minimal cervical spondylosis with preservation of overall alignment and disk heights without signs of facet joint arthrosis. T2 weighted magnetic resonance imaging (Figs. 47.3A and B) revealed focal single-level disease with a right sides C5–6 soft disk herniation and compression on the C6 nerve root.

Due to the patient's persistent clinical and radiographic findings concordant with C6 radiculopathy that has failed a trial of nonoperative management, the patient was identified as a candidate for surgery and elected to

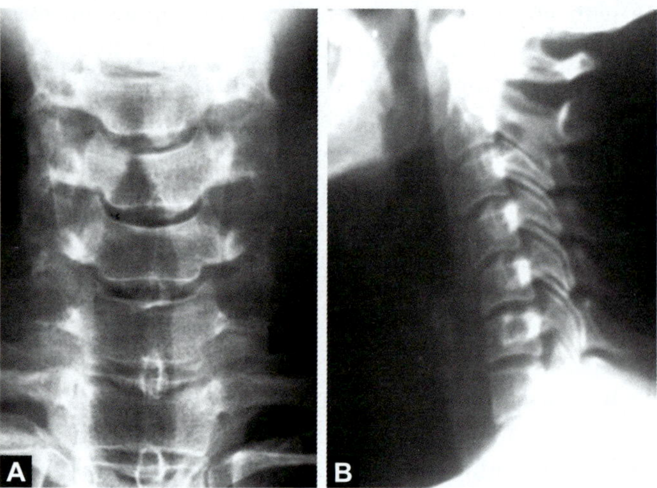

Figs. 47.2A and B: Anteroposterior and lateral cervical radiograph demonstrating minimal spondylotic degenerative changes.

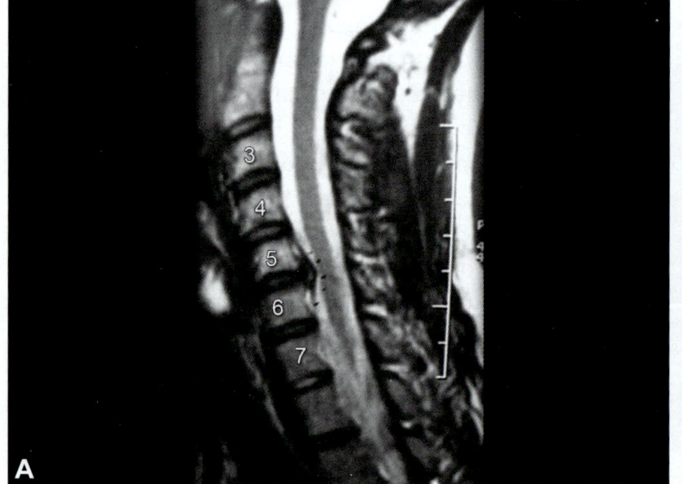

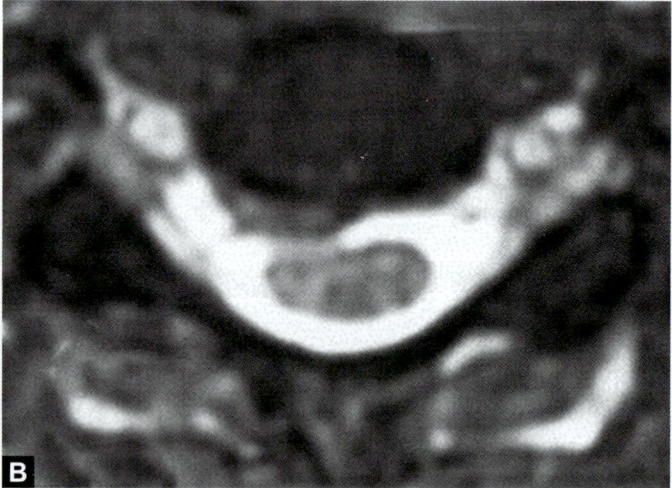

Figs. 47.3A and B: T2 weighted magnetic resonance imaging demonstrating right-sided C5–6 soft disk herniation with compression of C6 nerve root.

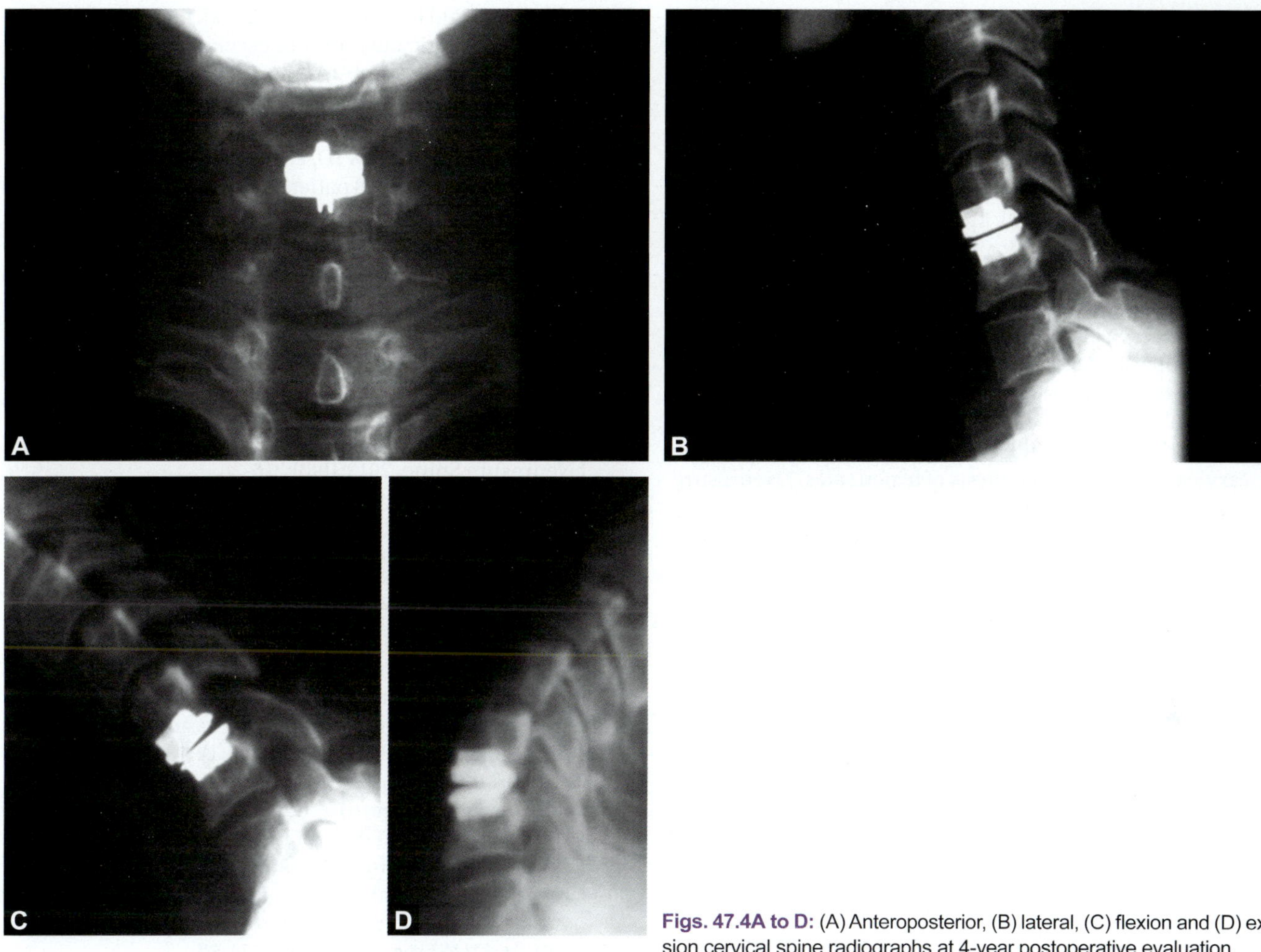

Figs. 47.4A to D: (A) Anteroposterior, (B) lateral, (C) flexion and (D) extension cervical spine radiographs at 4-year postoperative evaluation.

undergo C5-6 cervical arthroplasty. At 6-week postoperative follow-up, the patient was not on any pain medications, had a VAS neck score of 3/20, VAS arm score of 1/10, and an NDI score of 16/50. By 1-year, he was back to working full time with a VAS neck score of 2/10 and a VAS arm score of 0/10 with an NDI score of 6/50. By 2 years, he had no pain or disability with both neck and arm VAS scores of 0/10 and an NDI score of 0/50. These results, along with full neck ROM, were maintained at 4-year follow-up (Figs. 47.4 A to D).

REFERENCES

1. Chang UK, Kim DH, Lee MC, et al. Changes in adjacent-level disc pressure and facet joint force after cervical arthroplasty compared with cervical discectomy and fusion. J Neurosurg Spine. 2007;7(1):33-9.
2. Eck JC, Humphreys SC, Lim TH, et al. Biomechanical study on the effect of cervical spine fusion on adjacent-level intradiscal pressure and segmental motion. Spine. 2002;27(22):2431-4.
3. Hilibrand AS, Carlson GD, Palumbo MA, et al. Radiculopathy and myelopathy at segments adjacent to the site of a previous anterior cervical arthrodesis. J Bone Joint Surg Am Vol. 1999;81(4):519-28.
4. Gore DR, Sepic SB. Anterior discectomy and fusion for painful cervical disc disease. A report of 50 patients with an average follow-up of 21 years. Spine. 1998;23(19):2047-51.
5. Gore DR. Roentgenographic findings in the cervical spine in asymptomatic persons: a ten-year follow-up. Spine. 2001;26(22):2463-6.
6. Goffin J, Geusens E, Vantomme N, et al. Long-term follow-up after interbody fusion of the cervical spine. J Spinal Disord Techn. 2004;17(2):79-85.
7. Garrido BJ, Wilhite J, Nakano M, et al. Adjacent-level cervical ossification after Bryan cervical disc arthroplasty compared with anterior cervical discectomy and fusion. J Bone Joint Surg Am Vol. 2011;93(13):1185-9.
8. Nunley PD, Jawahar A, Cavanaugh DA, et al. Symptomatic adjacent segment disease after cervical total disc replacement: re-examining the clinical and radiological evidence with established criteria. Spine J. 2013;13(1):5-12.

9. Elsawaf A, Mastronardi L, Roperto R, et al. Effect of cervical dynamics on adjacent segment degeneration after anterior cervical fusion with cages. Neurosurg Rev. 2009; 32(2):215-24; discussion 224.
10. Reitman CA, Hipp JA, Nguyen L, et al. Changes in segmental intervertebral motion adjacent to cervical arthrodesis: a prospective study. Spine. 2004;29(11):E221-6.
11. Brodke DS, Zdeblick TA. Modified Smith-Robinson procedure for anterior cervical discectomy and fusion. Spine. 1992;17(10 Suppl):S427-30.
12. Bohlman HH, Emery SE, Goodfellow DB, et al. Robinson anterior cervical discectomy and arthrodesis for cervical radiculopathy. Long-term follow-up of one hundred and twenty-two patients. J Bone Joint Surg Am Vol. 1993;75(9): 1298-307.
13. Fraser JF, Hartl R. Anterior approaches to fusion of the cervical spine: a metaanalysis of fusion rates. J Neurosurg Spine. 2007;6(4):298-303.
14. Murrey D, Janssen M, Delamarter R, et al. Results of the prospective, randomized, controlled multicenter Food and Drug Administration investigational device exemption study of the ProDisc-C total disc replacement versus anterior discectomy and fusion for the treatment of 1-level symptomatic cervical disc disease. Spine J. 2009; 9(4):275-86.
15. Sasso R, Smucker JD, Hacker RJ, et al. Clinical outcomes of BRYAN cervical disc arthroplasty: a prospective, randomized, controlled, multicenter trial with 24-month follow-up. J Spinal Disord Techn. 2007;20(7):481-91.
16. Mummaneni PV, Burkus JK, Haid RW, et al. Clinical and radiographic analysis of cervical disc arthroplasty compared with allograft fusion: a randomized controlled clinical trial. J Neurosurg Spine. 2007(6):198-209.
17. Coric D, Nunley PD, Guyer RD, et al. Prospective, randomized, multicenter study of cervical arthroplasty: 269 patients from the Kineflex|C artificial disc investigational device exemption study with a minimum 2-year follow-up: clinical article. J Neurosurg Spine. 2011;15 (4):348-58.
18. Phillips FM, Lee JY, Geisler FH, et al. A prospective, randomized, controlled clinical investigation comparing PCM(R) cervical disc arthroplasty to anterior cervical discectomy and fusion: 2 year results from the US IDE clinical trial. Spine(Phila Pa 1976). 2013;38(15):E907-18.
19. Yu L, Song Y, Yang X, et al. C. Systematic review and meta-analysis of randomized controlled trials: comparison of total disk replacement with anterior cervical decompression and fusion. Orthopedics. 2011;34(10):e651-8.
20. Zigler JE, Delamarter R, Murrey D, et al. ProDisc-C and anterior cervical discectomy and fusion as surgical treatment for single-level cervical symptomatic degenerative disc disease: five-year results of a Food and Drug Administration study. Spine. 2013;38(3):203-9.
21. Sasso RC, Anderson PA, Riew KD, et al. Results of cervical arthroplasty compared with anterior discectomy and fusion: four-year clinical outcomes in a prospective, randomized controlled trial. Orthopedics. 2011;34(11):889.
22. Burkus JK, Haid RW, Traynelis VC, et al. Long-term clinical and radiographic outcomes of cervical disc replacement with the Prestige disc: results from a prospective randomized controlled clinical trial. J Neurosurg Spine. 2010;13(3):308-18.
23. Coric D, Cassis J, Carew JD, et al. Prospective study of cervical arthroplasty in 98 patients involved in 1 of 3 separate investigational device exemption studies from a single investigational site with a minimum 2-year follow-up. Clinical article. J Neurosurg Spine. 2010;13(6):715-21.
24. Zechmeister I, Winkler R, Mad P. Artificial total disc replacement versus fusion for the cervical spine: a systematic review. Eur Spine J. 2011;20(2):177-84.
25. Upadhyaya CD, Wu JC, Trost G, et al. Analysis of the three United States Food and Drug Administration investigational device exemption cervical arthroplasty trials. J Neurosurg Spine. 2012;16(3):216-28.
26. Pickett GE, Sekhon LH, Sears WR, et al. Complications with cervical arthroplasty. J Neurosurg Spine. 2006;4(2):98-105.
27. Riley LH, 3rd, Skolasky RL, Albert TJ, et al. Dysphagia after anterior cervical decompression and fusion: prevalence and risk factors from a longitudinal cohort study. Spine. 2005; 30(22):2564-9.
28. McAfee PC, Cappuccino A, Cunningham BW, et al. Lower incidence of dysphagia with cervical arthroplasty compared with ACDF in a prospective randomized clinical trial. J Spinal Disord Techn. 2010;23(1):1-8.
29. Tortolani PJ, Cunningham BW, Vigna F, et al. A comparison of retraction pressure during anterior cervical plate surgery and cervical disc replacement: a cadaveric study. J Spinal Disord Techn. 2006;19(5):312-7.
30. Chen J, Wang X, Bai W, et al. Prevalence of heterotopic ossification after cervical total disc arthroplasty: a meta-analysis. Eur Spine J. 2012;21(4):674-80.
31. McAfee PC, Cunningham BW, Devine J, et al. Classification of heterotopic ossification (HO) in artificial disk replacement. J Spinal Disord Techn. 2003;16(4):384-9.
32. Heller JG, Sasso RC, Papadopoulos SM, et al. Comparison of BRYAN cervical disc arthroplasty with anterior cervical decompression and fusion: clinical and radiographic results of a randomized, controlled, clinical trial. Spine. 2009; 34(2):101-7.
33. Golish SR, Anderson PA. Bearing surfaces for total disc arthroplasty: metal-on-metal versus metal-on-polyethylene and other biomaterials. Spine J. 2012;12(8):693-701.
34. Salari B, McAfee PC. Cervical total disk replacement: complications and avoidance. Orthop Clin N Am. 2012;43(1): 97-107, ix.
35. Pickett GE, Rouleau JP, Duggal N. Kinematic analysis of the cervical spine following implantation of an artificial cervical disc. Spine. 2005;30(17):1949-54.
36. Moatz B, Tortolani PJ. Cervical disc arthroplasty: pros and cons. Surg Neurol Int. 2012;3(Suppl 3):S216-24.
37. Robertson JT, Papadopoulos SM, Traynelis VC. Assessment of adjacent-segment disease in patients treated with cervical fusion or arthroplasty: a prospective 2-year study. J Neurosurg Spine. 2005;3(6):417-23.

38. Kim SW, Limson MA, Kim SB, et al. Comparison of radiographic changes after ACDF versus Bryan disc arthroplasty in single and bi-level cases. Eur Spine J. 2009;18(2):218-31.
39. Delamarter RB, Zigler J. Five-year reoperation rates, cervical total disc replacement versus fusion, results of a prospective randomized clinical trial. Spine (Phila Pa 1976). [published online ahead of print 2 Nov 2012].
40. Singh K, Phillips FM, Park DK, et al. Factors affecting reoperations after anterior cervical discectomy and fusion within and outside of a Federal Drug Administration investigational device exemption cervical disc replacement trial. Spine J. 2012;12(5):372-8.

CHAPTER

48

Lumbar Total Disk Replacement Surgery

Hiroyuki Yoshihara, John A Bendo

INTRODUCTION

Spinal arthrodesis is currently the standard operative care for symptomatic patients having degenerative disk disease (DDD). Fritzell et al. demonstrated that lumbar spine fusion significantly improved outcomes in patients with chronic low back pain when compared with nonsurgical modalities.[1] However, disadvantages of spinal fusion include elimination of normal spine anatomy, diminished range of motion (ROM), bone graft site morbidity, muscle necrosis or dysfunction, pseudoarthrosis, and adjacent segment degeneration. Adjacent segment degeneration can develop after lumbar spine fusion, occurring secondary to a combination of altered spinal biomechanics and hereditary predisposition. Surgically treating low back pain is complex: successful patients outcomes from lumbar spinal fusion range from 60% to 85%.[2] And, pain relief can be incomplete, even in patients with radiographic evidence of solid spine fusion. Despite its popularity, fusion may not be the best solution for low back pain resulting from DDD.

Lumbar total disk replacement (L-TDR) is a newer surgical option that may avoid some of the issues commonly associated with spinal fusion. L-TDR involves entirely replacing the diseased disk with prosthesis. The prostheses have been designed using principles from total hip and knee replacements, and aim to alleviate pain and restore functional motion at the level of the disk replacement.[2] The primary goal of L-TDR is to remove the pain generator, while restoring and maintaining disk height, alignment, spinal stability, and motion. In comparison with fusion, L-TDR has several purported advantages. By preserving motion, L-TDR may decrease the incidence of adjacent spine segment degeneration by reducing stress at adjacent spine levels. Pseudarthrosis and bone graft site morbidity are also removed as potential complications. And, because L-TDR does not require a posterior approach, muscular necrosis or dysfunction is also removed as potential complications.

INDICATIONS FOR LUMBAR TOTAL DISK REPLACEMENT

Lumbar total disk replacement is indicated for patients with low back pain from DDD (single level from L3-S1) who have failed a minimum of 6 months of nonoperative treatments.[3] In carefully selected cases, L-TDR can also alleviate neuroforaminal stenosis by restoring the intervertebral disk height and increasing the neuroforaminal height. Ideal candidates for L-TDR are between 18 years and 60 years old, optimally below 50 years old. L-TDR is currently approved by the Food and Drug Administration (FDA) for single level disease, although investigational device exemption studies have alluded to its effectiveness when used for two-level disease as well. Symptomatic DDD should ideally be demonstrated by objective evidence supported by computed tomography or magnetic resonance imaging, as well as by a positive provocative discogram performed by an independent radiologist or anesthesiologist. A positive discogram should demonstrate concordant pain reproduction and use at least one control level that is not painful and does not reproduce the patient's symptoms. Discography has been reviewed in Chapter 15.

There are many contraindications to L-TDR. Spine-specific contraindications include spondylolisthesis, spondylolysis, posterior element disease (facet joint arthritis or previous facet joint resection), central or lateral recess stenosis, fixed deformity, infection, osteoporosis, or herniated nucleus pulposus with radiculopathy that cannot be decompressed by way of an anterior approach.[4] Relative contraindications include psychosocial pathology, multilevel disease, and obesity. Many of these contraindications are common in patients with DDD. Huang et al. studied the prevalence of contraindications to L-TDR in a cohort of patients undergoing lumbar surgery.[5] In the fusion group, 56 of 56 patients had contraindications to L-TDR. In the nonfusion group, 39 of 44 patients had contraindications to L-TDR. Due to the high incidence of contraindications, predictions that L-TDR will replace fusion surgery are currently premature. As clinical experience with TDR grows, several contraindications may be eliminated.[4]

SURGICAL APPROACH AND TECHNIQUE

Lumbar total disk replacement utilizes an anterior surgical approach. The patient is positioned supine on a radiolucent table, and assurances of adequate C-arm fluoroscopy are confirmed. The "Da Vinci" position, with legs and arms spread, allows the surgeon to operate between the legs. A general or vascular surgeon assists in accessing the diseased level through an anterior retroperitoneal dissection. Skin incision varies depending on the level. A Pfannenstiel skin incision for the L5-S1 segment is suitable, but not for the upper lumbar levels, where a longitudinal (midline or paramedian) incision is necessary. After the disk space is exposed, radiography confirms the level. Retractors are placed to assure adequate working space and to protect critical neighboring structures. The annulus is incised, and the disk is removed using rongeurs, leaving the lateral annulus intact. It is important that the posterior annulus fibrosus is adequately released to allow correct positioning and function of the prosthesis. The cartilaginous end plates are carefully removed, making sure to preserve the integrity of the bony end plates to help preventing subsidence. Each implant system varies in specific technique. A sizing device is used to determine the appropriate component size. The proper size and lordotic angle are determined with anteroposterior/lateral fluoroscopy to ensure proper spinal implant placement before implanting the final prosthesis. From a height standpoint, it is important to keep the implants on the smaller size to avoid overstuffing the disk space and to help preserve motion. The largest footprint should be chosen to prevent subsidence of the implant.

PROSTHESES

Two prostheses, SB Charité III and ProDisc-L, have been approved by the FDA, with several other prostheses currently under the clinical trial (Table 48.1).

SB CHARITÉ III (FIGS. 48.1 AND 48.2)

The initial design of the SB Charité III was the first total disk prosthesis, developed by Dr Butter-Janz and Dr Schellnack at the Charité clinic in former East Germany. The SB Charité III disk became commercially available for the first time in the late 1980s and was first implanted in the United States in 2000, gaining FDA approval in November of 2004. The device has end plates manufactured from cobalt-chromium-molybdenum (CoCrMo) alloy with small fins projecting into the vertebral bodies, and an intervening ultrahigh molecular weight polyethylene (UHMWPE) sliding core. To assist bony ingrowth, the outer layer is porous-coated with plasma-sprayed titanium and calcium phosphate (TiCaP). A specific feature of the SB Charité III is the sliding, unconstrained biconvex polyethylene core, which is designed to allow for an instantaneous axis of rotation closely paralleling the natural motion of the native disk. However, there are potential disadvantages to the SB Charité III disk. Because it has two articulations, over time the Charité III is theoretically more prone to polyethylene wear and debris than are

Table 48.1: Properties of lumbar total disk arthroplasty prostheses

SB Charité III	CoCrMo UHMWPE	Metal on polymer	2	Unconstrained	Mobile	Small fins/bone ingrowth
ProDisc-L	CoCrMo UHMWPE	Metal on polymer	1	Semiconstrained	Fixed	Keel/bone ingrowth
Maverick	CoCrMo	Metal on metal	1	Semiconstrained	Fixed	Keel/bone ingrowth
FlexiCore	CoCrMo	Metal on metal	1	Fully constrained	Fixed	Small fins/bone ingrowth

(Courtesy of Deput Spine, Raynham, MA)
Source: Reprinted from Lin and Wang.[2]

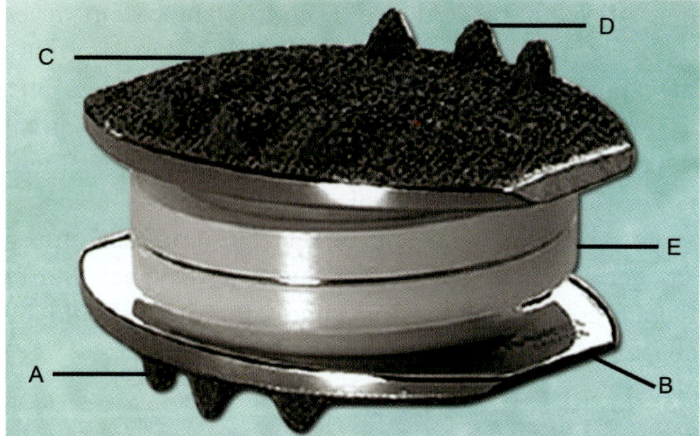

Fig. 48.1: SB Charité III artificial disk (oblique view). (A) anterior, (B) lateral, (C) CoCrMo alloy end plates, (D) fixation fins and (E) polyethylene core. *Source*: Reproduced with permission from Depuy Spine, Inc. Copyright Depuy Spine, Raynham, MA.

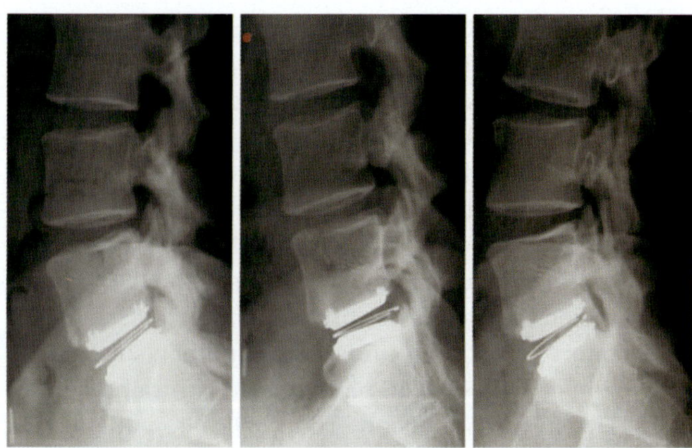

Fig. 48.2: Radiographic views of SB Charité III at L5–S1, at the 5-year follow-up time point, in (A) lateral, (B) flexion and (C) extension. *Source*: Reprinted from Guyer et al.[16]

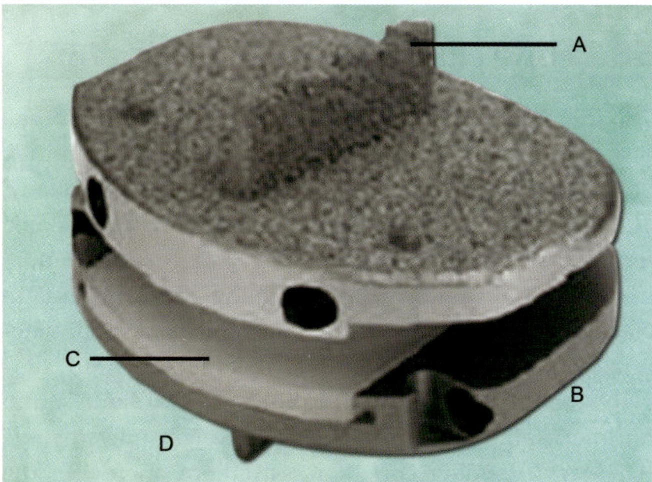

Fig. 48.3: ProDisc-L prosthesis (oblique view). (A) superior fixation keel, (B) lateral, (C) polyethylene core and (D) anterior. (Courtesy of Synthes, West Chester, PA).
Source: Reprinted from Lin and Wang.[2]

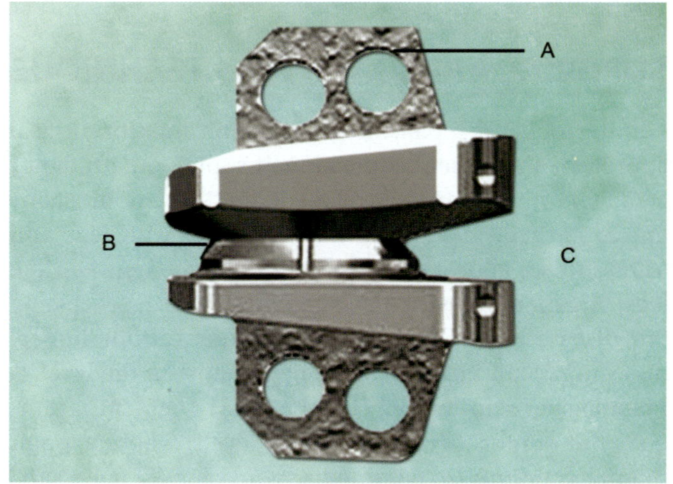

Fig. 48.4: Maverick artificial disk (lateral view). (A) superior fixation keel, (B) metal-on-metal articulation and (C) anterior. (Courtesy of Medtronic). *Source*: Reprinted from Lin and Wang.[2]

single-articulation designs.[2] As an unconstrained device, the risk of polyethylene extrusion is also greater, as is the risk of implant expulsion.

ProDisc-L (Fig. 48.3)

The ProDisc I, the initial design of the ProDisc-L, was developed by Dr Thierry Marnay in the 1980s and first implanted in 1990. The ProDisc-L has CoCrMo alloy end plates that are plasma sprayed with titanium, two vertical fins for fixation in the vertebral bodies, and a UHMWPE core. End plate fixation is assured by a single, large, porous-coated, midline sagittal keel. The polyethylene core is snap-fitted into the inferior end plate, resulting in a semiconstrained design, which should decrease the risk of extrusion. But, the fixed axis of rotation does not allow for coupled vertebral translation with flexion and extension.[2]

Maverick (Fig. 48.4)

The Maverick artificial disk was first implanted in Europe in early 2002. The characteristic feature of the Maverick prosthesis is its CoCrMo metal-on-metal bearing surface without a polyethylene component. Biomechanical and biomaterial research on articulating surfaces has shown that metal-on-metal bearings generate significantly fewer wear particles and stimulate less of an immune response than

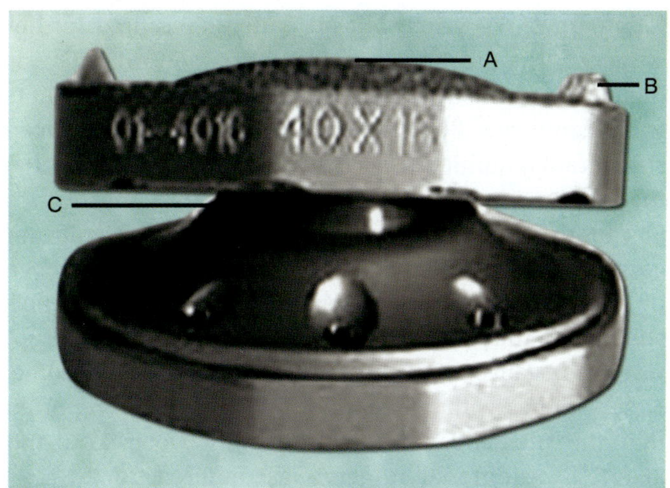

Fig. 48.5: FlexiCore implant (anterior view). (A) superior end plate, (B) lateral fixation fins and (C) metal-on-metal articulation. (Courtesy of Stryker Spine.)
Source: Reprinted from Lin and Wang.[2]

do metal-on-polyethylene bearings.[2] Like the ProDisc-L, the Maverick uses large, porous-coated central keels for fixation, producing a semiconstrained device with a fixed and slightly more posterior center of rotation.

FlexiCore (Fig. 48.5)

The FlexiCore artificial disk has a metal-on-metal (CoCrMo) articulating surface. The device is inserted as a single unit. The end plates, domed to fit into the concavities of the vertebral bodies, are coated with a titanium plasma spray to assist bone ingrowth fixation and have fins that affix to the vertebral bodies. The FlexiCore disk is a fully constrained design with a fixed center of rotation.

OUTCOMES

Clinical Outcome

Lemaire et al. reported the outcome of the SB Charité III with 11.3-year follow-up in 2005, finding that 90% of the patients had good or excellent clinical results in the Stauffer-Coventry Scale.[6] Several other prospective studies of the SB Charité III have also reported positive results, as well as Visual Analog Scale (VAS) improvement, Oswestry Disability Index (ODI) improvement, and patient satisfaction.[7-9] At an average of 8.7-year follow-up of the ProDisc I prosthesis, Tropiano et al. reported significant improvements in low back pain, radiculopathy, disability, and modified Stauffer-Coventry scores.[10] About 82.6% of Tropiano's patients were ''completely satisfied'' or ''satisfied'' with their results. In a 2-year follow-up study of the Maverick device by Huec et al. improvement was reported by the VAS for low back pain and leg pain (decreasing by 44 and 18 points, respectively), functional status improved by 25% in 75% of patients, and the average ODI score decreased by 20.7%.[11]

Accuracy of placement has been reported to affect the clinical outcome of L-TDR (Level I evidence).[12] Huang et al. reported that segmental ROM >5° was associated with a statistically significant but clinically modest better clinical outcome and a trend toward improved low back pain scores when compared with ROM ≤5° (Level III evidence).[13] One study found that reoperation at index level occurred in 1–28.6% of patients.[14] Putzier et al. published a retrospective study with a 17-year follow-up, finding reoperation to be necessary in 11% of patients.[15]

L-TDR vs Lumbar Fusion Surgery

There are four randomized controlled multicenter trials (Charité III, ProDisc-L, FlexiCore, Maverick) that studied the effectiveness of L-TDR compared with lumbar fusion surgery. However, the FlexiCore and Maverick trials were discontinued before completion.

The Charité trial randomized patients to either L-TDR with the Charité III disk or anterior interbody fusion with the Bagby and Kuslich, and tracked the outcomes for 5 years.[16] Outcomes on the composite score of clinical success showed that the Charité group was not inferior to the lumbar fusion group (57.8 vs 51.2%; $p < 0.04$). There were no statistically significant differences in functional impairment and pain intensity.

The ProDisc trial randomized patients to either L-TDR with the ProDisc-L device or to anterior lumbar circumferential fusion (using femoral ring allograft and posterolateral fusion with autogenous iliac crest bone graft in combination with pedicle screws) with a follow-up of 5 years.[17] Statistical success in the ProDisc group (53.7%) had reached similar levels as compared with the fusion group (50.0%) at 5-year follow-up. It was shown that L-TDR was noninferior compared with fusion with the two techniques showing similar improvement in ODI, SF-36, and VAS scores. There were no statistically significant differences between the groups.

The ProDisc trial was also performed for two-level L-TDR treatment, with patients being randomized similarly as in the one level ProDisc trial.[18] Clinical success was achieved in a significantly higher percentage of patients in the ProDisc group (73.2%) compared with the fusion group (59.7%) ($p < 0.05$).

The FlexiCore trial reported the initial result of patients from two clinics involved in a randomized multicenter controlled trial comparing the FlexiCore device versus anterior lumbar circumferential fusion with a 2-year follow-up.[19] Improvement in pain intensity (VAS –70 vs –62) and functional impairment (Oswestry –56 vs –46%) was slightly better in the FlexiCore group than in the fusion group. The Maverick trial randomized 405 patients into the lumbar disk arthroplasty group and 172 to control group receiving anterior lumbar interbody fusion. While both groups improved significantly from preoperative levels, the L-TDR group had statistically superior and significant results ($p < 0.05$) when compared VAS (53.4 vs 49), SF-36 (17.0 vs 14.3) and ODI (33.8 vs 29.2) improvement scores.[20]

Range of Motion

Shim et al. reported that the SB Charité III retained 11° of motion at a mean follow-up of 41 months.[21] Huang et al. retrospectively reported on the ProDisc I device at a mean follow-up of 8.7 years: 66% of prostheses retained >2° of motion at the implanted level.[22] McAfee et al. reported that accuracy of implant placement affects both clinical outcome and ROM after L-TDR.[12] Huang et al. reported that ROM >5° was associated with better clinical outcome when compared with ROM ≤5°.[13]

Facet Degeneration

Lemaire et al. reported 11% radiographic and 4% symptomatic facet degeneration at 10-year follow-up of the SB Charité III device.[6] Symptoms were developed in 36% of patients who had nonideal anterior positioning of the prosthesis. David et al. reported that 4.7% of patients required posterior fusion for symptomatic facet degeneration within 3–12 years after implantation of the SB Charité III.[23] Symptomatic facet degeneration accounted for 45.4% of index level reoperation. The development of symptomatic facet degeneration was also correlated with anterior placement of the prosthesis. van Ooij et al. reported a 40.7% incidence of facet joint degeneration among patients with unsatisfactory results from the SB Charité III.[24] Siepe et al. reported that the incidence was 20% at 53-month follow-up of the ProDisc II.[25]

Adjacent Level Degeneration

Huang et al. reported that the incidence of adjacent level degeneration (ALD) in their series was 24% at a mean follow-up of 8.7 years, but no patients required further surgery.[22] The prevalence of ALD after the ProDisc I was higher in patients with ROM <5°, suggesting that patients with significant ROM after L-TDR may have reduced risk of radiographic ALD.[26] However, Siepe et al. reported that the incidence of ALD was 10.2% in a trial with a 53-month follow-up of the ProDisc II, with no significant correlation between index level ROM and the occurrence of ALD ($p > 0.05$).[25] The degenerative changes in Siepe's study were mild, occurred late after surgery, and did not reveal a negative effect on postoperative clinical outcome. Other studies with >3 years of follow-up have reported that the incidence of ALD ranges between 17% and 28.6%.[15,21] Additional surgery was required for 2–3% of patients in two studies.[6,23]

COMPLICATIONS

Approach-related Complications

Approach-related complications include vascular injury, deep venous thrombosis, abdominal herniation, abdominal hematoma, and retrograde ejaculation. The reported rates of these complications have been similar to those reported for anterior lumbar interbody fusions and are clearly related to surgical technique and experience.[27,28] In a recent systematic review, the approach-related complication rate ranged from 2.1% to 18.7%.[14]

Short-term Implant-related Complications

Implant-related complications during the perioperative period include implant malposition, implant failure, vertebral body fracture, infection, and postoperative radiculopathy. The incidence of anterior migration or dissociation of the free-floating polyethylene core of the SB Charité III was 7% in early reports, but has become less common with increased surgeon experience and the introduction of a hydroxyapatite coating.[27] There have been rare reports of anterior liner subluxation of ProDisc II in the early postoperative period.[29,30] Vertebral body fracture during implantation or in the immediate postoperative period has also been rarely reported, and can be reduced by avoiding surgery on osteopenic patients and excessive distraction.[31-33] Postoperative radiculopathy has been attributed to iatrogenic herniation of nucleus pulposus or nerve root traction resulting from disk space distraction in patients with prior lumbar surgery and postoperative epidural fibrosis.[29,32,34] Postimplantation radiculopathy tends to improve without surgery.[33]

Long-term Implant-related Complications

Long-term implant-related complications include mechanical failure, osteolysis, and subsidence. The incidence of mechanical failure in the form of metallic end plate fracture was high in earlier L-TDR implants, and, however, has become less common with current metal technology.[33] Aseptic loosening, secondary to polyethylene wear and osteolysis, after implantation of polyethylene bearing L-TDR is currently rare. No significant data is available regarding metal wear or osteolysis of metal-on-metal L-TDR. Implant subsidence has been reported.[24,34] Cinotti et al. reported a 9% incidence of subsidence of the SB Charité III at a 2-year follow-up.[34] van Ooij et al. found that 67% of patients with unsatisfactory results after the SB Charité III had subsidence and believed that this was a significant contributor to poor outcomes.[24]

REFERENCES

1. Fritzell P, Hagg O, Wessberg P, et al. 2001 Volvo Award Winner in Clinical Studies: lumbar fusion versus nonsurgical treatment for chronic low back pain: a multicenter randomized controlled trial from the Swedish Lumbar Spine Study Group. Spine (Phila Pa 1976). 2001;26(23):2521-32; discussion 2532-4.
2. Lin EL, Wang JC. Total disk arthroplasty. J Am Acad Orthop Surg. 2006;14(13):705-14.
3. McAfee PC. The indications for lumbar and cervical disc replacement. Spine J. 2004;4(6 Suppl):177S-181S.
4. Frelinghuysen P, Huang RC, Girardi FP, et al. Lumbar total disc replacement part I: rationale, biomechanics, and implant types. Orthop Clin North Am. 2005;36(3):293-9.
5. Huang RC, Lim MR, Girardi FP, et al. The prevalence of contraindications to total disc replacement in a cohort of lumbar surgical patients. Spine (Phila Pa 1976). 2004;29(22): 2538-41.
6. Lemaire JP, Carrier H, Sariali el H, et al. Clinical and radiological outcomes with the Charite artificial disc: a 10-year minimum follow-up. J Spinal Disord Tech. 2005;18(4):353-9.
7. Regan JJ. Clinical results of charite lumbar total disc replacement. Orthop Clin North Am. 2005;36(3):323-40.
8. Ross R, Mirza AH, Norris HE, et al. Survival and clinical outcome of SB Charite III disc replacement for back pain. J Bone Joint Surg Br. 2007;89(6):785-9.
9. Gioia G, Mandelli D, Randelli F. The Charite III artificial disc lumbar disc prosthesis: assessment of medium-term results. J Orthoped Traumatol. 2007;8(3):134-9.
10. Tropiano P, Huang RC, Girardi FP, et al. Lumbar total disc replacement. Seven to eleven-year follow-up. J Bone Joint Surg Am. 2005;87(3):490-6.
11. Le Huec JC, Basso Y, Aunoble S, et al. Influence of facet and posterior muscle degeneration on clinical results of lumbar total disc replacement: two-year follow-up. J Spinal Disord Tech. 2005;18(3):219-23.
12. McAfee PC, Cunningham B, Holsapple G, et al. A prospective, randomized, multicenter Food and Drug Administration investigational device exemption study of lumbar total disc replacement with the CHARITE artificial disc versus lumbar fusion: part II: evaluation of radiographic outcomes and correlation of surgical technique accuracy with clinical outcomes. Spine (Phila Pa 1976). 2005;30(14):1576-83; discussion E388-90.
13. Huang RC, Girardi FP, Cammisa FP, Jr., et al. Correlation between range of motion and outcome after lumbar total disc replacement: 8.6-year follow-up. Spine (Phila Pa 1976). 2005;30(12):1407-11.
14. van den Eerenbeemt KD, Ostelo RW, van Royen BJ, et al. Total disc replacement surgery for symptomatic degenerative lumbar disc disease: a systematic review of the literature. Eur Spine J. 2010;19(8):1262-80.
15. Putzier M, Funk JF, Schneider SV, et al. Charite total disc replacement—clinical and radiographical results after an average follow-up of 17 years. Eur Spine J. 2006;15(2): 183-95.
16. Guyer RD, McAfee PC, Banco RJ, et al. Prospective, randomized, multicenter Food and Drug Administration investigational device exemption study of lumbar total disc replacement with the CHARITE artificial disc versus lumbar fusion: five-year follow-up. Spine J. 2009;9(5):374-86.
17. Zigler JE, Delamarter RB. Five-year results of the prospective, randomized, multicenter, Food and Drug Administration investigational device exemption study of the ProDisc-L total disc replacement versus circumferential arthrodesis for the treatment of single-level degenerative disc disease. J Neurosurg Spine. 2012;17(6):493-501.
18. Delamarter R, Zigler JE, Balderston RA, et al. Prospective, randomized, multicenter Food and Drug Administration investigational device exemption study of the ProDisc-L total disc replacement compared with circumferential arthrodesis for the treatment of two-level lumbar degenerative disc disease: results at twenty-four months. J Bone Joint Surg Am. 2011;93(8):705-15.
19. Sasso RC, Foulk DM, Hahn M. Prospective, randomized trial of metal-on-metal artificial lumbar disc replacement: initial results for treatment of discogenic pain. Spine (Phila Pa 1976). 2008;33(2):123-31.
20. Gornet MF, Burkus JK, Dryer RF, et al. Lumbar disc arthroplasty with Maverick disc versus stand-alone interbody fusion: a prospective, randomized, controlled, multicenter investigational device exemption trial. Spine (Phila Pa 1976). 2011;36(25):E1600-11.
21. Shim CS, Lee SH, Shin HD, et al. CHARITE versus ProDisc: a comparative study of a minimum 3-year follow-up. Spine (Phila Pa 1976). 2007;32(9):1012-8.
22. Huang RC, Girardi FP, Cammisa Jr FP, et al. Long-term flexion-extension range of motion of the prodisc total disc replacement. J Spinal Disord Tech. 2003;16(5):435-40.
23. David T. Long-term results of one-level lumbar arthroplasty: minimum 10-year follow-up of the CHARITE artificial disc in 106 patients. Spine (Phila Pa 1976). 2007;32(6): 661-6.

24. van Ooij A, Oner FC, Verbout AJ. Complications of artificial disc replacement: a report of 27 patients with the SB Charite disc. J Spinal Disord Tech. 2003;16(4):369-83.
25. Siepe CJ, Zelenkov P, Sauri-Barraza JC, et al. The fate of facet joint and adjacent level disc degeneration following total lumbar disc replacement: a prospective clinical, X-ray, and magnetic resonance imaging investigation. Spine (Phila Pa 1976). 2010;35(22):1991-2003.
26. Huang RC, Tropiano P, Marnay T, et al. Range of motion and adjacent level degeneration after lumbar total disc replacement. Spine J. 2006;6(3):242-7.
27. Griffith SL, Shelokov AP, Buttner-Janz K, et al. A multicenter retrospective study of the clinical results of the LINK SB Charite intervertebral prosthesis. The initial European experience. Spine (Phila Pa 1976). 1994;19(16):1842-9.
28. Zeegers WS, Bohnen LM, Laaper M, et al. Artificial disc replacement with the modular type SB Charite III: 2-year results in 50 prospectively studied patients. Eur Spine J. 1999;8(3):210-7.
29. Mayer HM, Wiechert K, Korge A, et al. Minimally invasive total disc replacement: surgical technique and preliminary clinical results. Eur Spine J. 2002;11 Suppl 2:S124-30.
30. Zigler JE, Burd TA, Vialle EN, et al. Lumbar spine arthroplasty: early results using the ProDisc II: a prospective randomized trial of arthroplasty versus fusion. J Spinal Disord Tech. 2003;16(4):352-61.
31. Lemaire JP, Skalli W, Lavaste F, et al. Intervertebral disc prosthesis. Results and prospects for the year 2000. Clin Orthop Relat Res. 1997(337):64-76.
32. Tropiano P, Huang RC, Girardi FP, et al. Lumbar disc replacement: preliminary results with ProDisc II after a minimum follow-up period of 1 year. J Spinal Disord Tech. 2003;16(4):362-8.
33. Huang RC, Sandhu HS. The current status of lumbar total disc replacement. Orthop Clin North Am. 2004;35(1):33-42.
34. Cinotti G, David T, Postacchini F. Results of disc prosthesis after a minimum follow-up period of 2 years. Spine (Phila Pa 1976). 1996;21(8):995-1000.

CHAPTER

49 Conventional, Microscopic and Endoscopic Surgical Treatment of Lumbar Disk Herniations

Bartosz Grobelny, Michael L Smith

HISTORY

Spinal pathology has been diagnosed and treated as early as 1550 BCE. Nonoperative treatments of spinal fractures used in those times such as immobilization and traction continue to be utilized to this day.[1] Surgical treatment of spinal disease, however, did not make much progress till the development of antiseptic techniques. Laminectomy was first described by MacEwen in 1886.[2]

Virchow first described traumatic lumbar disk herniation in 1857, and several surgeons described laminectomies and resections of "chondromas" in the early 1900s.[3,4] In 1934, Mixter and Barr associated lumbar disk herniation with the symptoms of sciatica. Surgical removal of herniated disk fragments was most often performed through a transdural approach until Love introduced the intralaminar-extradural discectomy approach in 1939.[5] The modern microsurgical approach for lumbar discectomy was introduced independently by Caspar and Yasargil in 1977, ushering the advances made in the coming years—techniques seeking to minimize tissue trauma while still treating the underlying pathology.[6,7] Currently, there are myriad of invasive surgical options for the treatment of symptomatic herniated lumbar disks, each with inherent advantages and limitations.

Nonoperative Management

While the purpose of this chapter is to address the effectiveness of the various surgical techniques, we would be remiss not mentioning conservative nonoperative management as the initial treatment of symptomatic lumbar intervertebral disk herniation, and as the standard against which to compare the effectiveness of interventions. The Maine Lumbar Spine Study showed that 75% of patients with sciatica from a lumbar herniated disk chosen for conservative therapy were able to avoid surgery.[8]

Current conservative management includes patient counseling and education, acupuncture, physical therapy, medications (NSAIDs, steroids, narcotics, or muscle relaxants), devices (braces/corsets, orthopedic pillows, and shoe inserts), and epidural steroid injections.[9] Conservative therapy is used for patients with nonemergent symptomatic herniated lumbar disks before referral for surgery of refractory symptoms.

MODERN TECHNIQUES

Laminectomy/Open Hemilaminotomy

Laminectomy and hemilaminotomy remain the mainstay for treating symptomatic lumbar intervertebral disk herniation. Laminectomy allows bilateral decompression of the thecal sac and nerve roots and bilateral access to the disk space. This is useful for broad disk herniation with central canal compromise and bilateral symptoms. Laminectomy is often the best approach for cauda equina syndrome, ensuring sufficient decompression. Laminectomy for decompression at a single disk level typically involves removal of the inferior two-third of the cephalad lamina and the superior one-third of the caudal lamina.

Hemilaminotomy is much more commonly performed for typical unilateral posterolateral disk herniation with ipsilateral leg pain. There is significantly less disruption of the muscular attachments, less exposure of dura, and no interruption of the posterior spinous process/interspinous ligament tension band system compared with full laminectomy. A small window is made in the inferior one-third of the ipsilateral cephalad hemilamina (Figs. 49.1A and B). The most common approach is that popularized by Caspar and Yasargil in 1977,[6,7] which involves the aid of the operative microscope to minimize exposure, though the surgery may also be performed under loupe magnification.

At our institution, this procedure is performed with the patient prone on a Wilson frame. For single level disease, a midline skin incision 3–4 cm long is made at the appropriate level and dissection is carried out with electrocautery through the fascia to the spinous processes. Subperiosteal dissection is performed on the side of the disk herniation to expose the hemilamina covering the involved disk space while leaving the facet capsule intact. A self-retaining retractor (e.g. Taylor or McCulloch) is placed and the microscope is brought in for the hemilaminotomy, which is performed with high-speed air drill and Kerrison rongeurs. The ligamentum flavum is pierced and resected, exposing the thecal sac and passing nerve root. The root is retracted medially to expose the disk and the fragment removed. The wound is closed in layers and the patient mobilized and discharged home same day provided there is no cerebrospinal fluid (CSF) leak.

Minimal Access Spinal Techniques

Minimally invasive surgery (MIS) techniques for lumbar disk were introduced in 1997 with the microendoscopic discectomy.[10] Using tubular retractors, MIS techniques potentially allow smaller incisions and less tissue trauma. Minimal access spinal techniques (MAST) may be a preferable term, emphasizing that the same surgical goal must ultimately be met, with the added benefit of decreased tissue injury from exposure. It also mitigates the improper suggestion that MIS may imply a less serious procedure or less prone to surgical complication. Though it began with the use of an endoscope to visualize the working area, MIS techniques are now most commonly performed with the operative microscope. There are various similar tubular retractor systems available from the major manufacturers, all offering tubes of various diameters and lengths (Fig. 49.2A). Expandable tubes are also available, although they have proven more useful for MIS fusion techniques than simple discectomy.

In our institution, the patient is placed prone on a Wilson frame and the appropriate level is identified with fluoroscopy. A vertical incision is planned 1.5 cm lateral to the midline centered on the disk space. Length of incision depends on the diameter of the tubular retractors one plans to use, but will generally be approximately 25 mm long for an 18 mm diameter tube. Sharp dissection and electrocautery are used to dissect through the dermis, fat, and fascia. Sequential dilators are inserted through the fascial defect and are used to dilate the subcutaneous tissues and dissect muscle from the lamina. We recommend against K-wires, as they can pass through the interlaminar space and cause dural or nerve root injury.

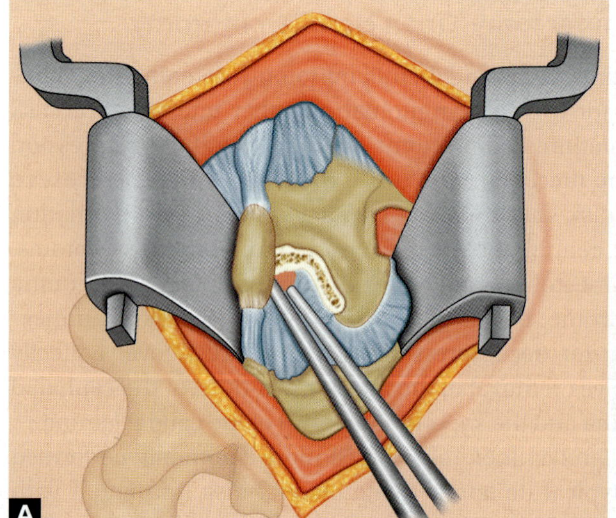

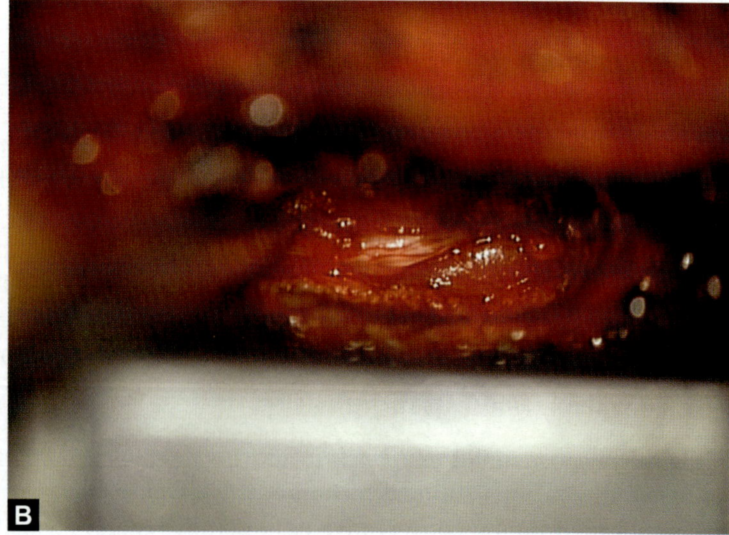

Figs. 49.1A and B: (A) Schematic representation of an exposure for an open hemilaminotomy. (B) Disk fragment seen compressing nerve root in an open hemilaminotomy exposure.

The tubular retractor is passed over the largest dilator and docked on the lamina over the disk space, fixed in place by a table-mounted arm (Figs. 49.2B and C). The microscope is brought in and the procedure is carried out as normal. Bayoneted instruments and fine drills help with visualization. Direct dural repair is difficult or impossible through small tubes, although persisting CSF fistula seems to be very rare, likely due to the very small dissection field and complete tissue collapse upon removal of the retractor. Closure of the wound is performed in layers and the patient may be discharged on the same day, barring any complications.

Percutaneous Mechanical Discectomy (Automated vs Endoscopic)

There are two forms of mechanical discectomy that do not involve direct exposure and visualization of the anatomy by the surgeon. With these, the instruments are either guided using a percutaneously inserted endoscope (Figs. 49.3A and B) or via fluoroscopy (Figs. 49.4A and B).

Under arthroscopic guidance, herniated disks can be removed via a posterolateral approach through percutaneous endoscopic discectomy (PED). Two portals are placed that allow for the use of suction and irrigation. This approach also allows for the inspection of the relevant anatomy and removal of most free fragments of disk material—the only exceptions being disk fragments that have migrated significantly in the cranial-caudal axis.[11] A solely radiographically guided approach [automatic percutaneous discectomy (APD)] does not allow for the removal of free disk fragments and is limited to central decompression of the nucleus pulposus by an automated suction nucleotome.

Both of these techniques can be performed with the patient in either a prone or lateral position with the patient under local anesthesia or mild sedation. Flexion of the

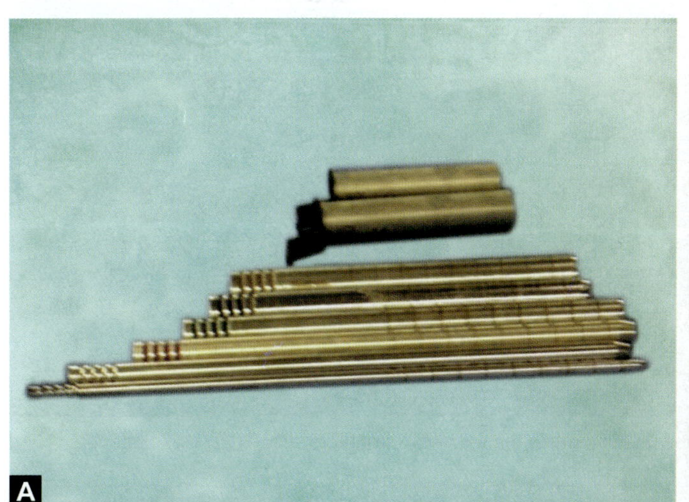

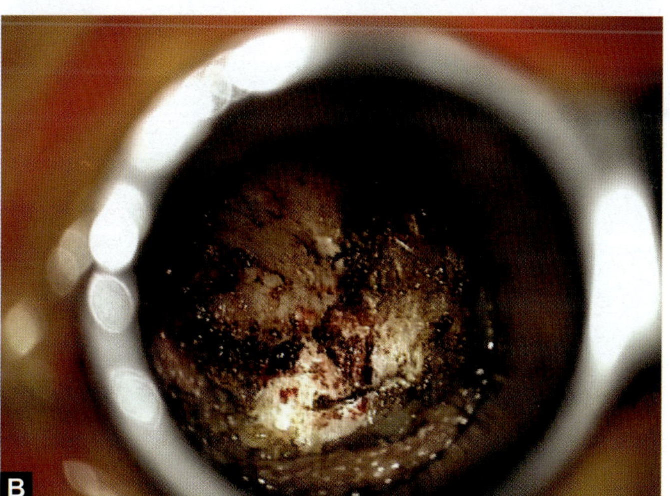

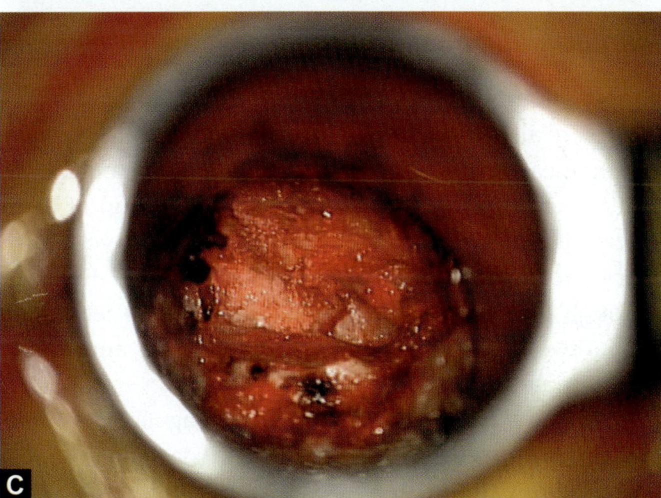

Figs. 49.2A to C: Minimally invasive surgery hemilaminotomy. (A) Dilators and tubes. (B) Exposure of the right hemilamina with the spinous process at the superior aspect of the figure. (C) Hemilaminotomy defect with exposed ligamentum flavum.

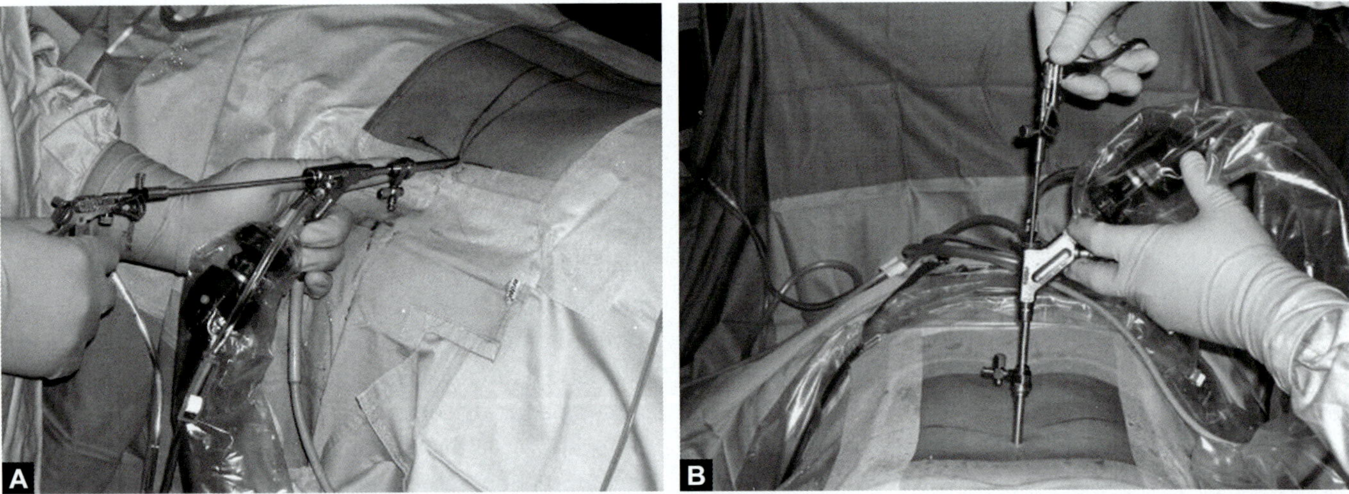

Figs. 49.3A and B: Approaches for percutaneous endoscopic discectomy. (A) Transforaminal and (B) interlaminar.
Source: Adapted from Ruetten et al.[29]

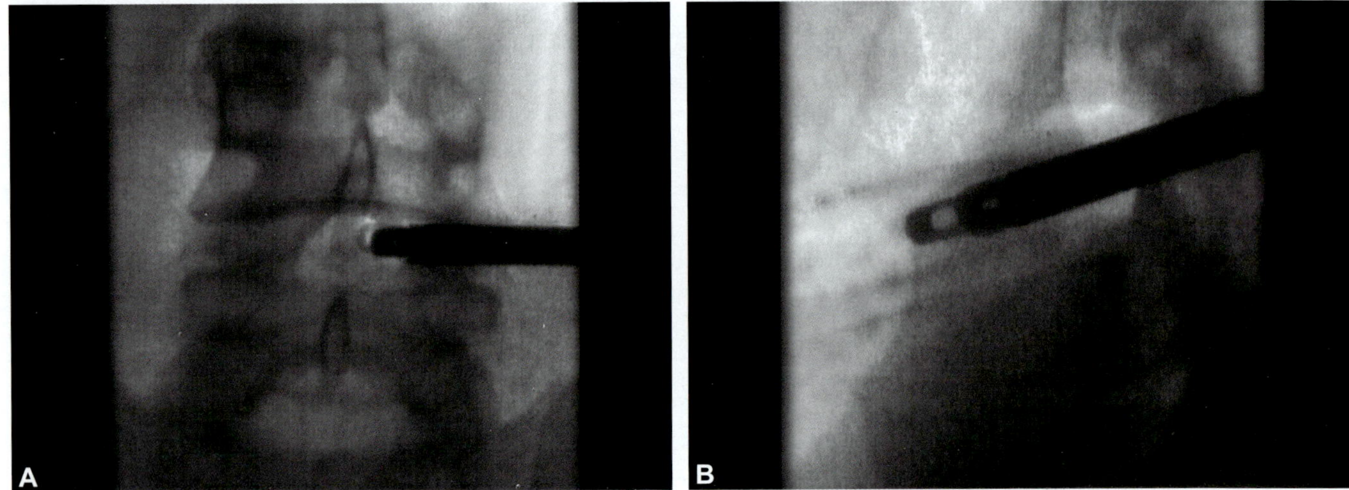

Figs. 49.4A and B: Fluoroscopic visualization of automatic percutaneous discectomy in the (A) anteroposterior and (B) lateral planes.
Source: Adapted from Jaikumar et al.[13]

hips reduces the lumbar lordosis and allows for a larger entry zone posteriorly. An 18-gauge, 25-cm, hubless, stainless steel trocar is inserted starting approximately 10 cm from midline and advanced obliquely, with fluoroscopic guidance, toward the posterior margin of the intervertebral disk, to reach the appropriate level. When the trocar is in the appropriate position, a 2.8-mm cannula with an internal, blunt-end, tapered dilator is placed over the hubless trocar. When the cannula and dilator are in the correct position, the dilator is removed. Annulotomy and discectomy are then carried out with appropriate tools and can be completed in 15–20 minutes.[11] In addition to this approach, a posterior interlaminar approach has been described.[12]

Percutaneous Laser Discectomy and Radio Frequency Thermocoagulation

There are also percutaneous methods that do not involve mechanical removal of the disk material. Percutaneous laser discectomy involves discectomy by action of short bursts of laser energy into the disk space.[13] This was introduced to lumbar disk surgery by Ascher and Heppner through their work with the CO_2 laser.[14] This technique is limited to reducing intradiscal pressure and is not appropriate for free disk fragments.

Similarly, radio frequency thermocoagulation is limited in its application. It is specifically designed to treat discogenic pain, with no use in decompressing disk herniations impinging on nerves or disk fragments. Intradiscal electrothermal annuloplasty (IDET) involves percutaneously threading a flexible heating electrode into the disk, such that the electrode passes circumferentially around the inner surface of the disk. The heating of the electrode denatures the collagen of the annulus (making it contract) and coagulates the pain fibers supplying the annulus, causing a nerve ablation without any discectomy.[13]

Chemonucleolysis

Chymopapain is derived from the latex of the fruit *Carica papaya*. Early animal work with similar compounds found that they were able to make the ears of rabbits droop. [15] An extension of this work by Smith et al. found that intradiscal injection in rabbits removed the nucleus pulposus without damaging the annulus fibrosus.[16] This, in turn, led to the attempted treatment of sciatica with intradiscal injections of chymopapain in 1963.[16] Collagenase, likewise, may be used for chemonucleolysis with identical indications, limitations, and contraindications.

The mechanism of action of chymopapain is through depolymerization of the proteoglycan and glycoprotein macromolecules in the nucleus pulposus responsible for the retention of water and turgidity, thus reducing disk height and bulge. It may also be involved in the inflammatory response in the affected nerve root.[13] For treatment patients are placed in a lateral or prone position for an extradural approach with a spinal needle under fluoroscopic guidance into the center of the nucleus pulposus. One to four thousands units are injected per disk space.[13,17]

Obvious limitations with this technique are sequestered disk fragments and "hard" disks. Age may also be a factor as older patients already have more significantly desiccated disks. Contraindications include allergies to papain, cauda equina syndrome, pregnancy, arachnoiditis, migrated disks, history of discitis, tumors involving the spinal cord, spinal canal compromise, and central or lateral recess stenosis, and diabetes mellitus with peripheral neuropathy.[13]

COMPARATIVE TRIALS

Numerous studies have been performed comparing the various treatments of symptomatic lumbar herniated disks with many of them being randomized controlled trials (RCTs). Open microdiscectomy, the standard in surgical treatment, has been the best studied in comparison with conservative treatment. The first RCT by Weber compared nonmicroscope-assisted discectomy with nonsurgical treatment. He found surgical patients fared significantly better at 1 year compared with the conservative management patients in terms of both patient and observer ratings, but this difference was lost after 4 and 10 years. However, 26% of those randomized crossed over to the surgical group.[18]

Despite the lack of long-term differences in outcome, Malter's analysis of Weber's data did show a gain of $29,000 in quality-adjusted life years in the surgical patients.[19] Similarly, in Greenfield's study the surgical group had a significant early improvement in outcome (12 and 18 months postsurgical) compared with the nonsurgical group, but this difference was no longer there at 24 months after the surgery.[20] The SPORT study compared open discectomy with conservative treatment. In actuality, there were two separate studies: an RCT and an observational study that allowed patients to elect surgical versus conservative treatment. Their surgeons were encouraged to use loupe or microscope magnification, though the precise breakdown is not known.

Again, like Weber's study, there was a significant amount of crossover, with small but insignificant differences in outcomes except the Sciatica Bothersomeness Index, which was significantly improved for the surgical intent-to-treat group throughout the 2-year follow-up.[9] In addition, the as-treated analysis showed strongly significant improvements in the surgical group over the conservative group at all time points extending 4 years of the study period.[9,21]

The observational cohort likewise showed strong results in favor of the patients who chose surgery.[22] Similarly, Buttermann compared open discectomy versus epidural steroid injection in symptomatic lumbar herniated disk patients and found an earlier improvement in pain and function in his operated patients, but this difference did not stay significant in late (2–3 year) follow-up. Those who crossed over into the treatment group did not have worse outcomes than those who were given surgery prior to injections.[23]

There are currently two prospective RCT comparing microscopic discectomy through a tubular retractor compared with conventional microdiscectomy. In the trial by Arts et al. the authors followed the two groups of patients for 1 year after their surgery at which point the tubular discectomy group was found to have statistically significant poorer functional status and visual analog pain scales than the conventional microdiscectomy. It should be noted, however, that the differences found in this study in the functional and visual analog scales were smaller than published minimally clinically important differences, thus this study could claim noninferiority between the two procedures with the exception of the finding that significantly fewer patients operated with tubular retractors reported good recovery (69% vs 79%). There were no differences in intraoperative complication rates, day of mobilization, mean hospital stay, or postoperative complications.[24]

Teli et al., however, compare three groups: endoscopic discectomy through a tubular retractor, discectomy with a Caspar retractor using microscope magnification, and the same using loupe magnification. While this trial shows no differences in functional outcomes across the three groups, it does show a trend for higher frequency of dural tears, root injury, and recurrent herniations in the endoscopic group compared with the other two cohorts.[25]

A particular concern for tubular discectomy is that the round tube inherently gives a more lateral view, usually the lateral half of the lamina and the medial facet. It is difficult to preserve as much of the facet with the tubular technique compared with conventional retractors, which allow a view directly down the spinous process. Postoperative CT scanning has tempered the senior author's enthusiasm for tubular microdiscectomy. The best candidate will be an operated level with a broad, flat hemilamina, without a large overlying or deviating spinous process. These subtleties are easily detected on preoperative axial MRI once one knows to look for them. L5-S1 is often suitable, L4-5 sometimes, while L3-4 or higher is almost never, due to the narrow interfacet distance at the higher levels.

Several RCTs compare percutaneous mechanical techniques with standard microdiscectomy. Chatterjee et al. compare APD using a nonflexible suction nucleotome with standard microdiscectomy in patients with contained lumbar disk herniations. They found that patients had significantly poorer outcomes at 6 months with APD than microdiscectomy.[26] Haines et al. showed that a combined group of automated percutaneous discectomy and endoscopic discectomy showed similar outcomes as microdiscectomy.[27] Similarly, Mayer et al. showed similar results for microsurgical and endoscopic discectomies.[28] However, both of the latter two trials were small ($n < 41$), so the conclusions that can be drawn are limited. A larger study by Ruetten et al., however, did also show similarly good long-term outcomes in both the percutaneous endoscopic and the microsurgical techniques. This study was not limited to contained disk herniations and allowed for the transforaminal and interlaminar endoscopic approaches to retrieve any disk fragments. There were fewer wound-related problems, lesser postoperative pain requirements, and a quicker return to work in the PED group. While acknowledging these advantages, the authors do emphasize the importance of the learning curve with the endoscopic procedure.[29]

Currently, there are no RCTs that compare percutaneous laser discectomy against any other form of treatment. There are studies that show that it can be effective in a well-selected population,[30] but currently more research needs to be done to establish its role. Similarly, there is very little data examining percutaneous radio frequency coagulation, with no trials comparing against accepted therapy or placebo.

Chemonucleolysis, although rarely done currently, does have multiple RCTs comparing against placebo to support its use.[31-35] The results from these are best synthesized in Gibson and Waddell's meta-analysis. This found that placebo was less likely to be effective than chymopapain intradiscal injections with an odds ratio of 0.24. Chemonucleolysis patients were also less likely to need open discectomy afterward with an odds ratio 0.41.[36] The same study analyzed several trials comparing chemonucleolysis against discectomy, which showed consistently worse outcomes with chemonucleolysis, though it was not found to be statistically significant.[36]

CONCLUSION

Radiculopathy from herniated lumbar disks can be excruciating and debilitating. Many patients will improve spontaneously in the first 4–8 weeks and their suffering eased with conservative measures. Surgery, however, remains the most powerful tool for providing rapid relief. The data in aggregate are insufficient to provide rigid guidelines. The patient must be treated as an individual, in alliance with his or her surgeon. The surgeon assesses the pathology and the likelihood of relief from surgery and the patient will relate his or her suffering and together a decision for surgical or nonsurgical management made. Microdiscectomy is a proven tool for decompression of nerve roots and relief of compressive symptoms with a low rate of complication. Minimally invasive techniques must be compared with this standard. Microscopic transtubular discectomy is essentially a microdiscectomy with a different retractor and a learning curve, but some data suggest worse clinical outcomes. Endoscopic techniques have a significant learning curve, with higher rates of complications and no solid proof of advantage. The appeal of the least invasive approaches (PED, APD, chemonucleolysis, and IDET) is made irrelevant by the lack of proven efficacy.

From all the studies performed to date, it is clear that there is a significant role for surgical intervention in the treatment of lumbar herniated disks. Emergent cases such as cauda equina syndrome would receive a rapid discectomy, most likely microscopic, for the decompression of the involved nerve roots. Nonemergent cases can be initially treated with a course of conservative treatment including pain medication, physical therapy, and epidural steroid injections with referral of refractory cases for surgical intervention. Although RCTs studying surgical treatment of lumbar disk treatment are burdened by high rates of crossover, there is strong evidence from the as-treated analyses and observational cohorts that surgical intervention does have a significant effect on patient outcomes.

The method of surgical intervention chosen does not appear to have significant effect on outcomes, for the most part. There is no clear advantage to performing the discectomy under any specific form of magnification or with any degree of "invasiveness" whether it is an open hemilaminotomy, one through tubular retractors, or an endoscopic approach. Though certain studies indicate there might be differences in complications based on technique, surgeon experience and comfort may be the most important factor in patient safety regardless of technique utilized. The only exceptions to this are automated percutaneous discectomy and chemonucleolysis that show poorer results than any of the other surgical interventions, especially since they cannot treat free disk fragments. Finally, there is still not sufficient data on laser discectomy and radio frequency coagulation, but they are not likely to find broad applications as they suffer the same limitations as automated percutaneous discectomy and chemonucleolysis.

REFERENCES

1. Knoeller S, Seifried C. History of spinal surgery. Spine (Phila Pa 1976). 2000;25(21):2838-43.
2. Ackerknecht E. Aus den Anfangen der Neurochirurgie. Schweizer Archiv fur Neurologie, Neurochirurgie und Psychiatrie. 1975;116:233-9.
3. Oppenheim H, Krause F. Uber Einklemmung bzw: Strangulation der cauda equina. Dtsch Med Wochenschr. 1909; 35:697-700.
4. Elsberg C. Experiences in spinal surgery: observations upon 60 laminectomies for spinal disease. Surg Gynecol Obstet. 1913;16:117-20.
5. Love J. Removal of protruded intervertebral disc without laminectomy. Proc Staff Meet Mayo Clin. 1939;14:800-5.
6. Yasargil M. Microsurgical operation of herniated lumbar disc. Adv Neurosurg. 1977;4:81.
7. Caspar W. A new surgical procedure for lumbar disc herniation causing less tissue damage through a microsurgical approach. Adv Neurosurg. 1977;4:74-7.
8. Atlas S, Keller R, Wu Y, et al. Long-term outcomes of surgical and nonsurgical management of sciatica secondary to a lumbar disc herniation: 10 year results from the Maine Lumbar Spine Study. Spine. 2005;30(8):927-35.
9. Weinstein J, Tosteson T, Lurie J, et al. Surgical vs nonoperative treatment for lumbar disk herniation: the Spine Patient Outcomes Research Trial (SPORT): a randomized trial. JAMA. 2006;296(20):2441-50.
10. Foley K, Smith M. Microscopic discectomy. Tech Neurosurg. 1997;3:301-7.
11. Kambin P. Arthroscopic microdiscectomy. Arthroscopy. 1992;8:287-95.
12. Ruetten S. The full-endoscopic interlaminar approach for lumbar disc herniations. Berlin: Springer; 2005.
13. Jaikumar S, Kim D, Kam A. History of minimally invasive spine surgery. Neurosurgery. 2002;51(Suppl 2):1-14.
14. Ascher P, Heppner F. CO_2-laser in neurosurgery. Neurosurg Rev. 1984;7:123-33.
15. Thomas L. Reversible collapse of rabbit ears after intravenous papain and prevention of recovery by cortisone. J Exp Med. 1956;104:245-52.
16. Smith L, Garvin P, Jennings R, et al. Enzyme dissolution of the nucleus pulposus. Nature. 1963;198:1311-2.
17. Burton AK, Tillotson KM, Cleary J. Single-blind randomised controlled trial of chemonucleolysis and manipulation in the treatment of symptomatic lumbar disc herniation. Eur Spine J. 2000;9(3):202-7.
18. Weber H. Lumbar disc herniation. A controlled, prospective study with ten years of observation. Spine. 1983;8(2): 131-40.
19. Malter A, Weinstein J. Cost-effectiveness of lumbar discectomy. Spine. 1996;21(24S):69-74S.
20. Greenfield K, Nelson R, Findlay G, et al. Microdiscectomy and conservative treatment for lumbar disc herniation with back pain and sciatica: a randomised clinical trial. Proceedings of the International Society for the Study of the Lumbar Spine. 2003:245.
21. Weinstein J, Lurie J, Tosteson T, et al. Surgical versus nonoperative treatment for lumbar disc herniation four-year results for the spine patient outcomes research trial (SPORT). Spine. 2008;33(25):2789-800.

22. Weinstein J, Lurie J, Tosteson T, et al. Surgical vs Nonoperative treatment for lumbar disk herniation the spine patient outcomes research trial (sport) observational cohort. JAMA. 2006;296(20):2451-9.
23. Buttermann G. Treatment of lumbar disc herniation: epidural steroid injection compared with discectomy: a prospective, randomized study. J Bone Joint Surg Am. 2004;86(4):670-9.
24. Arts M, Brand R, van der Akker E, et al. Tubular discectomy vs conventional microdiscectomy for sciatica: a randomized controlled trial. JAMA. 2009;302(2):149-58.
25. Teli M, Lovi A, Brayda-Bruno M, et al. Higher risk of dural tears and recurrent herniation with lumbar micro-endoscopic discectomy. Eur Spine J. 2010;19:443-50.
26. Chatterjee S, Foy P, Findlay G. Report of a controlled clinical trial comparing automated percutaneous lumbar discectomy and microdiscectomy in the treatment of contained lumbar disc herniation. Spine. 1995;20(6):734-8.
27. Haines S, Jordan N, Boen J, et al. Discectomy strategies for lumbar disc herniation: Results of the LAPDOG trial. J Clin Neuroscience. 2002;9(4):411-7.
28. Mayer H, Brock M. Percutaneous endoscopic discectomy: surgical technique and preliminary results compared to microsurgical discectomy. J Neurosurg. 1993;78:216-25.
29. Ruetten S, Komp M, Merk H, et al. Full-endoscopic interlaminar and transforaminal lumbar discectomy versus conventional microsurgical techniques. Spine. 2008;33(9): 931-9.
30. Zhao X, Fu Z, Xu Y, et al. Treatment of lumbar intervertebral disk herniation using C-arm fluoroscopy guided target percutaneous laser disk decompression. Photomed Laser Surg. 2012;30(2):92-5.
31. Dabezies E, Langford K, Morris J, et al. Safety and efficacy of chymopapain (Discase) in the treatment of sciatica due to a herniated nucleus pulposus. Results of a randomized, double-blind study. Spine. 1988;13(5):561-5.
32. Schwetschenau R, Ramirez A, Johnston J, et al. Double-blind evaluation of intradiscal chymopapain for herniated lumbar discs. Early Results. J Neurosurg. 1976;45:622-7.
33. Fraser R. Chymopapain for the treatment of intervertebral disc herniation. The final report of a double-blind study. Spine. 1984;9(8):815-8.
34. Javid M, Nordby E, Ford L, et al. Safety and efficacy of chymopapain (Chymodiactin) in herniated nucleus pulposus with sciatica. Results of a randomized, double-blind study. JAMA. 1983;249(18):2489-94.
35. Feldman J, Menkes C, Pallardy G, et al. Double-blind study of the treatment of disc lumbosciatica by chemonucleolysis. Rev Rhum Mal Osteoartic. 1986;53(3):147-52.
36. Gibson JN, Waddell G. Surgical interventions for lumbar disc prolapse. Cochrane Database Syst Rev. 2007;2:CD001350.

CHAPTER

50

Surgical Treatment of Lumbar Spinal Stenosis

Stephen P Maier II, Jane S Hoashi, Jeffrey D Klein

INTRODUCTION

Lumbar spinal stenosis is a clinical entity characterized by buttock and lower extremity pain and fatigue, typically precipitated by prolonged standing and ambulation. There is commonly lower back pain, and often-associated numbness and tingling in the lower extremities. Radiographically, lumbar stenosis refers to the absolute narrowing of the diameter of the spinal canal and neural foramen resulting in compression of the central neural elements as well as the exiting nerve roots. Although congenital forms of stenosis exist,[1,2] acquired spondylosis is the most common cause of lumbar stenosis, worsened by concurrent degenerative spondylolisthesis and scoliosis.

Aging individuals face inevitable degeneration of the spinal elements, thus predisposing them to lumbar spondylosis and the radiographic changes seen in lumbar stenosis. Ultimately, this renders them at increased risk for the development of the clinical symptoms of lumbar spinal stenosis. The process involves a cascade of events that begin as disk degeneration.[3] Disk desiccation leads to a loss of disk height accompanied by posterior bulging, resulting in increased stress on the facet joints. Stenosis of the canal is ultimately caused by hypertrophy of the facets, enlargement, and buckling of the ligamentum flavum, and osteophyte formation involving the vertebral endplates. Decreased disk height can also reduce foraminal height and cause compression of the nerve roots. Although the symptoms vary and depend on the areas and severity of compression, patients with stenosis commonly present with lower back pain along with variable activity-related symptoms into the lower extremities.

The natural history of mild-to-moderate stenosis is favorable, and progression is generally slow.[4,5] Although conservative measures are initially employed, symptoms can persist or worsen with age, and surgery is recommended in these cases. In fact, stenosis is the leading indicator for spinal surgery in adults aged 65 years and older.[6,7] A 2010 study estimated that nearly $1.65 billion was spent on over 37,000 lumbar spinal stenosis surgeries during 2007 among this age group.[8]

CLINICAL FEATURES

As previously noted, patients with lumbar stenosis typically present with lower back pain and bilateral buttock and leg pain in a pattern consistent with neurogenic claudication, radiculopathy, or a combination of the two.[9,10] Central stenosis is associated with neurogenic claudication, while lateral recess and foraminal stenoses give rise to radiculopathic symptoms.[3] Neurogenic claudication refers to a pain syndrome precipitated by walking and prolonged standing. It is characterized by pain and sometimes a burning sensation or paresthesias radiating from the back to the buttocks and to lower extremities. General weakness and fatigue of the lower extremities associated with ambulation are also common. These symptoms are alleviated by lumbar flexion such as occurs when sitting. This motion decreases the buckling of the ligamentum in the canal and reduces the compression of the neural elements contained both within the canal and the foramen (Figs. 50.1A and B). Patients describe the ability to walk longer distances while leaning over objects such as a stroller or a shopping cart.

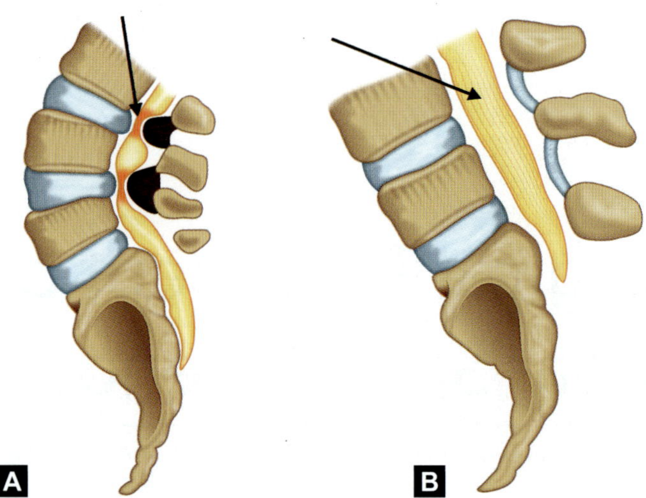

Figs. 50.1A and B: Schematic representation of painful effects due to lumbar stenosis in the (A) extended (standing) position, and (B) the flexed (seated) position. Pain is relieved during extension due to the flattening of the ligamentum flavum, which is the source of neural compression, and consequently, pain when it buckles.

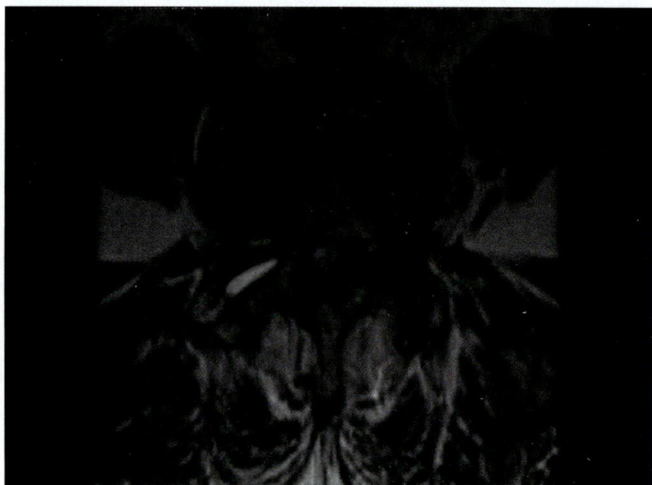

Fig. 50.2: T2-weighted axial image showing marked central stenosis and bilateral facet arthrosis with fluid in the right facet joint.

Radiculopathic pain is due to nerve root compression in either the lateral recess or neural foramen. These symptoms typically follow the dermatomal pattern of the affected nerve root. Symptoms can be unilateral or bilateral based on the location of the stenosis. It is not uncommon for symptoms to be unilateral despite imaging studies that reveal clear central and bilateral findings.

PHYSICAL EXAMINATION AND DIFFERENTIAL DIAGNOSIS

Pain radiating to the lower extremities can arise from conditions other than stenosis. Vascular disease, peripheral or diabetic neuropathy, neurologic disorders, hip or knee pathology, renal disorders, infection, and tumors can present with similar symptoms.[3,4] Therefore, a thorough physical examination is necessary to help reach an accurate diagnosis.

Motor and sensory deficits along dermatomal distributions should be noted, as they may reflect neural compression in the corresponding areas. Lumbar extension can elicit the patient's symptoms as this aggravates both central stenosis and foraminal narrowing. A thorough physical examination can also help rule out peripheral or diabetic neuropathy as well as other neurologic disorders. Signs of myelopathy should also be sought by observing the patient's gait and coordination as there is evidence that lumbar stenosis is associated with a predisposition for concomitant cervical stenosis.[11] The hip joint and greater trochanter should also be evaluated to rule out hip arthritis or trochanteric bursitis as sources of lower extremity pain.

One must carefully distinguish neurogenic claudication from the symptoms of peripheral vascular disease. Vascular claudication is due to reduced blood flow to the lower extremities and is characterized by lower extremity pain associated with ambulation. The pain of vascular claudication is typically more distal, while that from spinal stenosis is both proximal and distal. Patients may have diminished pulses and hair loss of their lower extremities.[4] In contrast to neurogenic claudication, the pain of vascular claudication is relieved only by rest and not by sitting or flexion of the lumbar spine.[12]

DIAGNOSTIC IMAGING

The standard radiographic modalities are utilized to confirm the clinical findings suggestive of stenosis on physical examination. Plain radiographs in anteroposterior and lateral views are used to assess for general coronal and sagittal alignment, spondylosis, associated spondylolisthesis, and scoliosis. Lateral flexion and extension films can be useful for identifying areas of instability. Magnetic resonance imaging (MRI) is the study of choice,[3] providing a clear image of disk degeneration, disk protrusion, ligamentum flavum thickening, osteophyte formation, and facet joint hypertrophy—all of which act in concert to create stenosis and compromise the neural elements (Fig. 50.2).[13] Computed tomography (CT) is quite helpful for bony detail and is commonly utilized in the setting of prior surgery where the anatomy has been distorted.

CT myelography is also useful when there is associated scoliosis. The deformity causes the spine to move in and out of the planes of the MRI study rendering it difficult to evaluate. The contrast column of the CT myelogram allows one to better assess the neural elements and any associated neural compression.[4]

ELECTRODIAGNOSTIC STUDIES

Though not routinely performed, electrodiagnostic studies, including electromyography (EMG), nerve conduction velocity (NCV) tests, and somatosensory evoked potentials (SSEP), may supplement radiographic imaging by helping to localize symptomatic levels. In addition, these techniques can help distinguish between radiculopathy and peripheral nerve issues such as neuropathy and nerve entrapment. Peripheral nerve disorders and radiculopathy may also coexist.

INDICATIONS FOR SURGERY

Conservative treatment is typically employed after the initial presentation of symptoms associated with spinal stenosis. Epidural steroid injections, nonsteroidal anti-inflammatory drugs (NSAIDs), physical therapy and exercise, and sometimes orthoses are utilized to manage these patients.[14] If symptoms persist or worsen and the patient deems them unacceptable, it is reasonable to consider surgical treatment in an effort to improve the impaired quality of life.

SURGICAL TREATMENT

Decompression

The objective in all lumbar spinal stenosis surgery is to decompress the compressed neural elements traversing or exiting the lumbar spinal canal. The canal has three distinct areas of potential compression: the central canal, the lateral recess, and the neural foramen. Decompressive surgery for any given patient must address each of these regions at all involved levels.

Central decompression requires resection of the medial portion of the lamina and the ligamentum flavum from each of the affected levels.[15] Lumbar stenosis is most commonly seen at the L4/5 level. This is typically due to bulging disks and ligamentum flavum hypertrophy and is 3–5 times more likely to occur in women than men.[16,17] In order to decompress the neural components, slightly >50% of the cephalad lamina and slightly <50% of the caudad lamina are surgically removed (Fig. 50.3).

Lateral recess stenosis is present in most, if not all, cases of lumbar stenosis necessitating thorough lateral decompression. Subarticular neural compression presents between the medial aspect of the hypertrophic superior articular facet and the posterior aspect of the vertebral body and disk.[18] Protruding disks, osteophytes, and synovial cysts emanating from arthritic facet joints can all act together to encroach upon the central and lateral canal with resultant neural compression (Figs. 50.4 and 50.5).

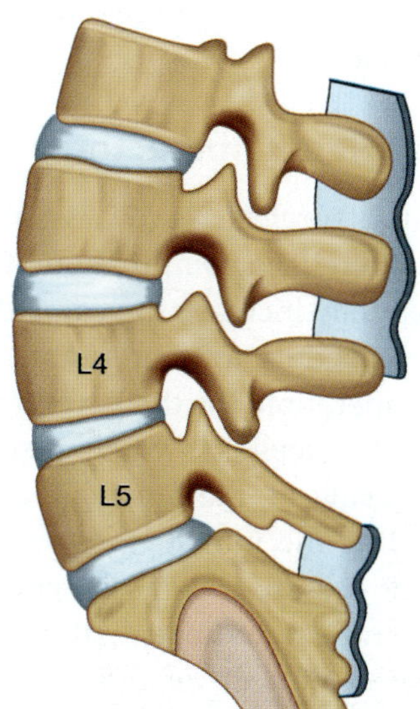

Fig. 50.3: An illustration depicting a laminectomy viewed laterally. Roughly half of the cephalad and caudad laminae are surgically removed allowing for the decompression of the spinal cord while maintaining stability of the spine.

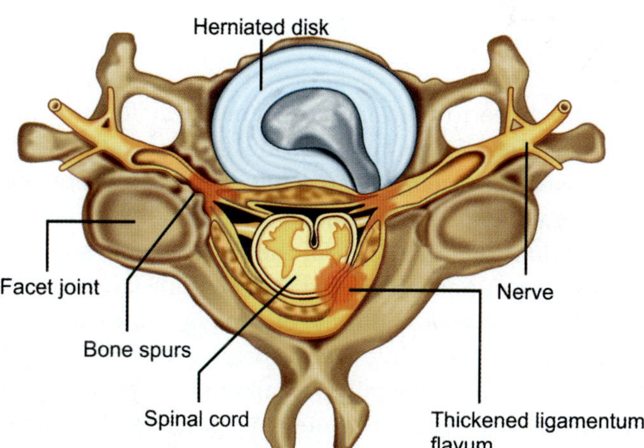

Fig. 50.4: There is ample room in a normal spinal canal for neurological elements to travel unhindered, but when the neural elements are compressed due to a protruding disk or hypertrophy of the ligamentum flavum, central canal stenosis or foraminal stenosis may result, respectively.

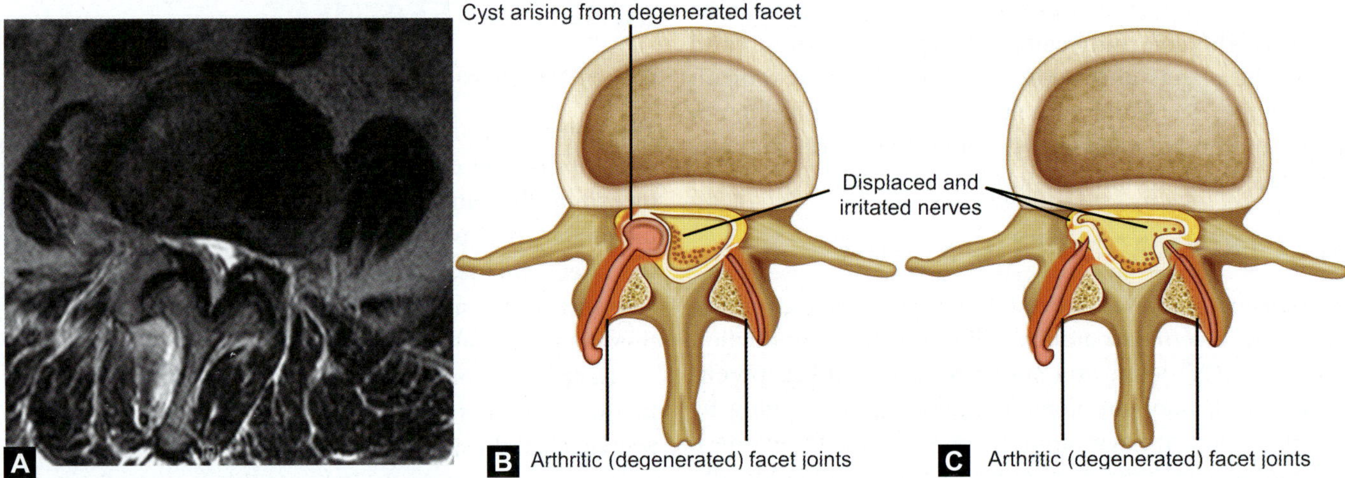

Figs. 50.5A to C: Arthritic degenerated facet joints may cause cyst formation within the canal that may impinge upon neural elements and contribute to spinal stenosis.

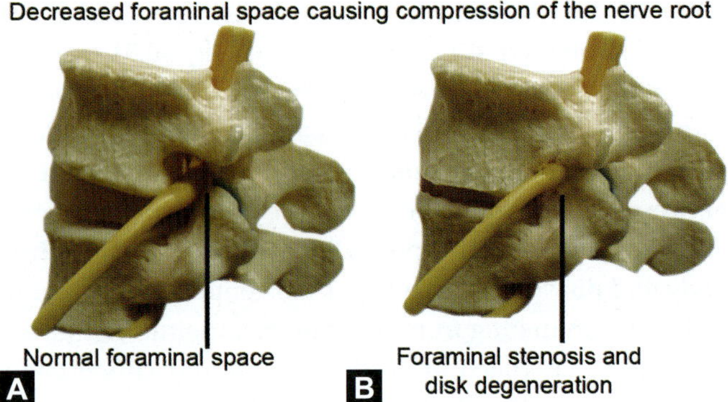

Figs. 50.6A and B: The neural foramen is the canal through which nerve roots exit the spinal canal. Stenosis may occur due to several factors, one such compression of these roots may be the result of disk degeneration, as shown in the figure.

Calcified hypertrophic lateral ligamentum flavum may also exacerbate the compression and the associated symptoms. Once the central canal has been decompressed, the lateral stenosis is addressed surgically by extending laterally and removing part of the hypertrophic superior articular facet and associated ligamentum flavum. One can directly visualize the nerve root in the recess and hence ensure complete decompression. At least 50% of the facet joint bilaterally and all of the pars should be maintained in order to avoid any potential iatrogenic instability.

Nerve roots exit the spinal canal through the neural foramen, and any compromise of the size of the foramen is an opportunity for compression of the exiting nerve root (Figs. 50.6A and B). Foraminal stenosis is more common in the lower lumbar levels as the nerve roots increase in size, while the foramen remains the same or decreases in size caudally.[19,20] Foraminal stenosis is most frequently caused by disk protrusion into the foramen and hypertrophy of the superior articular facet. Degenerative loss of disk height reduces the absolute dimensions of the foramen and is thus another important contributor to foraminal stenosis. The pars interarticularis and ligamentum flavum also border the nerve roots as they exit the spinal canal. Any alteration, ossification, swelling, or hypertrophy of these elements may lead to compromise of the neural foramen, associated neural compression, and consequently lead to sciatic pain.[21]

Laminectomy/Hemilaminectomy

Laminectomy, the surgical removal of the lamina and spinous process to relieve compression of the spinal elements and essentially increase the canal diameter, is the most common procedure to treat lumbar spinal stenosis (Fig. 50.7). This operation has the advantage of providing the surgeon with excellent working space and high visibility as a result of the removal of the posterior elements, including the interspinous-supraspinous ligament complex.[22] Lumbar stenosis commonly affects multiple levels and the indicated surgery thus involves the decompression of each of the involved levels. The muscle dissection starts in the midline and is taken out laterally with care taken to preserve the facet capsule. Disruption of the facet joints can lead to both degeneration and instability, and ultimately the need for a

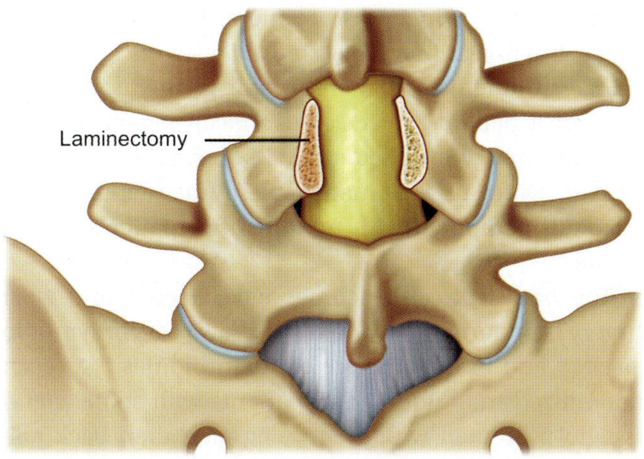

Fig. 50.7: Complete removal of both lateral laminae and the spinous process, called a laminectomy, relieves compression of the spinal components within the canal.

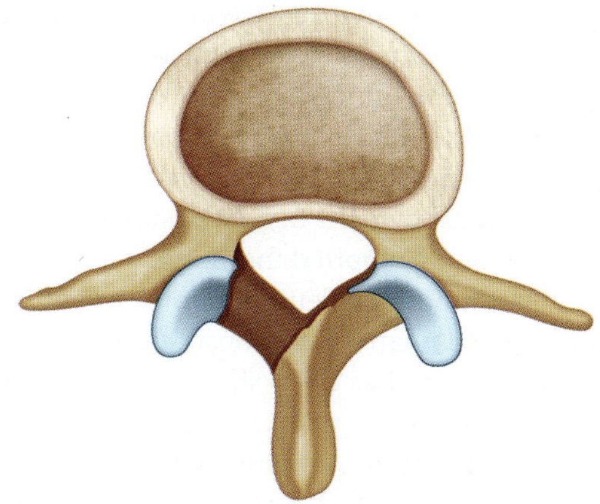

Fig. 50.8: Hemilaminectomy is performed for unilateral symptoms. Half of the caudad lamina of the superior vertebra and half of the cephalad lamina of the inferior vertebra are resected decompressing the spinal elements within.

fusion procedure in the future. The spinous processes within the confines of the chosen levels are resected. The laminectomy is begun centrally, gradually decompressing out laterally until the affected neural elements are determined to be relieved of compression. Care is taken to avoid an iatrogenic fracture of the pars interarticularis. Both disruption of facets, and compromise of the pars, can result in instability. In such cases, supplemental fusion may be required either at the time of surgery if anticipated or in the future as required. The role of fusion in treating patients with spinal stenosis has been debated. In general, when there are no radiographic signs of instability, such as spondylolisthesis, or coronal or sagittal plane deformity, a laminectomy without fusion can be performed.

Hemilaminectomy is a unilateral decompression in which the lamina and associated ligamentum flavum are removed unilaterally (Fig. 50.8).[23] This procedure is indicated for patients with specific unilateral symptoms, in which compressed neural elements are localized medially to one side of the spinal canal. The spinous process is retained, and along with >50% of the ipsilateral facet, the stability of the affected level is preserved. However, the intact spinous process and posterior ligaments create a restricted operating space that can make adequate access and decompression of the neural foramen technically more challenging than a complete bilateral laminectomy. However, the benefits to a minimal decompressive surgery such as hemilaminectomy include preservation of the contralateral neural arch and facet joints, increased posterior stabilization, and minimizing epidural scarring on the nonaffected side of the spinal canal.[24] This also leaves one side of the spinal canal untouched, which is helpful in the event future revision surgery is required.

Laminotomy and Foraminotomy

Laminotomy, foraminotomy, and laminoforaminotomy are classified as microdecompressive procedures in which the midline anatomy, as well as the bony structures not contributing to the stenosis, is left intact. In theory, these procedures allow for more stability, although the reported results are contradictory.[25-27] Laminotomy can be indicated in patients with primarily lateral recess stenosis as an alternative to hemilaminectomy and can be performed unilaterally or bilaterally.[3] In this procedure, a small fragment of the cephalad and caudad lamina are removed and the ligamentum flavum is resected (Fig. 50.9). Foraminotomy consists of a partial medial resection of the foramen to decompress the nerve root.[28] When combined with partial resection of the lamina, it is referred to as a laminoforaminotomy.[29]

In short, focal unilateral pathology is addressed by limited procedures designed to decompress a specific nerve root or roots. More generalized central stenosis involves a more extensive procedure in order to decompress both the central canal and the lateral neural elements.

SURGICAL OUTCOMES

Comparisons of the outcome of surgery to those of conservative treatment for lumbar spinal stenosis suggest surgery provides greater symptomatic improvement.[30-33]

Reported results show that 70–80% of surgical procedures have satisfactory outcomes.[34-36] Outcome measures of disability, pain, and function, using different outcome tools such as the SF-36, Oswestry Disability Index (ODI), the Japanese Orthopedic Association (JOA) score, and other scales have shown the benefit of surgery. The Maine Lumbar Spine Study reported that surgery may increase a patient's relative odds of definite improvement by up to 2.6 times when compared with nonsurgical treatment.[37]

Although surgery has been shown to provide greater immediate symptomatic relief than nonoperative treatment, the relative improvement in surgery appears to diminish over time.[30,33,34,37-39] Four-year and ten-year outcomes of the Maine Lumbar Spine Study reveal a decline in the condition of surgical patients during these intervals (Table 50.1).[30,37,38] Other studies corroborate the results of the Maine Group in terms of the regression of clinical improvement in the years following surgical intervention.[40]

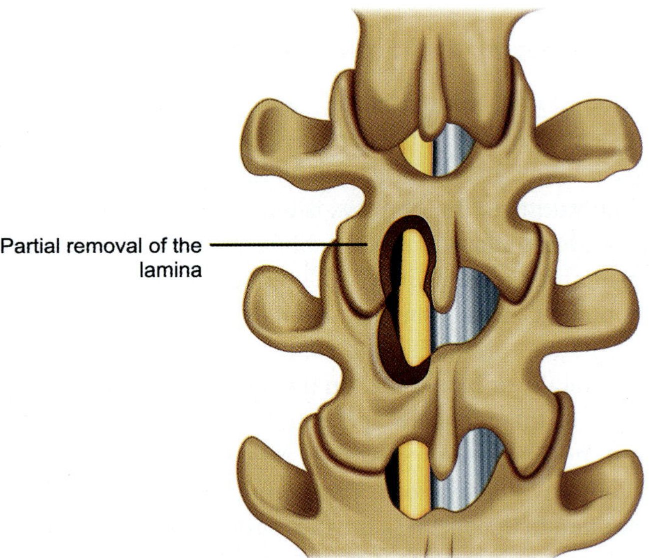

Fig. 50.9: An image depicting a laminotomy, in which only a partial resection of lamina is completed.

At 2-year follow-up, 63–67% of patients indicated excellent results, but 5-year outcomes showed a significant decline to 52%.[41] Nonetheless, there is still greater satisfaction in surgical patients versus nonsurgical patients.[33,40-42] In a randomized controlled trial, Malmivaara found that patients with surgical management maintained better outcomes compared with nonoperative patients at over 4 years.

The best surgical outcomes have been found when surgery is performed within the first few years of symptom onset[43,44] and in the absence of comorbidities.[43] A recent randomized trial[45] found that patients with spinal stenosis who presented with greater leg pain than back pain were more likely to benefit from surgery compared with nonoperative treatment. However, the strongest predictors of successful surgical outcome were found to be lower baseline ODI scores (less disability) and not smoking.[45]

Not every patient with symptomatic stenosis may be a surgical candidate. Many elderly persons have comorbidities that dramatically increase the risk of serious complications. In such cases, the risks of morbidity and mortality may be too great to proceed with a surgical intervention. These issues, as well as other lifestyle habits such as tobacco use, a negative prognostic indicator for healing and fusion, must all be considered before a patient undergoes surgery. A global approach, therefore, is necessary in order to effectively manage these patients both pre- and postoperatively.

INTERSPINOUS SPACER TECHNOLOGY

A less invasive surgical technique has been developed to treat lumbar spinal stenosis (Fig. 50.10). Interspinous spacer technology takes advantage of the fact that symptomatic relief is achieved with relative lumbar flexion in which posterior column distraction increases the diameter of the canal and foramen while stretching out redundant ligamentum flavum. Researchers have designed

Table 50.1: Percent of satisfied surgical and nonsurgical patients at 1-year, 4-year, and 10-year outcomes of the Maine Lumbar Spine Study

	1-year		*4-year*		*10-year*	
	Surgical	*Nonsurgical*	*Surgical*	*Nonsurgical*	*Surgical*	*Nonsurgical*
• Improvement in predominant symptom compared with baseline	54.6	27.8	70.2	52.3	54.2	41.7
• Improvement in low back pain compared with baseline	77.4	41.8	62.7	37.5	52.8	50.0
• Improvement in QOL, ≥moderate	80.6	48.9	63.5	48.8	–	–
• Satisfaction with current state	67.6	31.5	62.7	42.0	55.4	48.8

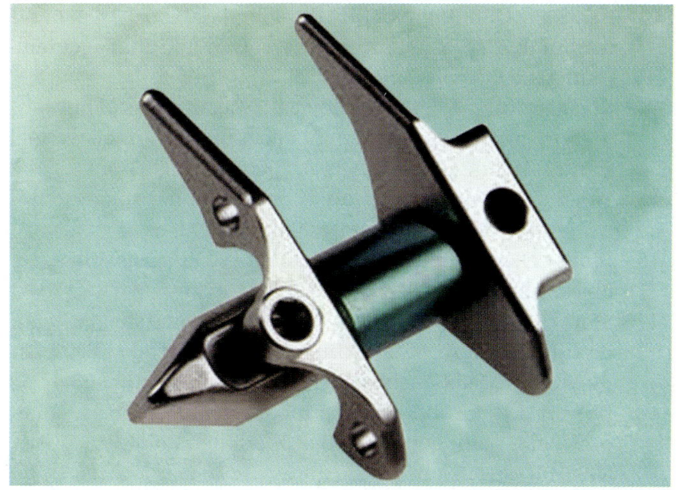

Fig. 50.10: The X-STOP implant is positioned intervertebrally and decompresses neurological elements that are being compressed.

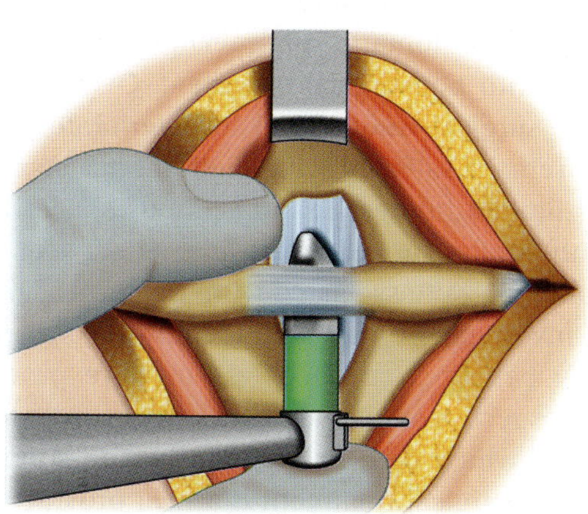

Fig. 50.11: The relatively minor incision required in the interspinous decompression technology, X-STOP implant.

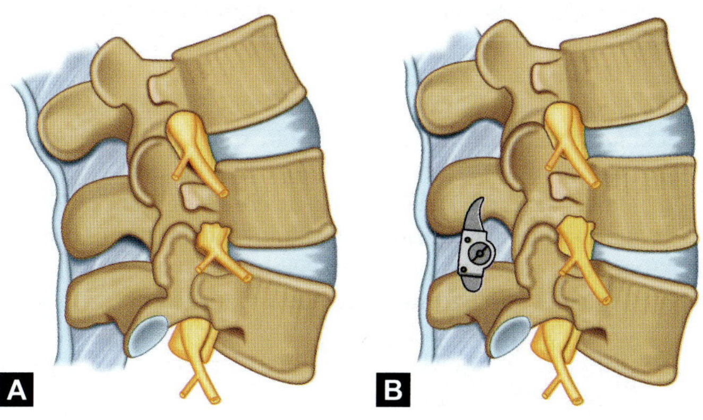

Figs. 50.12A and B: The schematic illustrates the sagittal positioning of the X STOP device between spinous processes of adjacent vertebrae (right) to alleviate the nerve root compression caused by foraminal constriction (left). The arms of the implant prohibit lateral and anterior migration of the spinal elements, while the ligament complex prevents posterior movement.

an implant that is placed between adjacent spinous processes called the X-STOP (Fig. 50.11). This system provides indirect decompression by blocking extension of the motion segment (Figs. 50.12A and B). It is used in mild-to-moderate stenosis, unless accompanied by limited direct decompression as well. Patients with classic neurogenic claudication who experience the greatest symptomatic improvement when seated benefit most from this procedure. X-STOP implantation and the surgery can be performed under local or general anesthesia. There is minimal disruption of muscle and the canal is not exposed, thus reducing the incidence of dural tears.

The surgical outcomes have been positive, similar to the short-term improvement in lumbar laminectomy. Two-year postoperative results showed 73% of patients expressing satisfaction with the procedure. At 4 years, the percentage of satisfied patients increased to 78%.[46,47] Another study reported comparable results in which 71% of patients had satisfactory results 1 year postoperatively, and 54% of patients reported significant clinical improvement in their symptoms. However, 29% of patients required additional caudal epidurals for recurrence of symptoms.[48] The X-STOP interspinous implant procedure has a higher surgical revision rate than lumbar decompression, particularly when used in degenerative spondylolisthesis. The X-STOP is contraindicated in patients whose symptoms are not relieved when seated and those with fixed neural deficits.

CONCLUSION

Although degenerative lumbar stenosis is a slowly progressive condition that is often managed conservatively in many patients, a significant number of these patients will progress to pain and discomfort that markedly affect their quality of life. Once deemed medically suitable, such patients are candidates for lumbar decompressive surgery. Still, many of these patients are over 65 years of age with comorbidities that place them at higher risk of complications from surgery. Reported results show immediate symptomatic improvement from surgery compared with nonsurgical treatment. Over a period of years, the surgical results tend to deteriorate, although patients remain satisfied with their surgical procedure. There is limited interest in interspinous spacer technology, with similar immediate results as surgical lumbar decompression but associated with higher revision rates. Further investigation may help identify specific patients who may benefit from such less invasive procedures. Future prospective studies are necessary in order to better understand which patients respond best to surgery and the types of surgical treatment that will provide optimal outcomes.

REFERENCES

1. Hsu WK. Lumbar degenerative disease. American Academy of Orthopaedic Surgeon. Orthopaedic Knowledge Update 10. 2011;10:599-610.
2. Arnoldi CC, Brodsky AE, Cauchoix J, et al. Lumbar spinal stenosis and nerve root entrapment syndromes. Definition and classification. Clin Orthop Relat Res. 1976;(115):4-5.
3. Patel CK, Truumees E. Spinal stenosis: pathophysiology, clinical diagnosis, and differential diagnosis. Rothman-Simeone (Ed). The Spine, 6th edition. 2011. pp. 1064-77.
4. Hilibrand AS, Rand N. Degenerative lumbar stenosis: diagnosis and management. J Am Acad Orthop Surg. 1999;7 (4):239-49.
5. Watters WC, 3rd, Baisden J, Gilbert TJ, et al. Degenerative lumbar spinal stenosis: an evidence-based clinical guideline for the diagnosis and treatment of degenerative lumbar spinal stenosis. Spine J. 2008;8(2):305-10.
6. Battie MC, Jones CA, Schopflocher DP, et al. Health-related quality of life and comorbidities associated with lumbar spinal stenosis. Spine J. 2012;12(3):189-95.
7. Deyo RA, Gray DT, Kreuter W, et al. United States trends in lumbar fusion surgery for degenerative conditions. Spine (Phila Pa 1976). 2005;30(12):1441-5; discussion 1446-7.
8. Deyo RA, Mirza SK, Martin BI, et al. Trends, major medical complications, and charges associated with surgery for lumbar spinal stenosis in older adults. JAMA. 2010; 303 (13):1259-65.
9. Arbit E, Pannullo S. Lumbar stenosis: a clinical review. Clin Orthop Relat Res. 2001(384):137-43.
10. Amundsen T, Weber H, Lilleas F, et al. Lumbar spinal stenosis. Clinical and radiologic features. Spine (Phila Pa 1976). 1995;20(10):1178-86.
11. Lee MJ, Garcia R, Cassinelli EH, et al. Tandem stenosis: a cadaveric study in osseous morphology. Spine J. 2008;8(6): 1003-6.
12. Porter RW. Spinal stenosis and neurogenic claudication. Spine (Phila Pa 1976). 1996;21(17):2046-52.
13. Issack PS, Cunningham ME, Pumberger M, et al. Degenerative lumbar spinal stenosis: evaluation and management. J Am Acad Orthop Surg. 2012; 20(8):527-35.
14. Koc Z, Ozcakir S, Sivrioglu K, et al. Effectiveness of physical therapy and epidural steroid injections in lumbar spinal stenosis. Spine (Phila Pa 1976). 2009;34(10):985-9.
15. Singh K, Samartzis D, Biyani A, et al. Lumbar spinal stenosis. J Am Acad Orthop Surg. 2008;16(3):171-6.
16. Binder DK, Schmidt MH, Weinstein PR. Lumbar spinal stenosis. Semin Neurol. 2002;22(2):157-66.
17. Storm PB, Chou D, Tamargo RJ. Lumbar spinal stenosis, cauda equina syndrome, and multiple lumbosacral radiculopathies. Phys Med Rehabil Clin N Am. 2002;13(3):713-33, ix.
18. Botwin KP, Gruber RD. Lumbar spinal stenosis: anatomy and pathogenesis. Phys Med Rehabil Clin N Am. 2003;14(1):1-15, v.
19. Hogan Q. Size of human lower thoracic and lumbosacral nerve roots. Anesthesiology. 1996;85(1):37-42.
20. Stephens MM, Evans JH, O'Brien JP. Lumbar intervertebral foramens. An in vitro study of their shape in relation to intervertebral disc pathology. Spine (Phila Pa 1976). 1991;16(5):525-9.
21. Cinotti G, De Santis P, Nofroni I, et al. Stenosis of lumbar intervertebral foramen: anatomic study on predisposing factors. Spine (Phila Pa 1976). 2002;27(3):223-9.
22. Matsudaira K, Yamazaki T, Seichi A, et al. Modified fenestration with restorative spinoplasty for lumbar spinal stenosis. J Neurosurg Spine. 2009;10(6):587-94.
23. Carlisle E, Fischgrund JS. Surgical management of lumbar spinal stenosis and degenerative spondylolisthesis. In Orthopaedic Knowledge Update 3, American Academy of Orthopaedic Surgeons 2006.
24. Mariconda M, Fava R, Gatto A, et al. Unilateral laminectomy for bilateral decompression of lumbar spinal stenosis: a prospective comparative study with conservatively treated patients. J Spinal Disord Tech. 2002;15(1):39-46.
25. Benz RJ, Garfin SR. Current techniques of decompression of the lumbar spine. Clin Orthop Relat Res. 2001(384):75-81.
26. Thomas NW, Rea GL, Pikul BK, et al. Quantitative outcome and radiographic comparisons between laminectomy and laminotomy in the treatment of acquired lumbar stenosis. Neurosurgery. 1997;41(3):567-74; discussion 574-5.
27. Aryanpur J, Ducker T. Multilevel lumbar laminotomies: an alternative to laminectomy in the treatment of lumbar stenosis. Neurosurgery. 1990;26(3):429-32; discussion 433.
28. Cirak B, Alptekin M, Palaoglu S, et al. Surgical therapy for lumbar spinal stenosis: evaluation of 300 cases. Neurosurg Rev. 2001;24(2-3):80-2.
29. Fu YS, Zeng BF, Xu JG. Long-term outcomes of two different decompressive techniques for lumbar spinal stenosis. Spine (Phila Pa 1976). 2008;33(5):514-8.
30. Atlas SJ, Keller RB, Robson D, et al. Surgical and nonsurgical management of lumbar spinal stenosis: four-year outcomes from the Maine Lumbar Spine Study. Spine (Phila Pa 1976). 2000;25(5):556-62.

31. Amundsen T, Weber H, Nordal HJ, et al. Lumbar spinal stenosis: conservative or surgical management?: A prospective 10-year study. Spine (Phila Pa 1976). 2000;25(11): 1424-35; discussion 1435-6.
32. Johnsson KE, Uden A, Rosen I. The effect of decompression on the natural course of spinal stenosis. A comparison of surgically treated and untreated patients. Spine (Phila Pa 1976). 1991;16(6):615-9.
33. Malmivaara A, Slatis P, Heliovaara M, et al. Surgical or nonoperative treatment for lumbar spinal stenosis? A randomized controlled trial. Spine (Phila Pa 1976). 2007; 32(1):1-8.
34. Weinstein JN, Tosteson TD, Lurie JD, et al. Surgical versus nonoperative treatment for lumbar spinal stenosis four-year results of the Spine Patient Outcomes Research Trial. Spine (Phila Pa 1976). 2010;35(14):1329-38.
35. Nath R, Middha S, Gupta AK. Functional outcome of surgical management of degenerative lumbar canal stenosis. Indian J Orthop. 2012;46(3):285-90.
36. Postacchini F. Surgical management of lumbar spinal stenosis. Spine (Phila Pa 1976). 1999;24(10):1043-7.
37. Atlas SJ, Deyo RA, Keller RB, et al. The Maine Lumbar Spine Study, Part III. 1-year outcomes of surgical and nonsurgical management of lumbar spinal stenosis. Spine (Phila Pa 1976). 1996;21(15):1787-94; discussion 1794-5.
38. Atlas SJ, Keller RB, Wu YA, et al. Long-term outcomes of surgical and nonsurgical management of lumbar spinal stenosis: 8 to 10 year results from the Maine Lumbar Spine Study. Spine (Phila Pa 1976). 2005;30(8): 936-43.
39. Katz JN, Lipson SJ, Larson MG, et al. The outcome of decompressive laminectomy for degenerative lumbar stenosis. J Bone Joint Surg Am. 1991;73(6):809-16.
40. Caputy AJ, Luessenhop AJ. Long-term evaluation of decompressive surgery for degenerative lumbar stenosis. J Neurosurg. 1992;77(5):669-76.
41. Postacchini F, Cinotti G, Gumina S, et al. Long-term results of surgery in lumbar stenosis. 8-year review of 64 patients. Acta Orthop Scand Suppl. 1993;251:78-80.
42. Chang Y, Singer DE, Wu YA, et al. The effect of surgical and nonsurgical treatment on longitudinal outcomes of lumbar spinal stenosis over 10 years. J Am Geriatr Soc. 2005;53(5): 785-92.
43. Jonsson B, Annertz M, Sjoberg C, et al. A prospective and consecutive study of surgically treated lumbar spinal stenosis. Part II: Five-year follow-up by an independent observer. Spine (Phila Pa 1976). 1997;22(24):2938-44.
44. Niggemeyer O, Strauss JM, Schulitz KP. Comparison of surgical procedures for degenerative lumbar spinal stenosis: a meta-analysis of the literature from 1975 to 1995. Eur Spine J. 1997;6(6):423-9.
45. Pearson A, Lurie J, Tosteson T, et al. Who should have surgery for spinal stenosis? Treatment effect predictors in SPORT. Spine (Phila Pa 1976). 2012;37(21):1791-802.
46. Zucherman JF, Hsu KY, Hartjen CA, et al. A multicenter, prospective, randomized trial evaluating the X STOP interspinous process decompression system for the treatment of neurogenic intermittent claudication: two-year follow-up results. Spine (Phila Pa 1976). 2005;30(12):1351-8.
47. Kondrashov DG, Hannibal M, Hsu KY, et al. Interspinous process decompression with the X-STOP device for lumbar spinal stenosis: a 4-year follow-up study. J Spinal Disord Tech. 2006;19(5):323-7.
48. Siddiqui M, Smith FW, Wardlaw D. One-year results of X Stop interspinous implant for the treatment of lumbar spinal stenosis. Spine (Phila Pa 1976). 2007;32(12):1345-8.

CHAPTER 51

Overview of Spinal Deformity Surgery

Justin Paul, Thomas Cheriyan, Anthony Petrizzo, Thomas J Errico

'L'Orthopedie, ou l'art de prevenir et de corriger dans les enfans, les difformites du corp'
English: 'Orthopedia, or the Art of Correcting and Preventing Deformities in Children'

— Nicolas Andry (Paris, 1741)

INTRODUCTION

Nicholas Andry derived the word orthopedics from the Greek phrase meaning "straight child". In his book, ''Orthopaedia'' published in 1741, he also illustrated the ''crooked tree'', which has been adopted as the symbol for the orthopedic discipline (Figs. 51.1A and B).[1,2]

Several Greek words form the foundation for diagnoses and descriptions of deformity of the spine. Scoliosis or ''crooked'' refers to a lateral deviation in the frontal (coronal) plane and is considered abnormal. However, kyphosis or ''hump'' and lordosis or ''bent backward'' refer to the lateral (sagittal) deviation and can be normal depending on the size of the curve and the location (Figs. 51.2A and B). Hippocrates and Galen of Pergamon were some of the first to use these terms in reference to spine disorders.[3-6]

Balancing the spine in the sagittal and coronal planes optimizes energy expenditure during standing and economy of movement during gait.[7-9] At birth, normal

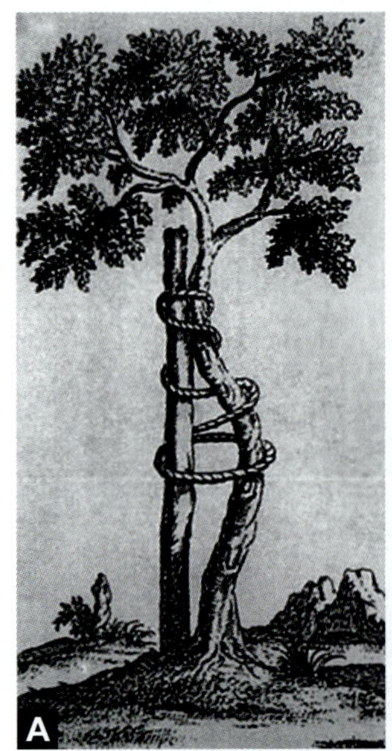

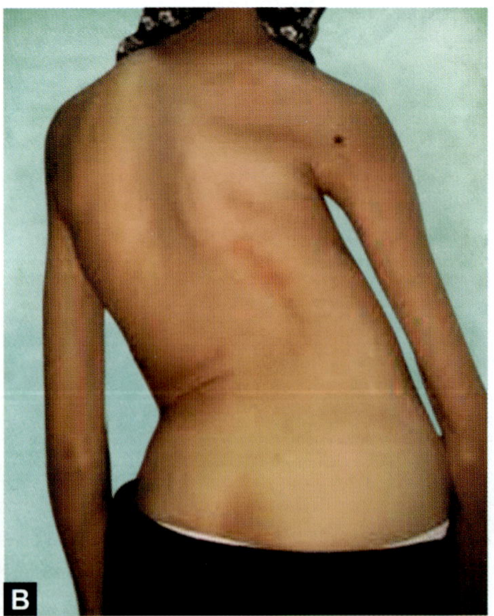

Figs. 51.1A and B: The Andry Tree, originally illustrated by Nicholas Andry, serves as a symbol for many orthopedic organizations. The straightening of a crooked tree with a straight post can be related to principles of spine deformity surgery.

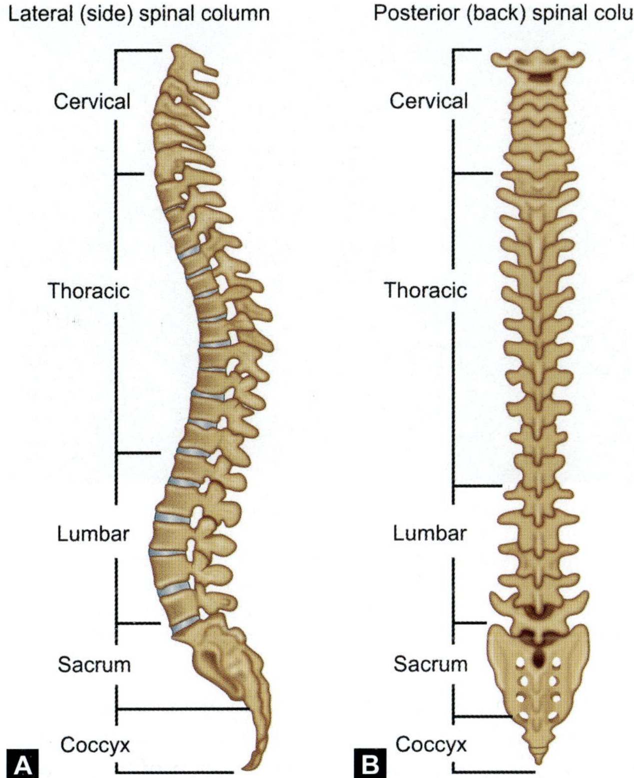

Figs. 51.2A and B: The normal spine viewed posteriorly appears straight, but viewed from the side has multiple normal curves.

curves in the sagittal plane include sacral kyphosis and thoracic kyphosis. Activation of the posterior paracervical musculature leads to development of upright head posture resulting in a position of cervical lordosis. Later, with ambulation and activation of the hip flexor musculature, the lumbar spine adopts its lordotic curve. While the spine provides a bony enclosure and protection for the spinal cord, it also serves the important function of transferring the weight of the head, trunk, and upper extremities to the pelvis. Regional or global deviations from proper alignment can result in abnormal weight distribution, resulting in long-term stresses. Based on the laws of biomechanics, deformity occurs in at least two and typically three planes (i.e. coronal, sagittal and axial/rotational) to varying degrees and significant asymmetry can lead to clinical manifestations of imbalance or pain.

A decision as simple as conservative or operative treatment of spine deformity requires a comprehensive understanding of the natural history of the specific deformity, spine biomechanics, and integration of these concepts with the goals and expectations of the patient and family. Early attempts to correct spinal deformity evolved over many years from the Hippocratic traction table to

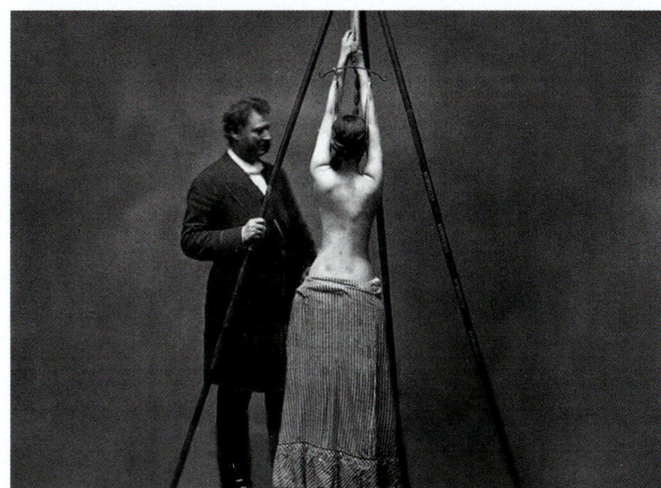

Fig. 51.3: Dr Sayre observes the change in the curvature of the spine in traction prior to being wrapped in a "plaster of Paris" cast.

immobilization in a plaster jacket.[10,11] This technique of wrapping a patient in plaster while suspended to reduce the deformity was developed by Dr Lewis Albert Sayre. Sayre was the first professor of orthopedics in the United States, serving the first academic orthopedic department at Bellevue Medical College in 1853 (Fig. 51.3).[12,13] In the 19th century, initial surgical attempts to correct scoliosis focused on the imbalanced paraspinal musculature with myotomies and tenotomies. Surgical intervention eventually progressed to fusion, reduction in deformity, and instrumentation.[14,15]

ANATOMY AND BIOMECHANICS

In order to understand the radiographic depiction of deformity, normal measures should be reviewed for each region of the spine. Using Cartesian coordinates to characterize deformity in the x-, y-, and z-axes, a reliable description of the deviation from normal spine alignment helps surgeons standardize diagnosis and treatment.[16-18] The sacrum is used as a reference point for positional translation and angulation in all planes with arbitrary designations of cephalad, anterior, and left of the centroid as positive (Fig. 51.4). In practice, Cartesian coordinates are less useful for global alignment and most appropriate for locally comparing vertebral segments.

The spine is normally without curvature in the coronal plane, with the result that any lateral deviation destabilizes the spine. When evaluating a patient with scoliosis, a plumb line dropped from the C7 vertebral body should bisect the sacrum.[19-21] If there is a deviation from midline, curves must be evaluated for the vertebrae defining the

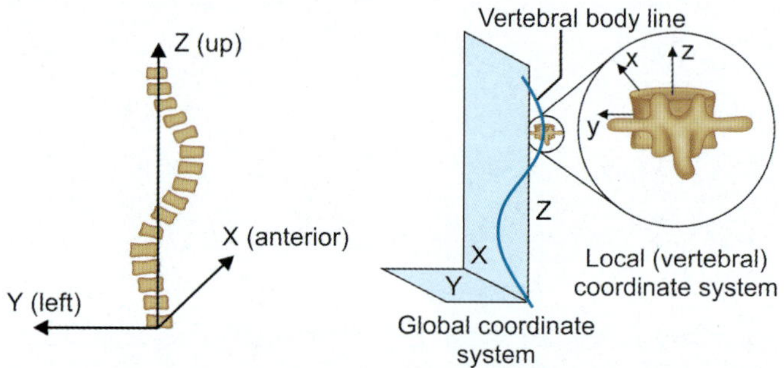

Fig. 51.4: Global coordinate system (left) is based on each vertebra (right), which defines its own coordinate system depending on its orientation.

upper, lower, and apical aspects of deformity. Identifying which vertebrae are in balance before surgery and which vertebral segments need to be incorporated into the fusion has long been a discussion among surgeons.

Harrington proposed that the fusion should extend caudally to a stable zone defined by parallel vertical lines through the lumbosacral facets.[22,23] King refined this theory describing the center vertical sacral line, which is a single line through the center of the sacrum, perpendicular to the iliac crests. The stable vertebra is bisected by this line (Fig. 51.5).[1,24]

In the sagittal plane, physiologic curves are essential for standing upright and distributing weight from the body to the pelvis.[1,3,5] In the cervical spine, a lordotic curve exists ranging from 25° to 50°. This region serves as the major contributor to flexion/extension, lateral bending, and rotation of the cranium. Motion decreases from the upper cervical spine toward the inflection point from lordosis to the kyphotic thoracic spine, usually at C7-T1. Loss of cervical lordosis can occur as the result of cervical degenerative changes; this process narrows the anteroposterior diameter of the spinal canal and can lead to spinal cord compression.

The thoracic spine is typically kyphotic (ranging from 20° to 50° in adults), with decreasing angulation toward the relatively neutral thoracolumbar junction. In the lumbar spine, lordosis ranges from 40° and 70° ending with the lumbosacral junction and transition to the kyphotic sacrum. Although the sacrum does little to contribute to trunk motion, it plays a very important role in transmitting the weight of the upper body to the pelvis and lower extremities. Understanding the parameters of the lumbosacral pelvis is important: it forms the basis for global sagittal alignment of the spine, with the goal of centering the head over the feet.

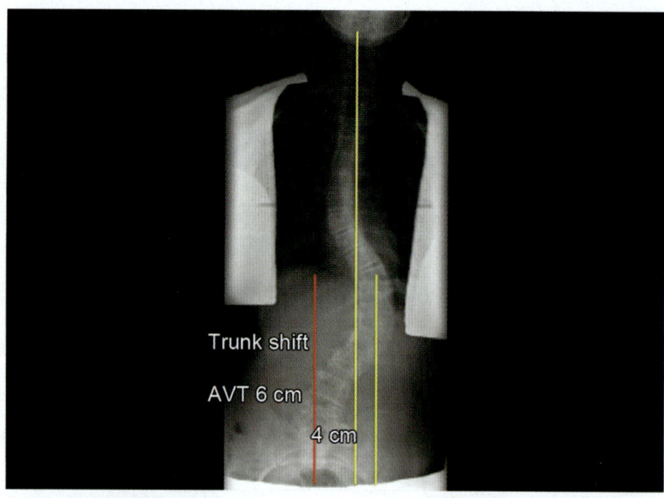

Fig. 51.5: Center vertical sacral line (CSVL) is shown in red; the translation from this to the line through the apex of the curve represents the apical vertebral translation. Trunk shift is the translation of C7 plumb line from CSVL. Stable vertebra is the inferior vertebra most closely bisected by the CSVL and in between Harrington's stable lines. Neutral vertebra has no rotation (pedicles appear symmetric).

The most important parameters involved in setting this foundation are sacral slope, pelvic tilt, pelvic incidence, and lumbar lordosis (Figs. 51.6A to D).[7,9,25] Of these, a parameter worthy of special attention is pelvic incidence, obtained from the angle between the line perpendicular to the sacral plate and the line from the midsacral plate to the hip-center axis. This is a morphologic measurement: it does not change from seated to standing and changes very little over one's lifetime. As pelvic incidence is fixed and the other angles are mathematically related to it, it can be thought of as the angle on which all other spinal curves are based.[10,26]

Despite seemingly adequate spinal alignment, without proper compensation from the lower extremities (e.g. hip or knee contractures), a patient can still have poor global alignment. The angle of the femurs with respect to the spine becomes relevant in patients with these contractures or who have had previous fusions and can no longer compensate in certain regions.

The notion of coupled motion is relevant to the multi-planar sense of deformity. This refers to the response to primary segmental motion with a secondary motion in another plane. For example, side bending in the coronal plane results in rotation into the convexity of the curve.[12,15,27,28] The secondary motion is subtle and results from the extensive ligamentous connectivity and changing orientation of facet articulations among vertebral levels. Although physiologic coupled motion is natural, pathologic coupled motion is apparent in cases

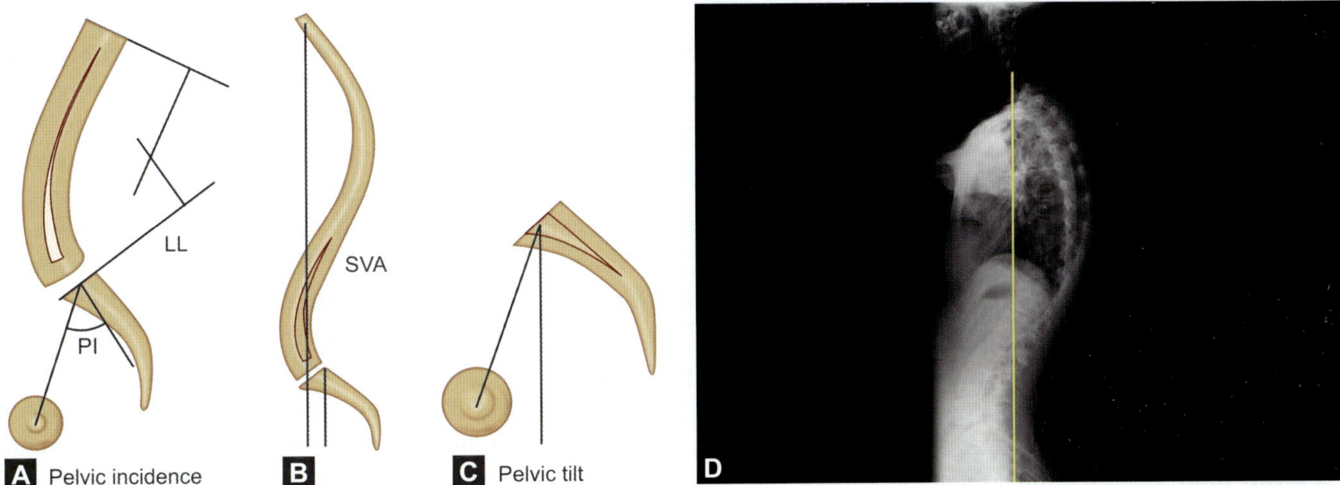

Figs. 51.6A to D: Sagittal parameters: (A) pelvic incidence (PI), lumbar lordosis (LL), (B) sagittal vertical axis (SVA), and (C) pelvic tilt, (D) lateral radiograph showing sagittal vertical axis yellow line.

of deformity. This is exemplified both radiographically and clinically. The prominence of the scapula and underlying rib rotation observed during the Adams forward bending test indirectly demonstrates the lateral curvature of the spine.

CLINICAL EVALUATION

Cases of spine deformity can present to the clinician's office through various sources, usually depending on the age of presentation. Congenital and juvenile deformities are frequently diagnosed early in life either as an isolated entity or as part of a syndrome. Adolescent deformity referral sources are often pediatricians or school screening programs where some degree of asymmetry in shoulder height, waist crease, or rib rotation may have been observed. Single curves can be easier to diagnose clinically than S-shaped double curves, where two balanced curves may give an overall illusion of symmetry. Consistent with many screening tools, false positives are common, but even subtle curves can worsen substantially during rapid growth. Younger patients are often free of symptoms with the exceptions of occasional parathoracic spasm with thoracic curves and lower back discomfort with thoracolumbar or lumbar curves. Older patients can complain of height loss or that clothes no longer fit properly. They may experience pain, fatigue, trunk shift, or decompensation with lateral list.[14,29,30]

In collecting the history, the severity, quality, and duration of symptoms are important. Although cosmetic complaints are more common, patients with focal deformity can be symptomatic with pain. For example, patients with Scheuermann's kyphosis may experience back pain in the apex of the curve.[16,18,31] Patients with local segmental deformity such as isthmic or degenerative spondylolisthesis can complain of a spectrum of nerve compression-related symptoms ranging from low back pain to neurogenic claudication. Questions about family history can be helpful in determining prognosis.

In addition to history, thorough physical examination is crucial to evaluating the patient with deformity. Careful attention to positions that produce pain or neurologic complaints is paramount. Head-to-toe physical examination should include evaluation of sensation, tone, strength, and reflexes and description of any associated features such as skin tags, tufts, or limb deformity. Musculoskeletal examination can reveal knee or hip degeneration, which can mimic or amplify spine pathology.

A plumb line can be used clinically to ascertain global coronal imbalance.[19,32] Truncal shift from large thoracolumbar and lumbar curves can be extremely unpleasant cosmetically for the patient. Judicious use of the physical examination provides important information about surgical correction. Typically a right-sided thoracic curve produces a right shoulder elevation. If the left shoulder is elevated, the surgeon should have high suspicion for a left thoracic curve, a double thoracic curve, or a left primary thoracolumbar curve.

RADIOLOGIC EVALUATION

As part of the patient encounter, standing radiographs should be obtained using a 36-inch cassette. The posteroanterior and lateral radiographs are standard and may be supplemented with dynamic studies such as side-bending films to evaluate the rigidity of the curve. These dynamic films assess the flexibility of the curve and distinguish structural from compensatory curves.

Improved digital imaging techniques allow for adequately large views of the entire spine with 36-inch film but do not allow for a more global perspective of alignment. Recent advances have made it possible to generate full-body radiographs. This is accomplished with collimation of the X-ray beam through a slit and scanning of the patient from head to toe.[22,33,34] The coupling of X-ray source and detectors in two planes simultaneously during acquisition allows for a three-dimensional (3D) reconstruction (Figs. 51.7A to C).[24]

Assessment of radiographs includes a global assessment of spinal balance and alignment in the coronal plane using the offset of the plumb line and Cobb technique to measure the degree of curvature. (Refer Chapter 11 for a more detailed description of radiological measurements.) In the sagittal plane, measurements of thoracic kyphosis and lumbar lordosis should be obtained. In addition, sagittal balance should be determined from the sagittal vertical alignment (Fig. 51.6). Ideally, on full-body images, the plumb line should bisect the femoral heads and malleoli. Although not necessary in the initial evaluation of deformity, computed tomography, magnetic resonance imaging, and myelography are options to evaluate neurologic symptoms or other associated pathologies.

CLASSIFICATION

Classification of spinal deformity is important for establishing accepted treatment guidelines and analyzing outcomes. Adolescent idiopathic scoliosis (AIS) represents the most commonly encountered deformity and thus early in its history of surgical treatment, surgeons adopted a stratification of deformity types to guide operative care. Adhering to the goal of fusing as few vertebrae as possible, King, Moe, and coworkers produced a classification system identifying a subgroup of thoracic scoliosis curves that could have a selective thoracic fusion.[1] This seminal work put forward several parameters correlating with satisfactory outcomes. The report emphasized the importance of identifying structural and compensatory curves and asserted that stable correction should include fusion of the most caudal segment centered over the sacrum. The implications were profound: selecting a thoracic-only fusion could reduce operative time and avoided long, motion-limiting fusions.

To improve the inter- and intraobserver reliability and incorporate sagittal plane deformity in the classification, Lenke et al. categorized all curve types into six major groups.[25] This expansion of the King classification system incorporated the sagittal plane with a lumbar modifier (Fig. 51.8). The system continued the motion-sparing theme, recommending selective fusions and avoiding fusion of nonstructural regions.

Focusing on accurately predicting the limits of deformity and extent of fusion necessary, Suk proposed a classification scheme of AIS consisting of four structural curves (single thoracic, double thoracic, double major, and thoracolumbar/lumbar), each with two subtypes that define the distal fusion levels depending on the relation between the end vertebra (EV) and the neutral vertebra (NV).[26]

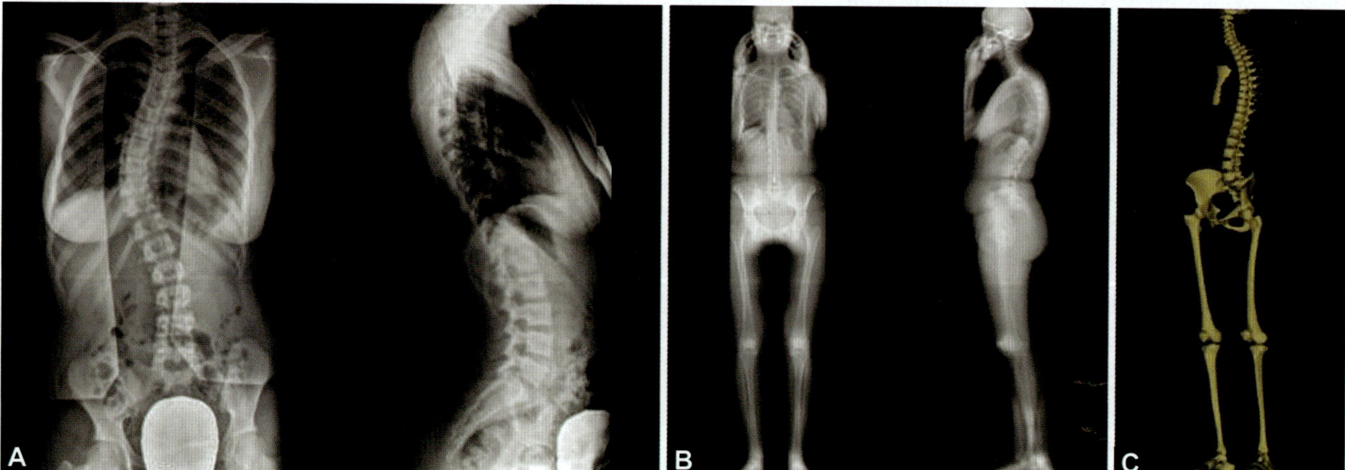

Figs. 51.7A to C: Difference between (A) 36-inch cassette and (B) full-body weight-bearing EOS image. (C) Skeleton modeling software generates a three-dimensional reconstruction from head to toe.

Deformities have been defined as either being coronal plane or sagittal plane, but surgeons now understand that while X-rays are usually taken in these two planes, the deformity is 3D (Figs. 51.9A to C). The Scoliosis Research Society (SRS), founded in 1966 with the burgeoning new field of surgical deformity correction, has recently recognized the need for 3D characterization of scoliosis and formed the 3D Scoliosis Committee to help guide these efforts. Although the classification systems proposed above consider the coronal plane deformity, the Lenke classification includes the sagittal plane in an attempt to define the 3D nature of the curve, but recent imaging advances may yet produce a more complete picture.

TREATMENT

The goals of each operation in spine deformity depend on the etiology and progression of the curve, symptomatology, and patient expectations. Current techniques are centered around the concepts of fusion to prevent further deformity, correction to restore balance, and preservation of as many motion segments as possible.[15,27,28]

Historically, the most common surgical procedure for the treatment of scoliosis has been instrumentation and fusion through a posterior approach to the spine.[35] Posterior transpedicle screw insertion provides fixation across all columns using the three-column model of stability (Figs. 51.10A and B). Approaching the spine anteriorly can be performed as a stand-alone procedure with release of soft tissues and/or fusion with instrumentation. Combine approaches are reserved for high-magnitude, rigid curves, and can be performed in a staged operation or all at once.

Neuromuscular forms of scoliosis present some of the most challenging cases due to anatomic complexity

Curve Type				
Type	*Proximal Thoracic*	*Main Thoracic*	*Thoracolumbar/ Lumbar*	*Description*
1	Non-structural	Structural (Major)*	Non-structural	Main thoracic (MT)
2	Structural	Structural (Major)*	Non-structural	Double thoracic (DT)
3	Non-structural	Structural (Major)*	Structural	Double major (DM)
4	Structural	Structural (Major)*	Structural (Major)*	Triple major (TM)$
5	Non-structural	Non-structural	Structural (Major)*	Thoracolumbar/Lumbar (TL/L)
6	Non-structural	Structural	Structural (Major)*	Thoracolumbar/Lumbar-Main Thoracic (TL/L-MT)

STRUCTURAL CRITERIA
(Minor Curves)

Proximal thoracic	- Side Bending Cobb ≥25°
	- T2-T5 Kyphosis ≥+20°
Main thoracic	- Side Bending Cobb ≥25°
	- T10-L2 Kyphosis ≥+20°
Thoracolumbar/ Lumbar	- Side Bending Cobb ≥25°
	- T10-L2 Kyphosis ≥+20°

*Major = Largest Cobb measurement, always structural
Minor = All other curves with structural criteria applied
$Type 4 - MT or TL/L can be major curve

LOCATION OF APEX
(SRS Definition)

Curve	*Apex*
Thoracic	T2-T11/12 Disk
Thoracolumbar	T12-L1
Thoracolumbar/Lumbar	L1/2 Disk-L4

Modifiers

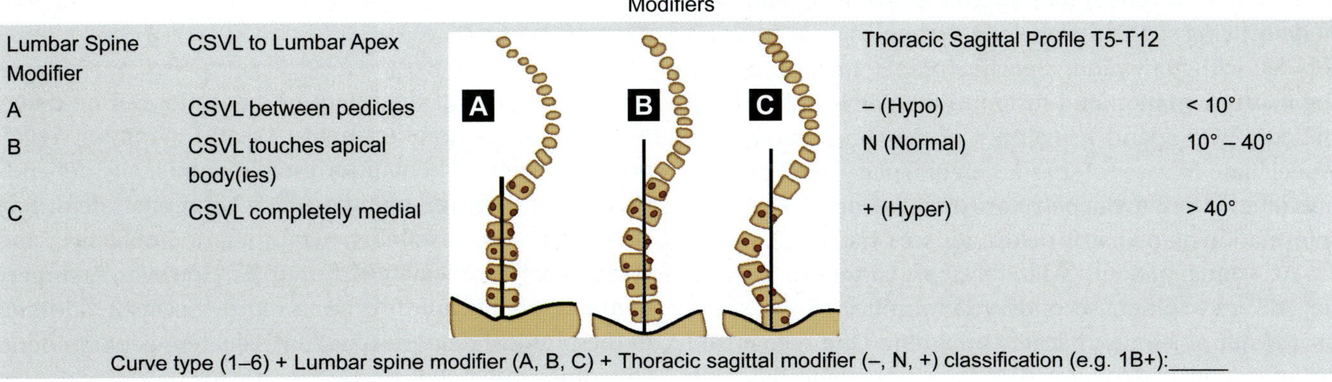

Fig. 51.8: Lenke classification of adolescent idiopathic scoliosis.

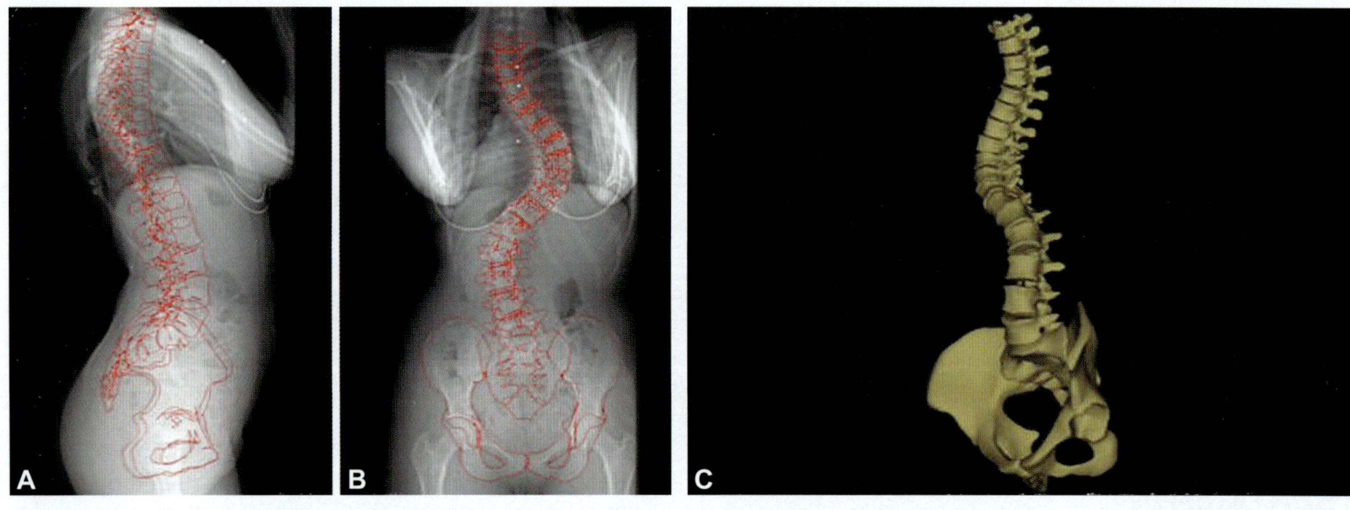

Figs. 51.9A to C: Plain radiographs showing (A) sagittal and (B) coronal perspectives, while (C) EOS software generated three-dimensional reconstruction showing the deformity has a rotational component that is not demonstrated adequately by the two traditional views.

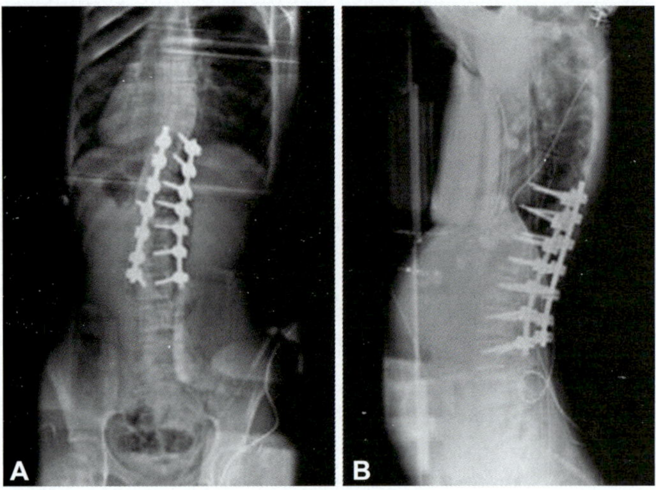

Figs. 51.10A and B: Posterior transpedicle screw-rod constructs stabilize the spine to facilitate solid bony fusion.

combined with social, caregiving, and rehabilitation issues.[31] Often the most important goal is optimizing activities of daily living such as propelling a wheelchair or bending for self-catheterization. Specific points include avoiding instrumentation and fusion to the pelvis in balanced patients who spend a majority of the time seated in a wheelchair. In cases of spastic cerebral palsy, rigid fixation and often fusion to the pelvis are often needed.[32] For more information on pediatric deformity, *see* Chapter 52.

As young patients who received corrective surgery for AIS grew older, secondary deformities of the spine as a result of surgery became apparent. One recognized complication of scoliosis surgery is iatrogenic flat-back syndrome.[33,34,36] This is a condition of sagittal imbalance typically caused by lengthening the posterior column in attempts to reduce the coronal deformity. This resulted in a different postural disorder manifested with forward inclination of the trunk, back pain, early fatigue during ambulation, and issues of cosmesis. Adult deformity is now recognized as a disease that can result not only from previous surgery but can also develop de novo (i.e. from degeneration) or from progression of adolescent scoliosis (Figs. 51.11A to D).[28,37]

The goals of treatment are to maintain horizontal gaze, restore erect posture, decrease asymmetric stresses on muscle groups, and improve lung function and body image. The mainstay is the posterior approach with vertebral wedge osteotomies stabilized with rigid fixation.[38] In the case of significant deformity in the sagittal plane with imbalance of >4 cm, a procedure with a combined anterior-posterior approach may be performed, either staged or in the same operative setting.[39-41] For more information on adult deformity, *see* Chapter 53.

OUTCOMES

Success of surgical treatment of deformity can be determined by radiographic measures and symptom relief, but the degree of benefit for the patient usually depends on the underlying pathology.[42,43] Untreated deformity can progress to instability, symptomatic imbalance, and stenosis in the concavity of the curves. However, as surgery demands significant direct and indirect costs in addition to the physical demands, patient selection is paramount. Outcomes research is needed to provide objective data to guide and inform this decision.

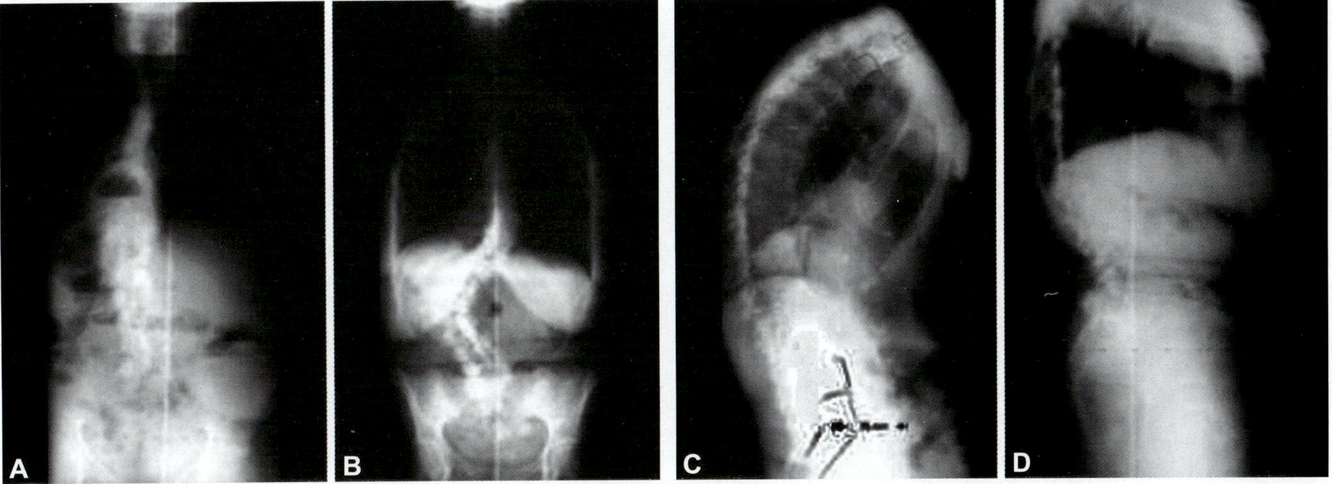

Figs. 51.11A to D: Adult deformity can occur de novo, progress from adolescence, or result from prior surgery.

Evidence-based clinical decision-making algorithms are based on masses of data collected from hospital stays and clinical encounters. Hospital systems are equipping database systems to collect information on perioperative morbidity, complications, length of stay, and cost for analysis.[44,45] State and national databases have been constructed but the limitations of surgical information increase along with the depth of the database.

Quality of life has become an essential factor in determining successful outcomes. For example, long-term results show AIS patients who have undergone fusion show satisfaction comparable with nondiseased counterparts with regard to work, marriage, and children.[46] These are not universally included as part of the clinical history and physical examination. Standardizing the questions asked of these patients at different surgical centers in each region of the country will help guide general trends in treatment. Functional limitations and perception of performance are also essential to global measures of quality of life. Measures of dynamic activities such as gait and functional range of motion are not part of a standard evaluation and there is limited data on the impact of fusion on physical activity. Ultimately, the impact of the deformity on the patient's life is the most important consideration.

Although there are validated instruments available to evaluate the disability from deformity, they vary in their ability to provide spine-specific information. For example, the Medical Outcomes Study (MOS) 36-Item Short Form Health Survey (SF-36)[47] is a generic survey that has broad usage in orthopedics but does not provide any information specific to spinal deformity. Conversely, the SRS has developed a questionnaire addressing the patient's self-perception, physical status, and even social limitations specifically relating to his or her spinal deformity. Beginning as the SRS-30, the most recent version involves 22 questions (SRS-22).[48]

Another metric that has been important for comparative cost-effectiveness research is the quality-adjusted life year, which quantifies disease burden by considering both the quality and the quantity of life lived. With large studies these data can be used to assess whether value is gained over time comparing surgical to nonsurgical intervention.[49] With the increasing wealth of reference data comparing profiles for patients with specific conditions, the goal of an international database of the economic and psychosocial impact of deformity surgery is increasingly within reach.

SUMMARY

Deformity of the spine can occur in both adult and pediatric populations, and these are conceptually separate pathologies requiring different strategies for surgical treatment. Rapidly evolving technology and an expanding analytical toolkit will help form a comprehensive biomechanical understanding and 3D classification of deformity, which can in turn be used to improve surgical planning for deformity correction in all three planes. These new tools and techniques for surgical management of deformity are now becoming supplemented by outcomes data. Integrating novel tools and outcomes measures will help guide the management of deformity surgery from a more objective standpoint.

REFERENCES

1. King HA, Moe JH, Bradford DS, et al. The selection of fusion levels in thoracic idiopathic scoliosis. J Bone Joint Surg Am. 1983;65(9):1302-13.
2. Rauschmann MA, Thomann KD. [200 years orthopedics. Images from the past]. Orthopade. 2000;29(12):1008-17.
3. Lafage V, Schwab F, Skalli W, et al. Standing balance and sagittal plane spinal deformity: analysis of spinopelvic and gravity line parameters. Spine. 2008;33(14):1572-8.
4. The genuine works of Hippocrates. Translated with a Priliminary Discourse and Annotations by Francis Adams. 2 Vols.
5. Lafage V, Schwab F, Vira S, et al. Spinopelvic parameters after surgery can be predicted. Spine. 2011;36(13):1037-45.
6. Goodrich JT. History of spine surgery in the ancient and medieval worlds. Neurosurg Focus. 200415;16(1):E2.
7. Legaye J, Duval-Beaupère G, Hecquet J, et al. Pelvic incidence: a fundamental pelvic parameter for three-dimensional regulation of spinal sagittal curves. Eur Spine J. 1998; 7(2):99-103.
8. Mahaudens P, Detrembleur C, Mousny M, et al. Gait in adolescent idiopathic scoliosis: energy cost analysis. Eur Spine J. 2009;18(8):1160-8.
9. Skalli W, Zeller RD, Miladi L, et al. Importance of pelvic compensation in posture and motion after posterior spinal fusion using CD instrumentation for idiopathic scoliosis. Spine. 200620;31(12):E359-66.
10. Schwab F, Lafage V, Patel A, et al. Sagittal plane considerations and the pelvis in the adult patient. Spine. 2009;34(17): 1828-33.
11. Sayre JW. Lewis Albert Sayre. Spine. 1995;20(9):1091-6.
12. Roozmon P, Gracovetsky SA, Gouw GJ, et al. Examining motion in the cervical spine. II: Characterization of coupled joint motion using an opto-electronic device to track skin markers. J Biomed Eng. 1993;15(1):13-22.
13. Zampini JM, Sherk HH, Lewis A. Sayre: the first Professor of Orthopaedic Surgery in America. Clin Orthop Relat Res. 2008;466(9):2263-7.
14. Jackson RP, Simmons EH, Stripinis D. Incidence and severity of back pain in adult idiopathic scoliosis. Spine. 1983; 8(7):749-56.
15. Majdouline Y, Aubin C-E, Robitaille M, et al. Scoliosis correction objectives in adolescent idiopathic scoliosis. J Pediatr Orthop. 2007;27(7):775-81.
16. Murray PM, Weinstein SL, Spratt KF. The natural history and long-term follow-up of Scheuermann kyphosis. J Bone Joint Surg Am. 1993;75(2):236-48.
17. Goldberg CJ, Moore DP, Fogarty EE, et al. Scoliosis: a review. Pediatric Surgery International. Springer; 2008;24(2):129-44.
18. Tribus CB. Scheuermann's kyphosis in adolescents and adults: diagnosis and management. J Am Acad Orthop Surg. 1998 Jan;6(1):36–43.
19. Schwab FJ, Smith VA, Biserni M, et al. Adult scoliosis: a quantitative radiographic and clinical analysis. Spine. 2002;27(4):387-92.
20. Mac-Thiong J-M, Transfeldt EE, Mehbod AA, et al. Can c7 plumbline and gravity line predict health related quality of life in adult scoliosis? Spine. 2009;34(15):E519-27.
21. Schwab F, Lafage V, Boyce R, et al. Gravity line analysis in adult volunteers: age-related correlation with spinal parameters, pelvic parameters, and foot position. Spine. 2006; 31(25):E959-67.
22. Deschênes S, Charron G, Beaudoin G, et al. Diagnostic imaging of spinal deformities: reducing patients radiation dose with a new slot-scanning X-ray imager. Spine. 2010;35(9):989-94.
23. Harrington PR. Treatment of scoliosis. Correction and internal fixation by spine instrumentation. J Bone Joint Surg Am. 1962;44-A:591-610.
24. Humbert L, De Guise JA, Aubert B, et al. 3D reconstruction of the spine from biplanar X-rays using parametric models based on transversal and longitudinal inferences. Med Eng Phys. 2009;31(6):681-7.
25. Lenke LG, Betz RR, Harms J, et al. Adolescent idiopathic scoliosis: a new classification to determine extent of spinal arthrodesis. J Bone Joint Surg Am. 2001;83-A(8):1169-81.
26. Suk S-I. Pedicle screw instrumentation for adolescent idiopathic scoliosis: the insertion technique, the fusion levels and direct vertebral rotation. Clin Orthop Surg. 2011;3(2):89.
27. Bridwell KH. Surgical treatment of idiopathic adolescent scoliosis. Spine. 1999;24(24):2607-16.
28. Bradford DS. Adult scoliosis. Current concepts of treatment. Clin Orthop Relat Res. 1988;(229):70-87.
29. Harrington PR. The history and development of Harrington instrumentation. Clin Orthop Relat Res. 1973;(93):110-2.
30. Cotrel Y, Dubousset J. [A new technic for segmental spinal osteosynthesis using the posterior approach]. Rev Chir Orthop Reparatrice Appar Mot. 1984;70(6):489-94.
31. Mercado E, Alman B, Wright JG. Does spinal fusion influence quality of life in neuromuscular scoliosis? Spine. 2007;32(19 Suppl):S120-5.
32. Boachie-Adjei O, Lonstein JE, Winter RB, et al. Management of neuromuscular spinal deformities with Luque segmental instrumentation. J Bone Joint Surg Am. 1989;71(4):548-62.
33. Kostuik JP, Errico TJ, Gleason TF. Techniques of internal fixation for degenerative conditions of the lumbar spine. Clin Orthop Relat Res. 1986;(203):219-31.
34. Booth KC, Bridwell KH, Lenke LG, et al. Complications and predictive factors for the successful treatment of flatback deformity (fixed sagittal imbalance). Spine. 1999;24(16): 1712-20.
35. Luque ER. Segmental spinal instrumentation of the lumbar spine. Clin Orthop Relat Res. 1986;(203):126-34.
36. Farcy J-P, Schwab FJ. Management of flatback and related kyphotic decompensation syndromes. Spine. 1997;22(20): 2452-7.
37. Bradford DS, Tay BK, Hu SS. Adult scoliosis: surgical indications, operative management, complications, and outcomes. Spine. 1999;24(24):2617-29.
38. Voos K, Boachie-Adjei O, Rawlins BA. Multiple vertebral osteotomies in the treatment of rigid adult spine deformities. Spine. 2001;26(5):526-33.
39. Noun Z, Lapresle P, Missenard G. Posterior lumbar osteotomy for flat back in adults. J Spinal Disord. 2001;14(4):311-6.

40. Kostuik JP, Maurais GR, Richardson WJ, et al. Combined single stage anterior and posterior osteotomy for correction of iatrogenic lumbar kyphosis. Spine. 1988;13(3): 257-66.
41. Bradford DS, Tribus CB. Current concepts and management of patients with fixed decompensated spinal deformity. Clin Orthop Relat Res. 1994;(306):64-72.
42. Dickson JH, Mirkovic S, Noble PC, et al. Results of operative treatment of idiopathic scoliosis in adults. J Bone Joint Surg Am. 1995;77(4):513-23.
43. Sponseller PD, Cohen MS, Nachemson AL, et al. Results of surgical treatment of adults with idiopathic scoliosis. J Bone Joint Surg Am. 1987;69(5):667-75.
44. Vavken P, Bianchi T. In Brief: cost-effectiveness analyses in orthopaedics. Clin Orthop Relat Res. 2011;469(8):2395-8.
45. Kepler CK, Wilkinson SM, Radcliff KE, et al. Cost-utility analysis in spine care: a systematic review. Spine J. 2012; 12(8):676-90
46. Takayama K, Nakamura H, Matsuda H. Quality of life in patients treated surgically for scoliosis: longer than sixteen-year follow-up. Spine. 2009;34(20):2179-84.
47. Ware JE, Sherbourne CD. The MOS 36-Item Short-Form Health Survey (SF-36). I. Conceptual framework and item selection. Med Care. 1992;30(6):473-83.
48. Asher M, Min Lai S, Burton D, et al. The reliability and concurrent validity of the Scoliosis Research Society-22 patient questionnaire for idiopathic scoliosis. Spine. 2003;28(1):63-9.
49. Abdullah KG, Benzel EC, Mroz TE. Comparative effectiveness research in spine surgery. Neurosurg Focus. 2012;33 (1):E2.

CHAPTER

52

Operative Management of Pediatric Deformities

Justin C Paul, Baron S Lonner, Courtney S Toombs

INTRODUCTION

The human spine is a flexible column with complex motion in three planes governed by articulations of each vertebra and the intervertebral disks. The erect spine has well-defined baseline curves in the sagittal plane and minimal curvature in the coronal plane (Figs. 52.1A to C). Deformity in the spine can develop in any plane, and in many cases all planes are affected. In addition to bending and curvature, vertebral bodies can "slip", or translate, away from normal alignment. This review divides pediatric deformity into three groups: scoliosis (curvature in the coronal plane), kyphosis (curvature in the sagittal plane), and spondylolisthesis (translational deformity).

SCOLIOSIS

Background/Etiology

Scoliosis is lateral deviation of the spine in the coronal plane. Idiopathic scoliosis affects 1–3% of boys and girls aged 10–18, with 0.1–0.3% of cases having curves > 30°.[1-3] Adolescent idiopathic scoliosis (AIS) accounts for approximately 80% of scoliosis curves occurring in adolescents aged 10–18, with adolescent girls more commonly affected than boys. AIS is a deformity distinguished from congenital scoliosis by having no clear identifiable defect in formation or segmentation of the vertebrae (Figs. 52.2 A to C).

Within congenital forms of scoliosis, the spectrum of clinical presentation ranges from mild curvature to spinal malformations that can facilitate relentless progression of spinal deformity.[4] These progressive curves can manifest in severe deformity and functional impairments. The pathology in this disease arises from a defect in formation, segmentation, or both (Figs. 52.3A and B).

Neuromuscular scoliosis arises from neurologic or muscular pathology with abnormal musculoskeletal support of the spinal column and is one of the most challenging spinal pathologies to treat.[5] Neurologic disorders that can lead to neuromuscular scoliosis include cerebral palsy, spinal muscular atrophy, and Friedreich's ataxia. Muscular diseases with the potential to generate spine deformity include muscular dystrophy, arthrogryposis, and myotonia. The often-severe curvature in both the sagittal and coronal planes that is seen in neuromuscular scoliosis is magnified by the accompanying pelvic obliquity. In addition, social issues are often at play as there commonly are cognitive defects to consider during rehabilitation, discussions of life expectancy and family values/expectations, and the need for exhaustive caregiving outside of the hospital. Table 52.1 provides an extensive list of etiologies of structural scoliosis.

ANATOMY/BIOMECHANICS

The ligamentous connectivity of the spinal column results in the phenomena of coupled motion where bending cannot occur without coupled rotation of the spine. In scoliosis, the ends of the curve are tilted with minimal rotation while the apical vertebrae undergo maximal rotation but neutral tilt. Coupled rotation results in the rib-hump on one side that is noted clinically when the patient bends forward; this is often considered by the patient to be the most unacceptable aspect of the deformity. AIS

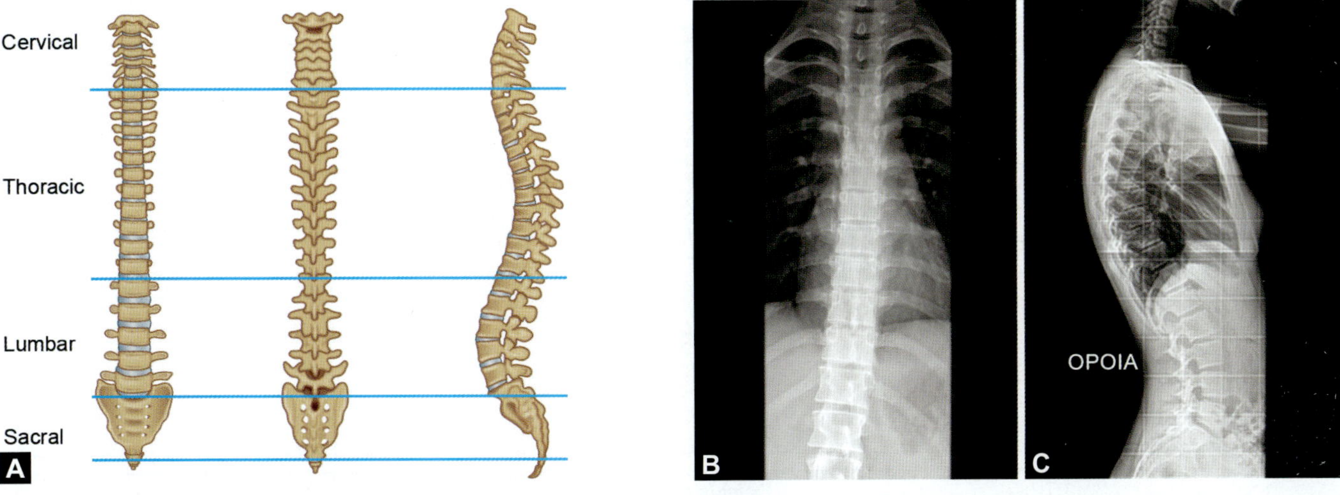

Figs. 52.1A to C: Normal spinal alignment in coronal and sagittal views.

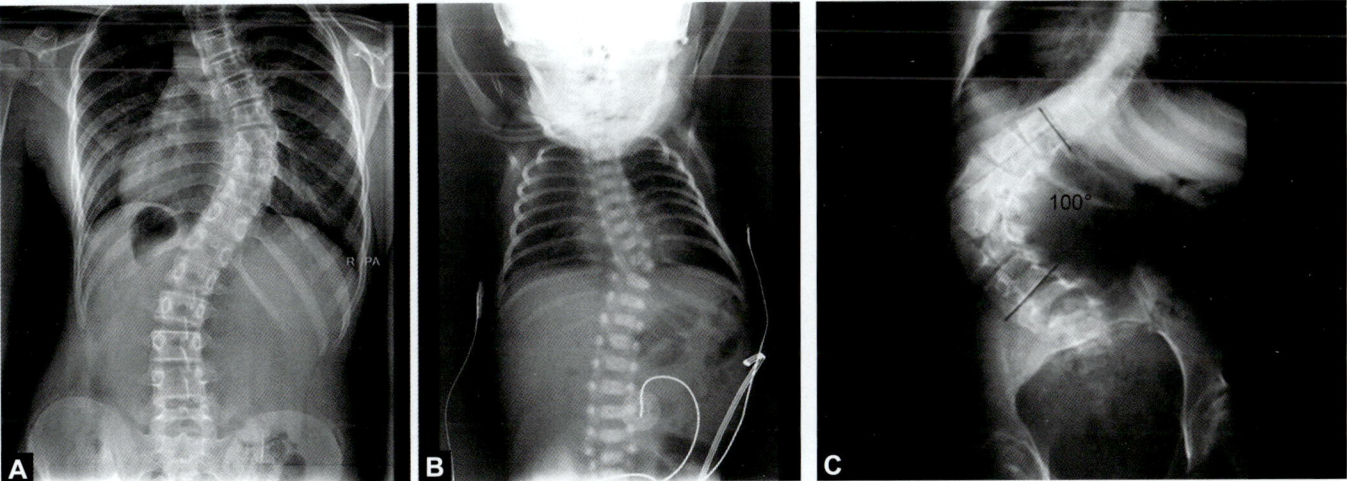

Figs. 52.2A to C: Pediatric scoliosis can be idiopathic with normal vertebrae in abnormal alignment or congenital, where malformed vertebrae result in deformity. Cerebral palsy is an example of neuromuscular etiology.

patients often have decreased kyphosis (hypokyphosis), hypothesized to be a result of anterior vertebral overgrowth leading to hypokyphosis, scoliosis, and axial rotation.[6]

CLINICAL EVALUATION

Clinical examination with an inclinometer (Figs. 52.4A to G) is a basic method for detection of truncal asymmetry resulting from scoliosis in school screening programs. Patients found to have truncal asymmetry may be subsequently referred to as spine specialist. In all initial patient evaluations, the clinician documents a thorough history including onset, presence of pain, and neurological symptoms. A general review of symptoms should include questions about the heart, lungs, kidneys, and eyes. A family history of scoliosis is common in patients with idiopathic scoliosis, although the inheritance pattern is not yet understood.

The initial survey includes inspection of the skin for café-au-lait spots (Figs. 52.4A to G) and inguinal or axillary freckling associated with neurofibromatosis. The back should be ruled out for midline nevus, sinus, or hair-patch, which may indicate underlying congenital spinal anomalies. Physical inspection includes a full neurological examination including testing of abdominal reflexes that if asymmetric may point to a spinal cord pathology such as syrinx. Other sometimes-subtle neurological findings include calf asymmetry and cavus foot deformity. In addition to measuring rib and lumbar prominence with an inclinometer, asymmetry of the shoulders (Figs. 52.4A to G), hips, and scapulae should also be assessed. The angle

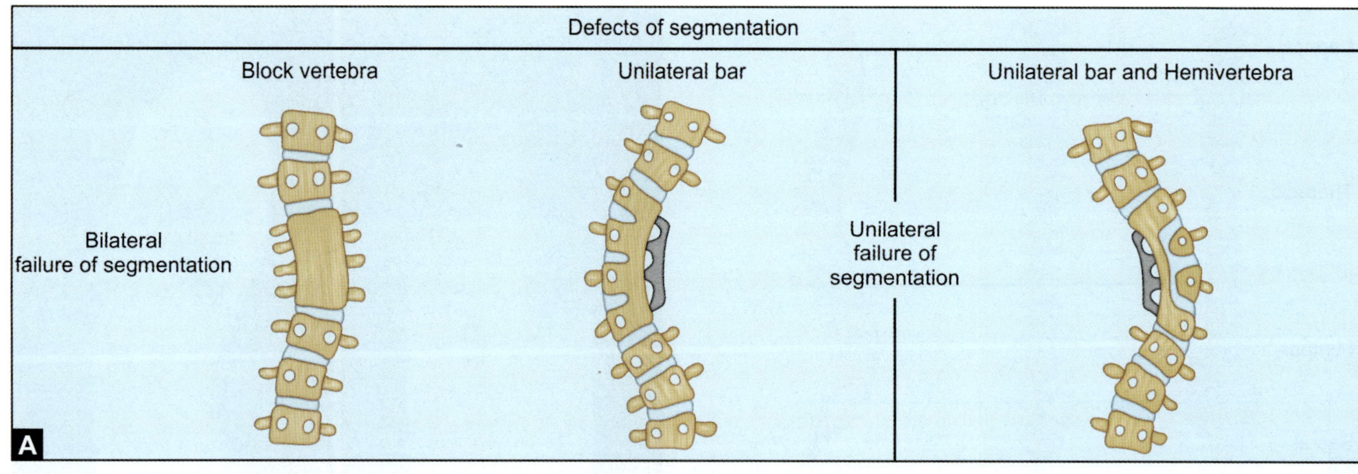

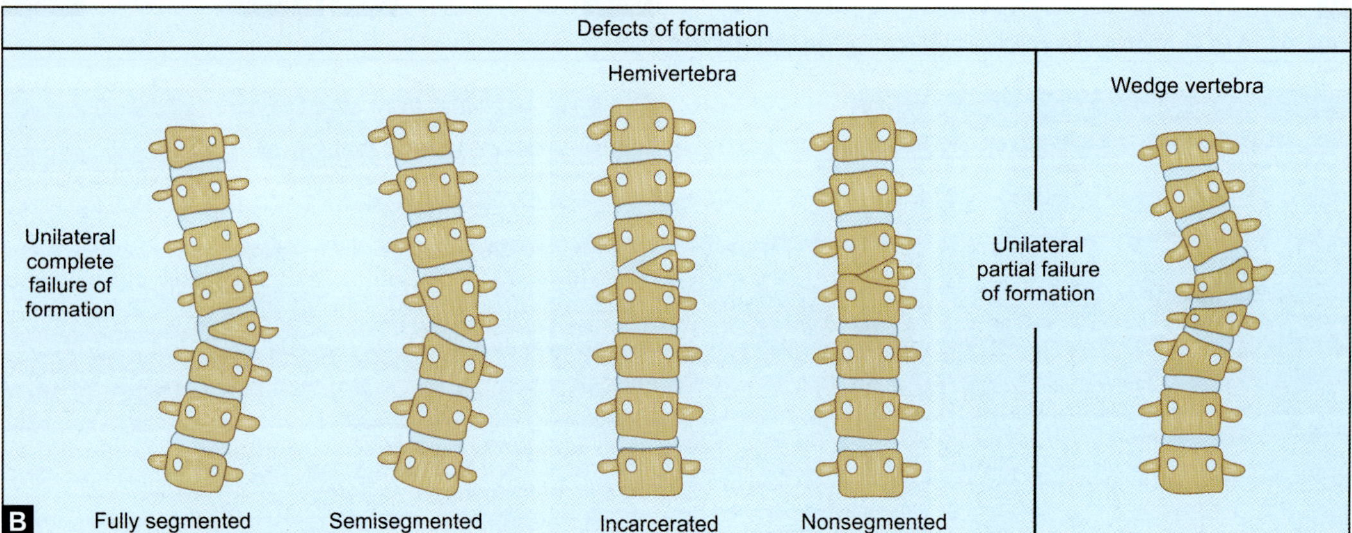

Figs. 52.3A and B: Defects of formation and segmentation.

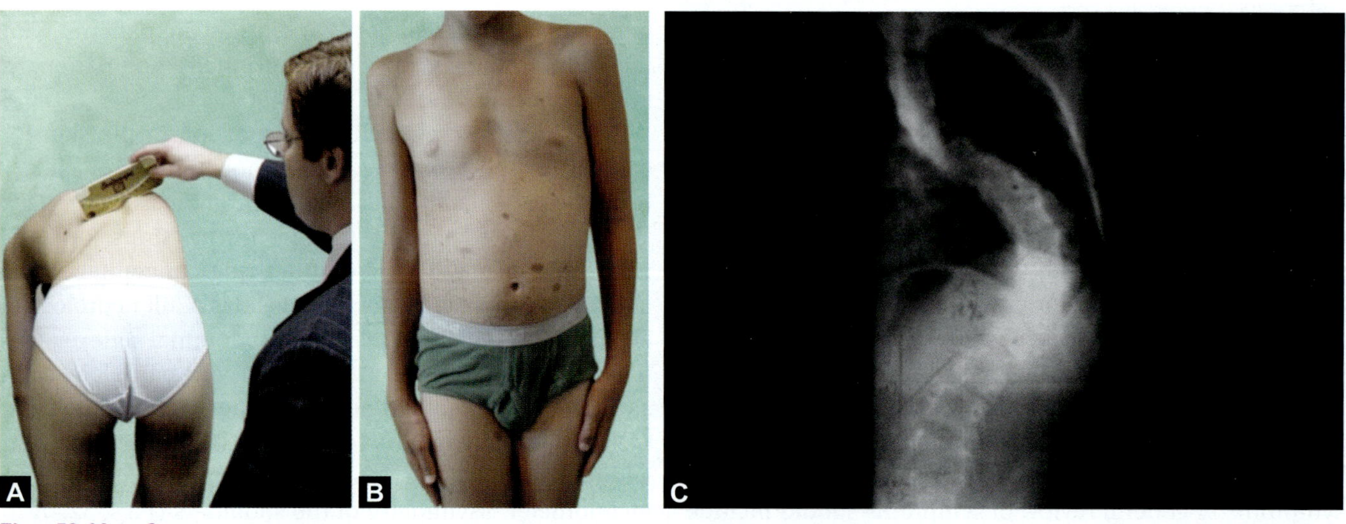

Figs. 52.4A to C

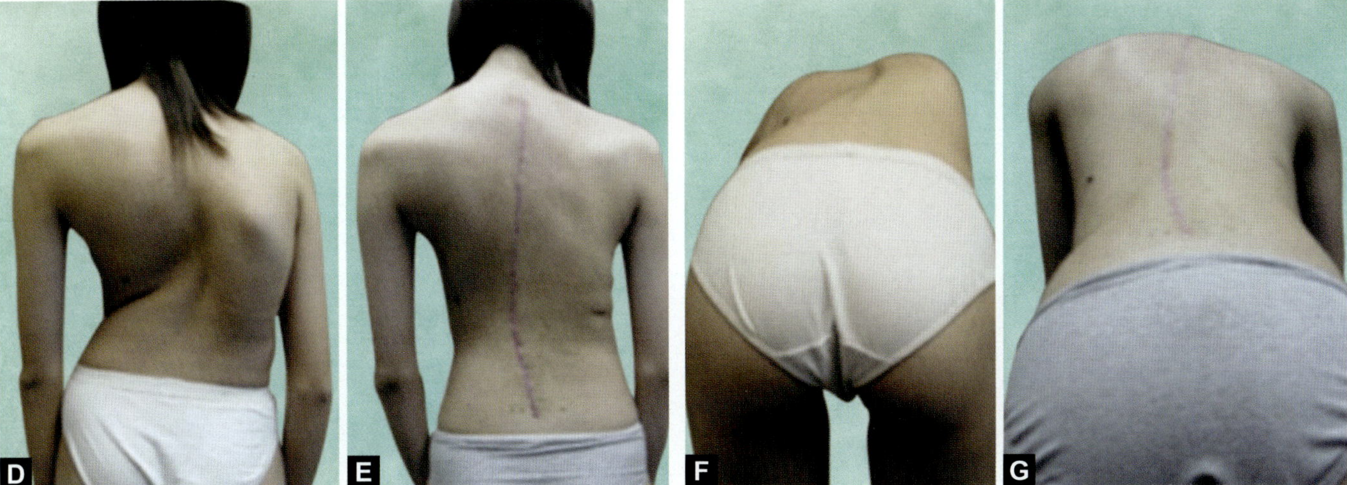

Figs. 52.4A to G: (A) Clinical examination with an inclinometer. (B) Café-au-lait spots noted over the abdomen. (C to G) Shoulder asymmetry is noted standing and on forward bend but is more pronounced for the patient on the left with a 101° curve than on the right (34°).

Table 52.1: Know etiologies of structural scoliosis
• Neuromuscular
– Cerebral palsy
– Poliomyelitis
– Spinal muscular atrophy (Werdnig-Hoffman, Dubowitz, Kugelberg-Welander)
– Dysraphism (Myelomeningocele, Spina bifida occulta, etc.)
– Familial Dysautonomia (Riley-Day Syndrome)
– Arthrogryposis
– Duchenne muscular dystrophy (DMD)
– Charcot-Marie-Tooth (CMT)
– Friedreich's ataxia
– Facioscapulohumeral dystrophy
• Congenital scoliosis (Hemivertebrae, etc)
• Connective tissue disorders (Neurofibromatosis, Ehlers-Danlos, Marfan's, etc.)
• Post-traumatic (Fracture, iatrogenic, irradiation, etc.)
• Skeletal Dysplasias [spondyloepiphyseal dysplasia (SED), etc.]
• Lumbosacral joint (spondylolisthesis)
• Tumor (osteoid osteoma, osteoblastoma, etc.)

of trunk rotation (ATR) is measured with an inclinometer: 7° is considered 83% sensitive and 86% specific for scoliosis (ATR of 5° is 100% sensitive and 47% specific).[7] Truncal shift, pelvic tilt, waist crease asymmetry, and rotational prominence on forward bend should all be documented. Leg lengths should also be measured (Figs. 52.5A to D). Pain localization is important and may present as intercostal neuralgia, rib tip syndrome, lumbosacral pain, or radicular pain—particularly in the adult patient disabling pain is much less common in pediatric patients and should raise a red flag to the possibility of underlying pathology such as syrinx, tethered cord, or neoplasm, such as osteoid osteoma.

Pulmonary function testing (PFT) has also become a useful tool in assessing the impact of AIS on pulmonary function, which is most common in early onset (under age 10 years) forms of scoliosis and severe curvature. Patients breathe into a device that measures forced vital capacity and forced expiratory volume in 1 second. Pulmonary function has been shown to decrease with increasing thoracic curve magnitude, as well as increased length of the curve and hypokyphosis, and is therefore PFT is an appropriate tool for assessing the operative patient.[8]

Predicting the rate of curve progression in an AIS patients has been largely based on parameters assessing growth potential, such as menarchal status, age, Risser sign (capping of the iliac apophysis), and bone age determinations; but these are coarse predictions based on percentages of the scoliotic population that have progression of curvature at a certain curve magnitude and Risser stage and therefore require serial longitudinal observation including X-rays.[9] More recently, a prognostic genetic test has become available that provides an individualized score. The ScoliScore saliva-based genetic test can be performed on AIS patients aged 9–13 of primarily Caucasian decent with scoliosis curves between 10° and 25°. The test identifies specific genes linked to scoliosis and provides a "score" that predicts a low, intermediate, or high likelihood of curve progression to >40° based on the genetic profile; these results can aid

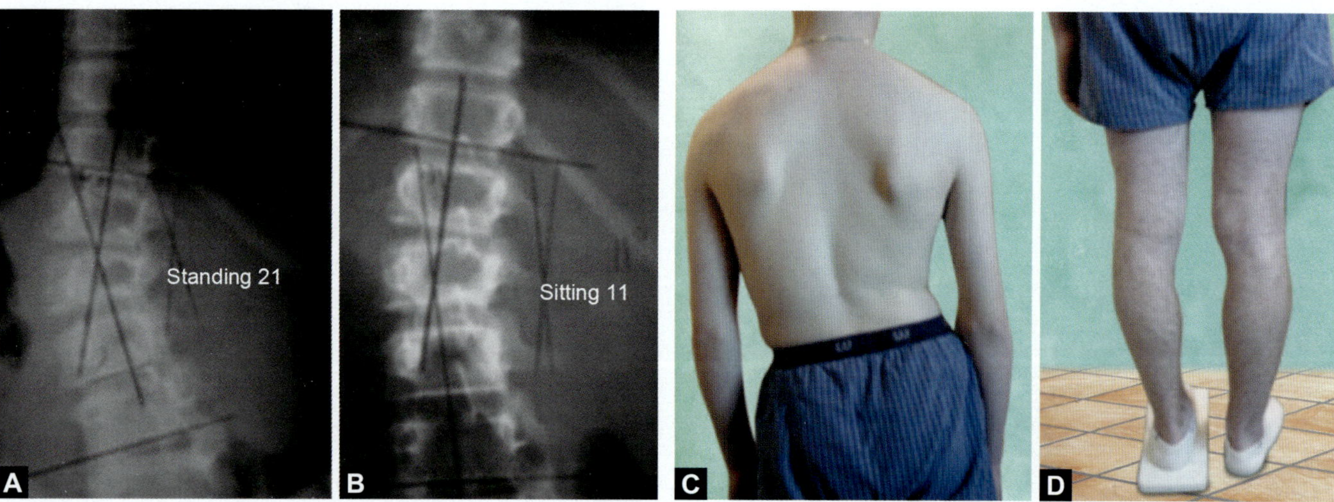

Figs. 52.5A to D: Observed spinal alignment can change on standing films when patients are standing on limbs of unequal length. Leg length discrepancy should be assessed and radiographs obtained with the shorter limb on a block of known height.

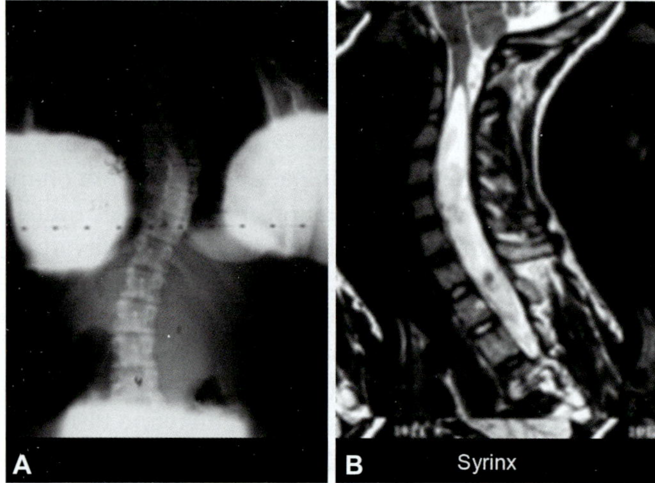

Figs. 52.6A and B: Syrinx formation diagnosed in a patient with a right-sided thoracic curve.

in determining follow-up intervals, making decisions on bracing and surgery, and counseling families with a child who has AIS.

In congenital scoliosis, a thorough history and physical examination with evaluation of possible syndromes or abnormalities of nonskeletal organ systems is necessary. Genitourinary and renal defects are present in up to 30% of congenital scoliosis cases, and cardiac defects are present in up to 10%. Overall, up to 61% of congenital scoliosis patients will have associated syndromes with other organ systems involved. The VATER and VACTERL acronyms involve Vertebral, Anorectal, Cardiac, Tracheo-esophageal fistula, Renal, and Limb (radial clubhand, thumb hypoplasia) deformities. As the neural axis and vertebrae develop simultaneously, associated anomalies may include diastematomyelia, syringomyelia (syrinx formation) (Figs. 52.6A and B), tethered cord, dural bands, cysts, lipoma with overall intraspinal anomaly rates ranging from 18% to 37%.[4,10]

RADIOLOGIC EVALUATION

Routine imaging includes standing posteroanterior and lateral radiographs. Patients with predominantly single plane (scoliosis or kyphosis) deformity can be followed clinically over time with a single X-ray instead of two views in order to minimize radiation exposure. MRI is not routinely indicated, but should be obtained for instances of refractory back pain, a left thoracic curve, rapidly progressive curvature, infantile or juvenile patients, neurological signs or symptoms, and infantile or juvenile idiopathic scoliosis and congenital anomalies for which surgery is being contemplated, as the likelihood of neural element abnormalities in these instances is elevated. CT is useful for defining skeletal anatomy in cases of congenital deformity, but should be used judiciously due to its significant associated radiation exposure.

The spinal deformity patient is evaluated and followed with X-rays to depict alignment and deformity.[11] Young female patients with spinal deformities are thus exposed to multiple doses of ionizing radiation, which includes radiation directed at the breast and pelvic region, potentially having adverse effects.[12-14]

Recent advances in the technology of spine radiography have produced the slot-scanning X-ray imager

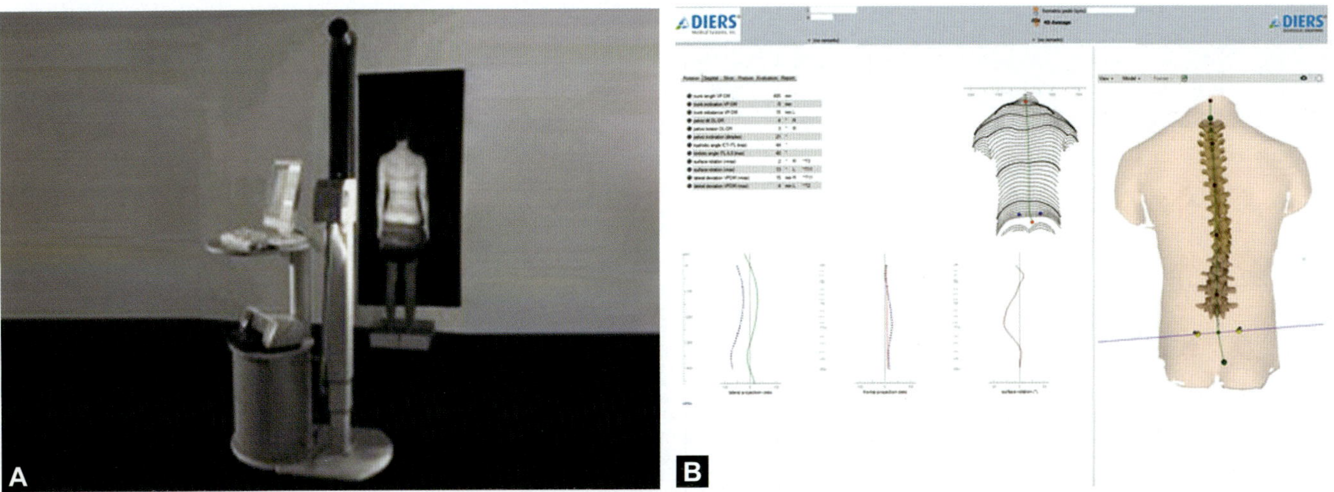

Figs. 52.7A and B: Diers® Formetric Scanner. (A) A patient exposes their back to the scanner, which maps specific spinal end points that allow the program to approximate the three-dimensional shape of the patient's spine and outer back surface. (B) The results of the scan provide valuable three-dimensional information about the patient's back as well as parameters traditionally measured on X-rays.

(EOS machine) that uses a low ionizing radiation dose X-ray.[15] The EOS imaging tool produces a biplanar, orthogonal image with sharp resolution of bony structures. The acquisition time for this radiograph is approximately 30 seconds, and charges are similar to those for standard radiographs. Radiation-free methods of assessing spinal curvature and three-dimensional back shape have also been recently introduced, including the DIERS Formetric Scanner (Figs. 52.7A and B). The Formetric Scanner shines a light on the patient's back while taking rapid and consecutive photographs, using landmarks such as the C7 prominence to digitally approximate the shape of the spine. The three-dimensional recreation of the patient's spine, as well as the topographical map of their back shape, produced by the Formetric Scanner is useful in replacing X-rays and providing clinical information about patients below the surgical range, and can serve as a radiation-free screening and observation tool.

CLASSIFICATION

Scoliosis can be classified descriptively by characteristics such as location (thoracic, thoracolumbar/lumbar, for example) and side of the apex, pattern (single or double), and magnitude (Cobb angle). AIS patients are most often females who present at 10 years of age or older with a right-sided thoracic apex curve. Curves > 10° are 1.4 times more common in females than in males; for curves > 30°, that ratio increases to 10:1. Juvenile scoliosis is defined as occurring between ages 3 and 10 years and is often highly progressive. Infantile scoliosis occurs between birth and age three.[16] Left thoracic curves usually predominate in the male population. While most AIS curves resolve, some can be malignant, or highly progressive.

Structural curves should be distinguished from compensatory curves on preoperative dynamic radiographs. The structural curve remains rigid despite bending in an attempt to straighten the curve, sometimes with the aid of bolsters, push-prone technique, or supine bending. In a landmark retrospective study of 405 patients, King et al. used the concept of structural and compensatory curves to posit that a structural thoracic curve can be fused without extending the fusion to lumbar segments.[17]

The classification described by King did not consider lumbar or triple curves, nor did it account for sagittal deformity. Classification schemes such as the Lenke classification sought to expand King's theory by categorizing the curve magnitude and orientation with curve type and two modifiers that address the deviation of the lumbar curve apex from the midline as well as the thoracic kyphosis.[18] The Lenke classification is currently the most commonly used classification for AIS (Fig. 52.8).

Scoliotic curves should be described by morphology, but with careful attention to patient characteristics and measures of growth potential. The patient's age, pubertal status (by Tanner stage or by age at menarche for females), and Risser grade are all important factors. The Risser grade is the percent of the iliac apophysis that has ossified as apparent on radiographs. Grade 1 represents 0-25% ossification (early puberty), grade 2 represents 25-50%, and so on until complete ossification signifying skeletal maturity (Fig. 52.9).

Curve Type (1–6)						
Lumbar spine modifier	Type 1 (Main thoracic)	Type 2 (Double thoracic)	Type 3 (Double major)	Type 4 (Triple major)	Type 5 (TL/L)	Type 6 (TL/L-MT)
A	1A*	2A*	3A*	4A*		
B	1B*	2B*	3B*	4B*		
C	1C*	2C*	3C*	4C*	5C*	6C*
Possible sagittal structural criteria (To determine specific curve type)	Normal	PT Kyphosis	TL Kyphosis	PT and TL Kyphosis	Normal	TL Kyphosis

*T5–12 sagittal alignment modifier: –, N, or +
–: <10°
N: 10–40°
+ : >40°

Fig. 52.8: The Lenke classification system characterizes the coronal and sagittal deformity with attention to the instability of caudal segments.

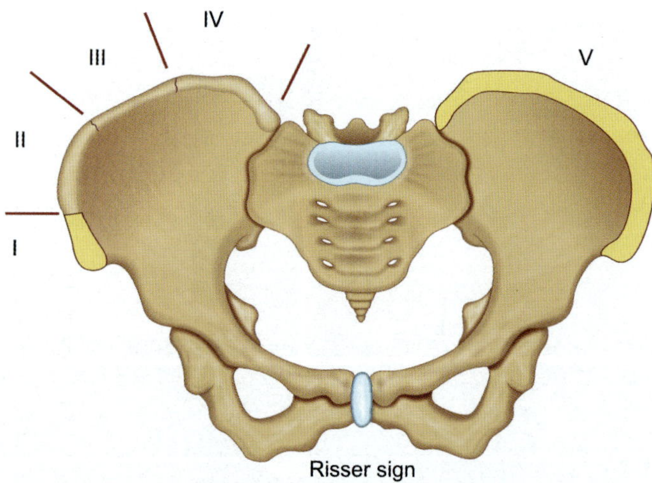

Fig. 52.9: Risser grading system uses the percent of the iliac apophysis that has calcified as apparent on radiographs. Increasing in increments of 25%, grade 1 represents 25% ossification (early puberty) and grade of 5 means 100% calcification at skeletal maturity.

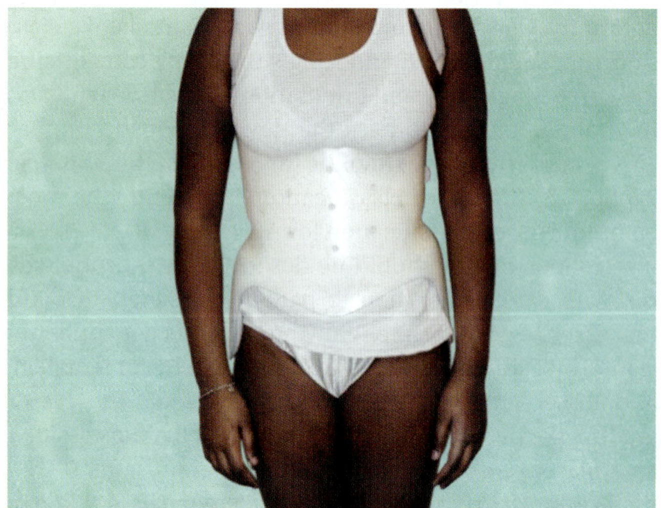

Fig. 52.10: Bracing is the most common nonoperative intervention used for growing patients with curves between 25° and 35°.

NONOPERATIVE TREATMENT

Although serial casting techniques have been used in cases of infantile and juvenile scoliosis, bracing is the most common nonoperative intervention used for growing patients with curves between 25° and 40° and a Risser score of 0–2 (Fig. 52.10).[19] The goal of bracing is to prevent progression of the deformity. Bracing rarely results in permanent correction of scoliosis, although chest wall molding of the thoracic prominence can be permanent. In bracing for kyphosis, permanent correction is more likely to occur. The AIS patient can be observed expectantly when presenting with curvatures of <20°. Radiographs may be obtained every 3–6 months during growth, with bracing employed if curve progression has occurred during prepubertal rapid growth.

Bracing is typically prescribed for 20–22 hours per day until the completion of growth, as the success of bracing has been tied to the number of hours the brace is worn. Because compliance with bracing can be challenging, part-time programs of 12–16 hours per day may be better tolerated. There are many brace types available, including the Milwaukee brace, Boston brace, Wilmington brace, and the Charleston brace; cessation of curve progression may be expected 75% of the time. The Charleston nighttime bending brace should be reserved for single lumbar or thoracolumbar curves of <35°.[20] Untreated AIS patients, or those treated with bracing, can present later in life with pain, disability, and worsening deformity resulting from degenerative cascade and curve progression in the sagittal and coronal plane and global imbalance.

Several indicators of maturity exist that can identify if a patient is near a growth spurt, which can alter treatment options for AIS.[21] Predicting the occurrence of the growth spurt or peak height velocity is important because they represent the time when AIS curves will progress the most. The "curve acceleration phase" is closely linked to rapidly increasing height.[22]

If the patient is in the period of peak height velocity and the curve acceleration phase, and has a significant curvature, surgery may be indicated. Conversely, if maturity markers indicate that a patient has completed their growth spurt, nonoperative management may be more appropriate, depending on the curve magnitude, clinical deformity, and location of the curvature.

OPERATIVE TREATMENT

Health-related quality of life (HRQOL), self-image, and body-image disturbances are important factors in the decision to operate for this disease. The natural history of untreated AIS can lead to deformity progression, pain, and, in severe cases, pulmonary disease. General indications for surgery include progressive curvature over 40° in the skeletally immature patient, and thoracic curvature over 50° or lumbar curvature over 40° in the skeletally mature patient. Curves in growing patients that have progressed (Risser 0–2) despite bracing are also an indication for surgery. Patients with significant lordosis or restrictive pulmonary disease are considered for surgery, even outside of the traditional parameters discussed above. Structural, progressive curvature of 20–35° in a growing adolescent can be considered for convex stapling procedures that encourage growth modulation to gradually straighten the spine. In some cases, considering the genetic profile (ScoliScore) can aid in the decision for surgery.

As the vertebrae appear individually normal despite the asymmetric growth during the growth spurt, AIS correction is best accomplished by arthrodesis (bony fusion) over the joint between two vertebrae (a segment) to prevent further deformity.[23] Pedicle screw and rod fixation of the spine is a well-defined and popular technique to correct the deformity, increase the rate of bony fusion, and minimize the need for bracing.[24] The goals of scoliosis surgery are to prevent curvature progression, correct deformity, preserve as many motion segments as possible, and minimize complications. Patients treated by posterior fusion may have an increase in pulmonary function up to 25 years after treatment.[25]

Adolescent idiopathic scoliosis patients treated with fusion into the lower lumbar segments are at risk of accelerated degeneration in caudal unfused segments in adulthood. Surgical plans to fuse distal segments often involve a decision of lower instrumented vertebra (LIV). A more proximal selected LIV should preserve motion and reduce the risk of long-term degeneration of distal unfused lumbar vertebral levels.[26,27]

Surgical indications for congenital scoliosis include the presence of high-risk deformity type (a bar or a bar with a contralateral hemivertebrae) and curve progression. The surgeon must consider age, remaining growth, truncal positioning (shoulder and neck imbalance), and cervicothoracic and thoracolumbar junctional deformities, as they can manifest in unsatisfactory deformities. In cases of thoracic insufficiency syndrome—a condition in which the thorax is unable to support normal respiration, which maybe due to congenital rib synostoses or fusions —expansion thoracoplasty may be performed with the vertical expandable prosthetic titanium rib (VEPTR, aka. titanium rib) device (Figs. 52.11A to E). The expandable prosthetic rib enlarges the constricted chest and thus straightens the spine indirectly without fusion and may improve pulmonary function.

In cases of neuromuscular scoliosis, the underlying neuromuscular condition guides the treatment strategy. Surgery is generally indicated for curvatures >50° in growing patients, but can be indicated for functional deterioration, pain, or cardiopulmonary compromise. Anterior and posterior instrumentation is often required, as are long fusions from the upper thoracic spine to the sacrum and pelvis, especially in nonambulators and those with significant pelvic obliquity (Figs. 52.12A to C).[5]

SURGICAL TECHNIQUE

Surgical technique should incorporate elements of the themes outlined in the classifications systems. The structurality of the curves inherent to the Lenke classification should be used to guide selection of structural major (largest) and compensatory curvatures. The nonstructural curve results as the spine compensates for the initial structural curve with another curve in the opposite direction. Selective fusion involves fusing the major curvature while leaving compensatory curvatures unfused; this is done to preserve postoperative motion.

Coronal and sagittal balance must be considered simultaneously so that kyphotic segments are included. Clinical features of the deformity should be considered.

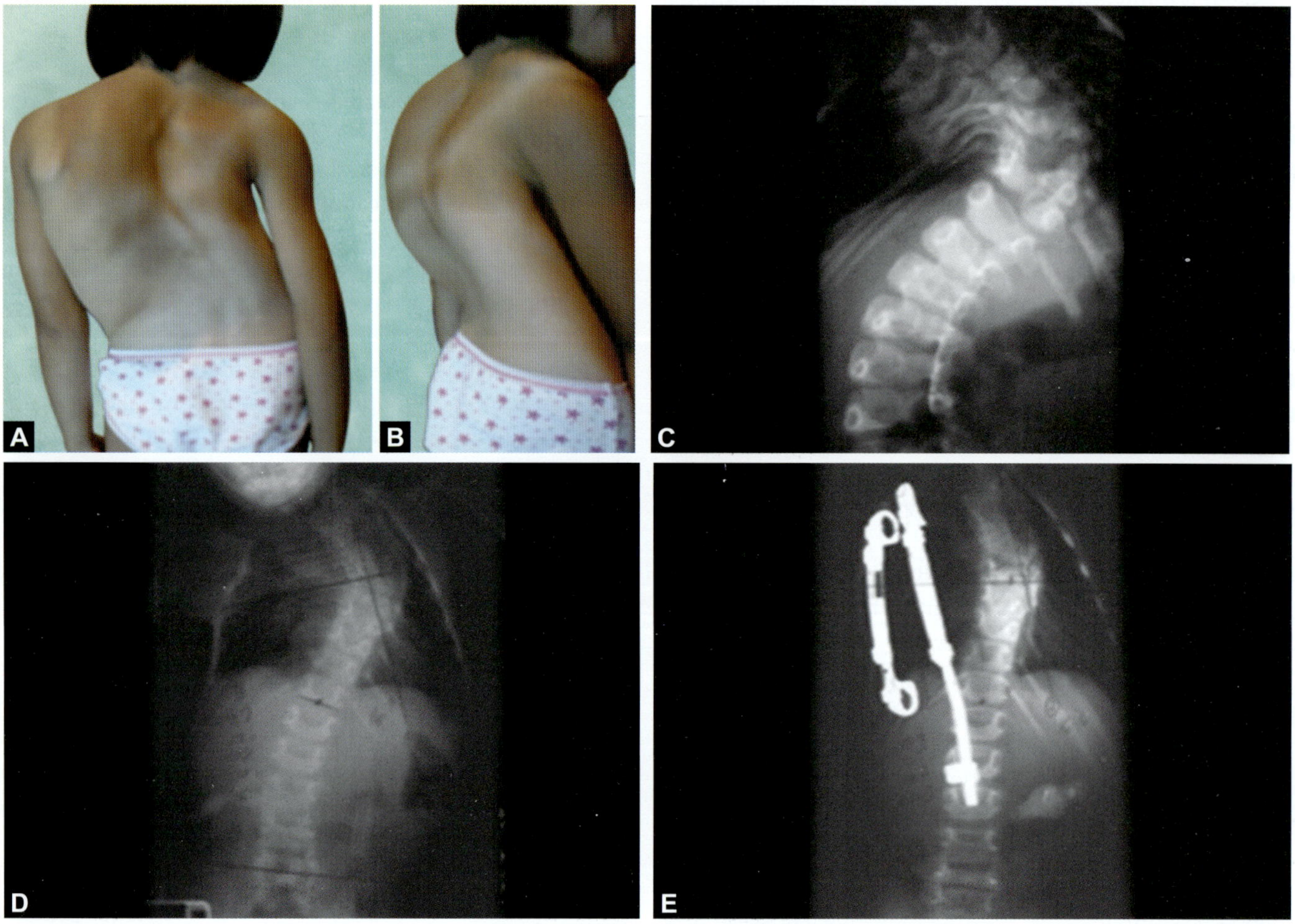

Figs. 52.11A to E: Gradual correction of congenital scoliosis with vertical expandable prosthetic titanium rib.

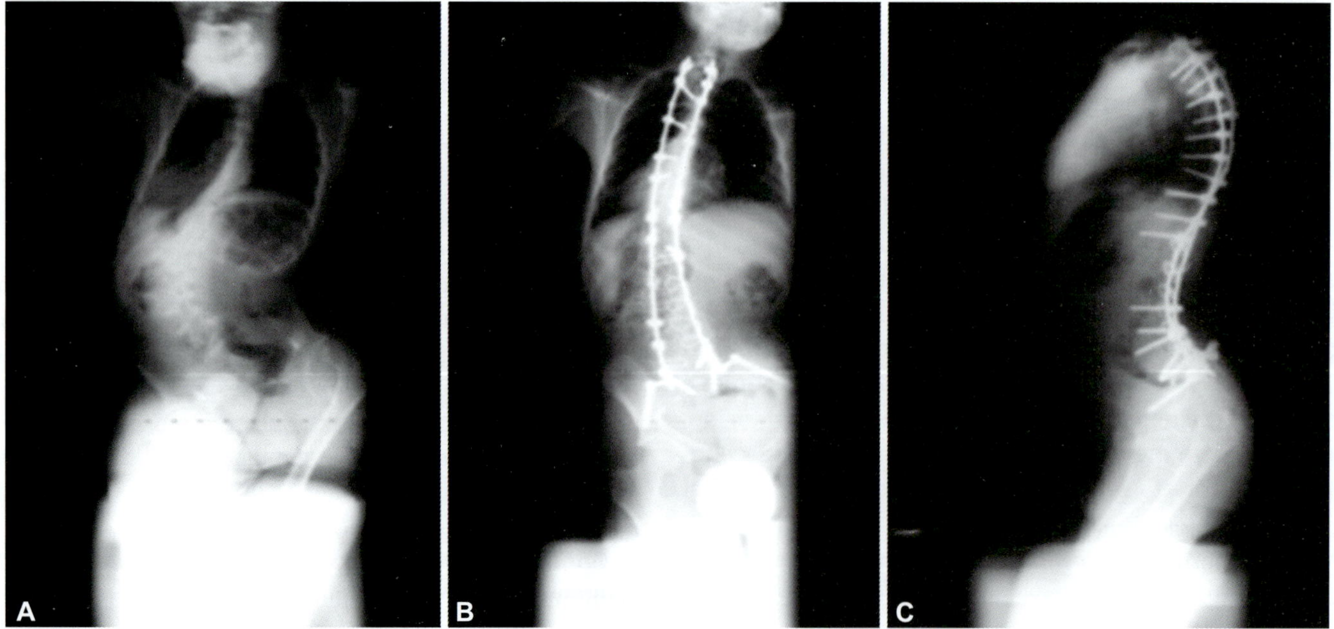

Figs. 52.12A to C: Neuromuscular deformity treated with fixation to the pelvis.

Rotational prominences of the scapula on forward bending should be corrected. The proximal thoracic curve should be addressed if one shoulder is elevated so as to restore shoulder symmetry.

There is an extensive history of attempted methods for correcting scoliosis and obtaining a spinal arthrodesis including wire, hook, and rod constructs, which have gained and lost favor over time. Considering the three-column model of spine stability, the surgical instrumentation of the spine using posterior segmental pedicle screw constructs is the only three-column fixation. Pedicle screws provide a very strong anchorage to the spine, rarely require revision in the pediatric population, and facilitate excellent three-dimensional correction of spinal deformity. Anterior dual-rod constructs have also been validated for thoracolumbar scoliosis, which may provide for fewer segments of fixation. Posterior transpedicular screws technique can be used for all curve types with or without anterior release in which intervertebral disks are removed to loosen up the spine and make it more flexible for purposes of correction. Posterior osteotomies, which involve cutting into the posterior spinal segments and removing bone, facilitate correction in three planes.

The first decision for the operative plan is to determine which surgical approach is appropriate. The posterior approach is considered the workhorse of scoliosis surgery, as all curves are amenable, more than one curve can be addressed, and osteotomies may be performed for large and rigid deformity. Anterior release can be performed with a posterior fusion for rigid coronal deformity of > 70° and for significant lordosis. Anterior fusion and instrumentation can be performed for a single thoracic curve of magnitude 40–70° and > 50% flexibility, instrumenting less than eight vertebrae.

In cases of hypokyphosis, approaching the spine anteriorly can be advantageous. The anterior approach for thoracic or thoracolumbar curves can spare motion levels, restore kyphosis, and can result in less junctional kyphosis after the fusion. Recently, anterior fusion has been used as stand-alone treatment in AIS. The thoracoabdominal anterior approach for thoracolumbar scoliosis with anterior spinal fusion and instrumentation has been used for its ability to correct apical trunk rotation correction, minimize blood loss, and may allow for shorter fusions than posterior approaches.[28]

In approaching the thoracic spine anteriorly, thoracoscopy can be considered in place of open thoracotomy as it results in reduced pain, improved pulmonary function, and spared shoulder function (Figs. 52.13A to D).[29] Thoracoscopy often provides enhanced visualization with the use of angled scopes, magnification, illumination, and multiple portals.[30] Cosmesis is also improved with little surgical scarring. Commonly known as video-assisted thoracoscopic surgery (VATS), this minimally invasive approach for anterior release and fusion in spinal deformities can have success in AIS with high-magnitude, kyphotic, rigid thoracic curves.[31] Combined approaches are reserved for rigid deformity usually > 60°; combined anterior and posterior technique helps in derotation for significant deformity axial plane deformity.

Despite successful outcomes with the treatments available, there is occasionally debate in selecting the most caudal level of spine fusion given the potential for adjacent level disease (ALD) and the desire to preserve motion and function. Correction of alignment of the spine can be accomplished at the expense of motion by fusing further segments—it is often more desirable to leave some residual curvature in order to maximize remaining motion segments. The decision to fuse to the fourth versus the third lumbar vertebrae is important to ensure motion preservation.[26]

An area of future research that addresses the concept of fusionless surgery, briefly mentioned above, has received increasing attention. Techniques and instruments in focus are surgical tethers (Fig. 52.14) and vertebral body stapling.[32,33] The question of when during the growth phase to use fusionless techniques remains unanswered.

OUTCOMES/COMPLICATIONS

Adolescent idiopathic scoliosis patients who have undergone surgery have life satisfaction scores comparable with their nondiseased counterparts.[34] Due to advancements in scoliosis surgery, patients can begin returning to full activity 3 months following surgery. Prospective study on the level of play that athletic individuals who have undergone AIS surgery partake in is ongoing.

Because spinal fusion prevents motion, adjacent nonfused levels may be prone to degeneration from the added stress (ALD).[35,36] It has been shown in AIS that lateral bending is increased postoperatively for unfused motion segments in the lumbar spine when a more distal instrumented vertebral level is fused.[27] However, with fusion levels of the third lumbar vertebrae or more cephalad, the adjacent level forces drop off significantly, as do concerns for early or intermediate term deterioration of motion segments.

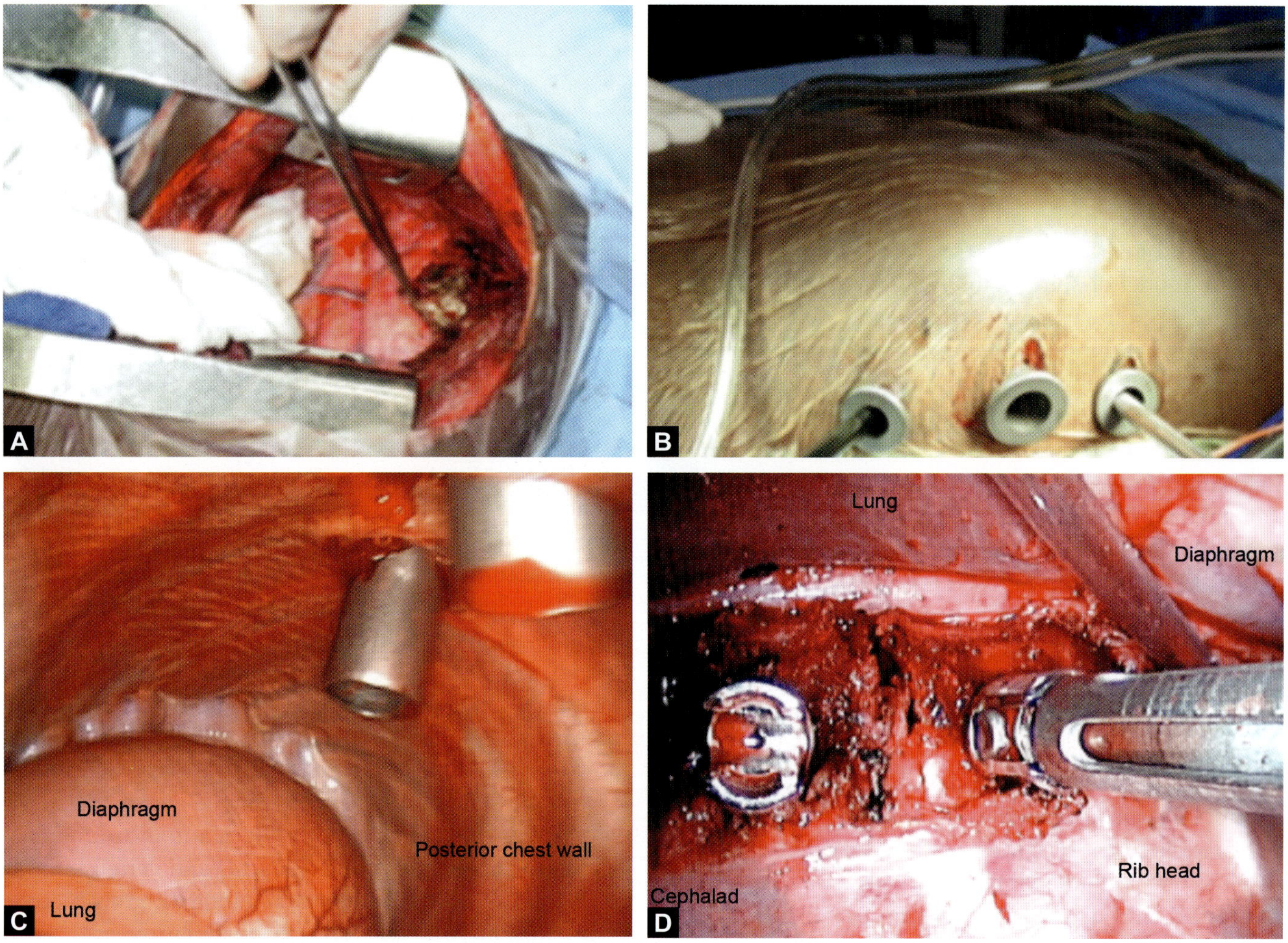

Figs. 52.13A to D: (A) Open thoracotomy versus (B) video-assisted thoracoscopic surgery. (C and D) Images from endoscopic cameras.

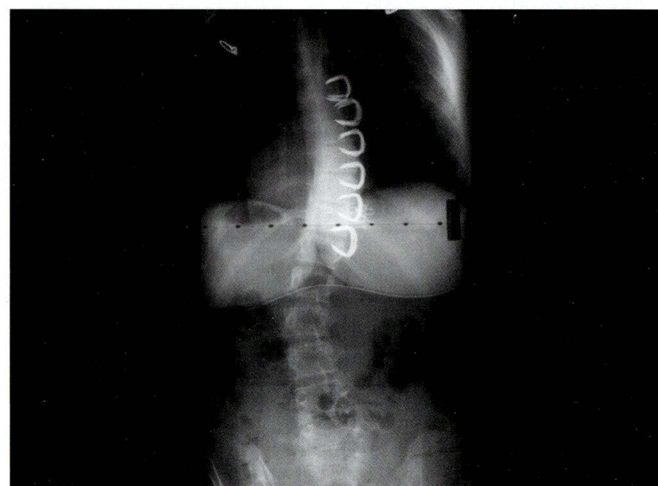

Fig. 52.14: Fusionless surgery with staples.

Fusion of the spine changes motion and gait parameters, significantly reducing lateral motion and flexion.[37-39] Mahaudens et al. showed that female AIS subjects lost up to 28% of pelvis, hip, and shoulder motion in the frontal plane and had similar losses in the transverse plane when compared with control subjects during gait—independent of Cobb angle—with reduced step lengths and stance phases.[40] Mahaudens' findings may not translate fully to modern techniques such as selective fusion, preservation of motion segments, and three-dimensional alignment preservation and should be further studied.

In an assessment of parents' and patients' concerns and preferences regarding scoliosis surgery, both groups ranked neurologic deficit as their greatest concern following surgery.[41] However, the rate of neurological complications is low, and permanent neurological complications are even more rare.[42] Recent research from the Scoliosis Research Society reported a 5.7% complications rate for AIS surgery, with the overall rate of neurological deficit ranging from 0.26% to 1.75% depending on surgical approach.[43]

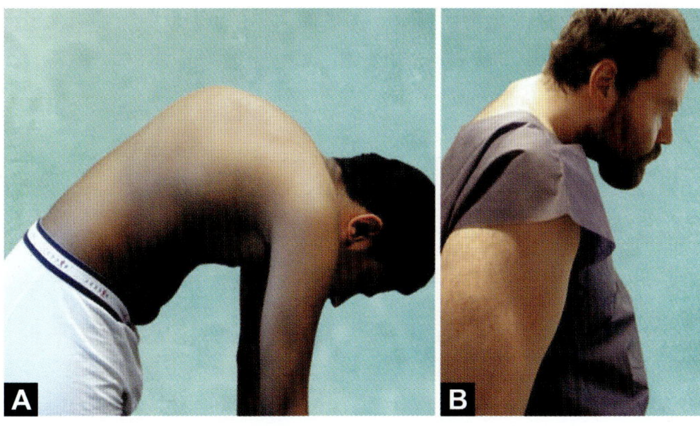

Figs.52.15A and B: Scheuermann's kyphosis.

Risks of neurological complications include severe curvature (over 80°) and the nature of the operative procedure. For example, a three-column resection or vertebral column resection for severe deformity carries elevated risk.

Sagittal alignment of the cervical spine depends on the thoracic spine. Thoracic hypokyphosis for example, which is typically present in patients with AIS and may persist if inadequately corrected at the time of surgery, is positively correlated with kyphosis in the cervical spine, which may result in premature disk degeneration.[44,45] Analogously, a lack of restoration of kyphosis results in a decrease in lumbar lordosis and may predispose the patient to disk degeneration and flatback.[46]

As the lower extremities attach to the spine through the pelvis, pelvic imbalance and compensatory tilt are often the result of over- or undercorrection of sagittal alignment (kyphosis and lordosis). Sagittal imbalance can lead to higher energy expenditure during ambulation or difficulty with tasks requiring bending down to the floor. Recently, impairment in HRQOL from sagittal deformity has been associated with static sagittal balance and pelvic alignment.[34,47]

KYPHOSIS

Background

With an incidence of 0.4–10%, the most common form of surgical hyperkyphosis is from Scheuermann's disease (Figs. 52.15A and B). First described in 1921, Scheuermann's kyphosis (SK) involves fixed thoracic kyphosis, wedged vertebrae, and endplate irregularities. In 1964 Sorensen described a kyphotic deformity characterized by three adjacent wedged vertebrae of five or more degrees; kyphotic deformities not meeting these criteria are termed structural idiopathic kyphosis. The deformity presents with a midthoracic, low thoracic, or thoracolumbar apex. Spondylolysis can be present in 10–12% of SK cases, and mild scoliosis is common.

Clinical Evaluation

Clinical evaluation of kyphosis should include a standard history and physical examination. Self-image and self-esteem from significant deformity are often an issue, though pain is variable. PFT should be ordered for any curve >90° because restrictive lung disease may be present.[48]

Standard radiographic analysis is imperative and should focus on obtaining adequate sagittal images. Close inspection may reveal anterior wedging (>5°) of three adjacent thoracic vertebrae. Wedging, in addition to irregularities in the vertebral endplates (called Schmorl's nodes), is typical of structural SK, which is different from a flexible postural kyphosis.

Health-related quality of life has also been observed to be negatively impacted in the SK population. SK patients have been shown to display worse HRQOL scores than AIS patients, and increasing kyphosis magnitude is negatively correlated with HRQOL scores, especially for self-image.[49]

Treatment

Scheuermann's disease can be treated nonoperatively with physical therapy, exercise, and bracing for curves from 55° to 70° in skeletally immature patients (Risser 0–3). The Milwaukee brace was the gold standard, but is no longer used due to its unacceptable appearance and psychosocial implications for the patient; lower profile braces are now favored. Operative treatment is reserved for SK with curvature of >70° in the thoracic spine (lower curve magnitudes in the thoracolumbar spine), refractory pain, or for issues of self-image and self-esteem related to spinal deformity that can have a significant impact on peer interactions and psychosocial development for the patient. Posterior fusion and instrumentation with pedicle screw-rod constructs are performed (Figs. 52.16 and 52.17). Anterior release in conjunction with posterior instrumented fusion was commonly performed for rigid kyphosis in the past, but anterior discectomy either via VATS or thoracotomy is now largely reserved for only significant disk herniations that would potentially compromise the spinal cord with corrective maneuvers performed posteriorly. The combined anterior and posterior approach is associated with more complications.[50] The pedicle subtraction osteotomy (Figs. 52.18A to F) is a powerful tool for correction of severe kyphotic deformity. Still, in an even more select group of patients, vertebral column resection may be performed (Figs. 52.19A to C).

The complication rate for operative treatment of SK has been detailed by the Scoliosis Research Society and is higher than that for AIS surgery: 14% of patients experienced a complication and 1.9% experienced an acute neurological complication. Of the 1.9% of patients with an acute neurological complication, 0.6% had a spinal cord injury.[51]

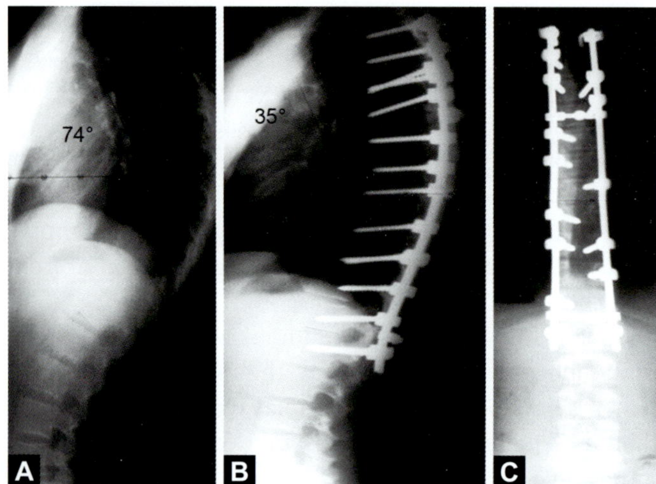

Figs. 52.16A to C: Posterior surgery for Scheuermann's kyphosis correction.

SPONDYLOLISTHESIS

Background

First described in 1782 by a Belgian obstetrician, Dr Herbinaux, isthmic spondylolisthesis, or anterior translation of the cephalad vertebra, is commonly diagnosed in young adolescent patients, while degenerative forms of spondylolisthesis are diagnosed with advanced age (Figs. 52.20A and B). Certain forms of spondylolisthesis can result from repetitive microfracture and stresses with elongation at the isthmus of the pars interarticularis. Lytic and acute forms of the disease are also possible. Spondylolisthesis has a hereditary component as well, as evidenced by the increased incidence in people of Inuit descent. High prevalence is noted in female gymnasts and football lineman due to the extreme hyperextension required for those activities, but the disease can affect any population.

Clinical Evaluation

The Wiltse-Newman classification of spondylolisthesis is based on the origin of the slippage (Fig. 52.21). Congenital

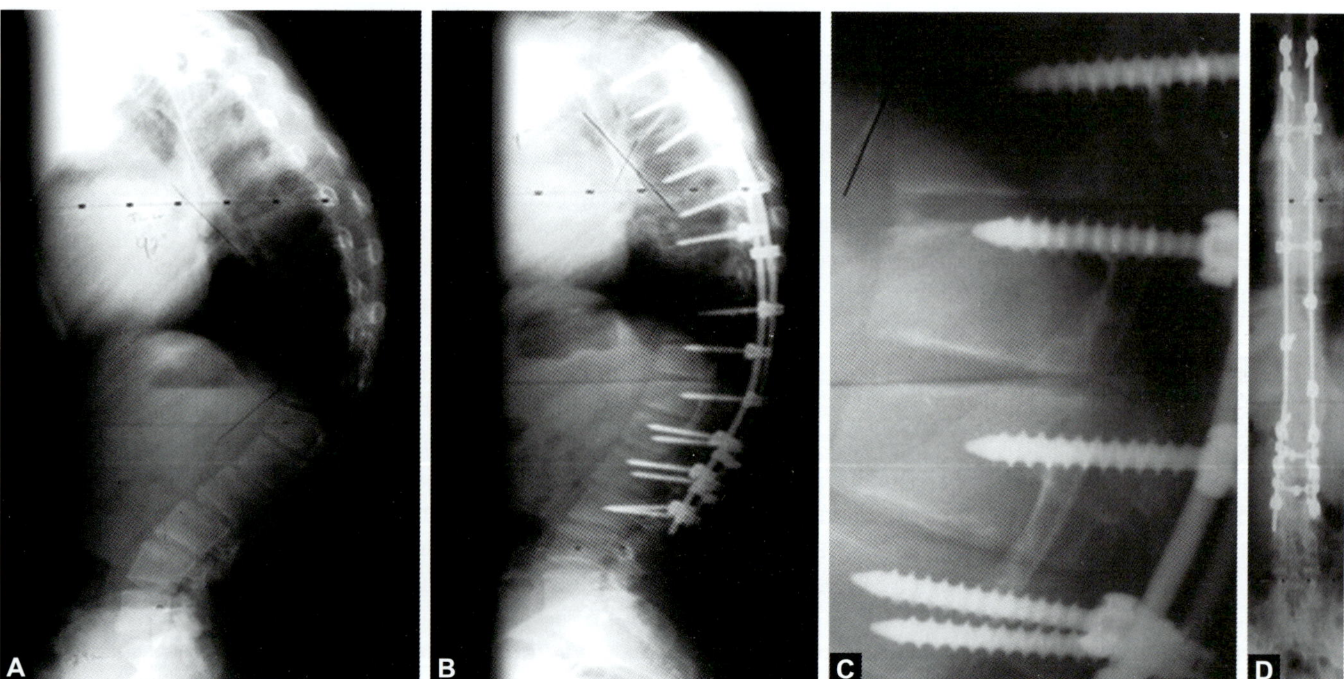

Figs. 52.17A to D: Mid-thoracic deformity correction.

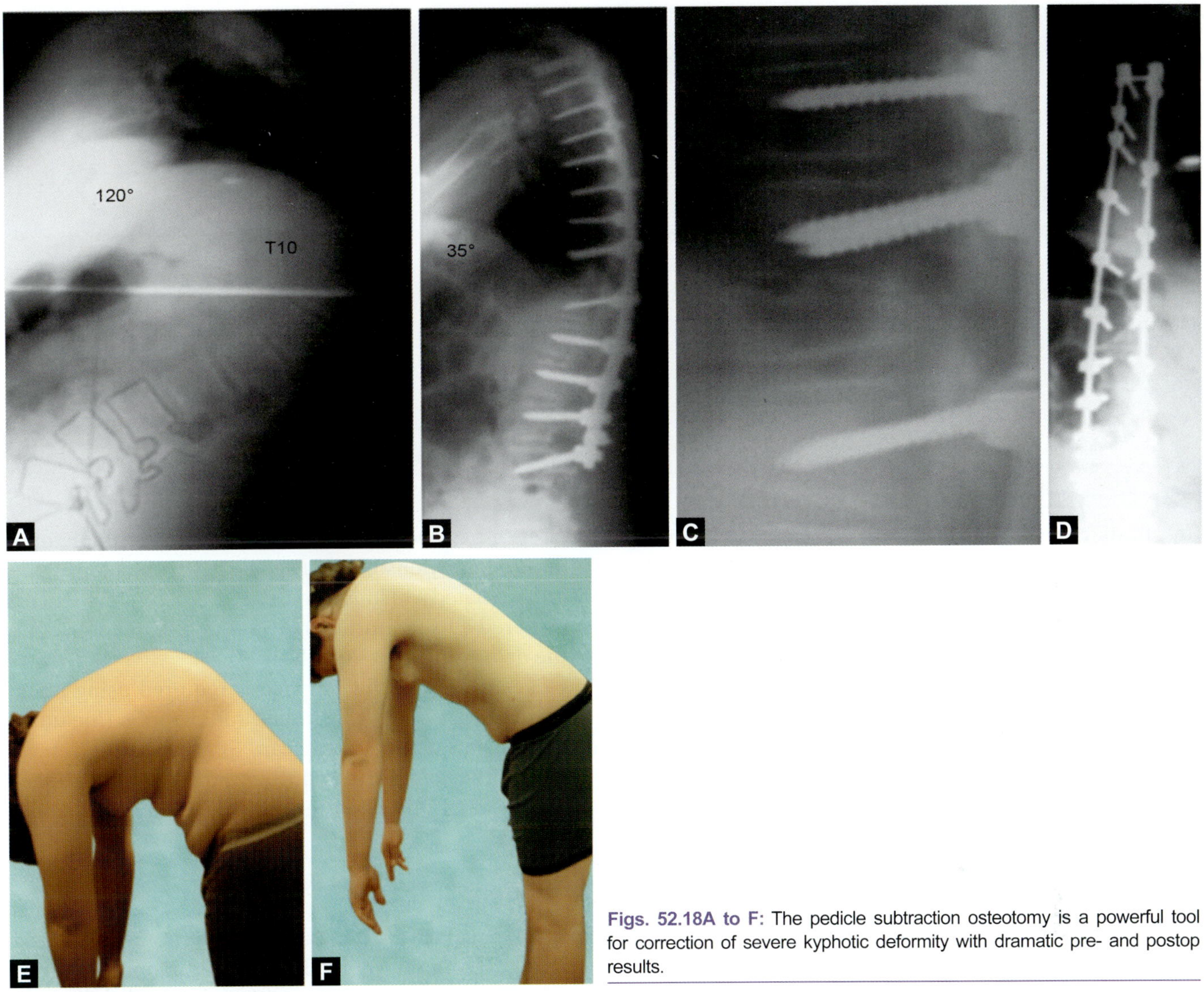

120°
T10
35°
A B C D E F

Figs. 52.18A to F: The pedicle subtraction osteotomy is a powerful tool for correction of severe kyphotic deformity with dramatic pre- and postop results.

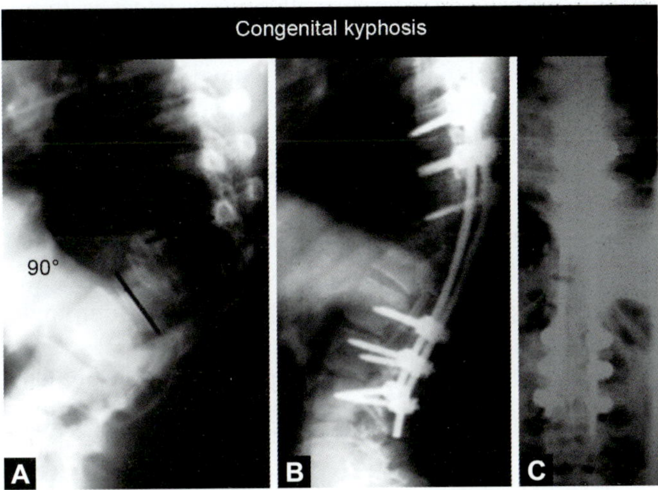

Figs. 52.19A to C: Congenital kyphosis treated with surgical reduction with a pedicle subtraction osteotomy along with posterior fusion and instrumentation.

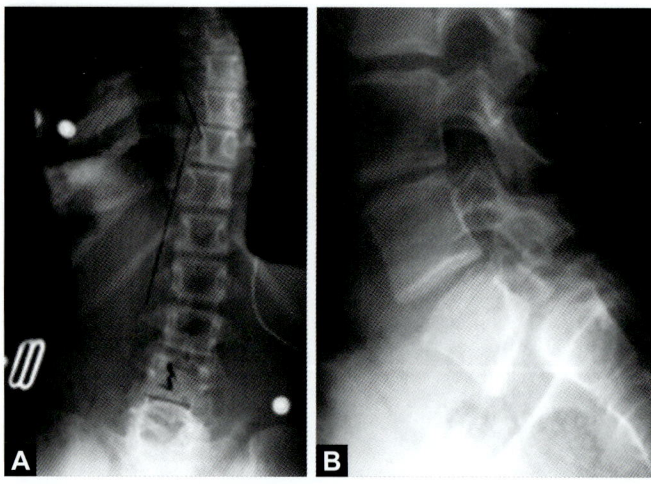

Figs. 52.20A and B: "Olisthesis" is the Greek term for slippage. In the lateral view, the L5 vertebra is translated anteriorly over S1 in this high-grade spondylolisthesis.

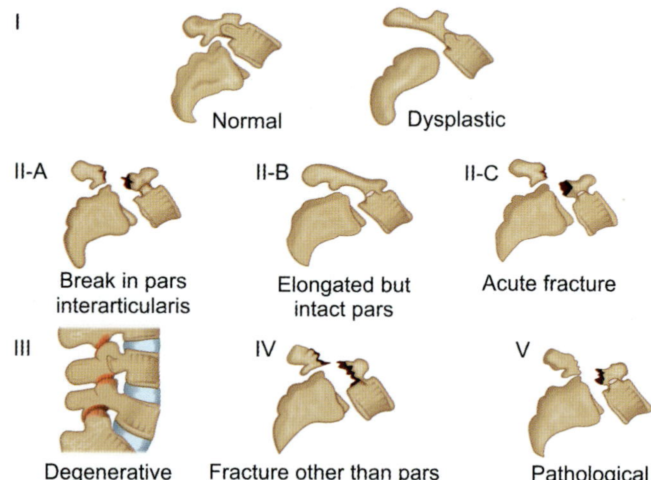

Fig. 52.21: Wiltse-Newman classification of spondylolisthesis.

(dysplastic) spondylolisthesis occurs early and is often severe, affecting females twice as often as males and is associated with spina bifida occulta. Isthmic spondylolisthesis, the most common form of spondylolisthesis (5–7% of occurrences), consists of a defect of the pars interarticularis, which is more common in females, especially in the high-grade form. Isthmic spondylolisthesis is also commonly associated with spina bifida occulta. In a typical case of isthmic spondylolisthesis, the cephalad vertebral body (usually L5) translates anteriorly, which is made more problematic by lumbosacral kyphosis occurring in the presence of a high-grade slip as opposed to the normal lordosis. Patients can present with generalized axial back pain and may complain of sciatica as the slip progresses and closes the space for the exiting nerve roots. Stiffening of the back and tightness of the hamstrings are common, with a resulting "waddle" during gait and limited forward flexion and straight leg raise (SLR). Symptoms of isthmic spondylolisthesis typically appear during the adolescent growth spurt, but most patients remain asymptomatic.

The Meyerding classification for spondylolisthesis measures the degree of translation by percentage of anterior translation over the caudad endplate surface. High-grade slips, grades 3–5, often present with neurologic deficits and cauda equina syndrome, which may be subtle with new-onset bed-wetting at night, e.g. necessitating a high degree of clinical suspicion. Local kyphosis progression can be quantified by the "slip angle", subtended by the lines across the cephalad aspect of L5 and perpendicular to a line drawn along the posterior border of the sacrum. An important determinant of sagittal alignment, pelvic incidence has been considered as a possible predictor of isthmic spondylolisthesis. Higher pelvic incidence has been associated with this disease, and as pelvic incidence is considered a fixed morphologic parameter, it contributes to the deforming forces involved.

Visualization of the slippage is required using imaging techniques such as standing radiographs (including coned-down lateral), bone scan, SPECT scan, CT scan, and MRI. The defect of the pars interarticularis can be seen on X-rays as a break in the so-called Scottie dog's neck (Fig. 52.22).

Treatment

Scoliosis occurs in 5–7% of patients with spondylolisthesis, with 30% of those spondylolisthesis patients requiring surgery. Nonoperative treatments or observation can be employed in young patients who are asymptomatic or who have low-grade slips. If a pars defect is found before the age of 10, regular X-rays every 6 months until growth is completed are recommended. If the slippage is <25% in an asymptomatic child, no activity restrictions are recommended; however, if the slippage is 25–50%, X-rays should be taken every 6 months and heavy labor and contact sports should be avoided. In symptomatic patients with <50% slippage, nonoperative treatment such as activity modification, NSAIDs, flexibility and strengthening exercises for the legs and abdominals, and immobilization by brace can be effective. However, in patients with a >50% slip and a spinal deformity with progression, surgery should be considered.

Surgical treatment can often provide relief of spondylolisthesis symptoms (Figs. 52.23A to G). Indications for

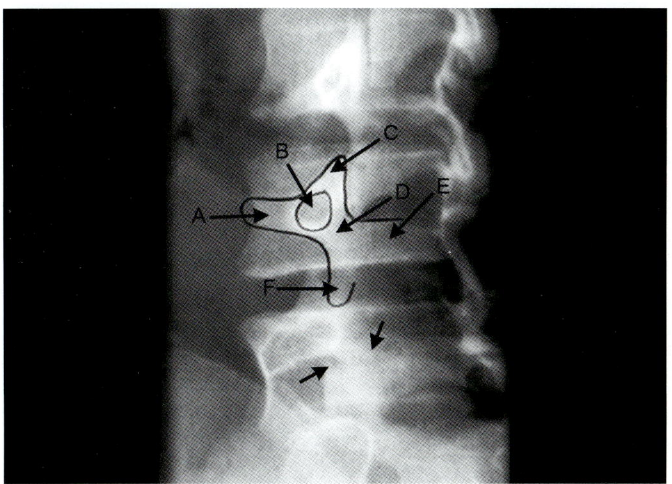

Fig. 52.22: The "Scottie dog's neck" is a representation of posterior elements of the vertebrae from an oblique radiograph. (A) "snout" representing the transverse process; (B) "eye" representing the pedicle; (C) "ear" representing superior facet; (D) "neck" representing the pars interarticularis/isthmus; (E) "body" representing lamina; (F) "foot" representing the inferior facet. Arrows below show disruption of the normal contour of the "neck" and thus injury to the pars.

surgery include persistence of major symptoms for >6 months despite nonoperative treatment methods, tight hamstrings, abnormal gait, postural deformities, or a neurological deficit. A lytic defect can be repaired or the segment can be fused in situ with a posterolateral fusion. Instrumentation improves the success rate of the actual fusion taking place and provides immediate stability. The decision of whether to reduce the deformity for high-grade slips or in the context of dysplasia should rely on careful consideration of slip angle (>35°), positive (forward) sagittal imbalance, clinical deformity, and deformity in the coronal plane (olisthetic scoliosis). There is an elevated risk of foot drop, usually transiently, following a reduction procedure.

CONCLUSION

Pediatric spinal deformity is composed of a number of conditions, most commonly AIS. Careful evaluation of

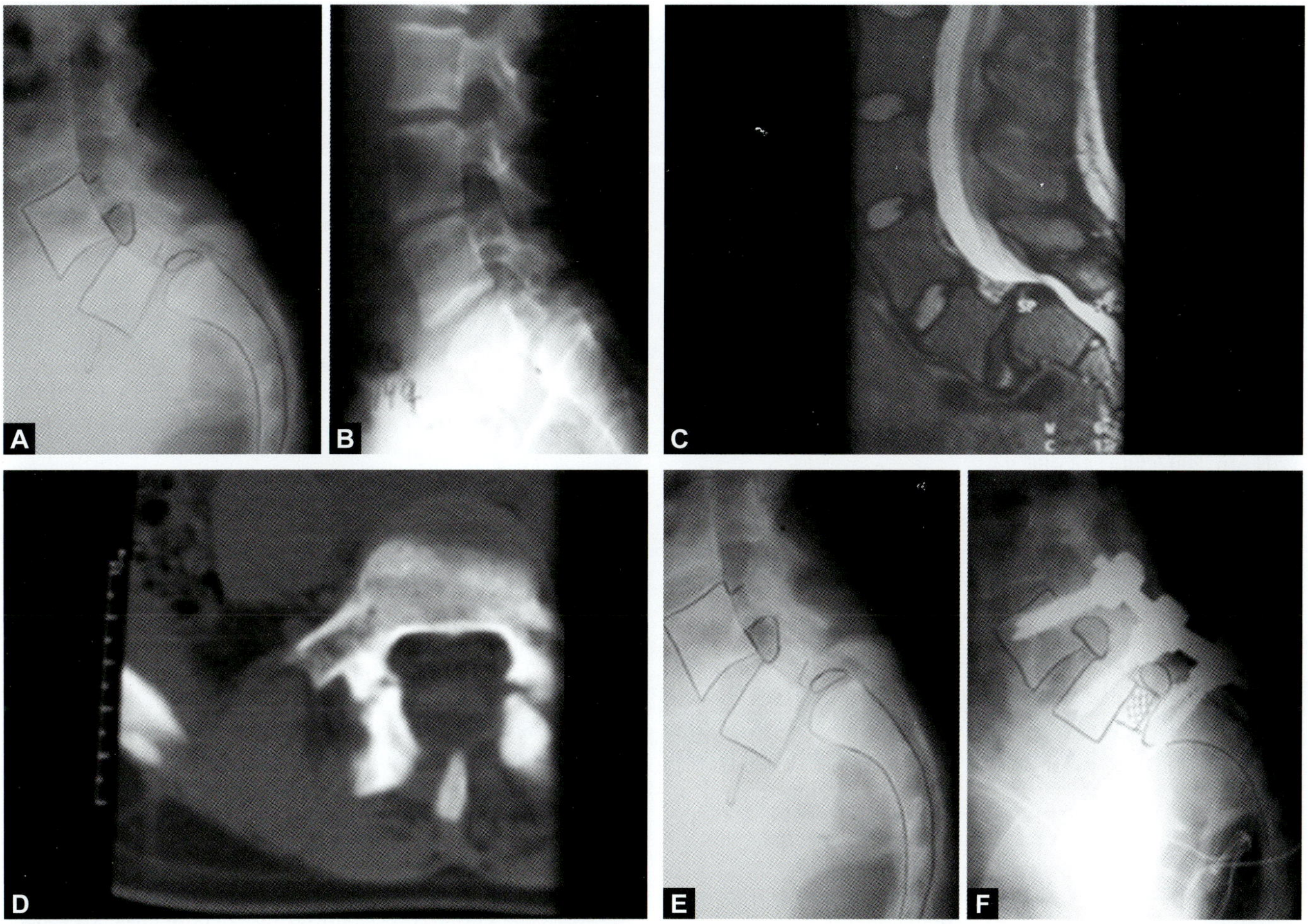

Figs. 52.23A to F

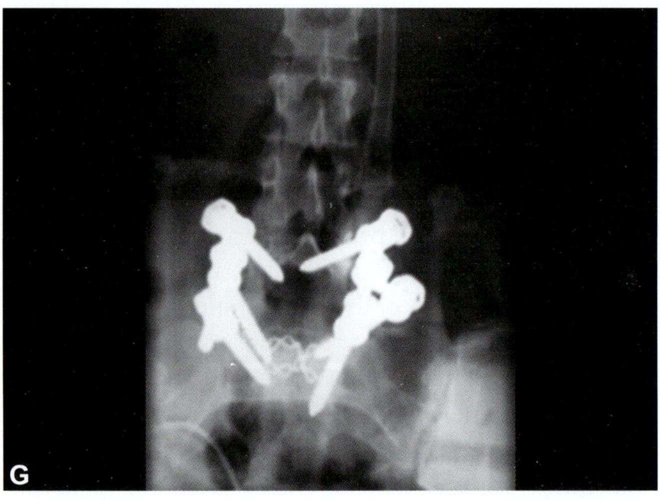

Figs. 52.23A to G: Spondylolisthesis treated with surgical reduction in the deformity and fusion with instrumentation of L4-S1 and intervertebral cage placement to augment fusion.

the patient, consideration of the individual's psychosocial disposition, and adherence to treatment approaches with the best evidence result in reliable outcomes for this diverse group.

REFERENCES

1. Peelle MW, Luhmann SJ. Management of adolescent idiopathic scoliosis. Neurosurg Clin N Am. 2007;18(4):575-83.
2. Donaldson S, Stephens D, Howard A, et al. Surgical decision making in adolescent idiopathic scoliosis. Spine. 2007;32(14):1526-32.
3. Stokes IA, Bigalow LC, Moreland MS. Three-dimensional spinal curvature in idiopathic scoliosis. J Orthop Res. 1987; 5(1):102-13.
4. Basu PS, Elsebaie H, Noordeen MH. Congenital spinal deformity: a comprehensive assessment at presentation. Spine. 2002;27(20):2255-9.
5. Sarwark J, Sarwahi V. New strategies and decision making in the management of neuromuscular scoliosis. Orthop Clin N Am. 2007;38(4):485-96, v.
6. Dickson RA. The etiology and pathogenesis of idiopathic scoliosis. Acta Orthopaedica Belgica. 1992;58 Suppl 1:21-5.
7. Huang SC. Cut-off point of the Scoliometer in school scoliosis screening. Spine. 1997;22(17):1985-9.
8. Newton PO, Faro FD, Gollogly S, et al. Results of preoperative pulmonary function testing of adolescents with idiopathic scoliosis. A study of six hundred and thirty-one patients. J Bone Joint Surg. American volume. 2005;87(9):1937-46.
9. Lonstein JE, Carlson JM. The prediction of curve progression in untreated idiopathic scoliosis during growth. J Bone Joint Surg. American volume. 1984;66(7):1061-71.
10. McMaster MJ. Occult intraspinal anomalies and congenital scoliosis. J Bone Joint Surg. American volume 1984;66(4): 588-601.
11. Bone CM, Hsieh GH. The risk of carcinogenesis from radiographs to pediatric orthopaedic patients. J Pediatr Orthop. 2000;20(2):251-4.
12. Nash CL, Jr., Gregg EC, Brown RH, et al. Risks of exposure to X-rays in patients undergoing long-term treatment for scoliosis. J Bone Joint Surg. American volume 1979;61(3): 371-4.
13. Gray JE, Hoffman AD, Peterson HA. Reduction of radiation exposure during radiography for scoliosis. J Bone Joint Surg. American volume 1983;65(1):5-12.
14. Goldberg MS, Mayo NE, Levy AR, et al. Adverse reproductive outcomes among women exposed to low levels of ionizing radiation from diagnostic radiography for adolescent idiopathic scoliosis. Epidemiology (Cambridge, Mass). 1998;9 (3):271-8.
15. Deschenes S, Charron G, Beaudoin G, et al. Diagnostic imaging of spinal deformities: reducing patients radiation dose with a new slot-scanning X-ray imager. Spine. 2010;35(9):989-94.
16. Wick JM, Konze J, Alexander K, et al. Infantile and juvenile scoliosis: the crooked path to diagnosis and treatment. AORN Journal. 2009;90(3):347-76.
17. King HA, Moe JH, Bradford DS, et al. The selection of fusion levels in thoracic idiopathic scoliosis. J Bone Joint Surg. American volume 1983;65(9):1302-13.
18. Lenke LG, Betz RR, Harms J, et al. Adolescent idiopathic scoliosis: a new classification to determine extent of spinal arthrodesis. J Bone Joint Surg. American volume 2001; 83-a(8):1169-81.
19. Sponseller PD. Bracing for adolescent idiopathic scoliosis in practice today. J Pediatr Orthop. 2011;31(1 Suppl):S53-60.
20. Nachemson AL, Peterson LE. Effectiveness of treatment with a brace in girls who have adolescent idiopathic scoliosis. A prospective, controlled study based on data from the Brace Study of the Scoliosis Research Society. J Bone Joint Surg. American volume 1995;77(6):815-22.
21. Duval-Beaupere G. [Maturation indices in the surveillance of scoliosis]. Revue de chirurgie orthopedique et reparatrice de l'appareil moteur 1970;56(1):59-76.
22. Nault ML, Parent S, Phan P, et al. A modified Risser grading system predicts the curve acceleration phase of female adolescent idiopathic scoliosis. J Bone Joint Surg. American volume 2010;92(5):1073-81.

23. Bridwell KH. Surgical treatment of idiopathic adolescent scoliosis. Spine. 1999;24(24):2607-16.
24. Majdouline Y, Aubin CE, Robitaille M, et al. Scoliosis correction objectives in adolescent idiopathic scoliosis. J Pediatr Orthop. 2007;27(7):775-81.
25. Pehrsson K, Danielsson A, Nachemson A. Pulmonary function in adolescent idiopathic scoliosis: a 25 year follow up after surgery or start of brace treatment. Thorax. 2001;56(5):388-93.
26. Auerbach JD, Lonner BS, Errico TJ, et al. Quantification of intradiscal pressures below thoracolumbar spinal fusion constructs: is there evidence to support "saving a level"? Spine. 2012;37(5):359-66.
27. Marks M, Newton PO, Petcharaporn M, et al. Postoperative segmental motion of the unfused spine distal to the fusion in 100 patients with adolescent idiopathic scoliosis. Spine. 2012;37(10):826-32.
28. Verma K, Auerbach JD, Kean KE, et al. Anterior spinal fusion for thoracolumbar scoliosis: comprehensive assessment of radiographic, clinical, and pulmonary outcomes on 2-years follow-up. J Pediatr Orthop. 2010;30(7):664-9.
29. Lonner BS, Auerbach JD, Estreicher M, et al. Video-assisted anterior thoracoscopic spinal fusion versus posterior spinal fusion: a comparative study utilizing the SRS-22 outcome instrument. Spine. 2009;34(2):193-8.
30. Lonner BS, Kondrachov D, Siddiqi F, et al. Thoracoscopic spinal fusion compared with posterior spinal fusion for the treatment of thoracic adolescent idiopathic scoliosis. Surgical technique. J Bone Joint Surg. American volume 2007;89 Suppl 2 Pt.1:142-56.
31. Lonner BS, Auerbach JD, Levin R, et al. Thoracoscopic anterior instrumented fusion for adolescent idiopathic scoliosis with emphasis on the sagittal plane. Spine J. 2009;9(7):523-9.
32. Newton PO, Upasani VV, Farnsworth CL, et al. Spinal growth modulation with use of a tether in an immature porcine model. J Bone Joint Surg. American volume 2008;90(12):2695-706.
33. Betz RR, Kim J, D'Andrea LP, et al. An innovative technique of vertebral body stapling for the treatment of patients with adolescent idiopathic scoliosis: a feasibility, safety, and utility study. Spine. 2003;28(20):S255-65.
34. Takayama K, Nakamura H, Matsuda H. Quality of life in patients treated surgically for scoliosis: longer than sixteen-year follow-up. Spine. 2009;34(20):2179-84.
35. Helgeson MD, Shah SA, Newton PO, et al. Evaluation of proximal junctional kyphosis in adolescent idiopathic scoliosis following pedicle screw, hook, or hybrid instrumentation. Spine. 2010;35(2):177-81.
36. Luhmann SJ, Lenke LG, Bridwell KH, Schootman M. Revision surgery after primary spine fusion for idiopathic scoliosis. Spine. 2009;34(20):2191-7.
37. Lenke LG, Engsberg JR, Ross SA, et al. Prospective dynamic functional evaluation of gait and spinal balance following spinal fusion in adolescent idiopathic scoliosis. Spine. 2001;26(14):E330-7.
38. Engsberg JR, Lenke LG, Uhrich ML, et al. Prospective comparison of gait and trunk range of motion in adolescents with idiopathic thoracic scoliosis undergoing anterior or posterior spinal fusion. Spine. 2003;28(17):1993-2000.
39. Engsberg JR, Lenke LG, Reitenbach AK, et al. Prospective evaluation of trunk range of motion in adolescents with idiopathic scoliosis undergoing spinal fusion surgery. Spine. 2002;27(12):1346-54.
40. Mahaudens P, Banse X, Mousny M, et al. Gait in adolescent idiopathic scoliosis: kinematics and electromyographic analysis. Eur Spine J. 2009;18(4):512-21.
41. Bridwell KH, Shufflebarger HL, Lenke LG, et al. Parents' and patients' preferences and concerns in idiopathic adolescent scoliosis: a cross-sectional preoperative analysis. Spine. 2000;25(18):2392-9.
42. Diab M, Smith AR, Kuklo TR. Neural complications in the surgical treatment of adolescent idiopathic scoliosis. Spine. 2007;32(24):2759-63.
43. Coe JD, Arlet V, Donaldson W, et al. Complications in spinal fusion for adolescent idiopathic scoliosis in the new millennium. A report of the Scoliosis Research Society Morbidity and Mortality Committee. Spine. 2006;31(3): 345-9.
44. Hilibrand AS, Tannenbaum DA, Graziano GP, et al. The sagittal alignment of the cervical spine in adolescent idiopathic scoliosis. J Pediatr Orthop. 1995;15(5):627-32.
45. Hwang SW, Samdani AF, Tantorski M, et al. Cervical sagittal plane decompensation after surgery for adolescent idiopathic scoliosis: an effect imparted by postoperative thoracic hypokyphosis. J Neurosurg Spine. 2011;15(5): 491-6.
46. Newton PO, Yaszay B, Upasani VV, et al. Preservation of thoracic kyphosis is critical to maintain lumbar lordosis in the surgical treatment of adolescent idiopathic scoliosis. Spine. 2010;35(14):1365-70.
47. Lafage V, Schwab F, Vira S, et al. Spino-pelvic parameters after surgery can be predicted: a preliminary formula and validation of standing alignment. Spine. 2011;36(13):1037-45.
48. Murray PM, Weinstein SL, Spratt KF. The natural history and long-term follow-up of Scheuermann kyphosis. J Bone Joint Surg. American volume 1993;75(2):236-48.
49. Lonner B, Yoo A, Terran JS, et al. Effect of spinal deformity on adolescent quality of life comparison of operative Scheuermann's kyphosis, adolescent idiopathic scoliosis and normal controls. Spine (Phila Pa 1976). 2013.
50. Lonner BS, Newton P, Betz R, et al. Operative management of Scheuermann's kyphosis in 78 patients: radiographic outcomes, complications, and technique. Spine. 2007;32(24):2644-52.
51. Coe JD, Smith JS, Berven S, et al. Complications of spinal fusion for Scheuermann kyphosis: a report of the scoliosis research society morbidity and mortality committee. Spine. 2010;35(1):99-103.

CHAPTER

53

Surgical Treatment of Adult Degenerative Deformity

Jeffrey B Knox, Justin Paul, Frank Schwab

INTRODUCTION

Adult degenerative spinal deformity represents a complex and challenging condition for the spine specialist. While the majority of deformity patients will not require surgical intervention, surgery has been shown to be superior to nonsurgical interventions in well-selected patients suffering from marked disability.[1-3] When considering a patient for surgical treatment of degenerative scoliosis, numerous factors must be considered in the decision to proceed with surgery, as well as planning the appropriate procedure to minimize complications and maximize patient benefit.

SURGICAL INDICATIONS

In contrast to pediatric deformity patients, back pain and functional disability are common complaints in adults with degenerative scoliosis. However, isolated back pain without neurologic compression or progressive deformity is rarely an indication for surgery, as such pain will often respond to conservative measures. It is important to but often challenging to isolate the source of pain in patients without neurologic compression or deformity—a task that is complicated by the potential interactions of disk degeneration, facet arthropathy, mechanical instability/subluxations, muscular fatigue, and myofascial pain, all of which often occur in patients with degenerative scoliosis. Intermittent mechanical pain that occurs during periods of activity and resolves with recumbency is often a result of segmental instability; such pain often carries a better potential for resolution with surgical stabilization.

It is important to realize that patients with notable spinal deformity, particularly in the sagittal plane, are burdened with significant disability, which arises from a variety of causes. Patients with sagittal imbalance compensate by retroversion of the pelvis and often knee flexion in order to maintain an upright posture. Because pelvic retroversion and knee flexion are energy inefficient, these compensatory measures often result in increased daily energy expenditure that may manifest clinically as thigh, buttock, hip, or knee pain, and fatigue. These compensatory mechanisms play a significant role in the development of disability associated with spinal deformity and should not be overlooked in the clinical evaluation of the deformity patient.

Neurologic dysfunction represents another common symptom and reason for surgical intervention in patients with degenerative scoliosis. Neurogenic claudication from central stenosis is a common complaint that is often due to a combination of facet hypertrophy and ligamentum overgrowth, with potential contribution from the deformity itself. Radiculopathy is also common and often results from foraminal compression within the concavity of the curve, but can also be a result of tension on the nerve root occurring on the convex side of the curve.

While curve magnitude and progression are important considerations, the decision to undergo surgical intervention should be based primarily on the patient's symptoms and functional status. Patients with large deformity but minimal symptoms have limited ability to benefit from surgical treatment. Deformity in the sagittal plane is the primary driver of symptoms and should be the focus of any discussion of surgical treatment for degenerative scoliosis.

PRESURGICAL CONSIDERATIONS

Degenerative scoliosis primarily affects patients with advanced age who often have multiple medical comorbidities and are at risk of complications after extensive surgical procedures. A comprehensive preoperative medical evaluation and coordination with the appropriate medical specialists and anesthesiologists is necessary to identify relevant comorbidities and to allow for medical optimization prior to any surgical intervention. Many medical complications are directly related to surgeon-controlled factors such as surgical time, blood loss, and the need for combined approaches. An experienced surgical team with a comprehensive surgical plan can minimize operative time and blood loss to lessen the potential for postoperative medical complications.

A patient's psychosocial factors such as expectations for treatment, social support following surgery, and psychiatric comorbidities are also important to consider prior to surgical intervention for spinal deformity, as they play a key role in patient satisfaction and surgical outcome.

Another important presurgical consideration is the patient's bone mineral density. As degenerative scoliosis disproportionately affects elderly females, osteoporosis is a common problem. Osteoporosis may itself contribute to pain due to progressive wedging and deformity of weak vertebral bodies, and treating osteoporosis may help slow this progression of deformity. Osteoporosis results in compromised screw purchase and can contribute to complications such as proximal junctional fracture or implant pullout with subsequent loss of correction.[4,5] Bone mineral density for at-risk patients and initiation of treatment prior to surgical intervention should be considered. The medication teriparatide is often useful in treating low bone mineral density. Teriparatide functions via an anabolic mechanism directly increasing bone formation and has been efficacious in improving spine bone mineral density, as well as pedicle screw fixation after lumbar fusions.[6,7]

SURGICAL PLANNING

Increasingly, the importance of presurgical planning is being emphasized in treatment of adult spinal deformity. The use of digital templating software enables the surgeon to simulate and visualize the results of differing types and locations of osteotomies, including the effects on overall sagittal and coronal alignment. Digital templating also allows for a more effective surgical strategy that can be tailored to the patient's specific anatomy to obtain more precise surgical results.[8] Additionally, with the use of a presurgical plan, the surgeon can be prepared for the necessary procedures with the appropriate equipment and blood management strategies.

Achieving satisfactory surgical results is based on several key goals of treatment. The first goal of surgery is to correct the deformity, particularly in the sagittal plane, which is the primary driver of symptoms in these patients. Once adequate reduction is obtained, the correction must be maintained with rigid fixation until a solid fusion can be obtained. Finally, selective decompression addresses any neurologic compression that often coexists with degenerative adult deformity.

Obtaining the appropriate degree of correction is critical for achieving favorable clinical outcomes.[8,9] While global sagittal alignment is a crucial component of the planning process, consideration of pelvic parameters is also of key importance to guiding the degree of correction. In particular, matching pelvic incidence to lumbar lordosis is an important consideration. Lumbar lordosis should be within 10° of pelvic incidence as failure to correct alignment within this range is associated with substandard postoperative outcomes despite the restoration of global sagittal alignment.[8]

SURGICAL TECHNIQUES

Decompression Alone

While the mainstay of treatment for degenerative scoliosis is spinal fusion with correction of deformity and selective decompression, performing isolated decompression without addressing the underlying deformity may be a viable alternative in selected patients. Isolated decompression is attractive option as it may avoid the inherent complications associated with spinal deformity correction and long-segment fusion; patients who receive isolated decompressions experience less blood loss, shorter hospital stays, and lower complication rates. But, isolated decompressions are associated with worse clinical outcomes compared with concomitant spinal fusion and deformity correction. Decompressing the spine without fusion can result in iatrogenic destabilization with progressive deformity, significant pain, and even recurrent stenosis. The use of isolated decompression strategy, therefore, should be limited to well-selected patients.[10]

Patients who are ideal candidates for isolated decompression are those with a primary complaint of radicular pain, numbness, or paresthesia with minimal axial back pain; an additional consideration is the underlying deformity. Patients with smaller deformities without significant sagittal imbalance are more likely to benefit without correction of the deformity. Also, stable deformities, which have not progressed over serial images, are less likely to be unstable and progressive after isolated decompression. The location of the decompression is important, as performing decompressions within the apex of the deformity carries a high risk of destabilizing the curve with deformity progression and should be avoided.

Osteotomies

Degenerative scoliosis is frequently associated with relatively rigid kyphosis and positive sagittal imbalance, thus treatment of this condition often necessitates osteotomies to adequately realign the spine. Careful planning of the appropriate type and location of an osteotomy allows for accurate deformity correction and minimization of the potential complications associated with the procedure.

The most basic type of osteotomy used to realign the sagittal plane is the Smith-Petersen osteotomy (SPO) or Ponte osteotomy (PO), both of which involve a chevron wedge resection of the posterior elements.[11,12] While these osteotomies are similar, the SPO was described in the setting of an autofused spine in ankylosing spondylitis while Ponte discussed correcting Scheuermann's kyphosis by performing multiple consecutive posterior osteotomies. As such, POs are the more accurate term for the osteotomy performed in the setting of adult degenerative deformity. As only the posterior elements are resected, the PO relies on a mobile anterior spine for correction and results in lengthening of the anterior column; this may result in undesired consequences such as gap formation in the anterior column with potential inhibition of arthrodesis, as well as potential for vascular or neurologic injury.[13-16] While a single PO provides only about 10° per segment, performing these osteotomies at multiple consecutive levels allows the surgeon to obtain gradual harmonious correction across a longer segment of the spine.[17] Utilization of multiple POs is safer than more extensive resections, with less blood loss and fewer complications than a single pedicle subtraction osteotomy.[17] Caution should be exercised when performing POs at levels with coronal deformity with significant rotation, as this can predispose toward a coronal shift into the concavity of the deformity with subsequent coronal plane decompensation.[17-19]

Another surgical option that is commonly used in treating degenerative scoliosis is the pedicle subtraction osteotomy. Pedicle subtractions involve a V-shaped osteotomy that extends through the vertebral body, resecting both pedicles and the posterior elements. Pedicle subtraction osteotomy hinges on the anterior cortex of the vertebral body and therefore does not lengthen the anterior column. The use of a pedicle subtraction osteotomy is a powerful tool to correct sagittal deformity, obtaining corrections of up to 30°–40° at a single level. While very effective, pedicle subtraction osteotomies have a relatively high complication rate.[17] The degree of bony resection combined with disruption of epidural veins results in potential for significant blood loss. The degree of resection and subsequent destabilization is associated with risk of pseudarthrosis. Additionally, retraction of the neural elements can result in early neurologic deficits, which are typically transient.

Extent of Fusion

Selecting which levels to fuse is an important consideration in obtaining the proper correction and minimizing potential complications. While maintaining motion at the maximum number of segments is desirable, such benefits must be carefully balanced against the risk of preserving potentially painful motion at segments, as well as the risk of future breakdown at these segments. Such adjacent disk degeneration can result in persistent pain and disability, as well as loss of sagittal balance and need for subsequent revision surgery.[20] In particular, motion segments between long, rigid segments are at particular risk of subsequent breakdown and should be avoided.

One example where the risk of subsequent breakdown is evident is in fusions that do not cross the thoracolumbar junction; while maintaining motion at this segment may appear desirable to preserve motion and avoid the difficulty of achieving fusion across this mobile area, this strategy is associated with significantly inferior outcomes. Numerous studies have demonstrated that long fusions including the L1 or L2 vertebra as the upper-instrumented vertebra (UIV) lead to a high rate of failure with poor clinical outcomes. Kim et al. demonstrated a rate of proximal adjacent segment failure of 50% in patients with a UIV between T11 and L2 versus 14% with a UIV of T9 or T10.[21] Similarly, Swank et al. reported only 10% good or excellent results among patients with fusions stopping distal to the thoracolumbar junction, with 18% of these patients requiring subsequent extension of their fusion across the thoracolumbar junction.[22]

While bridging the thoracolumbar junction is a desirable strategy, extension of fusion more proximally may be required in certain circumstances. Proximal extensions are associated, however, with increased complications. O'Shaughnessy et al. evaluated the outcomes of patients with fusions to the sacrum extending from either T3 or T10.[23] Patients in the study with a UIV of T3 experienced significantly higher complication rates (30% vs 15.8%), in particular a higher rate of pseudarthrosis (20% vs 5.3%) and required revision more frequently. Utilization of T10 as the UIV was associated with a higher rate of proximal junctional kyphosis (PJK) (18.4% vs 10%); however, such patients rarely required revision for this complication.

The status of adjacent disks and vertebrae should be considered when selecting the proper UIV. This includes the presence of degenerative disks, compression fractures, or areas of focal or regional kyphosis. Fusions ended adjacent to such areas have high rates of subsequent junctional breakdown and should be extended to bridge such areas when possible.

Selection of the lower instrumented vertebra (LIV) is a similarly important consideration in surgical planning. The lumbosacral junction represents a highly mobile area with significant challenges in obtaining fusion. While fusing short of the lumbosacral junction provides the advantage of decreased surgical time and trauma as well as decreased pseudarthrosis rates, doing so puts patients at significant risk of subsequent disk degeneration. An unfused lumbosacral junction adjacent to a long fusion segment experiences high levels of stress and motion that predisposes this level to accelerated degeneration. Eck et al. reported a 17% rate of subsequent degeneration in patients with a LIV of L4 or L5 with inferior results in pain and functional outcomes.[24] Similarly, Cho et al. reported a 58% rate of symptomatic adjacent segment degeneration in patients with a LIV of L5, 60% of which required revision. As is demonstrated, long fusions are generally recommended to include the sacrum, which provides more favorable and predictable long-term outcomes.

Pelvic Fixation

Although extensions of fusion to the sacrum are recommended, the lumbosacral junction represents a challenging area in which to achieve successful fusion. In addition to the mobility of the segment and the stresses placed on this level, obtaining adequate fixation into the sacrum can be challenging. Both L5 and S1 have large cancellous pedicles that poorly resist the forces placed on them at the end of a long fusion construct. Tricortical sacral fixation extending through the sacral promontory is recommended to improve fixation strength.[25,26] While tricortical sacral fixation provides superior biomechanics, the procedure may be insufficient to prevent loosening and subsequent pullout. One commonly utilized adjunct procedure to protect the distal fixation is the use of pelvic fixation.

While numerous strategies have been utilized, iliac screws represent a highly effective method of sacropelvic fixation. As iliac screws are divergent from the other fixation points in the spine, they offer significantly improved rigidity and resistance to pullout.[27] Additionally, the length of iliac screws allows them to gain purchase anterior to the axis of rotation of the pelvis, which further increases stability across the region. While iliac fixation can still be successfully utilized in patients with prior iliac crest harvesting, preoperative CT imaging can provide useful information for surgical planning if there is doubt about the ability of the ilium to provide sufficient purchase or if there is abnormal pelvic morphology, which may compromise the ability to place screws safely.[28]

Another useful technique for obtaining sacropelvic fixation is the S2-alar-iliac screw that was recently described.[11] The S2 screw begins at the S2 starting point, just lateral and distal to the S1 foramen, and extends through the sacroiliac joint and into the ilium. The S2 screw trajectory allows for a deeper and more medial starting point compared to traditional iliac fixation, which has the theoretical benefit of minimizing development of symptomatic hardware while also increasing the ease of connecting this fixation to the remainder of the construct. Despite the potential benefits, correct placement of the S2 screw can be technically challenging, and the consequences of hardware penetrating the sacroiliac joint are not yet clear.

While the use of adjunctive fixation within the sacrum has been utilized, such as S2 alar screws, these techniques do not obtain purchase into the ilium and have significantly less strength than fixation into the ilium. However, such fixation strategies do improve sacral fixation and can be useful as a salvage in patients where iliac fixation cannot be achieved.[29]

Interbody Fusion

An additional technique to improve fusion rates about the lumbosacral junction while protecting distal fixation is placement of interbody support. Interbody support is effective in obtaining fusion, as it places bone graft in an area of compression while also allowing for improving segmental lordosis. Interbody fusion can also be used at additional levels within a long fusion construct, allowing for improvement in segmental alignment and translation at these levels.[30] Interbody fusions can be performed via anterior or posterior approaches with good results, as well as through lateral approaches or other minimally invasive methods.[31,32]

Minimally Invasive Approaches

In an attempt to minimize morbidity and complications associated with extensive surgery for degenerative scoliosis, minimally invasive techniques are increasingly being developed. The use of lateral approaches is increasing, as they allow for interbody fusion through a minimally invasive approach. In patients with degenerative scoliosis, the spine is typically accessed through the concavity, which allows the surgeon to directly access and open collapsed disk spaces at the apex of the deformity; the procedure is then supplemented by posterior spinal fusion using either open or percutaneous techniques.

The minimally invasive technique allows for improvement in both coronal alignment and segmental lordosis; however, it has more limited effects on global sagittal balance and lumbar lordosis.[33,34] Minimally invasive strategies have also been shown to provide significant improvements in VAS, SF-36, and Oswestry Disability Index (ODI) scores.[34] Additionally, minimally invasive approaches have been associated with less blood loss, shorter lengths of stay, and lower infection and transfusion rates compared with standard open approaches. Major complication rates are low for minimally invasive techniques, with thigh dysesthesia representing the most common complication, which is typically self-limiting. But, long-term studies on fusion rates and long-term outcomes are lacking.[34-36]

STAGED OPERATIONS

Due to the extensive nature of the operation required to correct many deformities, procedures may sometimes be staged. While staging provides the benefit of limiting surgical duration during a single operative setting, staged procedures are associated with higher infection rates, malnutrition, and higher hospital costs as compared with single-stage procedures. Staging procedures should be avoided when feasible. In certain circumstances, which are often unplanned preoperatively, staging a procedure is necessary. Rhee et al. demonstrated that staged procedures can be performed safely in patients with complex deformity.[37]

COMPLICATIONS

Surgery for degenerative scoliosis is associated with a significant risk of complications in both the immediate and late postoperative period. While complication rates vary widely in the literature, a recent systematic review reported an overall complication rate of 41.2% among the studies reviewed.[38] However, the majority of complications are relatively minor, with the rate of major complications is much lower. Schwab et al. reported a rate of major complications of 8.4% in a recent large multicenter study.[39] In Schwab's series, the most common major complication was excessive bleeding, (defined as > 4 L), followed by deep infection, and finally symptomatic pulmonary embolus. Higher complication rates were associated with the use of staged procedures, as well as combined anterior/posterior approaches. Additional factors that have been associated with increased risk of complication including preoperative loss of lumbar lordosis, significant sagittal imbalance, osteotomies, and fusions that extend to the sacrum.[40] While the majority of complications occur in the early postoperative period, Bridwell et al. reported a 10% rate of complications between 3 years and 5 years after surgery; these late complications were most often due to pseudarthrosis, implant failures, or PJK.[41]

Multiple studies have documented significantly increased risk of complications among older patients.[40,42-44] Smith et al. reported a 71% complication rate among patients aged 65–85 with a 29% major complication rate in this age group. In contrast, patients between 45 years and 65 years demonstrated a 42% complication rate with only a 15% major complication rate.[43] Despite the increased risk of surgery in elderly patients, it is important to emphasize that these patients tend to be the patients with the worst preoperative functional status and have significant potential for improvement after surgical treatment.[43-45]

Proximal Junctional Kyphosis

An important and challenging complication after correction of degenerative scoliosis is PJK. PJK represents the common end point, which can occur as a result of a variety of mechanisms ranging from slow progression of proximal deformity to catastrophic subluxations, or fractures of the adjacent vertebral segment. While more benign forms of PJK are well tolerated, with few clinically significant consequences, a small subset of patients can develop more severe clinical course due to structural failure of the proximal adjacent segment.[46] Patients with severe proximal junctional failure tend to present with increased deformity, pain, and high risk of neurologic deficit.[47]

Many different factors have been shown to put patients at higher risk of developing PJK. Age is a factor in the development of PJK, as compromised bone mineral density can contribute to implant pullout and adjacent segment fracture.[46] Long rigid fusion constructs also contribute to development of PJK by transferring significant stresses on the adjacent segments. Fusions to the sacrum, segmental instrumentation, and circumferential fusions have been shown to increase the risk of PJK.[46,48]

Increased sagittal plane correction also places increased stress on the proximal adjacent level, thereby increasing the risk of PJK. Similarly, those with greater sagittal vertical axis (SVA) correction, greater LL improvement, and those undergoing more correction via PSO also had higher rates of PJK.[47,49] Additional factors that have been shown to contribute to increased risk of PJK include greater difference between lumbar lordosis and thoracic kyphosis, and increased mismatch of lumbar lordosis and pelvic incidence.[47,50]

Pseudarthrosis

Unlike pediatric deformity patients, patients undergoing surgical correction of degenerative scoliosis are at significant risk of pseudarthrosis. While pseudarthrosis rates are variable in the literature, Yadla et al. reported a pooled incidence of 12.9% in a recent systematic review.[38] Patients at increased risk include those with preoperative thoracolumbar kyphosis, postoperative positive sagittal balance >5 cm, concomitant hip osteoarthritis, and age >55 years old. The most common sites affected by pseudarthrosis are the thoracolumbar and lumbosacral junctions, with the majority affecting the thoracolumbar junction.[51] Diagnosis of pseudarthrosis can be challenging in many cases, due in part to the rigid segmental instrumentation. Patients may present with broken hardware, which can result in progression of deformity. Due to the rigidity of modern segmental instrumentation, hardware failure only occurs in a small subset of patients and may happen many years after surgery.[41,51]

OUTCOMES

While surgical correction of degenerative scoliosis is a challenging undertaking with significant complication rates, the procedure also has significant potential for improving patient outcomes. In a recent systematic review, Yadla et al. reported an average decrease in ODI of 15.7 points (range: 3.1–32.3) and average SRS score decrease by 23.1 points.[38] Both the ODI and Scoliosis Research Society (SRS) values represent significant improvements. One consideration that can affect surgical outcome is the degree of preoperative disability. Patients with higher degrees of disability prior to surgery tend to have the greatest potential for improvement after surgery.[2,40]

Patients with severe deformity also have a greater potential for improvement. Patients with loss of lumbar lordosis > 40°, SVA >120 mm, elevated pelvic tilt, and vertebral subluxations have been shown to have greater improvement in function after surgical intervention.[2] Compromised postoperative outcomes have been associated with elevated BMI, higher preoperative pain severity, and narcotic use, smoking, depression, and anxiety.[40,52]

Accurate restoration of alignment is a key factor in obtaining optimal postoperative outcomes, particularly in the sagittal plane. Multiple studies have emphasized the link between postoperative outcomes and restoration of the SVA and pelvic tilt; failure to accurately restore the sagittal plane is associated with persistent symptoms and poor surgical outcomes.[9,53-55]

CONCLUSION

Degenerative scoliosis represents a complex and challenging condition for the spine surgeon. Proper understanding of this disorder, as well as proper surgical planning, is crucial for obtaining surgical success. While surgical correction is associated with significant complications, particularly in the elderly, such treatments have the potential to provide significant benefits in properly selected patients.

REFERENCES

1. Smith JS, Shaffrey CI, Berven S, et al. Improvement of back pain with operative and nonoperative treatment in adults with scoliosis. Neurosurgery 2009;65(1):86-93; discussion 93-4.
2. Bridwell KH, Glassman S, Horton W, et al. Does treatment (nonoperative and operative) improve the two-year quality of life in patients with adult symptomatic lumbar scoliosis: a prospective multicenter evidence-based medicine study. Spine. 2009;34(20):2171-8.

3. Li G, Passias P, Kozanek M, et al. Adult scoliosis in patients over sixty-five years of age: outcomes of operative versus nonoperative treatment at a minimum two-year follow-up. Spine. 2009;34(20):2165-70.
4. Cloyd JM, Acosta FL, Jr., Ames CP. Complications and outcomes of lumbar spine surgery in elderly people: a review of the literature. J Am Geriatr Soc. 2008;56(7):1318-27.
5. Arlet V, Aebi M. Junctional spinal disorders in operated adult spinal deformities: present understanding and future perspectives. Eur Spine J. 2013;22 Suppl 2:S276-95.
6. Cosman F, Keaveny TM, Kopperdahl D, et al. Hip and spine strength effects of adding versus switching to teriparatide in postmenopausal women with osteoporosis treated with prior alendronate or raloxifene. J Bone Miner Res. 2013;28(6):1328-36.
7. Ohtori S, Inoue G, Orita S, et al. Comparison of teriparatide and bisphosphonate treatment to reduce pedicle screw loosening after lumbar spinal fusion surgery in postmenopausal women with osteoporosis from a bone quality perspective. Spine. 2013;38(8):E487-92.
8. Akbar M, Terran J, Ames CP, et al. Use of surgimap spine in sagittal plane analysis, osteotomy planning, and correction calculation. Neurosurg Clin N Am. 2013;24(2):163-72.
9. Schwab FJ, Patel A, Shaffrey CI, et al. Sagittal realignment failures following pedicle subtraction osteotomy surgery: are we doing enough? Clinical article. J Neurosurg Spine. 2012;16(6):539-46.
10. Transfeldt EE, Topp R, Mehbod AA, et al. Surgical outcomes of decompression, decompression with limited fusion, and decompression with full curve fusion for degenerative scoliosis with radiculopathy. Spine. 2010;35(20):1872-5.
11. O'Brien JR, Yu WD, Bhatnagar R, et al. An anatomic study of the S2 iliac technique for lumbopelvic screw placement. Spine. 2009;34(12):E439-42.
12. Smith-Petersen MN, Larson CB, Aufranc OE. Osteotomy of the spine for correction of flexion deformity in rheumatoid arthritis. CORR. 1969;66:6-9.
13. Bridwell KH, Lenke LG, Lewis SJ. Treatment of spinal stenosis and fixed sagittal imbalance. CORR. 2001(384):35-44.
14. McMaster MJ. A technique for lumbar spinal osteotomy in ankylosing spondylitis. J Bone Joint Surg. British volume. 1985;67(2):204-10.
15. Adams JC. Technique, dangers and safeguards in osteotomy of the spine. J Bone Joint Surg. British volume. 1952; 34-B(2):226-32.
16. Li F, Sagi HC, Liu B, et al. Comparative evaluation of single-level closing-wedge vertebral osteotomies for the correction of fixed kyphotic deformity of the lumbar spine: a cadaveric study. Spine. 2001;26(21):2385-91.
17. Cho KJ, Bridwell KH, Lenke LG, et al. Comparison of Smith-Petersen versus pedicle subtraction osteotomy for the correction of fixed sagittal imbalance. Spine. 2005;30(18):2030-7; discussion 2038.
18. Chen IH, Chien JT, Yu TC. Transpedicular wedge osteotomy for correction of thoracolumbar kyphosis in ankylosing spondylitis: experience with 78 patients. Spine. 2001;26 (16):E354-60.
19. Lagrone MO, Bradford DS, Moe JH, et al. Treatment of symptomatic flatback after spinal fusion. J Bone Joint Surg. American volume. 1988;70(4):569-80.
20. Cho KJ, Suk SI, Park SR, et al. Arthrodesis to L5 versus S1 in long instrumentation and fusion for degenerative lumbar scoliosis. Eur Spine J. 2009;18(4):531-7.
21. Kim JH, Kim SS, Suk SI. Incidence of proximal adjacent failure in adult lumbar deformity correction based on proximal fusion level. Asian Spine J. 2007;1(1):19-26.
22. Swank S, Lonstein JE, Moe JH, et al. Surgical treatment of adult scoliosis. A review of two hundred and twenty-two cases. J Bone Joint Surg. American volume. 1981;63(2):268-87.
23. O'Shaughnessy BA, Bridwell KH, Lenke LG, et al. Does a long-fusion "T3-sacrum" portend a worse outcome than a short-fusion "T10-sacrum" in primary surgery for adult scoliosis? Spine. 2012;37(10):884-90.
24. Eck KR, Bridwell KH, Ungacta FF, et al. Complications and results of long adult deformity fusions down to l4, l5, and the sacrum. Spine. 2001;26(9):E182-92.
25. Kato M, Taneichi H, Suda K. Advantage of Pedicle Screw Placement into the Sacral Promontory (Tricortical Purchase) on Lumbosacral Fixation. J Spinal Disord Tech. 2013. (E-pub ahead of print).
26. Orita S, Ohtori S, Eguchi Y, et al. Radiographic evaluation of monocortical versus tricortical purchase approaches in lumbosacral fixation with sacral pedicle screws: a prospective study of ninety consecutive patients. Spine. 2010;35 (22):E1230-7.
27. Tis JE, Helgeson M, Lehman RA, et al. A biomechanical comparison of different types of lumbopelvic fixation. Spine. 2009;34(24):E866-72.
28. Kuklo TR, Bridwell KH, Lewis SJ, et al. Minimum 2-year analysis of sacropelvic fixation and L5-S1 fusion using S1 and iliac screws. Spine. 2001;26(18):1976-83.
29. Koller H, Zenner J, Hempfing A, et al. Reinforcement of lumbosacral instrumentation using S1-pedicle screws combined with S2-alar screws. Oper Orthop Traumatol. 2013;25(3):294-314.
30. Li F, Chen Q, Chen W, et al. Posterior-only approach with selective segmental TLIF for degenerative lumbar scoliosis. J Spinal Disord Techn. 2011;24(5):308-12.
31. Crandall DG, Revella J. Transforaminal lumbar interbody fusion versus anterior lumbar interbody fusion as an adjunct to posterior instrumented correction of degenerative lumbar scoliosis: three year clinical and radiographic outcomes. Spine. 2009;34(20):2126-33.
32. Burneikiene S, Nelson EL, Mason A, et al. Complications in patients undergoing combined transforaminal lumbar interbody fusion and posterior instrumentation with deformity correction for degenerative scoliosis and spinal stenosis. Surg Neurol Int. 2012;3:25.
33. Acosta FL, Liu J, Slimack N, et al. Changes in coronal and sagittal plane alignment following minimally invasive direct lateral interbody fusion for the treatment of degenerative lumbar disease in adults: a radiographic study. J Neurosurg Spine. 2011;15(1):92-6.

34. Anand N, Baron EM. Minimally invasive approaches for the correction of adult spinal deformity. Eur Spine J. 2013;22 Suppl 2:232-41.
35. Mundis GM, Akbarnia BA, Phillips FM. Adult deformity correction through minimally invasive lateral approach techniques. Spine. 2010;35(26 Suppl):S312-21.
36. Berjano P, Lamartina C. Far lateral approaches (XLIF) in adult scoliosis. Eur Spine J. 2013;22 Suppl 2:242-53.
37. Rhee JM, Bridwell KH, Lenke LG, et al. Staged posterior surgery for severe adult spinal deformity. Spine. 2003;28(18): 2116-21.
38. Yadla S, Maltenfort MG, Ratliff JK, et al. Adult scoliosis surgery outcomes: a systematic review. Neurosurgical focus. 2010;28(3):E3.
39. Schwab FJ, Hawkinson N, Lafage V, et al. Risk factors for major peri-operative complications in adult spinal deformity surgery: a multi-center review of 953 consecutive patients. Eur Spine J. 2012;21(12):2603-10.
40. Schwab FJ, Lafage V, Farcy JP, et al. Predicting outcome and complications in the surgical treatment of adult scoliosis. Spine. 2008;33(20):2243-7.
41. Bridwell KH, Baldus C, Berven S, et al. Changes in radiographic and clinical outcomes with primary treatment adult spinal deformity surgeries from two years to three- to five-years follow-up. Spine. 2010;35(20):1849-54.
42. Acosta FL, Jr., McClendon J, Jr., O'Shaughnessy BA, et al. Morbidity and mortality after spinal deformity surgery in patients 75 years and older: complications and predictive factors. J Neurosurg Spine. 2011;15(6):667-74.
43. Daubs MD, Lenke LG, Cheh G, et al. Adult spinal deformity surgery: complications and outcomes in patients over age 60. Spine. 2007;32(20):2238-44.
44. Drazin D, Shirzadi A, Rosner J, et al. Complications and outcomes after spinal deformity surgery in the elderly: review of the existing literature and future directions. Neurosurg Focus. 2011;31(4):E3.
45. Smith JS, Shaffrey CI, Glassman SD, et al. Risk-benefit assessment of surgery for adult scoliosis: an analysis based on patient age. Spine. 2011;36(10):817-24.
46. Kim YJ, Bridwell KH, Lenke LG, et al. Proximal junctional kyphosis in adult spinal deformity after segmental posterior spinal instrumentation and fusion: minimum five-year follow-up. Spine. 2008;33(20):2179-84.
47. Hart RA, McCarthy I, Ames CP, et al. Proximal junctional kyphosis and proximal junctional failure. Neurosurg Clin N Am. 2013;24(2):213-8.
48. Yagi M, Akilah KB, Boachie-Adjei O. Incidence, risk factors and classification of proximal junctional kyphosis: surgical outcomes review of adult idiopathic scoliosis. Spine. 2011;36(1):E60-8.
49. Denis F, Sun EC, Winter RB. Incidence and risk factors for proximal and distal junctional kyphosis following surgical treatment for Scheuermann kyphosis: minimum five-year follow-up. Spine. 2009;34(20):E729-34.
50. Mendoza-Lattes S, Ries Z, Gao Y, et al. Proximal junctional kyphosis in adult reconstructive spine surgery results from incomplete restoration of the lumbar lordosis relative to the magnitude of the thoracic kyphosis. Iowa Orthop J 2011;31:199-206.
51. Kim YJ, Bridwell KH, Lenke LG, et al. Pseudarthrosis in adult spinal deformity following multisegmental instrumentation and arthrodesis. J Bone Joint Surg. American volume. 2006;88(4):721-8.
52. Smith JS, Shaffrey CI, Glassman SD, et al. Clinical and radiographic parameters that distinguish between the best and worst outcomes of scoliosis surgery for adults. Eur Spine J. 2013;22(2):402-10.
53. Glassman SD, Bridwell K, Dimar JR, et al. The impact of positive sagittal balance in adult spinal deformity. Spine. 2005;30(18):2024-9.
54. Lafage V, Schwab F, Patel A, et al. Pelvic tilt and truncal inclination: two key radiographic parameters in the setting of adults with spinal deformity. Spine. 2009;34(17):E599-606.
55. Schwab F, Patel A, Ungar B, et al. Adult spinal deformity-postoperative standing imbalance: how much can you tolerate? An overview of key parameters in assessing alignment and planning corrective surgery. Spine. 2010; 35(25):2224-31.

CHAPTER

54 Surgical Interventions in Osteoporosis and Compression Fracture

Peter G Passias, Andy Chang

INTRODUCTION

Osteoporosis is a major health concern around the world and is becoming increasingly prevalent with the increase in life expectancy. Approximately 10 million Americans are affected by osteoporosis with many more millions affected worldwide.[1] Osteoporosis is a systemic skeletal disease that results in decreased bone density and microarchitectural deterioration of bone tissue.[2] This usually occurs in the elderly and postmenopausal women. Because of the decrease in bone density, people who develop osteoporosis are at a higher risk of fractures. Osteoporotic fractures can occur anywhere in the body but the most common sites are in the hip, vertebrae, and distal radius.[2]

OSTEOPOROTIC COMPRESSION FRACTURES

Vertebral compression fractures are among the most common types of osteoporotic fractures.[2] Osteoporotic vertebral compression fractures (OVCFs) are characterized by pain, loss of height, and exaggeration of kyphosis.[3] Low-trauma or low-stress activities such as sneezing, coughing, laughing, or bending over to pick something up might result in a VCF in an osteoporotic patient.[4] Vertebral compression fractures typically occur at the thoracolumbar junction because at this zone, the rigid thoracic vertebrae transition into the more mobile lumbar segments.

Three types of compression fractures commonly occur: wedge, biconcave, and crush (Figs. 54.1A to C). The wedge fracture is the most common, affecting the anterior column of the vertebral body, forming the characteristic kyphotic hump seen in chronic osteoporotic patients. For biconcave fractures, only the central portion of the vertebral body is damaged, whereas in crush fractures the whole vertebral body is compressed.[5] Wedge fractures are usually asymptomatic because the neurological elements in the middle column remain undisturbed. Morbidities of OVCFs include back pain along with kyphotic spinal deformity, loss of height, and diminished ability to perform daily activities.[6]

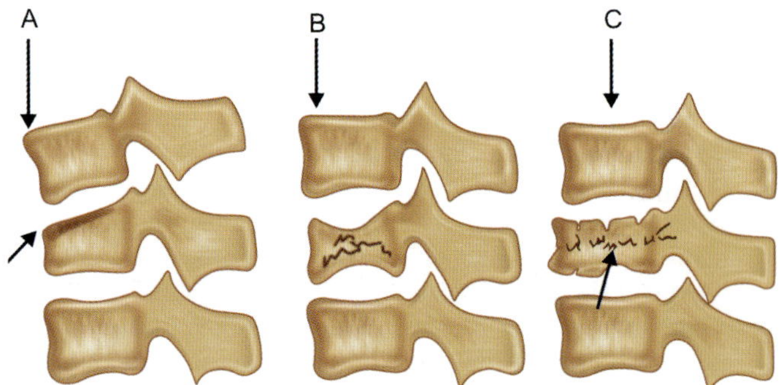

Figs. 54.1A to C: Basic patterns of compression fractures: (A) Wedge (B) biconcave and (C) crush.

CONSERVATIVE MANAGEMENT

Acute pain stemming from OVCFs usually resolves within 2–3 months after initial onset.[3] Therefore, OVCFs should be initially managed conservatively to relieve pain and achieve rehabilitation through analgesics, bed rest, and orthotics with eventual mobilization guided by associated pain intensity.[6,7] Analgesics such as acetaminophen, NSAIDs, and opioids are the first-line therapy used for pain relief. Side effects of NSAIDs include gastrointestinal (GI) bleeding, renal insufficiency, and an increase in cardiovascular risks. Opioids also have significant side effects including constipation, cognitive deficits, and respiratory depression.

In addition to using NSAIDs and opioids as analgesics, calcitonin has been reported to reduce pain while mobile and at rest for up to 4 weeks for acute pain associated with OVCFs.[8-10] However, there is currently insufficient evidence on the effect of calcitonin for chronic pain associated with OVCFs. Side effects for calcitonin treatment are mild, including enteric disturbances and flushing. In addition, bisphosphonates such as ibandronate and strontium ranelate are weakly recommended by the AAOS Clinical Practice Guideline summary to prevent additional symptomatic fractures after initial fractures.[11] Bisphosphonates may provide long-term pain relief but do not relieve pain from an existing fracture. Due to the side effects of each drug, individuals should be monitored and evaluated according to their level of pain as well as their past history to prevent ensuing comorbidities.[6]

Postural bracing with hyperextension orthosis has also been reported to reduce pain and increase quality of life. After a short period of bed rest, mobilization should occur as early as possible, pain permitting, to allow rehabilitation and strengthening of trunk muscles.[6] Use of orthotics should be discouraged when no longer needed, to avoid excessive immobilization and muscle atrophy.

SURGICAL TREATMENT

Surgical treatment is the next option if conservative treatment fails. Approximately 40% of conservatively treated patients with acute OVCFs continue to have disabling pain after 1 year of treatment with high class pain medication.[12] Surgical intervention is employed for fractures that are considered unstable. Although somewhat controversial, instability has been defined in both mechanical and clinical terms. Mechanically, compression fractures by definition will have preservation of the middle column. Inability of the vertebral segment to resist further deformation from continued loading will typically be secondary to progressive compressive forces anteriorly or tensile forces posteriorly. Although strict criteria for sagittal alignment and percentage of compression have not been found to be predictive, the greater segmental kyphosis and percentage of compression generally increase the mechanical loading seen anteriorly and tensile forces posteriorly. Additional factors, including strength and viability of the compressed bone and maintenance of the posterior osteoligamentous complex, also contribute to the ultimate result. Clinical instability, although not common with this type of injury, refers primarily to neurological status and ability to tolerate symptoms associated with the injury. Like conservative treatment, the goal of surgical intervention is to reduce pain and increase quality of life.

The two surgical procedures most widely performed for OVCFs are percutaneous vertebroplasty and kyphoplasty. Vertebroplasty involves percutaneous injection of bone cement such as polymethylmethacrylate into the compressed vertebrae. Kyphoplasty is a similar process with an additional step of first inserting an inflatable bone tamp to reduce the compressed vertebral body before injecting bone cement to stabilize the reduction. Both surgeries aim to provide immediate and future pain relief while potentially reversing height loss and increasing quality of life.

There is some evidence in the literature demonstrating a beneficial effect to vertebroplasty procedures. An observational study by DePalma et al.[13] reported that the vertebroplasty procedure reduced visual analog scale (VAS) pain scores immediately after surgery continuing up to 2 years postoperatively. Unblinded randomized control trials comparing vertebroplasty with conservative care reported results showing the benefits of vertebroplasty by reducing pain, improving mobility, and function as well.[14-17] However, the results were nonuniform from study to study because the follow-up times were not the same for each study. Although these trials found significant improvement in pain after vertebroplasty, the statistically significant reduction in pain when compared with conservative treatment did not last for the entirety of each follow-up study. For example, the pain after vertebroplasty was significantly different from conservative treatment after 2 weeks,[15] 1 month,[18] 12 months,[16,19] and 24 months.[17] Blasco et al. reported that patients treated with vertebroplasty had faster pain relief and greater improvement at 12-month follow-up.[16] Based on this, the literature appears to be inconsistent with regard to duration of pain relief following vertebroplasty.

However, two studies comparing patient outcomes for vertebroplasty and a sham procedure have questioned the validity and benefits of vertebroplasty.[20,21] The improvements reported in the vertebroplasty group were similar to the improvements in the control group undergoing a sham procedure. In the sham procedure, the subjects were prepared and treated as they were undergoing the vertebroplasty procedure until the 13-gauge needle insertion while not actually receiving treatment.[20,21] Although both groups showed a decrease in pain, the vertebroplasty group did not show a significant advantage in pain reduction and functional outcomes when compared with the sham procedure over the follow-up period. One of the studies, however, noted that there was a trend toward a higher rate of improvement in pain for the vertebroplasty group.[21] These two randomized, blinded, and controlled trials were the first trials to suggest that vertebroplasty is not as beneficial as initially thought. Further high-quality randomized control trials are required to compare the effectiveness of vertebroplasty to other treatment and controls. Based on current evidence, vertebroplasty is not recommended for patients with OVCFs.[11]

Focus has also recently shifted to determining the efficacy and safety of kyphoplasty because of its potential to reduce kyphotic wedge caused by compression fractures. However, there are fewer high-quality studies reporting on kyphoplasty as a treatment of OVCF than there are for vertebroplasty. A prospective nonrandomized controlled trial by Kasperk et al. reported that VAS pain scores improved significantly for the kyphoplasty group but not for the conservative treatment control group up to 6 months.[22] In addition, the midline vertebral height of the kyphoplasty treated vertebral bodies increased by 12.1%, while the control group showed a decrease in height by 8.2%.[22] A prospective randomized controlled trial by Wardlaw et al.[23] more recently reported similar results, with pain being reduced for the kyphoplasty group up to 12 months with the most significant improvement seen in the first few months. Like vertebroplasty, initial studies comparing kyphoplasty with conservative treatments have reported that kyphoplasty is beneficial to providing pain relief in patients with OVCFs.

Studies for OVCF comparing kyphoplasty and vertebroplasty have reported that mean pain scores decreased significantly from pre to postoperation.[7,24-26] There were no significant differences found between the VAS and Oswestry Disability Index (ODI) for the two surgical treatments up to 6 months[24,26] or 12 months.[7] Despite the similarities found in pain scores between the two treatments, one prospective nonrandomized study reported that kyphoplasty had a longer lasting effect for decreasing pain than the vertebroplasty group.[25] Pain for the kyphoplasty group remained low immediately after surgery up until 2 years while pain for the vertebroplasty group was low only up to 2 months and became less pronounced between 2 months and 2 years. It is hypothesized that the longer lasting pain reduction in kyphoplasty is due to its ability to reduce kyphosis and possibly have a correcting effect on sagittal balance while simultaneously reducing compensatory action by the back muscles.[25]

The majority of the studies on kyphoplasty were nonrandomized; higher quality randomized controlled trials are required in order to produce higher quality results. Also, since the two studies that reported no significant difference between the sham procedure and vertebroplasty,[20,21] the benefit of the kyphoplasty treatment can be questioned as well. The argument can be made that kyphoplasty may not provide the same benefit in pain reduction as originally thought because of the results of the comparative studies reporting that vertebroplasty pain scores are not significantly different from kyphoplasty pain scores. Nonetheless, until further higher quality randomized controlled trials are performed comparing kyphoplasty to sham or vertebroplasty, no definitive conclusions can be drawn from these inferences. Until then, kyphoplasty should only be performed if conservative treatment does not adequately reduce pain and improve quality of life.[11,27]

During kyphoplasty, two common approaches can be used to inject the cement into the damaged vertebral body—unilateral or bilateral. The bilateral transpedicular approach is the standard method used, enabling symmetric repositioning of the vertebral bodies.[28,29] The fracture is first reduced through traction under fluoroscopic guidance. Biopsy needles enter the damaged vertebra bilaterally through the pedicle. A K-wire is placed through the biopsy needle close to the anterior wall where it is then widened to form a cavity for placement of the balloons. The balloons are then positioned near the anterior wall and then inflated carefully without fracturing the end plates or posterior wall. After reduction, the cavity is filled with cement bilaterally.[28] The same transpedicular procedure can be performed unilaterally (Figs. 54.2 and 54.3).

For OVCFs in the thoracic spine, transpedicular kyphoplasty is difficult because the anatomy of the thoracic pedicles do not allow adequate placement of the balloons prohibiting adequate reduction.[28] Therefore, the unilateral extrapedicular approach is preferred, as it does not require pedicle perforation. Instead of access through the pedicle, the biopsy needle only perforates the lateral pedicle at the base.[28] A recent study by Wang et al. reported the average operating time and exposure to X-rays to be less in the unilateral kyphoplasty group than for the bilateral

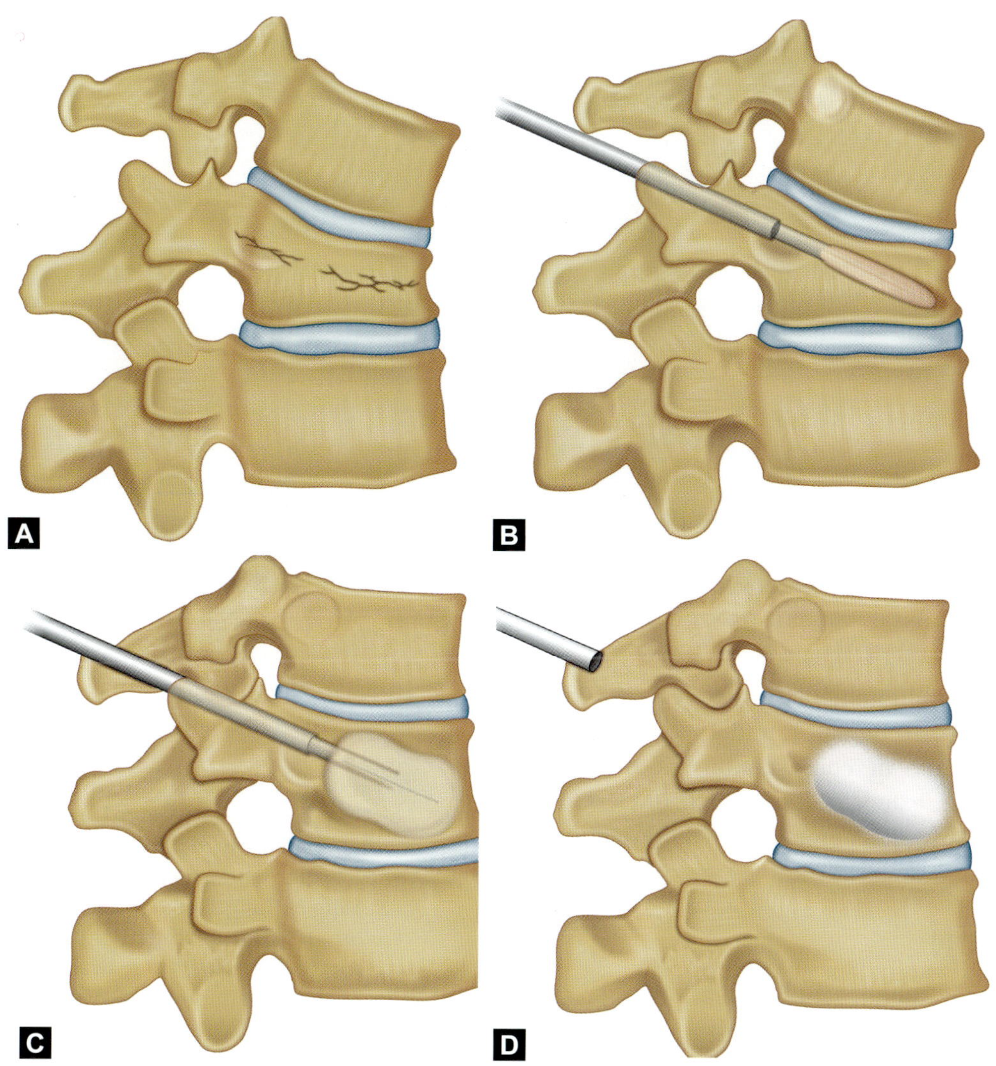

Figs. 54.2A to D: Schema of (A) lumbar compression fracture, (B) insertion of instrument through pedicle, (C) inflation of balloon with injection of filling material, and (D) hardening of filling material with removal of instrument.

group.[29] There was otherwise no significant difference in pain scores, vertebral height restoration, and cement leakage, suggesting that the unilateral approach should be used to reduce operation time and X-ray exposure. The kyphoplasty approach should be used at the discretion of the surgeon taking into account the anatomy of the patients through preoperative planning.

ADVERSE EVENTS FOR VERTEBROPLASTY AND KYPHOPLASTY

The reported complications for vertebroplasty include local cement leakage, pulmonary cement embolism, pyogenic spondylitis, and osteomyelitis.[30-37] Pulmonary cement embolism rate was reported in 23% of patients receiving vertebroplasty.[34] Cement leakage has been reported from 11% to 73% of vertebroplasty procedures.[33] However, the majority of the cases are not symptomatic cement leaks. For instance, the incidence of cement leakage is approximately 75% but symptomatic cement leaks are approximately 1.5% of all cases.[7,36] While cement leakage and pulmonary cement embolism are more common, pyogenic spondylitis and osteomyelitis are serious and rare complications that have been seen in a handful of cases.

The reported complications of kyphoplasty are local cement leakage and pulmonary cement embolism. Compared to vertebroplasty, there is a lower incidence of cement leakage complications for kyphoplasty.[36,37] The incidence of

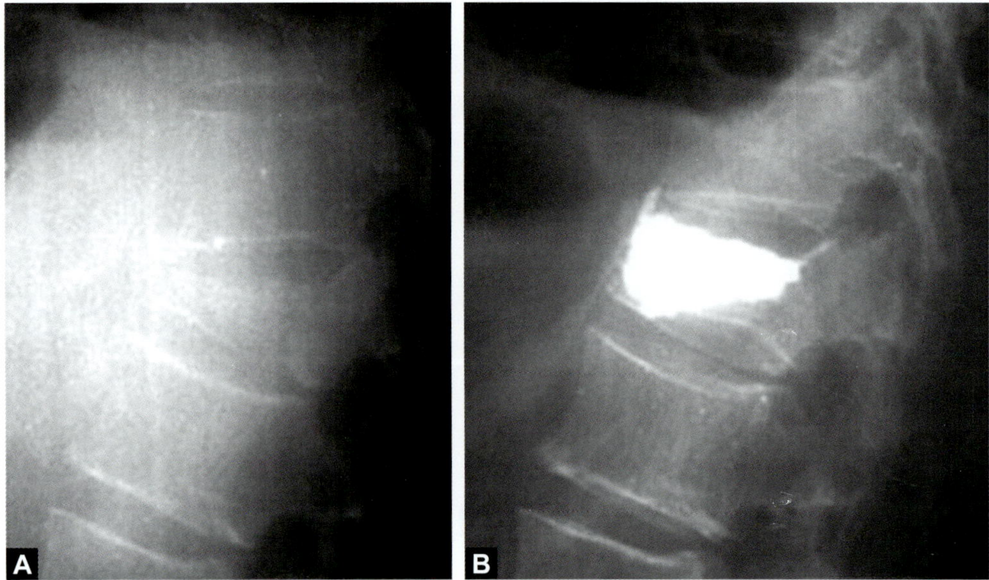

Figs. 54.3A and B: Plain radiographs of (A) collapsed vertebra prior to kyphoplasty with (B) restoration of vertebral height following kyphoplasty.

symptomatic and asymptomatic cement leaks for kyphoplasty was reported to be 0.04% and 14% respectively.[36] The lower incidence of complications is most likely attributed to more extensive experience in performing kyphoplasty because the procedure is more technically demanding.

CONCLUSION

Conservative care remains to be the initial approach to treating OVCFs. However, because of the growing elderly population, there will be more people who do not respond to conservative treatment who will require surgical care. More uniform study designs and high-level prospective, randomized, and controlled trials for kyphoplasty and vertebroplasty should be performed to produce more conclusive results about the benefits for each surgical treatment.

REFERENCES

1. Cummings SR, Melton LJ. Epidemiology and outcomes of osteoporotic fractures. Lancet. 2002;359:1761-7.
2. Genant HK, Cooper C, Poor G, et al. Interim report and recommendations of the World Health Organization Task-Force for Osteoporosis. Osteoporos Int. 1999;10:259-64.
3. Silverman SL. The clinical consequences of vertebral compression fracture. Bone. 1992;13 Suppl 2:S27-31.
4. Bono CM. Vertebral compression fractures what time destroys, methylmethacrylate may mend. Cleve Clin J Med. 2003;70:88-90.
5. Michael S Linn, Chol W Kim, Mark Valente. Compression fractures of the thoracic and lumbar spine. In: Zigler JE, Eismont FJ, Garfin S, Vaccaro AR (Eds). Spine Trauma, 2nd edition. AAOS; 2011. pp. 499-510.
6. Longo UG, Loppini M, Denaro L, et al. Conservative management of patients with an osteoporotic vertebral fracture: a review of the literature. J Bone Joint Surg Br. 2012;94:152-7.
7. Li X, Yang H, Tang T, et al. Comparison of kyphoplasty and vertebroplasty for treatment of painful osteoporotic vertebral compression fractures: twelve-month follow-up in a prospective nonrandomized comparative study. J Spinal Disord Tech. 2012;25:142-9.
8. Knopp-Sihota JA, Newburn-Cook CV, Homik J, et al. Calcitonin for treating acute and chronic pain of recent and remote osteoporotic vertebral compression fractures: a systematic review and meta-analysis. Osteoporos Int. 2012; 23:17-38.
9. Lyritis GP, Ioannidis GV, Karachalios T, et al. Analgesic effect of salmon calcitonin suppositories in patients with acute pain due to recent osteoporotic vertebral crush fractures: a prospective double-blind, randomized, placebo-controlled clinical study. Clin J Pain. 1999;15:284-9.
10. Lyritis GP, Paspati I, Karachalios T, et al. Pain relief from nasal salmon calcitonin in osteoporotic vertebral crush fractures. A double blind, placebo-controlled clinical study. Acta Orthop Scand Suppl 1997;275:112-4.
11. Esses SI, McGuire R, Jenkins J, et al. The treatment of symptomatic osteoporotic spinal compression fractures. J Am Acad Orthop Surg. 2011;19:176-82.
12. Venmans A, Klazen CA, Lohle PN, et al. Natural history of pain in patients with conservatively treated osteoporotic vertebral compression fractures: results from VERTOS II. AJNR Am J Neuroradiol. 2012;33:519-21.

13. DePalma MJ, Ketchum JM, Frankel BM, et al. Percutaneous vertebroplasty for osteoporotic vertebral compression fractures in the nonagenarians: a prospective study evaluating pain reduction and new symptomatic fracture rate. Spine (Phila Pa 1976). 2011;36(4):277-82.
14. Diamond TH, Bryant C, Browne L, et al. Clinical outcomes after acute osteoporotic vertebral fractures: a 2-year nonrandomised trial comparing percutaneous vertebroplasty with conservative therapy. Med J Aust. 2006;184:113-7.
15. Voormolen MH, Mali WP, Lohle PN, et al. Percutaneous vertebroplasty compared with optimal pain medication treatment: short-term clinical outcome of patients with subacute or chronic painful osteoporotic vertebral compression fractures. The VERTOS study. AJNR Am J Neuroradiol. 2007;28:555-60.
16. Blasco J, Martinez-Ferrer A, Macho J, et al. Effect of vertebroplasty on pain relief, quality of life, and the incidence of new vertebral fractures: a 12-month randomized follow-up, controlled trial. J Bone Miner Res. 2012;27:1159-66.
17. Farrokhi MR, Alibai E, Maghami Z. Randomized controlled trial of percutaneous vertebroplasty versus optimal medical management for the relief of pain and disability in acute osteoporotic vertebral compression fractures. J Neurosurg Spine. 2011;14:561-9.
18. Rousing R, Hansen KL, Andersen MO, et al. Twelve-months follow-up in forty-nine patients with acute/semiacute osteoporotic vertebral fractures treated conservatively or with percutaneous vertebroplasty: a clinical randomized study. Spine (Phila Pa 1976). 2010;35:478-82.
19. Klazen CA, Lohle PN, de Vries J, et al. Vertebroplasty versus conservative treatment in acute osteoporotic vertebral compression fractures (Vertos II): an open-label randomised trial. Lancet. 2010;376:1085-92.
20. Buchbinder R, Osborne RH, Ebeling PR, et al. A randomized trial of vertebroplasty for painful osteoporotic vertebral fractures. N Engl J Med. 2009;361:557-68.
21. Kallmes DF, Comstock BA, Heagerty PJ, et al. A randomized trial of vertebroplasty for osteoporotic spinal fractures. N Engl J Med. 2009;361:569-79.
22. Kasperk C, Hillmeier J, Noldge G, et al. Treatment of painful vertebral fractures by kyphoplasty in patients with primary osteoporosis: a prospective nonrandomized controlled study. J Bone Miner Res. 2005;20:604-12.
23. Wardlaw D, Cummings SR, Van Meirhaeghe J, et al. Efficacy and safety of balloon kyphoplasty compared with non-surgical care for vertebral compression fracture (FREE): a randomised controlled trial. Lancet. 2009;373(9668):1016-24.
24. De Negri P, Tirri T, Paternoster G, et al. Treatment of painful osteoporotic or traumatic vertebral compression fractures by percutaneous vertebral augmentation procedures: a nonrandomized comparison between vertebroplasty and kyphoplasty. Clin J Pain. 2007;23:425-30.
25. Grohs JG, Matzner M, Trieb K, et al. Minimal invasive stabilization of osteoporotic vertebral fractures: a prospective nonrandomized comparison of vertebroplasty and balloon kyphoplasty. J Spinal Disord Tech. 2005;18:238-42.
26. Liu JT, Liao WJ, Tan WC, et al. Balloon kyphoplasty versus vertebroplasty for treatment of osteoporotic vertebral compression fracture: a prospective, comparative, and randomized clinical study. Osteoporos Int. 2010;21:359-64.
27. McGuire R. AAOS clinical practice guideline: the treatment of symptomatic osteoporotic spinal compression fractures. J Am Acad Orthop Surg. 2011;19:183-4.
28. Robinson Y, Heyde CE, Forsth P, et al. Kyphoplasty in osteoporotic vertebral compression fractures—guidelines and technical considerations. J Orthop Surg Res. 2011;6:43.
29. Wang Z, Wang G, Yang H. Comparison of unilateral versus bilateral balloon kyphoplasty for the treatment of osteoporotic vertebral compression fractures. J Clin Neurosci. 2012;19:723-6.
30. Zhang JD, Poffyn B, Sys G, et al. Comparison of vertebroplasty and kyphoplasty for complications. Orthop Surg. 2011;3:158-60.
31. Walker DH, Mummaneni P, Rodts GE, Jr. Infected vertebroplasty. Report of two cases and review of the literature. Neurosurg Focus. 2004;17:E6.
32. Yu SW, Chen WJ, Lin WC, et al. Serious pyogenic spondylitis following vertebroplasty—a case report. Spine (Phila Pa 1976). 2004;29:E209-11.
33. Shapiro S, Abel T, Purvines S. Surgical removal of epidural and intradural polymethylmethacrylate extravasation complicating percutaneous vertebroplasty for an osteoporotic lumbar compression fracture. Case report. J Neurosurg. 2003;98:90-2.
34. Kim YJ, Lee JW, Park KW, et al. Pulmonary cement embolism after percutaneous vertebroplasty in osteoporotic vertebral compression fractures: incidence, characteristics, and risk factors. Radiology. 2009;251:250-9.
35. Choe DH, Marom EM, Ahrar K, et al. Pulmonary embolism of polymethyl methacrylate during percutaneous vertebroplasty and kyphoplasty. AJR Am J Roentgenol. 2004;183:1097-102.
36. Lee MJ, Dumonski M, Cahill P, et al. Percutaneous treatment of vertebral compression fractures: a meta-analysis of complications. Spine (Phila Pa 1976). 2009;34:1228-32.
37. Taylor RS, Taylor RJ, Fritzell P. Balloon kyphoplasty and vertebroplasty for vertebral compression fractures: a comparative systematic review of efficacy and safety. Spine (Phila Pa 1976). 2006;31:2747-55.

CHAPTER

55

Surgical Management of the Rheumatoid Spine

Ronald Moskovich, Jeffrey Knox

INTRODUCTION

Rheumatoid arthritis (RA) is a chronic inflammatory disorder, which affects up to 1–2% of the world's adults,[1] with significant geographic variability reflecting the multifactorial nature of the condition. While the exact etiology of RA remains uncertain, it is currently thought to be caused by exposure to an unknown environmental pathogen in a genetically susceptible host. The exposure exacts an aggressive systemic response from the host, leading to chronic synovial inflammation and progressive destruction of bone, cartilage, and ligaments, with subsequent symmetric erosive polyarthropathy. Although this chain of events primarily targets the joints of the appendicular skeleton, synovial articulations of the axial skeleton are also common targets, with spinal involvement a significant cause of morbidity and mortality.

RA of the spine is estimated to be present in 17–88% of patients with RA[2] and is the second most common site of involvement after the metacarpophalangeal joints. RA of the spine is primarily a disorder of the cervical spine, with the vast majority of cases involving the upper cervical vertebrae. This region is particularly susceptible due to the large number of synovial joints, which are the primary target of RA, rather than intervertebral disks.

SPINE MANIFESTATIONS

The most common and earliest manifestation of RA in the cervical spine is atlantoaxial subluxation (AAS), which accounts for >60% of rheumatoid cervical spine cases.[3] AAS is caused by erosion and instability of the synovial articulations about the dens, combined with damage to the transverse and accessory atlantoaxial ligaments. The majority of subluxations are anterior,[4] with approximately 20% of cases lateral and 7% posterior.[5] Despite their rarity, posterior subluxations may result in a higher rate of neurologic injury compared with anterior subluxations.[6] As the disease progresses, subsequent involvement of the alar and apical ligaments as well as the occiput-C1 and C1-2 articulations may occur, leading to superior migration of the odontoid, also known as pseudobasilar invagination. Although less common, this pattern of instability carries a poor prognosis and a high rate of neurologic injury due to direct compression of the brain stem or spinal cord by the odontoid or from kyphosis of the upper cervical spine or brain stem.[7] Paradoxically, as this superior migration progresses, the ring of C1(atlas) settles down on the conical odontoid process-C2 body (axis), which can result in pseudostabilization as the anterior atlantoaxial interval decreases and anteroposterior motion at the atlantoaxial articulation is reduced.

Involvement of the subaxial cervical spine is much less common than upper cervical involvement and is present in only 15–20% of rheumatoid patients. Subaxial subluxations occur as a result of rheumatoid destruction of the facet joints along with the discovertebral joints. This phenomenon may occur at multiple levels resulting in a so-called "staircase" deformity. Secondary changes may occur in response to chronic instability including posterior ligament thickening, osteophyte formation, and ankylosis. Subaxial involvement can exist in isolation but more commonly occurs in combination with upper cervical spine disease.

CLINICAL EVALUATION

Clinical evaluation of the rheumatoid patient with documented or potential spinal instability is often challenging due to the systemic nature of their disease. Peripheral joint involvement may result in joint pain and limited range of motion, which can mask early signs of myelopathy and make motor testing unreliable. Peripheral nerve entrapments commonly occur in patients with RA and can mask or mimic radicular pain. Despite the challenges, a thorough history and physical examination is key to the proper evaluation of these patients. Serial examinations are the best tool to identify subtle findings or evidence of progressive neurologic compromise.

The most common complaint with cervical spine involvement is neck pain, which is present in 50% of patients.[8] This pain is often localized to the upper cervical spine and may be associated with occipital headaches, due to compression of the lesser occipital (C1) or greater occipital (C2) nerves. Patients may also describe subjective feelings of instability, possibly associated with a palpable subluxation or "clunk" with flexion and extension of the neck. An electrical sensation that radiates down the neck into the limbs and trunk with neck flexion, Lhermitte's sign, if present, is an ominous indicator of cervical spinal cord compression.

Patients with cervical instability may present with a variety of neurologic complaints depending on the location and severity of compression. They may present as well with signs and symptoms of myelopathy, including gait instability, loss of manual dexterity, spasticity, weakness, and paresthesias. In the setting of superior migration of the odontoid, patients may present with brain stem symptoms and signs, such as tinnitus, vertigo, diplopia, dysphagia, or cranial nerve deficits, including the glossopharyngeal, hypoglossal, and trigeminal nerves. If patients present with such deficits, it is important to rule out other causes, as cranial nerve involvement is relatively uncommon in rheumatoid cervical instability.[9] Traditional neurological evaluation may be confounded by the musculoskeletal manifestations of advanced RA. The only indication of spinal cord compression may be a decrease in ambulatory ability or an emerging need for increased ambulatory support, such as a patient transitioning from using a cane to requiring a walker or wheelchair. Bowel and bladder incontinence are late findings and indicate severe neurologic compression and advanced disease.

Approximately 50% of patients with radiographic instability are clinically asymptomatic.[10] Routine imaging of asymptomatic patients should be considered to identify patients who may be at risk of neurological injury due to unrecognized cervical instability or spinal cord compression.

NATURAL HISTORY

Natural history of the rheumatoid cervical spine in untreated patients is relatively well described. Pharmacotherapy reduces disease activity and may prevent or slow disease progression and subsequent joint destruction. Early medical management has resulted in a reduction in patients with rheumatoid cervical spine instability as well as the number of patients progressing to require surgical intervention.

Cervical spine involvement begins early in the course of RA, often becoming evident within the first 2–5 years of diagnosis. Once cervical instability is present, it tends to progress. Pellicci et al. found that 80% of their patients with cervical spine involvement showed radiographic progression without treatment.[3] Reiter et al.[7] demonstrated patients who were at a higher risk of progression were male, had positive rheumatoid factor, and had more severe peripheral disease. The contribution of prolonged corticosteroid use to cervical spine disease progression has not been well defined.

The development of neurologic symptoms is ominous, as once these symptoms manifest patients exhibit a much poorer overall prognosis, with progression of neurologic symptoms and functional decline. The 1-year mortality for untreated patients may reach 50%.[11,12]

GRADING

While numerous classification systems exist, they are often challenging to implement in practice. The Ranawat classification[13] is commonly used for evaluation of patients' baseline functional status and follow-up. (Table 55.1) The American Rheumatological Association (ARA) classification system is another commonly used functional classification.[14] (Table 55.2)

IMAGING

Initial imaging should be comprised of plain radiographs with lateral flexion and extension views (Figs. 55.1A to C). These studies may be used to evaluate symptomatic

Table 55.1: Ranawat grading system

Class I	No neural deficit
Class II	Subjective weakness with hyper-reflexia and dysesthesia
Class III	Objective weakness and long tract signs
IIIA	Ambulatory
IIIB	Nonambulatory

Table 55.2: Functional classification of rheumatoid arthritis

Class I	Complete ability to carry on all usual duties without handicaps
Class II	Adequate for normal activities despite handicap of discomfort or limited motion at one or more joints
Class III	Limited to little or none of the duties of usual occupation or self-care
Class IV	Incapacitated, largely or wholly bedridden or confined to wheelchair, little or no self-care

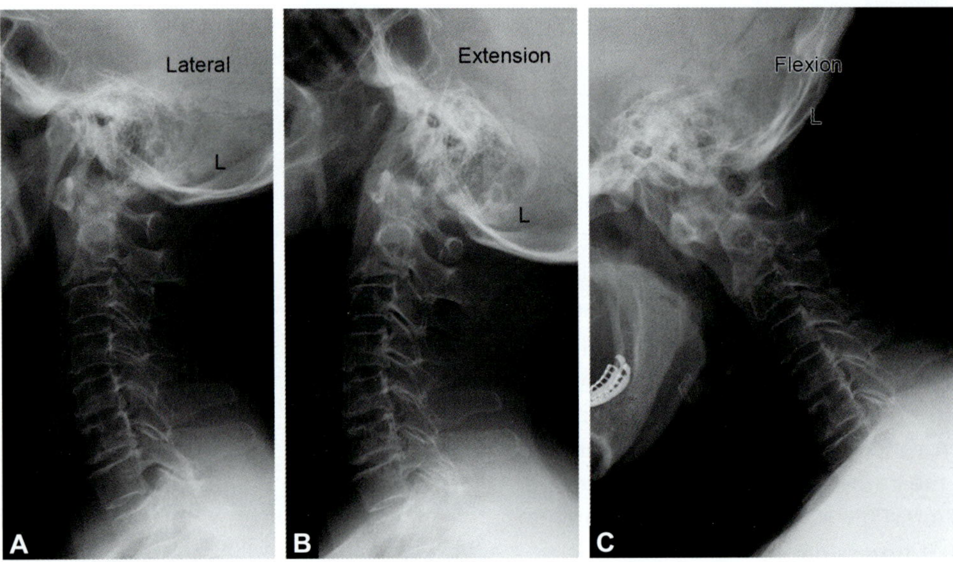

Figs. 55.1A to C: Lateral cervical radiograph of an 80-year-old woman with rheumatoid arthritis. Lateral extension and flexion views demonstrate unstable anterior atlantoaxial subluxation. Note the break in the spinolaminar line between C1 and C2 in all positions.

patients as well as screen asymptomatic patients. The primary measurements to evaluate AAS are the anterior atlantodental interval (AADI or ADI) and the posterior atlantodental interval (PADI), also referred to as the space available for the cord (SAC). The ADI is the distance between the posterior aspect of the anterior arch of C1 and the anterior aspect of the dens on the lateral radiograph. The normal adult value is <3 mm and is usually inversely proportional to the SAC. The ADI is commonly measured, however, this measurement has been shown to correlate poorly with development of neurologic symptoms and is unreliable in guiding treatment.[15] Alternatively, the PADI is a more reliable indicator of patients at risk for neurologic compromise. The PADI is defined as the distance between the posterior aspect of the dens to the anterior aspect of the C1 lamina and is equivalent to the SAC. Normal PADI is 14 mm at C2, and values < 14 mm are associated with an increased risk of neurologic injury.[15]

It is sometimes challenging to accurately assess superior migration of the dens, due to difficulty in visualizing the odontoid process on plain radiographs. Visualization is often compromised by bony erosions due to RA as well as decreased bone mineral density. The mastoid air cells overlie the dens on the lateral radiograph, further limiting accurate visualization of the dens. The clivus, hard palate, basion (anterior aspect of the foramen magnum), and the opisthion (posterior aspect of the foramen magnum), as well as the atlas, the pedicle, and lower endplate of C2, are important landmarks. Several indices have been described using these landmarks to evaluate superior migration of the odontoid. Some of the more common measurements and lines used in evaluation are described in Table 55.3 and illustrated in Figures 55.2 and 55.3.[16-22]

The ADI and Redlund-Johnell measurements generally use clearly visualized structures, resulting in reproducible measurements. Other indices may be compromised by an inability to accurately see the bony points or the need to estimate landmarks. By using a combination of the Clark, Redlund-Johnell, and Ranawat measurements, the reliability of diagnosing superior migration of the odontoid

Table 55.3: Commonly used measurements and lines used in evaluation of occipito-C1-C2 relationships

Measurement	*Description*	*Diagnostic criteria*
McGregor's line[16]	Line drawn from posterosuperior aspect of the hard palate to the most caudal (lowest) cortical margin of the occiput	Cranial settling is diagnosed when the apex of the dens rises >4.5 mm above this line
McRae's line[17]	Line drawn from foramen magnum from the basion to the opisthion (posterior rim of foramen magnum)	Protrusion of the tip of the dens above this line indicates cranial settling
Chamberlain's line[18]	Line drawn from posterior aspect of the hard palate to the opisthion	Protrusion of the tip of the dens >3 mm above this line indicates cranial settling
Wackenheim's line[19]	Line drawn along the superior surface of the clivus	Protrusion of the dens posterior to the projection of this line indicates settling
Fischgold-Metzger's line[20]	Line drawn between the tips of mastoid processes on the anteroposterior open-mouth odontoid view	Protrusion of the tip of the dens above this line indicates cranial settling
Ranawat index[13]	Center of the C2 pedicle and transverse axis of the atlas	(Normal range: males: 17 +/− 2 mm; females: 15 +/− 2 mm) Severity of settling relative to decreases in the distance measured
Redlund-Johnell measurement[21]	McGregor's line to the midpoint of the caudal margin of the C2 body	(Normal: males ≥34 mm; females ≥29 mm) Severity of settling relative to decreases in the distance measured
Clark Stations[22] (simplest method, relationships do not change in flexion, extension or neutral views)	Dividing the odontoid process into three equal parts, or stations, from superior to inferior. Assess which station of the odontoid process is level with (adjacent to) the anterior ring of the atlas	*Station I*: Anterior ring of atlas is level with superior third of odontoid process (normal) *Station II*: If the anterior ring of atlas is level with (adjacent to) the middle third of the dens (mild) *Station III*: When the anterior ring of atlas is level with (adjacent to) the caudal third of the dens (severe)

may be improved, with 94% sensitivity and a 91% negative predictive value for vertical subluxation.[23]

Due to the limitations of plain radiographs in rheumatoid disease, particularly in the upper cervical spine, advanced imaging is recommended in patients with documented or suspected instability. Computed tomography (CT) demonstrates bony compression and osseous anatomy, which aids in surgical planning. Myelography provides an assessment of neural compression in flexion and extension to evaluate dynamic compression.

Magnetic resonance imaging (MRI) is now the neuroanatomic study of choice and is recommended for all patients with evidence of cervical instability on plain radiographs or with neurologic deficits. MRI provides detail of soft tissues such as the periodontoid pannus, which often contributes to further reduction in the SAC that is not discerned on plain radiographs.[24] MRI directly pictures the neural elements, which can provide information about compression or deformity. One example is the cervicomedullary angle, between the anterior aspect of the cervical cord and the medulla. Normal measurements range between 135° and 175°, with angles <135° indicative of superior migration of the odontoid and correlation with myelopathy and neurologic injury.[25] The addition of dynamic views can add useful information in evaluating compressive pathology. Allmann et al. showed that the addition of flexion views revealed 12% of patients who had no compression on neutral imaging showed compression on flexion MRI (Fig. 55.4).[26]

TREATMENT

Understanding the natural history of rheumatoid cervical instability helps guide the clinician in treating this challenging disorder. As mentioned previously, these patients are at significant risk of progressive, irreversible neurologic deficits as well as sudden death from spinal cord or brain stem compression. Treatment should be focused on prevention of these catastrophic events whilst minimizing the morbidity associated with intervention. Nonoperative management should focus on aggressive medical management of the RA. Disease modifying anti-

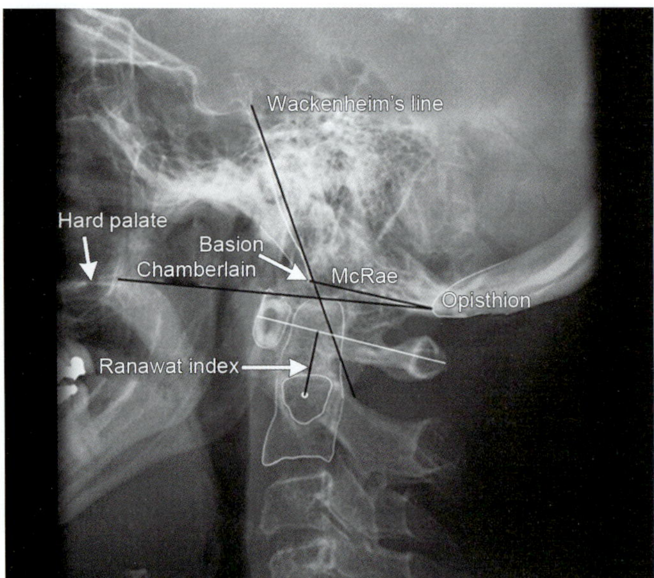

Fig. 55.2: Commonly drawn lines and measurements to assess occipito-C1–C2 relationships. The lines in this figure are somewhat arbitrary, as the center of the various landmarks must be estimated.[49]
Source: Reprinted with permission from Wasserman BR, Moskovich R, Razi AE. Rheumatoid arthritis of the cervical spine: clinical considerations. Bull NYU Hosp Jt Dis. 2011;69(2):136-48.

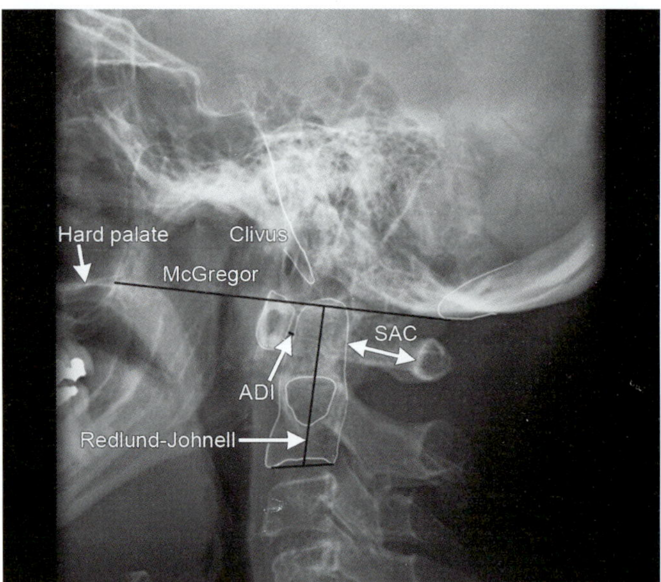

Fig. 55.3: Commonly drawn lines and measurements to assess occipito-C1–C2 relationships. These lines are based on clearly defined cortical landmarks.
Source: Reprinted with permission from Wasserman BR, Moskovich R, Razi AE. Rheumatoid arthritis of the cervical spine: clinical considerations. Bull NYU Hosp Jt Dis. 2011;69(2):136-48.

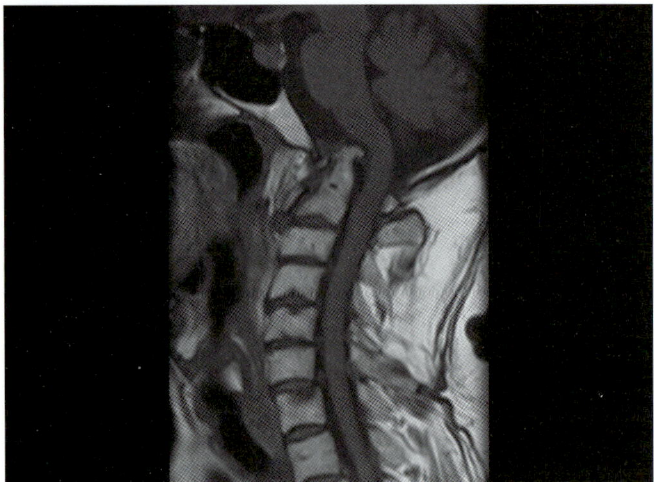

Fig. 55.4: Midline sagittal MRI of a 67-year-old woman with longstanding rheumatoid arthritis. The image demonstrates marked vertical subluxation of the dens. The tip of the dens impinges on the medulla and significantly reduces the functional cervicomedullary angle (normal range: 135° to 175°). The atlantodental interval paradoxically decreases and may fall into the "normal" range.

rheumatic drugs (DMARDs) have the potential to slow or halt progression of cervical spine instability and may also reduce the size of compressive pannus.[27] Symptoms can be managed with nonsteroidal anti-inflammatory drugs (NSAIDs), physical therapy, and a brief course of immobilization. While cervical collars may help with symptoms of neck pain, their use does not stabilize the cervical spine or prevent significant subluxation from occurring. Patients should be monitored with serial imaging, using lateral flexion and extension radiographs every 2–3 years to evaluate for asymptomatic progression. Progression of axial disease parallels peripheral disease activity, so that more frequent follow-up is recommended for this subset of patients. Nonoperative management with routine clinical follow-up is indicated for the majority of RA patients who have mild instability and are neurologically intact. Taking interval radiographs and tracking functional scores may provide a good indicator for operative intervention.

Surgery should be considered for all patients with a neurologic deficit in the presence of cervical instability, as untreated patients have increased rates of morbidity and mortality. Stabilization and/or decompression prevent further neurologic injury and often improve neurologic function. While the majority of patients can expect to improve one Ranawat class after surgery, the potential for improvement is less in more advanced disease. Once patients are Ranawat IIIB, only 20% of patients can be expected to achieve one Ranawat class of improvement.[28] Additionally, patients with more advanced disease and neurologic dysfunction experience much higher rates of postoperative complications, and higher mortality, making surgical intervention less appealing in such situations.[7] Surgical intervention also can be considered for patients who have pain refractory to extensive conservative management.

While numerous radiographic parameters have been proposed as surgical indications, treatment decisions should be made with consideration of the overall functional status of the patient, their physiologic reserve, and their treatment expectations. In the setting of asymptomatic AAS, surgical treatment is recommended if the SAC is < 14 mm. This amount of stenosis takes into account soft-tissue compression in addition to compression from instability. Additional surgical indications for asymptomatic AAS include a cord diameter < 6 mm on the flexion MRI as well as a cervicomedullary angle of 135° or less.[24] Asymptomatic patients with subaxial instability may also be considered for surgical intervention once the SAC becomes <13 mm. In contrast, surgical intervention for superior migration of the odontoid is less well defined in asymptomatic patients, but should be considered to prevent the need for subsequent more complex and dangerous salvage procedures.

SURGICAL OPTIONS

Surgical treatment of the rheumatoid spine is focused on restoring or preserving existing neurologic function by stabilizing the unstable segments and performing selective decompressions as necessary. This can be achieved through both fusion and nonfusion techniques.[30] While a large variety of techniques have been used, the primary goal remains to achieve and maintain stability at the affected levels.

Surgical treatment of AAS requires reduction, if possible, and immobilization of the C1–C2 articulation to achieve subsequent fusion. The atlantoaxial joint is a challenging motion segment to immobilize and fuse, as it is the most mobile spinal segment and largely dependent on soft-tissue restraints. A variety of techniques can be used to stabilize this articulation ranging from traditional wire fixation to more modern screw-based constructs. Brooks and Jenkins described a technique of bilateral sublaminar wire fixation using wires looped around the arch of the axis and the lamina of C2 bilaterally. The wires are then tightened over bilaterally placed wedges of iliac crest autograft positioned over the interlaminar space.[31] Gallie wiring or its modifications utilize a C1 sublaminar wire looped over a single, wide, notched iliac crest autograft and under the C2 spinous process to achieve fixation.[32] The increased risk of a dural tear and neurologic injury due to spinal cord compression engendered by simultaneous C1 and C2 sublaminar wire passage is thus reduced.[33-36] Wire constructs provide limited stability, mostly with respect to rotation and translation.[37] Adjunctive postoperative halo immobilization may be helpful for cases remaining unstable after final wire tightening.

Interlaminar clamp fixation with interposed bone graft provides benefits over wiring techniques. Atlantoaxial union in one study was achieved within 12 weeks in 80% of patients (20/25).[38] The clamp fixation was revised in two patients, with subsequent fusion. Three of 25 patients required revision surgery for nonunion due to loosening of the clamp. Nonunion is more likely to develop in patients with RA, with the pseudarthrosis generally between the posterior bone graft and the ring of C1. Both wire and interlaminar clamp techniques are still utilized, and while they remain good fallback options, they have been largely superseded by more stable, direct atlanto-axial fixation techniques.

The development of direct segmental screw fixation methods provides rigid fixation and increases fusion rates while obviating the need for postoperative halo immobilization. Transarticular C1–C2 screw fixation, described by Grob and Magerl, involves posterior passage of screws through the C2 pars interarticularis, transfixion of the C1–C2 facet joint, and C1 lateral mass screw purchase.[39] Supplementation with posterior Gallie wiring and grafting is necessary to increase flexion-extension stability. Posterior bone grafting is necessary to obtain a fusion. This technique provides rigid fixation[40] with high fusion rates. It is technically demanding and its use may be limited by patient anatomy. The presence of significant cervicothoracic kyphosis may make it very difficult, if not impossible, to line-up and safely advance screws across the C1–C2 facet joints. Additionally, up to 23% of patients have vertebral artery anatomy that precludes the use of this method of fixation.[41] Preoperative multiplanar imaging is essential to determine if a patient's anatomy is a contraindication to the use of transarticular screw fixation. (Figs. 55.5 and 55.6)

Segmental lateral mass fixation of C1 and C2 using the Harms technique involves screw placement into C1 and C2.[42] Screws are placed into the lateral mass of C1 and connected to screws placed into the C2 lamina, pedicle, or pars interarticularis of C2 and connected with rods. Such constructs have the advantage of avoiding injury to the vertebral artery even in patients with aberrant anatomy that precludes the use of transarticular screws.

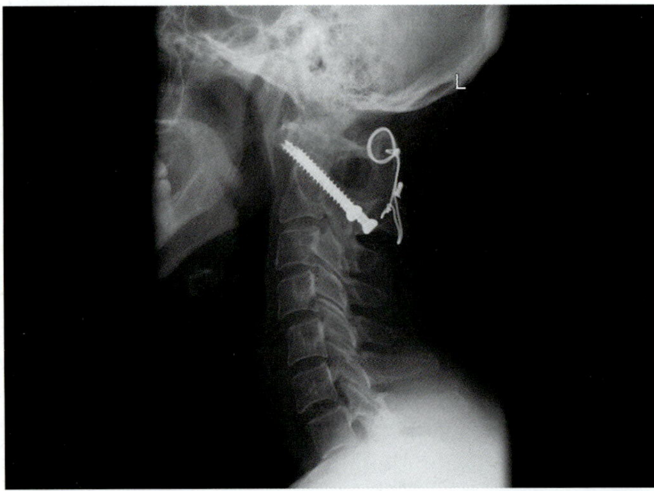

Fig. 55.5: Lateral cervical radiograph of a 55-year-old woman with a C1–C2 fusion. The arthrodesis was performed for rheumatoid atlantoaxial subluxation 9 years prior. There is no radiographic evidence of occipitocervical pathology nor signs of subaxial involvement. *Source:* Reprinted with permission from Wasserman BR, Moskovich R, Razi AE. Rheumatoid arthritis of the cervical spine: clinical considerations. Bull NYU Hosp Jt Dis. 2011;69(2):136-48.

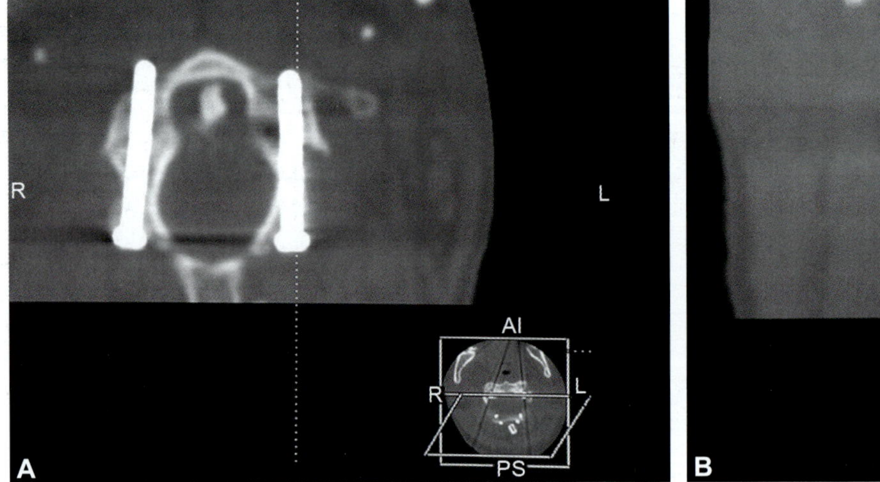

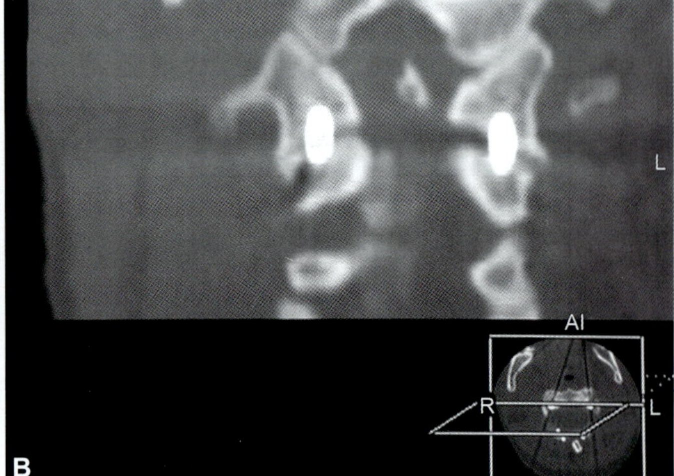

Figs. 55.6A and B: (A) Tilted axial CT reconstruction along the axis of the transarticular screws used for C1–C2 fixation. (B) Coronal reconstruction demonstrating passage of the screws across the C1–C2 facet joints bilaterally. Note that metal-hardening artifact makes the screw diameter appear larger than actual size.

If further C1-C2 reduction is needed beyond that achieved by initial patient positioning, it may be done after screw insertion by placing the rod and using the screws as an anchor to realign the vertebrae. The insertion of the C1 and C2 screws is possible using a relatively small access portal and is relatively independent of the degree of high thoracic kyphosis. Segmental fixation using C1 lateral mass and C2 pedicle screws is biomechanically equivalent to C1-C2 transarticular screw fixation.[43] For patients in whom adequate reduction cannot be achieved, concomitant C1 laminectomy may be required. A posterior C1-C2 arthrodesis using autograft bone should be performed to maximize the reliability of achieving a fusion. In the face of a pseudarthrosis, there is a high likelihood of implant fixation failure.

Surgical intervention for superior migration of the odontoid generally requires reduction of the deformity followed by occipitocervical arthrodesis. Reduction may be achieved using gradual cervical traction; however, this technique is often poorly tolerated by these patients.[44] Occipitocervical fixation using screw-rod systems may permit intraoperative realignment. Screw and rod or plate constructs are biomechanically superior to traditional wire constructs.[45-47] Transoral decompression followed by posterior wiring with a contoured occipitocervical rod has a high success rate in rheumatoid atlantoaxial vertical subluxation, even without bone grafting.[21] Its use, however, has largely been superseded by rigid segmental fixation and fusion techniques with the development of improved implant technology that facilitates reliable fixation in this vulnerable area. If rigid fixation is used it is imperative to achieve a bony fusion, or risk implant failure.

If adequate reduction cannot be obtained and compression persists, patients may require concomitant decompression using either posterior laminectomy and/or anterior decompression by transoral odontoid resection. Resection of the odontoid results in a significant risk of subsequent atlantoaxial instability, and concomitant posterior C1–C2 fusion is usually required to prevent this complication. In patients with mild-to-moderate cord compression from periodontoid pannus, successful posterior arthrodesis without direct decompression often results in spontaneous regression of the pannus.[27,48,49]

Subaxial instability can be managed using a number of techniques including both anterior and posterior procedures. Posterior instrumented arthrodesis is the primary treatment for the majority of patients. Standalone anterior procedures in rheumatoid instability of the subaxial spine may be insufficient to prevent progressive collapse in the face of advanced osteoporosis and deformity (especially kyphosis), and the addition of posterior fixation may improve the outcomes. Properly selected patients may be appropriately treated with anterior discectomy and arthrodesis. Prior to any surgical intervention, the clinician must be vigilant for signs of subtle instability at adjacent levels, as failure to recognize and include these levels in the stabilization may lead to later deterioration and the need for additional surgery. That being said, restoration of good lordotic sagittal alignment of the spine may minimize the risks of adjacent segment disease. Early intervention for C1-C2 and possibly subaxial instability may pre-empt the development of more severe deformity and neurological catastrophe.

REFERENCES

1. Lawrence RC, Helmick CG, Arnett FC, et al. Estimates of the prevalence of arthritis and selected musculoskeletal disorders in the United States. Arthritis Rheum. 1998;41(5):778-99.
2. Rawlins BA, Girardi FP, Boachie-Adjei O. Rheumatoid arthritis of the cervical spine. Rheum Dis Clin N Am. 1998; 24(1):55-65.
3. Pellicci PM, Ranawat CS, Tsairis P, et al. A prospective study of the progression of rheumatoid arthritis of the cervical spine. J Bone Joint Surg Am. 1981; 63(3):342-50.
4. Dreyer SJ, Boden SD. Natural history of rheumatoid arthritis of the cervical spine. Clin Orthop Relat Res. 1999(366):98-106.
5. Nguyen HV, Ludwig SC, Silber J, et al. Rheumatoid arthritis of the cervical spine. Spine J. 2004;4(3):329-34.
6. Lipson SJ. Cervical myelopathy and posterior atlanto-axial subluxation in patients with rheumatoid arthritis. J Bone Joint Surg Am. 1985;67(4):593-7.
7. Reiter MF, Boden SD. Inflammatory disorders of the cervical spine. Spine. 1998;23(24):2755-66.
8. Fujiwara K, Owaki H, Fujimoto M, et al. A long-term fol low-up study of cervical lesions in rheumatoid arthritis. J Spinal Disord. 2000;13(6):519-26.
9. Casey AT, Crockard HA, Geddes JF, et al. Vertical translocation: the enigma of the disappearing atlantodens interval in patients with myelopathy and rheumatoid arthritis. Part I. Clinical, radiological, and neuropathological features. J Neurosurg. 1997;87(6):856-62.
10. Collins DN, Barnes CL, FitzRandolph RL. Cervical spine instability in rheumatoid patients having total hip or knee arthroplasty. Clin Orthop Relat Res. 1991(272):127-35.
11. van Asselt KM, Lems WF, Bongartz EB, et al. Outcome of cervical spine surgery in patients with rheumatoid arthritis. Ann Rheum Dis. 2001;60(5):448-52.
12. Paus AC, Steen H, Roislien J, et al. High mortality rate in rheumatoid arthritis with subluxation of the cervical spine: a cohort study of operated and nonoperated patients. Spine. 2008;33(21):2278-83.
13. Ranawat CS, O'Leary P, Pellicci P, et al. Cervical spine fusion in rheumatoid arthritis. J Bone Joint Surg. American volume 1979;61(7):1003-10.
14. Steinbrocker O, Traeger CH, Batterman RC. Therapeutic criteria in rheumatoid arthritis. J Am Med Assoc. 1949; 140(8):659-62.
15. Boden SD, Dodge LD, Bohlman HH, et al. Rheumatoid arthritis of the cervical spine. A long-term analysis with predictors of paralysis and recovery. J Bone Joint Surg. American volume 1993;75(9):1282-97.
16. McGregor M. The significance of certain measurements of the skull in the diagnosis of basilar impression. Br J Radiol. 1948.
17. McRae DL, Barnum AS. Occipitalization of the atlas. Am J Roentgenol Radium Ther Nucl Med. 1953;70(1):23-46.
18. Chamberlain W. Basilar impression (platybasia). A bizarre developmental anomaly of the occipital bone and the upper cervical spine with striking and misleading neurologic manifestations. Yale J Biol Med. 1939; 11(5)487-96.
19. Wackenheim A. Disostosi chiro-lombare. Disostosi stenotica del canale vertebrale e brachichiria. Radiologia Medica. 1979;65(1-2):21-6. [Italian]
20. Fischgold H, Metzger J. Etude radiotomographique de l'impression basilaire. Rev Rheum Mal Osteoartic. 1952; 19:261-8. [French]
21. Redlund-Johnell I, Pettersson H. Radiographic measurements of the cranio-vertebral region. Designed for evaluation of abnormalities in rheumatoid arthritis. Acta Radiol Diagn (Stockh). 1984;25(1):23-8.
22. Clark CR, Goetz DD, Menezes AH. Arthrodesis of the cervical spine in rheumatoid arthritis. J Bone Joint Surg. American volume 1989;71(3):381-92.
23. Riew KD, Hilibrand AS, Palumbo MA, et al. Diagnosing basilar invagination in the rheumatoid patient. The reliability of radiographic criteria. J Bone Joint Surg. American volume 2001;83-A(2):194-200.

24. Dvorak J, Grob D, Baumgartner H, et al. Functional evaluation of the spinal cord by magnetic resonance imaging in patients with rheumatoid arthritis and instability of upper cervical spine. Spine. 1989;14(10):1057-64.
25. Bundschuh C, Modic MT, Kearney F, et al. Rheumatoid arthritis of the cervical spine: surface-coil MR imaging. AJR. 1988;151(1):181-7.
26. Allmann KH, Uhl M, Uhrmeister P, et al. Functional MR imaging of the cervical spine in patients with rheumatoid arthritis. Acta Radiol. 1998;39(5):543-6.
27. Yamaguchi I, Shibuya S, Arima N, et al. Remarkable reduction or disappearance of retroodontoid pseudotumors after occipitocervical fusion. Report of three cases. J Neurosurg Spine. 2006;5(2):156-60.
28. Peppelman WC, Kraus DR, Donaldson WF, 3rd, et al. Cervical spine surgery in rheumatoid arthritis: improvement of neurologic deficit after cervical spine fusion. Spine. 1993;18 (16):2375-9.
29. Casey AT, Crockard HA, Stevens J. Vertical translocation. Part II. Outcomes after surgical treatment of rheumatoid cervical myelopathy. J Neurosurg. 1997;87(6):863-9.
30. Moskovich R, Crockard HA, Shott S, et al. Occipitocervical stabilization for myelopathy in patients with rheumatoid arthritis. Implications of not bone-grafting. J Bone Joint Surg. American volume 2000;82(3):349-65.
31. Brooks AL, Jenkins EB. Atlanto-axial arthrodesis by the wedge compression method. J Bone Joint Surg. American volume 1978;60(3):279-84.
32. Dickman CA, Sonntag VK, Papadopoulos SM, et al. The interspinous method of posterior atlantoaxial arthrodesis. J Neurosurg. 1991;74(2):190-8.
33. Lundy DW, Murray HH. Neurological deterioration after posterior wiring of the cervical spine. J Bone Joint Surg. British volume 1997;79(6):948-51.
34. Smith MD, Phillips WA, Hensinger RN. Complications of fusion to the upper cervical spine. Spine. 1991;16(7):702-5.
35. Sudo H, Abumi K, Ito M, et al. Spinal cord compression by multistrand cables after solid posterior atlantoaxial fusion. Report of three cases. J Neurosurg. 2002;97(3 Suppl):359-61.
36. Geremia GK, Kim KS, Cerullo L, et al. Complications of sublaminar wiring. Surg Neurol. 1985;23(6):629-35.
37. Dickman CA, Crawford NR, Paramore CG. Biomechanical characteristics of C1-2 cable fixations. J Neurosurg. 1996; 85(2):316-22.
38. Moskovich R, Crockard HA. Atlantoaxial arthrodesis using interlaminar clamps. An improved technique. Spine. 1992; 17(3):261-7.
39. Grob D, Magerl F. [Surgical stabilization of C1 and C2 fractures]. Der Orthopade. 1987;16(1):46-54. [German]
40. Richter M, Schmidt R, Claes L, et al. Posterior atlantoaxial fixation: biomechanical in vitro comparison of six different techniques. Spine. 2002;27(16):1724-32.
41. Paramore CG, Dickman CA, Sonntag VK. The anatomical suitability of the C1-2 complex for transarticular screw fixation. J Neurosurg. 1996;85(2):221-4.
42. Harms J, Biederman L, Matthis W. The direct posterior C1/ C2 fusion as an alternative to the Magerl technique. Poster presented at: Cervical Spine Research Society, Twenty-Seventh Annual Meeting, Seattle, Washington December 16-18, 1999.
43. Melcher RP, Puttlitz CM, Kleinstueck FS, et al. Biomechanical testing of posterior atlantoaxial fixation techniques. Spine. 2002;27(22):2435-40.
44. Kolen ER, Schmidt MH. Rheumatoid arthritis of the cervical spine. Semin Neurol. 2002;22(2):179-86.
45. Abumi K, Takada T, Shono Y, et al. Posterior occipitocervical reconstruction using cervical pedicle screws and plate-rod systems. Spine. 1999;24(14):1425-34.
46. Sandhu FA, Pait TG, Benzel E, et al. Occipitocervical fusion for rheumatoid arthritis using the inside-outside stabilization technique. Spine. 2003;28(4):414-9.
47. Sutterlin CE, 3rd, Bianchi JR, Kunz DN, et al. Biomechanical evaluation of occipitocervical fixation devices. J Spinal Disord. 2001;14(3):185-92.
48. Grob D, Wursch R, Grauer W, et al. Atlantoaxial fusion and retrodental pannus in rheumatoid arthritis. Spine. 1997;22 (14):1580-3; discussion, 1584.
49. Goel A, Dange N. Immediate postoperative regression of retroodontoid pannus after lateral mass reconstruction in a patient with rheumatoid disease of the craniovertebral junction. Case report. J Neurosurg Spine. 2008;9(3):273-6.
50. Wasserman BR, Moskovich R, Razi AE. Rheumatoid arthritis of the cervical spine: clinical considerations. Bull NYU Hosp Jt Dis. 2011;69(2):136-48.

CHAPTER

56

Traumatic Cervical Spinal Fracture Surgery

Justin C Paul, Robert Norton, Themistocles Protopsaltis

INTRODUCTION

Vertebral fractures are common events, with >50,000 fractures occurring annually in the United States.[1] As the spine is a complex structure with many motion segments, alignment and stability are important clinical variables to consider. Although the integrity of bony and ligamentous structures must be determined, evaluating potential injury to the spinal cord and nerve roots is a priority. Traumatic injuries to the spine are a heterogeneous group with many treatment options ranging from activity modification, bracing with orthoses, and operative fixation through instrumentation. Such treatment heterogeneity precludes simple classification of a broad range of injuries. Thus, spine injuries are most easily divided by anatomical location, differentiating cervical, and thoracolumbar/sacral injuries. This chapter will detail cervical injuries and thoracolumbar/sacral injuries shall be discussed in Chapter 57.

Historically, conservative treatment of spine injuries often required long periods of immobilization with traction, which presented the risk of pneumonia, deep vein thrombosis, and decubitus ulceration. Spine surgery in the trauma setting has historically been associated with high mortality, although surgical decompression has been recorded by Paulus of Aegina dating as far back as the seventh century.[2] In 1646, the first documented open reduction in a spinal fracture was documented by Fabricius Hildanus.[2-7]

Surgical techniques were not universally accepted until the 1950s with the introduction of spinal instrumentation.[8] The stable environment provided by instrumentation enhanced bony fusion and offered earlier mobility, decreased complications from immobilization, and reduced risk for neurologic compromise from spinal instability.

CERVICAL SPINE

Approximately 40% of cervical spine trauma will have some neurological deficit, as opposed to 15–20% in thoracolumbar trauma. Spinal cord injury (SCI) has an incidence of 4.0–5.3 per 100,000, which has remained relatively unchanged over time according to previous estimates. Males have about four times higher incidence. Major causes include motor vehicle accidents (MVAs), accounting for about 45% of events. These occur primarily in the younger population, while falls in the older population account for 20%. Sports and violence are other major contributors.[9-11]

Age is an important consideration in cervical trauma. Adults constitute a much larger proportion of the cervical spine injury with only 2% of all spine traumas occurring in children or adolescents.[12] Level of injury also depends on age as children <8 years of age often present with fractures to C1, C2, or the occiput, while adults often have fractures lower than C3. There is higher risk of neurologic injury in children due to their relatively larger head, less muscular control, weaker ligaments, and more horizontally oriented facets (allowing more flexion and extension). They are vulnerable to spinal cord injury without radiographic abnormalities (SCIWRA).[13]

Anatomy and Mechanism of Injury

The mechanism of injury typically involves forced flexion or extension from unrestrained deceleration forces. These forces frequently produce some component of distraction or axial compression. Anatomic constraints limiting hyperflexion and distraction in flexion include the posterior longitudinal ligament (PLL), the ligamentum flavum, and the facet capsule. Constraints limiting hyperextension and distraction in extension include the anterior longitudinal ligament (ALL), the anterior annulus, and spinous process impingement (Fig. 56.1). Compressive loads are primarily borne by the intervertebral (IV) disk, the vertebral body, and the neural arch. The vertebral body and disk complex share approximately equal load through paired articular pillars.[14]

As articulations of the occiput, the atlas and axis are anatomically quite different from the remaining vertebrae. Grossly, they are ring structures with an anterior and posterior arch connected by lateral masses. The atlas revolves around the atlas and accounts for approximately 40% of total cervical flexion and extension and 60% of cervical rotation. Important stabilizers of these atypical vertebrae include the tectorial membrane, the cruciform ligament, and apical alar ligaments. The lower cervical vertebrae C3–C7 facilitate rotation through obliquely oriented facets. Rotation is coupled with ipsilateral bending. The uncovertebral joints are involved in this coupled motion guiding controlled translation with cervical flexion.

Initial Evaluation and Management

All blunt trauma patients should be placed in cervical spine immobilization in the field by emergency medical services (EMS). Immediate control of cervical motion involves immobilizing the neck in a rigid collar. Upon arrival to the hospital the patient should be processed via the standard ATLS trauma protocol with attention to airway, breathing, circulation, disability, and exposure (ABCDE). The head-tilt–chin-lift maneuver should be avoided and resuscitative measures to prevent hypoxia, and hypotension must be initiated immediately. The goals of spinal immobilization are to provide spinal stability and protect the spinal cord. Rigid cervical collar and sandbags or supportive blocks with a backboard/ straps are most effective in limiting motion of the cervical spine.[15] The pediatric patient sustaining cervical trauma, with a relatively large head circumference, less muscle control, and protective reflexes should inspire caution with positioning.[13] Ideal backboards have the head recessed to accommodate the head size to prevent relative flexion of the cervical spine.

The trauma patient should be treated with the assumption that the spine is unstable until proven otherwise.

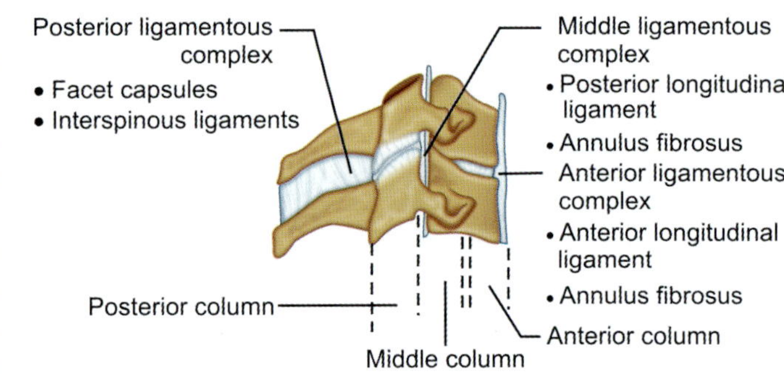

Fig. 56.1: Static and dynamic stabilizers of the cervical spine.

While addressing life-threatening injuries, trauma staff should not neglect maintaining rigid cervical immobilization. Rigid cervical orthoses provide stability in the coronal, sagittal, and axial planes. The collar secondarily provides a reminder to caregivers that the patient has a significant cervical spine injury.

Despite the need for careful attention to detail, cervical trauma often requires rapid measures of care since 18% of blunt trauma patients with proven cervical spine injuries required emergency intubation within 30 minutes of arrival to the emergency department.[16] As the airway is of prime importance, the cervical spine care is potentially overlooked. Traction for the sake of airway control can be dangerous as oral intubation of patients with unstable fractures showed axial traction resulted in significant distraction and even posterior subluxation at the fracture site.[17] A cadaver study further demonstrated manual stabilization is preferred over traction to avoid increased distraction forces.[18] Orotracheal intubation with manual in-line stabilization (MILS) has shown reduced motion compared with collar for intubation and overall safety is improved.[19]

When appropriate, cervical traction is accomplished with a variety of devices. Gardner-Wells tongs are available in many centers and should be applied carefully. Pins are placed one finger's width above the pinna of the ear in line with the external auditory meatus. For reducing facet dislocations, a slight anterior displacement will apply an extension force, whereas posterior displacement will apply a flexion force.

Steroid use is not effective for pure root lesions, but has been used extensively for cord injury. Steroids are historically believed to counteract the secondary inflammatory events of SCI. While the efficacy of SCI steroid protocols remain controversial, they are considered by many centers to be the standard of care.[20-24]

Methylprednisolone is typically administered with a 30 mg/kg bolus, then 5.4 mg/kg/h for 23–48 hours. It should be noted that there is minimal benefit from steroids if started > 8 hours after injury.[25]

When the patient is stabilized and lifesaving treatments have been initiated, proper evaluation of spine trauma includes a thorough physical and neurologic examination. Sensation (light touch and pinprick) and motor function should be assessed in all myotomes and dermatomes with careful attention to other injuries to the extremities. A rectal examination to test for perianal sensation, resting tone, and the bulbocavernosus reflex is essential (Figs. 56.2A and B). Non-intoxicated patients without symptoms of neck pain, paresthesias, weakness, or distraction injuries may be cleared of cervical injury with a normal examination. Importantly, these patients must demonstrate full range of motion of the cervical spine without pain.[26]

Radiologic Evaluation

Plain radiographs obtained on arrival to the emergency department constitute the first-line radiologic assessment. Radiographs must be obtained on all high-risk patients, such as those involved in high-velocity MVA or fall > 10 feet, or who present with a closed head injury, neurologic deficit, or pelvic and extremity fractures. Anteroposterior, lateral, and open mouth odontoid (OMO) views are obtained with careful attention to visualize from the occiput to first thoracic vertebrae T1 in order to evaluate the cervicothoracic junction (Figs. 56.3A to C). A swimmer's view can be used to better visualize this area if needed. Films should be inspected for subtle abnormalities such as soft tissue swelling, hypolordosis, disk-space narrowing or widening, and widening of the interspinous distances.

The lateral X-ray is indispensable for cervical spine evaluation. The anterior vertebral margin, posterior vertebral margin, spinolaminar junction (or Swischuk's) lines should be inspected for stepoffs. Also, the anterior atlantodental space should be measured with the normal value 2.5–3 mm in adults and up to 4.5 mm for pediatric patients.

Several radiographic evaluations exist for high-cervical injuries at the atlanto-occipital joint (Fig. 56.4). The Chamberlain line is drawn from the posterior margin of foramen magnum (opisthion) to the dorsal posterior margin of the hard palate. The odontoid should not be >3 mm above this line. McRae line is drawn across the foramen magnum from the anterior margin (basion) to the opisthion. The odontoid should be beneath this line and a perpendicular line at apex of odontoid normally intersects in ventral quarter of McRae line. The McGregor line drawn from the most caudal aspect of the occiput to the hard palate should cross the odontoid with <4.5 mm extending above. The power ratio can be used to detect anterior subluxation and should be less than one. Lines are drawn from basion to the midvertical portion of posterior laminar line of the atlas and from the opisthion to the midcervical portion of the posterior surface of the anterior atlas.

Many radiographic lines have been documented with varying degrees of sensitivity for cervical injury and these forms of evaluation can be difficult with inferior films or obscurities from the collar and other equipment. Therefore, a more reasonable approach may be to confirm that occipital condyles rest congruently in the C1 fossae and

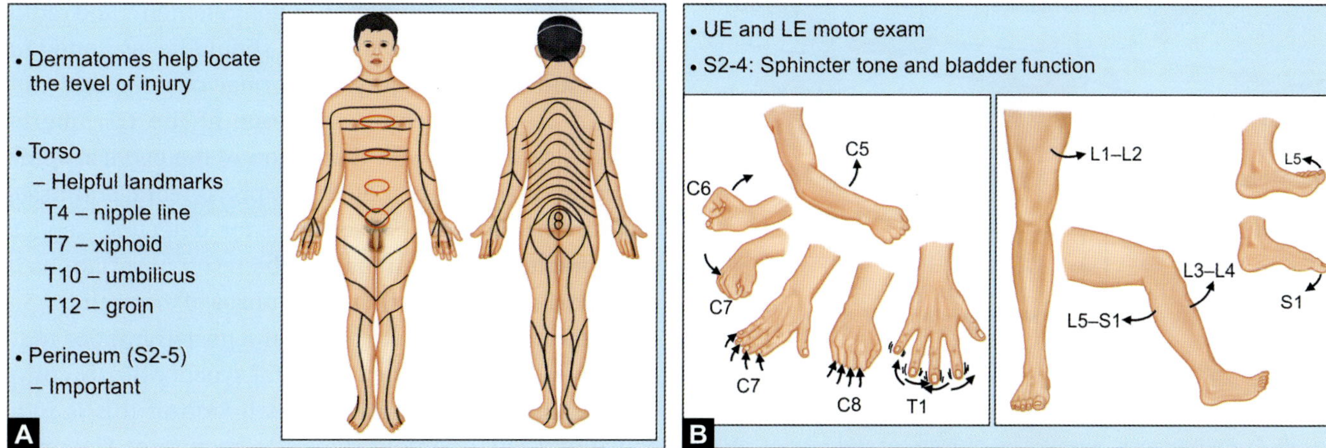

Figs. 56.2A and B: Sensory and motor examination. The dermatomes outlined in (A) are shown in detail in Figure 56.24.

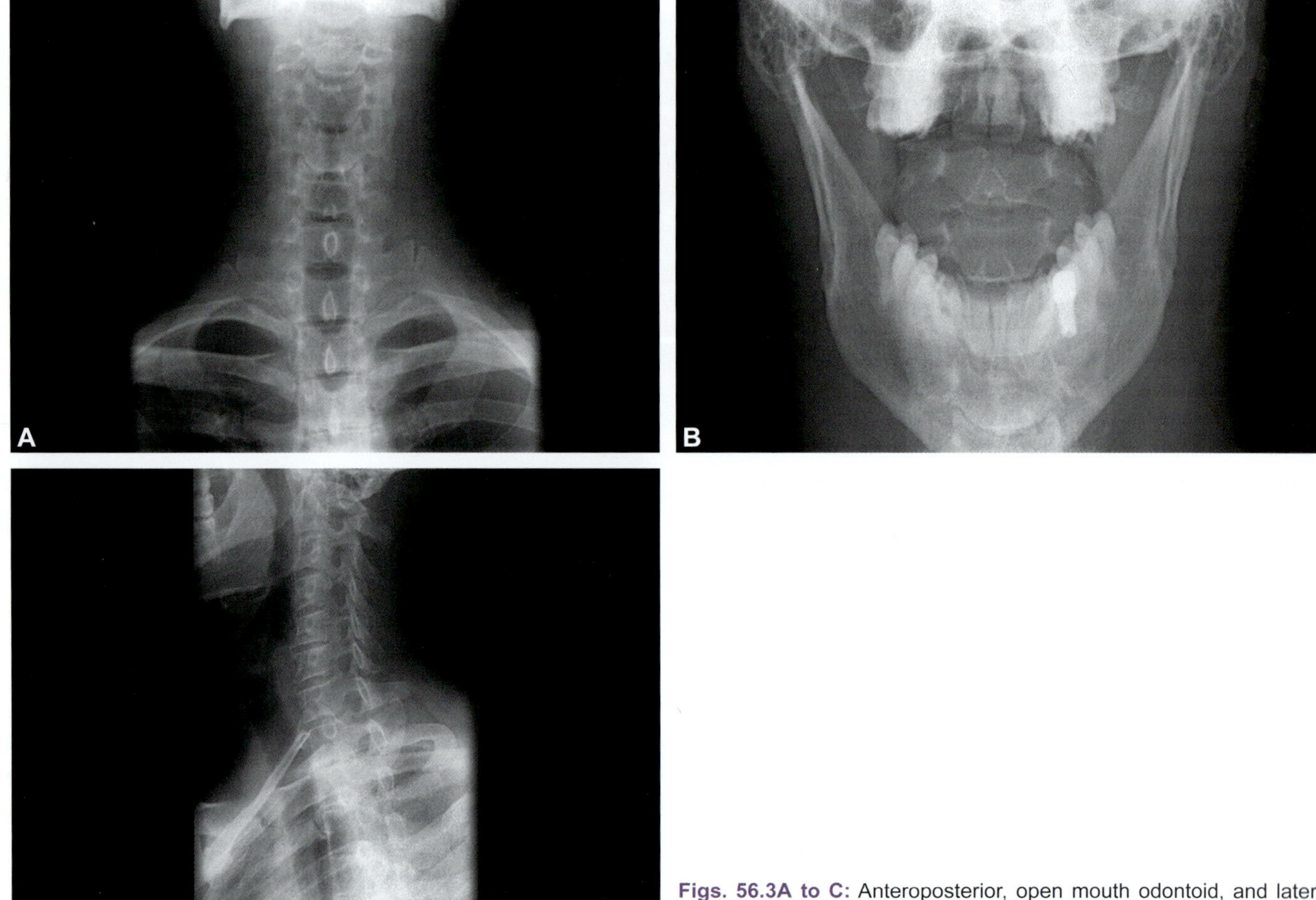

Figs. 56.3A to C: Anteroposterior, open mouth odontoid, and lateral views of the cervical spine (Wiki Commons).

Fig. 56.4: Radiographic evaluations of high-cervical injuries at the atlanto-occipital joint.

that the proper alignment of the foramen magnum and C1 spinolaminar line. Atlanto-occipital injury can be detected by a basion-dens distance >10 mm with a sensitivity of 50% or with a C2 body "posterior axial line" >12 mm from the basion with a sensitivity of 76–100%.

In addition to examination of bony elements and radiographic measurements, the films should be evaluated for soft tissue signs of injury. Abnormal contour and fullness of the prevertebral soft tissue at the C1 anterior arch are associated with disruption of the cervical spine. However, it should be noted that prevertebral soft tissue measurements are 64% sensitive for detecting cervical spine fractures,[27] which may be the result of variations in head position, body habitus, and phase of inspiration.

The Harris composite ring in the posteroinferior margin represents the C2 neurocentral synchondrosis cortex and foramen transversarium. Disruption of this is indicative of a low odontoid (type III) fracture or Hangman fracture (fracture of both pedicles or pars interarticularis of the axis vertebra). The OMO view is best to identify a C1 burst fracture (Jefferson fracture), odontoid fractures, and lateral flexion fractures of the axis. A single lateral radiograph is sensitive up to 74–86% for cervical spine injury, and with the added OMO view approaches 100%.[28] Despite this high degree of sensitivity, cervical spine computed tomography (CT) has become routine in many trauma centers for the evaluation of the stable patient with multiple blunt trauma cervical spine due to its fast acquisition and processing.

High-resolution CT scans with sagittal and coronal reformats (Fig. 56.5) enhance detection of minimally displaced fractures and retropulsed fragments. CT also shows the orientation of fractures and allows the detection of otherwise occult injury. Thus, a three-view cervical spine series can have a negative predictive value (NPV) of over 99% for spine fractures.

While CT and radiographs demonstrate excellent accuracy for osseous injury, soft tissue instability can cause catastrophic neurologic injury left untreated. This includes damage to ligamentous stabilizers, facets, capsules, and disks. Therefore, these must be evaluated even in the neurologically intact patient in the high risk or obtunded patient. The NPV of plain radiographs with normal flexion-extension radiographs is over 99%. However, the utility of flexion-extension radiographs for ligamentous integrity in awake patients is subject to controversy as pain and neck spasms may complicate the interpretation. Passive flexion-extension fluoroscopy in the anesthetized patient can risk neurologic embarrassment from iatrogenic SCI from disk herniation/epidural hematoma.[29]

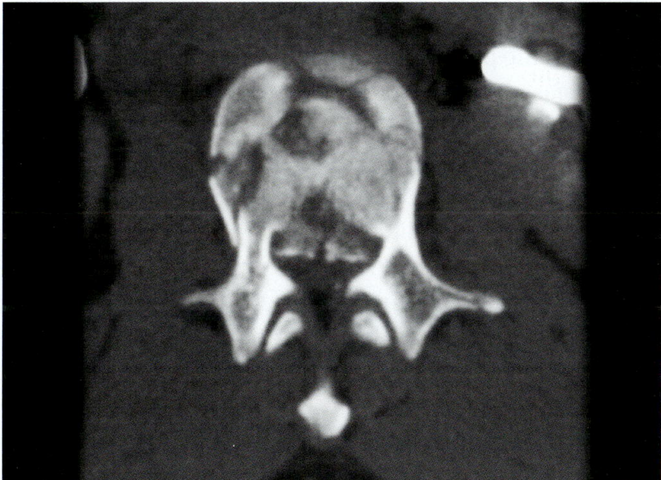

Fig. 56.5: High-resolution CT scan in axial plane showing burst fracture with compression of canal.

Magnetic resonance imaging (MRI) has the highest sensitivity for soft tissue injury as it is highlighted for the ability to assess epidural space for hematoma, bone fragments, disk, and osteophytes. Lack of radiation or contrast minimizes risk, and it is the best modality to inspect the cord for edema, hemorrhage, or laceration. Depending on the quality of the image, prognostic information for SCI may be interpreted. If arterial damage is suspected, magnetic resonance angiography (MRA) is available to identify blood flow defects.

The T1 sequence (Fig. 56.6A) outlines the basic anatomy. The cerebrospinal fluid (CSF) appears dark, the cord has intermediate signal, and the bright disk and prevertebral fat help outline the low signal ALL and anterior annulus. Ligamentum flavum is outlined well but CSF obscures the PLL and posterior annulus. The T2 sequence (Fig. 56.6B) emphasizes cord pathology and shows ligamentous disruption. The cord is intermediate signal and the CSF is bright forming a clear outline of the PLL, annulus, and ligamentum. A sagittal gradient echo (GE) (Fig. 56.6C) shows hemorrhage, and distinguishes osteophytes from disk material. The fat signal is reduced so vertebral bodies are darker, while disks and CSF remain bright for better visualization of the annulus and PLL. Clinicians should make use of a powerful diagnostic modality with MRA screening of the vertebral arteries for all patients with blunt cervical spine trauma >1 cm with a major dislocation or subluxation, fracture of the foramen transversarium, or neurologic deficits consistent with vertebral vessel insufficiency.[30] On a T1-weighted image, the flowing blood is dark (signal void) and bright on GE.

Limitations of MRI include the availability of the magnet and the time required to acquire the study. Also, the obtunded patient cannot answer questions about implanted or hidden metal, which could be hazardous to the patient and staff. The MRI may also be oversensitive for acute soft tissue injury as incidence of inconsequential abnormalities is reported as 25–40%.

The decision to order an MRI should be guided by clinical suspicion for SCI, occult vascular injury, hematoma, ligament tear, or disk herniation/extrusion.[31] In cervical trauma patients with clinical cord or root injury with negative radiographs and CT, MRI is the next step. Obtaining MRI before reduction in a facet subluxation or dislocation may be considered, but this is controversial as many of these herniations will not worsen canal compromise and delay of treatment is not recommended.[32]

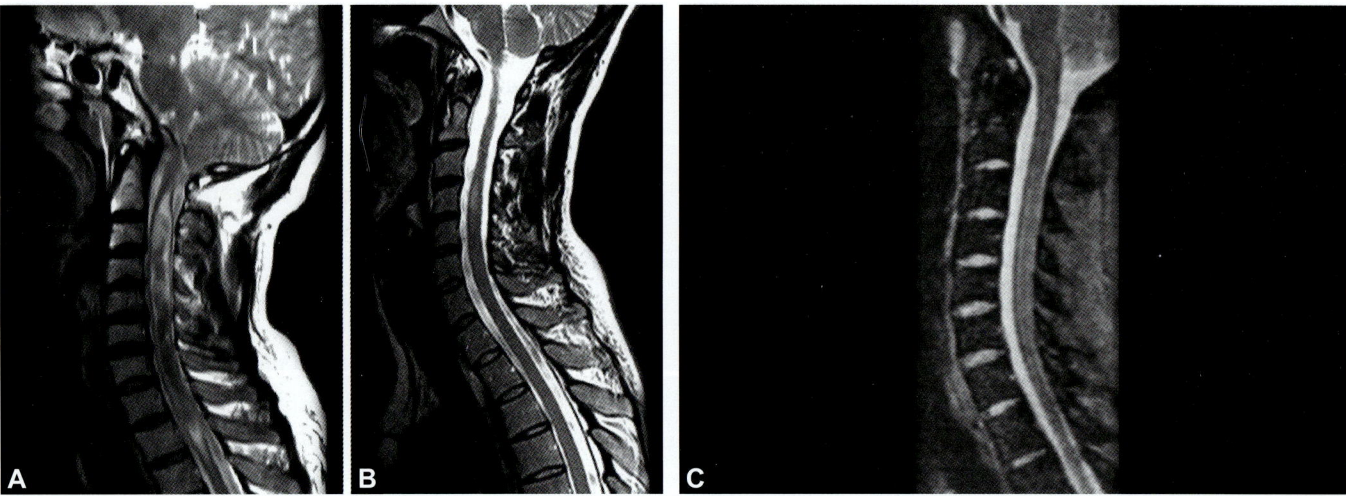

Figs. 56.6A to C: (A) Sagittal T1 is an excellent sequence for basic anatomy. The cerebrospinal fluid (CSF) is dark, the cord is intermediate signal, and the bright disk and prevertebral fat help outline anterior longitudinal ligament/anterior annulus that is low signal. The ligamentum is outlined well but the posterior longitudinal ligament (PLL)/posterior annulus can be obscured by CSF. (B) Sagittal T2 emphasizes cord and ligamentous pathology. The CSF is bright, the cord is intermediate, and vertebral bodies are less dark than T1 with less contrast to the disk. The PLL/annulus is dark and outlined by disk and CSF. The ligamentum is dark outlined by CSF. (C) Sagittal gradient echo provides detailed information on hemorrhage, osteophytes, and extrusion of disk material. The fat signal is reduced so vertebral bodies appear darker. The intervertebral disk and CSF are bright for better visualization of dark annulus/PLL and the cord is well seen as intermediate signal.

Patients can be divided into four major groups for guiding radiologic workup. First, the alert, awake patient without neurologic findings but with neck pain should have the standard radiographs (with OMO view for increased diagnostic yield). In light of equivocal studies, one must be conscious of a possibly reduced dislocation/subluxation. Flexion-extension views of the cervical spine may be considered. Second, the patient with an unreliable examination (obtunded, unconscious, or distracted from polytrauma) is the most difficult to diagnose. Radiographs are obligatory but may be adequate without further imaging if concomitant life-threatening injuries are to be treated. Although it is seldom performed, limited physiologic stress may be reproduced with a radiographic series obtained while erect.

Third, the question of when to forego radiographs is considered. No films are necessary in a nonintoxicated, neurologically intact patient with full painless range of motion who is able to follow complex commands and responds immediately. Any cervical tenderness or intoxication is an indication for films.[28] Lastly, children should be evaluated as a distinct demographic. Important considerations in the pediatric population take into account normal variants. The C2–C3 vertebrae may translate up to 3 mm, which is termed "pseudosubluxation". The atlantodens interval normally measures ≤ 4.5 mm in children, compared with 3 mm in adults. The synchondrosis between the cranial tip of the dens and body (often called a physis) closes between ages 3 and 6 years, which should not be mistaken for a fracture. The vertebral bodies below C2 are wedge-shaped until approximately age 8 years, lest they be mistaken for compression fracture.

CLASSIFICATION

In order to classify spine fractures and dislocations, a two-column theory of spinal stability was proposed by Holdsworth in 1970 (Fig. 56.7). This identified the anterior column as the biomechanical support for compression forces and the posterior column for resistance to tension.[33] The increased used of CT in the 1970s and 80s drew attention to fracture comminution and canal encroachment. Francis Denis then proposed a method to classify spine injury based on a three-column theory in 1983 to include a middle column delineated by the midvertebral body anteriorly and posteriorly by the posterior wall of the vertebral body, PLL, and the posterior annulus fibrosis.[34] The classification included compression type fractures, burst fractures, seat-belt injuries, and fracture-dislocations with graded instability based on mechanical and neurologic components.

More practical methods of classification begin descriptively with the specific vertebrae and continue classifying by fracture pattern. With high-cervical injury involving the base of the occiput, C1, and C2, several classification systems are employed depending on the fracture type and pattern.

Occipital Condyle and Atlanto-occipital Dissociation

Occipital condyle fractures are rare, occurring in <3% of head and neck trauma, are the result of high-energy trauma involving the head.[35,36] Skull base fractures and other high-cervical injuries may be present in these cases. Plain radiography often misses these injuries, but CT scan is highly effective for diagnosis. First classified by Anderson and Montesano[37] into type I, which is comminuted due to axial compression; type II with extension into the basilar skull; and type III with occipital condyle avulsion (Fig. 56.8). The type III avulsion is likely from the rotational force, where the condyle remains attached to the alar ligament. With any occipital condyle fracture, a high degree of vigilance is necessary. Occipitocervical dislocation or atlanto-occipital dissociation (AOD) must be ruled out as this has historically been a fatal injury through the associated intracranial injury as well as vertebral artery injuries, although recent advances in early recognition and stabilization have improved the mortality. The significance of this rare injury inspired several different methods of evaluating the joint radiographically using key landmarks such as the basion and dens: the Powers ratio[38] Harris measurements and the Rule of Twelve[39,40] Lee's lines (X-line method)[41] and the Dublin method (distance from the posterior mandible to the dens).[42]

C1 (Atlas) Ring

Fractures of the atlas can be through the anterior or posterior arches, the lateral masses. Bilateral burst fractures of the C1 ring with anterior, posterior, and lateral fracture lines are called ''Jefferson fractures'', often due to axial load (Fig. 56.9). The lateral mass displacement is an indicator of disruption of the transverse ligament, an important stabilizer. More than 7 mm suggests disruption of this ligament. There is adequate space for the cord so neurologic compromise is rare especially with the decompressive effect of this fracture.

C2 (Axis)

Traumatic spondylolisthesis of C2 results from bilateral pars fractures and is commonly referred to as the ''Hangman fracture'' (Fig. 56.10). This results from severe hyperextension, compression, and rebound flexion. Both the Francis and Effendi classifications use fracture displacement (<3.5 mm) and angulation (<11°) to decide on operative intervention. Similarly the system of Levine

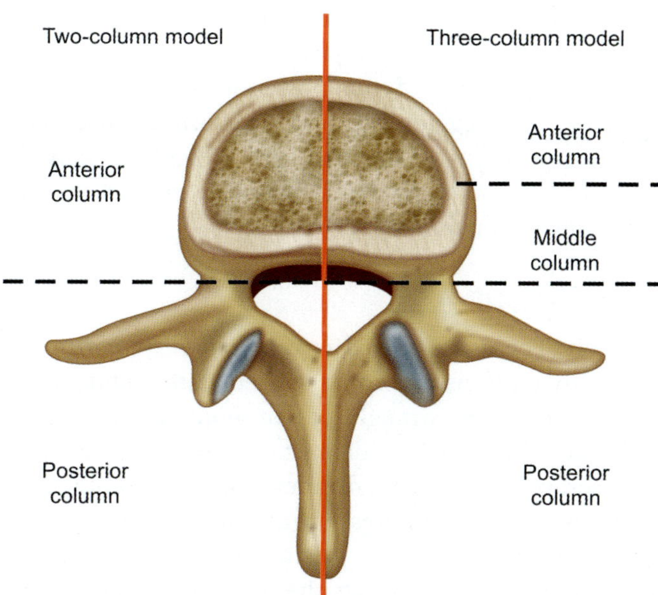

Fig. 56.7: Two- and three-column models used to classify instability of spinal injuries.

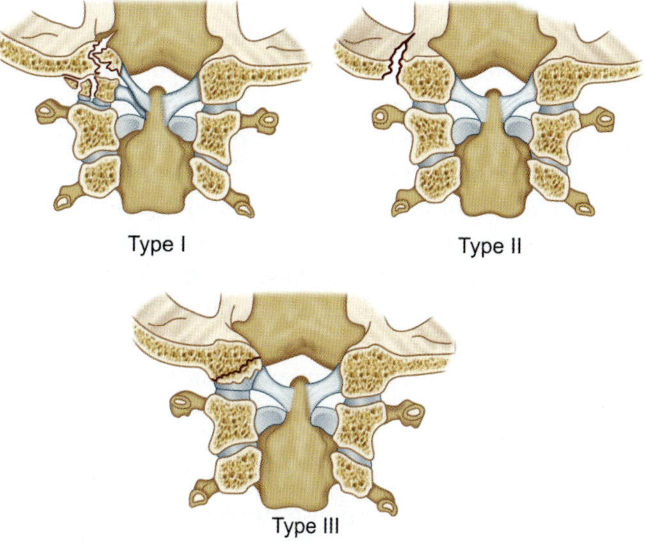

Fig. 56.8: Anderson and Montesano classification of occipital condyle fractures. Type I results from axial loading. Type II extends from a basilar cranial fracture. Type III can result from a combination of bending and rotation forces with condyle avulsion.

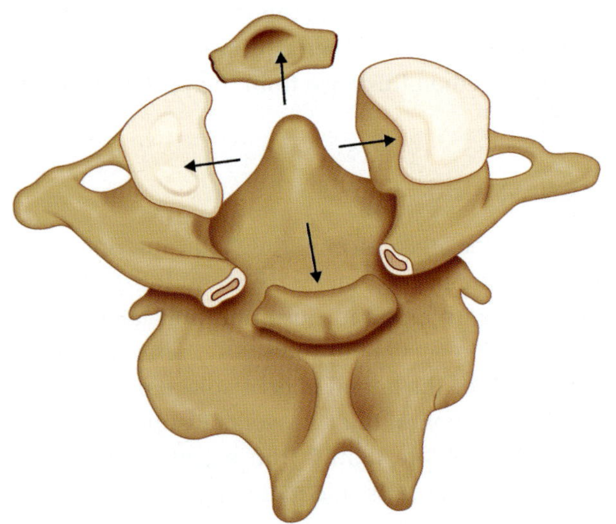

Fig. 56.9: Jefferson fracture.

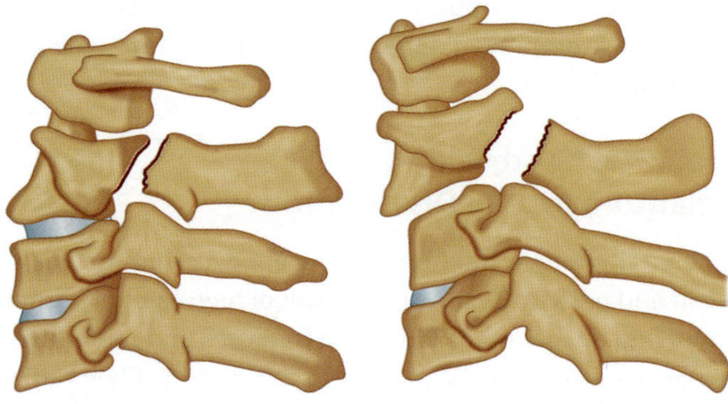

Fig. 56.10: Hangman fracture.

and Edwards outlines three types: type I is an injury with acceptable displacement and without flexion. Type II shows unacceptable displacement and flexion, while type IIa is flexion without translation. The rare type III is similar to type I but with bilateral facet dislocation.[43,44] Type II is the most common type and produces a highly unstable pattern due to disk and PLL disruption. Type IIa is inherently unstable with a more oblique fracture line producing more angulation than translation. One must avoid traction in the type IIa for fear of displacement.

As a relatively large process emanating from the anterior portion of the C2 ring, the odontoid (dens) may be fractured with bending forces. The Anderson classification grades injuries to the C2 odontoid typed one through three based on anatomic fracture level: type I is a tip avulsion, type II is a waist fracture, and type III is a fracture extending to the C2 vertebral body.[45] Type I fractures are very rare avulsion fractures at the apical ligament attachment. Notably, type II is the most common at the intersection with the body but is considered not to extend to the articulating portions of C2. Authors have proposed a subclassification of type II waist fractures accounting for fracture line orientation in addition to displacement and comminution. This is due to the variable methods of surgical fixation.[46]

As a final note on C2 fractures, the benign avulsion fracture of the small portion of the anteroinferior vertebral body is termed an "extension teardrop" fracture. This should not be confused with the flexion-compression teardrop fracture in the subaxial spine, which represents more significant injury.

Cervical Compression and Burst

The subaxial spine can be injured with anterior column compression or burst fractures, isolated posterior element injuries, and fracture-dislocations of the articulating facets. Compression fractures that maintain and intact the posterior wall of the vertebral body, the PLL and posterior elements are generally benign. However, the injury is called a compression burst fracture when axial loading produces compressive failure of the posterior barrier to bony retropulsion. These are unstable and commonly associated with SCI. The compression-flexion "teardrop" injury produces a characteristic pattern of injury with a large triangular bony fragment off the anteroinferior aspect of the vertebral body (Fig. 56.11). The severity of injury is variable depending on canal compromise from retrolisthesis of the vertebral body and retropulsion of fragments. The degree of injury is the sum of the combined tensile failure of the posterior osteoligamentous complex and degree of kyphotic deformity. Radiographic features are widespread and difficult to classify. Therefore, decision making is based on clinical presentation and estimation of stability.

Facet Disruption

Allen and Ferguson devised a classification system grouping injury patterns according to their static radiographic appearance, then arranging them along a spectrum of anatomic disruption. Six distinct classes are noted including compressive flexion, distractive flexion, compressive extension, vertical compression, distractive extension, and lateral flexion (Fig. 56.12). Distractive flexion often preserves the ALL and disrupts the posterior elements. The congruence and stability of the facets are a factor in these injuries and thus the class is further divided into stages

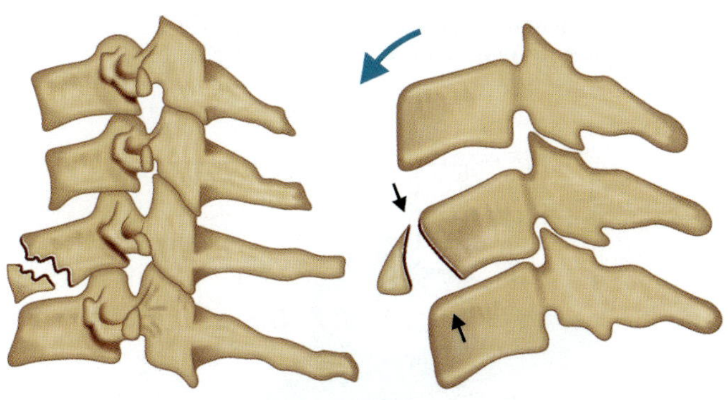

Fig. 56.11: Compression-flexion "teardrop".

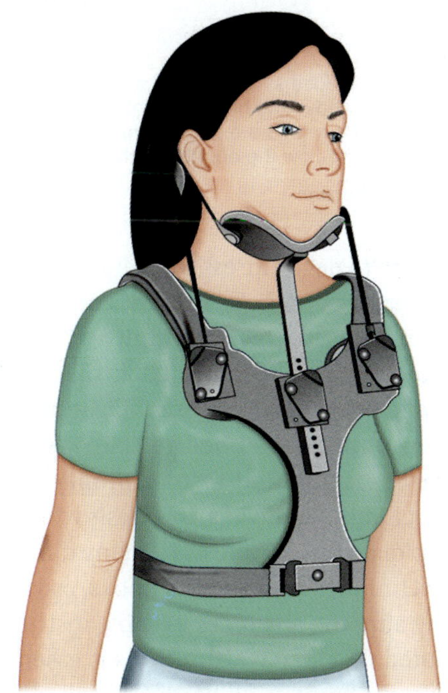

Fig. 56.13: Sternal occipital mandibular immobilizer brace.

of severity one through four denoting facet subluxation, unilateral facet dislocation, bilateral facet dislocation (>50% displacement), and complete dislocation, respectively. It should be noted that this classification rarely guides management but is a helpful tool for research.

NONOPERATIVE TREATMENT

The short-term goal of managing cervical fractures and dislocations is to limit the potential for catastrophic neurologic injury and stabilize injured segments with the most minimally invasive treatment. Long-term goals include preventing progressive deformity and chronic pain. Goals must be modified for concomitant medical comorbidities and focus on mobilization and aggressive rehabilitation.

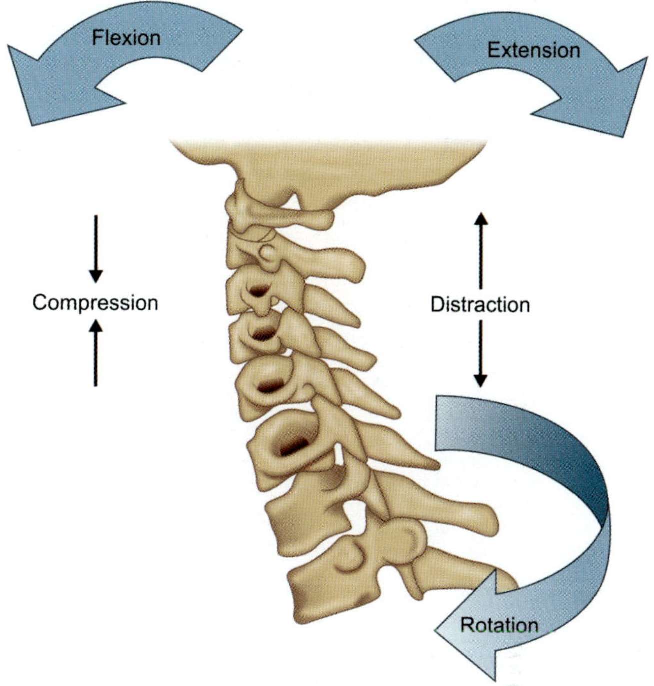

Fig. 56.12: Facet disruption classified by injury mechanism.

The alert patient with c-spine injury often requires traction or immobilization even without obvious canal compromise on X-ray as 25–33% of these patients have a herniated disk so the risk of extrusion of disk material with motion must be respected.

Various bracing options exist for the indirect stabilization of the spine. Stabilization with bracing involves the use of a cervical collar. Many collars are poor for rotational (axial) and lateral bending (coronal) stability.[47] The rigid collars placed in the field are often carefully replaced with well-padded, fitted collars such as Philadelphia, Malibu/Aspen, or Miami-J brands. Cervicothoracic orthoses such as 4-Poster Brace, Minerva brace, or sternal occipital mandibular immobilizer are more stable in rotation and lateral bending, which are ideal for fractures below C3 (Fig. 56.13).

The halo vest (Fig. 56.14) is the most rigid external immobilization in all planes with flexion/extension, lateral bending, and rotation limited by 90-99%.[48] However, this vest carries risks of discomfort, pin loosening, and pin site infection. In elderly patients, complications can be as dire as respiratory distress (10%), dysphagia (14%), and death (19–40%).[49] Though not a surgical procedure, halo vest application can be performed in the operating room instead of the emergency room setting. As always, caution for positioning is essential. First, the vest is removed with

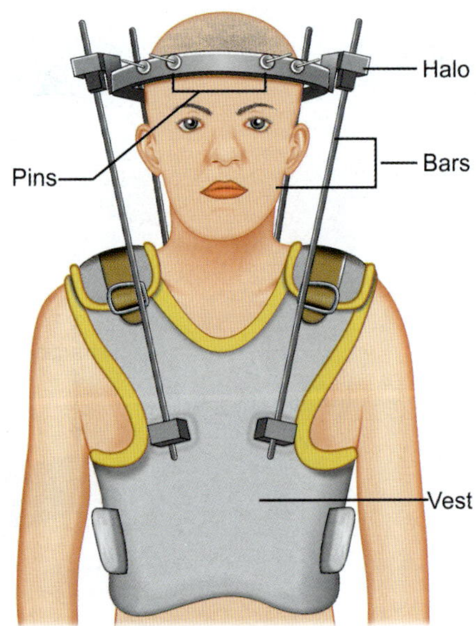

Fig. 56.14: Halo vest.

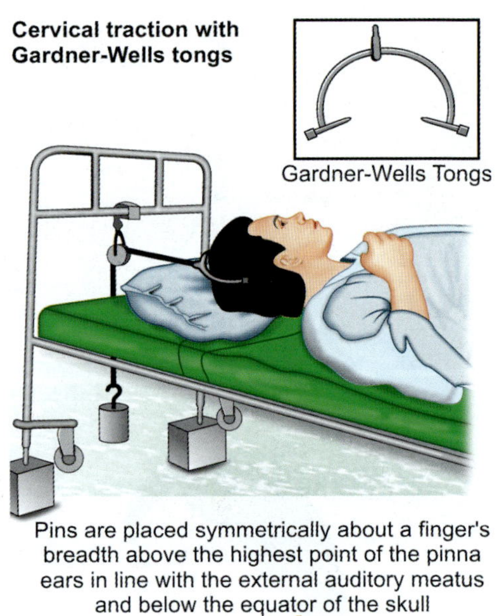

Fig. 56.15: Cervical traction.

the collar placed temporarily. Then, the patient is logrolled to a radiolucent table. The halo is initially secured to table with the available attachments.

The specific case of facet dislocation (''jumped facets'') or subluxation often requires immediate application of cervical traction. Bilateral jumped facets require cervical fusion, but a unilateral jumped facet may be treated definitively with immobilization. Initial closed reduction in jumped facets is safe and effective in the awake and alert patient. As discussed, prereduction MRI may delay treatment and is not always recommended.

General guidelines include beginning with 10 lbs (4.5 kg) with radiographs and neurologic examination after hanging weight (Fig. 56.15). Five-pound increments proceed every 30 minutes with a limit estimated at one-third of the body weight. Of note, the limit for high-cervical (C1–C2) pathology of 20 lbs (9 kg) is less than that for subaxial (C3–C7), which may be up to 50 lbs (22.7 kg). After reduction is confirmed by X-ray, the patient may be left with 20 lbs in extension using bumps or placed in a halo until definitive fixation. Failure of reduction after 3–6 hours, greater than 1 cm of distraction on X-ray, or any neurologic deterioration warrants cessation of traction. An MRI is required if the injury is irreducible and surgical treatment typically proceeds.

OPERATIVE TREATMENT

Timing of surgical intervention and type of surgical approach are still controversial for many injuries, but the overall goals are to decompress the neural elements when there is a neurologic deficit, restore stability to prevent future compression, correct deformity to prevent long-term sequelae such as chronic back pain and sagittal imbalance, and provide for early mobilization to avoid the complications of prolonged bed rest. To redistribute the stresses over the spine and restore proper alignment, a broad overarching scheme of arthrodesis with instrumentation is employed but manifests in many different procedures and techniques with various hooks, rods, wires, and screws. Early after the advances in spine instrumentation, surgeons noted that stable arthrodesis is essential to successful outcomes because all hardware will ultimately fail without bony fusion.[3,5]

Surgeons often advocate a posterior approach to the spine as the posterior ligamentous structures are mostly under tension and thus referred to as the ''posterior tension band''. Injury to this posterior tension band with distraction forces allows long-term deforming forces to produce kyphosis. Posterior instrumentation restores this biomechanical balance necessary to prevent deformity. Posterior instrumentation, often with lateral mass screws, typically provides this mechanical advantage and adequate fixation for bony fusion. Translation injuries such as fracture dislocations often necessitate circumferential (anterior and posterior) approaches to address the failure of the widespread tissue disruption. This is thought to be especially important in the areas of high-stress cervicothoracic junction.

Occipital Condyle and Atlanto-occipital Dissociation

The infrequency of this fracture makes studies difficult to conduct and treatment strategies vary. Nonetheless, 6–12 weeks in a stable orthosis is sufficient to treat non-displaced, impacted, and unilateral injuries. However, the mechanical instability demonstrated by displacement, avulsion, or bilateral occipital injury requires halo vest immobilization or surgical stabilization with posterior fixation extending to the occiput. Condylar or lateral mass translation >1 mm is considered abnormal. The type III occipital condyle fractures are inherently unstable and have been associated with lower cranial nerve injury (especially cranial nerve XII), and thus require occipito-cervical fusion. Type II fractures with CT showing delayed or nonunion on follow-up may benefit from this procedure as well. Rare bilateral type III occipital condyle fractures and AOD should be taken for occipitocervical fusion.[50,51] Surgical techniques involve arthrodesis and instrumentation of the occiput and the upper cervical spine via a posterior approach (Fig. 56.16).

C1 (Atlas) Ring

Fractures of the atlas have a high rate of spontaneous fusion and limited ligamentous instability. Therefore, they are treated surgically only when the lateral mass displacement is >7 mm as seen on an OMO view. The radiograph is used to assess the alignment of the lateral masses of C1 and C2 using the rule of Spence.[52] MRI can also show violation of the transverse ligament but this is less used for surgical decision making.[53] Fractures that meet these criteria are treated with C1 lateral mass screws (Figs. 56.17A and B), transarticular screws (screws through the C2 pars interarticularis, C1–C2 articulation, and into the lateral mass of C1 shown in Figures 56.18A and B), or wiring techniques (Fig. 56.19) because >7 mm suggests disruption of transverse ligament, which is a key soft tissue stabilizer. Craniocervical stabilization can be accomplished with the various rods, plates, and wire-loop constructs. Isolated anterior or posterior arch fractures, singular lateral mass fractures, and transverse process fractures may be treated in a halo. The C2 pars interarticularis or pedicle screws or C2 laminar screws can be extended to subaxial spine lateral mass screws for a more stable construct in cases of osteoporosis or poor screw purchase.

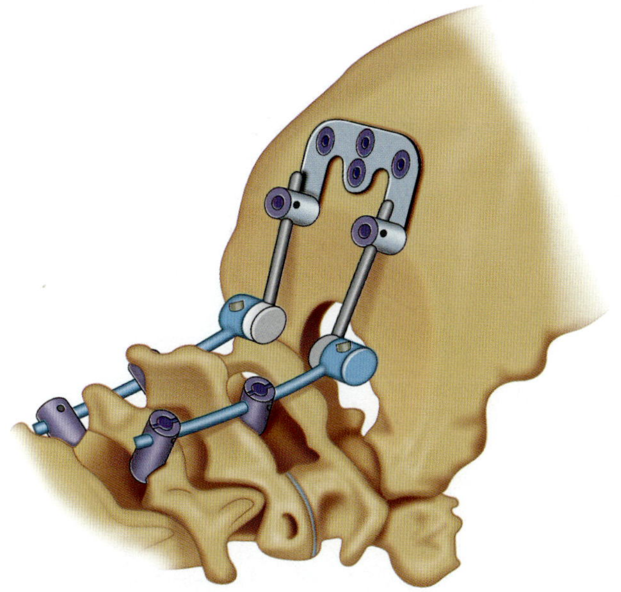

Fig. 56.16: Occipital-cervical fusion with instrumentation for atlanto-occipital dissociation. An occipitocervical loop construct is fixed with four screws to the dense midline ridge between the foramen magnum and the external occipital protuberance and attached to the cervical spine with a rod-screw construct.

C2 (Axis)

Hangman type IIa fractures should not have cervical traction applied as it may worsen displacement. By Levine and Edwards classification, types I and II may be treated with a halo, but type II and III with severe angulation or inability to maintain reduction require posterior fixation with C2 pars interarticularis lag screws, C1–C2 arthrodesis with transarticular screws, or Harms technique screw/rod constructs or multilevel posterior cervical arthrodesis and instrumentation. Another option is C2–C3 anterior cervical discectomy and fusion. When necessary, reduction maneuvers typically involve hyperextension. Hangman fractures can be successfully treated with collar or halo vest immobilization in over 90% of cases.[54]

Odontoid fracture healing rate depends on surface area and vascularity, both of which are deficient in the area of type II fractures at the waist. Therefore, treatment involves a cervical orthosis for type I and III, but the high nonunion rate of waist fractures warrants C1–C2 fusion surgery. Any fracture with >4–6 mm of displacement should be treated operatively. However, a halo vest may be attempted in young patients when nondisplaced.[55-58] Osteosynthesis with odontoid screw fixation (Figs. 56.20A to C) and posterior C1–C2 fusion techniques are the preferred methods of surgical treatment.

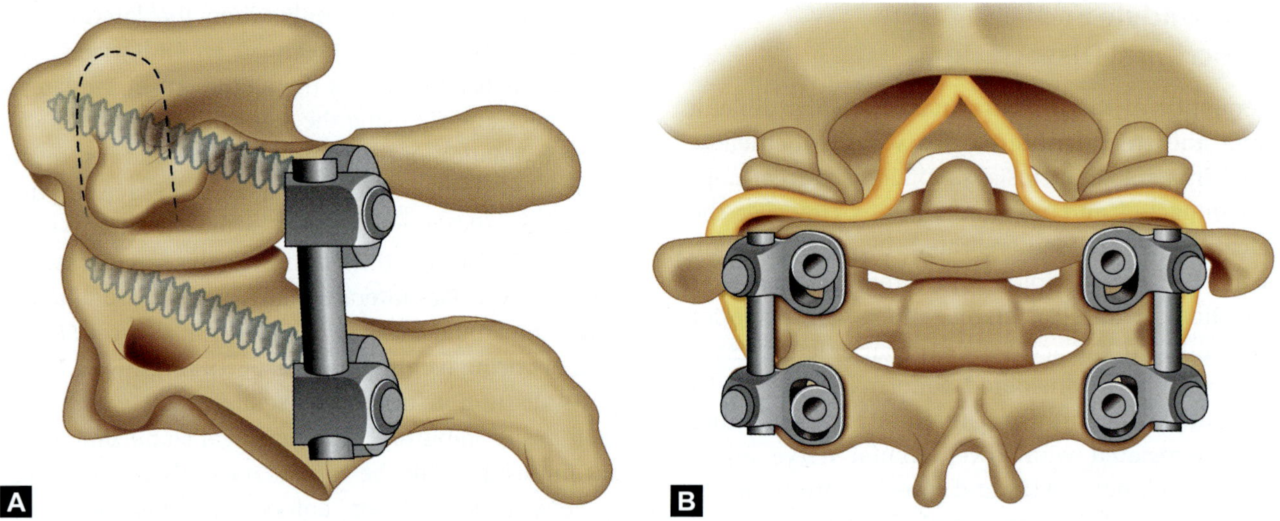

Figs. 56.17A and B: C1–C2 lateral mass screw with rod constructs, which can be supplemented with wiring and/or bone grafting to promote arthrodesis.

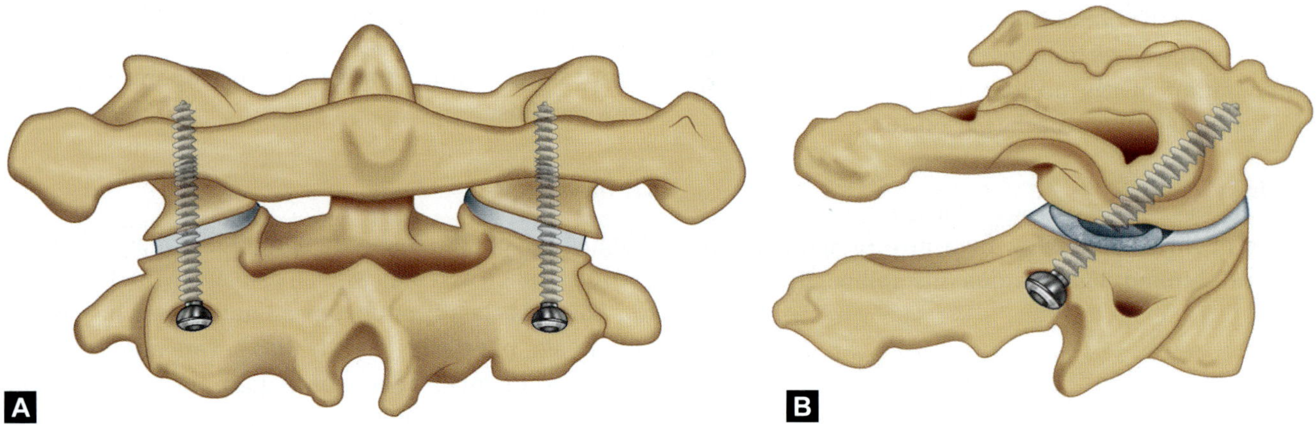

Figs. 56.18A and B: Illustration of C1–C2 transarticular screws (through pars interarticularis of C2, then the C1–C2 lateral mass joint and into the C1 lateral mass).

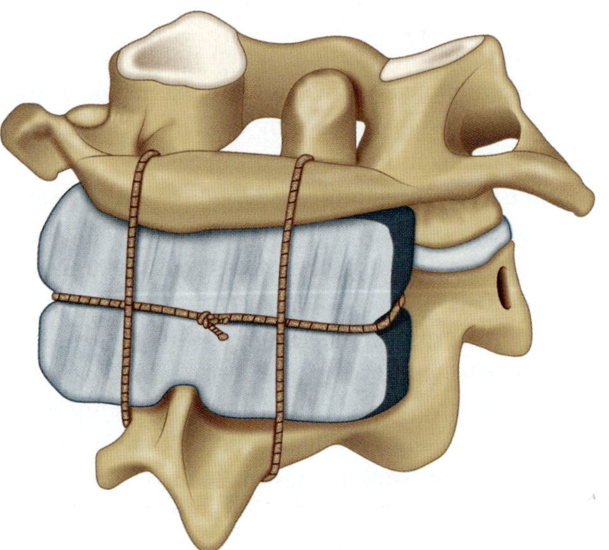

Fig. 56.19: Posterior wiring/bone graft technique for C1–C2 fusion (Sonntag fusion).

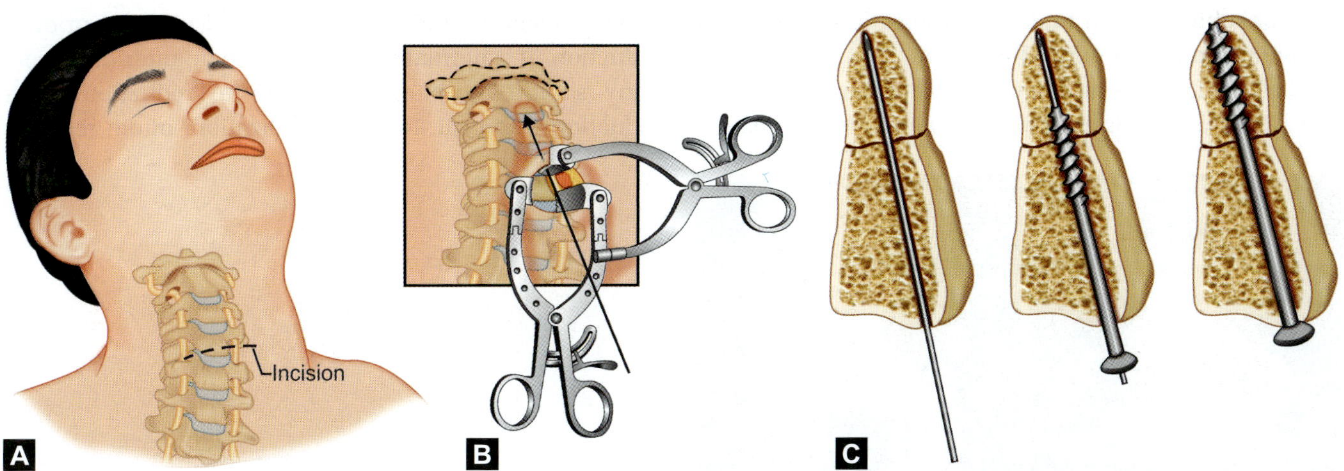

Figs. 56.20A to C: Anterior odontoid screw fixation. Left image shows positioning and exposure. Right image shows screw fixation.

Odontoid screw fixation involves placement of a lag screw across the fracture. Historically two-screw techniques have been used, but studies have shown equivalent results with one-screw techniques.[58,59] This technique preserves C1–C2 motion and the procedure is performed through an anterior approach, which is generally well tolerated, although there have been reports of severe dysphagia.[60,61]

The first attempts to treat odontoid fractures surgically used the posterior approach. The wire-loop method over the posterior arches was introduced in 1937 by Cone and Turner and improved upon by Gallie in 1939, in 1978 by Brooks', and in 1991 by Sonntag. These methods address the instability potentially at the expense of C1–C2 motion, although the subaxial spine should compensate to some extent.[62,63] Despite good fusion rates, a notable disadvantage to these methods is that months of stabilization with cervical orthoses are required postoperatively.

Although posterior wiring techniques remain an option, currently more popular options include Magerl transarticular screw technique and the Harms technique. C1–C2 transarticular screws[64] are technically challenging due to the close proximity of the vertebral artery to the path of the screw. Thus, a safer and more popular option is the C1 lateral mass combined with C2 pars or pedicle screws and rod instrumentation.[43] The added benefit is the ability to directly manipulate and reduce malalignment. Screw techniques increased fusion rates above 90% and reduced the need for external orthoses.

Cervical Compression and Burst

With pure cervical anterior column compression fractures, the canal is protected and the patient can be treated with an orthosis for 6–12 weeks. Cervical burst fractures however are commonly associated with incomplete or complete SCI due to retropulsion of fragments into the canal. As these fractures are difficult to classify, management guidelines are rather flexible. Prolonged traction and halo management have been used in the past, but severe cases will more likely benefit from surgery. Operative indications are based on neurologic status and estimated mechanical stability. Patients with neurologic deficits, loss of more than half vertebral body height, kyphosis or sagittal plane translation, and persistent pain can all benefit from operative fusion.[65] The reason sagittal deformity is treated is that cervical kyphosis tends to progress and leads to long-term sagittal imbalance.[66]

Retropulsed fragments and retrolisthesis often require anterior approach for fixation but may also require posterior fixation. Surgery to maintain alignment and restore mechanical stability to the anterior column involves anterior corpectomy with placement of iliac crest strut bone autograft or allograft, or placement of titanium mesh cages, which can be filled with osteoconductive and osteoinductive agents (Figs. 56.21A and B). Anterior plating can provide support to improve fusion rates, but plating also seems to reduce postoperative pain.[67,68]

Facet Disruption

Operative and nonoperative treatments of facet dislocations have changed over the years. Before 1987 nearly all patients underwent manipulation under anesthesia (MUA). Failure to reduce meant open reduction and posterior cervical fusion.[69,70] Rapid traction for the awake and alert patient is now generally agreed as safer than

MUA for subluxation or unilateral dislocation with closed immobilization as definitive treatment.

Bilateral dislocations require cervical fusion (Figs. 56.22 A to C). An irreducible facet dislocation with herniation must be taken to the OR for anterior discectomy prior to reduction. If a herniated disk is present, anterior discectomy should be performed prior to reduction. After reduction, surgical fusion stabilization often requires

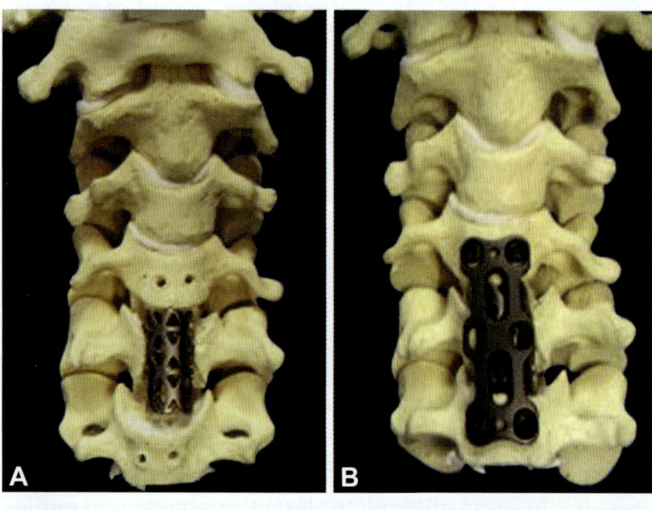

Figs. 56.21A and B: Lateral postoperative film of a C5 burst fracture treated with C5 corpectomy, titanium cage (A) and anterior cervical fusion (B).

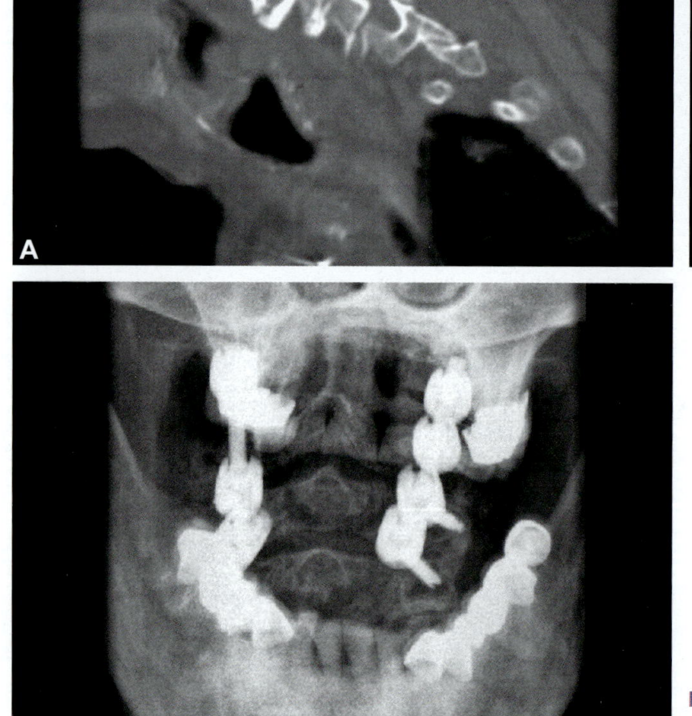

Figs. 56.22A to C: Treatment of cervical fracture-dislocation with laminectomy and posterior fusion of C1 through C4 levels with lateral mass screws.

anterior and posterior approaches to address procedure for the anterior column and the posterior tension band. Posterior instrumentation in the subaxial spine is most commonly accomplished using lateral mass screws in C3, C4, and C5. On the lower limb of the metallic construct, pedicle screws provide more secure anchoring and may be used in C6. This is preferable near the cervicothoracic junction to decrease the biomechanical stress and risk of instrumentation failure.

Postoperative Care

Postoperative care is typically in a monitored setting, especially in the context of polytrauma. The cervical trauma patient is prone to complications. Neurogenic shock and autonomic dysregulation must be anticipated, potentially with invasive monitoring (discussed in the SCI section). In the context of multiple surgeries for other traumatic injuries, clinicians should consider deferment of postoperative extubation. Sims et al. showed that 14 of 105 patients with cervical injury managed with halo fixation required emergent or semiemergent reintubation, and six patients had poor outcomes secondary to prolonged intubation attempts.[71]

Spinal Cord Injury

In the spectrum of traumatic neurologic injuries, spinal cord injury can produce some of the most devastating clinical outcomes. The bony limits to the space for the spinal cord and exiting nerves places these structures at high risk for injury (Fig. 56.23). Even if the cord is not directly contused or cut, small injuries can be worsened during patient transport or by hemodynamic instability and prolonged spinal cord hypoxia.

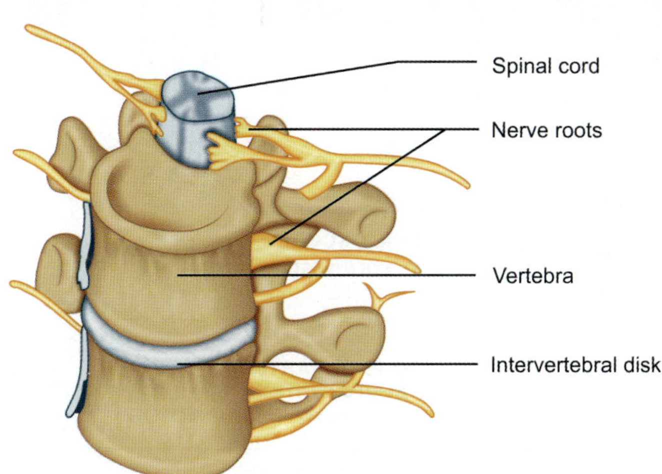

Fig. 56.23: Relationship of spinal cord/nerve roots to vertebral bodies.

The descriptions of the many resulting clinical phenomena involve defining several terms. Paraplegia is the impaired motor and/or sensory function in thoracic, lumbar, and sacral segments, while tetraplegia (or quadriplegia) additionally includes cervical pathology disabling both upper limbs. A complete injury refers to the patient with no spared motor or sensory function in the lowest sacral segments after the end of spinal shock. An incomplete injury refers to the partial preservation of motor or sensory function below the neurologic level, but also qualifies the period before sacral connectivity has returned as indicated by the bulbocavernosus reflex. Neurologic level is the lowest segment where motor and sensory function is normal on bilaterally.

Spinal shock is generally seen in the initial 24–48 hours after injury. The neurologic level cannot be determined during this time until return of the bulbocavernosus reflex, which marks the end of spinal shock. Neurogenic shock is a clinical circumstance whose mechanism is circulatory in nature manifesting as hypotension with paradoxic bradycardia. The pseudohypovolemia occurs as a result of functional sympathectomy and loss of peripheral vasoconstriction as cardiac accelerator fibers arise from T1 to T4. Vasopressors and colloids are useful with a goal to keep mean arterial pressure (MAP) > 85 mm Hg and PaO_2 > 60 mm Hg.

Specific Syndromes

Some incomplete cord injuries are named for their characteristic findings, although they do not represent all of the potential clinical presentations that may be encountered. Brown-Sequard involves hemisection of the cord and has the best prognosis. It is often due to penetrating trauma and results in ipsilateral motor and proprioception loss with contralateral loss of pain and temperature sensation. Central cord syndrome is the most common type of incomplete SCI, resulting from hyperextension with canal stenosis. The weakness of the upper extremities is greater than that of the lower extremities. The central gray matter has a high metabolic requirement and is therefore subject to ischemic insult.

Anterior cord syndrome refers to para- or quadriplegia with dissociated sensory loss. This is due to direct contusion of the cord by bony fragments or damage to the anterior spinal artery. Posterior column function may still be present as signified by ability to respond to pain and light touch. This has the worst prognosis for recovery of motor function, but proprioception and vibratory sensation are usually spared. A mixed syndrome is characterized by diffuse involvement of the cord and has a good prognosis for recovery. Early motor recovery is the best prognostic indicator. In patients with a neurologic level higher than T8, clinicians should be watchful for hypertension with dizziness, diaphoresis, and headache as this may represent autonomic dysreflexia. This is because T8 represents the beginning of splanchnic outflow of sympathetic fibers.

CLASSIFICATION

Traditionally, SCI has been classified according to severity of clinical disability. The Frankel scale popularized in 1970s by Hans Frankel but originally devised at Stoke Mandeville Hospital in 1930s formed the basis for the presently used ASIA (American Spine Injury Association) international classification of SCI published in 1982 (Fig. 56.24). While the Frankel scale A through E assesses the "usefulness" of the extremities, the ASIA classification relates A and B to the S4–S5 level and ASIA B and C are quantitative. Both ASIA and Frankel E imply that neurologic examination may not detect injury.

Grade A is a complete neurological injury with no clinically detectable motor or sensory function in sacral segments below the level of the injury. Grade B is incomplete with preserved sensation only below neurologic level and in sacral segments. This sensory function may be only partial and sacral sparing qualifies as preserved sensation. Grade C is incomplete with some preserved motor below the level of the injury, but is of no practical use to the patient. This means less than half of the muscle

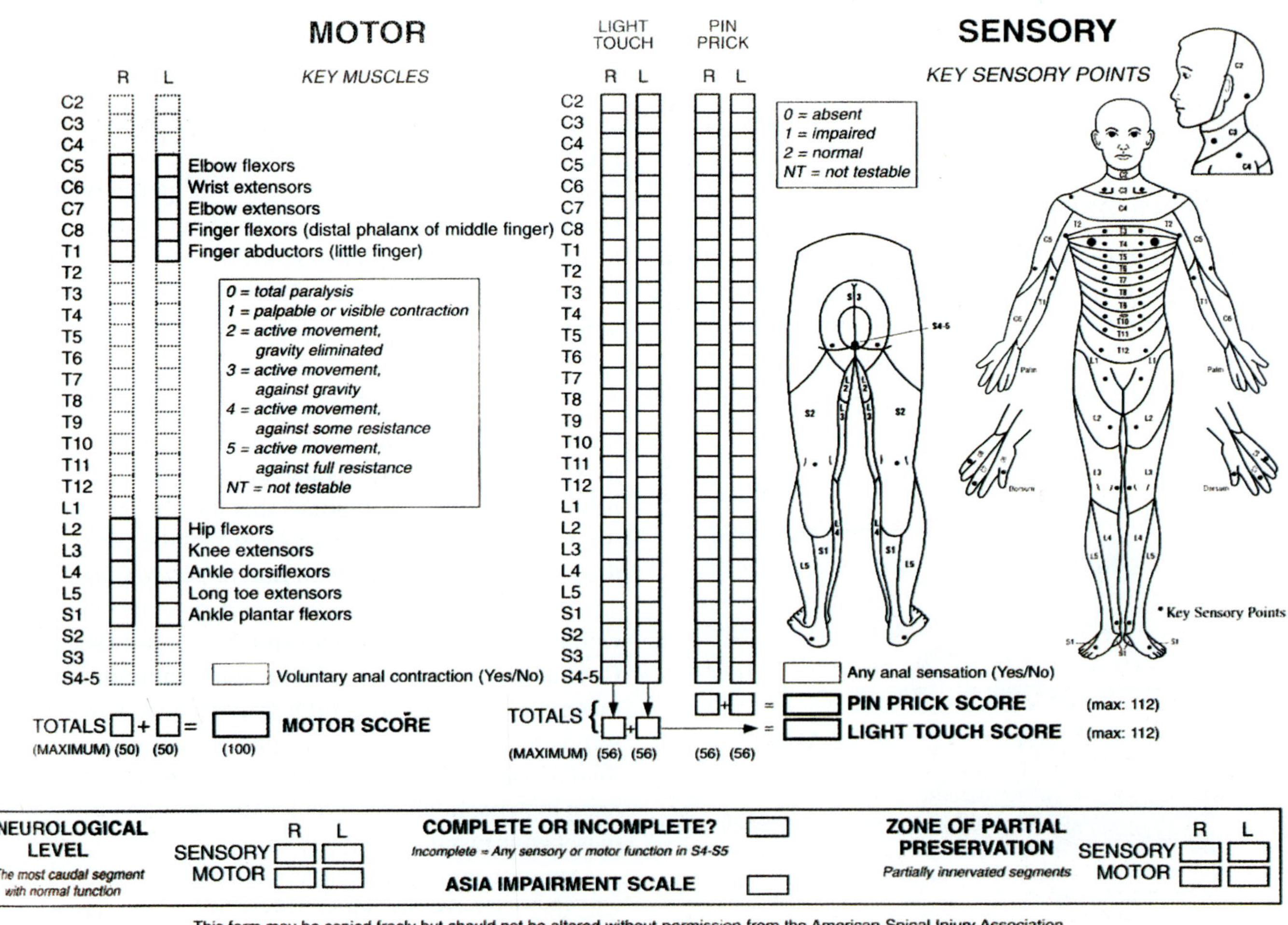

MOTOR

KEY MUSCLES

R L

C2, C3, C4
C5 Elbow flexors
C6 Wrist extensors
C7 Elbow extensors
C8 Finger flexors (distal phalanx of middle finger)
T1 Finger abductors (little finger)
T2, T3, T4, T5, T6, T7, T8, T9, T10, T11, T12, L1
L2 Hip flexors
L3 Knee extensors
L4 Ankle dorsiflexors
L5 Long toe extensors
S1 Ankle plantar flexors
S2, S3, S4-5

0 = total paralysis
1 = palpable or visible contraction
2 = active movement, gravity eliminated
3 = active movement, against gravity
4 = active movement, against some resistance
5 = active movement, against full resistance
NT = not testable

Voluntary anal contraction (Yes/No)

TOTALS ☐ + ☐ = ☐ MOTOR SCORE
(MAXIMUM) (50) (50) (100)

LIGHT TOUCH R L | PIN PRICK R L

C2–S4-5

TOTALS
(MAXIMUM) (56) (56) (56) (56)

SENSORY

KEY SENSORY POINTS

0 = absent
1 = impaired
2 = normal
NT = not testable

Any anal sensation (Yes/No)

PIN PRICK SCORE (max: 112)
LIGHT TOUCH SCORE (max: 112)

• Key Sensory Points

NEUROLOGICAL LEVEL — The most caudal segment with normal function — R L SENSORY ☐☐ MOTOR ☐☐

COMPLETE OR INCOMPLETE? ☐ — Incomplete = Any sensory or motor function in S4-S5

ASIA IMPAIRMENT SCALE ☐

ZONE OF PARTIAL PRESERVATION — Partially innervated segments — R L SENSORY ☐☐ MOTOR ☐☐

This form may be copied freely but should not be altered without permission from the American Spinal Injury Association.

Fig. 56.24: Neurologic (motor and sensory) examination recommended by the American Spinal Injury Association (ASIA).

groups below the level have more than three of five strengths. Grade D is incomplete with preserved useful motor function below the level of the injury and more than half the muscles have grade 3 or more strength. Grade E denotes a patient with no clinically detected abnormality in motor or sensory function and with normal sphincter function. Abnormal reflexes and subjective sensory abnormalities may be present.

OPERATIVE CARE TO OPTIMIZE FUNCTION

The surgeon must consider the overall function of the patient with SCI, which is directly related to the neurologic level. A patient with a C5 level will have maintained deltoid and biceps, which allow them to abduct shoulder and flex elbow. Surgical intervention to maximize function should follow a year of observation and aggressive physical therapy. The surgical goals for the C5 level include elbow extension, wrist extension, and key-pinch grip between the thumb and index finger. This can be accomplished with transfer of the posterior deltoid to the triceps for elbow extension, transfer of the brachioradialis (BR) to the wrist extensors for active wrist extension, and attachment of the BR to flexor pollicis longus and thumb interphalangeal joint fusion for pinch.

C6 level function allows for locomotion by wheelchair. The surgical goals for a patient who maintains wrist extension include restoration of lateral pinch and active grasp with similar procedures noted above. Transfer of pronator teres to flexor digitorum profundus can improve active cylinder grip.

The intact triceps in the C7 level function allows for more independent transfer and independent living. The surgical goals are for active thumb flexion, active finger flexion, and hand opening. This can be accomplished with the aforementioned procedures along with tenodesis of the extensors to the distal radius for hand opening with wrist flexion. The C8 level patient can perform fully independent transfers with improved finger strength and dexterity. The goals are to optimize finger and thumb flexors for grasp. Intrinsic muscles of the hand are usually weak producing claw hand deformity, which can be treated with capsulodesis of the metacarpophalangeal joints.

REFERENCES

1. Vaccaro AR, Silber JS. Post-traumatic spinal deformity. Spine. 2001;26(24 Suppl):S111-8.
2. Lifshutz J, Colohan A. A brief history of therapy for traumatic spinal cord injury. Neurosurg Focus. 2004;16(1):E5.
3. Omeis I, DeMattia JA, Hillard VH, et al. History of instrumentation for stabilization of the subaxial cervical spine. Neurosurg Focus. 2004;16(1):E10.
4. Deshaies EM, DiRisio D, Popp AJ. Medieval management of spinal injuries: parallels between Theodoric of Bologna and contemporary spine surgeons. Neurosurg Focus. 2004; 16(1):E3.
5. Singh H, Rahimi SY, Yeh DJ, et al. History of posterior thoracic instrumentation. Neurosurg Focus. 2004;16(1):E11.
6. Goodrich JT. Cervical spine surgery in the ancient and medieval worlds. Neurosurg Focus. 2007;23(1):E7.
7. Goodrich JT. History of spine surgery in the ancient and medieval worlds. Neurosurg Focus. 2004;16(1):E2.
8. Frankel HL, Hancock DO, Hyslop G, et al. The value of postural reduction in the initial management of closed injuries of the spine with paraplegia and tetraplegia. Spinal Cord. 1969;7(3):179-92.
9. Riggins RS, Kraus JF. The risk of neurologic damage with fractures of the vertebrae. J Trauma. 1977;17(2):126-33.
10. Keenen TL, Antony J, Benson DR. Non-contiguous spinal fractures. J Trauma. 1990;30(4):489-91.
11. Bohlman HH. Acute fractures and dislocations of the cervical spine. An analysis of three hundred hospitalized patients and review of the literature. J Bone Joint Surg. American volume. 1979;61(8):1119-42.
12. McGrory BJ, Klassen RA, Chao EY, et al. Acute fractures and dislocations of the cervical spine in children and adolescents. J Bone Joint Surg. American volume. 1993;75(7): 988-95.
13. Herzenberg JE, Hensinger RN, Dedrick DK, et al. Emergency transport and positioning of young children who have an injury of the cervical spine. The standard backboard may be hazardous. J Bone Joint Surg. American volume. 1989; 71(1):15-22.
14. Pal GP, Sherk HH. The vertical stability of the cervical spine. Spine. 1988;13(5):447-9.
15. Podolsky S, Baraff LJ, Simon RR, et al. Efficacy of cervical spine immobilization methods. J Trauma. 2006;23(6):461-5.
16. Criswell JC, Parr MJ, Nolan JP. Emergency airway management in patients with cervical spine injuries. Anaesthesia. 1994;49(10):900-03.
17. Bivins HG, Ford S, Bezmalinovic Z, et al. The effect ofaxial traction during orotracheal intubation of the trauma victim with an unstable cervical spine. Ann Emerg Med. 1988;17 (1):25-9.
18. Lennarson PJ, Smith DW, Sawin PD, et al. Cervical spinal motion during intubation: efficacy of stabilization maneuvers in the setting of complete segmental instability. J Neurosurg. 2001;94(2 Suppl):265-70.
19. Shatney CH, Brunner RD, Nguyen TQ. The safety of orotracheal intubation in patients with unstable cervical spine fracture or high spinal cord injury. Am J Surg. 1995;170(6):676-9, discussion 679-80.
20. Merola A, O'Brien MF, Castro BA, et al. Histologic characterization of acute spinal cord injury treated with intravenous methylprednisolone. J Orthop Trauma. 2002;16(3):155-61.

21. Carlson GD, Gorden CD, Nakazawa S, et al. Sustained spinal cord compression: part II: effect of methylprednisolone on regional blood flow and recovery of somatosensory evoked potentials. J Bone Joint Surg. American volume. 2003;85-A(1):95-101.
22. Hurlbert RJ. Methylprednisolone for acute spinal cord injury: an inappropriate standard of care. J Neurosurg. 2000;93(1 Suppl):1-7.
23. Coleman WP, Benzel D, Cahill DW, et al. A critical appraisal of the reporting of the National Acute Spinal Cord Injury Studies (II and III) of methylprednisolone in acute spinal cord injury. J Spinal Disord. 2000;13(3):185-99.
24. Short DJ, Masry El WS, Jones PW. High dose methylprednisolone in the management of acute spinal cord injury - a systematic review from a clinical perspective. Spinal Cord. 2000;38(5):273-86.
25. Sayer FT, Kronvall E, Nilsson OG. Methylprednisolone treatment in acute spinal cord injury: the myth challenged through a structured analysis of published literature. Spine J. 2006;6(3):335-43.
26. Anderson PA, Gugala Z, Lindsey RW, et al. Clearing the cervical spine in the blunt trauma patient. J Am Acad Orthop Surg. 2010;18(3):149-59.
27. Herr CH, Ball PA, Sargent SK, et al. Sensitivity of prevertebral soft tissue measurement of C3 for detection of cervical spine fractures and dislocations. Am J Emerg Med. 1998;16 (4):346-9.
28. Diliberti T, Lindsey RW. Evaluation of the cervical spine in the emergency setting: who does not need an X-ray? Orthopedics. 1992;15(2):179-83.
29. Cox MW, McCarthy M, Lemmon G, et al. Cervical spine instability: clearance using dynamic fluoroscopy. Curr Surg. 2001;58(1):96-100.
30. Giacobetti FB, Vaccaro AR, Bos-Giacobetti MA, et al. Vertebral artery occlusion associated with cervical spine trauma. A prospective analysis. Spine. 1997;22(2):188-92.
31. Klein GR, Vaccaro AR, Albert TJ, et al. Efficacy of magnetic resonance imaging in the evaluation of posterior cervical spine fractures. Spine. 1999;24(8):771-4.
32. Hadley MN. Initial closed reduction of cervical spine fracture-dislocation injuries. Neurosurgery. 2002;50(3 Suppl): S44–50.
33. Holdsworth F. Fractures, dislocations, and fracture-dislocations of the spine. J Bone Joint Surg. American volume. 1970;52(8):1534-51.
34. Denis F. The three column spine and its significance in the classification of acute thoracolumbar spinal injuries. Spine. 1983;8(8):817-31.
35. Noble ER, Smoker WR. The forgotten condyle: the appearance, morphology, and classification of occipital condyle fractures. AJNR. American Journal of Neuroradiology. 1996; 17(3):507-13.
36. Leone A, Cerase A, Colosimo C, et al. Occipital condylar fractures: a review. Radiology. 2000;216(3):635-44.
37. Anderson PA, Montesano PX. Morphology and treatment of occipital condyle fractures. Spine. 1988;13(7):731-6.
38. Powers B, Miller MD, Kramer RS, et al. Traumatic anterior atlanto-occipital dislocation. Neurosurgery. 1979;4(1):12-7.
39. Wholey MH, Bruwer AJ, Baker HL. The lateral roentgenogram of the neck; with comments on the atlanto-odontoid-basion relationship. Radiology. 1958;71(3):350-6.
40. Harris JH, Carson GC, Wagner LK, et al. Radiologic diagnosis of traumatic occipitovertebral dissociation: 2. Comparison of three methods of detecting occipitovertebral relationships on lateral radiographs of supine subjects. AJR. 1994;162(4):887-92.
41. Lee C, Woodring JH, Goldstein SJ, et al. Evaluation of traumatic atlantooccipital dislocations. AJNR. 1987;8(1):19-26.
42. Dublin AB, Marks WM, Weinstock D, Newton TH. Traumatic dislocation of the atlanto-occipital articulation (AOA) with short-term survival. With a radiographic method of measuring the AOA. J Neurosurg. 1980;52(4):541-6.
43. Harms J, Melcher RP. Posterior C1-C2 fusion with polyaxial screw and rod fixation. Spine. 2001;26(22):2467-71.
44. Effendi B, Roy D, Cornish B, et al. Fractures of the ring of the axis. A classification based on the analysis of 131 cases. J Bone Joint Surg. British volume. 1981;63-B(3):319-27.
45. Anderson LD, D'Alonzo RT. Fractures of the odontoid process of the axis. J Bone Joint Surg. American volume. 1974;56(8):1663-74.
46. Grauer JN, Shafi B, Hilibrand AS, et al. Proposal of a modified, treatment-oriented classification of odontoid fractures. Spine J. 2005;5(2):123-9.
47. Hughes SJ. How effective is the Newport/Aspen collar? A prospective radiographic evaluation in healthy adult volunteers. J Trauma. 1998;45(2):374-8.
48. Benzel EC, Hadden TA, Saulsbery CM. A comparison of the Minerva and halo jackets for stabilization of the cervical spine. J Neurosurg. 1989;70(3):411-4.
49. Majercik S, Tashjian RZ, Biffl WL, et al. Halo vest immobilization in the elderly: a death sentence? J Trauma. 2005;59 (2):350-6, discussion 356-8.
50. Vaccaro AR, Lim MR, Lee JY. Indications for surgery and stabilization techniques of the occipito-cervical junction. Injury. 2005;36 Suppl 2:B44-53.
51. Hanson JA, Deliganis AV, Baxter AB, et al. Radiologic and clinical spectrum of occipital condyle fractures: retrospective review of 107 consecutive fractures in 95 patients. AJR. 2002;178(5):1261-8.
52. Spence KF, Decker S, Sell KW. Bursting atlantal fracture associated with rupture of the transverse ligament. J Bone Joint Surg. American volume. 1970;52(3):543-9.
53. Dickman CA, Mamourian A, Sonntag VK, et al. Magnetic resonance imaging of the transverse atlantal ligament for the evaluation of atlantoaxial instability. J Neurosurg. 1991; 75(2):221-7.
54. Greene KA, Dickman CA, Marciano FF, et al. Acute axis fractures. Analysis of management and outcome in 340 consecutive cases. Spine. 1997;22(16):1843-52.
55. Sonntag VK, Hadley MN. Nonoperative management of cervical spine injuries. Clin Neurosurg. 1988;34:630-49.
56. Apuzzo ML, Heiden JS, Weiss MH, et al. Acute fractures of the odontoid process. An analysis of 45 cases. J Neurosurg. 1978;48(1):85-91.

57. Ekong CE, Schwartz ML, Tator CH, et al. Odontoid fracture: management with early mobilization using the halo device. Neurosurgery. 1981;9(6):631-7.
58. Hadley MN, Dickman CA, Browner CM, et al. Acute axis fractures: a review of 229 cases. J Neurosurg. 1989;71(5 Pt 1): 642-7.
59. McBride AD, Mukherjee DP, Kruse RN, et al. Anterior screw fixation of type II odontoid fractures. A biomechanical study. Spine. 1995;20(17):1855-9, discussion 1859-60.
60. Böhler J. [Screw-osteosynthesis of fractures of the dens axis (author's transl)]. Unfallheilkunde. 1981;84(6):221-223.
61. Apfelbaum RI, Lonser RR, Veres R, et al. Direct anterior screw fixation for recent and remote odontoid fractures. J Neurosurg. 2000;93(2 Suppl):227-36.
62. Dickman CA, Sonntag VK, Papadopoulos SM, et al. The interspinous method of posterior atlantoaxial arthrodesis. J Neurosurg. 1991;74(2):190-98.
63. Brooks AL, Jenkins EB. Atlanto-axial arthrodesis by the wedge compression method. J Bone Joint Surg. American volume. 1978;60(3):279-84.
64. Grob D, Magerl F. [Surgical stabilization of C1 and C2 fractures]. Der Orthopäde. 1987;16(1):46-54.
65. White AA, Johnson RM, Panjabi MM, et al. Biomechanical analysis of clinical stability in the cervical spine. Clin Orthop Relat Res. 1975;(109):85-96.
66. Panjabi MM, White AA, Johnson RM. Cervical spine mechanics as a function of transection of components. J Biomech. 1975;8(5):327-36.
67. Caspar W, Barbier DD, Klara PM. Anterior cervical fusion and Caspar plate stabilization for cervical trauma. Neurosurgery. 1989;25(4):491-502.
68. Epstein NE. Anterior cervical dynamic ABC plating with single level corpectomy and fusion in forty-two patients. Spinal Cord. 2003;41(3):153-8.
69. Lee JY, Nassr A, Eck JC, et al. Controversies in the treatment of cervical spine dislocations. Spine J. 2009;9(5):418-23.
70. Lee AS, MacLean JC, Newton DA. Rapid traction for reduction of cervical spine dislocations. J Bone Joint Surg. British volume. 1994;76(3):352-6.
71. Sims CA, Berger DL. Airway risk in hospitalized trauma patients with cervical injuries requiring halo fixation. Ann Surg. 2002;235(2):280-84.

CHAPTER 57

Thoracolumbar and Sacral Fracture Surgery

Robert Norton, Justin C Paul, Themistocles Protopsaltis

INTRODUCTION

Fractures involving the thoracic and lumbar segments of the spine have a wide spectrum of presentation and severity, ranging from low-energy pathologic vertebral compression fractures to high-energy fracture-dislocations with associated spinal cord injury. Approximately 90% of injuries occur at the thoracolumbar (TL) junction.[1] Management protocol has been controversial. In general, surgical treatment is indicated for unstable fracture patterns, progressive neurologic deterioration, and complete neurological deficits to facilitate rehabilitation.

ANATOMY AND MECHANISM OF INJURY

The thoracic spine is much more rigid and stable secondary to its articulations with the rib cage and coronal facet orientation. This is in contrast to the relatively more mobile lumbar spine with its sagittal oriented facet joints. The TL junction has a propensity for injury due to the sharp transition from a rigid, kyphotic thoracic spine to a more mobile, lordotic lumbar spine. Furthermore, this region serves as a neurologic transition, from the conus medullaris to the cauda equina, generally at the level of L1 (Fig. 57.1).

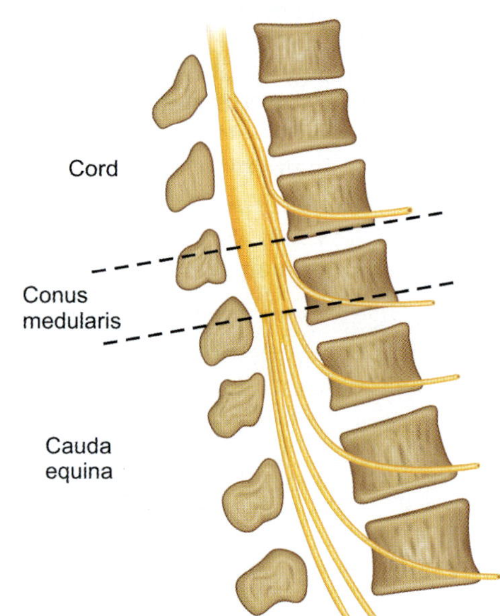

Fig. 57.1: Lumbar neuroanatomy.

CLINICAL EVALUATION

Clinical examination in a patient with a suspected spinal fracture always begins with the advanced trauma life support protocol. All organ systems and extremities should be evaluated for injury, as spinal fractures have a high incidence of related injuries and noncontiguous spinal fractures. The spine examination begins with inspection and palpation of the entire spine and a thorough neurological examination. A high degree of suspicion should be maintained for associated chest or abdominal trauma, as well as extremity injuries such as calcaneus fractures in the setting of a burst fracture. Neurologically intact patients with no TL spine pain with motion and palpation may be discontinued for lumbar spine precautions if distracting injuries are absent.

RADIOLOGIC EVALUATION

Traditionally, plain radiographs (anteroposterior and lateral views) have been recommended for initial evaluation;

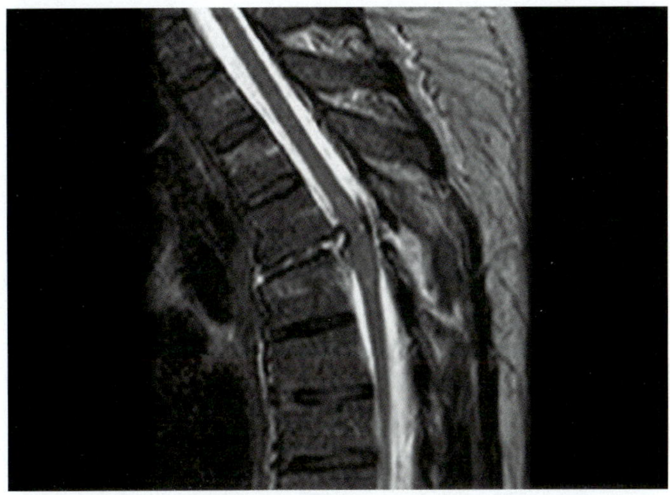

Fig. 57.2: MRI of lumbar spine showing significant cord injury.

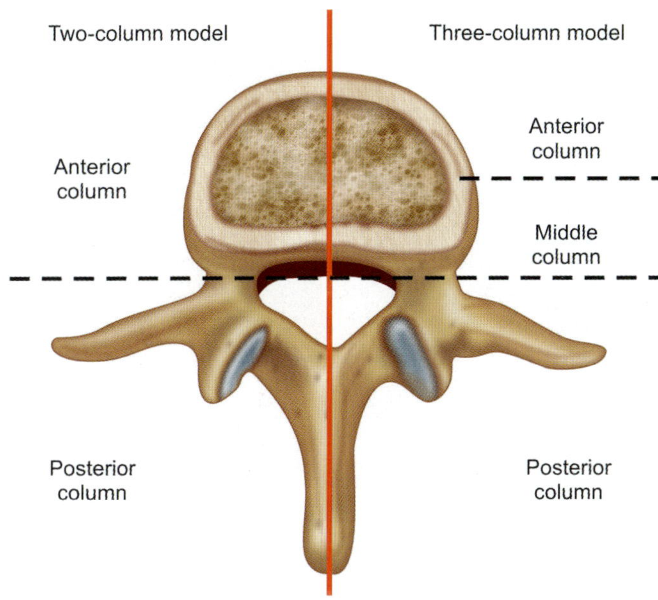

Fig. 57.3: Two- and three-column models used to classify instability of spinal injuries.

however, CT is often the study of choice in many trauma centers. Severe symptoms or altered mental state may necessitate CT or MRI. In practice, both are usually obtained with a minimum of full length anteroposterior/lateral radiographs of the entire spine to evaluate for noncontiguous injuries and dedicated CT imaging with reconstruction views of the injured area or any area of suspected injury that is not well visualized on plain radiographs. Coronal and sagittal reconstructions should be obtained in patients with a neurologic deficit. A neurologic deficit that cannot be explained by CT scan warrants further investigation with urgent MRI (Fig. 57.2). In addition to diagnosing all soft tissue injuries including disk herniations and damage to the posterior ligamentous complex (PLC), MRI aids in detecting an epidural hematoma, and injury to the cord, conus medullaris, and cauda equina.

CLASSIFICATION

The classification and treatment of TL spine fractures have undergone many permutations and have remained controversial. Classically, these injuries have been described by the mechanism of injury described by Ferguson and Allen,[2] or the anatomic three-column model as described by Denis[3] (Fig. 57.3). The important concept of the Denis classification was the addition of a middle column to Whitesides historic initial two-column concept. With the addition of the middle column, TL fractures could be differentiated on the pattern of injury and involvement of the middle column.[4,5]

An evolution to the Denis classification was introduced by McCormack[6] who took into consideration the load-sharing characteristics of fracture patterns in terms of vertebral comminution, degree of fragment displacement, and the amount of kyphotic deformity; all within the setting of the three-column model. They found that the fundamental principle of load sharing between long-bone fracture fixation and implant system is no different in the spine. With significant comminution or fracture displacement, load sharing and transfer are compromised. Furthermore, with a greater degree of kyphotic deformity, and therefore more anterior column disruption, pedicle screw instrumentation is subject to higher cantilever bending loads.

Most recently, the Thoracolumbar Injury Classification System (TLICS) has been proposed in an effort to categorize injuries by morphology, PLC disruption, and neurologic involvement rather than by anatomy or injury mechanism.[7] The TLICS is designed to grade and predict acute spine stability, risk of future deformity, and progressive neurologic compromise. In doing so, appropriate treatment recommendations may be facilitated. Reportedly, this system has demonstrated good inter and intra-observer reliability.[8]

COMPRESSION FRACTURES

Compression fractures have a bimodal distribution. They tend to occur in young individuals after sustaining a

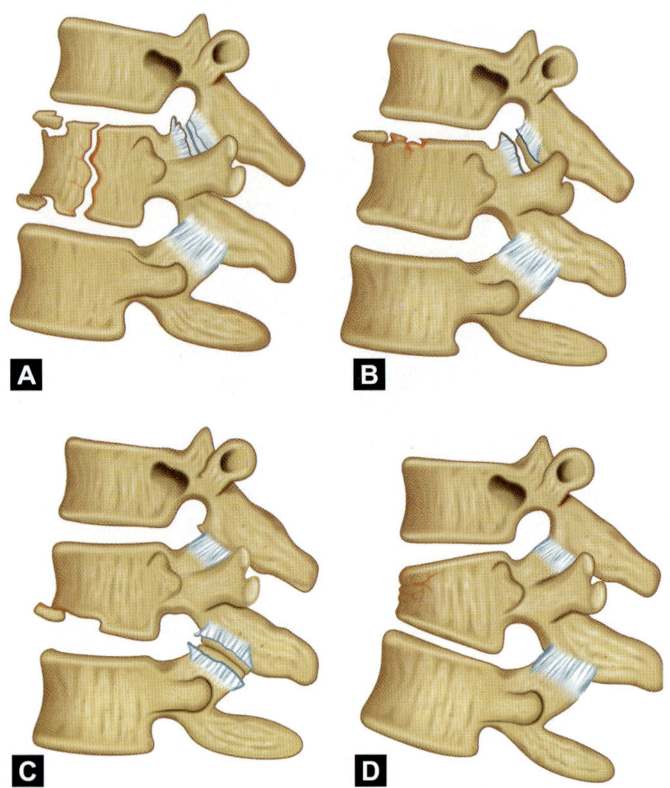

Figs. 57.4A to D: Denis classification for compression fractures: type A involves fracturing of both superior and inferior end plates; type B, which is the most common, involves failure of the superior vertebral end plate. Type C involves failure of the inferior end plate, and type D involves failure of the central aspect of the anterior vertebral body with relative preservation of the end plates.

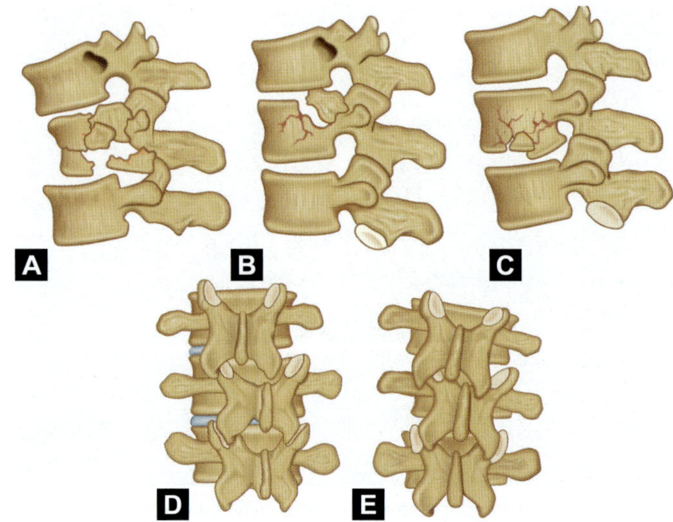

Figs. 57.5A to E: Denis classification system for burst fractures. Type A represents failure of both superior and inferior end plates. Type B, which is the most common, involves only the superior end plate. Type C is a fracture of the inferior end plate, type D is a burst rotation from a combined axial load and rotational injury, and type E is a burst fracture associated with lateral flexion injury.

high-energy injury or in elderly patients involved in low-energy mechanism injuries such as a fall from standing height. Four subtypes have been described by Denis (Figs. 57.4A to D); type A involves fracturing of both superior and inferior end plates, type B, which is the most common, involves failure of the superior vertebral end plate. Type C involves failure of the inferior end plate, and type D involves failure of the central aspect of the anterior vertebral body with relative preservation of the end plates.

The mechanism of action involves an axial directed compressive load to the spine resulting in simultaneous compression and flexion with failure of the anterior column in compression and preservation of the middle and posterior column height. This injury pattern is generally stable secondary to the maintained integrity of the PLC;[9] however, vertebral body height compression >50% is suggestive of PLC disruption and potential instability.[9-14] Because this injury pattern is usually isolated and stable without neurologic compromise, often it is treated nonoperatively.

Care must be taken to evaluate for pathologic causes of vertebral compression fractures, especially in the setting of low-energy injuries. Common causes of pathologic fractures include osteoporosis, metastatic cancer, primary sarcoma, and multiple myeloma. When suspected, appropriate workup, diagnosis, and management are paramount.

BURST FRACTURES

As with compression fractures, burst fractures also result from a fall or motor vehicle accident, but these are generally associated with a higher energy mechanism of injury. Supraphysiologic axial loading of the spinal column results in compression failure of the anterior and middle column. Again, the Denis classification system (Figs. 57.5A to E) is commonly used. Type A represents failure of both superior and inferior end plates. Type B, which is most common, involves only the superior end plate. Type C is a fracture of the inferior end plate, type D is a burst rotation from a combined axial load and rotational injury, and finally type E is a burst fracture associated with lateral flexion injury.

Characteristics of a burst fracture have been described, which contribute to instability; however, this is a subject of much controversy. Nevertheless, these characteristics include >50% loss of vertebral body height, >20° of initial kyphosis or progressive kyphosis, >50% of canal

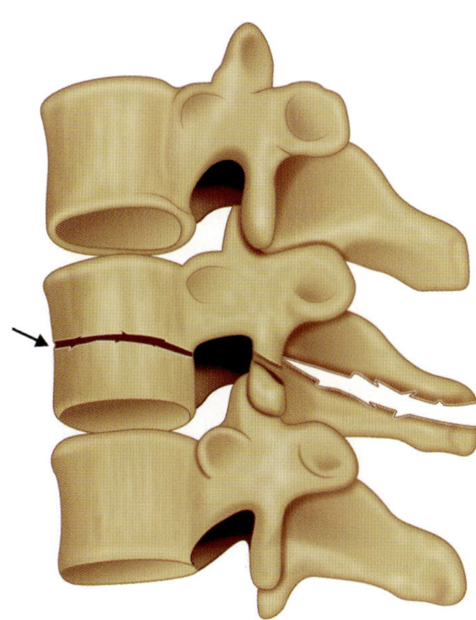

Fig. 57.6: Chance fracture.

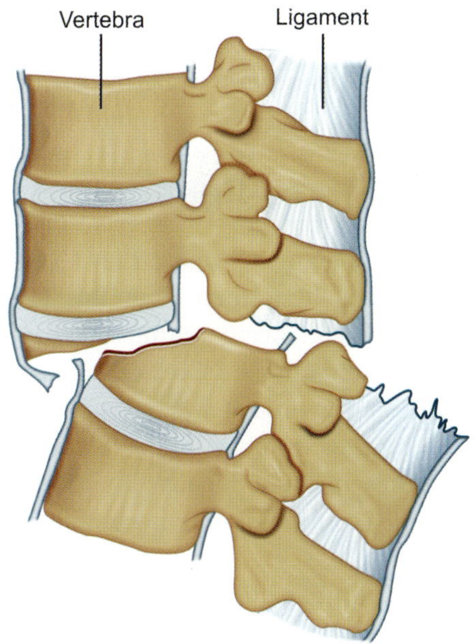

Fig. 57.7: Thoracic fracture dislocation, unstable injury pattern.

compromise, progressive neurological deficit,[15,16] and loss of integrity of the PLC.[17] Traditional teaching was that with a loss of >50% vertebral body height and/or kyphosis of >20°, or neurological deficit represented a high-energy unstable injury pattern with significant risk of collapse into further kyphosis and requirement for operative intervention. More recently, light has been shed on the importance of the PLC and its contribution to stability. In reality, determination of stability is multifactorial and dependent on all of the aforementioned injury characteristics; however, the relative contribution of these injury characteristics in determination of stability continues to be debated.

FLEXION-DISTRACTION INJURIES

Chance fracture (Fig. 57.6) is more commonly seen in young children and most often the result of a motor vehicle accident while using a lap belt only. These injuries occur when the primary force vector acts along an axis of rotation located anterior to the middle column. If the moment arm is in front of the anterior column, then the anterior column fails in tension. If the moment arm is within the anterior column, then it will fail in compression. In either situation, the middle and posterior columns fail in tension. In general, there are three types of Chance fractures: purely bony, purely ligamentous, or a combination of the bony and ligamentous injury.

This injury pattern is associated with a high rate of intra-abdominal injury to hollow viscus organs. Therefore, a high index of suspicions should be maintained with a low threshold for evaluation by the trauma team. Neurological injury may occur and is related to cord compression from the translated vertebral elements and/or epidural hematoma. Overall, the incidence of a major neurologic deficit has been reported to be 25%.[18]

FRACTURE-DISLOCATION INJURIES

These injuries are the result of a high mechanism injury with disruption of all three columns and represent an extremely unstable injury pattern (Fig. 57.7). Although they can occur anywhere throughout the spine, they have a heavy predilection for the TL spine due to the facet orientation. Similar to Chance injuries, a fracture-dislocation involves a flexion and distraction component that results in translation of the superior spinal segment relative to the inferior segment. Facet dislocations represent a continuum of injuries occurring from ligamentous disruption alone or with facet fracture. Combination mechanism injuries can also involve compression failure of the anterior and middle columns.

If the mechanism of injury imparted on the spine is predominantly of a shearing motion, then a translational and/or rotational force will ensue causing unilateral or bilateral facet fracture/dislocation with resulting energy dissipation proceeding horizontally via disk or vertebral body disruption. In either event, the result is a highly unstable injury with an extremely high rate of neurological injury.[19]

LOW LUMBAR INJURIES

The lower lumbar segments include L3–L5 and are less commonly involved in trauma than the TL region. A variety of injuries can occur within the lumbar spine depending on the directional forces acting on the injured spinal segments at the time of injury. As in the previously described TL injuries, lumbar injury characteristics can be classified based anatomically, mechanistically, or morphologically (compression, distraction, translation/ rotation).

Because the lumbar spine contains nerve roots as opposed to a spinal cord and because of the larger cross-sectional area of the canal within the lumbar spine compared with the thoracic spine, a greater degree of canal compromise can be tolerated. Thus, a larger canal-to-neural element ratio is tolerated with significant translational or burst fracture injury patterns. In this respect, if neurological compromise is observed, then a significant amount of energy was imparted, creating an unstable injury pattern.

TREATMENT GOALS

The primary treatment goals of any spinal injury are to prevent or limit neurological injury and to restore stability. Secondary goals include correction of deformity, facilitation of rehabilitation, and preservation of adjacent segment motion. Important factors to consider when deciding on management options include the neurological status, spinal stability, degree of deformity, and any associated injuries.

Nonoperative Management

The advantage of nonoperative treatment includes the obvious avoidance of perioperative morbidity. However, this option can only be entertained in the setting of a stable injury without significant deformity or neurological injury. The majority of isolated compression fractures and burst fractures are stable without neurological injury and as such can usually be treated without surgery. The key step is determining stability, which is generally agreed upon to be dependent on the integrity of the PLC, kyphosis <25–30°, anterior vertebral body height loss <50%, and most importantly, the neurologic status. Those injuries that are found to be stable may be managed in an external orthosis. Prior to ambulation, standing radiographs in the brace should be obtained with periodic radiographs thereafter to ensure maintenance of reduction within the brace. Studies have found no difference in functional outcome, pain scores, and degree of kyphosis correction in stable injury patterns without neurological deficit.[20-24]

Isolated flexion-distraction injuries which are of the pure bony injury variety are generally managed successfully with a hyperextension brace or orthosis unless unable to obtain and maintain a satisfactory reduction of the kyphosis. Those that have a combination of bony and ligamentous components or purely ligamentous injury pattern are best managed operatively.

In regard to isolated lumbar fractures, the general agreement is of nonoperative management for the majority of injuries even if there is an isolated root injury. Because the canal-to-neural element ratio is so large, in the setting of mild canal compromise without significant deformity or instability, further decompression operatively tends to not significantly alter neurological recovery.[14] Furthermore, the prognosis of neurological recovery from a root injury is improved compared to a cord injury. However, a severe neurological deficit with significant canal compromise or specific nerve root compression may be improved with direct operative decompression and fusion.

Operative Management

Surgical indications include progressive neurologic deficit, stable incomplete deficit in the setting of ongoing compression, complete deficit in an effort to facilitate rehabilitation, and previously described injury characteristics highly suggestive of instability. Anterior decompression and stabilization (Fig. 57.8) offer the most direct method of clearing the spinal canal with the highest rates of neurological recovery and inclusion of fewest motion segments compared with a posterior approach (Fig. 57.9). This may be accomplished with a corpectomy and structural graft. The disadvantage of an isolated anterior approach is the potential for higher failure rate in the setting of PLC disruption.[25] Furthermore, anterior column reconstruction allows for direct restoration of the vertebral body height, but at the expense of the associated morbidities and potential complications accompanying an anterior approach.

Posterior approach offers the advantage of avoiding the visceral and vascular structures associated with an

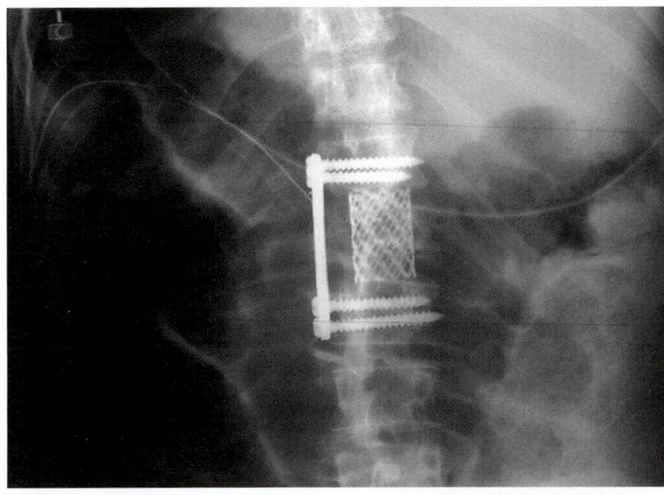

Fig. 57.8: Thoracolumbar burst fracture treated with anterior corpectomy and instrumentation with cross-linked rod-staple-screw construct. Cage contains salvaged fractured bone and allograft.

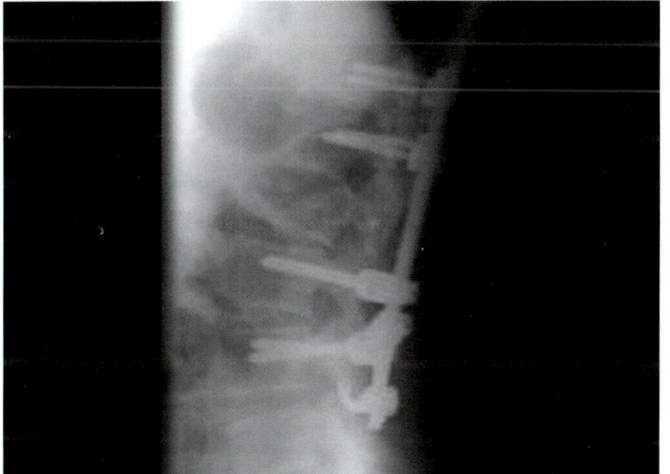

Fig. 57.9: Stability is achieved with posterior pedicle screw construct.

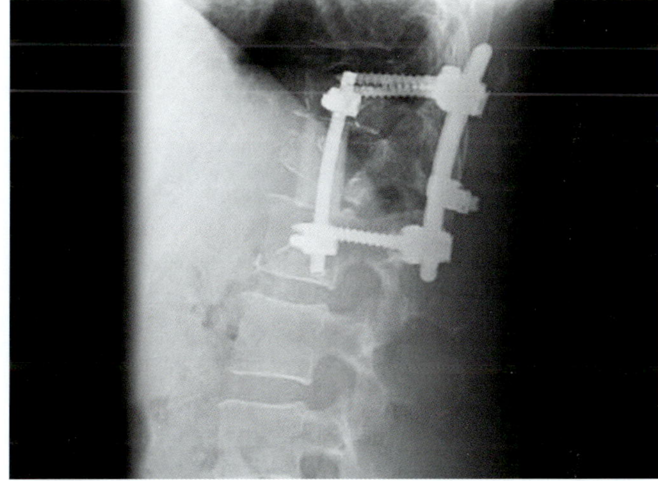

Fig. 57.10: Combined anterior and posterior approach provides the greatest degree stability.

anterior approach. If performed within 3 days of the injury and up to 2 weeks, fracture fragments may be indirectly reduced by an average of 15% via ligamentotaxis.[26] Otherwise, direct decompression may be performed through a transpedicular approach. Another advantage of the posterior approach is that laminectomy may be performed to directly reduce entrapped neural elements and repair traumatic dural tears associated with burst fractures and neurological injuries.[27] Posterior pedicle screw instrumentation may be accomplished using a short or long construct, depending on the severity of injury and integrity of the anterior column. In the setting of a compression or burst fracture and using the load-sharing classification,[6] a score of >6 points indicates a high rate of failure using short segment instrumentation (pedicle screws one level above and below injury level). In this scenario, a long construct (pedicle screws two to three levels cephalad and two levels caudal to the injury level) or a combined anterior and posterior fixation (Fig. 57.10) may be warranted.

In the setting of a purely ligamentous or combined flexion-distraction injury, a posterior approach is recommended to directly address the posterior tension band disruption with a PLC injury. Instrumentation should be limited to as few spinal segments as possible to allow for reconstruction of the posterior column with preservation of as many motion segments safely feasible. This type of injury can be treated with posterior short-segment instrumentation because the load bearing capacity of the anterior column generally is not significantly compromised.[28]

Finally, translational injuries, or fracture-dislocations are generally unstable and best managed operatively.

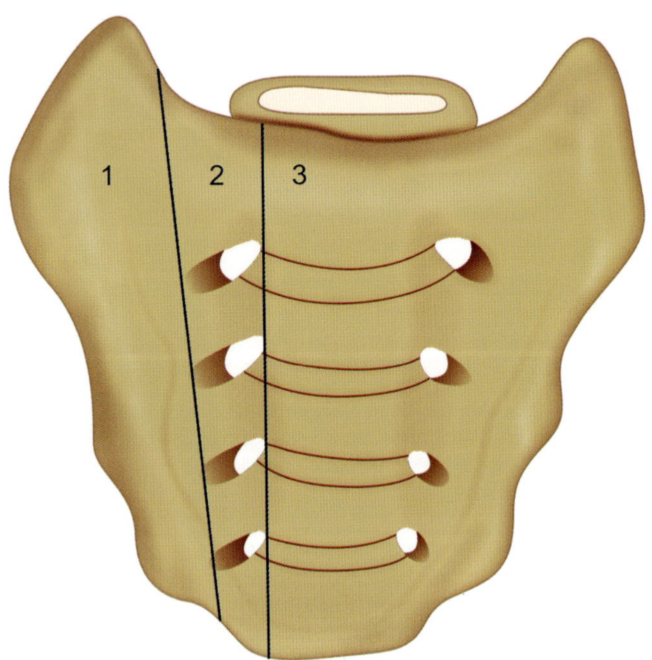

Fig. 57.11: Denis classification of sacral fractures.

Reduction is facilitated with a posterior approach and instrumentation. Severely unstable injuries with anterior column disruption may benefit from the addition of interbody fusion.[29]

As a brief note on sacral fractures, they are classified anatomically with the method proposed by Denis where zone I is a fracture lateral to neuroforamen, zone II is through neuroforamen, and zone III is medial (Fig. 57.11). Zone III fractures have the highest rate of neurologic deficit and are the least common, but may require spinopelvic fixation if there is vertical shear or an L5 transverse process avulsion fracture.

REFERENCES

1. Wood KB, Bohn D, Mehbod A. Anterior versus posterior treatment of stable thoracolumbar burst fractures without neurologic deficit: a prospective, randomized study. J Spinal Disord Techniques. 2005;18 Suppl:S15-23.
2. Ferguson RL, Allen BL. A mechanistic classification of thoracolumbar spine fractures. Clin Orthop Relat Res. 1984;(189):77-88.
3. Denis F. The three column spine and its significance in the classification of acute thoracolumbar spinal injuries. Spine. 1983;8(8):817-31.
4. Vaccaro AR, Kim DH, Brodke DS, et al. Diagnosis and management of thoracolumbar spine fractures. Instruct Course Lectures. 2004;53:359-73.
5. Spivak J, Vaccaro A, Cotler J. Thoracolumbar spine trauma: I. Evaluation and classification. J Am Acad Orthop Surg. 1995;3(6):345-52.
6. McCormack T, Karaikovic E, Gaines RW. The load sharing classification of spine fractures. Spine. 1994;19(15):1741-4.
7. Vaccaro AR, Lehman RA, Hurlbert RJ, et al. A new classification of thoracolumbar injuries: the importance of injury morphology, the integrity of the posterior ligamentous complex, and neurologic status. Spine. 2005;30(20):2325-33.
8. Harrop JS, Vaccaro AR, Hurlbert RJ, et al. Intrarater and interrater reliability and validity in the assessment of the mechanism of injury and integrity of the posterior ligamentous complex: a novel injury severity scoring system for thoracolumbar injuries. Invited submission from the Joint Section Meeting On Disorders of the Spine and Peripheral Nerves, March 2005. J Neurosurg Spine. 2006;4(2):118-22.
9. Panjabi MM, Oxland TR, Kifune M, et al. Validity of the three-column theory of thoracolumbar fractures. A biomechanic investigation. Spine. 1995;20(10):1122-7.
10. Panjabi MM, White AA. Basic biomechanics of the spine. Neurosurgery. 1980;7(1):76-93.
11. Brown T, Hansen RJ, Yorra AJ. Some mechanical tests on the lumbosacral spine with particular reference to the intervertebral discs; a preliminary report. J Bone Joint Surg. American volume. 1957;39-A(5):1135-64.
12. Plaue R. [Mechanics of vertebral compression fracture (static pressure studies in dead vertebrae)]. Zentralbl Chir. 1973;98(21):761-70.
13. Ching RP, Tencer AF, Anderson PA, et al. Comparison of residual stability in thoracolumbar spine fractures using neutral zone measurements. J Orthop. 1995;13(4): 533-41.
14. Zigler JE, Eismont FJ, Garfin SR, Vaccaro AR (Eds). Spine Trauma, 2nd edition. Rosemont, IL: American Academy of Orthopaedic Surgeons, 2011.
15. Holdsworth F. Fractures, dislocations, and fracture-dislocations of the spine. J Bone Joint Surg. American volume. 1970;52(8):1534-51.
16. McAfee PC, Yuan HA, Lasda NA. The unstable burst fracture. Spine. 1982;7(4):365-73.
17. Oner FC, van Gils AP, Dhert WJ, et al. MRI findings of thoracolumbar spine fractures: a categorisation based on MRI examinations of 100 fractures. Skeletal Radiol. 1999;28(8): 433-43.
18. Chapman JR, Agel J, Jurkovich GJ, et al. Thoracolumbar flexion-distraction injuries: associated morbidity and neurological outcomes. Spine. 2008;33(6):648-57.
19. Levine AM, Bosse M, Edwards CC. Bilateral facet dislocations in the thoracolumbar spine. Spine. 1988;13(6):630-40.
20. Weinstein JN, Collalto P, Lehmann TR. Thoracolumbar "burst" fractures treated conservatively: a long-term follow-up. Spine. 1988;13(1):33-8.
21. Shen WJ, Shen YS. Nonsurgical treatment of three-column thoracolumbar junction burst fractures without neurologic deficit. Spine. 1999;24(4):412-5.
22. Aligizakis A, Katonis P, Stergiopoulos K, et al. Functional outcome of burst fractures of the thoracolumbar spine managed non-operatively, with early ambulation, evaluated using the load sharing classification. Acta Orthopaedica Belgica. 2002;68(3):279-87.

23. Cantor JB, Lebwohl NH, Garvey T, et al. Nonoperative management of stable thoracolumbar burst fractures with early ambulation and bracing. Spine. 1993;18(8):971-6.
24. Wood K, Buttermann G, Butterman G, et al. Operative compared with nonoperative treatment of a thoracolumbar burst fracture without neurological deficit. A prospective, randomized study. J Bone Joint Surg. American volume. 2003;85-A(5):773-81.
25. Vaccaro AR, Lim MR, Hurlbert RJ, et al., Spine Trauma Study Group. Surgical decision making for unstable thoracolumbar spine injuries: results of a consensus panel review by the Spine Trauma Study Group. J Spinal Disord Techniques. 2006;19(1):1-10.
26. Willén J, Lindahl S, Irstam L, et al. Unstable thoracolumbar fractures. A study by CT and conventional roentgenology of the reduction effect of Harrington instrumentation. Spine. 1984;9(2):214-9.
27. Cammisa FP, Eismont FJ, Green BA. Dural laceration occurring with burst fractures and associated laminar fractures. J Bone Joint Surg. American volume. 1989;71(7):1044-52.
28. Finkelstein JA, Wai EK, Jackson SS, et al. Single-level fixation of flexion distraction injuries. J Spinal Disord Techniques. 2003;16(3):236-42.
29. Yadla S, LeBude B, Tender GC, et al. Traumatic spondyloptosis of the thoracolumbar spine. J Neurosurg Spine. 2008; 9(2):145-51.

CHAPTER

58

Tumors of the Spine

Donato Pacione, Irene Kim, Dimitris Placantonakis, Anthony Frempong-Boadu

INTRODUCTION

There are three main types of spine and spinal cord tumors based on their anatomical location in relation to the dura and spinal cord.

1. *Extradural*: The most common tumor type, which arises from the vertebral body or epidural space
2. *Intradural extramedullary*: The second most common type, which arises from the nerve roots or the leptomeninges
3. *Intramedullary*: The least common type, which arises from within the spinal cord

Of note, spinal metastases comprise the majority of all spinal tumors and can occur in all three anatomic spaces. This will be discussed in detail later in the chapter.

PRIMARY EXTRADURAL SPINAL TUMORS

The primary extradural spinal tumors may be divided into benign and malignant tumors.

Benign

Aneurysmal Bone Cyst

Aneurysmal bone cysts account for up to 20% of all primary spine tumors and may be primary or secondarily associated with other tumors such as osteoblastoma, hemangioma, or giant cell tumors.[1,2] On computed tomography (CT) imaging (Figs. 58.1A to E), they appear as multilobulated lytic lesions that may be significantly destructive and associated with pathologic vertebral body fractures.[3] Histologically, they are expansile osteolytic blood-filled lesions with a honeycomb appearance.[4] Patients may present with back pain secondary to bony destruction or instability, as well as neurologic symptoms secondary to spinal cord or nerve root compression as the tumor expands. Although these lesions are considered benign, recurrence rate is reported as high as 25% with partial resection or intralesional curettage.[5] En bloc excision is associated with the highest cure rate and best overall prognosis.[5,6] Due to their destructive nature and necessity for total resection, surgical intervention may require a combination of anterior and posterior approaches as well as stabilization (Figs. 58.1D and E). As these are significantly vascularized tumors, preoperative embolization is often utilized to decrease operative blood loss.[7] If the diagnosis is uncertain, a needle biopsy may be performed first with subsequent en bloc or curettage resection.

Hemangioma

Hemangiomas of the spinal column are benign lesions that account for approximately 3% of all spinal tumors with an incidence of 10–29% based on autopsy data.[3,8,9] These tumors exhibit a slight female predominance, occur more often in older patients, and are most often found in the vertebral bodies of the lumbar spine.[8] Only 0.9–1.2% of hemangiomas are considered symptomatic with the most common presenting symptom being back pain.[3,8] However, these lesions can result in neurologic symptoms secondary to compression of the spinal canal or neural elements if they are expansile in nature. Radiographically, hemangiomas have a distinctive honeycomb pattern on

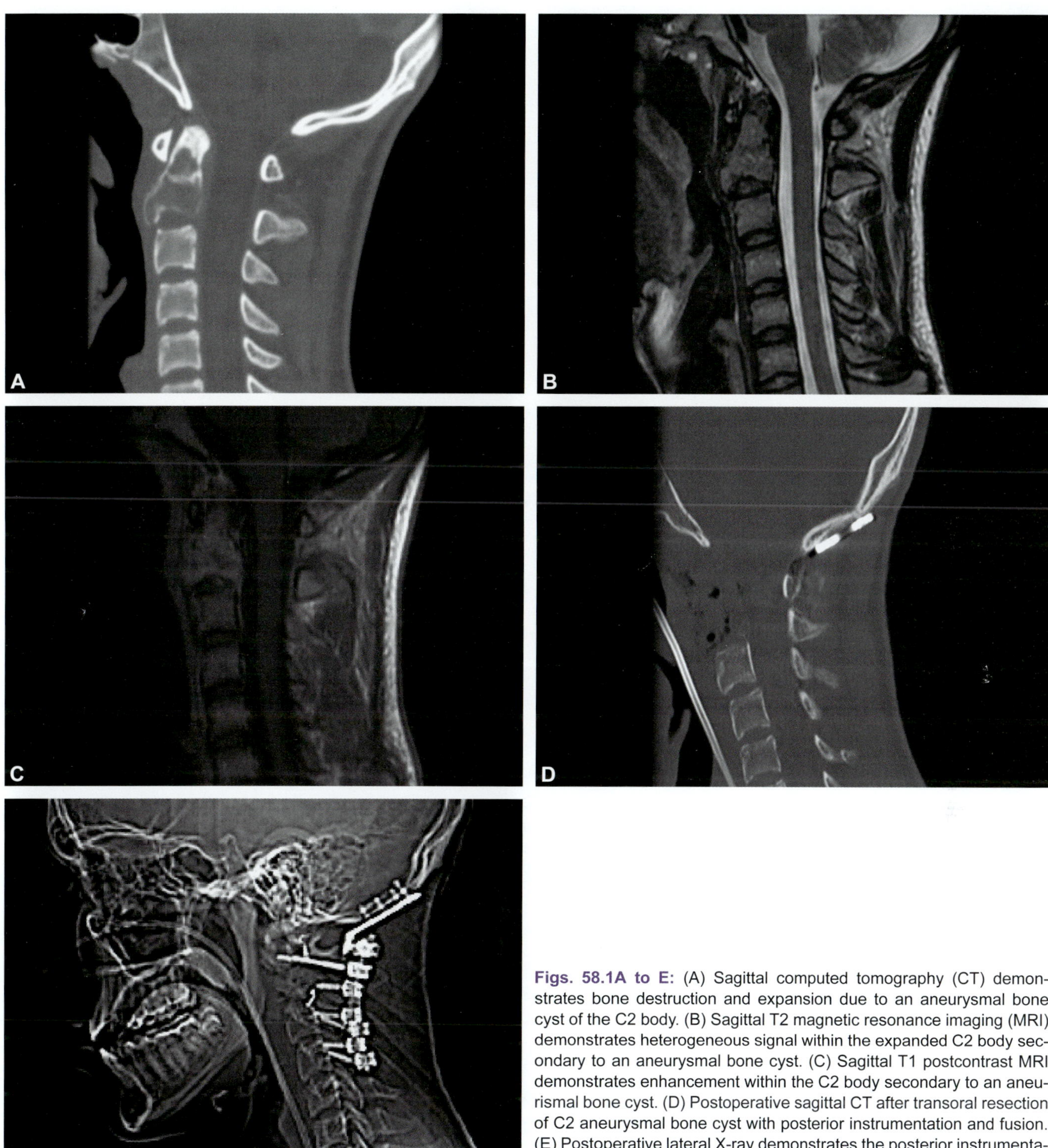

Figs. 58.1A to E: (A) Sagittal computed tomography (CT) demonstrates bone destruction and expansion due to an aneurysmal bone cyst of the C2 body. (B) Sagittal T2 magnetic resonance imaging (MRI) demonstrates heterogeneous signal within the expanded C2 body secondary to an aneurysmal bone cyst. (C) Sagittal T1 postcontrast MRI demonstrates enhancement within the C2 body secondary to an aneurismal bone cyst. (D) Postoperative sagittal CT after transoral resection of C2 aneurysmal bone cyst with posterior instrumentation and fusion. (E) Postoperative lateral X-ray demonstrates the posterior instrumentation utilized for stabilization after resection of C2 aneurysmal bone cyst.

CT imaging. Surgical treatment with decompression and stabilization may be necessary for symptomatic patients. In cases of back pain associated with pathologic fracture from the vertebral hemangioma, kyphoplasty or vertebroplasty has been demonstrated as an effective treatment method.[9]

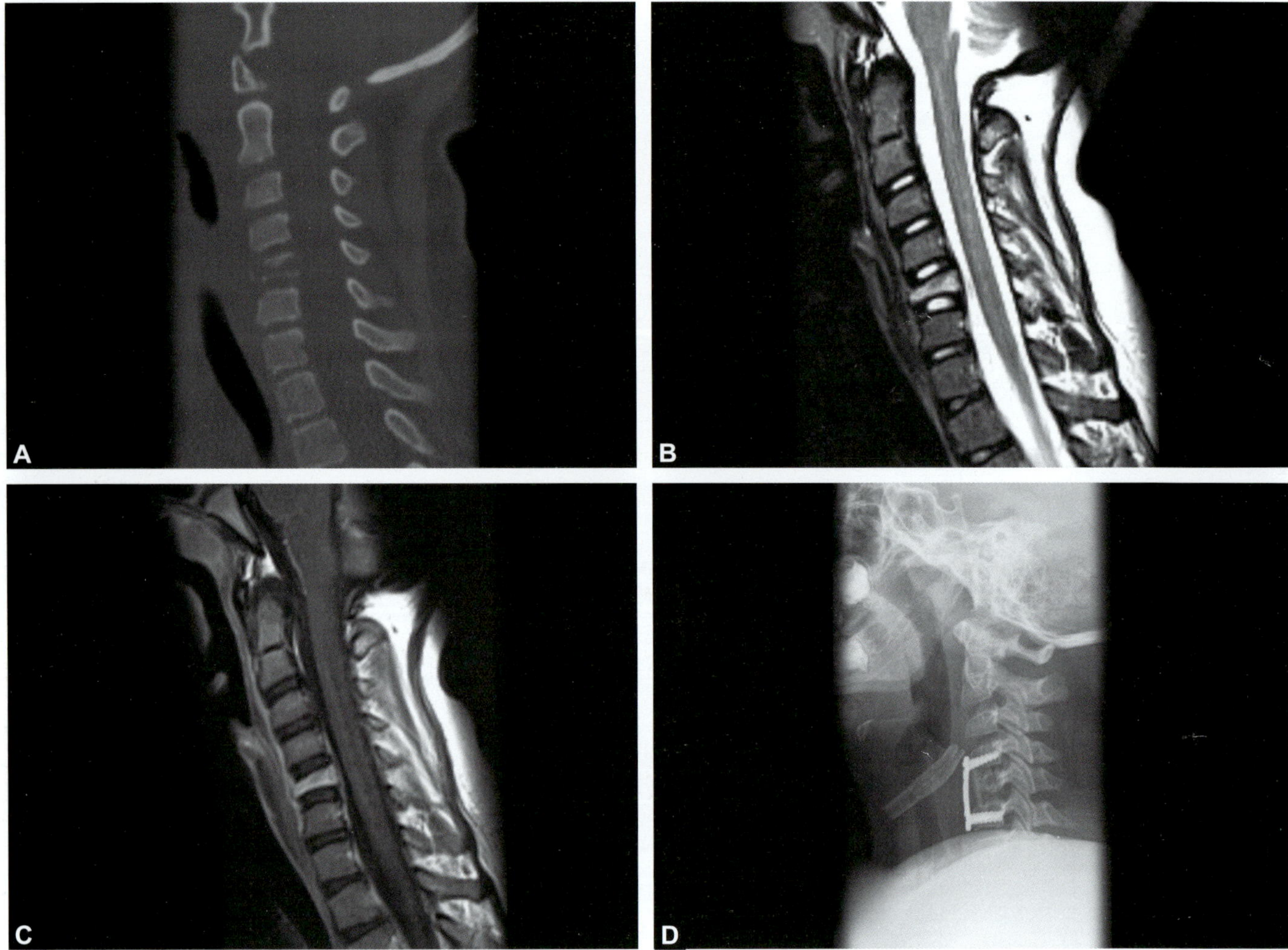

Figs. 58.2A to D: (A) Sagittal computed tomography (CT) demonstrates a lytic C5 eosinophilic granuloma with vertebral body collapse. (B) Sagittal T2 magnetic resonance imaging (MRI) demonstrates hyperintense signal within the C5 vertebral body secondary to eosinophilic granuloma. (C) Sagittal T1 postcontrast MRI demonstrates enhancement within the C5 vertebral body secondary to eosinophilic granuloma. (D) Postoperative lateral cervical spine X-ray after C5 corpectomy with placement of bone strut graft and plating construct.

Eosinophilic Granuloma

Eosinophilic granulomas are benign tumors that account for < 1% of all primary bone tumors.[10] Approximately 80% of spinal eosinophilic granulomas occur in children < 10 years of age.[3,10] They are the result of proliferation of Langerhans histiocytes and demonstrate the presence of Birbeck granules within the cytoplasm.[3] The presence of multiple lesions within the spine or elsewhere in the body is known as Langerhans cell histiocytosis that may be further subclassified as Hand-Schuller-Christian disease (exophthalmos, diabetes insipidus, and skull lesions) or Letterer-Siwe disease (disseminated lesions involving multiple organ systems).[3] The most common presenting symptom with spinal eosinophilic granuloma is neck or back pain, although patients can present with neurologic deficit.[10,11] Radiographically, eosinophilic granulomas present as lytic lesions of the vertebral body (Figs. 58.2A to D) and are the most common cause of loss of vertebral height also known as vertebra plana.[3,10] However, they can also involve the posterior elements as well as invade the spinal canal. Treatment is usually conservative and may involve intralesional corticosteroid injection, immobilization, or radiation.[3,10] Surgical decompression and stabilization is reserved for patients who are refractory to these treatments or who present with gross instability or neurologic deficit.[3]

Chondroma/Enchondroma

Chondromas are benign cartilaginous tumors that account for approximately 4% of all primary bone tumors.[12]

Enchondromas are chondromas that occur within the medullary cavity and may develop into expansile lesions that result in vertebral body destruction. Neurologic symptoms develop more often from periosteal chondromas that expand into the spinal canal and neural foramen.[3,12] Lesions may appear lytic with calcification. Chondromas are usually solitary but chondromatosis may be present in patients with Ollier or Maffucci syndrome.[12] The treatment of these lesions is surgical. There is a risk of sarcomatous degeneration and, as such, treatment is often gross total resection with concurrent stabilization when necessary.[3] Complete resection can be curable with a recurrence rate of < 10%.[13]

Osteoid Osteoma and Osteoblastoma

Osteoid osteomas are relatively small lesions that occur most often in male children and adolescents. Patients generally present with nocturnal pain that is responsive to aspirin. These lesions occur most often in the posterior elements of the lumbar spine.[14] Osteoid osteomas may present with severe scoliotic deformity out of proportion to the size of the lesion, secondary to muscle spasm from irritation.[15] Surgical intervention is generally reserved for lesions associated with neurologic deficit or significant deformity. The surgical treatment is usually en bloc resection or intralesional curettage, and stabilization if necessary.

Osteoblastomas are histologically similar but are usually larger than 2 cm and have the potential for malignant transformation.[3] Patients present with nocturnal back pain and may experience neurologic symptoms secondary to the large size and expansile nature of these lesions. Surgical treatment is recommended due to the likelihood of growth as well as the potential for malignant transformation.[15] En bloc resection should be performed when possible and stabilization is often necessary.

Benign Locally Aggressive

Chordoma

Chordomas are the most common benign primary spinal tumors with an incidence of 0.08 in 100,000 and a 2:1 male predominance.[16,17] They may occur anywhere along the neuroaxis, as they are derived from remnants of the notochord. However, the majority of spinal chordomas (52%) are located in the sacrum/pelvis.[16] Although generally slow growing, chordomas are locally aggressive and have a high recurrence rate, with a 5-year survival rate between 62% and 86%.[16] On CT imaging, chordomas demonstrate lytic bone destruction with a large associated soft tissue mass (Figs. 58.3A to F). Magnetic resonance imaging (MRI) tends to have a mixed signal with variable enhancement.[17,18] In many cases, a needle biopsy may be performed prior to radical surgical resection in order to confirm the diagnosis. The biopsy tract must be clearly marked and included in the surgical resection as there is a high tendency for recurrence along the biopsy tract.[19] Treatment of spinal chordoma is often a combination of surgical resection and radiation. Whenever possible, en bloc resection with wide margins should be performed, as this has been shown to increase disease-free survival (51 vs 17.5 months).[20] En bloc resection is not only technically challenging, but often requires sacrificing neurologic elements, which is better tolerated in the sacral region than in the cervical spine. En bloc spondylectomy may be performed through a combined anterior/posterior approach or through a posterior only technique depending on the extent of tumor invasion to the surrounding tissue.[21] All en bloc resections and the majority of piecemeal resection of spinal chordomas require reconstruction and stabilization.

Giant Cell Tumor

Giant cell tumors are primary bone tumors that rarely occur in the spine. The majority of giant cell tumors of the spine occur in the sacrum and are the second most common sacral tumor after chordomas.[17] The incidence of giant cell tumors in the mobile spine varies from 1% to 9% with the majority occurring in the cervical region.[22] Histologically, these tumors contain multinucleated giant cells that are osteoclastic and are interspersed with spindle cell stroma, which are the proliferative component of the tumors.[17] CT imaging demonstrates lytic expansile lesion that may involve the surrounding soft tissues. MRI demonstrates a hypointense lesion on T1 and T2 imaging with heterogeneous contrast enhancement.[17,22] Although giant cell tumors are technically considered to be benign lesions, they can be locally aggressive and in rare cases metastasize.[23] En bloc resection should be performed when technically and neurologically feasible as it has been demonstrated to yield a lower recurrence rate and a longer disease-free survival compared with intralesional resection.[22]

Malignant

Chondrosarcoma

Chondrosarcomas are rare malignant tumors of the spine that account for 7–10% of all primary spine tumors.[13] They

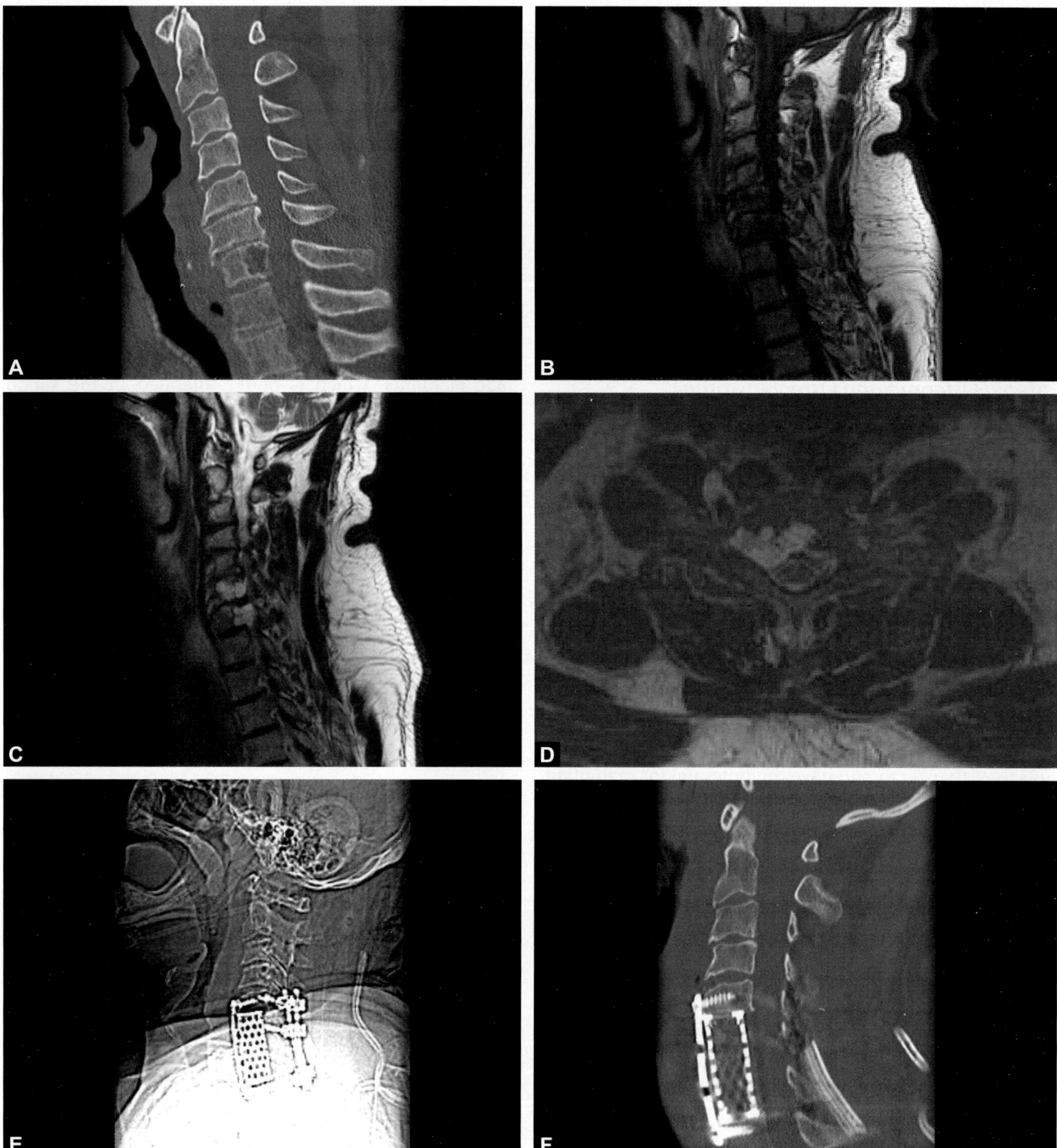

Figs. 58.3A to F: (A) Sagittal computed tomography (CT) demonstrates C6–C7 chordoma with lytic destruction of the vertebral body. (B) Sagittal T1 postcontrast magnetic resonance imaging (MRI) demonstrates the irregular enhancement of the C6–C7 vertebral bodies secondary to chordoma. (C) Sagittal T2 MRI demonstrates hyperintense signal within the C6–C7 vertebral bodies secondary to chordoma. (D) Axial T2 MRI demonstrates hyperintense signal within the C6–C7 vertebral bodies with extension to the foramen transversarium. (E) Axial T2 MRI again demonstrates hyperintense signal within the C6–C7 vertebral bodies with extension to the foramen transversarium. (F) Postoperative lateral X-ray demonstrates a combined anterior and posterior stabilization construct after C6–C7 corpectomy for resection of tumor. (G) Postoperative sagittal CT after C6–C7 corpectomy with placement of titanium cage and anterior plating as well as posterior instrumentation and fusion.

are the second most common malignant primary spine tumor (25%).[13,17] These tumors exhibit 2:1 male predominance and occur most frequently in the thoracic spine.[13,17] The most common presenting symptom is pain but up to 50% may present with a neurologic deficit. Chondrosarcomas are composed of cartilage-forming cells, and can develop as a primary lesion or as a secondary transformation of an osteochondroma.[17] They are classified from WHO grade I–IV, with a 10-year survival of up to 90% in low-grade lesions, and 30–40% in high-grade lesions.[13]

Ewing Sarcoma

Ewing sarcoma is a disease that affects children and young adults and most often involves the long bones.[17] Primary vertebral involvement is uncommon, occurring in only 3.5–15% of all cases, 50% of which involve the sacrum.[24,25] Patients may present with back pain or neurologic deficit depending on the size and location of the lesion. Lesions are usually lytic and demonstrate bony destruction on imaging studies.[24] Overall, 20% of patients will present with metastatic disease.[25] In general, the first-line treatment of Ewing sarcoma involves intensive chemotherapy and radiation. However, many patients with spinal lesions will require surgical decompression due to neurologic compromise and stabilization due to bony destruction of the vertebral column. There is debate regarding the efficacy of aggressive surgical resection with negative margins. Despite chemotherapy and radiation, there is a 20–25% failure of local control.[25] Some series suggest that there is prolonged survival with en bloc resection with negative margins versus piecemeal or intralesional curettage.[25,26]

Osteosarcoma

Osteosarcomas are the most common malignancy of bone and the third most common tumor of the spine.[17,25] They occur most often in adolescence and may be associated with hereditary retinoblastoma and Paget disease. They can occur anywhere in the spine and involve the vertebral body in 90% of cases.[17,25] As a result, patients often present with pain secondary to pathologic fracture as well as neurologic deficit due to canal compromise. On imaging, both osteolytic and sclerotic patterns are often seen. The treatment algorithm for these tumors involves neoadjuvant chemotherapy to initially shrink the tumor as well as to treat the likely systemic micrometastases. This is followed by en bloc spondylectomy with wide margins if possible followed by stabilization.[25,27] Conventional external beam radiotherapy (XRT) is relatively ineffective as a primary treatment of osteosarcomas and may be used for palliative cases with significant metastatic disease. However, case reports suggest that stereotactic radiosurgery may be effective for local control in situations in which en bloc resection cannot be performed.[28]

INTRADURAL EXTRAMEDULLARY SPINAL TUMORS

Schwannomas

Spinal schwannomas are benign slow growing tumors that arise from the myelin producing Schwann cells of nerve roots. They arise from the sensory rootlets in approximately 75–90% of cases, and their growth results in displacement of the axons of the associated nerve root.[29] Consequently, the most common presenting symptom of schwannomas is radiculopathy. However, larger tumors may also present with myelopathy secondary to spinal cord compression. The majority of these tumors occur sporadically. However, they may be associated with neurofibromatosis type II (NF2) and, less commonly, NF1. Patients with NF2 will often develop multiple schwannomas over their lifetime.

The majority of schwannomas are completely intradural. However, they are classically described as dumbbell tumors in which there is both an intradural and extradural component, depending on their location on the involved nerve root. In some cases, the dumbbell shape is secondary to constriction at the dural sleeve of the exiting root, whereas others achieve a dumbbell configuration due to constriction at the neural foramen. Approximately 8–23% of tumors are completely extradural and occur entirely within or lateral to the neural foramen.[30] In rare cases, up to 1.5% of schwannomas may be entirely intramedullary in location.[31] On MRI, schwannomas are discrete nodular lesions that are T1 isointense, T2 hyperintense, and avidly enhance with gadolinium contrast (Figs. 58.4A to C). The lesions may also contain areas of cystic degeneration.

Small asymptomatic schwannomas may be observed with serial imaging, as they are generally benign slow-growing lesions. Treatment of symptomatic spinal schwannomas is generally surgical and often curative, if complete resection is possible. Depending on the degree of nerve root involvement, patients may be at risk of new deficits. As a result, debulking and partial resection may be necessary.

Neurophysiologic monitoring is necessary for the resection of spinal schwannomas and may be helpful in

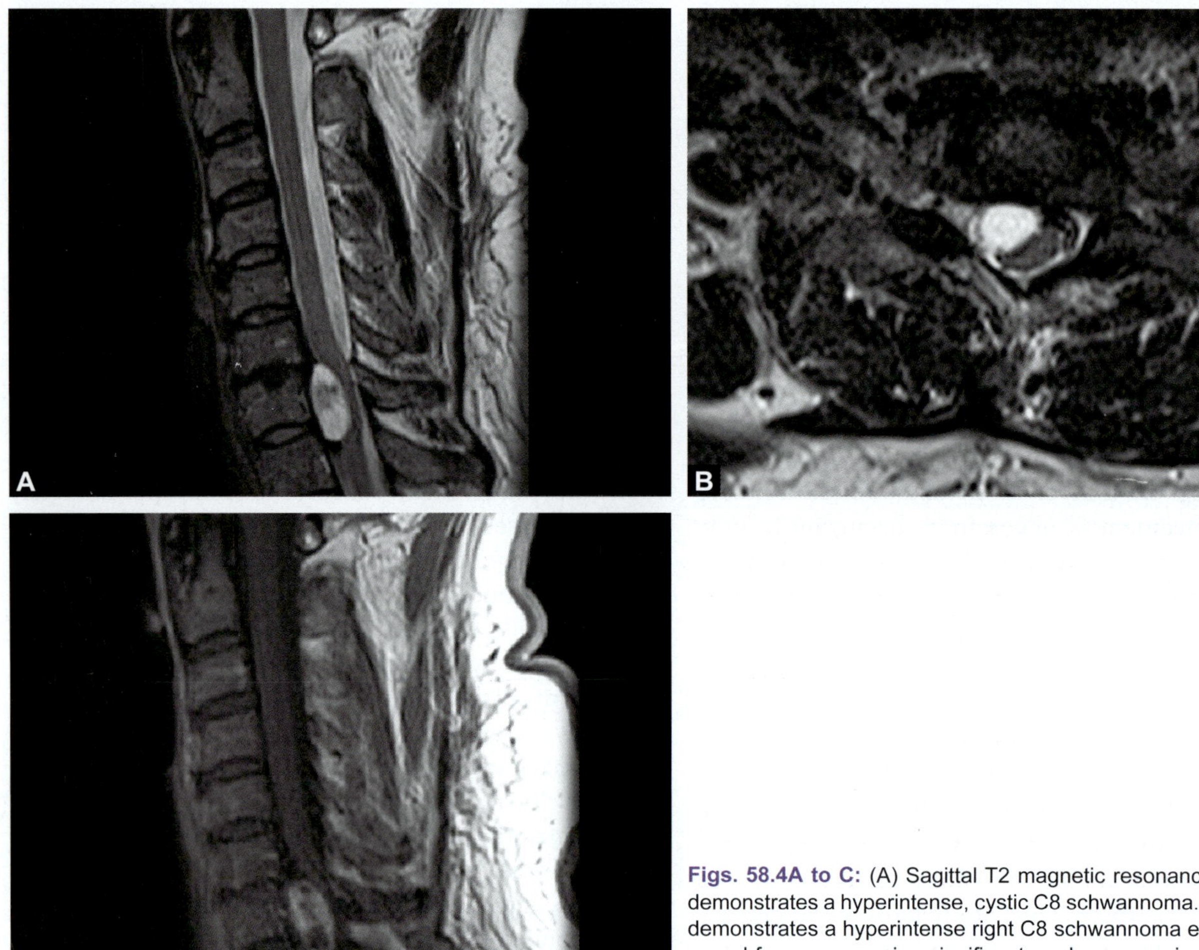

Figs. 58.4A to C: (A) Sagittal T2 magnetic resonance imaging (MRI) demonstrates a hyperintense, cystic C8 schwannoma. (B) Axial T2 MRI demonstrates a hyperintense right C8 schwannoma extending into the neural foramen, causing significant cord compression. (C) Sagittal T1 postcontrast MRI demonstrates an avidly enhancing C8 schwannoma.

determining the functionality of the involved nerve root distal to the tumor. In cases where the nerve root does not respond to motor stimulation, it may be sacrificed without significant risk of deficit. It is postulated that the nerve roots associated with the tumors are often no longer functional by the time a patient presents for surgical resection.[31,32] Postoperative deficits after sacrificing nerve roots are reported to be between 0% and 23% with no incidence of significant motor deficit.[31,32]

In general, schwannomas are resected through a standard posterior approach via a laminotomy or hemilaminotomy. Tumors with an extensive extradural component extending through the neural foramen may require a partial facetectomy. In rare cases, an anterior approach with corpectomy may be utilized.[33] The majority of cases do not require stabilization with instrumentation and fusion unless there is significant bone removal involving the facet joints.[31,34] Smaller tumors with nerve roots that can be sacrificed may be removed in an extracapsular fashion. However, larger tumors often require intracapsular debulking with an ultrasonic aspirator. In the majority of cases, gross total resection can be achieved if the nerve root involved is of minimal functional significance. Subtotal resection may be necessary in larger tumors with significant extension along the nerve root in the brachial plexus or lumbosacral plexus.[31,34] There is a higher rate of recurrence with a subtotal resection and despite gross total resection, there is still a 10% recurrence rate at 5 years.[31] Patients who are poor surgical candidates and who do not present with significant myelopathy secondary to spinal cord compression may be candidates for stereotactic radiosurgery. Stereotactic radiosurgery for schwannomas demonstrates high rates of control and tumor regression.[35] Cases of subtotal resection are not recommended for adjuvant radiosurgery treatment, but should instead be observed for regrowth.[36]

Neurofibroma

Neurofibromas are nerve sheath tumors that consist of axons or dendrites of immature neurons. As these tumors develop from neurons, they tend to encapsulate and engulf the involved nerve root. They may occur sporadically but are often associated with NF1. Patients with NF1 can have multiple neurofibromas involving several nerve roots that can coalesce to form plexiform neurofibromas. Although these are benign tumors, in cases of NF1, there is a potential for malignant transformation into malignant peripheral nerve sheath tumors. Patients often present with pain and radiculopathy secondary to nerve root involvement but may also develop myelopathy in larger lesions. On MRI, the lesions appear as round, T1 isointense, T2 hyperintense, and contrast-enhancing masses.

Asymptomatic lesions, especially in the case of NF1, should be followed with serial imaging. Symptomatic or growing lesions should be treated with surgical resection. As the nerve is often encapsulated and intimately involved with the tumor, complete resection may not be possible in functional nerve roots. Neurophysiologic monitoring with direct nerve root stimulation is necessary to determine the degree of functionality of the involved nerve root. Plexiform neurofibromas (Figs. 58.5A to D) encompass multiple nerve roots and as a result, complete resection is often not possible. Subtotally resected benign neurofibromas are observed with serial imaging and adjuvant treatment with radiation or chemotherapy is not recommended.[36] Patients with NF1 harbor a risk of malignant degeneration secondary to adjuvant radiation therapy.[37]

Surgical resection of neurofibromas is generally achieved through a laminectomy or hemilaminotomy. In the case of smaller tumors, a minimally invasive technique may be utilized.[38] Tumors with a significant extraforaminal component may require partial or complete facetectomy. Stabilization with instrumentation and fusion is often not required in the setting of a solitary neurofibroma. In patients with NF1, there is a higher rate of postsurgical instability secondary to associated dystrophic vertebral body changes and higher rates of kyphoscoliosis.[39] Stabilization with instrumentation and fusion (Fig. 58.5E) is recommended at the time of tumor resection in this population, in order to avoid progressive deformity.[39]

Meningioma

Spinal meningiomas account for approximately 25–40% of spinal tumors.[36,40] There is a significant female predominance with 80% of spinal meningiomas occurring in women.[36] Similar to intracranial meningiomas, spinal meningiomas arise from the arachnoid cap cells of the dura. As a result, they may occur anywhere in the spine, most frequently in the thoracic spine (80%).[36,40] Patients with NF2 are at risk of multiple intracranial and spinal meningiomas. The most common presenting symptoms are back pain as well as progressive myelopathy (motor dysfunction, sensory disturbances, and incontinence due to spinal cord compression. Radiographically, spinal meningiomas are avidly contrast enhancing on MRI (Figs. 58.6A to C). The T2 characteristics may be heterogeneous due to the presence of calcifications within the meningioma.

Spinal meningiomas tend to be slow growing benign tumors (WHO grade I) and asymptomatic lesions may be observed with serial imaging. Symptomatic tumors should be addressed with complete surgical resection. The recurrence rates after complete resection are 0–15%.[40,41] Resection of the involved dura and replacement with a dural patch graft has a similar rate of recurrence as coagulation of the dura with minimal dural resection.[40] Prior to surgical resection, a CT scan should be obtained to determine the degree of calcification as this is associated with a higher rate of surgical morbidity.[41] The dural attachment is most often located laterally or ventrolaterally in the spinal canal. In a recent series, 73% of the surgically resected spinal meningiomas had a dural attachment ventral to the dentate ligament.[41] Despite a ventral dural attachment, the majority of spinal meningiomas can be removed through standard posterior approach via a laminectomy or hemilaminotomy (Fig. 58.6D).[34,41] Extended facetectomy/pediculectomy in order to achieve a more lateral exposure or a ventral approach with corpectomy may require stabilization and fusion.[34] As with the majority of spinal cord tumors, these cases should be performed with intraoperative neurophysiologic monitoring. Patients with incomplete resection, tumor recurrence, or those deemed to be poor surgical candidates may be treated with either conventional external beam radiation therapy or stereotactic radiosurgery.[36,42,43]

INTRADURAL INTRAMEDULLARY SPINAL TUMORS

Ependymoma

Ependymomas are the most common type of intramedullary spinal cord tumor, accounting for 60% of all intramedullary tumors.[36,44,45] There is a slight male predominance

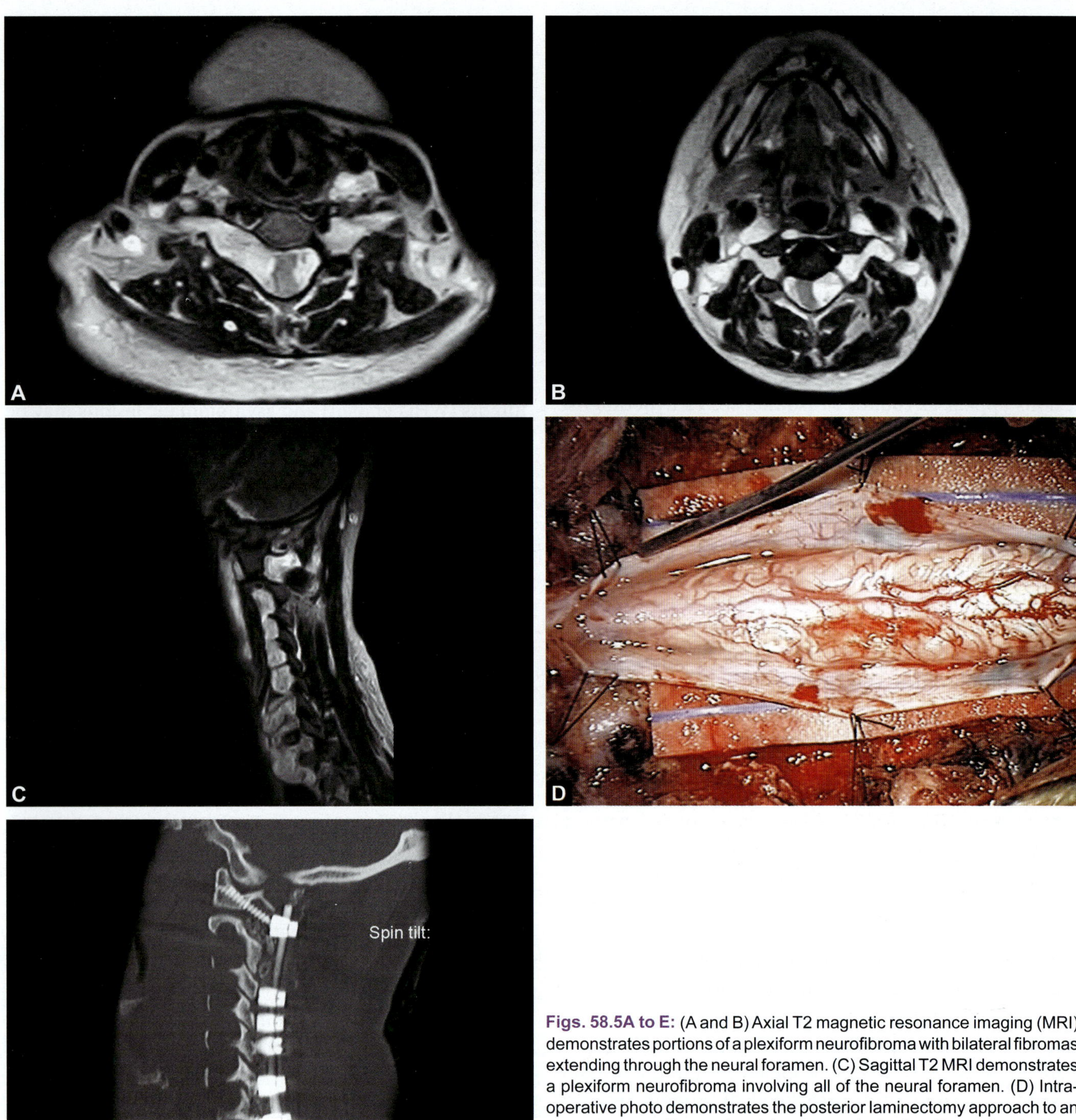

Figs. 58.5A to E: (A and B) Axial T2 magnetic resonance imaging (MRI) demonstrates portions of a plexiform neurofibroma with bilateral fibromas extending through the neural foramen. (C) Sagittal T2 MRI demonstrates a plexiform neurofibroma involving all of the neural foramen. (D) Intraoperative photo demonstrates the posterior laminectomy approach to an extensive neurofibroma involving the cervical spine. Due to its plexiform nature, the tumors were debulked to provide decompression of the spinal cord. (E) Postoperative sagittal computed tomography demonstrates the instrumentation placed for stabilization.

(56%) with spinal ependymomas.[44] There are two types of spinal ependymomas, cellular and myxopapillary, which are distinguished based on their cellular origin. Cellular ependymomas originate from the ependymal cells of the central canal of the cervical and thoracic spinal cord. They are slightly more aggressive and are often classified as WHO grade II or III. Myxopapillary ependymomas originate from cells of the filum terminale and are histologically

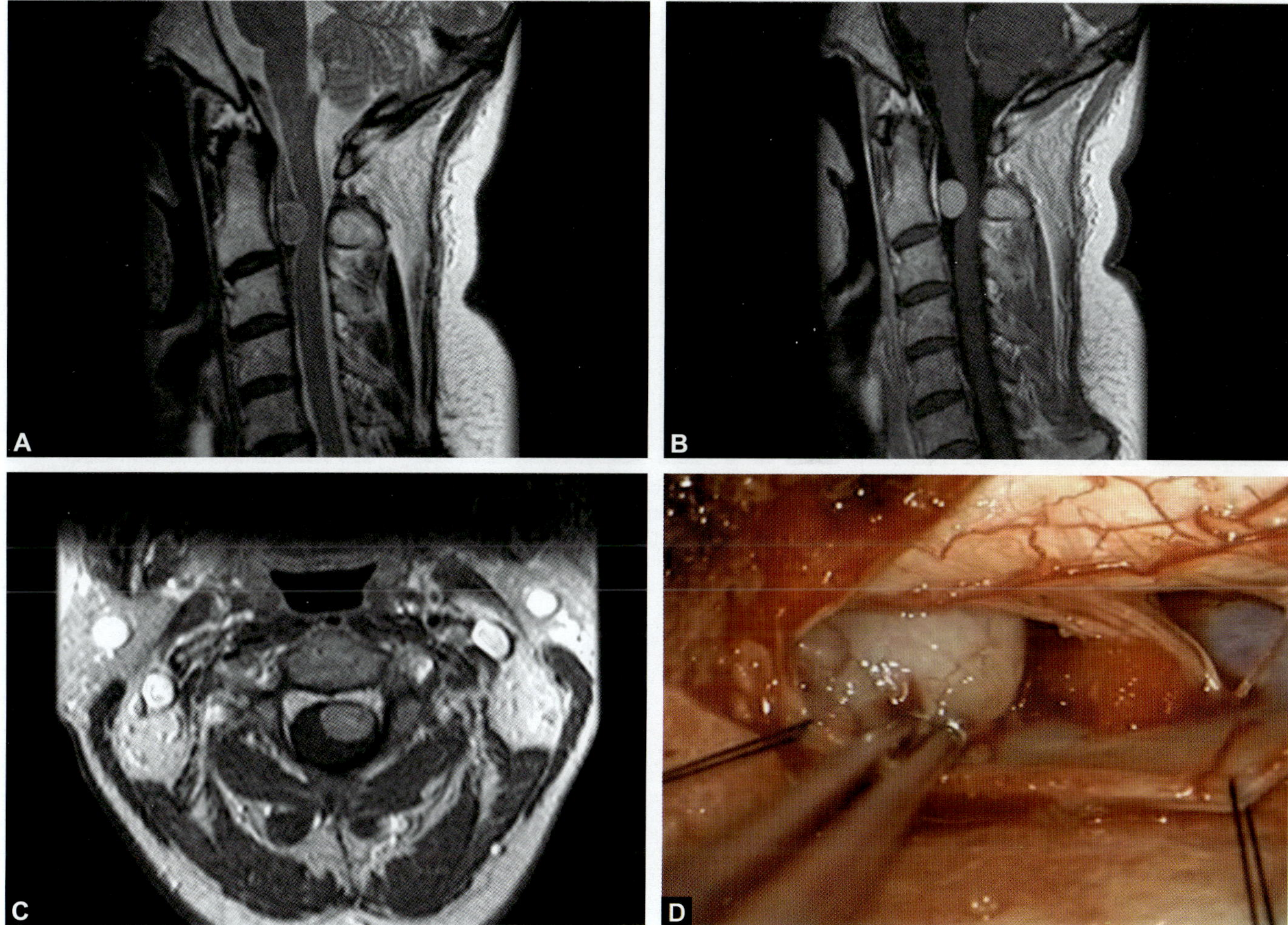

Figs. 58.6A to D: (A) Sagittal T2 magnetic resonance imaging (MRI) demonstrates a ventrolateral meningioma behind C2 causing spinal cord compression. (B) Sagittal T1 postcontrast MRI demonstrates an avidly enhancing C2 meningioma. (C) Axial T1 postcontrast MRI demonstrates an avidly enhancing meningioma located ventrolateral to the spinal cord. (D) Intraoperative photo demonstrates the standard posterior approach for the resection of a ventrolateral meningioma through a laminectomy.

benign tumors (WHO grade I).[36] On MRI (Figs. 58.7A to D), ependymomas are T2 hyperintense enlargements within the spinal cord and exhibit heterogeneous enhancement on T1 imaging.[36,46] There are rare case reports of extramedullary spinal ependymomas.[45] Due to the intramedullary nature of these tumors, patients often present with progressive myelopathy and sensory disturbances.

As the majority of these tumors are relatively benign in nature, complete surgical resection can be curative, especially in the case of myxopapillary ependymomas. Resection is generally performed through a posterior approach either through laminectomy or hemilaminotomy (Figs. 58.8A and B). There has also been a trend toward minimally invasive approaches for resection of smaller spinal ependymomas.[47] The tumor is usually accessed where it comes to the surface or through a midline myelotomy. Lateralized tumors may be approached through the dorsal root entry zone. Ependymomas often have a defined plane that facilitates resection. However, complete resection may be limited by the degree of spinal cord invasion. As with all spinal cord tumors, intraoperative neurophysiologic monitoring is necessary to assist in determining the limits of the resection. In a recent literature review, gross total resection was achieved in 77% of patients with a 5-year progression-free survival rate of nearly 100%.[36,44] Subtotal resection has been associated with a 5-year progression-free survival rate of 45%. The addition of adjuvant radiation therapy was shown to improve the 5-year progression-free survival rate to 65%.[44] As would be expected, subtotal resection is associated with higher grade tumors and lower rates of progression-free survival.

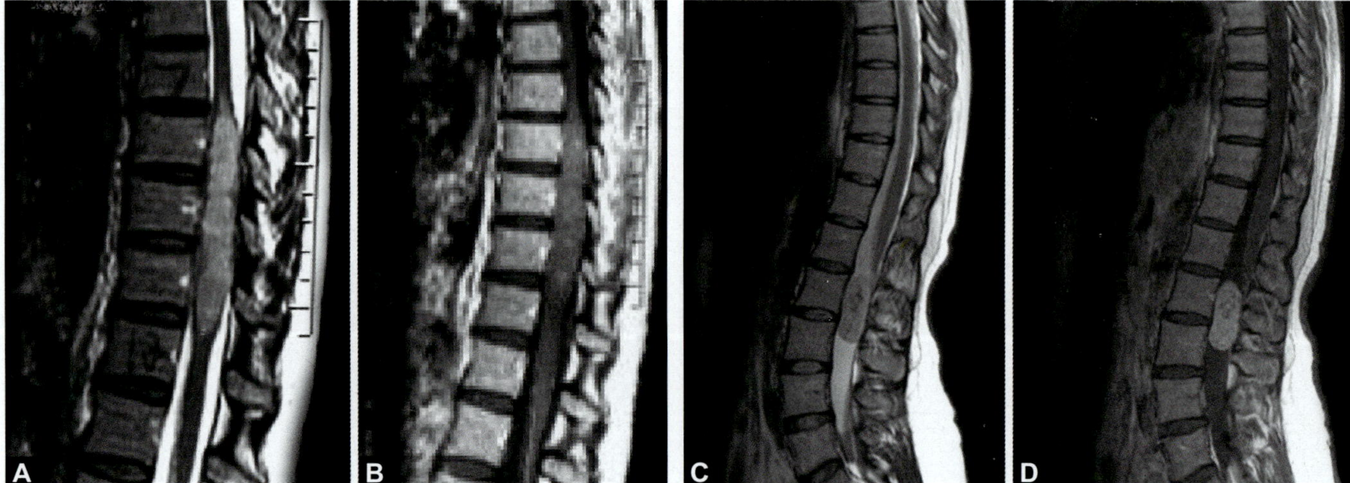

Figs. 58.7A to D: (A) Sagittal T2 magnetic resonance imaging (MRI) demonstrates hyperintense signal of an intramedullary thoracic ependymoma. (B) Sagittal T1 postcontrast MRI demonstrates an enhancing intramedullary thoracic ependymoma. (C) Sagittal T2 MRI demonstrates a myxopapillary ependymoma. (D) Sagittal T1 postcontrast MRI demonstrates enhancing myxopapillary ependymoma.

Astrocytoma

Astrocytomas are the second most common (20–40%) intramedullary spinal cord tumor.[36,48] However, they are the most common intramedullary tumor in children, accounting for 55% of tumors.[48] The majority of astrocytomas (75%), especially in children, are low-grade lesions, either pilocytic (WHO grade I) or fibrillary (WHO grade II). Less commonly, they may be WHO grade III or IV.[36,49] They may occur anywhere within the spinal cord with the majority occurring within the cervical and thoracic region.[49,50] On MRI imaging, they appear as T2 hyperintense lesions that diffusely infiltrate the spinal cord and often do not have a well-demarcated border (Figs. 58.9A and B). T1 postcontrast imaging demonstrates irregular contrast-enhancing borders and may also show intratumoral cysts.[36] Most patients present with motor or sensory deficits, depending on the level of cord involvement.[49,50]

Overall, the WHO grade is the most important prognostic factor for spinal cord astrocytomas.[36,49,50] Pilocytic astrocytomas, when compared with infiltrative astrocytomas, demonstrate significantly higher 5-year (85% vs 36%) and 10-year (78% vs 17%) survival rates.[49,51] Age is also linked to a better prognosis, with younger patients demonstrating longer progression-free and overall survival.[48-51] The role and extent of surgical resection in the treatment of these tumors is controversial. As these are infiltrative tumors, there is often no distinct plane between tumor and normal spinal cord. Gross total resection is often not possible without significant neurologic morbidity. A gross total resection is achieved more often with pilocytic tumors (up to 80% in some series) compared with infiltrative tumors (0–12%).[36,49-51] Multivariate analysis has demonstrated no association between progression free or overall survival and extent of surgical resection.[49,50] XRT for subtotal resection and recurrence has been linked to improved progression-free and overall survival.[51] Surgical resection is usually performed through a posterior approach and standard laminectomy or hemilaminotomy. Tumors that do not come to the surface of the spinal cord are accessed through a midline myelotomy or if significantly lateralized, through the dorsal root entry zone. Neurophysiologic monitoring is necessary and monitoring parameters often dictate the extent of resection. Resection of these tumors is not destabilizing and instrumentation and fusion is not necessary.

Hemangioblastoma

Hemangioblastomas are the third most common intramedullary spinal cord tumor, accounting for approximately 3% of intramedullary tumors.[36,52] The majority (75%) are solitary lesions, which occur sporadically, while 25% are associated with von Hippel-Lindau (VHL) disease and multiple CNS lesions.[52] They are more commonly found in males. Patients most commonly present with progressive sensory or proprioceptive deficits.[36,52]

Hemangioblastomas are benign lesions made up of stromal cells surrounded by a vascular matrix involving

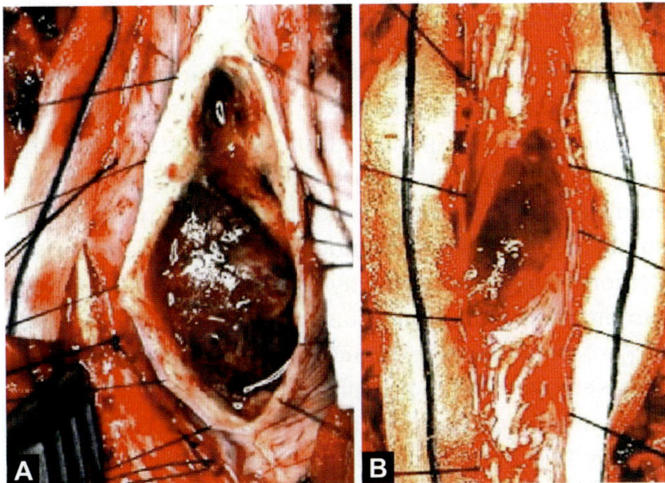

Figs. 58.8A and B: (A) Intraoperative photo demonstrates thoracic intraspinal ependymoma. (B) Intraoperative photo demonstrates myxopapillary ependymoma within the cauda equina.

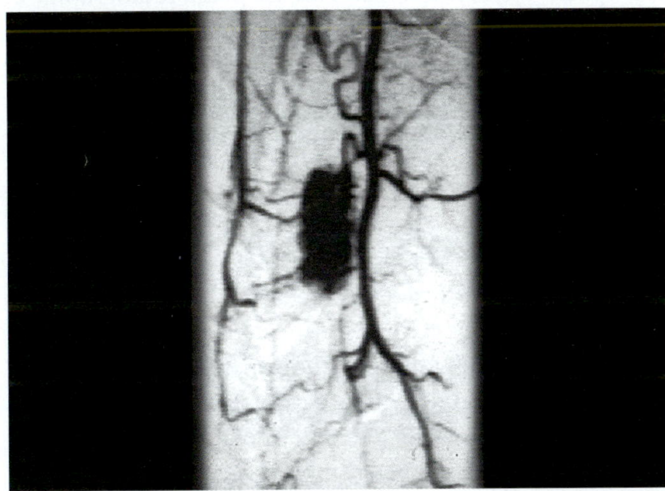

Fig. 58.10: Spinal angiography of a hemangioblastoma demonstrates large feeding vessels and draining veins.

feeding arteries and large draining veins, and usually occur dorsal to the dentate ligament.[52] MRI demonstrates a contrast-enhancing nodule that may be associated with a cyst or syrinx. Angiography will demonstrate the hypervascularity of the tumor with large feeding vessels and large draining veins (Fig. 58.10).

Hemangioblastomas are benign lesions. In cases of sporadic tumor development, complete surgical resection is curative. Patients with VHL are prone to recurrence or the development of new lesions throughout their lifetime and should be monitored with serial MRI's, despite gross total resection.[52] Surgical resection is usually carried out through a posterior approach via a laminectomy or hemilaminotomy. Care must be taken to identify the borders

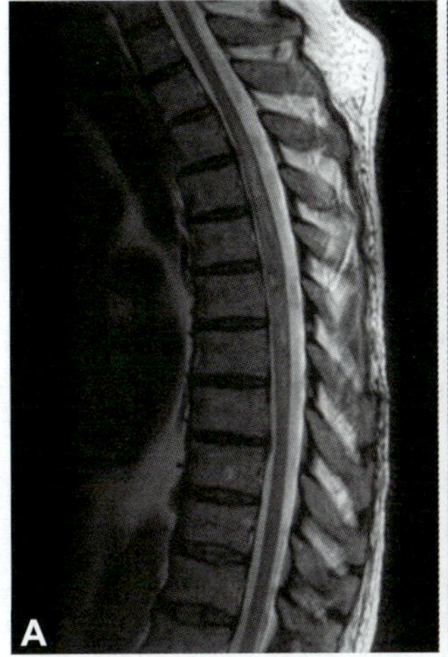

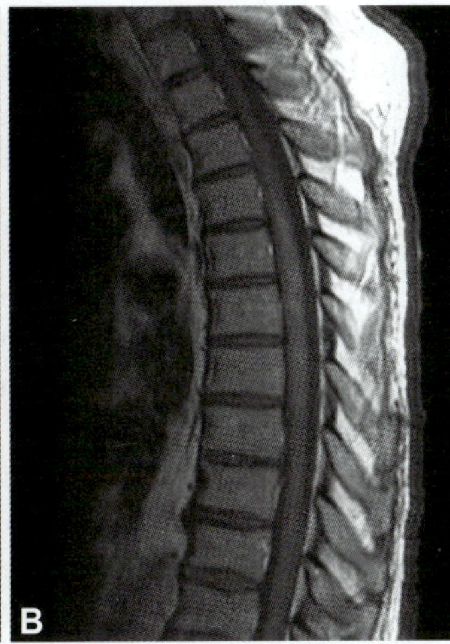

Figs. 58.9A and B: (A) Sagittal T2 magnetic resonance imaging (MRI) demonstrates diffuse heterogeneous signal with spinal cord expansion from T3 to T8 secondary to a low-grade astrocytoma. (B) Sagittal T1 postcontrast MRI demonstrates diffuse, patchy enhancement within the spinal cord secondary to a low-grade astrocytoma.

of the tumor and the associated vascular network. This network of feeding arteries and draining veins should be dissected and coagulated in order to decrease bleeding during dissection of the tumor plane. If the vascular anatomy is favorable, preoperative embolization may be performed in order to reduce intraoperative blood loss and facilitate maintenance of the tumor plane.[53]

Although rare, hemangioblastomas may be located in the ventral aspect of the spinal cord. Approach to these lesions through a standard posterior midline myelotomy or a posterolateral approach may result in neurologic deterioration or subtotal resection. Instead these lesions may be approached through a more direct anterior approach with a corpectomy and subsequent stabilization.[34,54]

Surgical resection is the primary treatment modality of hemangioblastomas and there is no role for chemotherapy or standard external beam radiation therapy. However, stereotactic radiosurgery may be an effective alternative for VHL patients with multiple lesions, recurrence, or those whose surgical resection may be associated with a high morbidity.[55]

Ganglioglioma

Spinal cord gangliogliomas are rare tumors that account for approximately 1% of all intramedullary tumors.[56,57] They are composed of a mixture of glial cells, usually astrocytes, and neurons, typically ganglion cells. These tumors are most often found in the pediatric population with 75% occurring in children < 16 years of age.[56] Gangliogliomas can occur anywhere in the spinal cord but have a predilection for the cervicothoracic region.[56] Patients often present with slowly developing symptoms of weakness and sensory disturbances. On MRI, these tumors appear as heterogeneous lesions with T2 hyperintensity and patchy contrast enhancement.[57]

Gangliogliomas are generally considered to be benign, slow growing tumors (WHO grade I). However, there are case reports of malignant transformation to anaplastic gangliogliomas (WHO grade III).[58,59] Anaplastic gangliogliomas are extremely rare and account for < 5% of gangliogliomas.[58] Surgical resection, with an attempt at gross total resection, is the first-line treatment of these lesions. In a large series, gross total resection was achieved in 82% of patients with a 50-year survival rate of 88% and progression-free survival rate of 67%.[56] Surgical resection of these lesions is through a laminectomy or hemilaminotomy. As with other intramedullary lesions, resection should be performed with the use of neurophysiologic monitoring. In the case of subtotal resection or recurrence, adjuvant chemotherapy or radiation may be utilized.

SPINAL METASTASES

It is estimated that 30–90% of all patients who die of cancer are found to harbor spinal metastases in cadaver studies.[60-64] Approximately 10% of all cancer patients will develop symptomatic spine metastases with nearly 50% requiring some form of treatment.[60,62] Symptoms associated with spinal metastasis may be the initial presentation in up to 10% of patients with undiagnosed cancer.[65] Surgical intervention is required in 5–10% of patients with symptomatic metastases.[60,66-68] The highest incidence is found in patients 40–65 years of age, as this group also has the highest incidence of cancer.[60,69] Men have a slightly higher rate of spinal metastasis than women as a result of the higher prevalence of lung cancer in men, as well as prostate cancer.[60,69] Overall, spinal metastatic disease is most likely to originate from breast (16.5%), lung (15.6%), and prostate (9.2%) cancer, and to a lesser extent renal cell carcinoma, melanoma, thyroid cancer, lymphoma, multiple myeloma, and colorectal cancer.[60,70-73] With improvements in medical treatment and increased life expectancy in cancer patients, there will be an increase in the number of patients treated for spine metastases in the future.

Diagnosis

The diagnosis and evaluation of suspected spinal metastatic disease may require multiple imaging modalities.

Plain Radiographs

Plain radiographs are insufficiently sensitive and specific to rule in or rule out suspected spine metastasis. Radiographic findings of spinal metastasis include lytic vertebral body erosion, blastic sclerosis, pedicle erosion, vertebral compression fractures, large paraspinal masses, and spinal deformities.[60,74] Standard spine radiographs will demonstrate an abnormality in 85–94% of patients with symptomatic spinal metastases.[75-78] In an autopsy study, 26% of patients were found to have spinal metastases that were not detected on plain radiographs.[63] Plain films accurately predict the level of metastatic cord compression in only 21% of patients.[79] In order to be visible on plain radiographs, at least 30–50% of the vertebral bone must be eroded. [74] As a result of these significant limitations, further imaging is often required in patients with suspected spinal metastases. The role of plain radiographs in obtaining new diagnoses of spinal metastases is diminishing, but plain films may have some utility for assessing alignment and stability as they are more readily performed in the upright, flexion, and extension positions than other radiographic modalities.

Bone Scan

Nuclear scintigraphy detects areas of increased metabolic and osteoblastic activity associated with metastatic disease, as well as inflammation or infection within the skeletal system. Bone scans are capable of detecting spinal metastases at an earlier stage than plain films. In several series, bone scans detected metastases in approximately 30% of patients with normal plain radiographs.[80,81] Scintigraphy has a sensitivity of 62–89% and a specificity of 78–81% in detecting vertebral metastases.[82,83] Because scintigraphy lacks specificity and has relatively poor resolution, further imaging with CT or MRI is necessary.

Single photon emission tomography (SPECT) is a three-dimensional form of nuclear scintigraphy, which is more sensitive and specific than conventional bone scans and provides superior resolution.[82,84] SPECT is also capable of distinguishing between metastatic and benign lesions.[82,85]

Positron Emission Tomography

Positron emission tomography with 18F-fluorodeoxyglucose (FDG-PET) measures the utilization of glucose and detects regions of high metabolic activity. FDG-PET has a higher sensitivity and specificity than scintigraphy at detecting vertebral metastatic lesions at an earlier stage.[83,86,87] With sensitivity and specificity > 90%, FDG-PET is a useful screening and surveillance tool,[83,87] particularly in the case of nonsclerotic metastases originating from solid tumors.[83,87,88] Similar to scintigraphy, FDG-PET is limited by its resolution and further imaging is necessary after a lesion is identified.

Computerized Tomography

Computed tomography allows for a detailed three-dimensional view of the bony anatomy of the spinal column and associated soft tissues. CT provides information regarding the degree of bone involvement and destruction by tumor, which is often needed for preoperative planning. Visualization of the spinal cord and neural elements with CT is significantly inferior to that seen on MRI. However, when combined with myelography, CT provides information regarding areas of neural compression that is comparable with MRI.[89] CT scans are often used in conjunction with MRI in the overall assessment of spinal metastases. In addition to visualizing the spinal lesion, CT scans of the chest, abdomen, and pelvis are also utilized as part of a complete workup to determine the extent of metastatic burden.

Magnetic Resonance Imaging

Magnetic resonance imaging is the most sensitive imaging modality for early detection of spinal metastases.[90,91] Because of its superior three-dimensional soft tissue imaging as well as detailed visualization of soft tissue-osseous interface, MRI is considered the gold standard in evaluation of spinal metastases.[90-92] MRI also provides high-resolution imaging of the spinal cord and neural elements and is a highly sensitive modality for identifying the area of neurologic compression. T1 sequences usually reveal bony metastases as hypointense lesions due to the replacement of fat in bone marrow with tumor cells. Axial T2 sequences can be used to assess the degree of epidural disease, spinal cord compression, and obliteration of the subarachnoid spaces. The addition of gadolinium contrast to T1 sequences provides further information as metastatic tumors are often avidly enhancing.[72] Gadolinium contrast is particularly useful in identifying intradural metastases and leptomeningeal involvement. Through the addition of diffusion-weighted imaging (DWI), MRI may be utilized to differentiate between benign and pathologic compression fractures.[93] The use of MRI is an imperative imaging modality for the evaluation of spinal metastasis and has been shown to alter therapeutic decision making.[94]

Angiography

The use of digital subtraction angiography is a valuable adjunct when dealing with spinal metastases that are known to have a high degree of vascularity. Primary lesions such as renal cell carcinoma, hepatocellular carcinoma, leiomyosarcoma, thyroid carcinoma, angiosarcoma, pheochromocytoma, and paraganglioma tend to develop highly vascular metastatic lesions. Angiography is used both as a diagnostic modality to provide information regarding the vascular supply of the tumor and therapeutically through embolization. Preoperative embolization of vascular spinal metastases reduces intraoperative blood loss, improves tumor resection, and shortens overall operative time.[95-99] Embolization may also be therapeutic for patients who are not considered surgical candidates.[99,100]

Percutaneous Biopsy

Spinal metastases are the initial presentation of malignancy in approximately 10% of patients.[65,101] The histologic tumor type is one of the most important factors influencing the treatment plan. Patients who are not immediate surgical candidates and have no other easily accessible lesion will need a percutaneous biopsy of the spinal tumor. Because biopsies are performed when the histology of the lesion is unknown, the lesion could represent metastatic or primary tumor, such as chordoma. Chordomas have the potential to seed or recur along the biopsy tract. As a result, surgeons should be involved in the biopsy planning to prepare for possible resection of the margins of the tract.[19,102] Percutaneous biopsy is performed using CT image guidance with a success rate of 80–90%, with biopsies of lytic lesions having a slightly higher yield than sclerotic lesions.[103-106] This procedure is often performed on an outpatient basis with most patients being discharged after a short observational period.[104]

Treatment Options

Overall the prognosis is poor for patients with spinal metastases and the median survival time can be as short as 3–6 months.[107,108] An increased survival time has been associated with preservation of ambulatory status, no evidence of systemic visceral disease or brain metastasis, single site of epidural compression, rate of onset of motor deficits, and radiosensitive tumors.[108] A patient's presenting motor function is the strongest predictor for ambulatory outcome.[108,109] Treatment of metastatic spinal disease is not curative for most types of metastases, and the goal is to improve pain, as well as maintain neurologic function and mechanical stability. The treatment of spinal metastasis is with surgery, radiation therapy, chemotherapy, or a combination of modalities.

Surgical Treatment

Surgical intervention is capable of addressing the major factors associated with spinal metastasis: neurologic compromise, improving pain, and maintaining mechanical stability. However, as an invasive treatment modality with significant associated morbidity (10–30%), it requires careful patient selection.[70,110] Due to the risks of surgery and recovery time, a patient should have a life expectancy of at least 3 months to be a candidate for surgery.[62,110,111] In the setting of neurologic compromise secondary to spinal metastasis, surgical intervention allows the most immediate decompression of neurologic structures. The landmark randomized prospective trial by Patchell et al. examined the difference between patients undergoing surgical resection, stabilization, and XRT with those patients treated only with XRT. Patients in the surgical treatment group were more likely to walk after treatment than those in the XRT group (84% vs 57%).[112] Those patients who were able to walk prior to treatment were more likely to retain that ability after surgical treatment rather than XRT (94% vs 74%) and those who could not walk before treatment were also more likely to regain that ability after surgery (62% vs 19%).[112] Patients in the surgical group retained the ability to walk for 122 days compared with 13 days in the XRT group.[112] There was also an improvement in survival in the surgical group (126 vs 100 days).[112] Conclusions from these results are limited by the exclusion of patients with highly radiosensitive tumors such as lymphoma, myeloma, and small cell lung cancer (Table 58.1). However, in the absence of radiosensitive pathology, surgical intervention provides superior sustained neurologic improvement. In the setting of solitary spinal renal cell carcinoma metastasis, en bloc surgical resection has been shown to improve disease-free survival.[113-115]

The most common site of metastatic spinal disease is in the vertebral body of the thoracolumbar spine, which is responsible for supporting up to 80% of the axial load.[116] Osteolytic activity of tumor within the vertebral body compromises the load capacity resulting in compression or burst fractures. Cadaveric studies demonstrate that strength reduction is proportional to the cross-sectional area of a lytic and, more recently, that fractures could be predicted from the CT cross-sectional area of intact bone and bone mineral density.[117] Others studies suggest that, in the thoracic spine, impending collapse is found with 50–60% destruction of the vertebral body alone or 25–30% involvement of the body with costovertebral joint destruction.[118] In the lumbar spine, collapse is predicted with 35–40% involvement of the vertebral body or 20–25% of the body and destruction of the posterior elements.[118] Involvement of the facet joints may predispose patients to translational instability, spondylolysis, and dislocation.

Surgical stabilization of metastatic lesions is performed in conjunction with decompression. A large review of the literature demonstrated a greater improvement in neurologic function with laminectomy and stabilization (64%) when compared with patients undergoing laminectomy alone (42%).[119] The addition of stabilization did not significantly alter the surgical mortality rate.[119] Anterior decompression and stabilization was found to have the best improvement in neurologic function (75%) but was also associated with a higher mortality rate (10% vs 5% for laminectomy and stabilization).[119] The combination of posterior decompression/stabilization to generate adequate tumor margins from the spinal cord and adjuvant image-guided intensity-modulated radiation therapy (IGIMRT) or spinal radiosurgery (SRS) provides excellent tumor control rates. This approach eliminates the need for aggressive surgical resections, including anterior approaches, which are associated with higher morbidity and mortality rates.

Once a patient has been deemed a surgical candidate, a decision must be made regarding the approach and necessity of stabilization. The surgical approach is often dictated by the location of the tumor, both the spinal segment and location within the vertebra. Histology of

Table 58.1: Radiosensitivity of primary tumors

Radiosensitive	*Moderately radiosensitive*	*Moderately radioresistant*	*Radioresistant*
Lymphoma	Breast	Lung	Renal cell carcinoma
Multiple myeloma	Prostate	Gastrointestinal	Melanoma
Small cell lung cancer			Sarcoma

the tumor may also play a role as there is evidence that patients with renal cell carcinoma may benefit from a complete spondylectomy.[62,115]

Because the majority of metastases originate in the vertebral body and extend to the ventral aspect of the spinal cord, an anterior approach may provide good decompression of neurologic structures in certain cases. Anterior approaches are associated with lower rates of wound breakdown, wound infection, and cerebrospinal fluid leak than posterior approaches.[120-123] For tumors located in the cervical spine, both anterior and posterior approaches are relatively straightforward and similar to those performed for degenerative disease. Posterior decompression and stabilization for metastatic disease to the cervicothoracic junction has been shown to produce excellent outcomes.[124]

Anterior Approach

With regard to anterior approaches, tumors within the cervicothoracic junction or upper thoracic spine (T1–T4) sometimes require a combination of anterolateral cervical approach, sternal window or sternotomy/manubriotomy, and possible thoracotomy.[68,125,126] This region is particularly challenging because of the presence of the great vessels that may prohibit direct anterior access to the tumor. For tumors of the mid-thoracic spine (T5–T10), anterior access is achieved via a right-sided thoracotomy in order to minimize injury to the aortic arch and great vessels.[68,120] A left-sided thoracotomy may be utilized if there is significant left-sided pathology. Anterior access to the thoracolumbar junction (T11–L1) often requires a left-sided approach, to avoid the liver. In such an approach, a combination of thoracotomy and retroperitoneal access may be used depending on the level of the crus of the diaphragm.[68,120] Tumors of the lumbar spine (L2-5) may be accessed through transpsoas, retroperitoneal, or trans-abdominal/transperitoneal approaches.[68,120] Sacral lesions may be accessed through a transperitoneal approach. Limitations of the anterior approach are associated with increased morbidity and mortality due to need for sternotomy, thoracotomy, retroperitoneal approaches, and mobilization of large vessels.[119,120,123]

Posterior Approaches

Because of the associated difficulties of the anterior approach to the cervicothoracic and thoracic lesions, a posterior transpedicular approach to ventral decompression is being increasingly utilized.[127] Based on a recent review of the literature, the Spine Oncology Study Group makes a strong recommendation of the use of the posterior or posterolateral approach (bilateral transpedicular, costotransversectomy, or lateral extracavitary) for lesions from T2 to T5.[123] Posterior approaches from T6 to L5 should also be performed as a preferred alternative to the anterior approaches (Figs. 58.11A to E).[123,128-130] The posterior surgical techniques used to access the vertebral body are more anatomically challenging.[123] Sacral lesions may be approached posteriorly, anteriorly through a transperitoneal approach, or a combined anterior-posterior approach.

Method of Stabilization

Once a surgical approach is chosen and a resection is performed, attention must be turned to stabilization of the spine. Anterior stabilization can be achieved through the use of autograft, allograft, titanium mesh cages, expandable titanium cages, polyetheretherketone (PEEK) cages, polymethylmethacrylate (PMMA) secured by Steinman pins, or PMMA-filled chest tube.[131,132] The anterior column support strut is usually covered with a plate or screw rod construct to span a level above and a level below the corpectomy site. If the anterior resection is at the cervicothoracic junction, thoracolumbar junction, involves two or more adjacent vertebral bodies, is associated with kyphosis, or there is involvement of the posterior elements, then posterior supplementation with pedicle screw fixation is recommended.[60,98,119] Anterior stabilization from the posterior only approach utilizes similar support devices with significant reliance on the expandable cage (Figs. 58.11D and E).[128,129] The posterior approach also relies on a combination of posterior fixation devices based primarily on pedicle screws, with hooks and wires becoming rapidly obsolete.[124]

Minimally Invasive Techniques

In addition to standard surgical approaches, there has been an increased utilization of minimally invasive and percutaneous surgical techniques. Video-assisted thoracoscopic surgery (VATS) allows for access and resection from T1 to T12 but has been limited by a steep learning curve, prolonged operative times, and substantial blood loss.[133,134] Minimally invasive retroperitoneal techniques, such as the extreme lateral and direct lateral approaches,

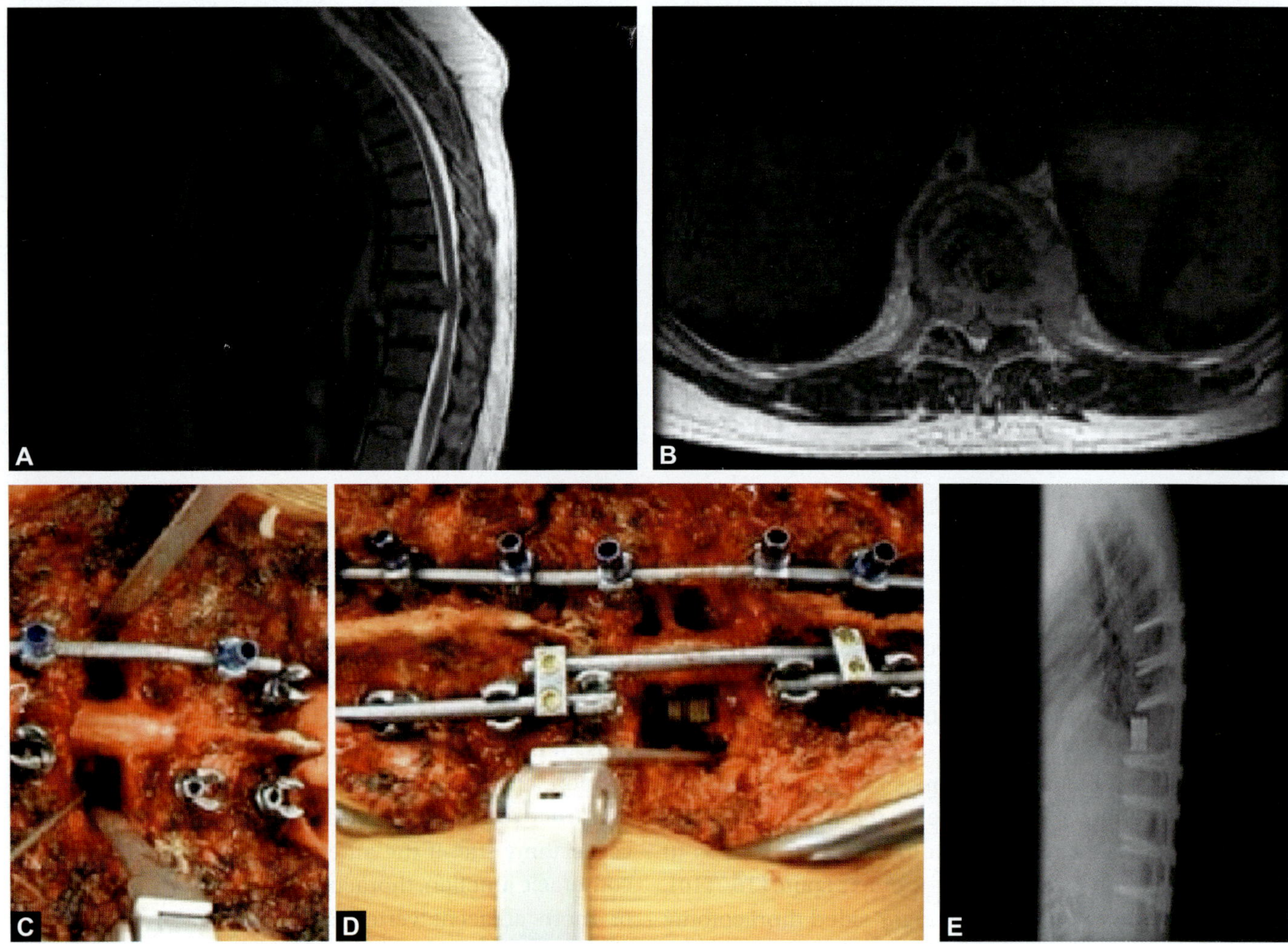

Figs. 58.11A to E: (A) Sagittal T2 magnetic resonance imaging (MRI) demonstrates pathologic T9 compression fracture. (B) Axial T2 MRI demonstrates grade 2 epidural disease from a pathologic T9 compression fracture. (C) Intraoperative photo of T9 lateral extracavitary vertebrectomy. (D) Intraoperative photo of T9 lateral extracavitary vertebrectomy after placement of expandable cage. (E) Postoperative lateral X-ray demonstrates T9 expandable cage and T7-L1 instrumentation and fusion.

have become increasingly popular in the realm of degenerative disease. This technology can be applied to gain anterior access to lumbar spinal metastases.[135,136] With the use of three-dimensional image guidance, there has been an increase in the placement of percutaneous thoracolumbar pedicle screws for posterior stabilization.[137,138] The advantage of all of the minimally invasive techniques is less destruction/disruption of tissue and decreased postoperative pain.[95,133,135,137,138]

Vertebroplasty and Kyphoplasty

Percutaneous vertebroplasty and kyphoplasty are minimally invasive techniques that may provide pain relief and stabilization in patients with pathologic compression fractures. Vertebroplasty is a radiographically guided injection of PMMA into the vertebral body.[139,140] Significant pain relief after vertebroplasty is observed in 63–97% of cases.[140-142] The hypothesized mechanism of pain relief from vertebroplasty is a combination of mechanical stabilization of microfractures as well as destruction of nerve terminals by the exothermic and chemical effects of PMMA.[141,143] In a recent review, the complication rate of vertebroplasty ranged from 0% to 17% per level treated, with the majority being minor complications.[140] Most complications are associated with cement extravasation with the majority of cement leaks being asymptomatic.[140,144] The major side effects of cement extravasation are through local compression of neurologic structures or the hematogenous spread resulting in pulmonary embolism.[145]

One of the limitations of vertebroplasty is the inability to restore height and improve kyphotic deformity. Kyphoplasty addresses this limitation and involves the placement of a balloon into the vertebral body, which is then expanded to create a cavity prior to injection of PMMA.[142] Pain relief in kyphoplasty is similar to vertebroplasty but with 42% restoration of height.[142] Kyphoplasty has been shown to have a lower propensity for cement extravasation due to the increased viscosity of the cement, lower injection pressure into the cavity created, and obliteration of potential bone or vascular pathways by the balloon tamp.[146,147] Vertebroplasty and kyphoplasty offer a minimally invasive treatment option for patients who are not surgical candidates and can be used in conjunction with radiation therapy for significant pain relief from pathologic fracture.[148]

Traditionally the presence of significant posterior cortical disruption or epidural cord compression is considered a relative contraindication for both kyphoplasty and vertebroplasty, as posteriorly displaced tissue, bone or cement may lead to neurologic compromise.[140] However, recentanecdotal evidence has challenged this notion.

An alternative to kyphoplasty is plasma-mediated radio frequency ablation combined with vertebroplasty. Plasma-mediated radio frequency ablation involves the percutaneous placement of a radio frequency wand into the vertebral body. Radio frequency energy is then applied to saline solution to create a focused plasma field at the tip of the wand. The energized particles in the plasma cause molecular dissociation converting the ablated tissue into gas at relatively low temperatures 40–70°C.[149] This results in the creation of a cavity with minimal heat transferred to the surrounding tissue.[150] Once a cavity is created, PMMA is then injected to fill that space. The advantage of radio frequency ablation is cavity creation through the ablation of tissue rather than the displacement of tissue, as in kyphoplasty. This technique may reduce the risk of epidural compression from posterior tissue displacement, as well as decrease the risk of cement extravasation by creating a directed clean cavity.[149]

Decision Making and Overall Management

Treatment of spinal metastatic disease is palliative with the goal of improving overall quality of remaining life through alleviation of pain and maintenance of neurologic function and mechanical stability. Decision making regarding treatment involves balancing the risks and side effects with expected survival. Many scoring systems and algorithms have been developed to help guide optimal treatment protocols. Tomita et al. developed a scoring system based on the grade of malignancy of the primary tumor, visceral metastases, and number of bone metastases (Table 58.2).[151] In this system more weight is given to the type of tumor as well as significant systemic disease.[151] With the Tomita scoring system a better prognosis is associated with a lower score. A score of 2–3 corresponds to a good prognosis and patients should be treated with a wide excision.[151] Patients with an intermediate prognosis (score of 4–5) should undergo an intralesional excision.[151] Palliative surgery should be undertaken in patients with a score of 6–7.[151] Those patients with a poor prognosis (score 8–10) should be treated with XRT.[151]

Tokuhashi et al. developed a scoring system based on performance status, number of extraspinal bone metastases, number of metastases in the vertebral body, visceral metastases, type of primary cancer, and degree of neurologic deficit (Table 58.3).[152,153] The primary cancer type was found to have the highest predictive value and is therefore weighted more in the Tokuhashi scoring system. According to the Tokuhashi score, aggressive surgical resection (i.e. anterior resection, combined anterior/posterior resection, en bloc resection) is recommended for patients with a good prognosis (score of 12–15) and expected survival of >1 year.[153] For patients with an intermediate prognosis (score of 9–12) and expected survival of 6 months to 1 year, a palliative surgery (i.e. posterior decompression, posterior stabilization) is recommended.[153] Patients with a poor prognosis (1–8) and expected survival of <6 months should have conservative treatment in the form of XRT.[153]

Beyond scoring systems, Bilsky and Smith developed a general decision-making framework based on the NOMS (Neurologic, Oncologic, Mechanical instability, Systemic disease) algorithm.[154] The neurologic factors include the degree of myelopathy and/or radiculopathy, as well as the radiographic extent of epidural metastatic disease.

Table 58.2: Tomita scoring system[151]

	Score 1	*Score 2*	*Score 3*
Primary tumor	Slow growth	Moderate growth	Rapid growth
Visceral metastases		Treatable	Untreatable
Bone metastases	Solitary	Multiple	

The extent of epidural involvement (determined by T2 MRI imaging) is divided into four grades based on the degree of subarachnoid space obliteration and epidural spinal cord compression: grade 0 involves only the bony elements with no impingement on the epidural spaces (Fig. 58.12A); grade 1 involves impingement on the subarachnoid space without spinal cord deformation (Figs. 58.12B to D); grade 2 demonstrates partial subarachnoid space obliteration and spinal cord deformation (Fig. 58.12E); and grade 3 is spinal cord deformation with complete obliteration of the subarachnoid space (Fig. 58.12F).[127,154] Grade 0 and 1 are considered low-grade lesions, whereas grade 2 and 3 are considered high grade. With the widespread use and availability of IGIMRT/SRS, this grading scale has been

Table 58.3: Tokuhashi scoring system[153]

	Score 0	*Score 1*	*Score 2*	*Score 3*	*Score 4*	*Score 5*
Karnofsky performance	10–40	50–70	80–100			
Extraspinal bone metastases	3 or more	1–2	0			
Vertebral metastases	3 or more	2	1			
Visceral metastases	Unremovable	Removable	None			
Primary site	Lung	Liver	Other	Kidney	Rectum	Breast
Palsy	Frankel A, B	Frankel C, D	Frankel E			

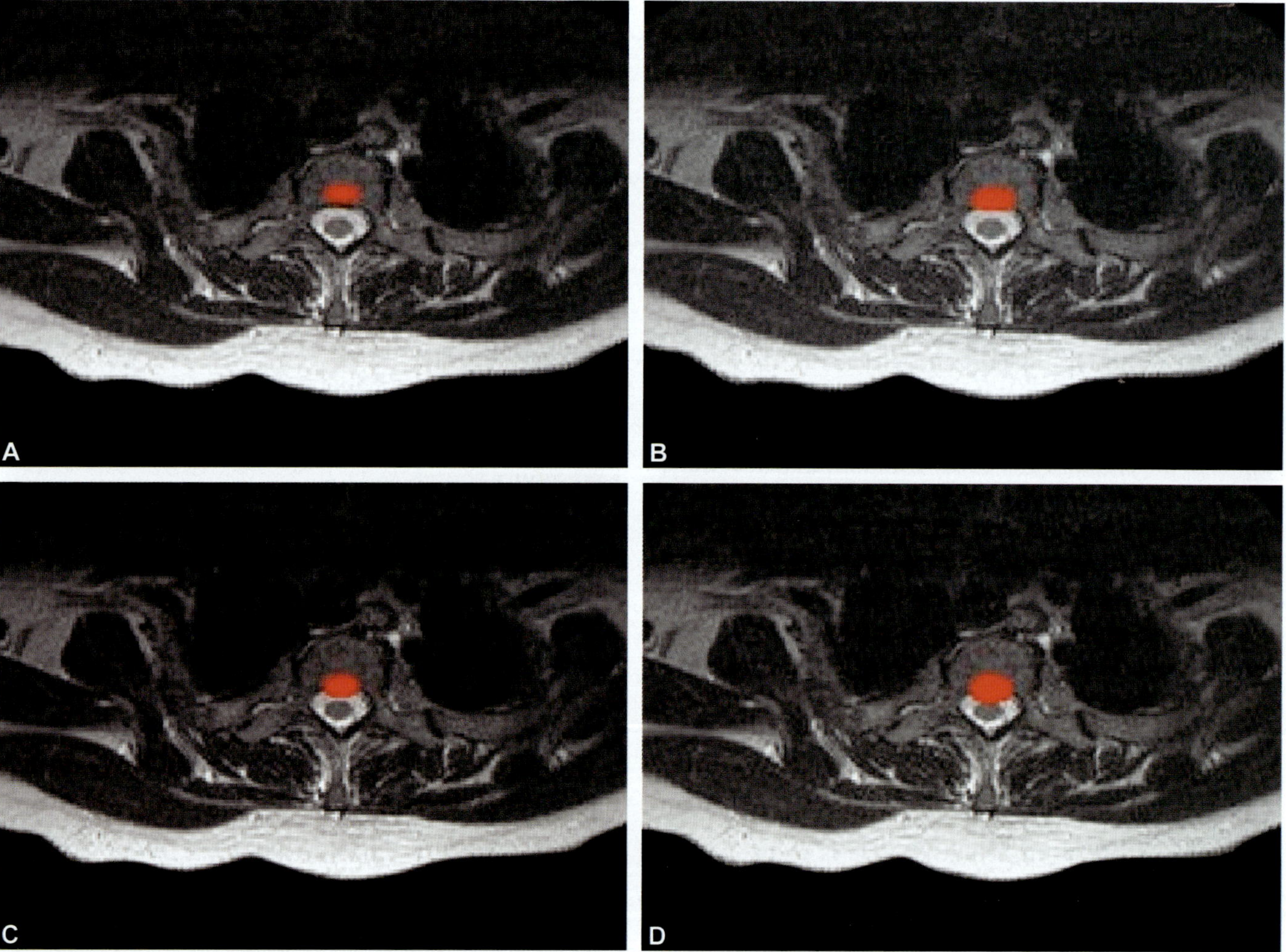

Figs. 58.12A to D

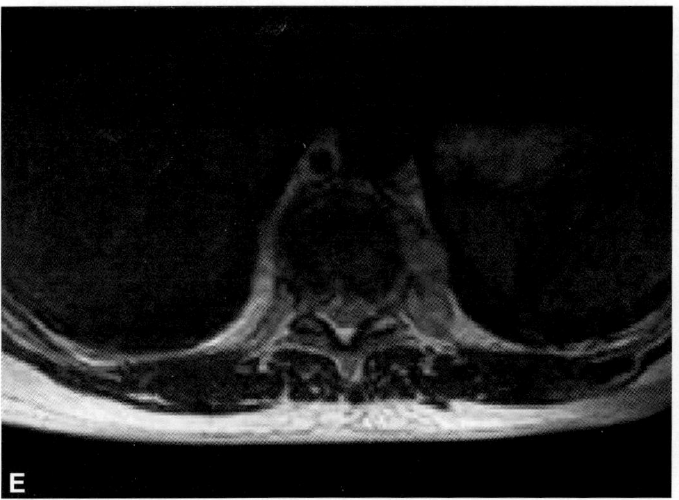

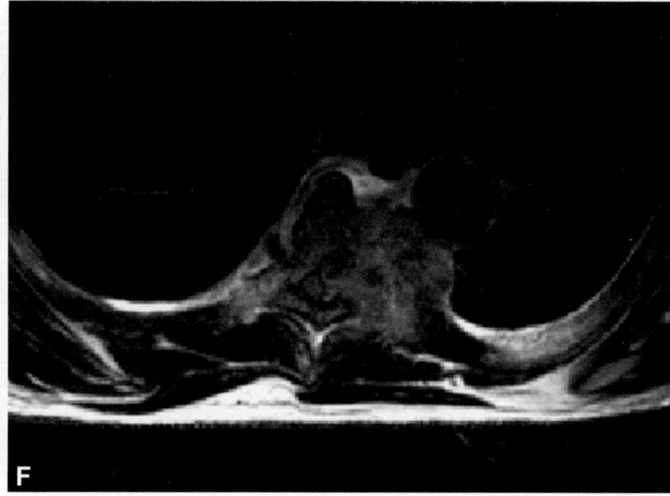

Figs. 58.12A to F: Axial T2 magnetic resonance imaging (MRI) at a thoracic level indicating the location of (A) grade 0 epidural disease, (B) grade 1a epidural disease, (C) grade 1b epidural disease, (D) grade 1c epidural disease, (E) grade 2 epidural disease, and (F) grade 3 epidural disease.

modified to include subclassifications of grade 1 disease to account for different degrees of epidural impingement and therefore assess risk of IGIMRT/SRS.[155]

Grade 1 a involves epidural impingement without deformation of the thecal sac (Fig. 58.12B).[155] Grade 1b involves epidural impingement with deformation of the thecal sac but without spinal cord abutment (Fig. 58.12C).[155] Grade 1c involves deformation of the thecal sac with spinal cord abutment but no spinal cord compression (Fig. 58.12D).[155] A grade 0, 1a, or 1b lesion may be treated with XRT or IGIMRT/SRS depending on the radiosensitivity of the tumor, without significant risk of radiation to the spinal cord. A grade of 1c, 2, or 3 requires surgical decompression and at least partial tumor resection prior to IGIMRT/SRS, in order to generate tumor/cord margins, in the case of radioresistant tumors. However, high-grade epidural disease caused by radiosensitive tumors can be treated with conventional XRT, as long as there is no extensive neurologic impairment that would respond better acutely to surgical decompression. Oncologic factors are related to the radiosensitivity of the primary tumor. Significantly radiosensitive tumors should be treated with traditional XRT. However, with the advent of IGIMRT/SRS, even the most radioresistant tumors can be treated nonsurgically as long as there is a spinal cord margin. Prior to IGIMRT/SRS, patients with a good Tokuhashi or Tomita score with solitary renal cell metastases were treated with en bloc spondylectomy with a recurrence rate of 7.5% at a median of 16 months.[156] However, IGIMRT/SRS for solitary renal cell carcinoma is associated with comparable recurrence rates.[156] Given the similar control rates, the treatment paradigm is shifting toward the less invasive IGIMRT/SRS approach instead of spondylectomy for solitary renal cell metastases.

Mechanical instability is related to pain associated with movement as well as radiographic evidence of instability. Systemic disease is related to the systemic tumor burden as well as medical comorbidities.[154] Overall, the NOMS framework is meant to address the factors that may be most influential in overall patient outcome.

Maintenance of mechanical stability is one of the major goals of the treatment of metastatic spinal disease. However, in deciding the need for surgical intervention, most scoring systems, except NOMS, do not take mechanical instability into account. The recently created Spinal Instability Neoplastic Score (SINS) is a classification system used to determine the likelihood of instability secondary to a neoplastic lesion (Table 58.4).[157] This system assigns a score based on location, mechanical pain, type of bone lesion (lytic vs blastic), spinal alignment, vertebral body collapse, and the degree of involvement of posterior elements. A score of 0–6 corresponds to stability, 7–12 is indeterminate, and 13–18 denotes instability likely requiring surgical stabilization. The most important prognostic factor for instability is the presence of subluxation or translation that is therefore weighted the most. This scoring system has demonstrated a near perfect intraobserver and interobserver reliability as well as a sensitivity

Flowchart 58.1: Suggested management and treatment algorithm for spinal metastases based primarily on NOMS paradigm.

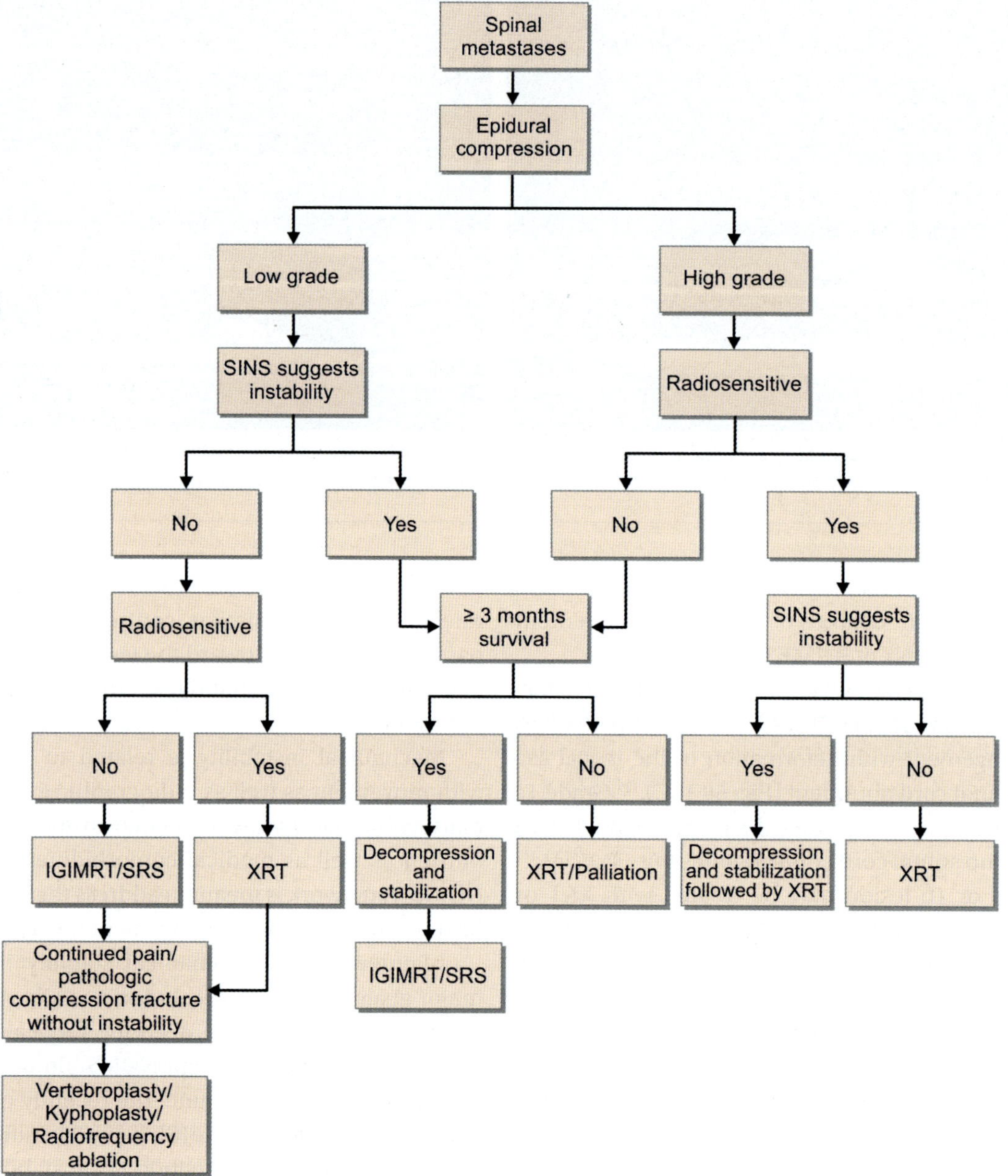

and specificity of 95% and 79%, respectively.[158] A recent analysis utilized the SINS criteria and found the presence of kyphosis/scoliotic deformity and the presence of lytic tumors as the most important factors associated with development or progression of vertebral compression fractures.[159]

Utilizing the above scoring systems and treatment recommendations, a suggested management algorithm, based primarily on the NOMS paradigm, is shown in Flowchart 58.1.

Conclusion

Spinal metastasis is a disease process with an increasing incidence. Treatment requires a multidisciplinary approach, including surgery and various XRT modalities, with a goal of maintaining quality of life and function. The decision-making process should take into account the histology of the primary tumor, the neurologic manifestations, the radiographic extent of epidural disease, and the systemic tumor burden.

Table 58.4: Summary table including all elements of the SINS

Element of SINS	*Score*
• Location	
- Junctional (occiput-C2, C7-T2, T11-L1, L5-S1)	3
- Mobile spine (C3-C6, L2-L4)	2
- Semi-rigid (T3-T10)	1
- Rigid (S2-S5)	0
• Pain relief with recumbency and/or pain with movement/loading of the spine	
- Yes	3
- No (occasional pain but not mechanical)	1
- Pain free lesion	0
• Bone lesion	
- Lytic	2
- Mixed (lytic/blastic)	1
- Blastic	0
• Radiographic spinal alignment	
- Subluxation/translation present	4
- De novo deformity (kyphosis/scoliosis)	2
- Normal alignment	0
• Vertebral body collapse	
- >50% collapse	3
- <50% collapse	2
- No collapse with >50% body involved	1
- None of the above	0
• Posterolateral involvement of the spinal elements (facet, pedicle or CV joint fracture or replacement with tumor)	
- Bilateral	3
- Unilateral	1
- None of the above	0

REFERENCES

1. Gasbarrini A, Cappuccio M, Donthineni R, et al. Management of benign tumors of the mobile spine. Orthop Clin N Am. 2009;40(1):9-19, v.
2. Martinez V, Sissons HA. Aneurysmal bone cyst. A review of 123 cases including primary lesions and those secondary to other bone pathology. Cancer. 1988;61(11):2291-304.
3. Ropper AE, Cahill KS, Hanna JW, et al. Primary vertebral tumors: a review of epidemiologic, histological, and imaging findings, Part I: benign tumors. Neurosurgery. 2011;69(6):1171-80.
4. Saccomanni B. Aneurysmal bone cyst of spine: a review of literature. Arch Orthop Trauma Surg. 2008;128(10):1145-7.
5. Liu JK, Brockmeyer DL, Dailey AT, et al. Surgical management of aneurysmal bone cysts of the spine. Neurosurg Focus. 2003;15(5):E4.
6. Boriani S, De Iure F, Campanacci L, et al. Aneurysmal bone cyst of the mobile spine: report on 41 cases. Spine. 2001;26(1):27-35.
7. De Cristofaro R, Biagini R, Boriani S, et al. Selective arterial embolization in the treatment of aneurysmal bone cyst and angioma of bone. Skeletal Radiol. 1992;21(8):523-7.
8. Barzin M, Maleki I. Incidence of vertebral hemangioma on spinal magnetic resonance imaging in Northern Iran. Pakistan J Biologic Sci.: PJBS 2009;12(6):542-4.
9. Hao J, Hu Z. Percutaneous cement vertebroplasty in the treatment of symptomatic vertebral hemangiomas. Pain Physician. 2012;15(1):43-9.
10. Rimondi E, Mavrogenis AF, Rossi G, et al. CT-guided corticosteroid injection for solitary eosinophilic granuloma of the spine. Skeletal Radiol. 2011;40(6):757-64.
11. Brown CW, Jarvis JG, Letts M, et al. Treatment and outcome of vertebral Langerhans cell histiocytosis at the Children's Hospital of Eastern Ontario. Can J Surg. Journal canadien de chirurgie 2005;48(3):230-6.
12. Fahim DK, Johnson KK, Whitehead WE, et al. Periosteal chondroma of the pediatric cervical spine. J Neurosurg Pediatr. 2009;3(2):151-6.
13. McLoughlin GS, Sciubba DM, Wolinsky JP. Chondroma/Chondrosarcoma of the spine. Neurosurg Clin N Am. 2008;19(1):57-63.
14. Kransdorf MJ, Stull MA, Gilkey FW, et al. Osteoid osteoma. Radiographics: A Review Publication of the Radiological Society of North America, Inc. 1991;11(4):671-96.
15. Thakur NA, Daniels AH, Schiller J, et al. Benign tumors of the spine. J Am Acad Orthop Surg. 2012;20(11):715-24.
16. Mukherjee D, Chaichana KL, Gokaslan ZL, et al. Survival of patients with malignant primary osseous spinal neoplasms: results from the Surveillance, Epidemiology, and End Results (SEER) database from 1973 to 2003. J Neurosurg Spine. 2011;14(2):143-50.
17. Ropper AE, Cahill KS, Hanna JW, et al. Primary vertebral tumors: a review of epidemiologic, histological and imaging findings, part II: locally aggressive and malignant tumors. Neurosurgery. 2012;70(1):211-9; discussion 219.
18. Sciubba DM, Chi JH, Rhines LD, et al. Chordoma of the spinal column. Neurosurg Clin N Am. 2008;19(1):5-15.
19. Bergh P, Kindblom LG, Gunterberg B, et al. Prognostic factors in chordoma of the sacrum and mobile spine: a study of 39 patients. Cancer. 2000;88(9):2122-34.
20. Hsieh CT, Liu MY, Su WF, et al. Spontaneous cerebrospinal fluid rhinorrhea: a rare initial presentation of clival chordoma. Neurology India. 2009;57(4):513-4.
21. Clarke MJ, Dasenbrock H, Bydon A, et al. Posterior-only approach for en bloc sacrectomy: clinical outcomes in 36 consecutive patients. Neurosurgery. 2012;71(2):357-64; discussion 364.
22. Boriani S, Bandiera S, Casadei R, et al. Giant cell tumor of the mobile spine: a review of 49 cases. Spine. 2012;37(1):E37-45.

23. Siebenrock KA, Unni KK, Rock MG. Giant-cell tumour of bone metastasising to the lungs. A long-term follow-up. J Bone Joint Surg. British volume 1998;80(1):43-7.
24. Ilaslan H, Sundaram M, Unni KK, et al. Primary Ewing's sarcoma of the vertebral column. Skeletal Radiol. 2004;33 (9):506-13.
25. Sundaresan N, Rosen G, Boriani S. Primary malignant tumors of the spine. Orthop Clin N Am. 2009;40(1):21-36, v.
26. Boriani S, Amendola L, Corghi A, et al. Ewing's sarcoma of the mobile spine. Eur Rev Med Pharmacol Sci. 2011;15 (7):831-9.
27. Kawahara N, Tomita K, Fujita T, et al. Osteosarcoma of the thoracolumbar spine: total en bloc spondylectomy. A case report. J Bone Joint Surg. American volume 1997;79(3):453-8.
28. Braccini AL, Bondiau PY, Litrico S, et al. Long term survival of an atlas osteosarcoma treated by surgery, chemotherapy and robotic stereotactic radiotherapy: a case report. Radiother Oncol. 2010;97(3):608-9.
29. Tryggvason G, Barnett A, Kim J, et al. Radiographic association of schwannomas with sensory ganglia. Otol Neurotol. 2012;33(7):1276-82.
30. Conti P, Pansini G, Mouchaty H, et al. Spinal neurinomas: retrospective analysis and long-term outcome of 179 consecutively operated cases and review of the literature. Surg Neurol. 2004;61(1):34-43; discussion 44.
31. Safavi-Abbasi S, Senoglu M, Theodore N, et al. Microsurgical management of spinal schwannomas: evaluation of 128 cases. J Neurosurg Spine. 2008;9(1):40-7.
32. Kim P, Ebersold MJ, Onofrio BM, et al. Surgery of spinal nerve schwannoma. Risk of neurological deficit after resection of involved root. J Neurosurg. 1989;71(6):810-4.
33. O'Toole JE, McCormick PC. Midline ventral intradural schwannoma of the cervical spinal cord resected via anterior corpectomy with reconstruction: technical case report and review of the literature. Neurosurgery. 2003;52(6): 1482-5; discussion 1485-6.
34. Angevine PD, Kellner C, Haque RM, et al. Surgical management of ventral intradural spinal lesions. J Neurosurg Spine. 2011;15(1):28-37.
35. Sachdev S, Dodd RL, Chang SD, et al. Stereotactic radiosurgery yields long-term control for benign intradural, extramedullary spinal tumors. Neurosurgery. 2011;69(3):533-9; discussion 539.
36. Chamberlain MC, Tredway TL. Adult primary intradural spinal cord tumors: a review. Curr Neurol Neurosci Rep. 2011;11(3):320-8.
37. Evans DG, Birch JM, Ramsden RT, et al. Malignant transformation and new primary tumours after therapeutic radiation for benign disease: substantial risks in certain tumour prone syndromes. J Med Genetics. 2006;43(4):289-94.
38. Tredway TL, Santiago P, Hrubes MR, et al. Minimally invasive resection of intradural-extramedullary spinal neoplasms. Neurosurgery. 2006;58(1 Suppl):ONS52-8; discussion ONS52-8.
39. Taleb FS, Guha A, Arnold PM, et al. Surgical management of cervical spine manifestations of neurofibromatosis type 1: long-term clinical and radiological follow-up in 22 cases. J Neurosurg Spine. 2011;14(3):356-66.
40. Bostrom A, Burgel U, Reinacher P, et al. A less invasive surgical concept for the resection of spinal meningiomas. Acta Neurochir. 2008;150(6):551-6; discussion 556.
41. Sandalcioglu IE, Hunold A, Muller O, et al. Spinal meningiomas: critical review of 131 surgically treated patients. Eur Spine J. 2008;17(8):1035-41.
42. Gerszten PC, Burton SA, Ozhasoglu C, et al. Radiosurgery for benign intradural spinal tumors. Neurosurgery. 2008;62 (4):887-95; discussion 895-6.
43. Gerszten PC, Quader M, Novotny J, Jr., et al. Radiosurgery for benign tumors of the spine: clinical experience and current trends. Technol Cancer Res Treat. 2012;11(2):133-9.
44. Oh MC, Ivan ME, Sun MZ, et al. Adjuvant radiotherapy delays recurrence following subtotal resection of spinal cord ependymomas. Neuro-oncology. 2013;15(2):208-15.
45. Guppy KH, Hou L, Moes GS, et al. Spinal intradural, extramedullary anaplastic ependymoma with an extradural component: case report and review of the literature. Surg Neurol Int. 2011;2:119.
46. Abul-Kasim K, Thurnher MM, McKeever P, et al. Intradural spinal tumors: current classification and MRI features. Neuroradiology. 2008;50(4):301-14.
47. Dahlberg D, Halvorsen CM, Lied B, et al. Minimally invasive microsurgical resection of primary, intradural spinal tumours using a tubular retraction system. Br J Neurosurg. 2012;26(4):472-5.
48. Kothbauer KF. Neurosurgical management of intramedullary spinal cord tumors in children. Pediatr Neurosurg. 2007;43(3):222-35.
49. Fakhreddine MH, Mahajan A, Penas-Prado M, et al. Treatment, prognostic factors, and outcomes in spinal cord astrocytomas. Neuro-oncology. 2013;15(4):406-12.
50. Garces-Ambrossi GL, McGirt MJ, Mehta VA, et al. Factors associated with progression-free survival and long-term neurological outcome after resection of intramedullary spinal cord tumors: analysis of 101 consecutive cases. J Neurosurg. Spine. 2009;11(5):591-9.
51. Minehan KJ, Brown PD, Scheithauer BW, et al. Prognosis and treatment of spinal cord astrocytoma. Int J Radiat Oncol Biol Phys. 2009;73(3):727-33.
52. Lonser RR, Weil RJ, Wanebo JE, et al. Surgical management of spinal cord hemangioblastomas in patients with von Hippel-Lindau disease. J Neurosurg. 2003;98(1):106-16.
53. Biondi A, Ricciardi GK, Faillot T, et al. Hemangioblastomas of the lower spinal region: report of four cases with preoperative embolization and review of the literature. AJNR Neuroradiol. 2005;26(4):936-45.
54. Pluta RM, Iuliano B, DeVroom HL, et al. Comparison of anterior and posterior surgical approaches in the treatment of ventral spinal hemangioblastomas in patients with von Hippel-Lindau disease. J Neurosurg. 2003;98(1):117-24.
55. Moss JM, Choi CY, Adler JR, Jr., et al. Stereotactic radiosurgical treatment of cranial and spinal hemangioblastomas. Neurosurgery. 2009;65(1):79-85; discussion 85.
56. Jallo GI, Freed D, Epstein FJ. Spinal cord gangliogliomas: a review of 56 patients. J Neuro-oncology. 2004;68(1):71-7.
57. Mechtler LL, Nandigam K. Spinal cord tumors: new views and future directions. Neurol Clin. 2013;31(1):241-68.

58. Schneider C, Vosbeck J, Grotzer MA, et al. Anaplastic ganglioglioma: a very rare intramedullary spinal cord tumor. Pediatr Neurosurg. 2012;48(1):42-7.
59. Winograd E, Pencovich N, Yalon M, et al. Malignant transformation in pediatric spinal intramedullary tumors: case-based update. Child's Nerv Syst. 2012;28(10):1679-86.
60. Sciubba DM, Petteys RJ, Dekutoski MB, et al. Diagnosis and management of metastatic spine disease. J Neurosurg Spine. 2010;13(1):94-108.
61. Cobb CA, 3rd, Leavens ME, Eckles N. Indications for nonoperative treatment of spinal cord compression due to breast cancer. J Neurosurg. 1977;47(5):653-8.
62. Sundaresan N, Digiacinto GV, Hughes JE, et al. Treatment of neoplastic spinal cord compression: results of a prospective study. Neurosurgery. 1991;29(5):645-50.
63. Wong DA, Fornasier VL, MacNab I. Spinal metastases: the obvious, the occult, and the impostors. Spine (Phila Pa 1976). 1990;15(1):1-4.
64. Jaffe HL. Tumors and tumorous conditions of the bones and joints. Philadelphia: Lea & Febiger; 1958.
65. Livingston KE, Perrin RG. The neurosurgical management of spinal metastases causing cord and cauda equina compression. J Neurosurg. 1978;49(6):839-43.
66. Bell GR. Surgical treatment of spinal tumors. Clin Orthop Relat Res. 1997(335):54-63.
67. Bilsky MH, Lis E, Raizer J, et al. The diagnosis and treatment of metastatic spinal tumor. Oncologist. 1999; 4(6):459-69.
68. Walsh GL, Gokaslan ZL, McCutcheon IE, et al. Anterior approaches to the thoracic spine in patients with cancer: indications and results. Ann Thorac Surg. 1997;64(6):1611-8.
69. Perrin RG, Laxton AW. Metastatic spine disease: epidemiology, pathophysiology, and evaluation of patients. Neurosurg Clin N Am. 2004;15(4):365-73.
70. Choi D, Crockard A, Bunger C, et al. Review of metastatic spine tumour classification and indications for surgery: the consensus statement of the Global Spine Tumour Study Group. Eur Spine J. 2010;19(2):215-22.
71. Brihaye J, Ectors P, Lemort M, et al. The management of spinal epidural metastases. Adv Tech Stand Neurosurg. 1988;16:121-76.
72. Jacobs WB, Perrin RG. Evaluation and treatment of spinal metastases: an overview. Neurosurg Focus. 2001;11(6):e10.
73. Ibrahim A, Crockard A, Antonietti P, et al. Does spinal surgery improve the quality of life for those with extradural (spinal) osseous metastases? An international multicenter prospective observational study of 223 patients. Invited submission from the Joint Section Meeting on Disorders of the Spine and Peripheral Nerves, March 2007. J Neurosurg Spine. 2008;8(3):271-8.
74. Gabriel K, Schiff D. Metastatic spinal cord compression by solid tumors. Semin Neurol. 2004;24(4):375-83.
75. Rodichok LD, Harper GR, Ruckdeschel JC, et al. Early diagnosis of spinal epidural metastases. Am J Med. 1981; 70(6): 1181-8.
76. Stark RJ, Henson RA, Evans SJ. Spinal metastases. A retrospective survey from a general hospital. Brain. 1982;105 (Pt 1):189-213.
77. Bach F, Larsen BH, Rohde K, et al. Metastatic spinal cord compression. Occurrence, symptoms, clinical presentations and prognosis in 398 patients with spinal cord compression. Acta Neurochir (Wien). 1990;107(1-2):37-43.
78. Cole JS, Patchell RA. Metastatic epidural spinal cord compression. Lancet Neurol. 2008;7(5):459-66.
79. Levack P, Graham J, Collie D, et al. Don't wait for a sensory level-listen to the symptoms: a prospective audit of the delays in diagnosis of malignant cord compression. Clin Oncol (R Coll Radiol). 2002;14(6):472-80.
80. O'Mara RE. Bone scanning in osseous metastatic disease. JAMA. 1974;229(14):1915-7.
81. McNeil BJ. Rationale for the use of bone scans in selected metastatic and primary bone tumors. Semin Nucl Med. 1978;8(4):336-45.
82. Han LJ, Au-Yong TK, Tong WC, et al. Comparison of bone single-photon emission tomography and planar imaging in the detection of vertebral metastases in patients with back pain. Eur J Nucl Med. 1998;25(6):635-8.
83. Peterson JJ, Kransdorf MJ, O'Connor MI. Diagnosis of occult bone metastases: positron emission tomography. Clin Orthop Relat Res. 2003(415 Suppl):S120-8.
84. Bushnell DL, Kahn D, Huston B, et al. Utility of SPECT imaging for determination of vertebral metastases in patients with known primary tumors. Skeletal Radiol. 1995;24 (1):13-6.
85. Even-Sapir E, Martin RH, Barnes DC, et al. Role of SPECT in differentiating malignant from benign lesions in the lower thoracic and lumbar vertebrae. Radiology. 1993;187(1):193-8.
86. Cook GJ, Houston S, Rubens R, et al. Detection of bone metastases in breast cancer by 18FDG PET: differing metabolic activity in osteoblastic and osteolytic lesions. J Clin Oncol. 1998;16(10):3375-9.
87. Yang SN, Liang JA, Lin FJ, et al. Comparing whole body (18) F-2-deoxyglucose positron emission tomography and technetium-99m methylene diphosphonate bone scan to detect bone metastases in patients with breast cancer. J Cancer Res Clin Oncol. 2002;128(6):325-8.
88. Laufer I, Lis E, Pisinski L, et al. The accuracy of [(18)F] fluorodeoxyglucose positron emission tomography as confirmed by biopsy in the diagnosis of spine metastases in a cancer population. Neurosurgery. 2009;64(1):107-13; discussion 113-4.
89. Helweg-Larsen S, Wagner A, Kjaer L, et al. Comparison of myelography combined with postmyelographic spinal CT and MRI in suspected metastatic disease of the spinal canal. J Neurooncol. 1992;13(3):231-7.
90. Algra PR, Bloem JL, Tissing H, et al. Detection of vertebral metastases: comparison between MR imaging and bone scintigraphy. Radiographics. 1991;11(2):219-32.
91. Avrahami E, Tadmor R, Dally O, et al. Early MR demonstration of spinal metastases in patients with normal radiographs and CT and radionuclide bone scans. J Comput Assist Tomogr. 1989;13(4):598-602.
92. Keogh C, Bergin D, Brennan D, et al. MR imaging of bone tumors of the cervical spine. Magn Reson Imaging Clin N Am. 2000;8(3):513-28.

93. Karchevsky M, Babb JS, Schweitzer ME. Can diffusion-weighted imaging be used to differentiate benign from pathologic fractures? A meta-analysis. Skeletal Radiol. 2008;37(9):791-5.
94. Colletti PM, Siegel HJ, Woo MY, et al. The impact on treatment planning of MRI of the spine in patients suspected of vertebral metastasis: an efficacy study. Comput Med Imaging Graph. 1996;20(3):159-62.
95. Olerud C, Jonsson H, Jr., Lofberg AM, et al. Embolization of spinal metastases reduces peroperative blood loss. 21 patients operated on for renal cell carcinoma. Acta Orthop Scand. 1993;64(1):9-12.
96. Roscoe MW, McBroom RJ, St Louis E, et al. Preoperative embolization in the treatment of osseous metastases from renal cell carcinoma. Clin Orthop Relat Res. 1989(238):302-7.
97. Sun S, Lang EV. Bone metastases from renal cell carcinoma: preoperative embolization. J Vasc Interv Radiol. 1998;9(2):263-9.
98. Sciubba DM, Gokaslan ZL. Diagnosis and management of metastatic spine disease. Surg Oncol. 2006;15(3):141-51.
99. Prabhu VC, Bilsky MH, Jambhekar K, et al. Results of preoperative embolization for metastatic spinal neoplasms. J Neurosurg. 2003;98(2 Suppl):156-64.
100. Gottfried ON, Schloesser PE, Schmidt MH, et al. Embolization of metastatic spinal tumors. Neurosurg Clin N Am. 2004;15(4):391-9.
101. Cahill DW. Surgical management of malignant tumors of the adult bony spine. South Med J. 1996;89(7):653-65.
102. Ruggieri P, Angelini A, Ussia G, et al. Surgical margins and local control in resection of sacral chordomas. Clin Orthop Relat Res. 2010;468(11):2939-47.
103. Kornblum MB, Wesolowski DP, Fischgrund JS, et al. Computed tomography-guided biopsy of the spine. A review of 103 patients. Spine (Phila Pa 1976). 1998;23(1):81-5.
104. Lis E, Bilsky MH, Pisinski L, et al. Percutaneous CT-guided biopsy of osseous lesion of the spine in patients with known or suspected malignancy. AJNR Am J Neuroradiol. 2004;25(9):1583-8.
105. Ghelman B, Lospinuso MF, Levine DB, et al. Percutaneous computed-tomography-guided biopsy of the thoracic and lumbar spine. Spine (Phila Pa 1976). 1991;16(7):736-9.
106. Babu NV, Titus VT, Chittaranjan S, et al. Computed tomographically guided biopsy of the spine. Spine (Phila Pa 1976). 1994;19(21):2436-42.
107. Loblaw DA, Laperriere NJ, Mackillop WJ. A population-based study of malignant spinal cord compression in Ontario. Clin Oncol (R Coll Radiol). 2003;15(4):211-7.
108. Rades D, Fehlauer F, Schulte R, et al. Prognostic factors for local control and survival after radiotherapy of metastatic spinal cord compression. J Clin Oncol. 2006;24(21):3388-93.
109. Constans JP, de Divitiis E, Donzelli R, et al. Spinal metastases with neurological manifestations. Review of 600 cases. J Neurosurg. 1983;59(1):111-8.
110. Cooper PR, Errico TJ, Martin R, et al. A systematic approach to spinal reconstruction after anterior decompression for neoplastic disease of the thoracic and lumbar spine. Neurosurgery. 1993;32(1):1-8.
111. Klimo P, Jr., Schmidt MH. Surgical management of spinal metastases. Oncologist. 2004;9(2):188-96.
112. Patchell RA, Tibbs PA, Regine WF, et al. Direct decompressive surgical resection in the treatment of spinal cord compression caused by metastatic cancer: a randomised trial. Lancet. 2005;366(9486):643-8.
113. Jackson RJ, Loh SC, Gokaslan ZL. Metastatic renal cell carcinoma of the spine: surgical treatment and results. J Neurosurg. 2001;94(1 Suppl):18-24.
114. Sundaresan N, Rothman A, Manhart K, et al. Surgery for solitary metastases of the spine: rationale and results of treatment. Spine (Phila Pa 1976). 2002;27(16):1802-6.
115. Tomita K, Kawahara N, Baba H, et al. Total en bloc spondylectomy for solitary spinal metastases. Int Orthop. 1994;18(5):291-8.
116. Magerl F, Aebi M, Gertzbein SD, et al. A comprehensive classification of thoracic and lumbar injuries. Eur Spine J. 1994;3(4):184-201.
117. Windhagen HJ, Hipp JA, Silva MJ, et al. Predicting failure of thoracic vertebrae with simulated and actual metastatic defects. Clin Orthop Relat Res. 1997(344): 313-9.
118. Taneichi H, Kaneda K, Takeda N, et al. Risk factors and probability of vertebral body collapse in metastases of the thoracic and lumbar spine. Spine (Phila Pa 1976). 1997;22(3): 239-45.
119. Witham TF, Khavkin YA, Gallia GL, et al. Surgery insight: current management of epidural spinal cord compression from metastatic spine disease. Nat Clin Pract Neurol. 2006;2(2):87-94; quiz 116.
120. Fourney DR, Gokaslan ZL. Anterior approaches for thoracolumbar metastatic spine tumors. Neurosurg Clin N Am. 2004;15(4):443-51.
121. Gokaslan ZL, York JE, Walsh GL, et al. Transthoracic vertebrectomy for metastatic spinal tumors. J Neurosurg. 1998;89(4):599-609.
122. Sundaresan N, Steinberger AA, Moore F, et al. Indications and results of combined anterior-posterior approaches for spine tumor surgery. J Neurosurg. 1996;85(3):438-46.
123. Polly DW, Jr., Chou D, Sembrano JN, et al. An analysis of decision making and treatment in thoracolumbar metastases. Spine (Phila Pa 1976). 2009;34(22 Suppl):S118-27.
124. Placantonakis DG, Laufer I, Wang JC, et al. Posterior stabilization strategies following resection of cervicothoracic junction tumors: review of 90 consecutive cases. J Neurosurg Spine. 2008;9(2):111-9.
125. Cohen ZR, Fourney DR, Gokaslan ZL, et al. Anterior stabilization of the upper thoracic spine via an "interaortocaval subinnominate window": case report and description of operative technique. J Spinal Disord Tech. 2004;17(6):543-8.
126. Sundaresan N, Shah J, Foley KM, et al. An anterior surgical approach to the upper thoracic vertebrae. J Neurosurg. 1984;61(4):686-90.
127. Wang JC, Boland P, Mitra N, et al. Single-stage posterolateral transpedicular approach for resection of epidural metastatic spine tumors involving the vertebral body with circumferential reconstruction: results in 140 patients. Invited submission from the Joint Section Meeting on Disorders of the Spine and Peripheral Nerves, March 2004. J Neurosurg Spine. 2004;1(3):287-98.

128. Hunt T, Shen FH, Arlet V. Expandable cage placement via a posterolateral approach in lumbar spine reconstructions. Technical note. J Neurosurg Spine. 2006;5(3):271-4.
129. Sciubba DM, Gallia GL, McGirt MJ, et al. Thoracic kyphotic deformity reduction with a distractible titanium cage via an entirely posterior approach. Neurosurgery. 2007;60(4 Suppl 2):223-30; discussion 230-1.
130. Snell BE, Nasr FF, Wolfla CE. Single-stage thoracolumbar vertebrectomy with circumferential reconstruction and arthrodesis: surgical technique and results in 15 patients. Neurosurgery. 2006;58(4 Suppl 2):ONS-263-8; discussion ONS-269.
131. Akeyson EW, McCutcheon IE. Single-stage posterior vertebrectomy and replacement combined with posterior instrumentation for spinal metastasis. J Neurosurg. 1996;85(2): 211-20.
132. Fourney DR, Abi-Said D, Lang FF, et al. Use of pedicle screw fixation in the management of malignant spinal disease: experience in 100 consecutive procedures. J Neurosurg. 2001;94(1 Suppl):25-37.
133. Huang TJ, Hsu RW, Li YY, et al. Minimal access spinal surgery (MASS) in treating thoracic spine metastasis. Spine (Phila Pa 1976). 2006;31(16):1860-3.
134. McLain RF, Lieberman IH. Endoscopic approaches to metastatic thoracic disease. Spine (Phila Pa 1976). 2000;25(14): 1855-8.
135. Muhlbauer M, Pfisterer W, Eyb R, et al. Minimally invasive retroperitoneal approach for lumbar corpectomy and anterior reconstruction. Technical note. J Neurosurg. 2000;93(1 Suppl):161-7.
136. Ozgur BM, Aryan HE, Pimenta L, et al. Extreme Lateral Interbody Fusion (XLIF): a novel surgical technique for anterior lumbar interbody fusion. Spine J. 2006;6(4):435-43.
137. Holly LT, Foley KT. Three-dimensional fluoroscopy-guided percutaneous thoracolumbar pedicle screw placement. Technical note. J Neurosurg. 2003;99(3 Suppl):324-9.
138. Nottmeier EW, Seemer W, Young PM. Placement of thoracolumbar pedicle screws using three-dimensional image guidance: experience in a large patient cohort. J Neurosurg Spine. 2009;10(1):33-9.
139. Weill A, Chiras J, Simon JM, et al. Spinal metastases: indications for and results of percutaneous injection of acrylic surgical cement. Radiology. 1996;199(1):241-7.
140. Halpin RJ, Bendok BR, Liu JC. Minimally invasive treatments for spinal metastases: vertebroplasty, kyphoplasty, and radiofrequency ablation. J Support Oncol. 2004;2(4):339-51; discussion 352-5.
141. Cotten A, Dewatre F, Cortet B, et al. Percutaneous vertebroplasty for osteolytic metastases and myeloma: effects of the percentage of lesion filling and the leakage of methyl methacrylate at clinical follow-up. Radiology. 1996;200(2):525-30.
142. Fourney DR, Schomer DF, Nader R, et al. Percutaneous vertebroplasty and kyphoplasty for painful vertebral body fractures in cancer patients. J Neurosurg. 2003;98(1 Suppl): 21-30.
143. Mathis JM, Barr JD, Belkoff SM, et al. Percutaneous vertebroplasty: a developing standard of care for vertebral compression fractures. AJNR Am J Neuroradiol. 2001;22(2):373-81.
144. Zoarski GH, Snow P, Olan WJ, et al. Percutaneous vertebroplasty for osteoporotic compression fractures: quantitative prospective evaluation of long-term outcomes. J Vasc Interv Radiol. 2002;13(2 Pt 1):139-48.
145. Choe DH, Marom EM, Ahrar K, et al. Pulmonary embolism of polymethyl methacrylate during percutaneous vertebroplasty and kyphoplasty. AJR Am J Roentgenol. 2004;183(4): 1097-102.
146. Belkoff SM, Mathis JM, Fenton DC, et al. An ex vivo biomechanical evaluation of an inflatable bone tamp used in the treatment of compression fracture. Spine (Phila Pa 1976). 2001;26(2):151-6.
147. Phillips FM, Todd Wetzel F, Lieberman I, et al. An in vivo comparison of the potential for extravertebral cement leak after vertebroplasty and kyphoplasty. Spine (Phila Pa 1976). 2002;27(19):2173-8; discussion 2178-9.
148. Rose PS, Laufer I, Boland PJ, et al. Risk of fracture after single fraction image-guided intensity-modulated radiation therapy to spinal metastases. J Clin Oncol. 2009;27(30):5075-9.
149. Georgy BA, Wong W. Plasma-mediated radiofrequency ablation assisted percutaneous cement injection for treating advanced malignant vertebral compression fractures. AJNR Am J Neuroradiol. 2007;28(4):700-5.
150. Chen YC, Lee SH, Saenz Y, et al. Histologic findings of disc, end plate and neural elements after coblation of nucleus pulposus: an experimental nucleoplasty study. Spine J. 2003;3(6):466-70.
151. Tomita K, Kawahara N, Kobayashi T, et al. Surgical strategy for spinal metastases. Spine (Phila Pa 1976). 2001;26(3):298-306.
152. Tokuhashi Y, Ajiro Y, Umezawa N. Outcome of treatment for spinal metastases using scoring system for preoperative evaluation of prognosis. Spine (Phila Pa 1976). 2009; 34(1): 69-73.
153. Tokuhashi Y, Matsuzaki H, Oda H, et al. A revised scoring system for preoperative evaluation of metastatic spine tumor prognosis. Spine (Phila Pa 1976). 2005; 30(19):2186-91.
154. Bilsky M, Smith M. Surgical approach to epidural spinal cord compression. Hematol Oncol Clin N Am. 2006;20(6): 1307-17.
155. Bilsky MH, Laufer I, Fourney DR, et al. Reliability analysis of the epidural spinal cord compression scale. J Neurosurg Spine. 2010;13(3):324-8.
156. Bilsky MHMD, Laufer IMD, Burch SMD. Shifting paradigms in the treatment of metastatic spine disease. Spine. 2009;34(22S)(Suppl):S101-S107.
157. Fisher CG, DiPaola CP, Ryken TC, et al. A novel classification system for spinal instability in neoplastic disease: an evidence-based approach and expert consensus from the Spine Oncology Study Group. Spine (Phila Pa 1976). 2010; 35(22):E1221-9.
158. Fourney DR, Frangou EM, Ryken TC, et al. Spinal instability neoplastic score: an analysis of reliability and validity from the spine oncology study group. J Clin Oncol. 2011;29(22):3072-7.
159. Cunha MV, Al-Omair A, Atenafu EG, et al. Vertebral compression fracture (VCF) after spine stereotactic body radiation therapy (SBRT): analysis of predictive factors. Int J Rad Oncol Biol Phys. 2012;84(3):e343-9.

CHAPTER

59

Intraoperative Monitoring in Spine Surgery

Thomas Cheriyan, Rachel N Rattenni, Jerry Cheriyan, Athena M Lolis, Thomas J Errico

INTRODUCTION

The objective of intraoperative neurophysiologic monitoring (IONM) is to reduce and/or prevent adverse events that may lead to permanent neurologic injury during spine surgery.[1] As spinal surgeries have become longer, more complex, and more extensive, the need for accurate and reliable neuromonitoring during surgery has become essential. IONM aims to inform the surgeon of impending neurological deficit, thus allowing modification of the operative strategy to minimize or reverse neurological insult. The common IONM modalities used include:

- Stagnara wake-up test
- Somatosensory evoked potential (SSEP)
- Motor evoked potential (MEP)
- Triggered electromyography (tEMG)/pedicle screw testing
- Spontaneous electromyography (sEMG)

This chapter gives a brief overview of the modalities

STAGNARA WAKE-UP TEST

The Stagnara wake-up test was among the first methods used for assessing intraoperative neurological function. The test involves gradually lightening anesthesia until the patient can move his or her extremities voluntarily. The Stagnara wake-up test gives an estimate of gross motor function, but does not assess fine motor or sensory function. Thus, potential devastating injuries may be missed. Other limitations of the wake-up test include one-time testing as opposed to continuous testing, risk of air embolism, self-extubation, recall of event, self-induced contamination, positional change, and lack of assessment of nerve root integrity.[2] The Stagnara wake-up test is no longer considered an adequate stand-alone technique, but can be considered to be an adjuvant to other more reliable modalities, like the SSEP or TcMEP.[2]

SOMATOSENSORY EVOKED POTENTIAL

Somatosensory evoked potentials have been used for IONM since its inception in the 1960s, and continue to be the most widely used IONM modality. The Scoliosis Research Society and the European Spinal Deformity Society advocated the use of SSEPs to limit neurologic damage during the correction of spinal deformities in a joint position statement issued in 1997.[3] SSEP monitors the dorsal column-medial lemniscus pathway, which mediates tactile discrimination, vibration sensation, form recognition, and joint and muscle sensation.[4] While SSEP monitoring provides a good indication of sensory spinal cord function, it does not provide information about motor or nerve root integrity.

Technique

Somatosensory evoked potential monitoring involves the electrical stimulation of mixed fibers caudal to the region of the spinal cord that is being assessed, with recordings of these signals rostrally, usually in the scalp.[5] The median nerve and the ulnar nerve are selected for monitoring in the upper limbs, while the posterior tibial nerve and the peroneal nerve are commonly used to monitor the lower extremities.

To ascertain the threshold of stimulation, peripheral responses can be recorded at the brachial plexus or the popliteal fossa for the upper and lower extremity, respectively; this can also help in identifying nerve compression or limb ischemia. However, these peripheral stimulations are less sensitive to anesthesia and can be used to distinguish these changes from those relating to surgical manipulation.[4]

When the upper extremity is stimulated, impulses are transmitted to the spinal cord through the peripheral nerve and brachial plexus where the Erb's point potential is generated. The N13 potential is seen at the fiber synapse in the dorsal column nuclei. The stimuli then pass through the medial lemniscus to the thalamus to generate the N20 potential. These stimuli reach the primary sensory cortex to generate the N20 and P22 potentials (Fig. 59.1A). In the lower extremity, SSEPs are transmitted through the peripheral nerves and the popliteal potential is generated before reaching the lumbosacral plexus; the impulses reach the cauda equina to generate the N21 lumbar potential. The action potentials are then transmitted along the dorsal root to enter the spinal cord posteriorly. Thus, the integrity of the dorsal column is best assessed when using this modality. The lower extremity stimulation produces the P37/P40 potential when they reach the cortex (Fig. 59.1B).

Warning criteria for SSEP have been established; an amplitude decrease of more than 50% or increased latency of more than 10% is considered significant.[2,4,5]

Limitations

A specificity of 95–100% and sensitivity of 28–92% has been reported.[4] SSEP recordings are also dependent on factors like halogenated anesthetic agents, nitrous oxide, blood pressure and temperature. Neuromuscular scoliosis, cerebral palsy, neuropathy, and myelopathy are among certain underlying pathologies that can affect SSEP responses.

MOTOR EVOKED POTENTIALS

Motor evoked potentials routinely used in IONM include transcranial motor evoked potentials (TcMEPs) and the corticospinal motor evoked potential. TcMEP has been used for the past several decades, and received FDA approval in 2002. TcMEP uses a train of high-voltage stimuli applied to the scalp to directly stimulate the corticospinal tract. The signals are recorded from motor contraction (muscle MEP) from the epidural space of the spinal cord. The corticospinal MEP [direct wave (D-wave)] is the evoked potential generated by direct stimulation of the motor cortex that is recorded from the epidural space of the spinal cord. These modalities evaluate the integrity of the entire motor pathway during high-risk spinal surgeries.

Technique

To obtain the corticospinal MEP response, the motor cortex is stimulated and a D-wave is generated from the direct activation of the axons of the corticospinal tract. Additionally, an indirect wave (I-wave) is also generated from the indirect activation of the corticospinal tract via synaptic activity.

Even though general anesthesia can limit the activity of anterior horn cell and interneurons of the spinal cord, the D-wave of the corticospinal tract is usually resistant to anesthetics as well as neuromuscular blockade. General anesthesia will cause the I-waves to be diminished when they reach the anterior horn cell. Thus, a sequential time locked train of stimuli is necessary, rather than a single

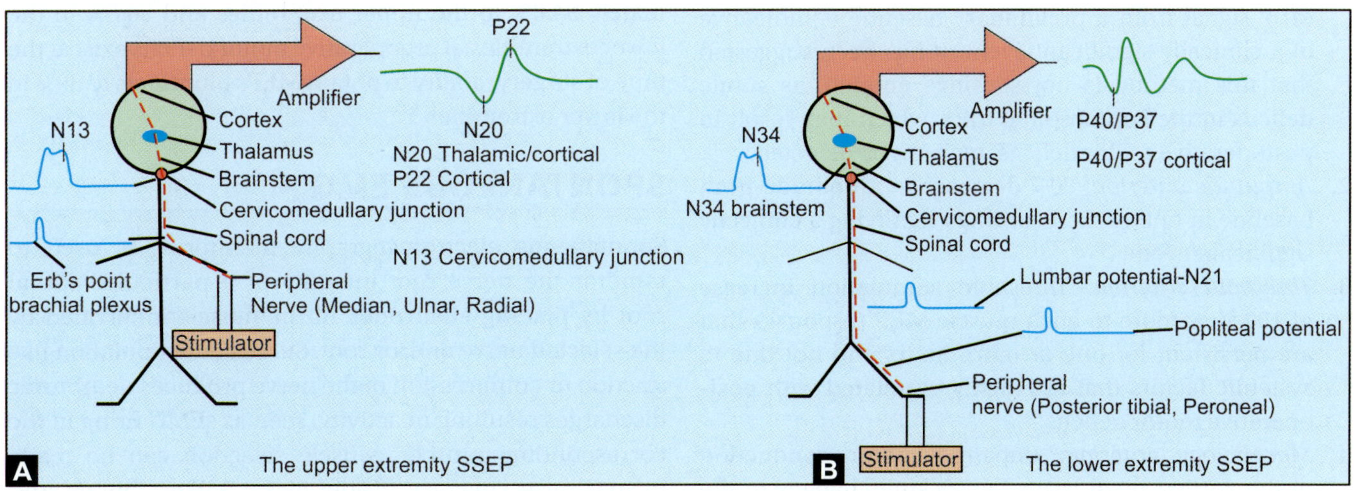

Figs. 59.1A and B: Schematic diagram of somatosensory evoked potential: (A) upper limb, (B) lower limb.

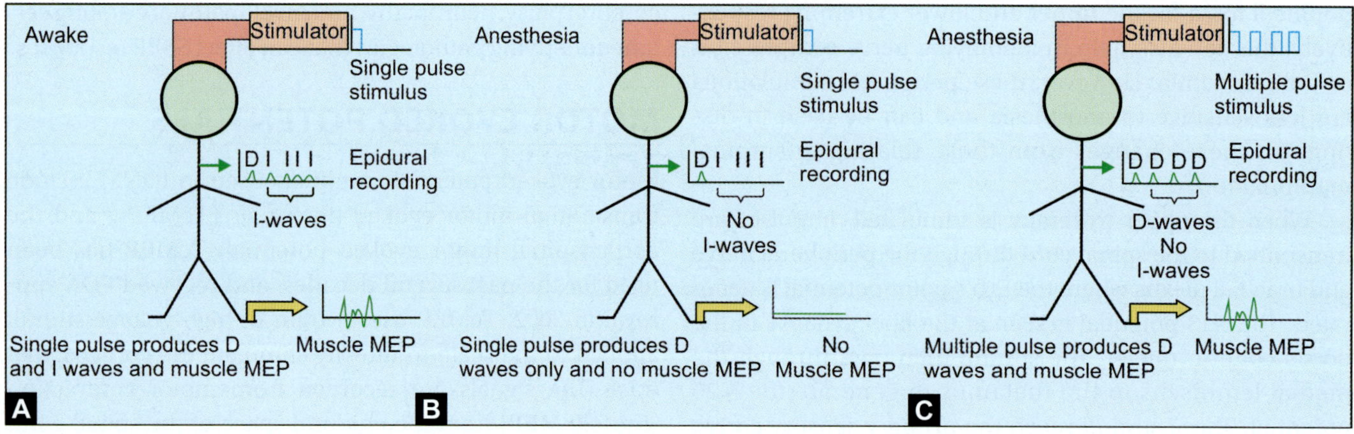

Figs. 59.2A to C: Schematic diagram of single stimulus TcMEP responses in (A) awake, (B) anesthetized and (C) multipulse transcranial motor evoked potentials (TcMEPs) stimuli response in anesthetized patient.

stimulus (Figs. 59.2A to C). Stimuli used range from 75 to 900 V in amplitude and currents up to 0.9 A, depending on the type of electrode used.[6]

Stimulating electrodes are usually placed over C3 and C4 or C1 and C2. While lateral placement might optimize stimulation, midline placement may facilitate better responses from the lower extremities. However, the point of stimulation with these placements is not the cortex but the corona that radiates in the deep white matter.[7]

A complete loss of D-wave amplitude during surgery is likely to result in permanent motor deficit, while a complete loss of MEP with 50% preservation of D-wave amplitude generally results in transient paraplegia. Muscle MEP responses are recorded from TcMEP stimulation. Muscle MEPs can be obtained from a single stimuli and provide instantaneous information. Currently, four methods of interpreting muscle MEP recordings are used:[4]

1. *All or nothing*: Most widely used; complete loss of MEP signal from a preliminary baseline is indicative of a clinically significant event. It has been suggested that this method is not sensitive enough, as subtle deficits in the corticospinal tract, which may result in postoperative motor deficits, may not be detected.
2. *Amplitude criterion*: 80% decrease in amplitude from baseline in one of six recordings signifying a clinically significant event.
3. *Threshold criterion*: Threshold stimulation increase of 100 V or more to elicit muscle MEP responses that are persistent for one or more hours and not due to systemic factors that are highly correlated with postoperative motor deficits.
4. *Morphology criterion*: Impaired motor conduction of the corticospinal tracts by tracking changes in the pattern and duration of MEP waveform morphology.

However, optimal warning criteria for TcMEP have not been established, and TcMEP has a relatively higher inter/intrauser variability than SSEP.[2] With a 70% reduction in amplitude as the warning threshold, the sensitivity and specificity of TcMEP at 95.0% and 90.9%, respectively, have been reported.[8]

Limitations

Optimal signal acquisition requires total intravenous anesthesia consisting of short-acting agents such as fentanyl or propofol. Nitrous oxide, muscle relaxants, and volatile agents should not be used. TcMEP recording also precludes the use of neuromuscular blockades. TcMEPs assess only 5% of the motor pathway and do not allow for continuous monitoring.[5] TcMEP is contraindicated in patients with deep brain stimulators or cochlear implants.

Current success rates for obtaining MEPs are approximately 94.8% in the upper extremities and 66.6% in the lower extremities; if preoperative motor deficits exist at the time of surgery, ability to obtain MEPs plummets to 39% in the lower extremities.[9]

SPONTANEOUS EMG

Spontaneous electromyography monitoring is used to monitor the nerve root integrity of a particular spinal root by placing electrodes in the muscle innervated by the selected nerve and/or root. Surgical manipulation like traction or compression of the nerve produces neurotonic discharges resulting in activity, seen as sEMG firing in the corresponding muscle. Muscle selection can be made to maximize coverage (Table 59.1). Spikes, bursts and trains signify neurological insult (Fig. 59.3). Spikes and bursts warn the surgeon of proximity to the nerve root. Trains signify excessive manipulation of the nerve and warn of impending nerve injury if manipulation is sustained. As with TcMEP, neuromuscular blockage precludes the use of sEMG. Also electrocautery, drills, and ECG leads may interfere with the sEMG recordings.[4] sEMG recording is highly sensitive for nerve root injury and combining with SSEP improves specificity. However, this modality has a high rate of false positives.

Table 59.1: Nerve root distribution of muscles frequently used in spontaneous electromyography

Root	*Muscle*	*Nerve*
C-3, C-4	Trapezius	CN XI
C-5, (C-6)	Deltoid	Axillary
C-5, C-6	Biceps brachii	Musculocutaneous
C-6, C-7	Triceps	Radial
(C-8), T-1	Abductor pollicis brevis	Median
C-8, (T-1)	Abductor digiti minimi	Ulnar
C-8, (T-1)	Abductor pollicis	Ulnar
C-8, (T-1)	First dorsal interosseous	Ulnar
T-7–12	External oblique	
T-7–12	Rectus abdominis	
L-2, L-3, (L-4)	Iliacus	Lumbar plexus
(L-2), L-3, L-4	Vastus lateralis/medialis	Femoral
(L-2), L-3, L-4	Rectus femoris	Femoral
(L-4), L-5, (S-1)	Semitendinosus/membranosus	Sciatic
L-4, L-5	Tibialis anterior	Peroneal
L-5, (S-1)	Extensor hallucis	Peroneal
L-5, (S-1)	Extensor digitorum brevis	Peroneal
(L-5), S-1	Gastrocnemius lateral	Tibial
S-1, (S-2)	Gastrocnemius medial	Tibial
S-1, S-2	Abductor hallucis	Tibial
S-3, S-4, S-5	External anal sphincter	Pudendal
S-3, S-4, S-5	External urethral sphincter	Pudendal

TRIGGERED EMG

Triggered electromyography is used to identify breach in the medial and inferior wall of the pedicle during pedicle screw placement. A breach in the medial or inferior wall can result in compression of neural elements.

Technique

When a screw is accurately placed in the pedicle, it is surrounded by bone, which acts as an insulator. Screw stimulation is performed by neurophysiologists and consists of stimulation of screws with increasing currents, while recording the compound muscle action potential (CMAP) responses, from muscles innervated by corresponding spinal segments.

Typically, a monopolar electrode is used to stimulate the top of the screw at increasing currents (Fig. 59.4). It is important to place the electrode on top of the screw and not the tulip, as these components are not fused and do not conduct current between each other. Needle electrodes are placed in appropriate innervated muscle groups to measure action potentials. An initial direct stimulus to the nerve root is given (<2 mA) to ensure muscle response; a stimulus of lesser current would be sufficient if there is a breach in the pedicle wall.

When the threshold stimulus is >20 mA, there is strong probability that there is no breach.[10] A response between 10 mA and 20 mA gives reasonable probability of no breach, with threshold >15 mA indicating a 98% likelihood of accurate screw positioning.[11] A threshold of >10 mA for screw stimulation and 7 mA for probe stimulation

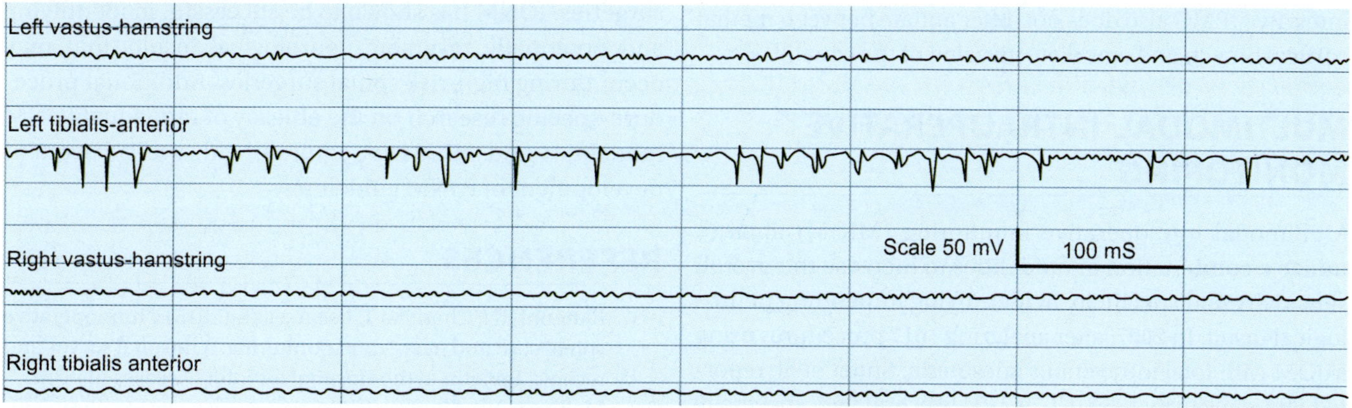

Fig. 59.3: Spontaneous electromyography recording showing train reading in left tibialis anterior.

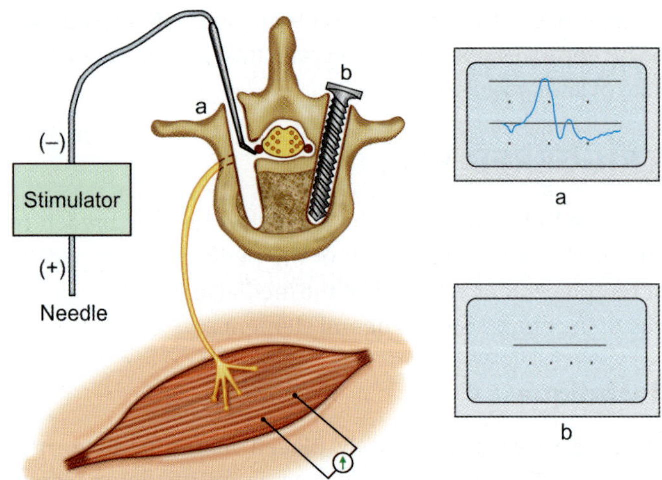

Fig. 59.4: Schematic diagram of triggered electromyography testing.

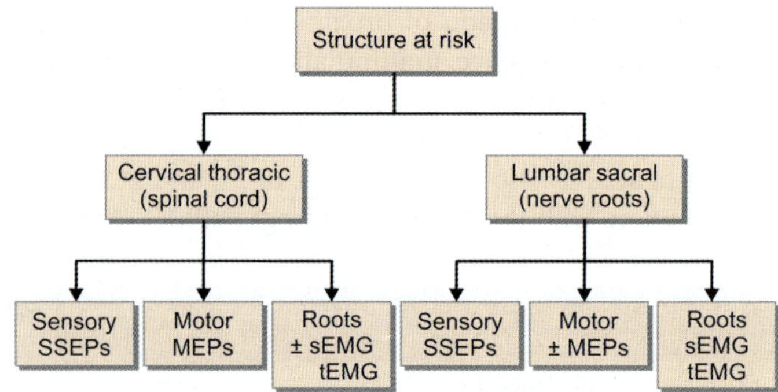

Fig. 59.5: Overview of multimodal intraoperative monitoring classified by spinal region at risk.

suggest a medical wall breach in lumbar pedicles.[12] Raynor et. al analyzed threshold values for 4857 lumbar pedicle screws and found that probability of medial wall breech increases with decreasing tEMG threshold with 0.31% for 8.0 mA, 17.4% for 4.0 to 8.0 mA, 54.2% for 4.0 mA, and 100% for 2.8 mA.[13] False negatives may occur due to use of muscle relaxants, current spread, and pre-existing nerve injury.[14] tEMG monitoring is highly sensitive for medial pedicle breach and is useful in minimally invasive surgery where anatomical landmarks may be challenging to visualize.

Limitations

Optimal alarm criteria have not been firmly established. tEMG may provide false-positive alarms in cases of multiple pedicle passes or if there is fluid present at the site of recording. This technique does not only directly assess nerve damage but also provide information regarding pedicle integrity.[5] tEMG also does not differ entiate between medial cortical breach and complete invasion of the canal.[15]

MULTIMODAL INTRAOPERATIVE MONITORING

Multimodal intraoperative monitoring (MIOM) aims to utilize a combination of modalities to increase the overall sensitivity and specificity in identifying impending neurological insult. In 2007, after analyzing 1017 procedures using MIOM with total intravenous anesthesia, Sutter et al. reported 89% sensitivity (95% CI 79.3–94.9%) and 99% specificity (95% CI 98.2–99.6%).[16] The development and research of safety enhancements in spine surgery is a major concern and is supported by several societies, such as the Spine Society of Europe (SSE), the Scoliosis Research Society (SRS), and the International Society of Intraoperative Neurophysiology (ISIN). MIOM is strongly recommended as a routine procedure in spine centers dealing with severe spinal disorders.[17] In 2010, Fehlings et al. reported the results of a 32-article meta-analysis of MIOM, noting that spine surgery has a 5% baseline for neurological complications, and that MIOM has a total sensitivity of 94.3% and specificity of 95.6%.[18] Though there is no consensus on which modalities are to be used for particular spine procedures, Gonazalez et al. suggested MIOM based on spinal region at risk, as shown in Figure 59.5.[1]

CONCLUSION

The objective of intraoperative electrophysiological neuromonitoring is to reduce the risk of adverse events leading to permanent neurological injury. Intraoperative monitoring of spinal cord and nerve root injury through SSEP, TcMEP, sEMG, and tEMG modalities is vital during spine surgeries. IONM has shown to be successful in identifying and potentially reversing neurological insults that may occur during high-risk spinal surgeries. Additional procedure-specific research on the efficacy of individual IONM modalities and MIOM is required, with the subsequent development of IONM guidelines.

REFERENCES

1. Rattenni RN, Cheriyan T, Lee A, et al. (2015). "Intraoperative spinal cord and nerve root monitoring: A hospital survey and review." Bulletin of the Hospital for Joint Diseases In print.
2. Malhotra NR, Shaffrey CI. Intraoperative electrophysiological monitoring in spine surgery. Spine. 2010;35(25):2167-79.

3. Peeling L, Hentschel S, Fox R, et al. Intraoperative spinal cord and nerve root monitoring: a survey of Canadian spine surgeons. Can J Surg. Journal canadien de chirurgie 2010;53(5):324-8.
4. Gonzalez AA, Jeyanandarajan D, Hansen C, et al. Intraoperative neurophysiological monitoring during spine surgery: a review. Neurosurg Focus. 2009;27(4):E6.
5. Lall RR, Lall RR, Hauptman JS, et al. Intraoperative neurophysiological monitoring in spine surgery: indications, efficacy, and role of the preoperative checklist. Neurosurg Focus. 2012;33(5):E10.
6. Stecker MM. A review of intraoperative monitoring for spinal surgery. Surg Neurol Int. 2012;3(Suppl 3):S174-87.
7. Journee H. Motor EP physiology, risks and specific anesthetic effects. In: Nuwer MR (Ed). Handbook of Clinical Neurophysiology. Amsterdam: Elsevier; 2008. pp. 218-134.
8. Tanaka S, Tashiro T, Gomi A, et al. Sensitivity and specificity in transcranial motor-evoked potential monitoring during neurosurgical operations. Surg Neurol Int. 2011;2:111.
9. Chen X, Sterio D, Ming X, et al. Success rate of motor evoked potentials for intraoperative neurophysiologic monitoring: effects of age, lesion location, and preoperative neurologic deficits. J Clin Neurophysiol. 2007;24(3):281-5.
10. Raynor BL, Lenke LG, Kim Y, et al. Can triggered electromyograph thresholds predict safe thoracic pedicle screw placement? Spine. 2002;27(18):2030-5.
11. Shi YB, Binette M, Martin WH, et al. Electrical stimulation for intraoperative evaluation of thoracic pedicle screw placement. Spine. 2003;28(6):595-601.
12. Calancie B, Molano MR. Alarm criteria for motor-evoked potentials: what's wrong with the "presence-or-absence" approach? Spine. 2008;33(4):406-14.
13. Raynor, Barry, L.; Lenke, Lawrence, G.; Bridwell, Keith, H.; Taylor, Brett, A.; Padberg, Anne, M., 2007: Correlation between low triggered electromyographic thresholds and lumbar pedicle screw malposition. Spine 32(24):2673-78.
14. Silverstein J, Basra S. Waveform window #21. Anomaly during pedicle screw stimulation. American journal of electroneurodiagnostic technology. Dec 2011;51(4):296-300.
15. de Blas G, Barrios C, Regidor I, et al. Safe pedicle screw placement in thoracic scoliotic curves using t-EMG: stimulation threshold variability at concavity and convexity in apex segments. Spine. 2012;37(6):E387-95.
16. Sutter M, Eggspuehler A, Grob D, et al. The diagnostic value of multimodal intraoperative monitoring (MIOM) during spine surgery: a prospective study of 1,017 patients. Eur Spine J. 2007;16 Suppl 2:S162-70.
17. Flynn JM, Sakai DS. Improving safety in spinal deformity surgery: advances in navigation and neurologic monitoring. Eur Spine J. 2013;22 Suppl 2:S131-7.
18. Fehlings MG, Brodke DS, Norvell DC, et al. The evidence for intraoperative neurophysiological monitoring in spine surgery: does it make a difference? Spine. 2010;35(9 Suppl): S37-46.

Index

Note: Page numbers followed by *f*, *t* and *b* indicate figures, tables and boxes respectively.

A

Acetaminophen, 147
Active release techniques, 162
Acupuncture
    applications of, 169–170
Acute cervical disk herniation, 38
Addiction
    addiction management, 152
    CAGE-AID questionnaire, 153*t*
    prevention of, 152
    scope of, 151
Addictive disorders, 173
Adjacent segment disease, 307
Adolescent idiopathic scoliosis (AIS), 61, 69
    classification, 67
    evaluation of, 62–67
Adult degenerative spinal deformity, 406
    complications, 410
    outcomes, 411
    presurgical considerations, 407
    surgical indications, 406
    surgical planning, 407
    surgical techniques, 407
Adult scoliosis, 71
Adult spinal deformity (ASD), 69, 73
    3D analysis, 78
    classification, 72, 72*f*
    coronal plane measurements, 75–76
    criticism of 2D measurements, 78
    curve measurement, 75
    evaluation, 69–72
    global alignment, 78
    imaging, 75
    sagittal plane measurements, 77
    spine related measurements, 71
Aggrecan, 6
Alendronate, 157
American College of Physicians (ACP), 44–45
    recommendations, 45*t*
American Pain Society (APS), 45
    recommendations, 45*t*
American Society for Testing and Materials, 16
Amyotrophic lateral sclerosis (ALS), 33
Anger spectrum emotions, 171
Ankylosing spondylitis, 27, 40, 127*f*
Annulus fibrosus, 26
Anterior cervical corpectomy, 326
Anterior cervical decompression and fusion (ACDF), 325, 345
Antitumor necrosis factor (TNF), 127
Anxiety, 171
Atlanto-occipital dissociation, 435
Axial neck pain, 26–27, 36
    anatomy, 36
    natural history, 36
    pathophysiology, 37
    prevalence, 36

B

Back pain, 27–28, 28*f*, 126
Biacuplasty, 261–262, 262*f*
Bone
    density testing, 132
    FRAX, 132
    scan, 98*f*
Botulinum toxin injections, 141

C

Calcitonin, 157
Carica papaya, 365
Cartilage injury, 213
Cell therapy, 9
Central sacral vertical line (CSVL), 66
Cervical and lumbar spine
    computed tomography, 88–95
    hypoechoic collection superficial to spine, 100*f*
    multilevel CT discography, 97*f*
    nuclear medicine, 95–100
    radiographs, 85, 85*f*
    ultrasound, 100
Cervical arthroplasty, 317
Cervical disk herniation
    anterior approach, 302–303
    complications, 306–307
    epidemiology, 301
    posterior approach, 303–304
    signs and symptoms, 301–302
    surgical options, 302
    treatment, 302
Cervical epidural steroid injections, 162
Cervical myelopathy, 33, 54, 160
Cervical pain, 39*f*
    referred, 54*f*
Cervical radiculopathy
    clinical presentation, 294
    double crush phenomenon, 297
    epidemiology, 294
    physical examination, 297
Cervical radiculopathy syndromes, 54, 56t–57*t*, 160, 294
Cervical spondylosis, 38, 324, 345
Cervical spondylotic myelopathy (CSM), 310–311
Cervical stenosis
    anterior approach, 314–317
    pathogenesis, 311
    posterior approach, 317
    posterior laminoforaminotomy, 320
    treatment options, 313
Cervical total disk replacement
    case example, 350–351
    complications, 349–350
    indications and contraindications, 347
    technical considerations, 346
Cervical traction, 162
Chondroitin sulfate (CS), 5
Chondrosarcomas, 459
Chronic low back pain, 48, 172
    aversion, 171
    central sensitization, 172
    chronic illness, 174
    countertransference, 175
    interpersonal and social factors, 173
    personality factors, 173
    psychiatric and psychological treatment, 174
    psychiatric comorbidity, 172–173
Chymopapain, 365
Cobb angle, 61*f*, 65–66, 76
    evaluation, 76
    measurements, 20
Cognitive-behavioral pain management, 182

Collagen, 15
fibers, 4*f*
Complex regional pain syndrome (CRPS), 30, 32
Computed tomography, 70
Conventional radiography, 70, 70*f*
Coronal alignment (CA), 76
Corticosteroid, 212
injections, 213*t*
Cyclobenzaprine, 149

D

Deep tendon reflex, 53*t*
Degenerative cervical disorders
complications, 329
surgical indications, 324
surgical options, 325
surgical outcomes, 328–329
Degenerative disk disease (DDD), 3
Degenerative end-plate, 114
Degenerative pain, 38
Degenerative scoliosis, 407
Denosumab, 158
Dermatomes, 52*f*
Diazepam, 149
Disability
functional assessment instruments, 81
objective tools, 81
Roland Morris questionnaire, 83
subjective tools, 83
Discitis/osteomyelitis, 40
Discogenic pain, 259
Discography
contraindications for, 124*t*
evidence, 124
indications, 124
Disk
herniation, 26
osteophyte complexes, 108

E

EOS machine, 70–71, 88
Epidural hematomas, 118
Epidural steroid injection, 140, 148, 193
caudal efficacy, 232
caudal procedure, 231
complications, 231
efficacy, 140, 228
interlaminar procedure, 229–230
transforaminal (TF) injections, 229
transforaminal procedure, 230
Evidence-based clinical decision model, 180*f*

F

Facet joint injections, 140
Ferguson method, 75
Fibromyalgia
clinical features of, 128
syndrome, 128
Flexion-distraction injuries, 451
Fluoroscopic aspiration, 237
Foraminal stenosis, 25
Fracture-dislocation injuries, 451
Free-standing anteroposterior radiograph, 76*f*
Fulcrum-bending radiographs, 65

G

Gait evaluation, 53
Gastrocnemius, 55
Genetic testing, 66
Gluteus maximus, 55

H

Hairy patches, 64
Hereditary factors, 61
Hereditary spastic paraplegias (HSPs), 33–34
Herpes zoster, 32
HRQOL score, 72

I

Ibandronate, 157
Infantile scoliosis, 61
Inflammatory arthritis, 40
Inflammatory bowel disease (IBD)-associated arthritis, 127
Inflammatory mediators, 7, 7*f*
International Association for the Study of Pain (IASP), 124
International normalised ratio (INR) value, 148
International Organization for Standardization, 16
Interspinous spacer technology, 374–375
Interventional diagnostic procedures
anatomy, 121
complications, 123
diagnostic nerve blocks, 120–121
discography, 121
disk degeneration and pain, 123
function of, 121
procedure, 123, 123*f*
Intervertebral disk (IVD), 3
cervical, 16*f*
etiology of, 5
morphologic changes, 4–5
morphology of, 3
Intra-articular facet injections
complications, 238
cyst intervention results, 238
diagnosis, 235–236
etiology and pathophysiology, 233
facet joint anatomy, 233
facet joint arthropathy, 235
imaging, 236
indications, 237
intra-articular facet, 237
treatment, 236
Intracranial tumors, 33
Intradiscal electrothermal therapy (IDET), 190
technique, 261*f*
Intradural extramedullary spinal tumors
astrocytoma, 466
ganglioglioma, 467
hemangioblastomas, 466
neurofibromas, 463
spinal meningiomas, 463
spinal schwannomas, 461

J

Joint Commission on the Accreditation of Health Organizations (JCAHO), 151

K

Keratin sulfate (KS), 5
Kyphoplasty, 472
Kyphosis, 399–400

L

Laminectomy, 274, 288*f*
Laminoplasty, 318, 327

Lhermitte's sign, 41
Lou Gehrig's disease, 33
Low back pain, 86*f*
  disability questionnaire, 83
Lumbar degenerative spondylolisthesis
  case example, 292
  electrodiagnostic studies, 299
  incidence, 286–287
  laminotomy, 288
  pathogenesis, 286
  presentation, 287
  surgical results, 300
  treatment, 299
Lumbar disk herniations
  chemonucleolysis, 365
  comparative trials, 365–366
  history, 361
  modern techniques, 361–365
Lumbar lordosis, 20
Lumbar myelogram, 97*f*
Lumbar neuroanatomy, 448*f*
Lumbar pain, referred, 55*f*
Lumbar spinal stenosis
  clinical features, 369–370
  diagnostic imaging, 370
  differential diagnosis, 370
  electrodiagnostic studies, 371
  surgical outcomes, 373–374
  surgical treatment, 371–373
Lumbar spine disorders
  cervical spine, 102–108
  lumbar spine, 108–119
Lumbar spine fusion
  discussion, 343
  indications, 337
  posterior approaches, 340–343
Lumbar total disk replacement surgery
  complications, 358
  flexicore, 357, 357*f*
  indications for, 354
  outcomes, 357–358
  prostheses, 355
  surgical approach and technique, 355
Lumbosacral radicular syndromes, 58*t*
Lumbosacral radiculopathies, 55, 58*t*

M

Magnetic resonance imaging (MRI), 31, 46, 70, 85, 102–103
Manual traction test, 53
Matrix metalloproteinase 3 (MMP-3), 5
McGill pain questionnaire, 83
Medial branch blocks (MBBs), 196
Medical Research Council (MRC), 50*t*
Micro-computed tomography, 134
Motion preservation technologies
  annulus repair, 336
  cell-based therapies, 333
  dynamic stabilization, 334
  facet replacement, 335
  interspinous distraction, 334
  nucleus replacement, 332
  synthetic nucleus replacement, 332
Multidisciplinary rehabilitation, 139
Multimodal intraoperative monitoring (MIOM), 486
Multiple sclerosis, 33
Musculoskeletal aspiration, 212
Myelopathy, 39

N

Narcotics
  "no ceiling effect", 145
National Institutes of Health National Center for Complementary and Alternative Medicine (CAM), 168
Neck, 54
  compression test, 54
  pain, 39
Nerve root distribution, 46*f*
Neural complications
  chemical injury, 249
  contrast dye, 250
  exacerbation of pain, 248
  vasovagal syncope, 248
Neuromechanical tests, 53
Neurotomy, 163
Neurotoxicity, 249
Nitrous oxide anesthesia, 33
Non-narcotic pharmaceutical intervention
  anticonvulsants, 148
  classification of, 148*t*
  gabapentin, 148
  muscle relaxants, 149
  nonopioid combination medication, 149–150
  nonsteroidal anti-inflammatory drugs, 147
  pregabalin, 148
  topical medications, 150
  tricyclic antidepressants, 149
Nonsteroid anti-inflammatory drugs (NSAIDs), 127, 162
Nontraumatic neck injuries, 161
Normal pressure hydrocephalus (NPH), 34
Novel management technique, 8
Nucleoplasty, 190, 260

O

Occupational work, classification of, 82*t*
Olympic weightlifters, 11
Opioid pharmacotherapy, 144
Oral steroid drugs, 162
Osteophyte formation, 234
Osteoporosis, 414
  aging, 155
  bone strengthening, 156
  calcium and vitamin D, 156
  diagnosing osteopenia, 132
  falling, 155
  laboratory testing, 133
  osteoporosis medications, 157*t*
  pathogenesis of, 132
  prescription medications, 156
  risk factors, 156*t*
  supplementation, 156
Osteotomies, 408
Oswetry disability index, 83, 83*t*

P

Pain
  axial, 26–27
  back, 27–28
  degenerative, 38
  local, 24
  radicular, 24
  referred, 24
  syndromes, 39
  types, 24
Pancoast tumor, 32
Patrick's test, 66*f*
Pediatric deformities
  anatomy/biomechanics, 388
  classification, 393
  clinical evaluation, 389
  inclinometer, 391*f*
  nonoperative treatment, 394

operative treatment, 395
outcomes/complications, 397–398
radiologic evaluation, 392–393
scoliosis, 388
surgical technique, 395–397
Pelvic fixation, 409
Pelvic incidence, 78
Pelvic tilt, 78
Pelvis, relative locations of, 21*f*
Percutaneous injection
intracyst distention, 237–238
Peripheral neuropathy, 31, 294
Plexopathy, 31
Positive test, 47
Positron emission tomography, 468
Postcontrast gadolinium imaging, 119
Pressure-related injuries
epidural abscess, 244
granuloma formation, 244
hematomas, 243
infections, 244
injectate associated, 243
meningitis, 244
osteomyelitis/diskitis, 244
vascular injury, 244–247
Protein growth factors, 8
Proteoglycans, 3
Prototypical noninflammatory pain syndrome, 128
Provocative tests, 53
Proximal junctional kyphosis, 410
Pseudarthrosis, 411
Pulmonary cement embolism rate, 417
Pulmonary function, 66

R

Radicular pain, 24
Radicular symptoms, 25
Radiculopathy
history, 49
myofascial release, 162
nonoperative treatment, 161–164
pathophysiology, 160
physical examination, 49
task force for, 159–160
Raloxifene, 157
Range of motion (ROM), 11
Red flags, 40, 57
Referred pain, 24
Reflex testing, 51
Rheumatoid spine
clinical evaluation, 421
grading, 421
imaging, 421–423
natural history, 421
spine manifestations, 420
surgical options, 425–427
treatment, 423
Reverse Lasègue test, 53
Rheumatoid arthritis (RA), 28, 40, 420
Rheumatologic disorders, 38
Rhizotomy
medial branch block, 254
Risedronate, 157
Rotatory subluxation, 76

S

Sacral fracture surgery
anatomy, 448
burst fractures, 450
classification, 449
clinical evaluation, 448
compression fractures, 449
low lumbar injuries, 452
radiologic evaluation, 448–449
Sacral slope, 78
Sacroiliac injections, 205
anatomy, 205
complications, 209–210
diagnosis, 205–208
injection technique, 208–209
Saddle anesthesia, 23
Sagittal vertical axis, 78
Saliva-based DNA sample, 67
Scoliosis curves, 61
Scoliosis patients, 62*f*
Scoliosis Research Society (SRS), 61
Scoliosis, 393
Scottie dog, 87*f*
Segment-pointer muscles, 50*t*
Selective nerve root blocks, 195
Selective serotonin reuptake inhibitors (SSRIs), 150
Sensory examination, tools used for, 52*f*
Shoulder abduction (Bakody) test, 53
Skin dimples, 64
Soft tissue injections
adverse effects, 213
corticosteroid preparations, 213*t*
indications, 213
injectables, 212
injection techniques, 216–217
platelet-rich plasma, 216
Somatic referred pain, 54
Spinal arthrodesis, 354
Spinal cord stimulators
complications, 268
indications, 265
neurogenic pain, 265
permanent implantation, 267–268
spine-related conditions, 265–266
technique, 266
trial/screening, 266–267
Spinal cord tumors, 456
Spinal corticosteroids, 249
Spinal curvature, 77
Spinal deformity, 20–21
anterior cervical instrumentation, 280
antibiotics, 277–278
decompression of, 274–276
deformity correction, 282–283
interbody fusion, 280
orthopedic instrumentation, 277–278
posterior cervical instrumentation, 280
stabilization of, 276
Spinal deformity surgery
anatomy and biomechanics, 379–381
classification, 382–383
clinical evaluation, 381
outcomes, 384–385
radiologic evaluation, 381–382
treatment, 383
Spinal degeneration, 233
Spinal disorders
adiculopathy *vs*. myelopathy, 30*t*
balance, stability and posture, 18–22
chronic pain syndromes, 24
conditions, 30–31
diagnostic studies, 41
differential diagnosis, 24
grading, 39, 41*t*
history, physical examination, 39
imaging studies, 41
prognosis, 23
risk factors, 23
threshold modulation, 24
Spinal epidural hematoma (SEH), 243
Spinal fracture surgery
cervical spine, 429
classification, 444–445
facet disruption, 436, 441

nonoperative treatment, 437
operative care, 445
operative treatment, 438
specific syndromes, 443
spinal cord injury, 443
Spinal infarction, 34
Spinal injections
complications and risks, 191
discograms, 193
epidural injections, 189
history, 187
peripheral joint injections, 189
sacroiliac injections, 188–189
spinal cord stimulators, 191
sympathetic nerve blocks, 189
trigger point injections, 187
Spinal injections complications
dural puncture, 241
intradiskal injections, 241
needle/injectate-related injuries, 240
pneumocephalus, 241
spinal cord trauma, 242
Spinal loading, 13
Spinal metastases
angiography, 469
diagnosis, 468
magnetic resonance imaging, 469
percutaneous biopsy, 469
surgical intervention, 470
Spinal neoplasms, 35
Spinal stenosis, 25
Spine biomechanics, 11
facet joint, 12
intervertebral disk, 12
spinal arthroplasty, 15–16
spinal motion, 13
uncovertebral joint, 12
Spine column, 11
longitudinal section, 12*f*
regions, 11*f*
Spine surgery intraoperative monitoring
motor evoked potentials, 483
somatosensory evoked potentials, 482
spontaneous EMG, 484–485
Stagnara wake-up test, 482
triggered EMG, 485
Spinopelvic parameters, 77*f*
Spondylolisthesis, 25, 114, 400
Spondylolysis, 25, 159
Spurling's test, 41, 298*f*
SRS-Schwab adult spinal deformity classification system, 72*f*
Steroids, 147
Straight-leg raise (SLR)
demonstration, 47*f*
test, 47
Subacute combined degeneration (SCD), 33
Subaxial spine, 37
Sympathetic nerve block (SNB), 189
clinical presentation, 222
complex regional pain syndrome, 221
CRPS management, 223
diagnosis, 223
Drucker's stages of causalgia, 226*t*
epidemiology, 221
lumbar sympathetic block, 224*f*
nociceptive and neuropathic pain, 221
pathophysiology, 221
pharmacological infusions, 225
prognosis, 223
stellate ganglion block fluoroscopy, 224
sympathetic block, 223
Synovial cysts, 235
Syringomyelia, 34
Systemic inflammatory disease, 40

T

T2-weighted sagittal images, 102*f*
Tendon reflexes, 52*t*
Teriparatide, 157
The medical outcomes study, 84
Thoracic kyphosis, 77*f*
Thoracic outlet syndrome (TOS), 32
Tizanidine, 149
Tokuhashi scoring system, 474*t*
Torticollis, 37
Total posterior arthroplasty system, 335
Transforaminal cervical epidural injection, 229*f*
Traumatic spondylolisthesis, 435
Trigger point injections, 141
diagnosis, 200–201
evidence, 203
indications, 201
preinjection block, 203
technique, 202
vasovagal syncope, 203
Tropical spastic paraparesis (TSP), 34

U

Ultrahigh-resolution MRI, 134
Ultrasound-guided injections, 210
Uncovertebral joint arthritis, 38
Unforeseen abnormalities, 247

V

Valsalva test (cough impulse test), 53
Vascular claudication, 26
Vertebral fracture assessments, 133
Vertebral squaring, 127*f*
Vertebroplasty, 472
Video-assisted thoracoscopic surgery (VATS), 471
Viscosupplementation, 214
Vitamin D receptor (VDR), 5

W

Whiplash type injuries, 37
Whiplash-associated disorders (WADs), 161
Wiltse-Newman classification of spondylolisthesis, 87*b*

Z

Zoledronic acid, 157
Zygapophyseal joint arthritis, 38